LEARNING TO CARE

·

Senior Content Strategist: Alison Taylor
Content Development Specialists: Katie Golsby and
Carole McMurray
Project Manager: Anne Collett
Designer/Design Direction: Maggie Reid
Illustration Manager: Nichole Beard

LEARNING TO CARE
THE NURSING ASSOCIATE

Ian Peate OBE, FRCN, EN(G) RGN, DipN(Lond), RNT B.Ed (Hons), MA, LLM
Head of School, School of Health Studies, Gibraltar Health Authority, Gibraltar;
Editor in Chief, British Journal of Nursing;
Visiting Professor, St George's University of London and Kingston University London;
Visiting Senior Clinical Fellow, University of Hertfordshire, UK
University of Gibraltar

FOREWORD BY

Professor Lisa Bayliss-Pratt
Chief Nurse and Interim Regional Director for London and the South East
Health Education England

ELSEVIER

Edinburgh London New York Oxford Philadelphia St Louis Sydney Toronto 2019

ELSEVIER

ISBN 978-0-7020-7605-3

Notices

Knowledge and best practice in this field are constantly changing. As new research and experience broaden our understanding, changes in research methods, professional practices, or medical treatment may become necessary.

Practitioners and researchers must always rely on their own experience and knowledge in evaluating and using any information, methods, compounds, or experiments described herein. In using such information or methods they should be mindful of their own safety and the safety of others, including parties for whom they have a professional responsibility.

With respect to any drug or pharmaceutical products identified, readers are advised to check the most current information provided (i) on procedures featured or (ii) by the manufacturer of each product to be administered, to verify the recommended dose or formula, the method and duration of administration, and contraindications. It is the responsibility of practitioners, relying on their own experience and knowledge of their patients, to make diagnoses, to determine dosages and the best treatment for each individual patient, and to take all appropriate safety precautions.

To the fullest extent of the law, neither the Publisher nor the authors, contributors, or editors, assume any liability for any injury and/or damage to persons or property as a matter of products liability, negligence or otherwise, or from any use or operation of any methods, products, instructions, or ideas contained in the material herein.

ELSEVIER your source for books, journals and multimedia in the health sciences

www.elsevierhealth.com

Printed in Great Britain

Last digit is the print number: 10 9 8 7 6 5 4 3 2

The publisher's policy is to use paper manufactured from sustainable forests

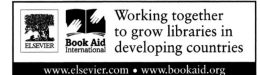

CONTENTS

This text is dedicated to my brother James Francis Peate, the eldest in a family of 11.

When the idea of the Nursing Associate was proposed in 2015, it was hard to imagine that in just three years the first cohort of trainees would be achieving their qualifications and joining the Nursing & Midwifery Council Register.

It's a huge achievement and a testament both to the dedication and hard work of the trainees themselves and to the health and social care partnerships across the country who seized the opportunity to innovate and develop this role.

So I am delighted to be invited to provide a Foreword for this text, the publication of which coincides with our first cohort of qualified Nursing Associates in January 2018. This first cohort are the pioneers, but there are many more to follow, now in training or about to join the programme, which is why *Learning to Care: The Nursing Associate* is both timely and an invaluable resource for current and future staff.

Whether you are a trainee on the programme, a qualified Nursing Associate about to embark on this exciting career, or a healthcare assistant thinking about a move into nursing, you will find the support and guidance you need in this book.

When HEE began developing this new role – the first in nursing for over 20 years – our vision was to ensure trainees gained a clear understanding of the needs of their local population and were confident and competent to work in a variety of health and care settings, in hospital, at home, or close to home; a vision supported by the breadth and scope of this text.

Covering all the key topics, and aligned to the curriculum framework, this comprehensive text will be an essential study support, especially for those new to formal academic work. Each chapter sets out a crucial element of the training and the knowledge and skills needed – from ethics to infection control – supported with a rich variety of clinical case studies to help link theory and practice, as well as helpful prompts to reflective learning.

Each chapter in the book, edited by Professor Ian Peate, has been provided by one or more contributors with experience in a variety of health and social care roles, some of whom are already working with trainee Nursing Associates either in a clinical or academic setting.

Whether the text is setting out a theoretical or practical topic, the Nursing Associate role is consistently placed in its appropriate context and relationship to that topic, which will be crucial in building an understanding of the role and how it will contribute to multi-disciplinary team working in health and care settings. The central importance of holistic, patient-centred care is also emphasised throughout.

For newly-qualified Nursing Associates, already embarked on their careers, there is clear and straightforward advice on continuing professional development and tips on preparing for revalidation.

Health and care assistants and clinical support workers will find Chapter 2 on the Care Certificate very helpful, while it also gives some guidance to Nursing Associates on how to support their HCA colleagues to complete this qualification.

So, on behalf of Health Education England, I would like to express our gratitude to Ian Peate for identifying the need for a specific text tailored to the academic and clinical learning needs of the trainee, not only to support them to become a qualified and registered Nursing Associate but to encourage them in life long learning.

I warmly commend this book to trainees, those considering the role and all those who work with and support them.

Lisa Bayliss-Pratt
September 2018

CONTRIBUTORS

Jaden Allan, MSc Ed, PG Dip, BSc
(Hons), RN Dip HE, SFHEA
Senior Lecturer
Department of Nursing, Midwifery and
    Health
Northumbria University, Newcastle,
United Kingdom

Janine Archer, PhD, PgCAP, MRes,
BSc(Hons), DPNS(MH)
Senior Lecturer (Nursing Associate)
School of Health & Society
University of Salford,
United Kingdom

Joanne Atkinson, RGN, MSc, PGDip,
BA (Hons)
Head of Subject Nursing, Midwifery and
    Health
Department of Nursing Midwifery and
    Health, Faculty of Life Sciences
Northumbria University, Newcastle,
United Kingdom

Stuart Baker, RN, BSc (Hons), PGCE,
FHEA, RNT
School of Care Sciences
University of South Wales, Pontypridd,
United Kingdom

Chris Barber, BSc (Hons), MEd, RN(LD)
Visiting lecturer (learning disability
    nursing)
School of Nursing and Midwifery
Birmingham City University, Birmingham,
United Kingdom

Carmel Blackie, MSc, BEd (Hons), RN,
SCM, HV, RNT, HVL, FIHV, SFHEA
Associate Professor
FHSCE Nursing
Kingston University and St George's
    University of London,
United Kingdom

Louise Bowden, BSc (Hons) Acute Child
Care
School of Health and Society
University of Salford,
United Kingdom

Rosemary Castle, BA (Hons), Social
Anthropology, MSc Nursing Studies
Faculty of Health and Social Care Sciences
    and Education
Kingston University and St George's
    University London, Kingston Upon
    Thames,
United Kingdom

Linda Castro, MSc Dermatology Skills
and Treatment
Clinical Nurse Specialist
Dermatology
Gibraltar Health Authority,
Gibraltar

Angelina Chadwick, RGN, RMN, Dip
BSc, PGCE, MSc SFHEA
Lecturer in Mental Health Nursing
School of Health and Society
The University of Salford
Greater Manchester,
United Kingdom

Jacqueline Chang, MA Medical Ethics
and Law, BSc Nursing
Senior Lecturer
School of Nursing
Kingston University, Kingston,
Surrey,
United Kingdom

Carl Clare, MSc, BSc
Programme Lead
Adult Nursing
University of Hertfordshire, Hatfield,
Hertfordshire,
United Kingdom

Julie Derbyshire, RGN, Dip Nursing, BA
(Hons) Education, MSc Practice
Education, Professional Doctorate in
Education
Faculty of Health and Life Sciences
Northumbria University, Newcastle,
United Kingdom

Paul Nicholas Deslandes, BPharm, PhD
Life Sciences and Education
University of South Wales, Treforest,
United Kingdom

Wyn Glencross, RGN, NMP, MA Medical
Law & Ethics
Tissue Viability Nurse Consultant
Medico Legal
GMS & Associates Ltd, Corby,
United Kingdom

Carrie Grainger, MSc Public Health, PG
Cert (Academic Practice), DipHE
Midwifery, RM, Fellow Higher Education
Academy
Lecturer in Health Promotion and Public
    Health
College of Nursing, Midwifery and
    Healthcare
University of West London, Brentford,
United Kingdom

Sigurd Haveland III, MCPara, BSc,
PGCETLHE, FdSc, DipION FHEA
Paramedic Science, Healthcare
Gibraltar Health Authority
St Bernard's Hospital,
Gibraltar

Barry Hill, MSc (Hons), PGCAP, PGCE,
BSc (Hons), DipHE
Senior Lecturer
Nursing, Midwifery and Health
University of Northumbria at Newcastle,
    Newcastle upon Tyne,
United Kingdom

Abby Hughes, RN, BN
Clinical Educator
University of Salford,
United Kingdom

Noleen Jones, BSc HC
School of Health Studies
Gibraltar Health Authority,
Gibraltar

Louise McErlean, BSc (Hons) Critical
Care Nursing, MA Teaching and
Learning
Senior Lecturer
Health and Social Work
University of Hertfordshire, Hatfield,
United Kingdom

Hamish MacGregor, RN, BA (Hons),
MSc
Director
Training and Consultancy
Docklands Training Consultants Ltd,
    London,
United Kingdom

Janet G Migliozzi, MSc, BSc (Hons), BSc,
PGDip ed, FHEA
Senior Lecturer
School of Health & Social Work
University of Hertfordshire, Hatfield,
United Kingdom

Christine Mullen, MBE, BSC, MSC
Skills for Health
Associate Consultant
Sector Skills for Healthcare, Bristol,
United Kingdom

Karen Louise Nagalingam, Masters in Health Care and Education, BSc in Nursing Studies, PGCert in Medical Simulation
Senior Lecturer in Nursing
Health and Social Care
University of Hertfordshire, Hatfield,
United Kingdom

Yvonne Needham, RN, RNT, OND, BSc(Hons), MA
Senior Fellow
Hull University,
United Kingdom

Sandra Netto, RN, PG Dip - Advanced Practice Infection (Diseases Prevention & Control)
Infection Prevention & Control Practitioner
Infection Prevention and Control
Gibraltar Health Authority,
Gibraltar

Laura Park, BSC (Hons)
Graduate Tutor
Nursing, Midwifery & Health
Northumbria University, Newcastle,
United Kingdom

Ian Peate, OBE, FRCN, EN(G) RGN, DipN(Lond), RNT BEd (Hons), MA, LLM
Head of School, School of Health
Studies, Gibraltar Health Authority,
Gibraltar
Editor in Chief British Journal of
Nursing
Visiting Professor St George's
University of London and Kingston
University London
Visiting Senior Clinical Fellow
University of Hertfordshire, UK
University of Gibraltar

Ben Pitcher, BSC, BN, PGCEd
Life Science and Education
University of South Wales, Pontypridd,
United Kingdom

Shirley Sardeña, MSc Library Information Management, BSc Information Science
Medical Librarian
Library
Gibraltar Health Authority,
Gibraltar

Karen Sumpter, MA, RGN, MA Management & Leadership, RN, FHEA, PGCert RNT
Senior Lecturer
Adult Nursing & Primary Care
University of Hertfordshire, Hatfield,
United Kingdom

Julie Swann, Dip COT, HCPC,
Independent Occupational Therapist
www.julieswann.com
Alsager,
United Kingdom

Kathy Whayman, RN, MSc Nursing; PGDip Healthcare Education
Senior Lecturer
Adult Nursing and Primary Care
University of Hertfordshire, Hatfield,
United Kingdom

Anthony Wheeldon, MSc Cardiorespiratory Nursing, PGDip Learning and Teaching, BSc (Hons) Nursing
Associate Subject Group Lead
Adult Nursing and Primary Care
University of Hertfordshire, Hatfield,
Hertfordshire,
United Kingdom

Karen Wild, MA, RN, HV, RNT
Registered Nurse
Cumbria,
United Kingdom

Rachel Wood, BSc Hons Dietetics
Highly Specialist Paediatric Dietitian
Therapy and Dietetics
Royal Manchester Children's Hospital,
Manchester,
United Kingdom

Simon Young, BPharm (Hons), PhD
Academic Subject Manager
Faculty of Life Sciences and Education
University of South Wales, Pontypridd,
Rhondda Cynon Taff,
United Kingdom

PREFACE

Learning to Care: The Nursing Associate is the first text that has been written specifically for you, the trainee Nursing Associate (NA). The focus will be on the provision of care to adults. The book has adopted a user-friendly approach as we wish to encourage you to become knowledgeable doers, with a curious mind that will lead you to discovery. Full colour illustrations, tables and boxes have been used to help you navigate the complexities that are associated with the provision of high quality, person-centred care.

The Care Certificate is a set of 15 standards that health and social care workers use as they deliver care and support and these 15 standards have been incorporated in chapters throughout the text. The Nursing and Midwifery Council (NMC) has taken on the responsibility to regulate the NA role; as it does this, it enhances protection for those people we have the privilege to offer care and support to. Regulation of the NA can ensure that standards are consistent across the board.

The NA has been designed to bridge the gap between healthcare assistants and registered nurses (RNs) in England. NAs will deliver care, freeing up RNs to spend more time using their skills and knowledge to centre on complex clinical responsibilities and to take a lead in the management of patient care. Learning to Care: The Nursing Associate has 39 chapters. The book will enable NAs to develop their caring skills, confidence and competence.

The contents of the book are based on key publications including, the NMC's Standards of Proficiency for Nursing Associates (NMC, 2018a) and Health Education England, Skills for Care and Skills for Health (2015). Each chapter has been written by skilled health and social care practitioners and experienced academics, with a keen interest in taking forward the role and function of the NA.

As the landscape of care provision is continually changing, this brings with it new roles and responsibilities in the health and social sectors. The NA is taking on much more in the line of direct care delivery, assuming many roles that the RN has traditionally undertaken and these include, for example, the management of medicines, wound care, urinary catheterization and observation and recording of a range of vital signs. The NA's scope of practice is varied, however, and will be determined by a number of factors including the context of care. Key to the scope of practice are the fundamentals of care and support; these essential elements of care provision are a key feature of this text.

As the NA is required to attend formal training and education as well as gaining essential hands on experience in care settings, they are required to be assessed theoretically and practically. *Learning to Care: The Nursing Associate* will help meet the educational needs of the NA in the classroom and in the care setting. The NA also has a responsibility for ongoing self and professional development (continuing professional development) to maintain their knowledge base through a commitment to life-long learning.

NAs will be required to engage in analytical thinking, to use information and/or evidence to provide care in a competent, confident and empathetic manner as they use their communication skills when working as key members of the care team. Where appropriate, the NA will be required to educate and support other health and social care workers with regards to the provision of high quality, effective care, as well as the individual recipient of care, families and communities. This text has a predominant clinical focus that reflects the NAs ability to offer direct and indirect individualized care to a variety of people in a range of settings; it engages the NA in reflective and analytical practice and encourages them in demonstrating processional and collaborative practice associated with the with Code (NMC 2018b).

A systems approach has been adopted for most of the text, whilst detailing the skills associated with care provision, primary care and community care also feature. Learning to care: The Nursing Associate is provided in two parts, bringing together anatomy and physiology, pathophysiology and care, providing the reader with all this information in one text, a one stop shop. There is an emphasis on:

- Knowledge: this concerns information and the understanding of that information to guide practice.
- Skills: the technical procedures and competencies that are required to care for people in a safe, compassionate and effective manner
- Attitudes: these are associated with behaviour and ways of thinking

Each of the 39 chapters begins with an aim and learning objectives, and a pre-test is provided to help you self-test and determine what your current knowledge base is. The chapters conclude with a looking back, feeding forward section. This provides a summary of what has been covered and encouragement for you to delve deeper and explore further.

Part one of the book lays down the fundamentals required to prepare for practice, Learning to Care. In part two, Providing Effective Care, each chapter is associated with a body system, introducing the anatomy and physiology of the system. This is accompanied by a selection of common conditions (pathophysiology), which addresses the diagnosis, care and treatment required. Various skills associated with those conditions are outlined and these are accompanied with boxed learning activities.

In order to enhance learning and to help the reader retain and apply the theory to practice, a range of interactive learning approaches have been used. Where appropriate, chapters will include a section that focuses on care in the home setting and/or the GP surgery; case studies are provided in order to help apply the theoretical component of the chapter to the art and science of caring; and the reader is also asked to stop and reflect. In part two of the text, most chapters have an OSCE (objective structured clinical examination) assisting the reader with regards to what might be expected of them when required to undertake an OSCE as part of their programme of study.

A feature called the medicine trolley is provided in table format which details a selection of medicines related to the conditions/system being discussed in the chapter. The detail includes the name of the drug (generic and trade name), the reason for administration, routes of administration, normal dose, side effects, contra-indications and specific nursing care required when caring for patients receiving medicines.

Boxed features include top tips and hints that the reader can use in the field (at work). Critical awareness boxes address a selection of critical issues that are related to the conditions/system under discussion, helping to improve knowledge and understanding. Chapters identify a 'community of care' and apply aspects of care to a specific community, for example, children, people with learning disabilities, people experiencing mental health problems and those who may experience inequality.

Throughout the text, discussion is underpinned by the best available evidence. Where appropriate, latest guidance is issued by reliable and valid sources (for example, National Institute for Health and Care Excellence (NICE); Scottish Intercollegiate Guidelines Network (SIGN); Department of Health and Social Care (DHSC), the various Royal Colleges and third and voluntary sectors)

We have very much enjoyed writing this text. The NA has always been the focus of each chapter, with an emphasis on helping you to help those you have the privilege to care for, who are very often the most vulnerable in our society. The NA is a key player in the health and social care work force, who very much has the potential to ensure that the patient is truly at the heart of all that is done. We hope you enjoy reading and using the contents of the book, just as we have enjoyed preparing it for you.

Ian Peate
March 2018

REFERENCES

Health Education England, Skills for Care and Skills for Health, 2015. The Care Certificate Framework Guidance Document. http://www.skillsforcare.org.uk/Document-library/Standards/Care-Certificate/Care-Certificate-Guidance-final—Feb-2015.pdf. (Last accessed March 2018).

Nursing and Midwifery Council, 2018a. Standards of Proficiency for Nursing Associates. https://www.nmc.org.uk/globalassets/sitedocuments/education-standards/nursing-associates-proficiency-standards.pdf. (Accessed November 2018.)

Nursing and Midwifery Council, 2018b. The Code Professional Standards of Practice and Behaviour for Nurses, Midwives and Nursing Associates. https://www.nmc.org.uk/globalassets/sitedocuments/nmc-publications/nmc-code.pdf. (Accessed November 2018.)

ACKNOWLEDGEMENTS

I would like to acknowledge the on-going encouragement of Jussi Lahtinen and Mrs Frances Cohen for their unfaltering presence.

I am grateful to my employers, Gibraltar Health Authority, who have offered me much support. They have provided me with a number of opportunities in my career, particularly Dr Ron Coram, the staff of the School of Health Studies library and my colleagues, a continual source of inspiration.

The staff at the Royal College of Nursing Library deserve a particular mention, as year on year, they provide me with exceptional professional services.

I would also like to thank Katie Golsby, development editor, as she helped me bring the manuscript to fruition.

Health and Social Care Provision

Karen Wild

OBJECTIVES

By the end of the chapter the reader will be able to:
1. Consider how health and social care has changed and evolved into its current provision
2. Have an understanding of the provision of healthcare within a range of National Health Service (NHS) settings
3. Be aware of the diverse settings for the provision of health and social care outside of the NHS
4. Understand the way in which health and social care is allocated locally and nationally
5. Understand the meaning of integrated health and social care services within the health and social care setting
6. Evaluate their understanding of health and social care in Britain

KEY WORDS

Healthcare
Social care
Integrated care
National Health Service (NHS)

Public health
Health Education England
Clinical Commissioning Groups (CCGs)

Patient choice
Welfare state
Brexit

CHAPTER AIM

The aim of this chapter is to support the Nursing Associate in their understanding of the way that health and social care is provided within the United Kingdom.

SELF TEST

1. Historically, health and social care in the UK has always been an integrated and seamless service. True or false?
2. What are the major events or discoveries that have shaped healthcare in your lifetime?
3. Are healthcare and social care the same or different? Make a list of what you think is provided in the UK under each heading.
4. When did public health funding become the responsibility of local authorities?
5. What health issues do you most commonly associate with individuals in prison?
6. What is the aim of intermediate care?
7. What does the term 'integrated care' mean to you?
8. What were the 'Five Giants' associated with the development of the welfare state?
9. Can you identify contemporary pandemics that impact upon the provision of health and social care in the UK?
10. What was the main focus of the 1999 Health Act?

INTRODUCTION

The Nursing Associate has a key role in the contribution of care to individuals and groups within the health and social care arena, and as such will benefit from a clear appreciation of the organizations and health and social settings in which they are employed. This chapter will explore those settings and help the Nursing Associate to appreciate how care is tailored to the health and social needs of local populations. Exploring the provision of health and social care within the three healthcare settings of *hospital*, *home* and *close to home* enables the Nursing Associate to appreciate their role in working across organizational boundaries, and in supporting the delivery of high-quality, person-centred, holistic care.

THE NHS – A POTTED HISTORY

The year 2018 marked 70 years of the National Health Service (NHS), which is being used more now than ever in its history of supporting the British public. The Health Service's founding principles – of care for all, on the basis of need not ability to pay – have stood the test of time. Change has always been a factor in the provision of health and social care, and as the current government moves to break away from the European Union, once again anxiety has been generated around the NHS and its future transformations. Brexit is one of the most vigorous recent debates that our country has seen, and the NHS has taken centre stage.

> 'The case for the NHS is straightforward. It does a good job for individual patients, offering high quality care for an ever-expanding range of conditions. It reduces insecurity for families, especially at times of economic uncertainty and dislocation, because access to care is not tied to your job or your income. And as one of the world's most cost-effective health systems, it directly contributes to the success of the British economy.' (Department of Health, 2017)

In 1942, Sir William Beveridge announced that 'Medical treatment covering all requirements will be provided for all citizens by a national health service' and in 1948, the National Health Service was created.

Assumed as free at the point of delivery, the cracks soon began to show, and as early as 1951, proposals were introduced to charge the public for prescriptions, dental care and spectacles. Table 1.1 highlights some of the events that have helped to shape the NHS and healthcare provision as we recognize it today.

REFLECTION 1.1

The information in this chapter is predominantly based on the present provision of health and social care in England.

There exists diverse provision of health and social care in Scotland, Wales and Northern Ireland. Throughout the chapter, as new themes are introduced, you can reflect on how the UK as a whole provides these vital services, and how the services can differ within the United Kingdom.

THE NHS AND HEALTHCARE REFORM

On 1 April 2013, the NHS saw its biggest reform in its 65-year history. Hundreds of NHS organizations were abolished and hundreds of others were created, transforming the provision, commissioning and regulation of healthcare. The reforms were designed to help ensure the long-term sustainability of the NHS, by achieving value for money and shifting care out of hospital and into the community.

Fig. 1.1 provides an overview of the health and care system from April 2013. It shows the statutory bodies that make up the system, centred around people and communities and where they will receive their local health and care services.

In 2013/14, the responsibility for the funding of public health services was handed over to local authorities.

In addition to the changes at NHS Trust level, local authorities now have a much larger role in the responsibility for budgeting public health activities. Health, social care, public health and children's services are integrated. Local authorities are charged with the role of working closely with health and care providers and to use their local knowledge to take on challenges such as alcohol and drug misuse, obesity and sexual health.

In 2014, the NHS presented its Five Year Forward View (DH, 2014), which set out a vision for change within the NHS. It recognized the needs of patients, deep-rooted health inequalities, new treatment emerging and the challenges of mental health, cancer care and the support of an ageing population.

The NHS is treating more patients than ever in its history, with a sharp increase in the number of emergency admissions, planned admissions, outpatient appointments and attendances at A&E departments.

The NHS is mainly paid for from general taxation and National Insurance contributions from the many. Fig. 1.2 shows from where the funding originates. According to the Department of Health (DH), spending on the NHS is due to rise from £123.7 billion in 2017 to £126.5 billion in 2020. Whilst this sounds like a good rate of growth, in real terms, it represents a slowing of the trend of spending on care while demands on the service are growing.

There are a number of factors that have influenced the increase in demand for the services provided by the NHS. One of the key drivers is the ageing population in the UK. Ageing brings with it a degree of associated physical and mental deterioration and the onset of more acute and long-term health problems. As a consequence, healthcare provision is continually adapting to better manage the provision of services for the older person. One example is the move to day case assessment, reducing the need for overnight admissions; this has been a main driver in the increase of elective admissions within the last decade.

REFLECTION 1.2

Apart from the ageing population making demands on the NHS, what other factors may increase the need for healthcare in your geographical area?

Within the last 30 years, the number of hospital beds has dropped by half. This dramatic decline has been attributed to medical development and shorter hospital stays. Forty years ago, a patient being treated for surgical hernia repair might expect to stay in hospital for 7–10 days after surgery, have a large abdominal wound, sutures or clips, and be recommended bed rest. Contemporary treatment sees the patient treated as a day case and home the same day after endoscopic surgery. This form of hospital admission has significantly increased, as has the occupancy level of the average hospital bed.

REFLECTION 1.3

What risks do you think are associated with the increased occupancy of a typical hospital bed? How might this impact on your role as a Nursing Associate in relation to person-centred care?

TABLE 1.1 Some Historical Events That Have Helped to Shape the Current NHS

1948 **NHS established**	The NHS is born on 5 July 1948 out of a long-held ideal that good healthcare should be available to all, regardless of wealth. For the first time, hospitals, doctors, nurses, pharmacists, opticians and dentists are brought together under one umbrella organization that is free for all at the point of delivery.
1952 **Prescription charges introduced**	Prescription charges of one shilling (5p) are introduced and a flat rate of a pound for ordinary dental treatment is also brought in on 1 June 1952. Prescription charges are abolished in 1965, and prescriptions remain free until June 1968, when the charges are reintroduced.
1954 **Smoking-cancer link established**	British scientist Sir Richard Doll begins research into lung cancer after incidences of the disease rise alarmingly. He studies lung cancer patients in 20 London hospitals, and issues a warning that smokers are far more likely than non-smokers to die of lung cancer.
1954 **Children get daily visits**	Until this point, children in hospital were often only allowed to see their parents for an hour on Saturdays and Sundays and were frequently placed in adult wards.
1958 **Polio and diphtheria vaccinations**	One of the primary aims of the NHS is to promote good health, not simply to treat illness, and the introduction of the polio and diphtheria vaccines is a key part of the NHS's plans. Before this programme, cases of polio could climb as high as 8,000 in epidemic years, with cases of diphtheria as high as 70,000, leading to 5,000 deaths. Everyone under the age of 15 is vaccinated, leading to an immediate and dramatic reduction in cases of both diseases.
1961 **The contraceptive pill is made available**	Initially, it is only available to married women, but this is relaxed in 1967. Between 1962 and 1969, the number of women taking the contraceptive pill increases dramatically, from approximately 50,000 to 1 million.
1962 **The Hospital Plan**	The Hospital Plan approves the development of district general hospitals for population areas of about 125,000.
1967 **The Salmon Report**	The report sets out recommendations for developing the nursing staff structure and the status of the profession in hospital management.
1968 **First NHS heart transplant**	Surgeon Donald Ross carries out Britain's first heart transplant at the National Heart Hospital in Marylebone, London.
1972 **CT scans introduced**	Computer tomography scans start to revolutionize the way physicians examine the body.
1978 **First test-tube baby**	In Oldham, Lancashire, Louise Brown is the world's first baby to be born as a result of in-vitro fertilization, which fertilizes the egg outside the woman's body before replacing it in the womb.
1979 **Bone marrow transplant**	Professor Roland Levinsky performs the UK's first successful bone marrow transplant for children with primary immunodeficiency at Great Ormond Street Hospital for Children.
1980s **MRI scans introduced**	Magnetic resonance imaging scanners prove more effective than CT scans in providing information about soft tissues, such as scans of the brain.
1980 **Black Report**	The report aims to investigate the inequality of healthcare that still exists despite the foundation of the NHS, i.e., differences between the social classes in the usage of medical services, infant mortality rates and life expectancy. Poor people are still more likely to die earlier than rich ones. The Whitehead Report in 1987 and the Acheson Report in 1998 reached the same conclusions as the Black Report. More recently, the Marmot Review of 2010 proposes an evidence-based strategy to address the social determinants of health, the conditions in which people are born, grow, live, work and age, which can lead to health inequalities.
1990 **NHS and Community Care Act**	Health authorities will manage their own budgets and buy healthcare from hospitals and other health organizations. In order to be deemed a 'provider' of such healthcare, organizations will become NHS Trusts, that is, independent organizations with their own managements.
1991 **First NHS Trusts established**	NHS trusts are established to make the service more responsive to the user at a local level. They aim to encourage creativity and innovation and challenge the domination of the hospitals within a health service that is increasingly focused on services in the community.
1998 **NHS Direct launches**	A nurse-led advice service provides people with 24-hour health advice over the phone. This service closes in 2014 and is replaced with the Call NHS 111 non-emergency number to access local healthcare services.
2000 **NHS walk-in centres**	NHS walk-in centres (WiCs) offer convenient access to a range of NHS services and are managed by Primary Care Trusts.
2002 **Primary care trusts launched**	The primary care trusts oversee 29,000 GPs and 21,000 NHS dentists. As local organizations, they are best positioned to understand the needs of their community, so they can make sure that the organizations providing health and social care services are working effectively.
2008 **Free choice is introduced**	Patients can choose from any hospital or clinic that meets NHS standards, according to what matters most to them, whether it is location, waiting times, reputation, clinical performance, visiting policies, parking facilities or patients' comments.

Continued

TABLE 1.1 Some Historical Events That Have Helped to Shape the Current NHS—cont'd	
2008 **The NHS at 60**	Since its launch in 1948, the NHS has grown to become the world's largest publicly funded health service.
2009 **New NHS Constitution**	For the first time in the history of the NHS, the Constitution brings together details of what staff, patients and the public can expect from the NHS. It aims to ensure the NHS will always do what it was set up to do in 1948: provide high-quality healthcare that is free and for everyone.
2009 **NHS Health Checks**	Primary care trusts begin implementing the NHS Health Check programme in April 2009 for adults in England between the ages of 40 and 74. It has the potential to prevent an average of 1,600 heart attacks and strokes and save up to 650 lives each year. It could prevent over 4,000 people a year from developing diabetes and detect at least 20,000 cases of diabetes or kidney disease earlier, allowing people to manage their condition better and improving their quality of life.
2009 **Care Quality Commission (CQC) launched**	The CQC is a new regulator for health, mental health and adult social care, and coordinates information from the monitoring and inspection of all health and social care services.
2009 **The Mid Staffordshire NHS Foundation Trust public inquiry**	An investigation into the apparently high mortality rates of patients admitted as emergencies to Mid Staffordshire NHS Foundation Trust since April 2005, and the care provided to these patients.
2011 **The Health and Social Care Bill**	Sets out the government's vision to create a modernized NHS built around patients, led by health professionals and focused on world-class healthcare outcomes.
2013 **The Health and Social Care Act (2012) takes effect.**	The act provides the most comprehensive reforms since the introduction of the NHS in 1948. Putting clinicians at the centre of commissioning care means that providers can become more innovative, supporting patient choice, and pushing the public health agenda forward.

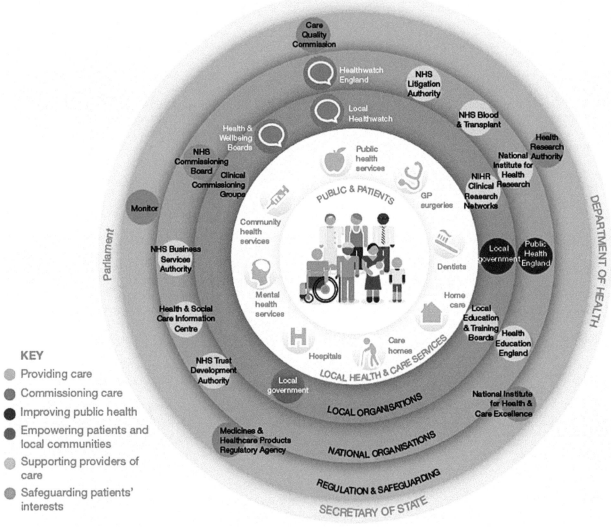

KEY
- Providing care
- Commissioning care
- Improving public health
- Empowering patients and local communities
- Supporting providers of care
- Safeguarding patients' interests

Fig. 1.1 An Overview of the Health and Care System from April 2013 (Department of Health. Contains public sector information licensed under the Open Government Licence v3.0).

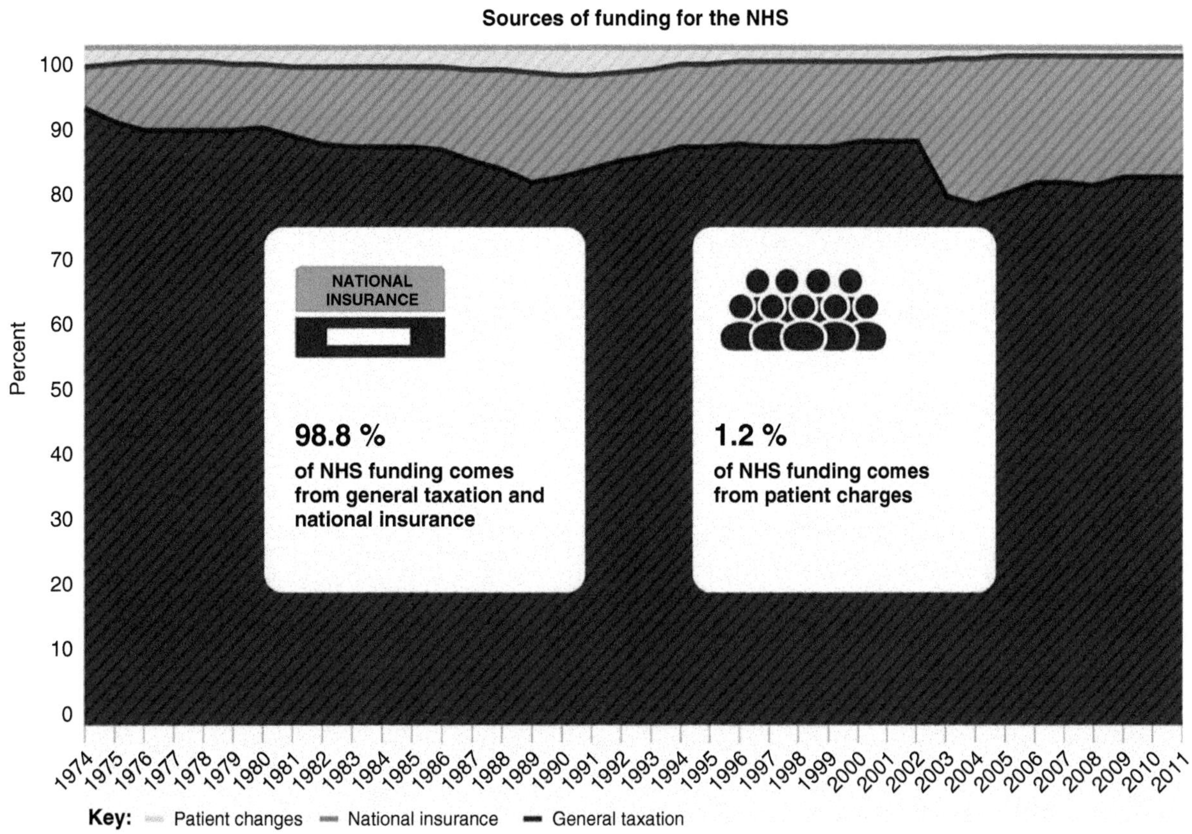

Sources of funding for the NHS

Fig. 1.2 Sources of Funding for the NHS (King's Fund, 2017).

Thelma, aged 76, is admitted to A&E following a fall at home. She has a history of alcohol misuse and has not been eating much for the last few weeks. She is confused about where she is, and is accompanied by her niece. Following assessment, there is an urgent need for Thelma to be admitted to the ward for treatment and rehabilitation. A search for a bed quickly shows that none are immediately available. The A&E trolley that Thelma has now been lying on for almost 5 hours is hard and unyielding. Thelma is at risk from obvious physical deterioration, and from the emotional trauma of the situation.

An occupancy level for overnight acute beds has risen from 87.1% in 2010 to 90.4% in 2017. According to information from the National Audit Office (2013), the risks of bed shortages, transfer times outside of the 4-hour standard from A&E, transfers outside of the patient's geographical area and healthcare-acquired infections, increase with bed occupancy levels over the 85% barrier.

As an employer, the NHS boasts just over one million full-time equivalent (FTE) staff. The number of nursing staff has slowly grown since 2013, with 286,020 FTEs in 2017. This slow growth fails to fully meet the demands of the service but is in part a reaction to the various reports on the quality of patient care within NHS establishments. Chapters in this text will explore the quality of care in detail. Health Education England has looked into the shortfall of nursing and estimates that by 2020, the deficit will be as much as 11.4%. Similar bodies exist in Scotland and Wales.

CLINICAL COMMISSIONING GROUPS (CCGs)

In their role of overseeing local geographical areas, CCGs commission most hospital and community NHS services in England. They are involved in deciding which health services are needed most for local populations and include general practice (GP) and dental services, in addition to many specialist hospital services. All GP practices belong to a CCG, along with other healthcare professionals. Typical commissions include:

- Elective hospital care
- Rehabilitation
- Emergency and urgent care 24-hours
- Most community health services
- Mental health and learning disability services.

The CCGs are expected to use their expertise and clinical knowledge to purchase the most efficient services to drive up competition and so improve quality and standards.

Patient choice

In April 2016, the government introduced the NHS Choice Framework (DH, 2016), which promotes the empowerment of patients in the choice and control over how they receive their healthcare. Included in the framework is the patient's right to the following:

- *Choice of which GP* service to register with.
- *Choice of where to go* for a first appointment as an outpatient.
- *Choice of clinical team* who will support care.

- *Opportunity to change hospitals* if patients wait longer than the maximum time of 18 weeks, or 2 weeks to see a specialist for cancer.
- *Choice of who carries out a specialist test.*
- *Choice of maternity services.* Women can opt for a home birth, birth in a midwife-led facility or in a hospital with maternity support.
- *Choice of services provided in the community.* Provided that the CCG has those services in place as part of its commissioning.
- *Choice to take part in health research.* Examples include clinical trials in medicines. Patients have the right to refuse to take part.
- *Choice to have a personal health budget.* Some individuals with long-term conditions can opt to have control about the way that care is planned and the way resources are allocated to provide appropriate care. This is a right extended to adults who are eligible for NHS continuing healthcare (CHC) and children who are eligible for continuing care (CC).
- *Choice of accessing treatment in another country in the European Economic Area.* This is a legal requirement set out in the NHS constitution and current EU law.

COMMON SERVICES PROVIDED BY THE NHS

The NHS is divided into primary, secondary and tertiary care, and the next section of this chapter will provide some common examples of how this operates within the UK.

Emergency care

In the UK, the 'Call 999' for serious and life-threatening illness or injury has long been in existence and triggers an emergency response. Paramedics attend and assess or triage individuals in an emergency.

The role of the nurse in urgent and emergency care can include handling more complex calls made to the 999 line; here they utilize advanced skills of communication and assessment. They can also assist other 999 call-handlers and be on hand to help when callers fail to follow instructions from call handlers. The 'Call 111' service is provided as a medical help and advice line for non-emergency or non–life-threatening situations. The call line can also be used to help people identify which service they may need for specific problems.

Primary care

Primary care is the most common point of contact for people engaging with NHS services, and accounts for around 90% of patient interaction. The services that are provided in primary healthcare are varied, and regularly include general practice, NHS dental healthcare, community pharmacies and optometry services.

GPs handle an estimated 300 million plus consultations every year. This is significantly more than visits to A&E departments. The introduction of GP-based clinical pharmacists is increasing, and the public are being increasingly encouraged to direct more common health complaints to clinical pharmacists before seeking advice and treatment from a GP.

The main aim of primary healthcare is to provide a focus on individuals rather than specific diseases, and this is reflected in the provision of healthcare that is generalist rather than specialist. GPs are a good example of this, and individuals can be referred from primary care to specialist practitioners for more detailed care. Primary care is focused on providing treatment for common illnesses, managing long-term conditions such as heart disease, the prevention of ill health and its consequences, screening for health associated with risk and immunization to prevent disease. Care is provided to all and involves the broadest scope of healthcare; many patients will tend to favour continuity of care with one group or individual GP practice. The introduction of digital primary care allows patients remote access to GP-based services.

COMMUNITIES OF CARE

Homeless People

'Pathway' is a charity that works to improve healthcare for people who are homeless. It does this by assisting the NHS to create teams of doctors, nurses and social care professionals to support approximately 3,500 homeless patients each year. Working closely with researchers from University College London, it recognizes that socially excluded groups like the homeless have mortality rates eight times higher than the population average for men, and almost twelve times for women.

An example of primary care is the 'Homeless Accommodation Leeds Pathway' in Leeds. In conjunction with the Leeds Community Health Care Trust, it runs the York Street Primary Health Care service for homeless people, and St George's Crypt, which support the homeless with emergency accommodation.

Visit the Pathway website www.pathway.org.uk for more examples of health and social care of homeless people.

Secondary care

Often referred to as hospital or community care, secondary care can be either planned (elective), for example hip replacement, or urgent and emergency care, such as triage following an accident. Other examples of secondary care include rehabilitative care, community health services, mental health and learning disability health services.

Access to secondary NHS care is normally through the primary care route; traditionally this has been thought of as '*gatekeeping*' where typically GPs authorize access to specialty care, hospital and inpatient referrals and diagnostic testing. The idea is that primary care opens the gate to specialist care where extra support and treatment is needed. Current debate around this method of healthcare introduces controversies such as the speed of referrals, meeting the needs of patient choice and the cost implications to CCGs (Greenfield, Foley & Majeed, 2016).

Secondary care is commissioned within Trusts by the CCGs, who allocate their substantial budgets to meet the secondary care need of specific populations. Depending on local commissioning arrangements, CCGs have a role in designing care pathways that deliver efficient and convenient patient services, with good communication between GPs and secondary care providers. Secondary care is often referred to as being the 'provider' of care. Under the new NHS Standards Contract for 2017–19, CCGs buy services from providers; this came into force on 1 April 2017 and will remain so until 31 March 2019. The NHS Standard Contract was updated in January 2018 to update the Contract in line with legislative and policy changes.

Patients can expect good communication and responses to their queries. Secondary care outcomes must be communicated to patients directly. When patients are discharged from secondary care, a discharge summary is sent to the GP within 24 hours of any care from A&E, inpatient or day-case treatment. In addition, arrangements for sufficient medication and shared care protocols on discharge remain the responsibility of the provider of secondary care. Clinical responsibility for shared care arrangements must be agreed by the CCG. Where existing care pathways are agreed this is not a problem; however, where new care is needed, the CCG will be required to commission that care. In the case study below, you can see how this can be established.

CASE STUDY 1.2 Brendan — Learning Difficulties

Brendon has Down syndrome, and now in his late 40s, is becoming increasingly dependent on the help of the support team of his supported living accommodation. Staff have noted how Brendan has become uncharacteristically untidy and is not attending to his hygiene. He has become angry and even aggressive when staff gently prompt him to take his cardiac medications. He has been found wandering late at night, inappropriately clothed, sometimes in his pyjamas.

The GP reviewed Brendan's current health and, knowing that a direct link exists between Down syndrome and dementia, referred him for secondary mental health care for assessment. A diagnosis of Alzheimer dementia was established.

Although a care package was in existence, the new diagnosis and subsequent need for a step up in care meant a review was necessary to provide the right services for Brendan as his dementia develops. In this situation, the CCG had to commission a new package of care to incorporate the need for ongoing mental health care.

Tertiary care

Tertiary care refers to highly specialized treatment, such as neurosurgery, transplants and secure forensic mental health services. Funded by the NHS via the Department of Health, it involves specific care for people needing complex treatments across a very broad range of specialist care. Individuals may be referred for tertiary care (for example, to a specialist stroke unit) from either primary care or secondary care.

CASE STUDY 1.3 Cancer Care

A 42-year-old woman is diagnosed with stage 2 breast cancer and is immediately referred following secondary care breast screening to the specialist tertiary oncology service. Here she receives more specialist analysis of the tumour and the surrounding lymph nodes. Surgical and treatment options are discussed.

The tertiary care in this scenario provides specialist surgical expertise with associated radiotherapy, hormone and chemotherapy, breast reconstruction options, counselling and follow-up screening services.

Maternity care

Maternity services in the UK can be divided into three broad areas:

- **Antenatal care** – primary care facility within the community setting; it involves the pregnant woman and her family, the midwife and the GP. Secondary care provides antenatal clinics with access to specialist screening, such as ultrasound scans, dieticians, mental health and help with smoking cessation. According to the Maternity Services Data Set (MSDS) of 2016, 11.6% of women at their antenatal booking appointment were smokers.
- **Intrapartum or intranatal care** – the care given during labour. According to NHS Digital, there were 636,401 deliveries in NHS hospitals during 2016–17, a decrease of 1.8% from 2015–16 (NHS England, 2017). Other options for women in labour are to give birth in a midwifery unit with minimal medical interventions, or to opt for a home delivery.
- **Postnatal care** – centres on the woman and her baby in the first 8 weeks following birth. Initially, the focus is on urgent care of the newborn and postpartum woman. In the primary setting, care supports infant nutrition, maternal physical and mental well-being, emotional support and adaptations to family life, contraception and immunization schedules.

COMMUNITIES OF CARE

Offender Healthcare

In the UK annually, there are approximately 100 prison births. Women offenders who give birth in prison can keep their baby for the first 18 months in a mother and baby unit.

The charity Birth Companions has introduced a Birth Charter for England and Wales stating that pregnant women in prison should:

1. have access to the same standard of antenatal care as other women in the community
2. attend antenatal classes and prepare for their baby's birth
3. be housed, fed and moved in such a way that the well-being of mother and baby are paramount
4. be informed that they have a place on a Mother and Baby Unit as soon as possible after they have been admitted to the prison
5. receive appropriate support if the woman opts for termination of pregnancy.

During childbirth, women should:

6. have access to a birth supporter of their choice
7. be escorted by officers who have received appropriate training and have been issued with clear guidance
8. be offered essential items for labour, as well as the early postnatal period
9. receive appropriate care while being transferred between prison and hospital.

Those women with babies in prison should:

10. be encouraged and supported in their chosen method of infant feeding
11. be supported in expressing, storing and transporting their breast milk safely, if these women are separated from their baby
12. be offered the same opportunities and support to nurture and bond with their babies as do women in the community
13. be allowed additional family visits.

All pregnant women and new mothers should:

14. be able to gain access to counselling when needed
15. receive appropriate resettlement services when released from prison.

(Adapted from *Birth Companions*, 2016)

Hospital at home

The principle here is that patients stay in their own homes, but they receive extra care and attention from the Hospital at Home team. The team works like a hospital ward team and has the same skills and clinical expertise. The team runs regular multidisciplinary meetings where they discuss the patients they are looking after. The service is designed to give patients extra support so that they do not have to be admitted to hospital or so that their admission is as short as possible. The patient may often stay under the supervision of the secondary or tertiary service with specialist nurses and consultant specialists providing remote supervision. The GP will be involved as part of a shared care arrangement.

COMMUNITIES OF CARE
Children and Young People

Whittington Health NHS Trust
'Our Hospital at Home service provides care for children and young people in Islington. Specialist community children's nurses work in partnership with acute paediatricians at Whittington Health and University College London Hospital to provide safe care at home for acutely unwell children and young people (0–18 years) enabling them to be discharged from hospital quicker or preventing admission.'

'A nurse-led team conduct home visits. They can administer IV antibiotics, monitor the trajectory of an acutely unwell child or young person and provide additional support to enable a carer to look after the child or young person within their home environment.'

'The service works closely with community paediatricians, GPs, midwives and other community health services.' https://www.whittington.nhs.uk/default.asp?c=20049

Intermediate care

Intermediate care exists to support people to be as independent as possible. It involves at-home care away from the hospital setting from a range of interdisciplinary professionals in health and social care. It can provide care as a means of preventing hospital admission or as a rehabilitation facility following hospital care. It aims primarily to help people make the move back into the community in a safe and timely way to prevent long-term hospital or residential care.

REFLECTION 1.4

Black and Minority Care
Mr Sastry is an 83-year-old Hindu who is admitted to intermediate care to support his rehabilitation following treatment for oesophageal cancer. As a member of the collaborative team in intermediate care, reflect on how you would apply the principles of a person-centred approach to help Mr Sastry.

The National Institute for Health and Care Excellence (NICE) guidelines (2017) describe the need for a person-centred approach to care and coin the phrase 'reablement' as a core principle of intermediate care. The Nursing Associate working within this environment will be part of a collaborative team who adopt a person-centred approach to care. In this way, individuals will receive care that optimizes their well-being and is sensitive of their cultural differences and preferences. According to NICE (2017) guidelines, intermediate care practitioners should:
* work in partnership with the person to find out what they want to achieve and understand what motivates them
* focus on the person's own strengths and help them realize their potential to regain independence
* build the person's knowledge, skills, resilience and confidence
* learn to observe and guide and not automatically intervene, even when the person is struggling to perform an activity, such as dressing themselves or preparing a snack
* support positive risk taking.

(NICE, 2017)

❗ HOTSPOT

The Nursing Associate working within the intermediate care setting will be part of a collaborative team, and as such will need to adopt a person-centred approach to care. In this way, individuals will receive care that optimizes their well-being and is sensitive of their cultural differences and preferences.

Integrated care

For care to be integrated, organizations and care professionals need to pull together all the different aspects of care that a person needs. Individuals benefit from an approach to care that is person-centred. In addition, they benefit from care that is co-ordinated within healthcare settings, across physical and mental health, bridging health and social care. Integrated care takes many different forms. In some circumstances, integration may focus on primary and secondary care, and in others, it may involve health and social care.

Typically, a person's care may be provided by several different health and social care professionals, across different providers. Fragmentation of the services and difficulty in accessing care not based around their (or their carers') needs can occur as a result of this. However, according to the government (2015) good integrated care can reduce:
* confusion
* repetition
* delay
* duplication and gaps in service delivery
* people getting lost in the system

(GOV.UK, 2015)

In the following case study, an example of good integrated care can be seen.

SOCIAL CARE: A POTTED HISTORY

The beginnings of contemporary social care can be attributed to the 1948 National Assistance Act and the creation of the welfare state. But the origins of social care go way back in history to Elizabethan poor law, the workhouse and insurance provision to support care via the mutual and friendly societies of the 19th and 20th centuries.

CASE STUDY 1.4 Ruben

Ruben is 83 years old, and apart from visiting the dentist and optician, he could not remember the last time he used the NHS. 'I had just turned 80 and my daughter persuaded me to go and see the doctor because of pain in my knee joints, I couldn't remember ever going to the doctor.' Ruben's GP records showed no evidence of any consultations since he was a teenager.

Ruben was prescribed nonsteroidal antiinflammatory drugs for his joint pain and referred to the practice nurse for routine health screening. 'That was the turning point for me, until then, I had felt that I was well!' reports Ruben.

Routine screening revealed that Ruben had type 2 diabetes. Over the past 3 years, Ruben has really got to know the diabetic team that monitors his health, and despite feeling at times that he is on a merry-go-round of appointments, the service provides him with support and advice from the specialist dietician, annual retinal screening from the ophthalmic services, referrals to the podiatry service and meetings with specialist nurses to review his blood glucose levels and adjust his medications accordingly.

Six months ago, Ruben was admitted to hospital with acute retention of urine caused by enlargement of his prostate. While there, he developed a urinary tract infection and was really disoriented for a number of days. Communication from the primary care setting meant that nursing and medical staff in hospital were able to compare his normal state, review his care package and organize intermediate care as a step down from hospital. Here, the liaison District Nurse was able to review his case, discuss the prospect of a trial without catheter (TWOC) with the urologist, and as a result, speed Ruben's return home. He was assessed by the Occupational Therapist who came home with him on discharge to gauge his need for adjustments to his home environment.

He is now the proud owner of a perching stool in his kitchen, an adapted chair for his shower, a rail to help him in and out of bed and a quad walking stick.

His care is now managed between the GP and the specialist diabetic care team, and he has a range of drug therapies, which the GP-based clinical pharmacist arranges and delivers in blister packs that are easy to read and help ensure the right dosage of drug is administered at the right time. This is supported by an electronic talking drug reminder device.

Most importantly, Ruben feels involved in the decisions about his care and he is able to express his anxieties about his prostate problem. Communication and information about who and when to contact the service for help have supported Ruben's transition from semi-dependency within the intermediate care setting, to independency within his own home.

(Adapted from Peate & Wild, 2018)

The evolution of the welfare state as we know it today was based on the desire to overcome the 'Five Giants' of want, disease, squalor, ignorance and idleness identified by William Beveridge (Fig. 1.3). To enable this, the Beveridge Report (1942) called for a radical change to the way that society supported health and social care. The wide range of suggestions included the setting up of universal benefits that would support those in old age, unemployment and sickness. It asked for a comprehensive and free at the point of delivery national health service, as well as free and universal secondary education. In addition, the report highlighted the need for an overhaul of spending to improve and create more public-sector housing, and an ambitious target of employment for all.

The post-war Labour government of 1945 set the ball in motion to establish a welfare state that is still recognizable today. Table 1.2 provides a brief overview of some of the key historical events that have helped to shape current social care in this country.

The following data serve as a salient reminder of the current social services provision in England. According to the Department of Health corporate plan 2014 to 2015:

- in England, there are over 17,500 care and nursing homes
- over 410,000 people live in residential care or nursing homes
- there are 220,000 state supported users in residential care
- 1.1 million people received community-based services from councils in 2012–13
- there are 720,000 state supported users of community services
- there are 1.63 million adult social care jobs in England
- there are estimated to be over 5.4 million informal carers
- local councils fund 60% of adult social care.

(DH, 2014)

LOOKING BACK, FEEDING FORWARD

Health and social care in the UK has been shaped by an eclectic mix of historical, political, scientific and technological developments. The public has emerged as a savvier consumer of care and, as such, expectations of the way that care is organized and delivered has come under intense scrutiny. Demographics have

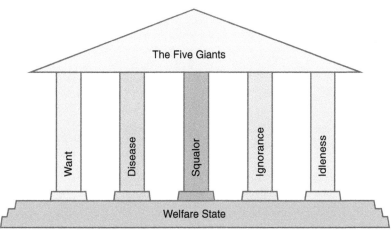

Fig. 1.3 The Five Giants.

TABLE 1.2	Some Historical Events that Have Helped to Shape Current Social Care
1948 National Assistance Act	Sets out a framework for an insurance-based system for a health service and unemployment support. Selective social support is provided on a means-tested basis, and charges applied for residential and non-residential services. The NHS is created.
1959 Mental Health Act	Community-based services for people with mental health needs, alongside the beginnings of a reduction of long stay psychiatric hospital provision.
1968 The Seebohm Report	'One door to knock upon' recommended the establishment of a family social service.
1973 NHS Reorganisation Act	The establishment of Health Authorities, coinciding with the reorganization of local government. Alignment of health authorities and local authorities was attempted.
1975	The development of a white paper, *Better Services for the Mentally Ill*, which sets the scene for an expansion of local authority social services and the provision of specialist mental health services through local general hospitals.
1977	The parallel provision of Joint Finance and Joint Care Planning Teams supports the notion of joined-up care.
1978 A Happier Old Age	A consultative document aims to highlight the debate around the well-being and dignity of elderly people (DHSS, 1978). The 1981 white paper, *Growing Older*, focuses on the need for services to 'help people to care for themselves'.
1980 Health Service Act	Establishes District Health Authorities from 1982 and sees a demise of joined-up care in some areas (DHSS, 1980).
1988	Sir Roy Griffiths publishes his report Community *Care; Agenda for action* (Griffiths, 1988).
1990 NHS and Community Care Act	Emphasizes the need, where possible, to support the care of people in their own homes. The independent sector is promoted, with the provision phased in over a 3-year period. In 1996, The Carers Act takes this further by introducing cash payment in lieu of services that service users can purchase independently.
1999 The Health Act	Introduces integrated provision between NHS and Social Services, with pooled budgets and commissioning arrangements.
2000	The NHS Plan launches, which introduces intermediate care as a stage between hospital and home.
2003 The Community Care Act	Requires Social Services and the NHS to communicate about the discharge of patients from hospital. It builds in a reimbursement provision where councils are responsible for delays in discharging patients if they cannot facilitate care.
2006	White paper, *Our Health, Our Care, Our Say: A new direction for community services*. The key policy areas are: better prevention; more choice; tackling inequalities; support for people with long-term needs (DH, 2006).
2010	White paper, *Building the National Care Service is* presented by the Labour government, it sets out the proposal to build a comprehensive National Care Service for all adults in England with an eligible care need, free when they need it.
2014 The Care Act	Includes funding reforms, achieves royal assent.
2017	The Chancellor announces £2 billion extra funding for adult social care in the March budget and a further £350 million boost to support winter care in the NHS in his November budget statement. Adapted from *The origins and development of social care*, The Kings Fund https://www.kingsfund.org.uk/sites/default/files/Securing_Good_Care_Chapter_1.pdf

changed too, with people living longer and presenting with many complex health and social care needs. New pandemics, such as diseases related to alcohol misuse and the increasing incidence of obesity, bring fresh challenges to the services. Data from the Department of Health corporate report of 2014 revealed the following information:

- England has one of the highest rates of obesity in the developed world – two-thirds of adults are overweight or obese, a leading cause of type 2 diabetes and heart disease.
- The gap between highest and lowest life expectancy based on area is around 12 years.
- Smoking still claims over 80,000 lives a year.
- More than one in five adults in England, or 9 million people, regularly drink alcohol at levels that could damage their health and more than 20,000 people die from alcohol-related causes each year.
- Around 665,000 people in England have dementia.
- The NHS Health Check programme is now being delivered in every local authority across England (Source: Public Health England).

(DH, 2014)

The *Next Steps NHS Five Year Forward View* (NHS 2017) sets out a radical plan to address the needs of the population and to uphold the initial principle of the NHS at its inception 70 years ago, that is, 24-hour care 7 days a week, available for all UK citizens who are in need.

REFERENCES

Beveridge, W.H.B., 1942. Social Insurance and Allied Services: Report by Sir William Beveridge. HM Stationery Office, London.

Birth Companions, 2016. Birth Charter for women in prisons in England and Wales. https://www.birthcompanions.org.uk/media/Public/Resources/Ourpublications/Birth_Charter_Online_copy.pdf.

Department of Health (DH), 2006. Our Health, Our Care, Our Say: A New Direction for Community Services. DH, London. https://www.gov.uk/government/uploads/system/uploads/attachment_data/file/272238/6737.pdf.

Department of Health (DH), 2014. Corporate Report. Department of Health Corporate Plan 2014 to 2015. DH, London. https://www.gov.uk/government/publications/department-of-health-corporate-plan-2014-to-2015.

Department of Health (DH), 2014. Five Year Forward View. DH, London. https://www.england.nhs.uk/wp-content/uploads/2014/10/5yfv-web.pdf.

Department of Health (DH), 2016. The NHS Choice Framework: What Choices Are Available to Me on the NHS? DH, London. https://www.gov.uk/government/publications/the-nhs-choice-framework.

Department of Health (DH), 2017. Next Steps on the NHS Five Year Forward View. DH, London. https://www.england.nhs.uk/wp-content/uploads/2017/03/NEXT-STEPS-ON-THE-NHS-FIVE-YEAR-FORWARD-VIEW.pdf.

Department of Health and Social Security (DHSS), 1978. A Happier Old Age: A Discussion Document on Elderly People in Our Society. The Stationery Office. Dept. of Health and Social Security, Great Britain. Welsh Office, Great Britain.

Department of Health and Social Security (DHSS), 1981. Growing Old. White Paper. HMSO, London.

GOV.UK, 2015. Delivering better integrated care. https://www.gov.uk/guidance/enabling-integrated-care-in-the-nhs.

Griffiths, R., 1988. Community Care: Agenda for Action. A Report to the Secretary of State for Social Services. HMSO, London.

Greenfield, G., Foley, K., Majeed, A., 2016. Rethinking primary care's gatekeeper role. Br. Med. J. 354.

King's Fund, 2017. The NHS in a Nutshell. https://www.kingsfund.org.uk/projects/nhs-in-a-nutshell/hospital-activity.

National Audit Office, 2013. Emergency Admissions to Hospital: Managing the Demand. DH, London.

NHS England, 2017. Maternity Services Monthly Statistics, England – April 2017, Experimental statistics. https://digital.nhs.uk/catalogue/PUB30071.

National Institute for Health and Care Excellence, 2017. Intermediate care including reablement. NICE guideline [NG74]. www.nice.org.uk.

Peate, I., Wild, K., 2018. Nursing Practice, Knowledge and Care, second ed. Wiley, Chichester.

The Care Certificate

Ian Peate

OBJECTIVES

By the end of the chapter the reader will be able to:
1. Understand the inception of the Care Certificate
2. Discuss the standards that make up the Care Certificate
3. Relate the Care Certificate to their daily working lives
4. Identify ways in which the Care Certificate can help support staff offer compassionate, safe and high-quality care and support
5. Align the Care Certificate to any course or programme of study the Nursing Associate and the healthcare assistant is undertaking
6. Consider competence and assessments of skills

KEY WORDS

Care	Benchmarks	Courage
Safety	Respect	Responsibility
Communication	Competence	
Standards	Confidence	

CHAPTER AIM

The aim of this chapter is to introduce the Care Certificate.

SELF TEST

1. What is the role of the Care Quality Commission in England?
2. What are the equivalent independent regulatory bodies in the other three countries of the UK?
3. How many standards make up the Care Certificate?
4. Is the completion of the Care Certificate a compulsory requirement?
5. In England, when and why was the Care Certificate introduced?
6. What resources might you use to complete the standards in the Care Certificate?
7. What does the term 'competency' mean?
8. How can you help to ensure that healthcare assistants remain competent in their place of work?
9. As a Nursing Associate, you must be aware of your own learning needs; how will you identify the learning needs of the healthcare assistant?
10. What form of appraisal (sometimes called an individual personal review) is implemented in the place where you work?

INTRODUCTION

The introduction of the Care Certificate was suggested by Camilla Cavendish (Cavendish, 2013), who was appointed to look into the role of the healthcare assistant after the Francis Inquiry (2013) into unacceptable standards of care at Mid-Staffordshire National Health Service (NHS) Foundation Trust and after serious challenges in other health and social care settings were identified. Applying only to England, the Certificate sets out the minimum standards that should be covered in induction training prior to staff starting work in health and social care settings. It describes the required values, behaviours and competencies that a new carer has to learn and demonstrate within their first 12-week period of employment. Nursing Associates (NAs) work with and support healthcare assistants as they work through the Care Certificate.

The Care Certificate is not a compulsory requirement for a healthcare assistant or an NA to complete. However, organizations that have responsibility for regulating services, such as the Care Quality Commission, will expect that new staff (such as the Nursing Associate) in workplaces regulated by the Commission will achieve the competencies that are set out in the Certificate as part of their induction to the service. The Certificate is an example of good practice. The NA's programme of study will incorporate the standards of the Care Certificate.

BOX 2.1   **The 15 standards in the Care Certificate**

1. Understand your role
2. Your personal development
3. Duty of care
4. Equality and diversity
5. Work in a person-centred way
6. Communication
7. Privacy and dignity
8. Fluids and nutrition
9. Awareness of mental health, dementia and learning disability
10. Safeguarding adults
11. Safeguarding children
12. Basic life support
13. Health and safety
14. Handling information
15. Infection prevention and control

(Reprinted With Permission From Skills for Health, Health Education England and Skills for Care.)

BOX 2.2   **Some examples of assessors**

- Health Professional e.g. Nurse, Occupational Therapist, Physiotherapist, Dietician, Social Worker
- NVQ or QCF Diploma in Health and Social Care at Level 2, 3 or 5
- NVQ in Health or QCF Diploma in Clinical Healthcare Support or QCF Diploma in Allied Health Professional Support or QCF Diploma in Maternity and Paediatric Support
- Registered Manager Award

(Reprinted With Permission From Skills for Health, Health Education England and Skills for Care.)

There are 15 standards associated with the Care Certificate (see Box 2.1). The overarching aim underpinning the Certificate is to ensure standardized training associated with the fundamentals of care and to help support staff in acquiring the vital skills and knowledge required to offer safe, high-quality and effective care. All 15 standards must be achieved in knowledge and practice and evidence of completion provided by compiling a portfolio. The portfolio then becomes a 'passport' across healthcare settings in England (Gilding, 2017).

Irrespective of where the support staff work, be it in cardiac care or mental health or residential care, if they have completed the Care Certificate they will have a common standard of initial training, and this will be reflected in the way they work. The Care Certificate provides some consistency to care provision across the health and social care sectors.

TEACHING AND ASSESSING THE CARE CERTIFICATE

Johnson and Buzzi (2016) note that there should be corresponding teaching delivered alongside completion of the Care Certificate that addresses all the knowledge elements. The teaching can be delivered in-house or by an external provider. Staff should be provided with opportunities to practise and develop their skills in a classroom environment; however, most of the assessed evidence has to be collected during real work activity. Some of the assessment criteria will only test knowledge; others, however, test knowledge as well as practical competence. Once the Care Certificate competencies have been successfully achieved, this should be recognized by other employers (Peate, 2015).

Skills for Care (2015) points out that the Care Certificate applies across health and social care and links to competences associated with National Occupational Standards and units that result in qualifications. The standards cover what is necessary to work as a carer, and they aim to equip staff with the fundamental skills required to provide quality care. They also offer a

basis from which staff can further develop their knowledge and skills as their careers progress.

It is intended that the Care Certificate will offer a clear indication to patients, employers and those who receive care and support, that the person who is providing care has been trained and developed against a particular set of standards and that they have been assessed for the skills, knowledge and behaviours required to provide compassionate and high-quality care and support. However, currently there is limited literature available to healthcare professionals on the reality of implementing the Care Certificate and the impact it might have on care outcomes.

As the employer delivers the learning required for staff to meet the outcomes of the Care Certificate, it is they who have the responsibility for deciding what approach is to be used. It is the member of staff's responsibility to complete the outcomes and to demonstrate competence.

On completion of the skills and knowledge aspects of the 15 standards, the Care Certificate is awarded by the employer. Employers can use their own template as there is no one set style.

The Certificate has been designed to be portable. If a member of staff has completed the Care Certificate elsewhere, there is no need for them to redo it if they change job. There is, however, an expectation that employers should help staff retain their knowledge and competencies. The employee is also expected to update knowledge and competences.

The assessor has responsibility for deciding whether the person being assessed has met the standards set out in the Care Certificate. The role of assessor is not something that should be undertaken lightly as it involves judging whether or not someone is competent to provide care and support to often very vulnerable people.

The assessor can be anybody who is competent both in the skills and the knowledge of the competencies being assessed; however, there is an expectation that they will have had some training in the assessment process. No specific qualifications are required to assess – this will vary from employer to employer. Skills for Care (ND) has produced an assessor document, and it is made clear by Skills for Health (ND) that the assessment of the Care Certificate has to be as rigorous as the assessment of any formal qualification.

Box 2.2 provides examples of the types of people who may be able to assess the Care Certificate. This is not an exhaustive list.

On completion, staff are assessed against all 15 of the standards and awarded the Certificate if there is sufficient evidence that they meet the required standards. Evidence of prior learning is not accepted, with the exception of the standard on basic life support (standard 12). Johnson and Buzzi (2016) note that assessment of knowledge and understanding is prefixed with verbs such as:

- Describe
- Explain
- Define
- List
- Identify

Confirmation can be based upon written or verbal evidence, such as a workbook, written questions, case studies or sound files. Evidence of performance is prefixed with words such as:

- Demonstrate
- Take steps to
- Use
- Show

Unless the use of simulation is allowed, assessment must be undertaken in the workplace during the learner's real work activity and has to be observed by the assessor. The employer has a responsibility to maintain records of staff training, required for inspection purposes, for example by the Care Quality Commission.

Understanding the rationale underpinning the introduction of the Care Certificate and its standards may help you to consider how you offer care and support, as well as putting you in a better position to help those you work with to achieve competence in the 15 standards. The rest of this chapter will provide an overview of each individual standard as outlined by Skills for Health (2015).

Standard 1: understanding your role

Understanding your role and the role and function of others is essential if care and support offered to people is to be safe and effective. Understanding role function can also help to reduce duplication of work, as well as reducing the risk of omissions. This is important whether you are a Nursing Associate, a healthcare assistant or a Registered Practitioner.

Job description

The ways in which all care workers practise will differ; regardless of this, the contribution that they make to the health and well-being of people should never be undervalued. There is no one core job description for health and care workers; nevertheless, each member of staff will have been provided with a job description or role descriptor (sometimes called a person specification).

REFLECTION 2.1

Find your job description (person specification, role descriptor) and make a comparison between your role and function and the role and function of a healthcare assistant. Think about the similarities between the two roles, but also think about the differences.

There has to be an understanding of role and function: the ways in which people are required to work that have been agreed on with the employer. When you have an understanding of your role, then you can begin to understand the role of others you work with. You will appreciate what is expected of you and what is expected of others, and this can help to improve working relationships, enhance the ways of working in partnership and improve the provision of care.

Knowing what is not expected in your role and the roles of others is as important as knowing what is included. There is no job description that would be able to provide details of every aspect of your work; however, it should provide a good idea of what your role is about.

Being a Nursing Associate is only one part of you. You bring to the role a range of experiences, attitudes and beliefs that are essential aspects of who you are. We come from different backgrounds and we all have a variety of experiences, attitudes and beliefs. These will impact on how you think, what you do and how you do it – for better or worse. You have to bear in mind that this is also true of others; for example, the healthcare assistant.

⚠ HOTSPOT

It must always be remembered that all of us, including those who provide care and those we provide care to, have different life experiences, attitudes and beliefs, and because of this there will always be potential for conflict.

Codes and standards

In order to practise safely, the Nursing Associate has to work within the confines of a Code of Conduct (Nursing and Midwifery Council (NMC), 2018a) and within agreed ways of working (often called standards and protocols). Codes and standards can be seen as benchmarks against which the Nursing Associate may be judged or called to account for their actions or omissions (see also Chapter 4). This may not be the same for other colleagues, such as the healthcare assistant. Codes and standards can help staff perform their role safely and effectively. In England, Skills for Health (2013) has produced the Code of Conduct ('the Code') (see Box 2.3), which contains the moral and ethical standards that are expected of all health and social care workers. Within the Code are the behaviours and attitudes that these staff are expected to demonstrate; it is seen as a model of best practice. It helps provide safe, compassionate care and support to people.

BOX 2.3 The Code of Conduct for Healthcare Support Workers and Adult Social Care Workers in England

As a Healthcare Support Worker or Adult Social Care Worker in England you must:
1. Be **accountable** by making sure you can answer for your actions or **omissions**.
2. **Promote** and **uphold** the privacy, **dignity**, **rights**, health and **well-being** of people who use health and care services and their carers at all times.
3. Work in **collaboration** with your colleagues to ensure the delivery of high quality, safe and compassionate healthcare, care and support.
4. Communicate in an open and **effective** way to promote the health, safety and well-being of people who use health and care services and their carers.
5. Respect a person's right to confidentiality.
6. Strive to improve the quality of healthcare, care and support through **continuing professional development**.
7. Uphold and promote equality, **diversity** and inclusion.

(Reprinted With Permission From Skills for Health, Health Education England and Skills for Care.)

When the guidance set out in the Code is followed, it will help ensure that the care provided is safe and compassionate and of a high standard. The public should expect to be treated with dignity, respect and compassion at all times by all staff.

REFLECTION 2.2

Access the Codes of Conduct for the following professional groups:
- Nurses, Midwives and Nursing Associates
- Doctors
- Dentists
- Paramedics

Now reflect on the content of two of them and identify the moral and ethical standards that are expected of those healthcare workers.

In order to work together as a team and function effectively, it is imperative that roles and functions are understood. When striving to ensure that staff have the right skills, knowledge and attitude, there is a need to identify gaps in skills and to work towards filling those gaps.

Standard 2: your personal development

Personal and professional development are the hallmarks of a professional. The Care Certificate emphasizes that personal development should occur throughout the health and social care worker's career. The healthcare assistant should be encouraged and required to engage in lifelong learning, and the Nursing Associate may be required to help develop staff who are currently working through the Care Certificate.

Deciding on what personal development is required begins in the workplace with an agreement, usually with the line manager, about the member of staffs' aims and objectives, as well as thinking about their strengths and any development needs. When this is agreed, goals are set so the objectives can be met. This approach is very much like the nursing process (a systemic approach to care provision), assessing patient needs and setting goals and objectives concerning care needs.

A personal development plan (PDP), an action plan, can help with organization. The PDP identifies the learning and development required to help staff do their job better or assist in career progression. It can also help track progress. Compiling a personal development plan, assessing skills, and receiving feedback from supervisors, managers and colleagues, as well as those being cared for, helps staff recognize if there are any skills gaps and improve areas of weakness.

Taking time to invest in a PDP is important and this can be used to monitor progress at set review points and identify any development needs. Through the PDP, staff can agree with employers how long it will take to complete the Care Certificate. Working with the employer, targets can be set and learning needs identified. Developing new skills and abilities may involve further training, attendance at specialist courses and the gaining of new qualifications.

The internet has a number of websites where training and development can be undertaken online at the person's own pace and location. Face-to-face and non–web-based materials can also assist in providing learning opportunities. It is not possible to complete the Care Certificate through the undertaking of eLearning or completing a workbook alone (Skills for Health, 2015), although eLearning can be used to enhance learning and demonstrate and assess aspects of the Care Certificate.

The Care Certificate should be thought of as a combination of skills and knowledge acquisition.

CRITICAL AWARENESS

Beware of rogue websites that purport to offer training or courses online that can lead to recordable qualification. Access this article:

Bradley, P. (2015) How to do the Care Certificate Standards in 10 Hours for £36. *British Journal of Healthcare Assistants*. 9 (11), 530–533.

Read the content of the article and think about the issues that are being discussed. One key issue to consider is that the Care Certificate can only be undertaken face-to-face.

Standard 3: duty of care

Duty of care is a legal obligation and can be applied in many ways. The Code of Conduct (Skills for Health, 2013) is all about duty of care. Chapter 5 of this book considers duty of care and the role of the Nursing Associate.

Duty of care is a legal requirement, you cannot choose whether or not to accept it. As soon as someone receives care or treatment, then a duty of care is owed. Legal action can be taken if this requirement is broken. A duty of care means promoting well-being and making sure that people are kept safe from harm, abuse and injury.

A duty of care is also owed to other people, for example, doctors, registered nurses, laboratory technicians, caterers, housekeepers, cleaners and technical/maintenance workers. If you are a home care worker you will probably work alone in a variety of homes, but there may well be other people on the premises, as well as whoever you are there to support. Your duty of care is to each individual and to the other workers you come into contact with in the community.

REFLECTION 2.3

In what ways do you think a healthcare assistant owes a duty of care to a person they offer care to? What duty of care does the Nursing Associate owe to staff who work in the laboratory where specimens are analysed?

Incidents, errors and near misses

Unfortunately, mistakes can happen when care is being provided. This might be the result of a lack of knowledge, ineffective communication, failure to share information, stress, negligence or the healthcare worker not focusing on what is happening or being done. All health and social care workplaces involve workers collaborating with regard to the well-being of those needing care or support. Table 2.1 lists mistake categories.

When errors do happen, it is essential that they are reported and recorded. Local policy and procedure must be implemented when acting upon and reporting errors. Usually there is a form to be completed (this may be hard copy or electronic). Addressing the immediate needs of the individuals involved is paramount; therefore the priority after something has gone wrong is to ensure patient safety and the well-being of the individual involved.

TABLE 2.1   Incidents and Errors

Category	Description
Adverse events	Action, or lack of action, leading to unexpected, unintended and preventable harm.
Errors	Not doing something as it should have been done, for example, as a result of poor time management, bad planning or being forgetful.
Near misses	Situations where an action could have harmed a person, but by chance or purpose, this was averted.
Incidents	Specific negative events. In health and social care, serious incidents are described as events that need investigation as they caused severe harm or damage to either the person receiving care or the organization.

(Reprinted with permission from Skills for Health, Skills for Care and Health Education England. https://www.skillsforcare.org.uk/Documents/Learning-and-development/Care-Certificate/Standard-3.pdf)

CRITICAL AWARENESS

Do you know what to do in your workplace if an error or incident occurs? Where can you find the policy and procedures related to these issues?

Complaints

Everybody using the health service has a right to complain or to comment on their care. When complaints are made they should be dealt with quickly. Complaints should be taken seriously and explored with the intention of learning from them. Each organization will have its own complaints procedure, and this policy must be adhered to.

CRITICAL AWARENESS

In England, the Department of Health has published the NHS Constitution (DH, 2015b), which provides guidance to help deal with and resolve complaints.

Standard 4: equality and diversity

Implementing good equality and diversity practices means that everyone will be afforded equal opportunities, irrespective of their abilities, background or lifestyle choices.

Equality and diversity are key elements of health and social care, ensuring that the services provided are fair and accessible. People should be treated as equals; they should expect to receive care that is based on dignity and respect and have their differences celebrated. Equality and diversity should never be seen as an 'added extra', a bonus to care provision; they should be seen as essential components. Whilst the terms 'equality' and 'diversity' are occasionally used interchangeably, they are not the same.

Equality

Equality is about the creation of a fairer society, where everybody can contribute and has the opportunity to fulfil their potential. It focuses on treating everyone fairly and equally, allowing no tolerance of discrimination or harassment (Talati, 2016). By eliminating prejudice and discrimination, services that are

BOX 2.4   The 9 Protected Characteristics (The Equality Act 2010)

1. Age
2. Race
3. Sex
4. Gender reassignment status
5. Disability
6. Religion or belief
7. Sexual orientation
8. Marriage and civil partnership status
9. Pregnancy and maternity

delivered will be personal, fair and appropriate. This will help create a society that is healthier and happier. When an equalities approach is adopted, it is recognized that who we are, based on social categories such as gender, ethnicity, disability, age, social class, sexuality and religion, will impact our life experiences.

Diversity

In contrast, or in addition to, equality, diversity recognizes individual as well as group differences, treating people as individuals and placing a positive value on diversity (difference) in the community and in the workforce. Diversity means that staff appreciate the differences between people and treat people's values, beliefs, cultures and lifestyles with respect.

Individual and group diversity has to be taken into consideration to ensure everybody's needs and desires are understood and responded to. Both patients and staff should be treated fairly, irrespective of their backgrounds and circumstances.

The Equality Act 2010 legally protects people from discrimination in the workplace and in wider society and has replaced previous anti-discrimination laws with a single Act. Its purpose is to prevent discrimination and unfair treatment. See Box 2.4 for an overview of the nine protected characteristics.

REFLECTION 2.4

Does your workplace have an equality and diversity policy? What does the policy say and how you might use it in practice to provide care that is fair and respectful?

Standard 5: working in a patient-centred way

The essence of this book, the preparation of the Nursing Associate, and the implementation of the Care Certificate are about ensuring that the patient is at the centre of all that is done.

The Royal College of Nursing (2017a) suggests that being person-centred means focusing care on the needs of the person as opposed to the needs of the service. More and more of those who require healthcare are no longer content to just passively allow healthcare staff do what it is that they think is best. Patients have their own views on what they think is best for them and their own priorities in life. As a result, healthcare workers have to adopt a more flexible approach to meeting needs. The systems and approaches we use have to suit the patient, rather than the other way round.

The patient becomes an equal partner in the planning of their care and their opinions are important, valued and respected. Staff have to take into consideration and act on what people want when care is being planned and delivered. Being person-centred means that we always put the safety, comfort and well-being of the patient central in all we do. Much can be done to promote safety and enhance comfort; for example, listening to what the patient says, anticipating needs and being aware that things we are doing or not doing may cause discomfort.

Person-centred care also requires an awareness of an individual's emotional and spiritual well-being. Spiritual care reflects a person's values, relationships and need for self-expression; it is not only about religious beliefs and practices.

The provision of care is at its best when it is centred round the needs, convenience and choices of people and their families and carers. Individuals often have multiple needs that can cross organizational boundaries. The patient's experience of care and support services should be as seamless as possible.

Putting patients and their families and carers at the centre of their care can only happen by listening to what they want, providing them with information, involving them in planning and decision-making, treating them with dignity and respect and enabling them to have choice and control over their lives and the services that they receive.

REFLECTION 2.5

Think about a person you have looked after and reflect on the care you provided. Did you:
- listen to what that person wanted
- provide them with information
- involve them in planning and decision-making
- treat them with dignity and respect
- enable the person to have choice and control?

Standard 6: communication

Chapter 9 is dedicated to effective communication skills. Communication is at the heart of everything we do, and is particularly important when care is being offered. Those to whom we offer care may feel vulnerable, alone and scared. To help alleviate these feelings, effective communication is required. Communication is essential within the care team to ensure that care is safe, coordinated and effective.

Standard 7: privacy and dignity

Dignity is also central to all we do. Recognizing and enabling an individual's right to privacy and dignity are essential aspects of best practice and accepted as a right by those who use healthcare services. The Equality Act places the responsibility on the healthcare organization to prevent discrimination and to demonstrate how it ensures equitable services. Providing care that safeguards the dignity of those who use health services demonstrates a respect for the diversity of the population and the individual needs of those users. This shows how care providers are meeting the requirements of the Act.

All staff, not just those who have direct patient-care interactions, must display values and behaviours that promote privacy, dignity and respect to recipients of care and to other members of staff. Upholding these values means treating people in a manner that makes them feel valued and respected and acting in a way that maintains their privacy and dignity.

According to the Royal College of Nursing (RCN) (2008) a working definition of dignity considers it to be concerned with how people feel, think and behave in relation to the worth or value of themselves and others. To treat someone with dignity, therefore, is to treat them as being of worth in a way that is respectful of them as individuals. When providing care, dignity can be promoted or diminished by:
- the physical environment
- organizational culture
- the attitudes and behaviour of nurses and others
- the way in which care activities are performed.

When dignity is evident in care provision, people will feel in control. They will be valued, confident, comfortable and capable of making decisions for themselves. However, when dignity is lacking, this can make people feel devalued. They lack control and feel discomfort. If they lack confidence, then they may be unable to make decisions for themselves. They can feel humiliated, embarrassed or ashamed (RCN, 2008).

Standard 8: fluids and nutrition

Food and drink is vital for us to function effectively. People require a diet that meets their nutritional needs and is safe. Eating and drinking the right things can make us feel good and can help us recover from surgery or illness. A working knowledge of the issues associated with nutritional needs is essential for all those who provide care. This also includes an understanding of food safety.

Many health problems arise as the result of poor diet. In some countries, obesity is increasingly common, whereas in others, malnutrition is widespread (Waugh and Grant, 2018).

Food provides nutrients; some of these are broken down to provide energy, whilst others are needed for growth, cellular metabolism, and to maintain health. It is acknowledged that good nutrition at all stages of life is important to develop, maintain and sustain health and well-being. The relationship between nutrition, diet and aging is multifaceted; there are many health conditions that can come about as a result of a poor diet, including coronary heart disease, diabetes, liver disease, constipation and osteoarthritis.

There are other conditions that require dietary modification (see Box 2.5).

REFLECTION 2.6

Choose two of the conditions in Box 2.5 and think about the dietary modifications that may be needed to alleviate them. How might you assist the person you are caring for to ensure that these dietary modifications are provided?

Food allergies

Food allergies and intolerances are life changing. They affect around 8% of children and 2% of adults in the UK (Food Standards Agency, 2017). In December 2014, the law on how allergen information is provided by food businesses changed. This can make it easier to identify allergens when buying food or eating

> **BOX 2.5 Some Conditions That Require Dietary Modification**
>
> - Diabetes mellitus
> - Diverticula disease
> - Coeliac disease
> - Acute renal failure
> - Liver failure
> - Lactose intolerance

> **BOX 2.6 Some General Food Hygiene Principles**
>
> - Remove all rings and jewellery prior to preparing food
> - Wash your hands
> - In between use, wash equipment in hot water
> - Make sure that food is cooked thoroughly
> - Store food in sealed containers and keep cooled
> - Food that is stored in a fridge should be labelled, dated and kept at a temperature of 5°C
> - In a fridge, store raw meat below cooked food
> - Raw and cooked foods should be stored separately
> - Wash equipment in hot soapy water or, if available, in a dishwasher

out. This law also applies to hospitals, clinics, care homes and all places where healthcare is provided.

Food allergy is a serious and potentially life-threatening medical condition. Sometimes allergy symptoms are mild, whereas other times they can be severe. All allergic symptoms must be taken seriously. Mild and severe symptoms can lead to a more serious allergic reaction called anaphylaxis. This reaction often involves more than one part of the body and can quickly become worse. Anaphylaxis must be treated immediately because it can cause death.

Anaphylaxis is treated with epinephrine. This is a safe medicine that comes in an easy-to-use device known as an auto-injector (EpiPen). The symptoms of an anaphylactic reaction occur shortly after contact with an allergen. In some people, there may be a delay of 2 to 3 hours prior to symptoms first appearing.

Food safety

Not all substances and objects that may result in harm or illness to people are visible. People can become ill from eating food that may taste normal and look safe. You should make sure that the food you prepare, including snacks, such as a sandwich, is safe to eat. Those serving food have to comply with food hygiene law.

Precautions must be taken to ensure that food is safe to eat. Failure to adhere to food-handling safety can result in serious gastrointestinal infections, for example:

- Enteric fever
- Escherichia coli
- Campylobacter food poisoning
- Dysentery
- Gastro enteritis

Where food is provided to individuals, it has to be handled, stored, prepared and delivered in a way that adheres to the Food Safety Act 1990 requirements. If, as part of your role, you are required to prepare or handle food, you have to possess the knowledge and skills to do this safely.

There are some basic principles that need to be kept in mind to protect people when food is being handed, stored or prepared (see Box 2.6).

For all those who receive care, an assessment of nutrition and hydration needs is required. The assessment should consider food allergies, food preferences (including any cultural needs), whether any support is required to eat and drink, and if the person has dentures or not. You should also determine the following:

- If the person needs help to cut up food or open packages, such as portions of butter or cheese
- If the person needs to be reminded to eat and drink
- If the person has a visual impairment that may necessitate some help with eating and drinking

- If they have preferences regarding the foods that they eat, such as if they are vegetarian or vegan
- If there are any foods they should not have because of medication or health conditions.

Fluids and hydration

Unless restricted for medical reasons, people should have access to fluids at all times and be encouraged to drink throughout the day. Thirst is an early sign of dehydration, therefore patients should not wait until they feel thirsty. Offer drinks to patients and encourage and support them to drink to ensure they are drinking enough. Regularly refresh drinks and place them within easy reach, especially for those who may have issues with mobility.

If there are any concerns about a patient's fluid intake, make sure these are reported to a senior member of staff. Concerns should be documented in the patient's care plan.

Standard 9: awareness of mental health and learning disability

There is stigma associated with living with a mental health need, dementia or learning disability, and this can generate feelings of loneliness or of being socially isolated. Focusing on the abilities and skills of someone who is living with a mental health condition or a learning disability can be positive, and people can be supported to live well.

It is important that you demonstrate a positive attitude towards people living with mental health needs, dementia and learning disabilities. You can help reduce the stigma by ensuring people are not isolated in social situations, promoting well-being, building on an individual's skills and abilities and creating opportunities for people to feel empowered and in control.

The boundary between physical and mental health is blurred, and one can have a profound effect on the other. There is much focus now on how best to integrate physical and behavioural care to achieve positive health outcomes that matter to patients.

Mental health conditions can include psychosis, depression, mood disorder and anxiety. Further specialist training should be provided to you if you are working with people with mental health conditions, dementia or learning disabilities. This will help extend your knowledge and develop your skills and capacity to meet the needs of the people you offer care to.

Whilst you may not be working in a role that directly supports these individuals, it is important to have awareness in any health or social care role. This is so that any signs and symptoms that you notice are passed on to other workers and that you show compassion and understanding when you experience any behaviour that you find difficult.

All of us are individual and unique; we all have different dispositions, life histories and experiences. The care and support we require has to be built on our individual needs and abilities. For example, if an individual with a learning disability can be provided with the support to use and develop their abilities they will become more independent.

Standards 10 and 11: safeguarding adults and children

The abuse of vulnerable adults is a major concern. Protection of vulnerable adults through safeguarding is a key requirement for all healthcare staff. Several chapters of this book address the important issue of adult safeguarding.

Safeguarding children

The child's welfare is paramount. Their best interests override other considerations, such as confidentiality, consent and the carer's interests. Where there is an immediate risk of serious harm to a child, act immediately. As of 31 October 2015, healthcare professionals have a mandatory duty to report female genital mutilation (FGM) in girls under 18 years (DH, 2015a).

Staff who work with children (any person up to the age of 18 years) have a responsibility to keep them safe and to protect them from harm. Just as with adults, safeguarding children is everyone's responsibility. Children should be protected from harm and abuse and there are some children who are in particular need of safeguarding. This chapter does not address child safeguarding further, and the reader is advised to research this issue in more depth.

Safeguarding adults

Safeguarding in the context of healthcare regulation means acting in the best interests of people when they are using or need to use the services of nurses, midwives and other healthcare professionals. Outside healthcare regulation it has a wider meaning that relates to protecting vulnerable adults from abuse and neglect, as well as actively promoting their welfare.

Safeguarding is about understanding various types of abuse and neglect, being able to identify the signs and what to look for, knowing what steps to take if there is a suspicion of abuse and knowing what to do if an adult discloses abuse. It is important to understand the safeguarding agenda and how the organization where you work responds to allegations of abuse.

A vulnerable adult has been described by the Care Standards Act 2000 as a person who is aged over 18 years who has a condition of the following types:
- A learning or physical disability
- A physical or mental illness, chronic or otherwise, including addiction to alcohol or drugs
- A reduction in physical or mental capacity

If you are working directly with vulnerable persons, you should be able to recognize the different types of abuse, identify the signs, and to know where to go for help. Most importantly, you must ensure that you keep accurate records.

Types of abuse

The main types of abuse are described in Box 2.7.

Other categories of abuse as listed in the Care Act 2014 are outlined in Box 2.8.

Healthcare workers have a central role to play in the protection of vulnerable adults. It has to be acknowledged that abuse can occur in a variety of environments. These include the NHS, as well as voluntary organizations, private care homes and patients' personal residences. Safeguarding the vulnerable adult means understanding the different types of adult abuse, recognizing the related signs and symptoms, and ensuring that any abuse is reported appropriately.

Standard 12: basic life support

Understanding how to deliver adult basic life support (BLS) out-of-hospital, or as a single rescuer or first responder in

---

BOX 2.7 Main Types of Abuse (British Geriatrics Society, 2009)

- Physical abuse may involve physical violence, misuse of medication, inappropriate restraint or sanctions.
- Sexual abuse.
- Psychological abuse, including emotional abuse; threats of harm or abandonment; deprivation of contact; humiliation; blaming; controlling; intimidation; harassment; verbal abuse.
- Financial or material abuse, including theft; fraud; exploitation; pressure in connection with wills, property, inheritance, or financial transactions; misuse or misappropriation of property, possessions, or benefits.
- Neglect and acts of omission, including ignoring medical or physical care needs; failure to provide access to appropriate health, social care or educational services; withholding medication, adequate nutrition or heating.
- Discriminatory abuse, including racist or sexist abuse, or abuse based on a person's disability.

BOX 2.8 Other Categories of Abuse (Gibson et al., 2016)

- Domestic abuse, includes psychological, physical, sexual, financial, emotional abuse, and so-called 'honour'-based violence.
- Modern slavery, includes slavery, human trafficking, and forced labour and domestic servitude.
- Organizational abuse, includes neglect and poor care practice within an institution or specific care setting, such as a hospital or care home.
- Self-neglect, includes a wide range of behaviours such as neglecting to care for personal hygiene, health or surroundings, and behaviours such as hoarding.

CRITICAL AWARENESS

It is essential that you understand how to raise concerns if there is, or if you suspect there is, a safeguarding issue. You must know how to raise concerns and what steps to take in the raising awareness process.

As well as understanding this from a patient's perspective, you should also think about yourself and how you can raise awareness if you think you are being abused.

hospital, can help save lives. Basic life support refers to maintaining airway patency and supporting breathing and the circulation without the use of equipment, other than a protective device. It is essential that those who may be present at the scene of a cardiac arrest should have learnt the appropriate resuscitation skills and be competent to be able to put them into practice.

Chapter 19 is concerned with first aid and includes a discussion of BLS, as well as information concerning choking and the use of an automated external defibrillator.

Standard 13: health and safety

Health and safety legislation exists to protect people at work and those who are affected by work activities. There is much legislation relating to general health and safety in a health or social care workplace. Being aware of the legislation can help you prevent harm to yourself, patients, visitors and staff. It is expected that staff are able to describe the main points of health and safety policies and procedures that have been agreed with the employer.

Regardless of where you work, your role, your function or your grade, everyone, from the newly employed member of staff to the longest serving employee, has a responsibility to keep the workplace safe. However, it is the employer who assumes the greatest responsibility, and as such, they have the most authority concerning health and safety issues. For your own safety, you have to understand your role and function.

Understanding the legislation makes all parties (managers and healthcare workers) accountable for their actions or omissions. There are certain workplace tasks that staff should not be permitted to undertake until they have received special training. The employer has to provide this training and give employees access to any additional support and information concerning health and safety that is considered necessary so that they are kept safe as they carry out their duties.

> **! HOTSPOT**
>
> You should never undertake any task that you have not received training for.

Legislation related to health and safety is vast; Table 2.2 outlines some of it. Policies and procedures in the workplace are derived from legislation. Rules and guidance aim to decrease the risk and hazards to a person's physical and emotional well-being while working.

Workplace hazards

Healthcare workers face a number of workplace hazards (in hospitals, clinics, GP surgeries or in the patient's own home). These include blood-borne pathogens and biological hazards (microorganisms, toxins); exposure to chemicals, drugs, waste, and anaesthetic gas; respiratory hazards; ergonomic hazards as a result of lifting and repetitive tasks; laser hazards; workplace violence; hazards associated with laboratories; and radioactive material and x-ray hazards.

Safety hazards are common and can be present in any workplace environment. They include unsafe conditions that could result in injury or death (such as floor spills), trip hazards (such as trailing cords), unguarded machinery and electrical hazards.

Working with people and infectious materials are biological hazards. Health workers in nursing homes, residential care facilities, another person's home, hospitals and so forth, can be exposed to biological hazards including:
- Blood and blood products
- Body fluids (urine, vomitus)
- Bacteria
- Viruses
- Fungi
- Any chemical that has the ability to cause harm.

TABLE 2.2 Some Aspects of Legislation Concerning Health and Safety at Work

Element of legislation	Description
Health and Safety at Work Act 1974	Describes how employers have a legal duty to assess all risks to the health and safety of employees.
Management of Health and Safety at Work Regulations 1999	Relate to how health and safety is managed within the workplace, including risk assessment and training.
Manual Handling Operations Regulations 1992	Provide information on lifting and handling. Addresses the transporting or supporting of any load and how to perform this safely and how to prevent injury.
Lifting Operations and Lifting Equipment Regulations 1998	Demand that all equipment used for lifting is fit for purpose, appropriate for the task, suitably marked and subject to statutory periodic thorough examination.
Provision and Use of Work Equipment Regulations 1998	Concerned with all work equipment from office furniture through to complex machinery. Also applicable if a company allows a worker to use their own equipment in the workplace and how this is to be used safely.
Control of Substances Hazardous to Health Regulations 1999	Information and training needs regarding hazardous chemicals used. The regulation requires employers to control substances that are hazardous to health.
The Regulatory Reform (Fire Safety) Order 2005	Details how every workplace must prevent/protect against fire.
Reporting of Injuries, Diseases and Dangerous Occurrences Regulations 1995.	Explains that employers have a duty to report to the enforcing authorities certain accidents befallen by employees.
Facilities for First Aid Under the Health and Safety (First Aid) Regulations 1981	Employers have to provide adequate and appropriate equipment, also ensuring that employees receive immediate attention if they are injured or taken ill at work.
Personal Protective Equipment at Work Regulations 1992	Employers must provide Personal Protective Equipment (PPE) to staff. The employee has a duty to use PPE in accordance with training and instruction given by their employer.

Every day we are exposed to hundreds of different chemicals; it is impossible to avoid such exposure to substances – hazardous or otherwise. Chemical hazards in the workplace can be in any form: liquid, solid or gas. The following can be considered hazardous:

- Anaesthetic and medical gases
- Solvents
- Vapours and fumes
- Flammable materials
- Disinfectants
- Bleach
- Pharmaceutical substances
- Cytotoxic drugs
- Laboratory chemicals.

Ergonomic hazards

These are related to the type of work a person does. Long-term exposure to these hazards can result in serious chronic illness and diminished mobility. Ergonomic exposure can include the following:

- Improperly adjusted workstations and chairs
- Frequent lifting
- Poor posture
- Awkward movements
- Repetitive movements.

Chapter 18 considers moving and manual handling.

Risk assessment and reporting of health and safety hazards

Risk assessments are carried out to identify if the workplace is safe, and to suggest actions to be taken to safeguard staff and visitors against hazards. We all have a part to play in reducing risks, and it is important that you know what you need to do if you identify a hazard. If there is something in the workplace that you think may be hazardous, then report it immediately to your manager.

Risk assessment is the process of identifying what hazards exist or could exist that are likely to cause harm. A risk assessment is a legal requirement (Management of Health and Safety at Work Regulations 1999). Areas of risk include the following:

- Electrical safety
- Fire safety
- Manual handling
- Hazardous substances.

! HOTSPOT

Being a responsible employee means that you are required to understand procedures for responding to accidents and sudden illness. You must only act within the sphere of your competence (see Chapter 19, First Aid).

Standard 14: handling information

To maintain the rights of patients, it is important to have secure systems for recording and storing information in a healthcare setting. Any information about patients and staff in a place of work has to be protected from access by unauthorized persons. Legislation and codes of practice exist with regard to the recording, storage and sharing of information in health and social care (see Table 2.3).

Professional bodies, such as the Nursing and Midwifery Council and the General Medical Council, provide guidance for various codes of practice. The Skills for Care (2013) guidance in the Code provides advice concerning the management of information and the importance of confidentiality. The Code (Skills for Care, 2013) states that all information about people who use health and care services and their carers must be treated as confidential.

All healthcare workers have a responsibility to ensure that any personal information is safeguarded. This responsibility extends to how personal information about other workers is managed. The employer has to have systems in place that meet the legal requirements concerning the storage of information and all staff have to act within the employer's agreed ways of working.

A number of chapters in this book explicitly discuss the management of information from a professional and legal perspective.

Standard 15: infection prevention and control

Hospital- and community-acquired infections are a major safety concern for those who provide healthcare, as well as for patients. Considering morbidity, mortality, increased length of stay and cost, efforts should be made to make care areas as safe as possible by preventing such infections.

Infection prevention must be seen as a priority in any setting where healthcare is delivered. Infection prevention and control is required to prevent the transmission of communicable diseases. This demands a fundamental understanding of the epidemiology of diseases, risk factors that increase patient susceptibility to infection, and the practices, procedures and treatments that may result in infection.

TABLE 2.3 Legislation Related to the Recording, Storage and Sharing of Information in Health and Social Care

Act	Description
Data Protection Act 1998	Concerns how information about individuals is used. Considers eight principles under which personal data must be protected and collected (see Box 2.9). The Act says that patient information must be confidential and can only be accessed with their consent. Patients must know what records are being kept and why the data is kept.
Freedom of Information Act 2000	The Freedom of Information Act gives individuals the right to ask organizations for all the information they have about them. Some information might be withheld to protect various interests. If that is the case, the individual must be made aware of it. Information about individuals will be handled under the Data Protection Act.
Data Protection Act 2018	This Act updates data protection laws in the UK. Its main intention is to implement the European Union's General Data Protection Regulation (GDPR).

BOX 2.9   The 8 Principles Associated With the Data Protection Act 1998

1. Personal data shall be processed fairly and lawfully and, in particular, shall not be processed unless:
   (a) at least one of the conditions in Schedule 2 is met, and
   (b) in the case of sensitive personal data, at least one of the conditions in Schedule 3 is also met.
2. Personal data shall be obtained only for one or more specified and lawful purposes, and shall not be further processed in any manner incompatible with that purpose or those purposes.
3. Personal data shall be adequate, relevant and not excessive in relation to the purpose or purposes for which they are processed.
4. Personal data shall be accurate and, where necessary, kept up to date.
5. Personal data processed for any purpose or purposes shall not be kept for longer than is necessary for that purpose or those purposes.
6. Personal data shall be processed in accordance with the rights of data subjects under this Act.
7. Appropriate technical and organizational measures shall be taken against unauthorized or unlawful processing of personal data and against accidental loss or destruction of, or damage to, personal data.
8. Personal data shall not be transferred to a country or territory outside the European Economic Area unless that country or territory ensures an adequate level of protection for the rights and freedoms of data subjects in relation to the processing of personal data.

Contains public sector information licensed under the Open Government Licence v3.0.

The risk of acquiring a healthcare-associated infection is linked to the mode of transmission of the infectious agent, the type of patient-care activity and the procedure that is being performed, as well as the patient's underlying immune defences. It is also important to ensure that healthcare workers are vaccinated against preventable diseases, for example, hepatitis B.

According to the Royal College of Nursing (2017b) infection prevention and control is the clinical application of microbiology. Infection or disease may be caused by bacteria, fungi, viruses or prions, and can result in a wide range of infections. Understanding how infections occur and how different microorganisms act and are transmitted, is key to fighting infection. See Chapter 16, which is dedicated to infection prevention and control, for more detailed information about this very important topic.

LOOKING BACK, FEEDING FORWARD

This chapter has addressed the Care Certificate. The 2013 Cavendish Review concluded that the preparation of healthcare assistants and social care support workers for their roles in providing care was variable across England. The report recommended the development of a Certificate of Fundamental Care – the 'Care Certificate'. This is a set of 15 standards for health and social care workers that aim to standardize introductory skills, knowledge and behaviours to ensure compassionate, safe and high-quality care.

The Nursing Associate Standards of Proficiency (NMC, 2018b) and the Curriculum Framework (Health Education England, 2016) incorporates all 15 standards, which can be cross referenced or mapped to the curriculum framework. The primary audience for the Care Certificate is new healthcare support workers or adult social care workers to be delivered as part of their induction. This includes healthcare assistants, assistant practitioners, care support workers and those who provide support to clinical roles in the NHS where there is any direct contact with patients.

It will help the Nursing Associate to understand the rationale for, content of, and assessment of the Care Certificate as they embark on their programme of study. Furthermore, understanding can also help healthcare assistants, for example, who, in the future, may draw on the support of the Nursing Associate to complete their Care Certificate.

REFERENCES

Bradley, P., 2015. How to do the Care Certificate Standards in 10 Hours for £36. Br. J. Healthc. Assist. 9 (11), 530–533.

British Geriatrics Society, 2009. Safeguarding Vulnerable Older People (Abuse and Neglect). Available from: http://www.bgs.org.uk/good-practice-guides/resources/goodpractice/safeguarding-vulnerable-older-people-abuse-and-neglect.

Cavendish, C., 2013. The Cavendish Review: An Independent Review into Healthcare Assistants and Support Workers in the NHS and Social Care Settings. Available from: https://www.gov.uk/government/uploads/system/uploads/attachment_data/file/236212/Cavendish_Review.pdf.

Department of Health (DH), 2015a. Female Genital Mutilation (FGM) Mandatory Reporting Duty. Available from: https://www.gov.uk/government/uploads/system/uploads/attachment_data/file/525405/FGM_mandatory_reporting_map_A.pdf.

Department of Health (DH), 2015b. NHS Constitution for England. Available from: https://www.gov.uk/government/publications/the-nhs-constitution-for-england/the-nhs-constitution-for-england.

Food Standards Agency, 2017. Allergy and Intolerance. Available from: https://www.food.gov.uk/science/allergy-intolerance.

Francis Inquiry, 2013. Report of the Mid Staffordshire NHS Foundation Trust Public Inquiry. Available from: http://www.midstaffspublicinquiry.com/report.

Gibson, J., Nicol, B., Royane, E., et al., 2016. Safeguarding adults in primary care: making a safeguarding adults referral. Br. J. Gen. Pract. 66 (647), e454–e456. doi:10.3399/bjgp16X685525.

Gilding, M., 2017. Implementing the care certificate: a developmental tool or a tick-box exercise? Br. J. Healthc. Assist. 11 (5), 242–247.

Health Education England, 2016. Nursing Associate Curriculum Framework. Available from: https://www.hee.nhs.uk/sites/default/files/documents/Curriculum%20Framework%20Nursing%20Associate.pdf.

Johnson, R., Buzzi, G., 2016. Handy guide to the care certificate. Br. J. Healthc. Assist. 10 (12), 602–605.

Nursing and Midwifery Council, 2018a. The Code. Professional Standards of Practice and Behaviour for Nurses, Midwives and Nursing Associates. https://www.nmc.org.uk/globalassets/sitedocuments/nmc-publications/nmc-code.pdf. (Last accessed November 2018).

Nursing and Midwifery Council, 2018b. Standards of Proficiency for Nursing Associates. https://www.nmc.org.uk/globalassets/sitedocuments/education-standards/nursing-associates-proficiency-standards.pdf. (Last accessed November 2018).

Peate, I., 2015. Care certificate standards 1 and 2: your role and your personal development. Br. J. Healthc. Assist. 9 (10), 496–501.

Royal College of Nursing (RCN), 2008. Defending Dignity – Challenges and Opportunities for Nursing. Royal College of Nursing, London.

Royal College of Nursing (RCN), 2017a. What Patient Care Means. Available from: http://rcnhca.org.uk/sample-page/what-person-centred-care-means/.

Royal College of Nursing (RCN), 2017b. Infection, Prevention and Control. Available from: https://www.rcn.org.uk/library/subject-guides/infection-prevention-and-control-subject-guide.

Skills for Care, ND. The Care Certificate Framework. Assessor Document. Available from: http://www.skillsforhealth.org.uk/images/projects/care_certificate/Care%20Certificate%20Framework%20(Assessor).pdf?_ga=2.112061191.2062581306.1506103455-2066035274.1506103455.

Skills for Care, 2015. The Care Certificate Standards. Available from: http://www.skillsforhealth.org.uk/standards/item/216-the-care-certificate.

Skills for Health, 2013. Code of Conduct for Healthcare Support Workers and Adult Social Care Workers in England. Available from: http://www.skillsforhealth.org.uk/images/services/code-of-conduct/Code%20of%20Conduct%20Healthcare%20Support.pdf.

Skills for Health, 2015. Care Certificate Update Shared Statement. Available from: http://www.skillsforhealth.org.uk/news/latest-news/item/256-care-certificate-update-shared-statement?_ga=2.80707732.2062581306.1506103455-2066035274.1506103455.

Talati, S., 2016. What are equality and diversity? Dent. Nurs. 12 (8), 430–431.

Waugh, A., Grant, A., 2018. Ross and Wilson Anatomy and Physiology in Health and Illness, thirteenth ed. Elsevier, Edinburgh.

3

Learning to Learn

Stuart Baker

OBJECTIVES

By the end of the chapter the reader will be able to:
1. Appreciate the importance of learning to learn
2. Understand the various methods of teaching and learning
3. Consider several learning styles
4. Know their own learning style
5. Identify and describe some key study skills
6. Apply study skills to meet their needs

KEY WORDS

Teaching

Learning styles

Assessing

Communication

Confidence

Competence

Study skills

Techniques

Practice learning

Problem solving

CHAPTER AIM

The aim of this chapter is to promote effective study skills.

SELF TEST

1. What do academic levels and credits mean?
2. What do you understand by study skills?
3. What is your learning style?
4. How do you identify your learning needs?
5. In the place where you are learning, where can you find resources to help you with your learning?
6. What human and material resources are available to help you learn?
7. What do you understand by the term mentor?
8. What are the potential barriers to learning?
9. When on placement, how do you think you can make the best use of learning resources?
10. Describe what you understand lifelong learning to mean

INTRODUCTION

The Nursing Associate studies both theory and practice. Studying for a Foundation Degree (FdSc) in Health or an equivalent qualification provides the student with appropriate knowledge that will support their skills in both areas. The Nursing Associate has to blend academic study skills and work-based learning skills, and develop these skills and strategies to enable them to study effectively, while at the same time working as an employee.

LEARNING TO LEARN

To learn effectively, there is a need to learn how to learn. Everyone learns in different ways and this important fact has to be acknowledged. Some people will have recently undergone a period of study, for example, at school, in a college of further education or even through a distance learning course, such as an access to a nursing course. Others will not. There are many reasons why people study: some for a sense of personal achievement (because they want to), some in order to be considered for a job or a course and some to improve the way they work and maybe increase their chance of climbing a career ladder. The subjects people study are also different: some study subjects that have no relationship to their work (often these people study just because they can). Others study with a specific reason in mind, for example, so they meet the criteria to be accepted on to a course or as part of a requirement by a professional body, such as is required by the Nursing and Midwifery Council (NMC) to be admitted to the professional register.

QUALIFICATION LEVELS AND ACADEMIC CREDIT

Most higher education programmes of study (e.g., a Foundation Degree in Healthcare) are made up of a number of individual units or modules. Programmes of study that are more than 1 year long span a number of levels. Credit is assigned to individual units or modules and to whole programmes. In England, Wales and Northern Ireland, the qualifications system is the same, whereas in Scotland, it is different. Table 3.1 shows higher education level qualifications.

A number of credits is normally allocated to each unit or module, which indicates the amount of learning undertaken, while a specified credit level indicates the relative depth of learning involved. Together, these are known as the 'credit value' (Quality Assurance Agency (QAA) (2009)). To receive the award, academic credits have to be earned and accumulated (see Table 3.2).

Once a module or unit is studied and successfully passed, credits are awarded in recognition of the amount and depth of learning achieved. Credits are then added together towards the total credit required for a programme of study and a qualification, for example, a Foundation Degree.

Health Education England (HEE) (2016) has decreed that the Nursing Associate should be educated to academic level 5; this is usually a Diploma of Higher Education or a Foundation Degree (this is known as the 'outcome award'). The NMC has set its required minimum outcome award for a pre-registration nursing education programme as a degree in nursing. Registered Nurses have to be educated to level six (this is usually a Bachelor of Science (Honours)) (NMC, 2010).

PERSONAL TUTOR

Now that you have an understanding of the credits and levels that are aligned with the course, one important person's role needs to be explained before addressing any other topic in this chapter. You will be allocated to a personal tutor at the commencement of your studies who will be your consistent point of contact throughout the duration of your course. Much of the role of a personal tutor is to be a signpost for you to other support services, such as student study skills, student finance, etc. Other parts of the role include the following:
- Discussing, monitoring and deciding issues regarding progression with the course
- Meeting either individually or as a group with other students to discuss general progress
- Initial discussions about unsatisfactory progress
- Acting as a referee

This list is not exhaustive, but getting to know and building a relationship with your personal tutor is very important. They are not just your point of contact whilst you are in university, they are available when you are on placement and can still be contacted either by email or telephone or indeed by visiting the university during times of clinical placement.

LEARNING STYLES

To achieve any academic award, it is helpful for students to know how they learn best. For some, this will be by reading textbooks and journal articles, for others by attending lectures and yet others through practical learning by doing tasks, completing simulated learning activities or web-based learning. A learning style questionnaire is a good way to find out what learning style best suits you, such as the very popular one developed by Honey and Mumford (1986). The student answers a number of questions and the output identifies with one of four different learning styles that fits the student's preferred style of learning:
1. Activist
2. Theorist
3. Pragmatist
4. Reflector

Activists are students who learn by doing. Activists can be summed up as those who learn by getting their hands dirty, who dive in with both feet with a sink or swim attitude. Activists have an open-minded approach to learning, immersing themselves fully and openly in new experiences. Activists learn least when listening to a lecture, reading lengthy textbooks and following precise instructions.

Theorist learners like to understand the theory behind the actions. They need models, concepts and facts to engage in the learning process. They prefer to analyse and synthesize, drawing new information into a systematic and logical 'theory'. Activities for theorists need to be very precise and supported by a concept or model. Theorists learn least when emotions and feelings are required and emphasis is placed on the use of these attributes.

TABLE 3.1 Higher Education Level Qualifications

Level	Award
Level 4 qualifications	Certificate of higher education (CertHE)
	Higher apprenticeship
	Higher national certificate (HNC)
	Level 4 award
	Level 4 certificate
	Level 4 diploma
	Level 4 National Vocational Qualification (NVQ)
Level 5 qualifications	Diploma of higher education (DipHE)
	Foundation degree
	Higher national diploma (HND)
	Level 5 award
	Level 5 certificate
	Level 5 diploma
	Level 5 NVQ
Level 6 qualifications	Degree apprenticeship
	Ordinary degree e.g., Bachelor of Arts (BA), Bachelor of Science (BSc) without honours Degree with Honours
	Graduate certificate
	Graduate diploma
	Level 6 award
	Level 6 certificate
	Level 6 diploma
	Level 6 NVQ

TABLE 3.2 Academic Credits

Level	Credits	Total credits	Award
Level 4	120	120	Certificate of higher education
Level 5	120	240	Diploma of higher education or Foundation Degree
Level 6	120	360	BSc, BSc (Hons)

When activities are organized without precision or any apparent underpinning principle, the theorist is not comfortable.

Pragmatist students need to be able to see how to put the learning into practice in the real world. They find it hard to grasp abstract concepts unless they can see a way to relate to them or put the ideas into action in their lives. This group of students could be seen as experimenters, trying out new ideas, theories and techniques to see if they work and if they are applicable to their current learning. For example, the pragmatist student who returns from a course may want to implement changes in their workplace to practices relating to what they have been taught. The situation where a pragmatist would learn the least is probably where they perceive that what they are being taught would only work in theory and they cannot see the practical application.

Reflectors learn by observing and thinking about what has happened. They may avoid leaping in and prefer to watch on from the periphery and absorb the material being presented to them. They often prefer to stand back and view experiences from a number of different perspectives, collecting and collating data and taking the time to work towards the conclusion. Having to do things that they feel unprepared for and working towards tight, structured deadlines are the most unsuitable learning situations for a student with this learning style.

In order for all students to choose the learning activities that are most suited to their style of learning, the course of study would need to be very flexible as each student would require a course almost tailor-made for them. A more practical approach is that knowing which learning style a person possesses allows them to develop and strengthen other styles so that they can become more of an all-round student. A student can have more than one learning style, either naturally or because they have developed other styles. Knowing the preferred learning style can also help the student and the personal tutor when seeking tutorial support.

Now is a good time to complete the learning style questionnaire (see Reflection 3.1).

> **REFLECTION 3.1**
>
> Using the internet, complete a Honey and Mumford learning style questionnaire and find out what your preferred method of learning is. Reflect on this and whether it has highlighted the style you expected.

LEARNING INVENTORIES

A learning inventory addresses how you prefer to learn. The most frequently used inventory is the VARK inventory developed by Fleming and Mills (1992). The four preferences are visual, auditory, read/write and kinaesthetic. The student who has a preference for visual learning can best recall learned material that has been represented in a visual format, perhaps through charts and graphs, rather than just being presented verbally. Auditory preference refers to those students who learn best by listening, those who can recall information that has been presented to them verbally. Read/write students prefer to learn by taking notes or reading presentations, such as PowerPoint slides in a lecture or by digesting sections of a textbook. The kinaesthetic student prefers to learn through a 'hands on' approach, such as simulations and work-based learning. One analogy that may help you identify which of these methods best describes you is to consider how you might assemble flat-pack furniture. The visual student will perhaps watch a video on the assembly, whereas the read/write student will read all the instructions completely before starting the assembly process. The kinaesthetic student will put the instructions to one side and simply start the assembly, whereas the auditory student would prefer to listen to someone else reading the instructions and then proceed with the assembly.

Understanding the way you learn best and your preferred manner of learning can enhance your learning experience and enable you make the most of your time studying to be a Nursing Associate.

> **REFLECTION 3.2**
>
> Using the internet, complete a VARK questionnaire and find out what your preferred method of learning is. Reflect on this and whether it has highlighted the method you expected.

TIME MANAGEMENT

For students on a course such as the Nursing Associate where there is a mixture of theory and clinical work, the concept of managing time must be addressed. Assignments will be due for completion during periods of clinical placement and this requires the student to be able to concentrate on both their academic studies and their clinical work at the same time, as both have equal importance. In this section, several tips about time management are provided to help equip you to succeed. We will consider time management in the clinical environment and how to get the most out of your clinical placements first, then look at time management applied to the theory element of the course.

Your placement

Benjamin Franklin famously said that if you fail to prepare then you must be prepared to fail. This is no different with clinical placements. Some simple preparatory steps can lead to a very successful placement experience. Before you go on placement, look at the profile of the clinical area you are going to. What sort of ward is it or which part of the community does it serve? If possible, talk to students who have already been to that area and find out what the needs of the patients tend to be. For example, if you are allocated to a surgical ward, is it vascular, gynaecology or general? Once you have this information, allocate some time in your schedule to look at ways that you could meet the nursing needs of patients in that area.

You will have received practice assessment documentation to complete while you are on placement. This may be in the form of a number of objectives that your allocated mentor will complete and sign to confirm that you have met the required standard or it may be a comment that you are working towards that objective and the mentor on the next ward can sign this off. It is essential that you are familiar with this documentation and the objectives you have outstanding and need to complete on placement.

Tips for a successful clinical placement experience

- Make contact with the department a week or two before the placement commences to find out what day and time to arrive, and where you should report to. Remember the first day of a placement may not be the first shift that you work as you will be allocated, wherever possible, to a shift pattern similar to that of your mentor.
- Make sure you know how to get there, and if you use public transport, ensure you know the times of the transport before and after the shift.
- If you drive, can you park at the placement? If there is a charge, make sure you have money with you.
- Carry a small notebook to jot down things like abbreviations, conditions, procedures, drugs, etc. to revise and read up about later.
- Take your ID badge.
- Remember that other Nursing Associates, nurses, healthcare support workers, receptionists and other people in the clinical areas can also be great resources. If your mentor is not on duty, you can still have a good experience.
- If there is something happening on the ward that you have not seen before, ask if it is possible to observe or participate.
- Finally, it is really worth remembering that while you are on placement and away from the university you are not alone. If you have any difficulties, contact your personal tutor. They would much prefer to deal with any issues as they arise and not wait until you come back in to the university, by which time the issue may well have escalated.

CRITICAL AWARENESS

Personal Tutor

It is very important that you keep in touch with your personal tutor throughout your clinical experience, especially if you have any queries. Do not leave those queries until you are next in university.

Know the course requirements

Ensure that you are familiar with the course structure and the individual module requirements, such as assignment due dates and the mechanisms the university (or the institution where you are studying) has for extensions (although it is not recommended that you plan in advance to have an extension) or how to submit extenuating circumstances. Each module will have a number of credits attached to it. Realistically, a 40-credit module requires twice the study time of a 20-credit module; therefore it is essential when planning module study-time to ensure a realistic time allowance. Each module and assignment will have learning outcomes and objectives. It is crucial that these are known so that when answering the assignment brief and writing essays it is clear that you are meeting the required outcomes and objectives.

It is good practice to plan ahead and create a schedule that includes all your commitments relating to study, clinical placement and other work, as well as personal or social life, over the coming few months. It is recommended that a total of 100 hours study is allowed for each 10 credits of a module; therefore a 20-credit module should be allotted 200 hours. Some of this time will be in face-to-face contact time, perhaps 50 hours for a 20-credit module, leaving only 150 hours to be allocated to independent study time. This may seem a lot, but reading, essay writing, academic supervision and other such activities will soon add up. For example, if 3 hours a day are allocated for study, a 20-credit module will require 50 study days.

If you are required to sit examinations, you should ensure you understand the structure of the exam. Some exams will be in a multiple-choice format, where you are asked a question and shown a number of possible answers and you are required to choose the answer that you think is correct. Another exam format may require you to answer a question that has been set around a certain topic. Your lecturer will have told you the topic to revise, but not the particular question format or slant that it will have in the exam. There are other formats too, such as labelling diagrams. In an anatomy and physiology exam, for example, you may be given a picture of the brain with five blank labels to complete.

The importance of understanding the course and the module is critical.

CRITICAL AWARENESS

Spider Diagrams

There are many ways in which you can prepare for an examination. We all have our own ways of doing this – what works for one person may not work for another.

Often with exams, the problem is not that we do not know the answer, but that we cannot recall the right things at the right time. For essay writing in particular, there is a need to be able swiftly to look over all that could be said and pick out the most pertinent parts, while leaving plenty of mental space for the crafting of a structured argument.

Spider diagrams are an excellent tool to aid the memory and create an overview. They can help condense complex topics onto a single memorable page by using a branching spatial organization, colour and images.

To create a spider diagram put the essence of the subject in pictorial form in the centre of the page; make it bright and visually distinctive. Next, divide the overall subject into sections, and radiate a branch for each section from the centre. It does not matter exactly *how* you slice and dice the subject, only that you do so.

Next add 'twigs' for the key facts and information. Each of these twigs can subdivide again, with the focus on a different subtopic each time.

What results from following this process is that each branch and twig provides a compact but accessible overview of a complex, interconnected subject.

The final form of exam that is particularly relevant to most health-related courses, such as the Nursing Associate course, is the Objective Structured Clinical Examination (OSCE) (or equivalent). This is a practical exam assessing the skills that have been taught on the course. The student often has one or more practices before the final OSCE, but again, the importance of understanding the requirements of the course and the module has to be stressed. This exam will be used to assess a student's competency at performing the required skills. Before the assessment, it is important to read and have an understanding of the skills that might be tested.

CRITICAL AWARENESS

Preparing for OSCE

Just as you would prepare for a written examination, you should also give some thought to how you will prepare for OSCE.

The OSCE is designed to assess your ability to competently apply your professional nursing skills and knowledge in relation to a given activity. This is set at the level expected of a Nursing Associate at their particular year of study. This means that you must show that you are capable of applying knowledge to the care of patients at the level expected of a Nursing Associate.

The examination tests your ability to apply knowledge to the care of patients rather than how well you can remember and recite facts. The scenario(s) and any related questions refer to current best practice and you should answer them in relation to published evidence and not according to local arrangements.

Prior to the examination, ensure that you have made use of any opportunities to practise – remember, practice makes perfect.

You should comply with local regulations, make sure you know where the venue is and give yourself plenty of time to get there. If required, make sure you have your examination number, a black pen and a watch with a second hand.

When you enter the room, be certain to read the examination scenario carefully for each station. Always adopt a professional approach: remember that an OSCE is a formal examination.

Note that sometimes OSCEs can be called OSCAs (Objective Structured Clinical Assessments).

Study patterns

It is often suggested that you should undertake the most difficult work when your concentration is strongest, which is usually at the start of the day. If this is the time that you study best, consider not checking social media or emails at this point and save this for a reward later in the morning. Remember to take regular breaks, perhaps every hour, as studying should not be a punishment, but something that you enjoy. Do small stints of studying, regularly. If you wait until the end of the module to revise and then try to cram all your studying into a few weeks, it will feel like a chore and definitely not an enjoyable experience.

Like many things in life, see this as cyclical. Make sure that you reflect on whether your study pattern is successful. For example, if you are getting less done in the evenings than you hoped, try something different, perhaps by studying in the early morning.

Where to study

Another important aspect that will help you is to have somewhere that you can study. If you can leave your books, articles and folders open in an office space at home this will make it easier when managing time as you will be able to pick up almost immediately where you left off. However, if you are using the kitchen table, for example, and cannot keep all your study material to hand, this is not too much of an issue. It may just mean that the first 5 minutes and last 5 minutes of each study session are taken up with opening and unpacking books and so forth. But

it does give you the opportunity to ensure that your workspace is organized with only articles and books that are most relevant at hand to help you focus on the given task. Also remember your preferred learning style. Additional places or times to study may include walking to university or work and listening to a relevant podcast or simply thinking, or making time to watch relevant videos.

One tip when considering time management is that you approach each study session with clarity and decide what that day's goal is. It could be working towards a long-term goal; for example, today's study session will increase your understanding of a certain aspect of the module or course, or could be a short-term goal, such as completing an assignment. All goals should be SMART, that is they should be Specific, Measurable, Achievable, Realistic and Timely. If you have a 3-hour study session, for instance, then your goal may be to write 300 words for your assignment. This is specific as you know what you have to do, you have set a measurement to attain (300 words), it is achievable for you, it is a realistic target – 100 words an hour allowing for coffee breaks, for example – and finally, it is timely as you have a clear time frame that you are using.

This goal-setting approach to study will help you to remain focused and achieve more in your study sessions.

Using Covey's time management matrix

Perhaps the biggest challenges to effective time management are distractions and procrastination, such as putting off the inevitable essay by doing something that does not really need doing now. Covey's time management matrix (see Table 3.3) can help you set your priorities. For example, completing an assignment that has to be submitted in 2 weeks' time would go into Quadrant I, whereas reading your favourite novel might go into Quadrant IV. When you have a holiday or are feeling particularly stressed or on a break from study, looking at a Quadrant IV item can be a good way of relaxing.

An important part of learning is learning when to switch off and relax.

There are some distractions that are not easy to put into Covey's time management matrix, such as giving attention to a child, but care still needs to be taken that these distractions to not become prolonged and just another form of procrastination.

One tip for avoiding distraction is to include setting goals, but within these goals, to also set targets; for instance, after 30 minutes, I will make a coffee, or after 1 hour, I will hang the washing out. Try to minimize or avoid distractions, such as reading emails or interacting with social media before starting work, as you will find those really important posts or emails will take longer to read and respond to than you think and eat into your study time. Turn your mobile phone to silent, if possible, and

TABLE 3.3 Covey's Time Management Matrix (Data from Covey, 1999)

Quadrant I: Urgent & Important	Quadrant II: Not Urgent & Important
Quadrant III: Urgent & Not Important	Quadrant IV: Not Urgent & Not Important

either let the house phone ring or use an answer phone to field calls. Do not become a hermit and stop socializing, but make a deal with yourself. For example, if you are invited out on Saturday night, go out rather than study, but offset it by dedicating more time on Sunday to your course studies.

Ultimately, time management is a very personal thing and what works for one student does not necessarily work for another. Do not be afraid to experiment, but remember to spend time reflecting on your effectiveness in these periods of study and think whether they can be improved.

REFLECTION 3.3

What things do you think may interfere with your ability to plan your time in an effective way? Make a list of these and reflect on the ways you can address, or at least minimize, the negative impact they may have on your time management.

BARRIERS TO LEARNING

Barriers to learning occur for all students, to some extent, and some of the issues already discussed in this chapter could represent such barriers. These can be barriers that make it harder for students to commence an educational course, to complete their studies or to achieve their full potential as a student. Broadly these can be categorized as:

- Educational barriers
- Institutional barriers
- Societal barriers.

Educational barriers

Many educational barriers have a direct link to institutional barriers. An example might be a student with a severe spelling difficulty. As well as being an educational barrier that may prevent the student developing their full potential, this can also be an institutional barrier if the institution does not have sufficiently robust measures in place to support a student and clearly advertised ways in which the student can access this support.

It is important to acknowledge that barriers to learning exist, understand what those barriers are, and know who has the responsibility to help overcome them, as well as find solutions as to how these barriers can be overcome. Another example of an educational barrier could be a lack of confidence in one's own ability to learn. This is often seen in mature students (Canning, 2010), but is not exclusive to this group. It may, for instance, be due to poor educational experiences in the past. Although this is not always an easy barrier to overcome, shared responsibility has to be seen as part of any solution. The institution will provide personal tutors, academic supervisors and also a department that can help meet any deficit the student may feel they have with their study skills, but the student also has a responsibility to access the services offered in order to reduce the negative impact barriers can have on their performance.

This is by no means a definitive list of educational barriers and indeed the later section looking at learning technologies addresses another educational barrier. However, the principle remains the same that the student needs to identify what the barrier is and then strive to overcome it.

Institutional barriers

One institutional barrier has already been addressed, as well as the fact that it is often hard to differentiate completely between an institutional barrier and an educational barrier. Institutional barriers include access and parking issues. Perhaps a student has a disability that requires them to park close to the lecture theatre, use a lift rather than climb stairs or sit at the front of a lecture theatre rather than the back, and there are many more examples that could be included. When these barriers are made known, the institution has a responsibility to overcome them, ensuring that the student is not penalized. The institution is required to make reasonable adjustments (Equality Challenge Unit, 2010).

Societal barriers

One large societal barrier has already been addressed, that of distractions and time management (a crossover with educational barriers exists here). Demands on your time probably forms a large part of this category: family wanting attention, friends suggesting that you go out, demands from a community group you are part of, such as amateur dramatics. To overcome these barriers consider compromises, for instance, you could go out every other weekend with friends, and while you are studying, you could consider being a part of the chorus line or backstage staff rather than the leading actor with all that that entails. Do not ignore your family, but explain to them the importance of your studies and the need to respect the fact that you will need time to study.

Whatever the learning barrier, it is important to your studies that these are either overcome or at least minimized so that you can become a more effective student.

LEARNING TECHNOLOGIES

Most university courses are delivered requiring some degree of computer literacy. As a minimum, assignments are usually word processed using readily available word processing packages. There will be no requirement for a specific package to be used as there are a number of commercially available products, such as Microsoft Word and many free applications, such as Open Office. Many universities offer free online software to enable the student to complete their assignments, view PowerPoint presentations and research using the internet. On completion, assignments and essays are usually submitted via an online portal. All assignments in UK universities are submitted this way and analysed to ensure there is no plagiarism. Thus, if two students at opposite ends of the country were to submit the same essay, then the similarity would be highlighted and the universities would have academic processes to follow to investigate likely plagiarism. Feedback is given via this tool as well, and it is important to read the feedback given (and not just look at the mark) as taking the feedback on board can improve your next submission.

The Nursing Associate commences at level 4 and then proceeds to level 5. This step up between levels can be made easier by the utilization of constructive feedback.

University courses are supported by Virtual Learning Environments (VLEs), such as Moodle, BlackBoard or Canvas. The VLE allows the lecturer to make the lecture slides available online rather than printing off lots of copies for students, who may not want the handouts anyway according to their preferred learning style. There are various facilities within the VLE to host formative quizzes, which enable the student to test their understanding of a subject, and also Multiple Choice Quizzes (MCQs), which are often used to both test understanding and grade the module being studied. Another common function in VLEs are discussion boards, which are similar to chat rooms or forums found on some websites where like-minded people post articles and comments of interest. The VLE enables the student to email other students or lecturers within the module and it allows the lecturer to publish announcements regarding the module.

As collaborative learning is advantageous for students, the VLE may contain Wiki pages and blogs so that group work can be facilitated. A group can work together on a Wiki looking at different aspects of a topic, such as caring for a patient with a certain condition. Each student can blog with their thoughts and reflections on a particular aspect of the course or indeed their feelings as they make the transition from an existing role to being a Nursing Associate. There are other specific functions in each individual VLE that will be explained and described by the institution, but, as discussed previously, it is important that the VLE and the use of technology does not create a barrier to learning. It should be remembered that it is very difficult for a student to 'break' the VLE, so experimentation must be encouraged, but the institution also has a responsibility to support students with the use of technology.

This barrier can therefore be overcome both at an educational level and at an institutional level. At a societal level, the barriers may be caused by factors such as financial hardship leading to limited access to IT equipment. This can be overcome by using computers at the institution or in local libraries. Most universities now have open access computer laboratories and indeed some universities offer schemes where students can buy discounted computers. There are also a number of charitable organizations around the UK that recycle and refurbish used computers.

Finally, it would be remiss not to mention the value of social media and other online platforms. A large proportion of the population, and most organizations, have websites and accounts on such platforms as Facebook and Twitter. There is a wealth of educational literature to be found on these sites and also updates from professional bodies, such as the NMC. For visual learner students who prefer videos, obviously there is a wealth of material on such sites as YouTube, but the authenticity and validity of the information being presented is not always obvious; therefore, universities will often have their own video-hosting channels and will also embed pertinent videos within their VLE.

The NMC (2017) has produced guidelines that must be adhered to with regard to the use of social media. The guidance is not intended to cover every social media situation that a Nursing Associate may face; however, it sets out broad principles that will enable them to think through issues and act professionally, ensuring public protection at all times.

Some lecturers will use learning aids, such as backchannelchat and Socrative websites that allow instant feedback from students using mobile devices. None of the technologies described in this section should be seen as barriers to learning, but as opportunities to enhance the learning experience.

LOOKING BACK, FEEDING FORWARD

A number of facets of learning have been addressed in this chapter and hopefully you have made use of the opportunity to discover your own learning style and preference. This chapter has highlighted the fact that there are a number of barriers that can impinge on people's ability to learn; however, it is important to realize that these can be overcome and then you can engage with the lifelong learning process.

REFERENCES

Canning, N., 2010. Playing with heutagogy: exploring strategies to empower mature learners in higher education. Journal of Further and Higher Education. 34 (1).

Covey, S., 1999. Seven Habits of Highly Successful People. Simon & Schuster, London.

Equality Challenge Unity, 2010. Managing Reasonable Adjustments in Higher Education http://www.ecu.ac.uk/wp-content/uploads/external/managing-reasonable-adjustments-in-higher-education.pdf.

Fleming, N.D., Mills, C., 1992. Helping students understand how they learn. The Teaching Professor 7 (4).

Health Education England, 2016. Nursing Associate Curriculum Framework https://www.hee.nhs.uk/sites/default/files/documents/Curriculum%20Framework%20Nursing%20Associate.pdf.

Honey, P., Mumford, A., 1986. The Manual of Learning Styles. Peter Honey Associates.

Nursing and Midwifery Council (NMC), 2010. Standards for Pre - Registration Nursing Education. https://www.nmc.org.uk/globalassets/sitedocuments/standards/nmc-standards-for-pre-registration-nursing-education.pdf.

Nursing and Midwifery Council, 2017. Guidance on Using Social Media Responsibly. https://www.nmc.org.uk/globalassets/sitedocuments/nmc-publications/social-media-guidance.pdf.

Quality Assurance Agency, 2009. Academic Credit in Higher Education England – an Introduction. http://www.qaa.ac.uk/en/Publications/Documents/Academic-credit-in-higher-education-in-England—an-introduction.pdf.

Professional and Regulatory Bodies

Christine Mullen

OBJECTIVES

By the end of the chapter the reader will be able to:

1. Understand the meaning and impact of professional regulation
2. Describe the principles and processes underpinning good standards of regulation
3. Describe the key bodies involved with, and responsible for, regulating professions
4. Have knowledge of the code of conduct for nurses, midwives and Nursing Associates (Nursing and Midwifery Council (NMC), 2018a).
5. Describe the standards and values outlined in the NMC Code for nurses, midwives and Nursing Associates (NMC, 2018a) and the NMC Standards of Proficiency for Nursing Associates (NMC, 2018b).
6. Demonstrate how to ensure, and provide evidence of, continual learning and development of the required standards

KEY WORDS

Professional values	Behaviour	Health
Professional standards	Patient-centred care	Well-being
Proportionate risk	Diversity	Patient safety
Quality assurance	Teamworking	Professional indemnity
Responsibility	Leadership	
Attitudes	Duty of care	

CHAPTER AIM

The aim of this chapter is to introduce the reader to 'regulation' – what it means for practitioners and the wider impact of being regulated in terms of employment and public expectations.

SELF TEST

1. Describe the meaning of being a regulated professional.
2. Outline the principles underpinning regulation.
3. Describe the code of conduct for nurses, midwives and Nursing Associates (NMC, 2018a).
4. Describe accountability as a registered practitioner.
5. Describe the 'platforms' of practice as determined in the Nursing Associate Standards of Proficiency (NMC, 2018b).
6. Describe the role of employers in supporting registered practitioners to maintain their registration, ensure their practice is up to date, and continually improve patients' quality of care.
7. Outline how you will maintain, record and demonstrate how you meet the required annual learning and development criteria for maintaining your fitness to practise as a Nursing Associate.

INTRODUCTION

The key purpose of regulating professionals is to assure the public that practitioners meet and improve upon the mandated required standards of practice and behaviours expected by the regulators and the public.

BACKGROUND TO THE DEVELOPMENT OF THE NURSING ASSOCIATE (NA) BECOMING A REGULATED PROFESSION

This section will examine the background to how the NA role came into being and its development into a regulated role.

Healthcare assistants/support workers (HAs) across health and social care have, up until now, not been regulated by any regulatory body. The question of regulation, however, has been around for many years. In England, it began in earnest early in 2000 with the drive for workforce modernization, including the creation of new roles, such as the Assistant Practitioner (Skills for Health, 2009), and new ways of working. However, despite some serious attempts, regulation did not progress. The catalyst for change came following a number of events: the

Mid Staffordshire NHS Foundation Trust enquiry (Sir Robert Francis QC, 2013), an independent review by Camilla Cavendish (Cavendish, 2013) and a review of the future education and training of nursing for registered nurses and care assistants by Lord Willis called *Raising the Bar* (Lord Willis, 2015). The Willis report made a number of important recommendations relevant to all assistants and to the Nursing Associate role in particular (see Box 4.1).

The developments described in Box 4.1 and the above-mentioned reports led to a number of publicized documents for employers to use as guides to understanding the minimum standards required in practice when employing and developing healthcare assistants and care assistants. The main ones are:

1. The Care Certificate Standards (Skills for Care, April 2015)
2. Code of Conduct for Healthcare Support Workers and Adult Social Care Workers in England (Skills for Care, March 2013)
3. Core Standards for Assistant Practitioners (Skills for Health, 2009).

Health Education England (HEE) encourages employers to use these guides as part of their workforce policies for recruiting, training, retaining and developing their healthcare assistants. However, there is no legal requirement for employers to use these codes and/or standards, but they do provide employers and care assistants with an outline of standards of 'best practice' and 'behaviours' expected as a minimum baseline for the roles. The Assistant Practitioner standards development was part of the workforce modernization agenda between 2004 and 2009.

BOX 4.1 Some Relevant Recommendations Associated with Various Roles (Lord Willis, 2015)

- Health Education England (HEE) should evaluate the impact of the Care Certificate on care outcomes and patient experience.
- Subject to the outcome of recommendation three, any future government should ensure that the Care Certificate is a mandatory requirement.
- HEE should implement the Higher Care Certificate.
- HEE should set the competency standards for care assistants (NHS bands 1–4) in both health and social care, and work with employers to ensure the workforce is trained to meet those standards.

Recommendations Indirectly Linked to the Nursing Associate

- HEE should explore with others the need to develop a defined care role (NHS Agenda for Change band 3) that would act as a bridge between the unregulated care assistant workforce and the registered nursing workforce.
- Care assistants should be offered Accreditation of Prior Experiential Learning (APEL) that could account for up to 50% of the undergraduate nursing degree.
- HEE, in collaboration with employers and Higher Education Institutes (HEIs), should support the development of more innovative work-based learning routes. Those learning routes should be standardized to allow care assistants to move easily into the nursing profession without having to give up their employment, as they study and train for their nursing degree and registered nurse status.

These were driven by employers, and Skills for Health provided its support and expertise to develop national standards of practice for this high-level role. The previously-mentioned standards/codes relate specifically to England – Scotland, Northern Ireland and Wales have all developed their own standards and codes for their healthcare support workers.

In addition to these developments, over the past 3 to 4 years, there has been increasing concern about shortages of staff, in particular nursing staff. These shortages caused problems in recruitment and impacted on services. There are a number of factors contributing to the difficulties. In particular, poor retention rates, pay freezes, increasing service demand, financial pressures across providers and reductions in overseas recruitment (in part due to the insecurity of Britain's decision to leave the European Union (EU)) have culminated in the supply of nurses not matching demand.

As a result of pressures on the service, the Cavendish report (Cavendish, 2013) and *Raising the Bar* recommendations (Lord Willis, 2015), the idea of a 'new high level' assistant role for nursing was launched and consultation began in 2016.

Background to the Nursing Associate role

The Nursing Associate role was accepted by leaders across nursing and by the public, and to date the outcomes of relevance are:

- November 2016 – the Nursing Associate role curriculum was released by Health Education England
- November 2016 – the NMC was invited and agreed to regulate the role
- January 2017 – the first cohort of trainee Nursing Associates started across 11 sites in England
- April 2017 – a second wave of trainees began across 24 sites in England.
- October 2018 – the NMC amends the code of conduct (NMC, 2018a) and introduces Standards of Proficiency for Nursing Associates (NMC, 2018b).

ISSUES REGARDING A CODE FOR NURSING ASSOCIATES

The current situation in relation to the NA and the Code of Conduct was discussed at the NMC's council meeting in July 2017 (Nursing and Midwifery Council, 2017a) (see Fig. 4.1). The NMC's approach aimed to formally engage and consult with key stakeholders during 2017 on a code for the NA. The NMC's intention is to give trainee NAs, employers and education providers a year's notice of the likely requirements NAs will need to register as practitioners. Once agreed and in place, NAs will be bound by the principles of a code. The NMC Council aims to approve the final versions between April and October 2018.

The current NMC Code will potentially provide the framework for the NA Code using the concept of 'proportionality' and 'enabling nursing/career progression' to inform the discussions. There may, therefore, be some adaptations/amendments to the Code to reflect the level of the NA role. NAs would be well advised to ensure they are familiar with the Code in the context of their practice. Further detail on the importance of regulation once employed as an NA is discussed in the following sections.

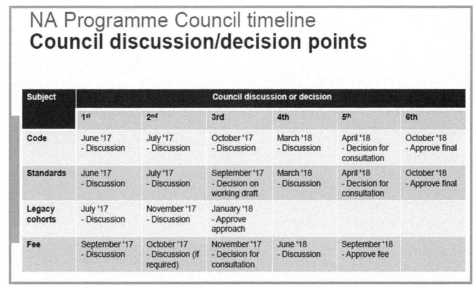

Fig. 4.1 NA Programme Council Timeline (Nursing and Midwifery Council, 2017a. Reproduced with permission of the NMC).

THE REGULATING BODIES, SYSTEMS AND PRINCIPLES

This section will provide an overview of the two key regulatory bodies and the employers' role in regulating the NA role. The two bodies are:
- The Professional Standards Authority
- The Nursing and Midwifery Council

The Professional Standards Authority

The Professional Standards Authority for Health and Social Care (PSA) is the current body with responsibility for health and social care regulation (PSA, 2016a). It replaced the previous body, the Council for Healthcare Regulatory Excellence (CHRE) in 2014.

In 2015, the PSA published a paper on 'rethinking regulation' (PSA, 2015b). They reassessed the role of regulation in promoting safety and quality, followed by a deliberate and considered redesign of the institutions and processes of regulation. The objectives they set out in the document align considerably with the government's intentions, and these are as follows:
- A shared 'theory of regulation' based on right-touch thinking
- Shared objectives for system and professional regulators and greater clarity of roles
- Transparent benchmarking to set standards
- A rebuilding of trust between professionals, the public and regulators
- A reduced scope of regulation so it focuses on what works
- An appropriate risk-assessed model of who and what should be regulated put into practice through a continuum of assurance
- Breaking down boundaries between statutory professions and accredited occupations
- Making it easier to create new roles and occupations within a continuum of assurance
- A drive for efficiency and reduced cost, which may lead to functional mergers and deregulation

- Placing real responsibility with the people who manage and deliver care.

Accredited Occupations Registers (Adapted from PSA, 2015a)

Accredited registers (AR) are applicable to those working in health and care occupations that have not been regulated by the state. The PSA have devised a Quality Mark that embodies standards they have established. Some examples of AR: Academy for Healthcare Science (AHCA); Complementary and Natural Healthcare Council (CNHC). The aim of the AR is to protect the public ensuring that they can access health and care practitioners from those registers that have been independently assessed and vetted by the PSA and who they permit to exhibit the PSA unique Quality Mark. This can provide the public with peace of mind when they access or use the services of someone on an Accredited Register. There are currently 17 Accredited Registered occupations.

A shared 'theory of regulation' would encompass a common purpose, common objectives and a shared understanding of the differences between regulation, inspection and quality improvement.

The Professional Standards Authority went on to produce a follow-up report, Regulation Rethought 2016 (PSA, 2016b). The PSA adopted three principles to test their proposed way forward, which are that regulation should be:
1. Proportionate to the harm it seeks to prevent (further expanded later)
2. Simple to understand and operate
3. Efficient and cost-effective.

Proportionate right-touch regulation

The concept of right-touch regulation is outlined in a document from the PSA (PSA, 2015c). It is an approach to regulatory decision-making defined by the PSA.

Using this definition, a decision on regulation is made against a series of questions used to assess what regulation, if any, is required for any given role. The different levels of regulation start with employer controls, credentializing and voluntary registration and move to statutory registration.

The PSA determines a role's level of regulation based on six principles:

1. Proportionate: Regulators should only intervene when necessary. Remedies should be appropriate to the risk posed, and costs identified and minimized.
2. Consistent: Rules and standards must be joined up and implemented fairly.
3. Targeted: regulation should be focused on the problem and minimize side effects.
4. Transparent: Regulators should be open, and keep regulations simple and user-friendly.
5. Accountable: Regulators must be able to justify decisions, and be subject to public scrutiny.
6. Agile: Regulation must look forward and be able to adapt to anticipate change.

These principles provide the foundation for thinking on regulatory policy in all sectors of society. The PSA sees the application of these six principles as bringing together a commonly agreed approach to good regulation and understanding of the sector and a quantified and qualified assessment of risk of harm. In other words, getting the balance right between regulation and risk.

CRITICAL AWARENESS

NAs need to understand the concept and application of 'proportionate' risk in the context of regulation and its relevance to practice.

The work of the PSA

The PSA promotes the health, safety and well-being of patients, service users and the public by raising standards of regulation and voluntary registration of people working in health and care. It aims to be a strong independent voice for patients in the regulation of health professionals throughout the UK. The PSA has four core regulatory functions that it uses to monitor all the regulatory bodies, including the NMC (see Box 4.2).

A recent document from NHS England on its shared commitment to quality (NHS England, July 2016), refers to key areas of responsibilities in relation to 'assurances' of services to patients, people who use services, carers and their advocates, professional staff, providers, commissioners and funders and national bodies. The two areas of relevance to regulation and to you as a registered practitioner are stated as follows:

- Professional staff: 'As skilled professionals you should be consistently supported to put quality at the centre of all you do… Where you see a need, you should feel empowered and supported to make changes to improve care…You will feel able

---

BOX 4.2   Professional Standards Authority Core Functions (PSA, 2016a)

1. Setting and promoting guidance and standards for the profession(s)
2. Setting standards for and quality assuring the provision of education and training
3. Maintaining a register of professionals
4. Taking action where a professional's fitness to practise may be impaired.

---

to work with people who use services as partners in their care and partners in driving service improvement.'
- Employers: '…your service will be well led in continually striving to improve care. Existing ways of understanding quality, including safety, effectiveness and positive experience will be considered alongside the efficient and equitable use of resources…'

The PSA uses a number of sources of information about the performance of the regulator and analyses how and if the information demonstrates how a regulator, for instance the NMC, is meeting each of the required standards. An overview of what the PSA expects of regulators in each of the four core areas (prioritize people, practise effectively, preserve safety and promote professionalism and trust) is provided later.

! HOTSPOT

Record an event in practice where you have worked with a patient and their family to help them understand the patient's care and treatment plan and to ascertain if any changes are needed to ensure the plan meets their needs.

All regulators are responsible for publishing and promoting standards of competence and conduct. These are the standards for safe and effective practice which every health professional and social worker should meet to become registered and to maintain their registration. They set out the quality of care that patients and service users should receive from health professionals in the UK and social workers in England (Wales, Scotland and Northern Ireland have a different process for social workers). Regulators also publish additional guidance to address specific or specialist issues. These complement the regulator's standards of competence and conduct. The standards reflect the following:
- Up-to-date practice and legislation
- Prioritization of patient and service user safety
- Patient and service user-centred care.

Education and training

The regulator (in this case the NMC) has a role in the following:
- Ensuring that students and trainees obtain the required skills and knowledge to be safe and effective
- Ensuring that standards of education and training are linked to 'standards for registrants' referred to earlier
- Ensuring that once registered, registrants remain up to date with evolving practices and continue to develop as professionals.

The regulators quality assure and, where appropriate, approve educational programmes that students must complete in order to be registered. For nursing and midwifery, the NMC has a publicly available list of approved providers.

Standards of good regulation in relation to registration

In order for a health professional to practise legally in the UK and a social worker to practise legally in England, they must be registered with the relevant regulator. The regulators only register those professionals who meet their standards. The regulator (NMC) is required to keep up-to-date records of all the professionals it has registered. The register should include a record of any action taken against a registrant that limits their entitlement to practise.

Standards of good regulation relating to registration that the PSA require are as follows:

- Only those who meet the regulator's requirements are registered.
- The registration process, including the management of appeals, is fair, based on the regulator's standards, efficient, transparent, secure and continuously improving.
- Employers are aware of the importance of checking a health professional or social worker's registration. Patients, service users and members of the public can find and check a health professional or social worker's registration.
- Risk of harm to the public and of damage to public confidence in the profession related to non-registrants using a protected title or undertaking a protected act, is managed in a proportionate and risk-based manner.
- Through the regulator's continuing professional development (CPD)/revalidation systems, registrants maintain the standards required to stay fit to practise.

Regulators that are monitored and assessed by the PSA

The PSA oversees the work of nine statutory bodies, which are shown in Box 4.3. In January 2017, the NMC formally agreed to a request from the Department of Health to be the regulator for the new Nursing Associate role.

The PSA undertakes an annual assessment of all nine regulatory bodies. Their report on the Performance Review Standards framework (PSA, 2016a) states their values as committed to be:

- focused on the public interest
- independent
- fair
- transparent.

BOX 4.3 The Nine Statutory Bodies Governed by the PSA (PSA, 2016a)

1. General Chiropractic Council
2. General Dental Council
3. General Medical Council
4. General Optical Council
5. General Osteopathic Council
6. General Pharmaceutical Council
7. Health and Care Professions Council
8. Nursing and Midwifery Council
9. Pharmaceutical Society of Northern Ireland.

The Nursing and Midwifery Council role

The NMC is the independent regulator for nurses, midwives and, as of 2017, the new Nursing Associate role. The NMC covers the whole of the UK; however, the NA role is currently for England only.

The NMC was established in 2001 and came into being on 1 April 2002. It is governed by a council of twelve members selected through open competition and comprises an even number of lay people and registered professionals. Council meetings are open to the public and available on the NMC website.

As an organization the NMC is:

- accountable to Parliament through the Privy Council and participates in an annual accountability hearing with the Health Select Committee of the UK Parliament
- performance reviewed annually by the PSA against its standards for good regulation, and publishes its findings
- a registered charity.

The NMC works in collaboration with key partners across health and care organizations, employers, other regulatory bodies, funders and commissioners. Its role is to protect patients and the public through efficient and effective regulation.

There are three core functions that will apply to the systems of assurance in relation to the NA role (see Box 4.4).

It is important to note that the NMC also requires student nurses or midwives to comply with its codes of practice and behaviour (NMC, 2009). This will most likely also apply to trainee NAs. The process of registration is described as a cycle, starting with registration through to ensuring fitness to practise; this is illustrated in Fig. 4.2.

The NMC Code of Professional Standards of Practice and Behaviour

The 'Code' is the document that all registered practitioners need to abide by in order to practise. The code encompasses four key themes that together with a section on public protection, signifies good nursing and midwifery practice (see Fig. 4.3).

The four themes have 'headed sub-themes' under which are a number of stated standards. A summary outline of the four sub-themes is provided here (the full Code is available from the NMC website https://www.nmc.org.uk/globalassets/sitedocuments/nmc-publications/nmc-code.pdf).

Prioritize people – five key headings

1. Treat people as individuals and uphold their dignity.
2. Listen to people and respond to their preferences and concerns.
3. Make sure that people's physical, social and psychological needs are assessed and responded to.
4. Act in the best interests of people at all times.
5. Respect people's right to privacy and confidentiality.

Practise effectively – seven key headings

1. Always practise in line with the best available evidence.
2. Communicate clearly.
3. Work cooperatively.
4. Share your skills, knowledge and experience for the benefit of people receiving care and your colleagues.
5. Keep clear and accurate records relevant to your practice.
6. Be accountable for your decisions to delegate tasks and duties to other people.

BOX 4.4 The Nursing and Midwifery Core Functions (Nursing and Midwifery Council, 2016. Reproduced with permission of the Nursing and Midwifery Council)

1. Maintaining a register of those eligible to practice as nurses or midwives in the UK
2. Setting standards to join the register and remain on the register
3. Acting when there are concerns about the conduct or practice of a nurse or midwife.

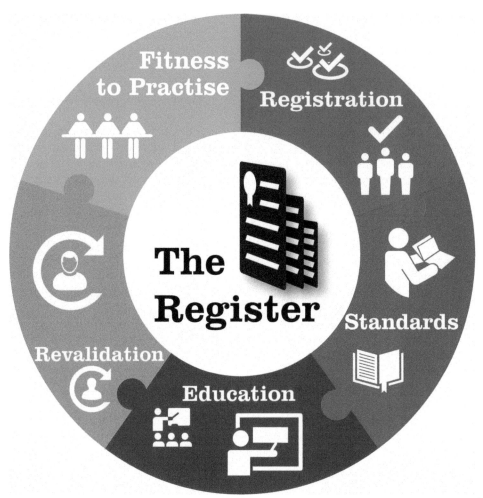

Fig. 4.2 NMC Functions. The NMC's functions work together to ensure the integrity, meaning and usefulness of the register (Nursing and Midwifery Council, 2016. Reproduced with permission of the NMC).

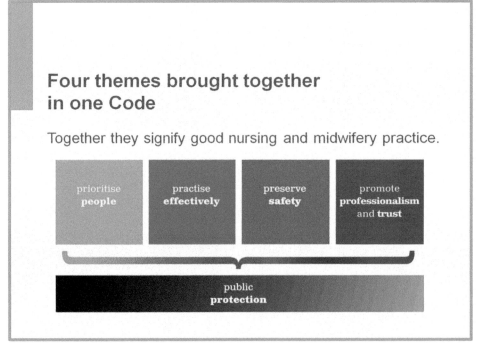

Fig. 4.3 The Four Key Themes of the NMC Code (Nursing and Midwifery Council, 2016. Reproduced with permission of the NMC).

7. Have in place an indemnity arrangement which provides appropriate cover for any practice you take on as a nurse or midwife in the UK

Preserve safety – seven key headings

1. Recognize and work within the limits of your competence.
2. Be open and candid with all service users about all aspects of care and treatment, including when any mistakes or harm have taken place.
3. Always offer help if an emergency arises in your practice setting or anywhere else.
4. Act without delay if you believe that there is a risk to patient safety or public protection.
5. Raise concerns immediately if you believe a person is vulnerable or at risk and needs extra support and protection.
6. Advise on, prescribe, supply, dispense or administer medicines within the limits of your training and competence, the law, our guidance and other relevant policies, guidance and regulations.
7. Be aware of, and reduce as far as is possible, any potential for harm associated with your practice.

Promote professionalism and trust – six key headings

1. Uphold the reputation of your profession at all times.
2. Uphold your position as a registered nurse or midwife.
3. Fulfil all registration requirements.
4. Cooperate with all investigations and audits.
5. Respond to any complaints made against you professionally.
6. Provide leadership to make sure people's well-being is protected and to improve their experiences of the healthcare system.

> ### ❗ HOTSPOT
> Registered practitioners have to ensure that they understand the Code of Conduct that governs their practice. They must at all times act in the best interests of patients.

It is recommended that NAs obtain a copy of the Code from the NMC website and reflect on their developing practice in the context of each of these themes.

The NMC website provides lots of information for registrants, employers and the public, such as guidance, advice, a variety of reports (including 'fitness to practise' outcomes), videos and various communications. One useful NMC document for the NA to read and understand is 'NMC professional indemnity arrangement' (Nursing and Midwifery Council, 2014) written following a new legal UK government Health and Associated Professions (Indemnity Arrangements) Order 2014 requirement. By law, nurses and midwives must have in place an appropriate indemnity arrangement in order to practise and provide care. Whilst the arrangement does not need to be individually held by the nurse or midwife, it is their responsibility to ensure that appropriate cover is in force. The NMC Code was updated to include indemnity as part of the required standard for practice.

> ### REFLECTION 4.1
> Having considered the regulatory code of practice, reflect on how you think you might help a service user/patient/client with a learning disability to navigate the various systems when they wish to make representation to a professional body.

TABLE 4.1 The Key Areas of Relevance in the Employer's Role (NHS Employers, 2011)

Key Area	Description

Recruitment	• Clear expectations, the use of employment checks and induction. These include:
	  • Verification of identity checks
	  • Right to work checks
	  • Professional registration and qualification checks
	  • Employment history and reference checks
	  • Criminal record checks
	  • Occupational health checks.

Supervision	Systems in place to provide supervision to individuals, where appropriate, and for the overall care being delivered to patients.
Continuing Professional Development	To ensure all staff continue to meet the requirements of the role they are employed to undertake.
Clear standards, expectations and boundaries	To ensure appropriate delegation and ensure individuals do not operate beyond their scope of competence.
Appraisal	Using the many different tools available to support the assurance process.
Policies	Embedded into practice that support staff to challenge issues of concern and deal with unacceptable behaviour or poor standards of care in an appropriate way.

The employer's role

Employers have a role to play in supporting all their staff and specific areas of particular importance for registered practitioners. In a document from NHS Employers (NHS Employers, 2011) they outline their key responsibility as employers is to deliver high quality care and ensure there are strong governance processes in place to assure the board that the quality of care and experience not only meets the desired standard, but is also continually improving. This is achieved through a variety of employment and workforce practices. There are several priority areas for the employer which, when reviewed against the expectations of the service, can provide assurance of the competence of their whole workforce.

Once in employment, it is important for NAs to find out about and understand these practices and policies as they directly support and relate to the enabling of registered practitioners to continue to work and stay in practice. The key areas of relevance are shown in Table 4.1.

Employers should ensure that they have in place the mechanisms and policies appropriate to fulfil their duties. It is important, therefore, that you fully understand your employer's human resource policies and conform to them. In the case of a concern being raised at work, your employer should undertake a thorough investigation of the issues to potentially resolve them or determine the need to report the incident to the NMC as a matter of regulatory concern.

Further practical aspects of regulation as described earlier is expanded on in the next section.

REGULATION OF THE NURSING ASSOCIATE – PRACTICAL ASPECTS TO REGISTERING AND REGULATION

This section will examine the implications of regulation in the context of the NA role and the Code (NMC, 2018a).

NA educational programme, standards and the potential code

The Standards of Proficiency for the NA (NMC, 2018b) are the minimum standards required for England. The framework provides the educational standards for the NA role. The proficiencies describe the required standards of practice and the expected behaviours and values for the NA role (NMC, 2018b). A summary of the eight domains used by health Education England (2016) are provided in Box 4.5.

REFLECTION 4.2

Describe how you effectively communicated with colleagues outside your organization for one of your patients in order to effect their transition to self-care and go home.

Learning outcomes and their relevance to the code being developed

The NMC Standards of Proficiency describe NA attitudes and behaviours as compassionate, competent and confident. These reflect the values in the nursing and midwifery framework for England (NHS England Chief Nursing Officer, 2016) where the six C's of compassion, care, commitment, courage, competency and communication provide the foundation of practice. The Standars of Proficiency make clear that on successful completion of the programme, the NA will have the knowledge, skills, attitudes and behaviours relevant to employment as a NA. They are also featured in the code of conduct (NMC, 2018a).

NAs are advised to consider the Standards of Proficiency (NMC, 2018b) and the Code of Conduct (NMC, 2018a) identifying where the Code of Conduct and the proficiencies meet and support each other in defining the roles and responsibilities of the NA.

CRITICAL AWARENESS

Trainee NAs must make themselves aware of the NMC Code and the Standards of Proficiency in the context of their practice and behaviour.

NAs must ensure that they adhere to the tenets of code as they offer care and support to people.

⚠ HOTSPOT

It is advisable to regularly access the NMC website (https://www.nmc.org.uk/) so as to keep up to date with developments that are occurring within the profession.

BOX 4.5 HEE NA Curriculum Framework Domains (Adapted from Health Education England, 2016)

Domain 1: Professional Values and Parameters of Practice
'Exercise personal responsibility and work independently within the defined parameters of practice, taking appropriate initiative in a variety of situations and performing a range of clinical and care skills consistent with the roles, responsibilities and professional values of a nursing associate.'

Domain 2: Person-Centred Approaches to Care
'Exercise those skills, attitudes and behaviours that support the planning, delivery and evaluation of high quality person-centred care.'

Domain 3: Delivering Care
'Work across organizational boundaries in a range of health and care settings and apply, in practice, the range of clinical and care skills appropriate to their parameters of practice.'

Domain 4: Communication and Inter-Personal Skills
'Communicate effectively across a wide range of channels and with a wide range of individuals, the public, health and social care professionals, maintaining the focus of communication on delivering and improving health and care services and … possess those inter-personal skills that promote clarity, compassion, empathy, respect and trust.'

Domain 5: Duty of Care, Candour, Equality and Diversity
'Explain the principles underpinning duty of care, equality and diversity and the need for candour and will consistently demonstrate the application of those principles in and across a range of settings across life-course.'

Domain 6: Supporting Learning and Assessment in Practice
'Exercise those skills, attitudes and behaviours that support personal development and life-long learning together, as well as those associated with the development of others.'

Domain 7: Teamworking and Leadership
'Explain the principles underpinning leadership frameworks and associated teamworking and leadership competencies and demonstrate a range of those competencies, attitudes and behaviours required of a nursing associate.'

Domain 8: Research, Development and Innovation
'Demonstrate the importance of being research aware, research and innovation, and their own role in this, across the health and care landscape in improving the quality of patient safety and care and in addressing the challenges faced within the context of rising public expectations.

'More specific learning outcomes sit under each of the domains outlined above and all are expected to be included in any programme devised from this framework document. With the overarching categorisation indicated by the domains means that there is an inherent degree of overlap and/or repetition in some of the areas. For example, holistic, person-centred care, managing/prioritising workloads, sound and improving digital literacy, the effective use and championing of existing and emerging technologies all cross domains and should be an integral part of each. In devising programmes and communicating outcomes to trainees, necessary overlap and repetition and the integrated nature of many of the learning outcomes should be explained and made explicit.'

BOX 4.6 Definitions Relating to Required Standards and Behaviours of Practice from the NA Curriculum (Health Education England, 2016)

Abuse: Includes physical abuse; domestic violence and/or coercive control; sexual abuse; psychological abuse; financial/material abuse; modern slavery; discriminatory abuse; organizational abuse; neglect/acts of omission; self-neglect.

Accountability: To be responsible for the decisions you make and answerable for your actions.

Autonomy: The freedom to make binding decisions within the parameters of practice that are based on professional ethics, expertise and clinical knowledge.

Duty of care: The legal obligation to: (1) Always act in the best interests of individuals and others; (2) Not act or fail to act in a way that results in harm; (3) Act within your competence and not take on anything you do not believe you can safely do.

Diversity: Celebrating difference, valuing people and recognizing them for their skills, talents and experiences, accepting that everyone is different and respecting those differences.

Equality: Treating everyone fairly and providing equal opportunities for everyone regardless of their race, gender, disability, age, sexual orientation, religion and belief.

Holistic: Concerning the whole person. A holistic approach to nursing considers the physical, social, economic psychological, spiritual and other factors when assessing, planning and delivering care.

Parity of esteem: Valuing mental health equally with physical health.

Person-centred care: Treating everyone fairly and providing equal opportunities for everyone regardless of their race, gender, disability, age, sexual orientation, religion and belief.

Responsibility: In connection with tasks or areas of work that have been assigned to an individual or individual, responsibility means that the individuals are expected to carry out those tasks, and that they are the owners of a task, event or area of work. Responsibility differs from accountability in that responsibility can be shared, but accountability cannot. Being accountable means not only being responsible for something, but ultimately being the person answerable for actions.

Unwarranted variation: Variations in health and care which can be changed if we choose to. They can be a sign of poor-quality care, missed opportunities and waste and can result in poorer outcomes, poorer experience and increased expense.

It is important to embrace the proficiencies and embed them into your clinical and personal practice. A number of terms are defined in the NMCs Standards of Proficiency for the NA (NMC, 2018b) that you would be wise to be fully aware of and apply in practice. Some key definitions are useful to consider in the context of your responsibilities and behaviours as a registered NA (see Box 4.6).

❗ HOTSPOT

The registered practitioner is, first and foremost, accountable to the patient.

REGULATION PROCESSES IN PRACTICE

There are several steps in the process of being regulated you will need to understand and comply with. These are:

a. Registration
b. Revalidation or re-registration
c. CPD
d. Indemnity

An overview of each of these processes (as known at the time of writing) is discussed in the following sections, highlighting some of the important points and actions that you will need to understand and action.

Registration

The current process for newly qualified nurses and midwives to register with the NMC is:

- Step one – Once the training programme has been completed the university sends the course details and personal information of the participants (such as name, address and date of birth) who were successful to the NMC's database.
- Step two – After confirming their qualification details, the NMC informs the registrant by post within 7–10 working days.
- Step three – The university is also required to send the NMC a declaration confirming a participant's good health and character. The NMC's standards for registration state that it may take up to 10 working days to receive, verify and allocate it to the registrant's application.
- Timeframe – The NMC aims to assess completed applications in 2–10 working days, meaning that the time between the university sending the declaration to the NMC and applications being assessed will be a maximum of 20 working days. As with all applications, the NMC will always aim to process these as quickly as possible.
- Advise – the NMC advises registrants to join the NMC register by creating an account with the NMC Online. At this point, registrants are required to declare any police cautions or criminal convictions to the NMC. Information on how to do this is provided by the NMC and is called 'declaring cautions and convictions'.
- Fee – A registration fee is payable and an online application form must be completed. The Nursing and Midwifery Council have approved the registration fee for the NA to be £120 this is the same fee for registered nurses. The first cohort of Nursing Associates qualify in 2019 and will therefore be required to register with the NMC as planned.
- Completion – once all the required information has been provided, a registration officer reviews the documents. If everything is completed correctly, applications are processed and registrants are put on the NMC register within 2–10 working days. Registrants can check on the NMC's website to see if their application has been accepted, as well as download and print a statement of entry.

It is important to note that your registration details need to be kept up to date in accordance with any changes in your personal life. The most common reason for a lapsed registration (and illegal practice) is a failure to keep the NMC updated of your contact details.

The NA registration process will reflect this process. During your training your education provider will keep up to date with the registration progress and will support you once you have completed your training programme.

! HOTSPOT

Registered practitioners must take responsibility for registering with the NMC and maintaining their ongoing registration.

Revalidation

Revalidation for nurses and midwives is a system introduced by the NMC in 2016 and requires nurses and midwives to revalidate their registration every 3 years.

Revalidation (Nursing and Midwifery Council, 2017b, 2017c) is the responsibility of the nurse or midwife.

Revalidation is:

- a process that nurses and midwives are required to follow to maintain their registration with the NMC
- a demonstration of their continued ability to practise safely and effectively
- a continuous process that they must engage with throughout their career.

Revalidation is not:

- an assessment of a nurse or midwife's fitness to practise
- a new way to raise fitness to practise concerns (any concerns about a nurse or midwife's practice will continue to be raised through the existing fitness to practise process)
- an assessment against the requirements of current/former employment.

The requirements currently involved in revalidation are as follows:

- A minimum of 450 hours of practice
- 36 hours of CPD, of which 20 hours must be participatory learning
- Five pieces of practice-related feedback
- Five written reflective accounts on the CPD and/or practice-related feedback and/or an event or experience in their practice and how this relates to the Code
- Reflective discussion with another nurse or midwife
- Health and character declaration
- Professional indemnity arrangement.

These requirements are used to 'assure' the NMC that nurses and midwives are up-to-date practitioners able to provide safe and effective care. This is especially important today with the ever-increasing advancements in healthcare knowledge, skills and technology. The cycle for revalidation is shown in Fig. 4.4.

Consideration of 'proportionality and risk', as discussed earlier, has determined the most appropriate approach for the NA role with regards to CPD. The previous system for nurses and midwives called Post Registration Education and Practice (PREP) has now been replaced by revalidation. NAs are required to provide evidence of their on-going personal and professional development just as the registered nurse and registered midwife are required to do.

It is worth noting that the revalidation process requires nurses and midwives to start the process of collating and validating the requirements 12 months before the date of renewal.

In summary, revalidation will be in place once you qualify as an NA. The process will require you to register on the NMC website through a personal online account/portal. You will be required to provide evidence that you have undertaken CPD since you last registered and you must comply with the NMCs requirement concerning revalidation. Failure to comply with these requirements may put your registration with NMC at risk and you will be unable to practice.

Continuing professional development (CPD)

CPD is described as:

> 'The way in which a worker continues to learn and develop throughout their career, keeping their skills and knowledge up to date and ensuring that they can work safely and effectively.' (Health Education England 2016 Page 65).

The NMC Standards of Proficiency for Nursing Associates (NMC, 2018b) sets out the knowledge, understanding, skills and competences, attitudes and behaviours a trainee Nursing Associate will need in order to become a NA. The proficiencies have been developed in partnership with a range of stake holders so as to support national consistency and coherence in the delivery of the education and training model for NAs.

The Standards of Proficiency (NMC, 2018b) and the NMC Code (NMC, 2018a) together form the basis for public expectation, quality and safety of care provided by NAs. In order to both register and continue as a registered practitioner, you will need to be able to demonstrate that you have maintained and developed the required standards, behaviours and attitudes.

Continuing professional development – the role of employers and practitioners

This section covers two key areas:

1. The employer's role.
2. The practitioner's role.

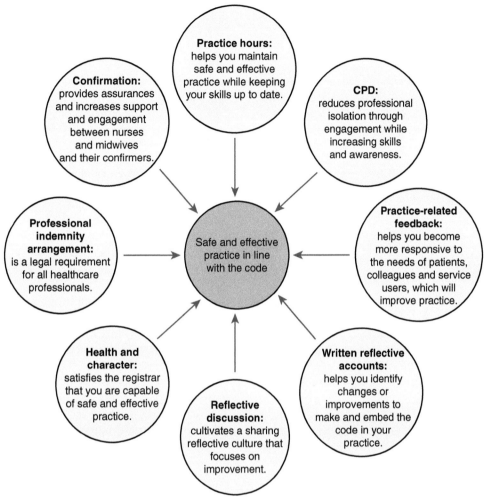

Fig. 4.4 Safe and Effective Practice In Line with the Code (Nursing and Midwifery Council, 2017b. Modified with permission of the NMC).

The employer's role. Employers' responsibilities in relation to CPD are to enable you, as a practitioner, to practise safely, to support you to maintain and improve your skills and knowledge and to support you to re-register. Two key areas are discussed further:
- Quality assurance and the employer's role
- CPD and the employer's support.

> **⚠ HOTSPOT**
>
> Registered practitioners are responsible for keeping their practice, knowledge and skills up to date and are ultimately accountable to the people they serve that they are competent practitioners.

Quality assurance – the employer's role. Employers need to assure their board, the public and the commissioners that the quality of care and patient experience not only meets the desired standard, but is continually improving. One of the main 'assurances' that directly links to CPD, requires employers to provide assurance of the competence of their whole workforce. They need to demonstrate this through a number of key areas (outlined on the NHS employers' website http://www.nhsemployers):
- Recruitment: clear expectations, the use of employment checks and induction.

- Supervision: systems in place to provide supervision to individuals, where appropriate, and for the overall care being delivered to patients.
- CPD: to ensure all staff continue to meet the requirements of the role they are employed to undertake.
- Clear standards, expectations and boundaries: to ensure appropriate delegation and assure individuals do not operate beyond their scope of competence.
- Appraisal systems: using the many different tools available to support the assurance process.
- Policies: embedded into practice that support staff to challenge issues of concern and deal with unacceptable behaviour or poor standards of care in an appropriate way.

Policies related to these areas are important and help to create a local system that puts patient safety at the heart of employment practice. There is evidence that shows a direct link between high levels of staff engagement and overall organizational effectiveness. The actions organizations take need to be underpinned by a set of behaviours that create a culture of patient safety and continual improvement in quality.

This requires:
- strong leadership
- an environment where staff are happy to raise concerns

- a system of staff engagement opportunities and systems on service delivery
- effective teamworking and a team ethos to delivering care.

CRITICAL AWARENESS

As a practitioner, you need to understand the employer's duty of assurance towards ensuring the competence of required standards and to encourage and support improvements in service quality and patient experience.

Boundaries of Practice

You need to have a clear understanding of your role, the role description and your boundaries of practice (sometimes called 'scope of practice') as a professional and within your employment role.

REFLECTION 4.3

Having considered your scope of practice, reflect on how you respond, or would respond, to a team member asking you to undertake a task that is outside your area of practice.

The employer's role and your role as a practitioner. The employer's role in enabling you to undertake CPD is very important. The main areas in which employers need to support you as a practitioner are through providing and/or having the following:

- Enabling resources – ensuring availability of required resources, in particular time and funding, to participate in CPD (formal and informal)
- Organizational policies and functions – employer policies of relevance to you as a practitioner are the following:
  - Registration policy on initial registration data and in relation to your responsibilities in maintaining your registration.
  - Policy on mentorship for students and staff.
  - Supporting staff and students, e.g., mentoring students, preceptorship requirements for newly qualified staff, and induction of new staff policy.
  - Partner policies/systems, e.g., Unison, Royal College of Nursing (RCN), the appraisal system.
  - Learning and development policies and systems, e.g., provision of mandatory health and safety programmes, learning and development systems (for example, in-house programmes), affiliations with education providers.
  - Creating a 'learning organization' culture – having an encouraging and supportive learning environment; having a 'no blame' culture; innovation; staff engagement events/systems; opportunities to share ideas to improve services and the patient experience; acknowledging risk, and supporting multidisciplinary teams learning and working together.

As a practitioner, you will need to take the initiative and find out about your employer's systems and policies to maximize the opportunities available to you.

CPD in practice

There are a number of ways you can update your practice and, indeed, many of you will have been involved in updating events

in your earlier role as a support worker. As a registered practitioner, CPD needs to formally become part of your everyday life and practice. These are examples of some ways in which structured learning activities could/should be undertaken:

- Formal learning that is face-to-face, physical and/or virtual/online
- Reading/study periods
- Self-directed learning – physical/online, etc.
- Educational supervision/mentoring
- Assessment activities
- Teaching within the workplace
- Action learning sets
- Informal learning, e.g., blogs, social media, etc.
- Simulation
- Shadowing.

Learning at work and for work does not have to always be 'a course'. Work-based learning is often 'an opportunity lost', especially if the culture of the team does not recognize the value of learning in work. One example of using work activities to proactively support patients has been developed in the Midlands promoted by NHE England. They have developed the concept of 'Making every contact count' (East Midlands Trainer Hub, 2008) and developed a 'tool' that they and other organizations can use to train practitioners in health and well-being. The programme advocates using all patient contacts to encourage and support patients to 'stay well and live healthy'. In addition to this, some additional opportunities are available in your day-to-day 'practice' at work and in your organization generally.

⚠ HOTSPOT

Registered practitioners need to proactively undertake CPD opportunities, both formally and informally, as part of their requirement to maintain and improve their practice.

Learning in practice

- As a front-line practitioner working with patients, many opportunities occur where listening to patients' experiences provides interesting insights about the care and service they have received, which are often not 'captured' or recognized as 'live service feedback' in action. This is particularly important when working with patients with chronic conditions where the patients often become 'experts' in their own condition. Capturing these events could be used as part of reflective learning and/or to stimulate ideas for improving services and/or care to patients.
- Working with teams, including multidisciplinary staff, to share and learn from each other the different care/treatment that each person provides, can enhance your understanding of the 'whole patient pathway'.
- Learning from 'critical events' through team post-event discussion, e.g., the death of a patient, or a cardiac arrest where there is often a 'post-event' conversation/discussion held in the work area.
- Participating in audits of your area of work to seek evidence to underpin the effectiveness of care and/or to demonstrate if a patient's pathway and/or treatment could be improved.

REFLECTION 4.4

Consider a critical incident that occurred in your area of work and how you and the team supported each other, sharing feelings, actions and thoughts about the event and what the outcome from the discussions was.

The organization you work in:

- Make sure you are aware of the supervision and mentorship system so that you have a supervisor and mentor.
- Contribute to staff and/or service quality improvement events: Many organizations have a system enabling staff to submit ideas for improving services. As a practitioner, your work experience often triggers ideas/suggestions to improve services. Taking the time to submit your ideas and possibly develop them could then be written up to form part of your CPD evidence.
- Education and learning development staff/team: Making sure you are aware of and understand the organization's education and learning development team and work so that you can access as much of it as is relevant to you. Some of this may include online learning updates, e.g., mandatory health and safety modules, etc.
- Partner organizations: Most organizations work with partner organization, e.g., RCN, Unison, etc., and have 'union representatives' in the organization. Some of the representatives have trained to be 'learning representatives', often called a Union Learning Representative (ULR). Unionlearn (Unionlearn with the TUC, 2011) describe the URL roles as helping to 'open up learning opportunities for union members and also support them during their learning. They also help to develop a learning culture in companies and other workplaces.'
- Most registered practitioners are members of a partner organization and they usually have a variety of learning and development opportunities that you can access and use as part of CPD: events, modules, articles, journals, guides on practice, etc.
- Some bigger employers have research forums/clubs you could join/attend, e.g., virtual learning networks, peer group forums, patient groups, practitioner networks. These forums could enable you to link your practice to evidence-based learning and enhance your skills in research and enquiry.

Here are some general tips on what you could/should do to help your CPD:

- Join a library (some organizations have their own) for access to books and journals.
- Read clinical journals regularly.
- Keep a record of your learning through a portfolio of practice, and/or using a diary of learning and reflection.
- Actively engage with learning at work at every opportunity.

As a practitioner, your role requires that you ensure you keep records of your learning day to day, for instance by using a portfolio of practice or a diary, and that you keep any study certificates of attendance/completion, etc., so that when the time for revalidation/registration is due, all the material required is available at your fingertips.

CRITICAL AWARENESS

There are many ways to continuously update and improve your practice. It is important that you are aware of the opportunities in your organization, with your patients in everyday practice, and with key partners, e.g., union partners, educational providers, etc.

REFLECTION 4.5

Reflect an activity you undertook with a patient in practice that was influenced and changed as a direct result of a CPD learning event you undertook.

The following case studies provide you with some recent examples of nursing practitioners' revalidation and CPD experiences. They are taken from the NMC website (reproduced with permission from the NMC), and may be useful to you in the future.

CASE STUDY 4.1 Marcela

Marcela is a practice nurse at a GP surgery. She also works some weekends as a band 5 nurse in accident and emergency (A&E).

When Marcela first heard about revalidation she wanted to learn as much about it as she could. 'I am from a different country so when something new comes up it's important to get it right, especially with the language – we might understand it differently,' she explains. 'Before, I just had all my certificates and reflections together and hoped for the best. But now, with the guidance and templates, I understand clearly what is needed.'

Reflective accounts – Marcela found the form for reflective accounts particularly helpful. Whereas before she might have just scribbled down a few notes about a training course or something she'd experienced in her practice, it now feels much more structured. 'To have all the questions in front of you helps you to think, yes, I have done something good and yes, I have learnt something,' she says. 'It was straight to the point.'

Reflective discussion – When it came to discussing her reflective accounts, Marcela chose to have this conversation with a nurse from another GP practice who she hadn't worked with before. 'We spent about an hour doing it, which was lovely,' she says. 'She was interested in what I'd learnt and how it had changed me as a practitioner. I felt like I got a lot out of it, and to have that conversation with someone who doesn't know me at all was amazing. She made me critique what I have actually achieved.'

Confirmation – A few days later Marcela had her confirmation discussion with her line manager, who is the senior nurse at her practice. Together they went through Marcela's portfolio, and Marcela describes this part of the process as 'much more on a professional level'. She adds: 'Someone is checking to make sure that I have done what I'm supposed to have done.' Immediately after the confirmation, Marcela went online to submit her application.

CPD – Revalidation wasn't without its challenges, though, as Marcela explains. 'I was always used to undertaking CPD in A&E – you're teaching students, you're attending seminars, you're learning all the time. But the participatory part of it I do find more challenging in GP land.' She recognizes that there are opportunities; reps will come in and run learning sessions at the regular practice meetings, for example. But it can be hard as a practice nurse, especially if you are working part-time, to take advantage of these opportunities.

Marcela has chosen to view revalidation as a way of turning this situation around, though. 'You know now that every 3 years someone will be checking your progress,' she says. 'You can say to them, 'What are you going to do to help me as a practitioner? How are you going to value me as a professional?' Revalidation is the best thing that could have happened to nurses. It encourages them to push, to be a bit braver. It will give nurses the power to be able to say, "This is what needs to be done".' (Data from www.nmc.org.uk. Accessed 18/7/17)

CASE STUDY 4.2 Carol

Carol is a registered nurse who manages a care home for 80 residents on the west coast of Scotland.

Preparing for revalidation – Carol admits that when she first heard about revalidation she had concerns. She wasn't sure what she would have to do, and as a manager of other nurses, she knew it would be important for her to understand the process so that she could lead by example. She started to prepare by putting together a portfolio. 'I already had a folder that I kept my certificates from training in, but they were in no particular order,' she explains. 'I'm not that great on the computer so I just set up a folder with some dividers, all my bits of evidence and the NMC forms.'

Practice hours – As a home manager, Carol doesn't have timesheets, so she used her pay slips and P60 as evidence that she had done her 450 practice hours. 'It was all quite straightforward, really,' she says. 'I've heard nurses saying before "Oh gosh, I hope they don't ask for my portfolio because mine is a mess!" But if you're in the habit of keeping these things you won't find it too complicated at all.'

Feedback – For some people it's the new feedback requirement that seems the most daunting, but Carol actually found this to be one of the easiest aspects. 'It's something we as care home staff have had to do for quite a long time,' she explains. 'What I like is that you can get feedback from residents and relatives. I like that; it might make people feel a wee bit more confident about themselves.'

As Carol explains, you don't necessarily have to ask for feedback face-to-face – there are lots of types of feedback you can use. 'As a manager, I could use thank you letters, I could use the questionnaires that we put out, and I was able to use the Care Inspectorate grades as well. There's lots of information that you can use to prove that you're doing a good job, and to learn about yourself as a practitioner.'

Reflective accounts – Carol chose to write one of her reflective accounts about the Care Inspectorate grades; for another reflection, she focused on some training she had done. She found the NMC form helpful in understanding what she was being asked to do. 'They aren't looking for reams and reams of paper,' she says. 'As long as you're capturing the important parts, reflecting on it, and linking it back to the Code, that's enough.'

Reflective discussion – When it came to discussing her reflective accounts, Carol found it really just formalized what she was already doing with her line manager, who is another registered nurse. 'We meet monthly and do a one-to-one so I am having those conversations regularly,' she explains. 'We just sat down together and discussed my five reflections one by one.'

Confirmation – Carol also had her confirmation with her line manager, and in that meeting they went through her whole portfolio together. 'She went through my learning hours, my reflective accounts, the NMC forms. It was quite self-explanatory really,' Carol says. 'I'll be a confirmer for my deputy, and possibly for some of the staff nurses too. We're doing their appraisals and supervisions already and I think confirmation will fit in with that quite nicely.'

Carol has some wise words for all those nurses and midwives getting ready for revalidation now: be prepared: 'As I've said to all my nurses – get your NMC Online account opened, find out when you need to revalidate, and get yourself organized. If you get a system up and running that suits you now, it means that when the time comes there's going to be very little work for you to do.'

And how does she feel about revalidation now that she's been through the process? 'I know we're already professionals,' she says. 'But I think revalidation is going to make nurses that wee bit more accountable. At the end of the day it's going to benefit our residents.'

'What I like is that you can get feedback from residents and relatives. I like that it might make people feel a wee bit more confident about themselves.'

(Data from www.nmc.org.uk. Accessed 18/7/17)

CRITICAL AWARENESS

You need to proactively engage in CPD opportunities in work, at work and for work.

You need to record your CPD activities as they happen so that your record is a 'live document' of your practice.

Professional indemnity

'Indemnity cover' is the term used to describe the financial backing available to cover the costs of a clinical negligence claim against you. Employers in the NHS and the independent sector's employers (including in General Practice) have what is known as 'vicarious liability' for the actions of their employed staff. This means that employers have legal responsibility for tasks carried out or actions taken by their employees, connected with their employment. Should an incident occur where a patient is injured, the patient's claim would therefore ordinarily be directed to the employer if an employee makes a mistake. Providers arrange to have 'cover' through insurance, which in the NHS is through the Clinical Negligence Scheme. Likewise, employers in the independent sector will make similar arrangements through an insurance company.

Nurses or midwives must have an appropriate indemnity arrangement in place. The large majority of nurses and midwives will meet the new requirement when they:

- work exclusively for the NHS, as the employers already have an appropriate indemnity arrangement
- work in an employed environment in the independent sector where their employer provides them with indemnity cover
- are self-employed and make their own professional indemnity arrangements.

If a nurse or midwife is self-employed they need to arrange their own cover. This could be done:

- as part of a membership of a professional body or trade union
- by direct cover from a commercial provider
- as a combination of both.

Further detailed guidance can be found in the NHS Litigation Authority, NHS Indemnity document.

Obtaining appropriate cover

The NMC guide on indemnity (Nursing and Midwifery Council, 2014) describes appropriate cover as

> '…an indemnity arrangement which is appropriate to your role and scope of practice and its risks. The cover must be intended to be sufficient to meet an award of damages if a successful claim is made against you.' (Nursing and Midwifery Council, 2014, p. 3)

Determining what appropriate cover is for you will be influenced by the following:

- What your job involves and where you work
- Who you provide care to and the level of care you provide.
- The risks involved with your practice

The NMC does not provide advice about the level of cover that an individual registrant needs. As a practitioner, you are said to be in the best position to determine, with your indemnity provider, the level of cover appropriate for your practice. Advice to inform your decision should be sought, as appropriate, from your professional body, trade union or insurer. The NMC document goes on to explain that you will need to be able to demonstrate that you fully disclosed your scope of practice and are able to justify your decisions if asked to do so.

If your circumstances change while you are registered with the NMC, you must ensure that your indemnity arrangements are still appropriate for the risks of your practice.

CRITICAL AWARENESS

You must ensure that you have indemnity insurance either from your employer or through an insurance company.

REFLECTION 4.6

Find out about your employer's indemnity policy so that you fully understand how it works and the scope of cover it provides.

LOOKING BACK, FEEDING FORWARD

The move towards regulation of a role that is a 'support role' to registered practitioners has been a long journey and advocated by many, including healthcare support staff themselves. The importance of patient safety, confidence and protection is at the heart of regulation. The PSA uses a framework based on proportionality of the risk associated with a role to determine if and at what level regulation is required for a role.

The Nursing Associate is a new role and the first 'support role' to be formally regulated. It will be subject to analysis and review of the impact and effectiveness of the role and how being regulated influences the role and role holders.

As a Nursing Associate you will be legally required to conform to the NMC Code and Standards required for the NA role. As a professional registrant, the standards and behaviours apply while you are in work and outside work. As this is a new role, there is an additional need for you to gain the confidence of the public, your nursing colleagues and the wider clinical team with whom you work in your role.

Once you become a registered practitioner you are required to keep your practice up to date. To do this you will need to engage in relevant learning opportunities and to maintain a record of your learning. It is also your responsibility to ensure your personal and professional information is kept up to date in order to remain on the NMC register and to satisfy your employer.

The regulation of Nursing Associates is a major milestone in the history of support staff development. The NA role is an explicit recognition of the valuable contribution support staff have made over many years in the provision of care and treatment. The NA is the first support role to be registered and will be closely monitored in terms of its impact on patients and services. Therefore the NA role is leading the way and will hopefully act as a catalyst to further develop and recognize all support staff.

REFERENCES

Cavendish, E., 2013. The Cavendish Review. NHSE, London.
East Midlands Trainer Hub, 2008. An Implementation Guide and Toolkit. Trent Publications, Trent.
Health Education England, 2016. Nursing Associate Curriculum Framework. HEE, London.
Lord Willis, 2015. Raising the Bar. Shape of Caring: A Review of the Future Education and Training of Registered Nurses and Care Assistants. Health Education England, London.
NHS Employers, 2011. Enhancing employment practice to increase quality and safety. NHSE, London. www.nhsemployers.org/.
NHS England Chief Nursing Officer, 2016. Leading Change, Adding Value. NHSE, London.
NHS England, 2016. Shared Commitment to Quality. NHSE, London.
Nursing and Midwifery Board Ireland, 2015. Scope of Nursing and Midwifery Practice Framework. NMBI, Dublin.
Nursing and Midwifery Council, 2009. Guidance on Professional Conduct for Nursing and Midwifery Students. NMC, London.
Nursing and Midwifery Council, 2014. NMC Professional Indemnity. NMC, London.
Nursing and Midwifery Council, 2016. Strategy 2015–2020 Dynamic Regulation for a Changing World. NMC, London.
Nursing and Midwifery Council, 2017a. NMC Council Papers. NMC, London.
Nursing and Midwifery Council, 2017b. The Revalidation Process. Requirement and Process. NMC, London.
Nursing and Midwifery Council, 2017c. How to Revalidate Booklet. NMC, London.
NMC, 2018a. The Code. Professional Standards of Practice and Behaviour for Nurses, Midwives and Nursing Associates. London: NMC. https://www.nmc.org.uk/standards/code/.
NMC, 2018b. Standards of Proficiency for Nursing Associates. London: NMC. https://www.nmc.org.uk/globalassets/sitedocuments/education-standards/nursing-associates-proficiency-standards.pdf.
Professional Standards Authority for Health and Social Care (PSA), 2015a. Accredited Registers Report. PSA, London.
Professional Standards Authority for Health and Social Care (PSA), 2015b. Rethinking Regulation. PSA, London.
Professional Standards Authority for Health and Social Care (PSA), 2015c. Right-Touch Regulation. PSA, London.
Professional Standards Authority for Health and Social Care (PSA), 2016a. The Performance Review Standards: Standards of Good Regulation. PSA, London.
Professional Standards Authority for Health and Social Care (PSA), 2016b. Regulation Rethought. PSA, London.
Skills for Health, 2009. Core Standards for Assistant Practitioners. SFH, Bristol.
Francis, Sir Robert QC, 2013. Report of the Mid Staffordshire NHS Trust Foundation Public Enquiry. London Stationery office, London.
Skills for Care & Skills for Health, 2013. Code of Conduct for Healthcare Support Workers and Adult Social Care Workers. Skills for Care & Skills for Health, London.
Skills for Care, Skills for Health & Health Education England, 2015. The Care Certificate Standards. Skills for Care, Skills for Health & Health Education England, London.
Skills for Health, 2009. Core Standards for Assistant Practitioners. Skills for Health, Bristol.
Unionlearn with the TUC, 2011. Working for Learners, third ed. Unionlearn, London.

The Law and the Nursing Associate

Chris Barber

OBJECTIVES

By the end of the chapter the reader will be able to:

1. Describe the meaning of the word 'law'
2. Be aware of the differences between law, policies, guidelines and ethics
3. Be aware and understand how laws are made
4. Discuss law as it applies to negligence, consent and mental capacity
5. Discuss the impact that confidentiality and discrimination as legal issues will have on your work as an NA
6. Understand how legal accountability and the Nursing and Midwifery Council (NMC) professional standards and code of conduct will impact upon their work as an NA

KEY WORDS

Law

Ethics

Policies

Guidelines

Negligence

Consent

Mental capacity

Safeguarding

Discrimination

Confidentiality

CHAPTER AIM

The chapter aims to introduce the reader to the law and legal issues as they relate to nursing practice and the role and person of the Nursing Associate (NA).

SELF TEST

1. What do you understand by the word 'law'?
2. What do you understand to be the differences between law, policy, guidelines and ethics?
3. Can a law ever be unethical?
4. What is the British legal system?
5. Describe the legal implications of negligence.
6. Describe the legal implications of consent.
7. What is mental capacity and how do you assess it?
8. As a Nursing Associate you must be aware of how the law impacts upon your work. How do you ensure you do this when working with a patient or service user?
9. What do you understand by the terms 'Code of Professional Conduct' and 'legal accountability'?
10. How would you apply legal accountability to the issue of confidentiality?

INTRODUCTION

The aim of this chapter is to provide the reader with a basic understanding of law and its impact upon the role and work of the Nursing Associate (NA). It is important for the NA to have a comprehensive understanding of the law as it relates to healthcare if the care provided is to be safe, appropriate and effective, regardless of the clinical and care environment (Dimond, 2015).

A range of issues that the NA will encounter in their professional lives, including negligence, consent to treatment, confidentiality, mental capacity and discrimination, will serve as a backdrop to an exploration of the meaning of law, the differences between law, policies, guidelines and ethics and the impact of law on the working lives of NAs. It is not the intention here to turn NAs into 'mini-lawyers or barristers' but for the NA to engage in caring for the patient or service user in a legally safe, knowledgeable and mindful manner.

WHAT IS LAW?

The word 'law' can have several meanings, for instance:
- The system of rules that a particular country or community recognizes as regulating the actions of its members, and which it may enforce by the imposition of penalties.

- An individual rule as part of a system of law, more commonly known as an Act of Parliament: for example, 'a new law (Act of Parliament) was passed to make divorce easier and simpler'.
- Something regarded as having binding force or effect on a person or group of people.

These 'definitions' and others similar to these can be found in many online dictionaries such as https://en.oxforddictionaries.com/definition/law and both generic and legal/law dictionaries.

In somewhat more colloquial or idiomatic usage, a person may be seen as 'a law unto himself' (to behave in a way that is independent and does not follow the usual rules for a situation, or one who ignores laws or rules or one who sets his own standards or behaviour). Bad luck is often seen as 'sod's law' or 'Murphy's law' (if something or anything *can* go wrong, it will), sometimes seen as being mocked by fate!

The rule of law is the legal principle that law should govern a nation, as opposed to being governed by arbitrary decisions of individual government officials or the military (martial law). It primarily refers to the influence and authority of law within society, particularly as a constraint upon behaviour, including the behaviour of government officials. The phrase can be traced back to 16th-century Britain and many online dictionaries will give examples of these.

There are different sources of law:

- *Statute*: The body of law contained in Acts of Parliament.
- *Common*: A system of law originating from the middle to late-12th century arising from the traditional and inherent authority of courts to define what the law is. Examples include most criminal law and procedural law before the 20th century and, even today, most contract law and the law of tort. Examples of common law usage you might be familiar with include 'common land' (land owned and used in common by the people) and 'common-law wife/husband'.
- *Ecclesiastical/canon*: Church law, particularly relating to the Anglican/Church of England and the Roman Catholic Christian denominations.
- *Judge made law/case law*: The body of law set out in decisions made by judges (as distinct from statute law). These are known as 'law reports' and are used for reaching the same decision in subsequent cases in other, usually lower, courts.
- *International law*: The system of law regulating the interrelationships of sovereign states and their rights and duties to one another.

Just as there are different sources of law, there are different forms of law, including among others:

- *Natural law*: Originating from ancient Greece and Greek philosophy and is the permanent underlying basis of all law.
- *Criminal law*: Refers to the body of law in the jurisdiction of the UK, the vast majority of which is set out in Acts of Parliament, such as the Theft Act, and the Offences Against the Person Act, which deal with crimes (acts and offences against the community as a whole rather than against an individual person) and their consequences in terms of penalties or punishments (fines, prison sentence).
- *Civil law*: A body of rules, originating from ancient Roman legal systems that delineate private rights and remedies, and govern disputes between individuals in such areas as contracts, property, and family law; distinct from criminal or public law.
- *Law of tort*: A body of rights, obligations and remedies that is applied by courts in civil proceedings to provide relief for persons who have suffered harm from the wrongful acts of others. Three elements must be established in every tort action:
  1. The accused person (the defendant) was under a legal duty to act in a particular way.
  2. The plaintiff (the person bringing the case to court) must demonstrate that the defendant breached this duty by failing to conform their behaviour accordingly.
  3. The plaintiff must prove that they suffered injury or loss as a direct result of the defendant's breach.

The meanings, forms, types and origins of law can be quite complex in nature and require a lot for the NA to make sense of them. However, everything that the NA will do is governed by such laws, particularly the law of tort and its links to and relationship with codes of professional conduct, such as that governing the conduct of NAs and nurses. The law of tort and specific statute law will form the focus of much of the remainder of this chapter.

DIFFERENCES BETWEEN LAW, PARLIAMENTARY BILLS, ACTS OF PARLIAMENT, WHITE AND GREEN PAPERS, POLICY, GUIDELINES AND ETHICS

There can sometimes be confusion between law and ethics and what is meant by law (as in Act of Parliament), White and Green Papers, policy and guidelines. This section will very briefly explore the meanings, similarities and differences between these forms of documents and processes (UK Parliament, 2017).

The brief definition of 'law' given earlier is a useful starting point as it is an 'umbrella' term that encompasses a range of different forms of rule systems. Some of these rule systems (such as statute and common law and law of tort) almost certainly will be applicable to the working lives of NAs, whilst others (such as ecclesiastical/canon law) will not be.

Parliamentary Bills

A Parliamentary Bill is a proposal for a new law, or a proposal to change an existing law, that is presented for debate in Parliament.

Bills are introduced for examination, discussion and amendment in either the House of Commons by Government Ministers who propose Public Bills or back-bench MPs who propose Private Members' Bills, or in the House of Lords by peers.

When both Houses have agreed on the content of a Bill, it is then presented to the reigning monarch for approval (known as royal assent). Once royal assent is given a Bill becomes an Act of Parliament and is law.

Acts of Parliament

An Act of Parliament is a document that has been passed by both Houses of Parliament and signed by the sovereign (royal assent) and which sets out legal and enforceable rules. Acts of

Parliament (Parliamentary Acts) can either be permissive (such as the Abortion Act (1967) which permits abortion on certain grounds) or prohibitive in nature.

Acts of Parliament (UK Parliament 2017) are classified as either:

- Public general Acts (the vast majority of Acts)
- Local Acts where their operation is confined to specific areas or regions of the UK
- Personal Acts which are confined to specific private individuals.

White Papers and Green Papers

White Papers and Green Papers, known as Command Papers, are documents created by Parliament. A White Paper contains a statement of policy (such as the *Valuing People* White Paper in 2001, which was a policy statement regarding services for those with a learning disability) or explanation of proposed legislation, such as a Parliamentary Bill. A White Paper is not law and, therefore, cannot be legally enforced; it has no legal power. However, a White Paper can lead to a proposed law being drafted. Green Papers are consultation documents produced by the government to allow people both inside and outside Parliament to give feedback on its policy or legislative proposals.

Policies

Policies are courses of action followed by governments, political parties or businesses, intended to influence and determine decisions, actions and other matters – guiding principles or procedures considered to be of benefit to others. Policies are a set of ideas or a plan of what to do in situations that have been agreed to officially by a group of people, such as an employing organization. Within the workplace, examples could include policies on manual handling, medicine administration, staff sickness and grievance.

Guidelines

Guidelines are statements by which to determine a course of action. A guideline aims to streamline particular processes according to a set routine or sound practice. By definition, following a guideline is never mandatory. Guidelines are not binding and are not enforceable, but may be issued and used by any organization (governmental or private) to make the actions of its employees or divisions more predictable.

Ethics

The standards of right and wrong, good and bad in respect of character and conduct within the individual person or within any given social structure or community are called ethics. Such individuals could include NAs, medical doctors and nurses and structures could include medicine (medical ethics) and nursing (nursing ethics). The term 'ethics' could also mean the usually academic formal enquiry into and study of the philosophy of right and wrong, good and bad within individuals and social structures. What is seen as good and right ethical behaviour expected of professionals will often find its way into codes of professional conduct, such as that issued by the NMC to all registrants.

Whilst there may, in some cases, be overlaps in meanings and functions, as can be seen from the previous discussion, there are major differences in the roles and functions of these documents and concepts. These differences can be explained as follows:

- Statute laws, most policies and ethical expectations and standards (as set out in professional codes of conduct) are enforceable and there are likely to be sanctions (punishments) if these laws, policies and expectations/standards are breached.
- White and Green Papers (Command Papers) and guidelines are not legally enforceable and therefore do not carry any sanctions if they are breached. However, guidelines are in place for a reason and employing organizations can take a rather 'dim view' if these guidelines are breached.
- Legality does not necessarily also tally with everyone's idea of being ethical. For instance, some people may consider the provision of abortion/termination of pregnancy under the terms of the Abortion Act 1967 as being unethical.
- Conversely, what some people may consider to be ethical may be illegal (such as assisted suicide).

THE LEGAL SYSTEM

The UK, as it is now, only came into being in 1922 with the partition of Ireland into Northern Ireland and the Republic of Ireland, so at the time of writing, the UK is less than 100 years old! The UK consists of four semi-autonomous countries:

- England
- Scotland
- Wales
- Northern Ireland.

Each of these four countries has law-making structures (legislatures or parliaments) and, whilst some laws/Parliamentary Acts will apply across the whole of the UK, laws originating and intended for one or two of these countries may not be applicable within the remaining countries. Indeed, Scotland has a long and proud history of having its own laws and legal system.

The Queen is the Head of State, although in practice the supreme authority of the Crown is exercised by the government of the day, which is headed by the Prime Minister, supported by the Cabinet (a group of senior ministers) and other ministers.

The UK Parliament consists of the House of Commons and the House of Lords. The House of Commons is made up of 650 Members of Parliament (MPs) elected by simple majority vote in a general election every 5 years. The House of Lords has more than 700 members: life peers (the largest group), hereditary peers and Anglican bishops. Most life peers are appointed on the recommendation of the Prime Minister or the House of Lords Appointments Commission.

As Scotland, Wales and Northern Ireland have their own legislatures (parliaments) that are separate from England, so too Scotland and Northern Ireland have court systems that are similarly separate from England and Wales. England and Wales share the same court system.

In Scotland, the principal law officer is the Lord Advocate. The Court of Session is the supreme civil court, its findings being subject to appeal to the Supreme Court in London. Most civil cases are dealt with in the sheriff courts. The supreme criminal court is the High Court of Justiciary, and the lower courts are the sheriff courts and district courts.

Northern Ireland has its own court structure, largely replicating that of England and Wales and the final court of appeal is the UK Supreme Court.

Swift (2015) and the UK Supreme Court (undated) provides much that is helpful in understanding the legal systems as they pertain to the four countries of the UK. Boxes 5.1 and 5.2 present the court systems within the four countries of the UK. At the top of all three legal systems is the Supreme Court which hears appeals from all four countries. The Supreme Court was established in 2009 to separate the judiciary (judges) from the legislature (Parliament). Prior to the establishment of the Supreme Court, the highest court of appeal in the UK were the Law Lords. However, all judges who currently serve in the Supreme Court are also Law Lords (Dimond, 2015).

Given that the forms of law that are likely to apply to the work and conduct of the NA are criminal law and the law of tort, any contact the NA has with the legal system will probably be the County, Crown and Magistrates Courts in England, Wales and Northern Ireland and the Sherriff's Court and the Justice of the Peace Courts in Scotland.

HOW LAWS ARE MADE

The journey from an idea to an Act of Parliament can take anything from a few weeks to many months and even years, and many Parliamentary Bills never make it onto the statute books to become law. This can be for a variety of reasons, usually because the Bill and its proposer run out of time or the Bill is rejected by Parliament.

Most Parliamentary Bills follow the same journey and it may be helpful to highlight the course of a specific Bill, the Autism Bill 2009, as it went through Parliament and eventually became the Autism Act 2009 (UK Parliament 2017).

The Autism Bill 2009 was influenced by the National Autistic Society's *I exist* campaign that focused on the experiences and needs of adults who were on the autism spectrum. This was a Private Members' Bill and was sponsored by Cheryl Gillan MP with the backing of 14 autism charities. It was chosen to go forward as it was drawn first in the Private Members' Bill ballot, a procedure to decide which of the many proposals gets some time to be debated in Parliament.

First Reading (House of Commons): The Autism Bill was introduced to the House of Commons by Cheryl Gillan MP (its sponsor) on 9 February 2009. This took a matter of minutes as there is no debate at this stage. The short title of the Bill was read out and followed by an order for the Bill to be printed and placed in the library of the Houses of Parliament.

Second Reading: This usually takes place around 2 weeks after the first reading. The debate is opened by the sponsor of the Bill and is the first opportunity for MPs to debate its general contents. At the end of the debate, the Bill is voted on and, if passed, proceeds to the Committee stage. The Autism Bill received its second reading on 27 February 2009.

Committee stage: The Autism Bill passed through to this stage and received a detailed examination by MPs and acknowledged experts in the field of autism. Here, each clause of Bill is rejected, amended or accepted. If there are amendments (proposals for change), the amended Bill is then printed and takes the place of the original Bill.

Report stage: This stage gives MPs an opportunity, on the floor of the House of Commons, to consider further amendments to the Bill. The Autism Bill went to the Report Stage on 19 June 2009.

BOX 5.1 Court System in England, Wales and Northern Ireland

Tribunals: the lowest civil courts in the UK. Hear and adjudicate on matters of civil law.

County Courts: hear and adjudicate on civil law cases sent to it by Tribunals. Family law cases are dealt with directly by the County Court and not by Tribunals. County courts do not hear criminal cases (except in Northern Ireland).

Magistrates Courts: the lowest criminal courts in the UK. Hear and decide on criminal, civil and family law cases. Magistrates, commonly known as Justices of the Peace (JPs), are members of the public who receive basic training in law, are supported and advised by trained lawyers and have powers to impose limited fines and/or prison sentences on those appearing before them.

Crown Court: hears and adjudicates on criminal law cases and cases referred from the magistrate's court.

High Court: hears and decides on criminal law cases sent to it by the Crown Court, County Court and Magistrates Court.

Court of Appeal: hears and decides on civil, criminal and family law and cases sent to it by the High Courts, Crown Courts, County Courts and Tribunals.

BOX 5.2 Court System in Scotland (Judiciary of Scotland 2017)

Tribunals: hear and adjudicate on less serious civil matters and cases.

Justice of the Peace Courts: hear and adjudicate on less serious criminal matters and cases. Similar to the Magistrates Courts in England, Wales and Northern Ireland.

Sheriff Courts: hear the majority of cases unless they are of sufficient seriousness to go to the Supreme Court in the first instance. Criminal cases are heard by a sheriff and a jury (solemn procedure). Civil matters are also heard by a sheriff sitting alone. Similar to the Crown and County Courts in England, Wales and Northern Ireland. The Sheriff Appeal Court was established on 22 September 2015 to hear appeals arising out of summary criminal proceedings from both the sheriff and justice of the peace courts.

Court of Session: Scotland's highest civil court. It deals with all forms of civil case, including civil wrongs (referred to as 'tort' in other jurisdictions), contract, commercial cases, judicial review, family law and intellectual property.

High Court of Justiciary: Scotland's supreme criminal court. When sitting at first instance as a trial court, it hears the most serious criminal cases, such as murder and rape. The High Court also hears and adjudicates on cases referred to it by the Sherriff Court and the Justice of the Peace Court.

Third Reading: Immediately following the Report stage, MPs debate the Bill in its entirety. At the end of the debate, MPs vote on whether to accept the Bill along with any amendments. In the case of the Autism Bill it was accepted on 19 June 2009.

Having completed all the stages in the House of Commons, the Bill then goes to the House of Lords.

First Reading (House of Lords): This stage takes place without debate and the name of the Bill is read out by the peer who has responsibility for the Bill in the Lords.

Second Reading: The Second Reading is opened by the peer who is responsible for the Bill in the Lords. Members of the House of Lords debate the key principles and main purpose of the Bill and raise any concerns or specific areas where they think that amendments are needed. The Autism Bill went through with no amendment on 10 July 2009.

Committee stage: Here a Bill is taken apart, line by line, and closely examined. Each clause is voted on and either accepted, amended or rejected by the peers who make up the committee. Any amendments will be printed and published.

Report stage: During the Report stage, the findings of the Lords committee are reported back and detailed examination continued. Any member of the Lords can take part and votes on any amendments may take place.

The Autism Bill did not have a committee stage or report stage in the Lords – the order of commitment was discharged as there were no amendments.

Third Reading: This is the chance for members to 'tidy up' a Bill, concentrating on making sure the eventual law is effective and workable, without loopholes. Unlike the House of Commons, amendments can be made at the third reading in the House of Lords. The Autism Bill received its third reading on 22 October 2009.

Amendment stage: Here, each House (Commons and Lords) considers the amendments made to a Bill by the opposite House. The exact wording of the Bill must be agreed upon by both Houses and the Bill 'ping-pongs' between the two Houses until agreement had been reached.

Royal Assent: Once the Autism Bill had successfully passed all its parliamentary stages in both Houses, it was presented to the Queen as Head of State for her acceptance and signature. Once signed and declared to the Houses of Parliament, the Bill became an Act on 12 November 2009.

LAW AND NEGLIGENCE

CASE STUDY 5.1   Joe and Zoe

Joe, who has Asperger syndrome (an autism spectrum condition) and depression, is in his late 50s and is a full-time carer for his wife, Zoe. Zoe has multiple physical health conditions, including cerebral palsy, diabetes, myasthenia gravis and atrial fibrillation and depression, and was recently discharged from an acute hospital after attempting an overdose. Prior to the hospital admittance, Joe and Zoe received little more than basic support from health and social care providers. This has not changed since Zoe was discharged following her overdose.

Joe believes that the health and social care providers were negligent and that this negligence contributed to his wife's mental ill-health and overdose.

REFLECTION 5.1

Consider Joe and Zoe in Case Study 5.1. They have a range of health and social care issues:

- Joe's Asperger syndrome (autism spectrum condition) and depression
- Zoe's physical disabilities and health issues
- Zoe's mental ill-health and attempted overdose.

Now reflect on the following points:

- Does Joe have a valid point when he claims that health and social care professionals have acted negligently towards him and his wife through not providing appropriate and ongoing support?
- What would be the legal basis for such a view?
- What would be the counter arguments for such a view?
- If Joe has a valid argument, what possible actions or remedies are open to him?

CARE IN THE HOME SETTING

There is a growing trend to care for people with long-term conditions in community settings, such as the person's own home. To care effectively for people in the home-care setting requires a significant new way of thinking with regard to the way long-term care and support are currently organized, managed, funded and delivered. The move needs to be away from care delivered away from home, for instance in a hospital setting, towards a community-based, responsive, adaptable, flexible service. Good chronic-disease management provides the Nursing Associate and other healthcare providers with opportunities for improvements in patient care and service quality, as well as a reduction in costs.

A publication by the mental health charity, Mind (Mind, 2013), provides much useful information in relation to possible negligence on the part of health and social care providers.

The following brief conversation between Joe, Ana (a mental health nurse) and Lauren (a trainee NA) may help to tease out whether negligence has occurred.

Ana: Given that negligence involves a breach of a legal duty of care owed to one person by another with this breach leading to damage to the person, a range of issues arise. To begin with: do health and social care professionals owe Joe and Zoe a legal duty of care and has there been a breach in this legal duty?

Joe: Surely, the answer to the first part of this question must be yes! The very fact that healthcare professionals such as Nursing Associates, nurses and doctors provide a range of clinical services to Zoe implies a contract and such a contract implies a legal duty of care on the part of the healthcare providers working with Zoe...

Lauren: And, I am assuming, to a certain extent, yourself.

Ana: Is this the case, though? Granted that the Nursing Associates, nurses and doctors who work with Zoe owe her a legal duty of care, does such a duty of care extend to you, Joe?

Joe: I see what you mean, Ana. Although some may disagree with this, I believe that as both Zoe's care giver and a person who is on the autism spectrum, the nursing and medical team have a responsibility to ensure that I am cared for safely and appropriately.

Lauren: Does this mean that you have a legal duty of care to Zoe, Joe?

Joe: Yes, I do, and sometimes I may technically be in breach of that duty of care if I fail her in some way or do not come up to expectations. This is something that I am acutely aware of. But that is a different issue to breaches of a duty of care that healthcare professionals are guilty of towards both Zoe and me due to either a lack of funding or a mistaken belief that we can cope, or both.

Lauren: Can you explain what you mean by 'ability to cope' and 'breaches of care' and whether such breaches of care, if any, amount to negligence?

Ana: Before you do, Joe, would I be right in thinking that negligence due to breaches of care is the real issue here?

Joe: Thank you Ana, and yes, you are right. Given Zoe's physical and mental health issues – issues that are well known to a range of healthcare professionals, I feel that we have been left to fend for ourselves, that these healthcare professionals have largely wiped their collective hands of us. I believe that the implicit message that we are receiving, that we can cope and that we do not need supporting, is inherently unsafe and could lead to a worsening of Zoe's physical and mental health and that my own health could suffer as a result.

Lauren: Is this negligence?

Joe: Yes. Negligence is the breach of a legal duty of care owed by care professionals to Zoe and me which results in damage being caused to either or both of us by a lack of support by care professionals. Negligence is caused by the care professionals ignoring us and not providing appropriate support which will allow Zoe to live at home and which will allow me to support her.

Ana: Where do you go to from here, Joe?

Joe: A formal complaint to the various healthcare providers who are supposed to be supporting Zoe and me would be a good place to start followed, if necessary, by taking the relevant healthcare provider to either a civil law tribunal or to the County Court, given that the negligence is a civil rather than a criminal issue.

Lauren: Just to summarize, here. Clinical negligence has occurred as a result of damage caused to Joe and Zoe through a lack of care and support by care professionals…

Ana: And that this negligence is an example of the law of tort and can be remedied through appropriate recourse to the civil courts.

Joe: Got it!

LAW AND CONSENT

CASE STUDY 5.2 Brenda

Brenda is a 55-year-old woman with a mild learning disability who lives by herself with support from a variety of health and social care professionals. Brenda has arrived on the surgical word of a large district general hospital for a pre-planned hysterectomy (surgical removal of the uterus and ovaries) due to the growth of fibroids (non-cancerous growths) within the uterus.

'It is a fundamental principle of health law, as well as being at the heart of medical and nursing ethics, that you cannot treat an individual unless you have obtained their consent. The patient's consent is required for all healthcare interventions, whether undertaken by Nursing Associates, nurses, medical practitioners, healthcare support workers and physiotherapists.' (Cox, 2015).

Consent can be given and obtained orally, in writing, gesturally or implicitly through the actions or behaviour of the patient or service user (Dimond, 2015). For example, Brenda rolling up her sleeve and presenting her arm in preparation for the blood pressure cuff at her GP surgery without having to be asked to do so implies consent to the measuring and monitoring of her blood pressure.

The NA must be clear as to what informed consent is and is not. For consent to be valid, it must be voluntary and informed, and the person consenting must have the capacity to make the decision. These terms are explained here (NHS Choices, 2016a):

- **Voluntary:** the decision to either consent or to not consent to treatment must be made by the person themselves, and must not be influenced by pressure from medical staff, friends or family. Any consent made under duress is invalid.
- **Informed:** the person must be given all of the information in terms of what the treatment involves, including the benefits and risks, whether there are reasonable alternative treatments and what will happen if treatment does not go ahead. Information must be presented in ways that the person (patient or service user) can understand and accept. Some people may be better at processing information visually, others verbally. The way that information is presented may work for one person but not for another. For example, some people may find reading difficult (may be only 'functionally literate'), may not be able to read English as English is not their first language or may not be able to read at all. To give written information to people who experience difficulties in reading will not be helpful and is unlikely to meet the 'informed' aspect of the criteria for giving a valid consent.
- **Capacity:** the person must be capable of giving consent, which means they understand the information given to them, and they can use it to make an informed decision, whether that decision is 'right' or 'wrong'. A person must not be deemed incapable of giving consent just because he or she chooses not to consent to treatment. Problems exist where the person is either unconscious, under the influence of alcohol or drugs or in a state of psychological or emotional shock.

For any form of intervention, informed consent must be obtained from Brenda. Brenda must be assumed to have the ability to give consent and it is the responsibility of the care professional to prove that Brenda does not have the ability to consent rather than Brenda's responsibility to prove that she does have the ability to consent. Prior to being admitted to hospital, areas of consent must include:

- Agreeing to being seen by her GP.
- The GPs original examination and administration of diagnostic procedures.
- The various options that Brenda has in terms of pain management and treatment.
- Where and when and how she wants to receive that treatment.

Attendance at the GP surgery does not imply a negation of the freedom and right that Brenda has to choose between therapeutic management options, including the option to do nothing.

Likewise, once Brenda has been admitted onto the surgical ward, informed consent must be obtained prior to any nursing or medical intervention. Even the seemingly most mundane of interventions, such as assisting Brenda with her personal hygiene, assisting her to get dressed or assisting her at mealtimes, should not be done without her consent. Here, the easiest way to gain that consent is to ask her permission (RCN, 2017).

The use of 'hospital passports' is an increasingly popular and relatively easy way for Brenda to express who she is, the important people in her life, her likes and dislikes and how she would like to be treated by nursing and medical staff. Such passports are readily available from the learning disability liaison nursing team and can be adapted to meet the communication needs of patient groups who may find verbal and/or written communication difficult. Other ways of communicating and obtaining consent for such groups could include the use of visual means, for instance simple line drawings or photographs indicating the procedure (such as washing or taking medicines) that is required to be undertaken. Close observations of Brenda's body language and facial expressions are important in determining her consent to whatever procedure is being proposed. Such observations are likely to be crucial if Brenda is unable to verbally communicate her wishes and consent (or refusal or withdrawal of such consent) (NHS Choices, 2015).

The issue of consent for 'minors' (people under the age of 18 years) has often been fraught with difficulties. When we are trying to decide whether a child is mature enough to make their own healthcare decisions, the issue of whether a child is 'Gillick competent' or whether they meet the 'Fraser guidelines' is often raised. Gillick competency and Fraser guidelines refer to a legal case that looked specifically at whether doctors should be able to give contraceptive advice or treatment to under 16-year-olds without parental consent. But since then, they have been more widely used to help assess whether a child has the maturity to make their own decisions and to understand the implications of those decisions. It is not enough that the child should understand the nature of the advice that is being given: he or she must also have a sufficient maturity to understand the consequences of what is involved (NHS Choices, 2016b).

LAW AND MENTAL CAPACITY

CASE STUDY 5.3   Josh

Josh is a young married man in his mid-thirties with two young children. Josh experiences mental health problems in the form of severe depression and suicidal thoughts, but refuses to accept the advice of his GP in relation to the management and treatment of this depression in terms of anti-depressant medication and possible hospital admission.

In the previous section relating specifically to law and consent, the idea of consent to treatment and/or medical and/or nursing intervention was introduced. It was noted that consent was an agreement to do something or to allow something to happen only after all the relevant facts are disclosed in a way that the patient or service user can understand and process (Dimond,

2015). Any such consent must be based on the mental capacity to give that consent.

To enable the NA to assist Josh in deciding whether or not to accept therapeutic interventions, a basic understanding of the Mental Capacity Act 2005 along with guidelines from the General Medical Council (2017) may be helpful.

For Josh, according to Sections 2 and 3 of the Mental Capacity Act 2005, such mental capacity is based on the following criteria:
- Understanding information given to him about a particular decision (in this case, Josh's decision to reject the use of anti-depressants or to receive hospital treatment), the consequences of accepting or not accepting the proposed treatment.
- Retaining that information long enough to be able to make his decision.
- Weighing up the information available to make the decision.
- Communicating that decision.

To determine whether Josh has the ability to make his own decisions regarding his mental healthcare, a basic understanding of the Mental Capacity Act 2005 and how it relates to Josh is crucial.

Section 2: For the purposes of this Act, Josh lacks capacity in relation to healthcare treatment and management if at the material time he is unable to make a decision for himself in relation to his treatment because of an impairment of, or a disturbance in the functioning of the mind or brain. It does not matter whether the impairment or disturbance is permanent or temporary. However, a lack of capacity cannot be established merely by reference to a person's age or appearance or a condition he has or an aspect of his behaviour that might lead others to make unjustified assumptions about his capacity. Josh must be presumed to have mental capacity unless it is proved otherwise.

It must be established that Josh, because he is currently experiencing severe depression and has expressed thoughts of suicide, has a mental impairment that prevents him from taking a decision for himself regarding his healthcare.

If Josh needs life-saving interventions and is unable, due to his mental state, to either accept or refuse the intervention, the nursing and medical team must act in Josh's best interests. This means that, under Section 4, the medical and nursing team must consider, so far as is reasonably ascertainable:
- Josh's past and present wishes and feelings (and specifically any relevant written statement made by him when he had capacity)
- The beliefs and values that would be likely to influence his decision if he had capacity
- Other factors that he would be likely to consider if he were able to do so.

The medical and nursing team must take into account, if it is practicable and appropriate to consult them, the views of:
- Anyone named by Josh as someone to be consulted on the matter in question or on matters of that kind. (It must be stressed here that Josh's next of kin or family does not have the right to decide for him, but they do have the right to be consulted and to have their views listened to and taken seriously.)

- Anyone engaged in caring for Josh or interested in his welfare.
- Any person holding a lasting power of attorney granted by Josh (Sections 9–14). A lasting power of attorney is where Josh confers on another person (usually a family member or friend) authority to make decisions about his personal welfare, property and affairs and which includes authority to make such decisions in circumstances where Josh no longer has mental capacity.

Sections 4a and 4b set out the conditions under which Josh can legally be restrained, usually so that life-saving interventions can be carried out. However, the need and reason for the use of physical restraint must be set out in his care plans and any form of physical restraint used must be in accordance with accepted best practice and only used when necessary for his and other people's safety.

If Josh loses mental capacity for whatever reason, he may need to consider the use of advanced directives (Sections 24–26) which records his right to refuse medical and nursing treatment.

LEGAL ACCOUNTABILITY AND CODE OF CONDUCT

Over recent years there has been debate, sometimes acrimonious, about whether healthcare assistants (HCAs) should be regulated and if so, the nature of such regulation and by whom. Much of this debate has been aired in a variety of nursing journals. The reason for this debate is in part due to the expanded and extended roles that many HCAs enjoy within their workplaces. Indeed, many HCAs now perform tasks that 50 years ago would have been the main if not the sole preserve of those in the medical profession, for instance the monitoring of blood pressure.

In line with most other health and social care staff groups, NAs are expected to understand and comply with a set of proficiency standards and codes of professional conduct. Perhaps the most relevant of these standards and professional conduct codes here are those that NAs and registered nurses are required to abide by.

The Department of Health invited the NMC to regulate the new role, to set up a part of the nurses' register for NAs and to devise a set of regulatory standards for the role, an invitation that was accepted in January 2017 and Standards of Proficiency for Nursing Associates were published in October 2018 (NMC, 2018). Whilst the term and role of 'nurse' is not protected under law, it must be made clear that the standards, and therefore the professional code that the NA will have to abide by, are the same as those that apply to registered nurses.

At the point of inclusion onto the Nursing Associate part of the NMC register, an NA will (NMC, 2018):

1. Be accountable for their practice and actions and act always in the best interests of their patient or service user in a manner that is safe, person-centred and compassionate.
2. Promote health by supporting patients and service users to make informed choices and maintain and improve their mental, behavioural, cognitive and physical health and well-being.
3. Provide and monitor care and support and deliver appropriate nursing interventions as delegated by the registered nurse,

actively considering the personal situations, characteristics, experiences, expertise, preferences and wishes of people, their families and carers when providing that care.
4. Work in teams and play an active role in multidisciplinary teams of professionals, collaborating and communicating effectively with colleagues, and with people and families to help them to manage their own care.
5. Improve safety and quality of care by making a contribution to continually improve the quality of care and treatment given, and improve people's experience of care through identifying, assessing and reporting risks to patient or service user health and well-being.
6. Contribute to integrated care through engaging with a variety of healthcare and other allied agencies and professionals.

SPECIFIC LEGAL ISSUES

1. Discrimination

> ## CASE STUDY 5.4   Emma
>
> Emma is a 50-year-old Nursing Associate working on a medical ward of her local general hospital. Emma has Asperger syndrome (an autism spectrum condition), experiences periods of depression and is the main caregiver for her 81-year-old father who is living with Alzheimer disease. Emma believes that she has been discriminated against by her ward managers on the grounds of her disability and being a caregiver in relation to shift patterns and access to professional development opportunities.

Equality, diversity and discrimination are legal as well as social, economic and political issues and may well impact upon both the working and personal lives of many health and social care professionals, including NAs. The Equality Act 2010 updated and expanded the Disability Discrimination Act 1997, the purpose of the new law being to:

- have regard to the desirability of reducing socio-economic inequalities
- reform and harmonize equality law
- restate the greater part of the enactments relating to discrimination and harassment related to certain personal characteristics
- prohibit victimization in certain circumstances; to require the exercise of certain functions to be with regard to the need to eliminate discrimination and other prohibited conduct
- increase equality of opportunity.

To make concrete these aims, the Equality Act 2010 establishes a number of 'protected characteristics':

- Age
- Disability (where the impairment has a substantial and long-term adverse effect on a person's ability to carry out normal day-to-day activities)
- Gender reassignment
- Marriage and civil partnership
- Pregnancy and maternity
- Race
- Religion or belief
- Sex
- Sexual orientation.

Direct discrimination under section 13 of the Act, is where Emma would be treated less favourably than another person as a direct result of her Asperger syndrome and that she is an 'informal carer' for her father. Preventing access to appropriate professional development opportunities and giving Emma shift patterns that negatively impact upon her carer role at home could be seen as examples of direct discrimination. Indirect discrimination (Section 19) is where Emma would be placed at a disadvantage when compared with a person who did not have Asperger syndrome or was not a carer and that the ward/hospital manager cannot show it to be a proportionate means of achieving a legitimate aim.

Emma's employing NHS Trust has a duty under Sections 20–22 of the Equality Act to recognize that Emma may need additional support in the form of making 'reasonable adjustments' to Emma's work environment. In relation to Emma, this duty comprises the following requirements.

- Where a provision, criterion or practice of the Trust and its management puts Emma at a substantial disadvantage in comparison with persons who do not have a disability, to take such steps *as it is reasonable* to have to take to avoid the disadvantage. This could include shift patterns that take into consideration Emma's caregiver responsibilities at home.
- Where a *physical feature*, such as sound and lighting levels and the use of overhead strip lighting puts Emma at a substantial disadvantage due to her sensory processing difficulties (a key element in Asperger syndrome) in comparison with persons who are not disabled, to take such steps *as it is reasonable* to have to take to avoid the disadvantage.

The key words here are '*as it is reasonable*'. This phrase is not defined in law and is thus open to interpretation. What to one person may be reasonable may be unreasonable to another.

2. Confidentiality

Confidentiality is any information, no matter what form this information takes or where it came from, that is meant to be kept secret and private and is not for public consumption whether it is labelled as such or not. This could include but, is not limited to:

- patient or service user information
- information regarding colleagues
- information about one's employer
- any information that could identify your employer
- colleagues or patients/service users.

Thus, the NA must not disclose confidential information or details that could identify people or organizations or post it on social media platforms such as Facebook or LinkedIn. Health professionals should not talk about work situations while sitting in hospital cafeterias, public places or on the top deck of the bus on the way home in case of being overheard by someone who should not be privy to such information. For those who disregard this advice, be it accidental or intentional, the possible consequences could include suspension from work, formal investigation, dismissal and being referred to the NMC with an allegation of professional misconduct.

If a patient or service user says that what is being shared is confidential, but then goes on to disclose that he or she is being abused or information relating to a criminal activity, the NA must inform the patient or service user of their duty of care to that person. The information regarding abuse or criminal activity must be shared with their line manager in accordance with organizational policies on safeguarding. Confidentiality is not an absolute and you have a common law duty of care to the patient or service user to report any abuse that is being disclosed to you. All employing organizations will have policies regarding this and it is part of your role to read and understand these policies.

If a relative of a patient or service user asks the NA to disclose information regarding the care of that person, general and factual information such as 'Priya is having a good day today and has enjoyed her lunch' is acceptable. Anything regarding the specific care that Priya has received should be referred to the ward, home or team manager. The same applies if the NA is visiting a friend or family member who is in hospital. The NA does not have the right to access or look at the person's nursing, care or medical notes. However, there may be situations where it is appropriate, such as when the person is being discharged home and there is a need to access certain information in planning appropriate care packages for that person. What information is given should be at the discretion of the care team in consultation with the patient or service user.

LOOKING BACK, FEEDING FORWARD

This chapter has sought to introduce the NA to the often highly complex area of UK law. Far from being on the periphery of health and nursing care practice, an understanding of how the various health and social care laws can impact upon the work of the NA and on the provision of high-quality care to the patient or service user is crucial. The impact the law will have is constantly evolving due to both the complexity and range of care that the NA will exercise and the addition of new pieces of legislation onto the statute books.

As a frontline care professional working in myriad of health and social care environments, the NA role is key in patient advocacy. An understanding of current and future health and social care law is vital for this role. Caring effectively for people requires that knowledge acquired be applied in an appropriate manner. The ability to apply that knowledge confidently can help those we have the privilege to care for to make well-informed decisions that are based on reliable evidence and to maintain their independence whilst doing so.

REFERENCES

Cox, C., 2015. Law of consent in healthcare. J. Diabetes Nurs. 19, 314–317. http://www.thejournalofdiabetesnursing.co.uk/media/content/_master/4340/files/pdf/jdn19-8-314-7.pdf.

Dimond, B., 2015. Legal Aspects of Nursing, seventh ed. Pearson Education, Harlow.

General Medical Council (2017) Consent guidance: legal annex-legislation. http://www.gmc-uk.org/guidance/ethical_guidance/consent_guidance_legislation.asp.

Judiciary of Scotland (2017) Court structure. http://www.scotland-judiciary.org.uk/16/0/Court-Structure.

Mind (2013) Clinical negligence. https://www.mind.org.uk/information-support/legal-rights/clinical-negligence/#.WfkqjIXXLIV.

NHS Choices (2015) Going into hospital with a learning disability. https://www.nhs.uk/Livewell/Childrenwithalearningdisability/Pages/Going-into-hospital-with-learning-disability.aspx.

NHS Choices (2016a) Consent to treatment. https://www.nhs.uk/Conditions/Consent-to-treatment/Pages/Introduction.aspx.

NHS Choices (2016b) Consent to treatment (children). https://www.nhs.uk/conditions/consent-to-treatment/children/.

Nursing and Midwifery Council (NMC) (2018) Standards of Proficiency for Nursing Associates. London: NMC. https://www.nmc.org.uk/globalassets/sitedocuments/education-standards/nursing-associates-proficiency-standards.pdf.

Royal College of Nursing (2017) Consent. https://www.rcn.org.uk/get-help/rcn-advice/consent.

Swift, H. (2015) Update: a guide to the UK legal system. http://www.nyulawglobal.org/globalex/United_Kingdom1.html.

UK Parliament (2017) Making laws. https://www.parliament.uk/about/how/laws/.

UK Supreme Court (undated) Supreme court and the UK's legal system. https://www.supremecourt.uk/docs/supreme-court-and-the-uks-legal-system.pdf.

Legislation

Autism Act 2009 https://www.legislation.gov.uk/ukpga/2009/15/contents

Data Protection Act 1998 https://www.legislation.gov.uk/ukpga/1998/29/contents

Equality Act 2010 https://www.legislation.gov.uk/ukpga/2010/15/contents

Mental Capacity Act 2005 https://www.legislation.gov.uk/ukpga/2005/9/contents

6

Professional Issues

Abby Hughes, Angelina Chadwick

OBJECTIVES

By the end of this chapter the reader will be able to:

1. Understand the professional issues relating to the role of the Nursing Associate
2. Define key issues related to professionalism
3. Describe the knowledge, behaviours and skills required to address professional issues
4. Understand the issues that underpin safe delegation
5. Appreciate the role of Nursing Associate in relation to advocacy, autonomy, accountably and confidentiality
6. Discuss how acting in a professional manner can impact on patient care

KEY WORDS

Professional

Abuse

Conduct

Responsibilities

Boundaries

Raising concerns

Social media

Practice

Delegation

Documentation

CHAPTER AIM

The aim of this chapter is to provide the reader with an understanding of the professional issues relating to the role of the Nursing Associate (NA).

SELF TEST

1. What is your understanding of what constitutes a professional issue?
2. When might you advocate for a patient?
3. What does practising autonomously mean?
4. What are you accountable for as a Nursing Associate?
5. In what circumstances might you breach patient confidentiality?
6. What is meant by professional boundaries?
7. Does the Nursing and Midwifery Council (NMC) promote the use of social media?
8. What issues do you need to consider when delegating a task?
9. How would you recognize abuse?
10. What would be deemed as unprofessional behaviour at work?

INTRODUCTION

In this chapter, a variety of professional issues will be discussed in relation to the role of the Nursing Associate (NA). It is important for the NA to have a good understanding of various professional issues and how these can impact on patient care.

ADVOCACY

The first professional issue to be explored is that of advocacy, which must be defined in order to consider the implications for the NA in terms of professional practice. Advocacy has many connotations and is derived from the term 'advocate'. The Health Education England curriculum (HEE, 2017) defines an advocate as a 'person or group or organization that supports and champions individuals or groups, ensuring that their views are considered and their rights upheld'. Advocacy is the practice of being an advocate, which for the NA involves supporting or representing an individual in terms of their views, rights and opinions relating to care and/or services. The HEE curriculum further outlines person-centred care as one of the eight domains relating to the development of the NA. Domain 2 identifies person-centred approaches to care and describes the attitudes and behaviours expected of an NA, to include the ability to 'act as an advocate for the holistic care of individuals'. Principle D in the Royal College of Nursing (RCN) publication *The Principles of Nursing Practice* (RCN, 2010) supports the theme of person-centred care where nursing staff support patients and their families to make informed choices and decisions about their treatment and care. The NMC's Standards of Proficiency also make clear the roles and responsibilities of the NA with regards to advocacy (NMC, 2018b). Therefore, as an NA, you are expected to represent the patient in respect of any need; this should be accepted as part of your person-centred care approach.

The Royal College of Nursing (RCN, 2008) defines advocacy as 'speaking on behalf of another' and being an integral part of the nurse's role. The NMC Code (2018a) further supports this and clearly states that all registered nurses must act in the best interest of people at all times, which requires balancing between the best interest of the patient and respecting their wishes. This implies that, as an NA, advocacy will be a part of professional practice, while supporting the registered nurse in providing care for individuals and acting in the best interest of individuals. The NA must first assess the need for advocacy for an individual, which will involve the ability to ask and listen, since individuals may not want the NA to advocate for them. The individual will require the provision of necessary information to enable them to make their own choices and to be supported in this process. However, be aware that at times it will create challenges when individuals choose not to accept or to refuse the care and treatment planned for them. Here the NA must respect the individual for their choices, whether in agreement or disagreement, never forcing opinions onto them.

Mind (2015), a mental health charity, supports the approach discussed earlier and outlines the skills and behaviours required to be an advocate (see Table 6.1).

It is important to note that, in certain circumstances, individuals may be legally entitled to professional advocates known as Independent Mental Health Advocates (IMHAs) or Independent Mental Capacity Advocates (IMCAs). These are formal roles and differ from the advocacy role of the NA.

CRITICAL AWARENESS

You are expected to be the patient's advocate. However, there may be occasions when this may not be appropriate due to a conflict of interests. In this situation, you would need to signpost the patient to an appropriate advocate to assist.

AUTONOMY

Autonomous practice relates to the ability to practise independently, making decisions based on the practitioner's own thoughts and ideas. This does not mean that the professional is free from the limits of practice, for example the law or the NMC, but it does mean that the professional can independently make decisions relating to some elements of patient care. An example of this could be when an NA decides how often to take a patient's physiological observations based upon an assessment of the patient. As a former healthcare assistant, or within a trainee role,

TABLE 6.1 Skills and Behaviour Required to Be an Advocate

What an advocate can do:	An advocate will not:
Listen to views and concerns	Give you their personal opinion
Provide information to make informed decisions	Solve problems and make decisions for you
Help/signpost to relevant people on the individual's behalf	Make judgements about an individual

(Data from Mind, 2018.)

the decision of monitoring frequency will usually have been made by the registered nurse. However, autonomous practitioners will decide the frequency themselves based on their skills, knowledge and decision-making abilities. They may use previous clinical experience, the patient's previous blood pressure, clinical signs and limitless other factors to make the decision, but the overall decision about this element of patient care will be made without reference to others. Practising autonomously may also mean that the professional acts upon the results of the physiological observations, within the limits of their practice. For example, recognizing a low blood pressure, elevating the patient's legs, summoning a registered nurse or doctor and making the decision to increase the frequency of subsequent physiological observations.

Healthcare workers have different levels of autonomy; some highly skilled professionals are able to make advanced decisions and have high levels of independent decision-making within their work. This may be the level of a nurse specialist, who independently cares for and manages patients with specific medical conditions or issues. Registered nurses, in order to become registrants, must pass specific domain competencies, which require them to practise autonomously (NMC, 2010). Registered nurses are expected to practise autonomously in the nursing care of patients while recognizing the limits of their competence. NAs will have some degree of autonomy in their practice but not to the level of a registered nurse. The Nursing Associate curriculum (HEE, 2017) states that NAs are not expected to act autonomously in certain circumstances, for example when changing plans of care. It also states that NAs will be working with registered nurses and will be guided and led by them, but that NAs will have some autonomy within their practice.

During the NA training, there will be a transition period towards more autonomous practice. The knowledge and skills developed during training will permit, once trained, some decision-making that will directly affect patient care within the limits of competence, local policy and the NMC Code of Conduct. The development of decision-making skills and professional judgement while training will support autonomous practice. The NA should remember that any decisions made in conjunction with a patient about their care should be based on the highest level of evidence available at the time. During training, there will be learning related to finding relevant evidence, critiquing it and applying it to clinical practice.

⚠ HOTSPOT

The Nursing Associate must always remember that there are limitations to their level of autonomous practice and they should escalate issues outside their remit, skills or knowledge to the registered nurse.

ACCOUNTABILITY

Accountability is a term regularly used by many healthcare professionals and is often associated with delegation, which will be explored later in this chapter. HEE (2017) defines accountability as taking 'responsibility for the decisions you make' and being 'answerable for your actions.' In order to be accountable in professional practice, the Royal College of Nursing (2015) states that an individual must have the knowledge and skills to perform an activity or intervention, accept the responsibility for doing the activity and have the authority to perform it within their role, through delegation while working within the confines of organizational policies. Therefore, the NA needs to ensure that they are fully competent to carry out any nursing duties and tasks and be fully conversant with what is being asked of them by the registered nurse. To ensure the NA is competent, they must consider the NMC's code of conduct and keep up to date. The Code, Professional Standards of Practice and Behaviour for Nurses, Midwives and Nursing Associates (NMC, 2018a) states that nurses must always practise in line with the best available evidence, and to achieve this, the nurse must do the following:

- Make sure that any information or advice given is evidence based, including information relating to using any healthcare products or services
- Maintain the knowledge and skills required for safe and effective practice.

The NA will be accountable to the patient and registered nurse, contractually to their employer, the law (through statute) and to the NMC, as their professional body. Therefore, they must acknowledge any limitations in terms of knowledge and skills and raise these concerns immediately to the appropriate person. This may be a registered nurse, doctor or register allied health professional depending on the context of the situation. It is vital that the NA has the ability to recognize the added responsibility and personal accountability associated with their role. Failure to acknowledge deficits in knowledge or skills and accepting responsibility when lacking the required insight and understanding can impact negatively on patient care. This can also apply when failing to act in the best interest of the patient. If errors are made, these could put the patient, the team and the service all at risk. Furthermore, the NA's registration and job could also be at risk; therefore, always practise within professional boundaries, recognizing the parameters of the role. The level of accountability of an NA will obviously be higher than that of a nursing assistant or support worker. The NA will be independently delivering care, under the direction of a registered nurse, but not always under direct supervision. This independent practice will require professional judgements to make decisions about patient care, using contemporary evidence. This increased responsibility will result in personal accountability.

CRITICAL AWARENESS

You need to think about some of the decisions you will be required to make in practice regarding patient care and consider what evidence you will need to support this clinical decision-making as part of your autonomous practice.

CONFIDENTIALITY

As a professional, people disclose sensitive and personal information with additional access to more private information via patient notes or electronic systems. To uphold the trust in the nursing and medical professions and to stay within the realms of the law, it is essential that such information is kept confidential. The important principle of confidentiality in healthcare is set

BOX 6.1   Caldicott Principles (Adapted from DH, 2013)

1. Justify the purpose for using confidential information
2. Don't use confidential information unless it is absolutely necessary
3. Use the minimum amount of confidential information necessary
4. Access to confidential information should be on a need-to-know basis
5. Everybody with access to confidential information should be aware of their responsibilities
6. Comply with the law
7. The duty to share information can be as important as the duty to protect patient confidentiality

out in the NHS Code of Practice (DH, 2003) and in the NMC Code (NMC, 2018a), as well as in case law. The NMC is very clear that it expects registrants to maintain patient confidentiality in all forms (NMC, 2018a).

The Caldicott principles were introduced to improve how patient information was managed across the NHS (DH, 2013) (see Box 6.1). Practically, patient notes and documents of a sensitive nature, such as admission sheets, should be kept securely and not left at patient's bed spaces or in unsecured unsupervised notes trolleys. Professionals should carry a minimum amount of documents on their person and only transport what is required to the patient home, leaving the documents locked in the car boot and not on display. Computer screens containing patient information, such as medication charts or test results, should be locked immediately after use.

As a professional, the NA may need to share or disclose information from a patient. In most circumstances, the patient's consent is required to share this information. For example, if a patient informed you they were struggling to prepare meals, you may want to refer them to social services for help; in order to do this, you would need to share their personal details, such as name and address, and health and care related details, such as their mobility. The patient should be fully informed of the information to be shared and their full consent should be gained in advance of sharing any information. Any questions or queries about this should be answered fully by the professional before the information is shared. Under special circumstances, however, professionals are required to share information and break their code of confidentiality. These situations include where there is concern for the public interest, for example where there has been a serious crime, or to prevent a serious crime, for national security, or where there is risk of harm to the patient or others, such as child abuse. A professional in these circumstances is required to disclose confidential information. When this is required, senior professional support should be sought immediately and the information disclosed should be relevant to the public protection issues and should be limited only to the details relevant to the issue.

A common situation is the dilemma of what information to disclose over the telephone, including those telephone enquiries made by a patient's concerned relatives. When not dealing face to face, the recipient's identity cannot be confirmed and therefore the potential for a breach of confidentiality is high. It is important for the professional to identify the caller as best as possible. Some hospitals set up password systems with relatives; some staff choose to call back relatives on the telephone number stored in the patient's records. After confirming the identity of the caller, the professional still needs to ensure that the patient has given their consent to that person having access to the information they are requesting. If in any doubt, senior advice, for example from the nurse in charge, should be sought before disclosing any information over the telephone.

Other issues concerning confidentiality arise surrounding the use of computers and technology. Always locking the computer screen and not sharing passwords are two ways to protect confidential information, but there are also concerns over mobile technology. To protect confidential information, storing and carrying any form of it on memory sticks and laptops should be avoided and, where possible, password protected. There is potential for misdirected emails just from misspelling an address; it is therefore best practice not to send any confidential information, but set up password-protected shared drives. Where this is not possible, sending encrypted or password-protected files would ensure any stray emails are not going to breach confidentiality rules.

AT THE GP SURGERY

Maintaining confidentiality at the GP surgery can sometimes be difficult, for instance patients providing personal details at reception. Professionals see many patients from the same area and those who know one another; some patients may ask about others in conversation, which can inadvertently breach confidentiality. In the storage and transfer of case notes, patient identifiable information needs to be considered in terms of maintaining confidentiality.

COMMUNITIES OF CARE

Children

For the professional, the rights and abilities of a child to keep information from their parents is often a contested area. Children under 16 years should be able to access the same degree of confidentiality as adults if they are presumed to be competent to consent to a treatment. Children are assessed using Gillick competence to determine if they have the required knowledge and maturity to consent to treatment.

(Adapted from CQC, 2016)

MAINTAINING PROFESSIONAL BOUNDARIES

It is essential that the NA ensures that they maintain professional boundaries. For the NA this will include knowing and working within the limits of their professional practice and having a clear understanding of their role within the healthcare team and when working with patients, carers or other professionals. This will include not undertaking duties normally performed by a registered nurse. As an NA you will undertake many aspects of patient care, performing intimate tasks or procedures on patients or spending time in developing long-term relationships with them. It is vital to be aware of inadvertent subtle ways of breaching your professional boundaries with patients; some examples include: becoming friends; meeting a patient socially outside working hours; accepting a friend request on social media; and receiving gifts. Other serious breaches include not having clear professional boundaries with patients, former patients or their relatives (NMC, 2018a).

CARE IN THE HOME SETTING

Professional boundaries can sometimes be difficult to maintain when caring for patients and their families at home. Requests from patients to attend family events or accept gifts can pose a conflict for the professional. A balance is required to maintain the therapeutic relationship and avoid potentially damaging this. Acceptance of gifts and attendance at family events can cause these boundaries to be blurred. Remember to maintain your professional boundaries at all times and if in doubt, speak to your manager.

APPROPRIATE USE OF SOCIAL MEDIA

Since its relatively recent introduction, social media has become widely popular both socially and professionally. It offers the power to connect with widespread audiences and change professional and personal landscapes. As such it can be a useful resource for professionals to develop working relationships, share ideas and network. Popular social media platforms include websites such as Twitter, LinkedIn and Facebook. These sites can all be used successfully by the NA, providing certain barriers are not crossed and NMC guidance is adhered to. Some registrants have unfortunately failed to follow such guidance and found their actions on social media brought into question by the NMC, resulting in registrations being removed or sanctions imposed (NMC, 2017). In addition to following the NMC Code (NMC, 2018a) at all times, the NMC also produced specific guidance to the use of social media (NMC, 2016) for its registrants. It could be argued that the most important factor to remember when using all social media is that anything that is added to these sites is permanent. Once posted, the user no longer has control over its use or who may see it. Therefore, it is crucially important to carefully consider the nature of any posts to social media, the potential impact and conformance with professional behaviour before uploading anything. As an NA you should act professionally at all times – this includes on social media sites.

When using social media, a primary consideration is confidentiality. No posts made to social media should ever discuss patients, be it positively or negatively, who are, or have been, in the care of the NA (NMC, 2016). No post should identify a patient, such as photographs of a colleague with the patient name board in the background. Even if photographs have been anonymised, the large audience that social media reaches means that confidential information could still be easily identified. Avoid discussing any professional matters, such as colleagues or organizational issues on social media.

NAs should uphold the values of the nursing profession at all times. This includes ensuring that any of their social media accounts present a professional image. Carefully consider which images to upload: provocative images or images taken when intoxicated, for example, do not portray the professional image expected of registrants. Other behaviour viewed as unprofessional may be bullying or intimidation via social media, and discrimination or inciting hatred (NMC, 2016). Any comments that do not uphold the professional values of the NMC should never be posted on social media. When considering what to share via a social media platform the NA should always uphold the tenets enshrined within the code of conduct (NMC, 2018a). If identifying yourself as an NA on social media, you will need

BOX 6.2   Principles of Delegation (RCN, 2015)

- Delegation must always be in the best interest of the patient and not performed simply in an effort to save time or money.
- The delegatee must have been suitably trained to perform the intervention.
- Full records of training given, including dates, should be kept.
- Evidence of competence assessment should be recorded, preferably against recognized standards, such as National Occupational Standards (www.skillsforhealth.org.uk).
- There should be clear guidelines and protocols in place so that the delegatee is not required to make a 'stand alone' clinical judgement.
- The role should be within the delegatee's job description.
- The team and any support staff need to be informed that the activity has been delegated (for example, a receptionist in a GP surgery or ward clerk in a hospital setting).
- The person who delegates the activity must ensure that an appropriate level of supervision is available and that the delegatee has the opportunity for mentorship. The level of supervision and feedback provided must be appropriate to the activity being delegated. This will be based on the recorded knowledge and competence of the delegatee, the needs of the patient/client, the service setting and the activities assigned (RCN, 2012).
- Ongoing development to ensure that competency is maintained is essential.
- The whole process must be assessed for the degree of risk.

BOX 6.3   The Five Rights of Delegation

1. Right task
A task that, in the professional judgement of the registered nurse, is appropriate for the patient.

2. Right circumstances
The person possesses the skills and knowledge to safely delegate, available resources, and other relevant factors considered.

3. Right person
The right person is delegating the right activity to the person with the right skills and knowledge to assist the right patient.

4. Right communication
Clear, concise description of the activity to be undertaken, including the objective, and expected outcomes.

5. Right direction
Appropriate supervision, evaluation, intervention – as needed, and feedback.

(Adapted from the Nursing Council of New Zealand, 2011)

to carefully consider offering any professional advice and do not act outside your professional boundaries or competence (NMC, 2016). If you choose to identify as an NA on social media, you must recognize that people may view your comments as professional advice and you must act in the knowledge of this at all times. Therefore, you must ensure, as in your practice, that any advice provided is evidence based and within the appropriate role boundary and level of expertise. Carefully consider who to link with on social media: current patients, previous patients, relatives, students may all try and link with you. It is important for the NA to be very clear about their professional boundaries when such a request to connect is received. Developing non-professional relationships via social media with people who are or have been in your care, or using social media to pursue such relationships, would be inappropriate (NMC, 2016).

! HOTSPOT

If in any doubt, don't post it, share it or tag it.

DELEGATION

Delegation was mentioned earlier in this chapter, since it is inextricably linked with accountability. Delegation can be described as 'the handing over of specific tasks or areas of responsibility while retaining accountability for those tasks/areas of work' (HEE, 2017). This can be applied whether it is the NA being delegated tasks by a registered nurse or the NA delegating tasks to another, for example to a support worker or a peer. Delegation of tasks can be both clinical and non-clinical. A clinical example would be to delegate the assessment of a patient's wound; non-clinical could be the ordering of meals.

The RCN (2015) have developed principles in relation to delegation, which must be considered by the NA (see Box 6.2)

The application of the principles to delegation involves knowing that the person to be delegated to is competent and able to carry out the task. It requires clear communication about the task being delegated, with confirmation of understanding by the person that they fully understand the task and agree to the responsibility of this being delegated to them. Delegation is an important aspect of nursing practice in terms of organizing the service and delivering effective patient care and should always be done in the best interest of the patient. The NA must be aware that they will be accountable for their actions once they have accepted a delegated task.

If you are delegated a task and agree to it without having the sufficient knowledge and/or skills to carry out the task competently, then you will not only put your registration at risk, but could also result a negative outcome for the patient or the service. Prior to delegating a task to someone the NA must also check if that person is competent to undertake it and if they fully understand and agree to it. In this situation, the NA remains responsible for the management of the delegated task. The five rights of delegation should be considered (see Box 6.3).

CASE STUDY 6.1   Amira

Amira, a 32-year-old woman, has recently undergone a mastectomy and is 2 days post operation. Amira has a pyrexia of 37.4°C and pulse of 82 beats per minute.

You are working as a Nursing Associate on a surgical ward. You are dealing with the relatives of an unwell patient, when the healthcare assistant you are working with tells you that Amira reports that her wound is leaking. You ask the healthcare assistant to 'check out the wound and let you know'.

Later on, you discover Amira has a new dressing in situ, but that dressing is not correct for her wound. You have to re-dress Amira's wound again, which causes her distress. The dressing change is painful for Amira as the incorrect dressing has adhered to the wound.

CRITICAL AWARENESS

Successful delegation is critical to enable you to manage your workload; however, you need to develop an understanding of the skills and knowledge of the team you are working with and how this may differ between shifts.

REFLECTION 6.1

In Case Study 6.1, what were the professional issues that arose?

What went wrong in the care of Amira in this case study?

Using the principles you now know about accountability and delegation, what should have happened in this case study?

SAFEGUARDING

Safeguarding in the context of healthcare regulation means acting in the best interests of people when they are using or needing the services of nurses and midwives (HEE, 2017). Safeguarding is also concerned with protecting vulnerable people and promoting their welfare, ensuring that they lead safe lives. Safeguarding is the responsibility of everybody, regardless of job title, experience, specialism or amount of involvement with the patient. You may be the most junior person within the team, on your first day, and have only met the patient for 5 minutes, but if you have any safeguarding concerns it is your responsibility to act on them in the correct way immediately and seek senior advice.

Safeguarding can be applied to both children and adults, but different legislation applies to children. The Care Act (2014) covers statutory responsibilities to and the legal framework for safeguarding adults and replaces *No Secrets* (DH, 2000). Key statutory documents for children's safeguarding includes *Working Together to Safeguard Children* (DH, 2015) and The Children's Act 2004. Most NHS trusts have a safeguarding team and a nominated safeguarding lead. This team will usually offer training to all staff about safeguarding and is a source of information and support when required. An 'at risk' or vulnerable person is someone at risk of abuse due to the actions or neglect of another (Office of the Public Guardian, 2017). The person may be at risk for many different reasons. Sometimes it is because they cannot understand that a certain action or behaviour is wrong; this may be due to their age (e.g., young children may not always be able to distinguish what actions are wrong), or cognitive impairment due to dementia, brain injury, acute mental health illness or a learning difficulty. Some people may be vulnerable and at risk as they cannot protect themselves, or stop unwanted behaviour. This may be due to a physical impairment, such as paraplegia, or frailty in older adults. Some people may be unable to summon help or report abuse, for instance because of dysphasia, stroke or unconsciousness. Some people may be vulnerable as they have more than one of these issues.

There have been some high-profile safeguarding cases. Examples include Baby P, who died in 2007 (Local Safeguarding Children Board Haringey, 2007) after suffering months of abuse by his mother and her boyfriend, and Winterbourne View (DH, 2012), a care home for adults with learning difficulties where six members of staff were jailed in 2011 for abuse and neglect. The Mid Staffordshire Enquiry (Francis, 2013) examined multiple failings at Mid Staffordshire Hospital, including widespread neglect. These high-profile cases raised concerns about the role of professionals in safeguarding.

Safeguarding is concerned with many types of abuse. Physical abuse, such as hitting, kicking, slapping; verbal abuse, such as being called derogatory names, including online; and financial abuse, such as taking or withholding money from a person.

Other forms of abuse include sexual abuse, emotional abuse, institutional abuse and fabricated illness. Neglect is also a form of abuse; the criminal offence of wilful neglect by a healthcare professional came into force in 2015. A custodial sentence can be given to professionals found guilty of the neglect or ill treatment of people in their care. Many other issues can come under the safeguarding umbrella, including domestic violence, female genital mutilation (FGM) and modern slavery.

It is important that the NA is trained to recognize signs and symptoms of abuse, such as bruising, withdrawal and disengagement or overdependence on healthcare professionals. It is the NA's individual responsibility to act on any concerns and report these immediately through the correct local channels, which often lie within social services or safeguarding teams. It is not the role of the NA to confront any patient or relative about whom accusations may have been made, but always to act in a non-judgemental manner. Concerns over possible repercussions from reporting a concern that is later found not to be abuse, should never prevent the NA from raising concerns that would be deemed to be acting in the best interest of a patient and acting to preserve their safety. Local policy about escalating concerns and summoning help should always be followed. In extremis, this may involve dialling 999 for immediate assistance.

It is essential in any safeguarding situation that much attention is paid to ensuring that local and national policy is followed with regard to documentation. The NA must ensure clear verbal and written communication between healthcare professionals for continuity of patient care. The NA's documentation may also be called upon for evidence in an investigation. Therefore, it is important that any concerns are documented factually in accordance with local record-keeping guidance and in alignment with guidance issued by the NMC (NMC, 2018a). Ensuring that any event is documented immediately ensures that you do not miss important facts. If evidence needs to be collected (e.g., clothing may need to be kept for the police if recent sexual abuse has been alleged), the NA should seek senior advice. Communicating concerns and actions to other professionals involved in the care of the patient is crucial and should follow confidentiality guidance previously discussed in this chapter.

! HOTSPOT

If you have any concerns about a patient's safety, escalate these concerns immediately to the appropriate person. This may be the line manager, safeguarding lead, or by calling '999'. Any concerns should be reported through the correct local channels

PROFESSIONAL BEHAVIOUR AT WORK

Many areas have been explored within this and other chapters that relate to professional behaviour at work. The NMC Code clearly articulates the standards of practice and behaviour expected of nurses. One of the four main principles in the NMC Code (NMC, 2018a) is to 'promote professionalism and trust'. The Code sets out the following standards relating to this section:

'You uphold the reputation of your profession at all times. You should display a personal commitment to the standards of practice and behaviour set out in the Code. You should be a model of integrity and leadership for others to aspire to. This should lead to trust and confidence in the profession from patients; people receiving care, other healthcare professionals and the public.'

The Nursing Associate must uphold the reputation of the profession at all times. To achieve this, you must:

- Keep to and uphold the standards and values set out in the Code
- Act with honesty and integrity at all times, treating people fairly and without discrimination, bullying or harassment
- Be aware at all times of how your behaviour can affect and influence the behaviour of other people
- Keep to the laws of the country in which you are practising
- Treat people in a way that does not take advantage of their vulnerability or cause them upset or distress
- Stay objective and have clear professional boundaries at all times with people in your care (including those who have been in your care in the past), their families and carers
- Make sure you do not express your personal beliefs (including political, religious or moral beliefs) to people in an inappropriate way
- Act as a role model of professional behaviour for students and newly qualified nurses and midwives to aspire to
- Maintain the level of health required to carry out your professional role
- Use all forms of spoken, written and digital communication (including social media and networking sites) responsibly, respecting the right to privacy of others at all times.

Nursing Associates registering with the NMC will be expected to uphold the standards as set out by them. This will include maintaining professional behaviour at all times, representing the role, the wider nursing profession and the organization they work within. Any breach of these would also result in action being taken by the employer in terms of breaching the workplace contract. Professional behaviour at work includes within the department and anywhere within the organization and encompasses any actions or omissions that could negatively impact on patient care or service delivery. Professional behaviour incorporates verbal actions, for example using appropriate language and avoiding derogatory terms about patients or anyone within the service while using appropriate tone and pitch and when speaking to patients, carers or staff. Giving consideration to non-verbal communication is fundamental; for example, avoid rolling of the eyes, tutting and disengaging or disinterested behaviours when listening to patients, carers or staff. The conduct of the NA with wider professional groups, team members, patients, carers and visitors must demonstrate professionalism at all times. However, it should be acknowledged that this might at times be challenging, especially when dealing with distressed or challenging patients or carers. Equally difficult is interacting with members of the wider service and even colleagues who may question the NA's practice, contradict advice and create conflict within the team. Professional behaviour is not just confined to negative aspects of interacting with individuals; it also applies to demonstrating fairness and equality to all those in contact with the NA, not displaying favouritism to friends within the team or to patients and others. Remember that the NA has the responsibility of being a role model to others.

Further examples of professional behaviour at work include informing staff if intending to leave the unit/ward or department for any reason, since any absence not being communicated could negatively impact on patient care and the service as a whole. Time keeping is another essential aspect of nursing practice; therefore, arriving on time for the start of a designated shift is expected, otherwise this could impact on the nursing handover, thus delaying aspects of patient care. Mobile phone usage is increasingly common in almost everyone's life. As part of the NAs' professional practice, mobile phone use should be kept for break times and emergencies only and must not interfere with clinical work.

Similarly, the NA will have to consider their professional behaviour outside of the workplace. The NMC Code (NMC, 2018a) states that 'You uphold the reputation of your profession at all times'. While this is currently aimed at registered nurses, Nursing Associates registering with the NMC will also be required to adhere to the Code. This means that the NA will need to think about their behaviour and conduct at all times, and not bring the profession into disrepute; otherwise, this could result in sanctions being applied by the NMC.

CASE STUDY 6.2   Amy and Tina

You are caring for Amy who has been experiencing severe postnatal depression and was been admitted to your inpatient ward 3 weeks ago for assessment and treatment. Her partner Tina has been very involved in her care and has been visiting the ward every day. One evening after your shift caring for Amy, you get home and find that Tina has sent you a friend request on Facebook. You accept the request, and she then messages you and asks how Amy's mood and behaviour has been and what medication is she is on.

REFLECTION 6.2

What are the professional issues that have arisen in Case Study 6.2?
Using the principles and guidance concerning the use of social media, professional boundaries and confidentiality, what should the Nursing Associate have done in this case study?

DUTY OF CANDOUR

Duty of candour refers to being open and honest (NMC, 2015). It may seem obvious and expected that healthcare professionals are open and honest with patients; however, prior to its formalization there were many instances of poor duty of candour. Following the Francis Report, the Government introduced new, legally enforceable expectations around duty of candour in November 2014 (General Medical Council and Nursing Midwifery Council, 2015). Duty of candour has now become a key professional value and duty, recognized as such by its inclusion in the NMC code of conduct. The Code (NMC, 2018a) emphasizes the importance of duty of candour within the patient safety domain and states that professionals must 'be open and candid with all service users about all aspects of care and treatment, including when any mistakes or harm have taken place.'

Duty of candour is most commonly applied when something has unfortunately gone wrong in healthcare. Common examples include developing pressure ulcers, falls or medication errors.

The patient must be informed of any mistakes as soon as possible and an apology offered. This is not an admission of fault. Any possible solutions to correct the mistake must be offered and carried out as appropriate and the patient must be made aware of any short- and long-term consequences from the mistake. (GMC, 2015; NMC, 2018a). In the event of a mistake, the NA must ensure they escalate it to the appropriate healthcare professional, who may be a senior nurse or consultant, describing what has happened and any action that has been taken to preserve the safety of the patient. The NA would need to ensure that they document all events and complete a local incident report. The multi-disciplinary team (MDT) will need to consider who the most appropriate healthcare professional is to discuss the incident with the patient as the professional may need to answer any patient questions that may arise.

Healthcare professionals also have a role in being open and honest within their organizations to promote patient safety and develop safe working cultures. It is important for NAs to report any incidents or near misses via the local reporting system. This will alert senior staff and allow incidents to be monitored and learned from. The NHS combines all incident reports across the UK via the National Reporting and Learning System (NRLS) to monitor incidents across the country and develop NHS-wide learning.

CASE STUDY 6.3 Fred

You are caring for Fred, who has been a resident in your care home for the last year. You have noticed that over the last few weeks, despite appropriate interventions, he has developed a pressure ulcer on his sacrum. Using the principle of duty of candour, what actions must now be taken?

LOOKING BACK, FEEDING FORWARD

This chapter has discussed many professional issues that should be considered by the NA. Those transitioning from former healthcare roles and others taking up the role of Nursing Associate will need to fully appreciate the many professional issues concomitant with registration. The NA will need to be a role model, demonstrating best practice while maintaining professionalism at all times. They will need to advocate for patients and practise with increased accountability and responsibility. Professional issues surrounding social media and boundaries will require the NA to ensure they understand the key issues and modify their behaviour in line with professional standards. Whilst not new, other issues, such as safeguarding and confidentiality, require the NA to possess competent decision-making skills, up-to-date knowledge and adhere to policies and procedures, for the protection of the patient and the service. This chapter has served as an introduction to professional issues that the NA needs to further explore as part of ongoing professional development.

REFERENCES

Care Act, 2014. http://www.legislation.gov.uk/ukpga/2014/23/pdfs/ukpga_20140023_en.pdf.

Care Quality Commission, 2016. Brief Guide, Capacity and Competence in under 18s. https://www.cqc.org.uk/sites/default/files/20151008%20Brief%20guide%20-%20Capacity%20and%20consent%20in%20under%2018s%20FINAL.pdf.

Department of Health, 2000. No Secrets: Guidance on Developing and Implementing Multi-Agency Policies and Procedures to Protect Vulnerable Adults from Abuse. Crown Copyright, London.

Department of Health, 2003. Confidentiality NHS Code of Practice. London, DH.

Department of Health, 2012. Transforming care: A national response to Winterbourne View Hospital final report. https://www.gov.uk/government/uploads/system/uploads/attachment_data/file/213215/final-report.pdf.

Department of Health, 2013. Information: To share or not to Share – Government response to the Caldicott review.

Department of Health, 2015. Working Together to Safeguard Children: A Guide to Inter-Agency Working to Safeguard and Promote the Welfare of Children. Crown Copyright, London.

Francis, R., 2013. Report of the Mid Staffordshire NHS Foundation Trust Public Inquiry. The Stationery Office, London.

General Medical Council & Nursing Midwifery Council, 2015. Openness and honesty when things go wrong: the professional duty of candour. https://www.nmc.org.uk/globalassets/sitedocuments/nmc-publications/openness-and-honesty-professional-duty-of-candour.pdf.

Health Education England, 2017. The Nursing Associate Curriculum Framework. HEE, Leeds.

Local Safeguarding Children Board, Haringey, 2007. Serious Case Review: Baby Peter. http://www.haringeylscb.org/sites/haringeylscb/files/executive_summary_peter_final.pdf.

Mind, 2018. Advocacy in mental health. https://www.mind.org.uk/media/23456559/advocacy-in-mental-health-2018.pdf.

Nursing Council of New Zealand, 2011. Guideline: delegation of care by a registered nurse to a health care assistant.

Nursing Midwifery Council, 2010. Standards for Pre-Registration Nurse Education. NMC, London.

Nursing Midwifery Council, 2016. Guidance on Using Social Media Responsibly. NMC, London.

Nursing Midwifery Council, 2017. What is our sanctions guidance? https://www.nmc.org.uk/ftp-library/sanctions/what-is-our-sanctions-guidance/.

Nursing and Midwifery Council, 2018a. The Code. Professional Standards of Practice and Behaviour for Nurses, Midwives and Nursing Associates. London: NMC. https://www.nmc.org.uk/standards/code/.

Nursing and Midwifery Council, 2018b. Standards of Proficiency for Nursing Associates. London: NMC. https://www.nmc.org.uk/globalassets/sitedocuments/education-standards/nursing-associates-proficiency-standards.pdf.

Office of the Public Guardian, 2017. Safeguarding Policy, Protecting Vulnerable Adults. https://www.gov.uk/government/publications/safeguarding-policy-protecting-vulnerable-adults/sd8-opgs-safeguarding-policy.

Royal College of Nursing, 2008. The Principles to Inform Decision Making: What Do I Need to Know, second ed. RCN, London.

Royal College of Nursing, 2010. The Principles of Nursing Practice: Principles and Measures Consultation Summary Report for Nurse Leaders. RCN, London.

Royal College of Nursing, 2012. Position Statement on the Education and Training of HCAs. RCN, London.

Royal College of Nursing, 2015. Accountability and Delegation: A Guide for the Nursing Team. RCN, London.

7

Documentation

Noleen P. Jones

OBJECTIVES

By the end of this chapter, the reader will be able to:

1. Understand the relevance of documentation to the nursing/caring role
2. Discuss the significance of documentation in the maintenance of the professional code
3. Explore the problems associated with inaccurate or incomplete documentation
4. Understand the legal requirements related to record-keeping
5. Be familiar with some of the types of documentation they may come across during a patient's journey in healthcare
6. Establish what kinds of information are needed to ensure records are comprehensive and how certain data should be entered

KEY WORDS

Record-keeping	Management of information	Communication
Accountability	Data protection	Evidence
Standards	Confidentiality	
Duty of care	Accuracy	

CHAPTER AIM

The aim of this chapter is for the reader to understand the reasons why nursing documentation is important, why accuracy and care is required when information about patients is recorded, and what are the professional and legal obligations with regard to record-keeping.

SELF TEST

Try to be as honest as possible with yourself and consider if any of the statements below apply to you. This should give you a good idea of how you feel about documentation. After you read this chapter, it may be useful to you to take the test again to see if your feelings have changed.

1. Most documentation is unnecessary and takes away my patient contact time
2. I write notes to cover my back
3. I feel record-keeping empowers my professional practice
4. I could explain the Caldicott principles to a new staff member in my department
5. I would be willing for anyone to audit/review my records
6. I inform my patients what I have written about them
7. I consciously remember to keep patient records out of sight to protect their privacy
8. I know what my organization's policies state about how to write my records
9. I am aware of all the implications for my patients and me if my documentation is incomplete
10. I review my organization's policies to update myself on changes at least once a year

INTRODUCTION

Documentation in a health and social care setting is a crucial communication tool. It provides detailed information about patients that can be used for reference to describe and justify plans or goals in patient care, monitor standards and pass on relevant information to individual patient's extended interprofessional team.

Two other reasons for maintaining accurate records are to promote professional integrity and demonstrate accountability. It is the responsibility and obligation of every healthcare professional to be answerable to the patient, the general public, their profession and their employer for their actions. The expectation from the Nursing and Midwifery Council (NMC) and the Department of Health (DH) is that every aspect of health and social care provision is of high quality, thus accurately completing documentation is a mandatory requirement for all staff in health and social care.

The following discussions on documentation concern both transcribed and computerized accounts. There is a growing trend in most organizations towards becoming 'paperless', prompted by the progress and integration of technology in care over the last three decades. This drive means that many nursing/healthcare records are now managed online. Contemporary nurses must therefore also understand and develop some computer literacy to meet these newer organizational demands.

A number of advantages and disadvantages will also be considered with each form of documentation and examples given.

DEFINITION OF DOCUMENTATION

Documentation in healthcare and nursing comprises all written and/or electronic records (Data Protection Act 1998) which reveal plans or accounts of patient care, evidence of the nature of the services provided and evaluations of the interventions put into place. The following list is not exhaustive, but types of documentation include:
- electronic medical records
- blood results
- vital signs charts
- emails
- imaging (such as x-rays)
- photographs
- audio or video communications.

THE PURPOSE OF DOCUMENTATION

Documentation exists to provide a description of the services required or given to the patient in care. It serves to deliver the goals of care and to justify the actions undertaken by the Nursing Associate (NA), or other healthcare professionals, in the administering of interventions. Patient reactions to interventions must also be included so that care plans may be altered, if required.

There are many other reasons why documentation is necessary; however, some stand out more than others:
1. To improve communication between the interprofessional team
2. To uphold good standards of care
3. To meet professional and legal standards.

Improve communications between the interprofessional team

It is through good record-keeping that nurses and other healthcare professionals provide the most detail about the care given to patients. Comprehensive written communication facilitates consistency, avoids confusion and decreases the potential for delays in treatment, repeated therapies or errors (Beach & Oates, 2014). See Box 7.1 for an example of the situation, background, assessment and recommendation (SBAR) communication tool in use.

CASE STUDY 7.1 Ms Ensum – Using an Interprofessional Communication Tool (SBAR)

Ms Ensum is a 76-year-old woman who was admitted to your surgical ward after suffering a fall. She was found to have a right hip fracture and underwent corrective surgery 2 days ago. An open reduction internal fixation (ORIF) was performed on her right leg and her immediate postoperative recovery proved uncomplicated. However, when you go to take her vital signs this morning, you notice that she is short of breath, has a rattly cough and her respiration rate is 22 breaths per minute. Her oxygen saturations are 93% on air. A tympanic temperature reading is elevated at 38.5°C. Her blood pressure is normal, but she is also a little tachycardic at 110 beats per minute.

REFLECTION 7.1

You are looking after Ms Ensum this morning and are concerned about the changes in her condition. Use the SBAR communication tool to summarize your assessment of the situation. How would you report your concerns to her doctor?

Uphold good standards of care

The quality of a nurse's record-keeping can be indicative of the standard of care given to patients: accurate, clearly written records that demonstrate how care was provided is a skill required by a nurse who embraces the accountability that comes with the role. Imprecise records can point to doubts about the quality of a nurse's work, as well as weakening the nurse's argument for provided care if things go wrong.

BOX 7.1 Examples of Effective Documentation: SBAR Communication Tool

A structured tool, such as SBAR, helps nurses to apply focused communication of care or concerns during handover to other nurses or members of the extended interprofessional team.

The World Health Organization (WHO) (2007) advocated the SBAR technique to promote 'standardized communication' during handovers. SBAR stands for:
- **SITUATION**: Who and where are you? What is the situation? Why are you calling the doctor? What is happening at the present time? What is the acute change? Explain in the fewest words possible what the situation is.
- **BACKGROUND**: What is relevant background information? What are the patient's vital signs and history? What were the circumstances leading up to this situation?
- **ASSESSMENT**: What is your assessment of the problem/What do you think the problem is?
- **RECOMMENDATION**: Have you applied any interventions? What action/response do you propose?

Example of SBAR in use

Patient's name and hospital ID
Situation:
Dr Warren, this is Jane from Seacole Ward. I'm calling about your patient, Ellie Francis, in the isolation bay. She had been afebrile for the last 24 hours but has suddenly spiked a temperature of 40°C and has significantly dropped her blood pressure.

Background:
Mrs Francis is an 82-year-old lady who was admitted under your care with community acquired pneumonia 48 hours ago. She is frail and has a history of emphysema. Her oxygen saturations have been stable for the last day or so, around 96% on 24% Oxygen via nasal cannula. Her blood pressure has been improving with slow intravenous fluids but has now dropped to 90/45 mmHg. Her pulse is also elevated.

Assessment:
I think Mrs Francis may be developing sepsis. She was changed onto oral antibiotics from intravenous this morning. I think this may have precipitated this change.

Recommendation:
I think we should increase the fluids we are giving Mrs Francis. She may need to have another chest x-ray and have her antibiotics reviewed and given intravenously. I would like her to be seen in the next few minutes, please.

Meet professional and legal standards

As professionals, nurses accept a duty of care for their patients. The Royal College of Nursing (RCN) (2017a) explains '...the law imposes a duty of care on a health care practitioner in situations where it is "reasonably foreseeable" that the practitioner might cause harm to patients through their actions or omissions.' Nurses neglecting documentation can therefore be considered as breaching the law.

The main aim of the NMC (2017a) is to protect the public. They set standards for nursing conduct, training and performance, among other regulations. The NMC 2018 Code singles out record-keeping for special consideration in clause 10 under *Practising Effectively*, pointing out that accurate and relevant documentation is an integral part of a nurse's duty. Substandard record-keeping accounted for at least 53 of the allegations being examined by the NMC in the first three months of 2017, 13% of the total cases of poor practice being investigated.

Records of health and social care are also classed as legal documents (Information Government Alliance, 2016) and can be recalled as evidence in certain situations, such as the following:

- Fitness to practise/disciplinary panels
- Criminal proceedings
- Coroners inquests.

The Access to Health Records Act 1990 states that the nurse has '... a duty to protect the confidential data of your patients and civil monetary penalties can be imposed for serious contraventions of the act.' Confidentiality clauses are compulsory in most professional contracts to protect clients from the unnecessary disclosure of information between people. It is vital that nurses develop a relationship of trust with their patients. Breaking confidentiality will not only prevent this from happening, but also contravene the nurse's employment contract. The law therefore obligates the nurse to comply with the responsible management of data and information pertaining to individuals in their care.

CRITICAL AWARENESS

The nurse should be discreet about what information is being shared, verbally and in writing, about any patient. This includes conversations over the phone. They should ensure that they cannot be overheard and that they have been able to verify who the person at the other end is. Any communications must be recorded in the patient's case notes for reference.

However, history indicates that healthcare professionals are not always as diligent as they should be in protecting patient data. In 1997, fears about lax accessibility to patient information and poor security were brought to light by the press and instigated the Caldicott Report (1997). The investigation proposed that a number of general principles be applied by health and social care organizations when exchanging patient information.

The principles are further supported by other relevant legislation, such as the Human Rights Act 1998 and the Data Protection Act 1998. The primary purpose of the Data Protection Act 1998 is to set out mandates for the handling of information pertaining to individuals. Records which relate to physical or mental health are regarded as being particularly sensitive and require additional care, over and above the main eight common-sense doctrines that form the backbone of the Act. The Act emphasizes that patients must issue consent before their personal information is shared. Additionally, the Human Rights Act 1998 points out that privacy and confidentiality is a fundamental human right.

Justification for the disclosure of information becomes more stringent if it is especially delicate. Patients must have the capacity to understand and weigh up the risks and benefits involved when consent is obtained. Where consent from the patient is not possible (for example, if the patient is unconscious), the data that is shared must be with the patient's best interests in mind (Caldicott, 2013, p. 11).

REFLECTION 7.2

Provide answers for the following questions. If you cannot answer assertively, or are not sure if you are right, consider how or where you can obtain the information you need.

1. One of your patients requests access to his health records.
2. You have a patient in your care under police custody and the officer asks for their medical details.
3. A physiotherapist aide requests the notes of a patient in your care.

Think about the types of information about yourself that may be out there in the public domain, perhaps on places like social media.

Have you engaged privacy locks to protect that information? How distressed would you be if that policy failed to protect your data?

TYPES OF PATIENT DOCUMENTS

Although documentation may vary from organization to organization, most patient records will consist of a similar assortment, described in Table 7.1.

Medical information about patients can be held in a number of places, including GP and dental practices and private clinics or hospitals (NHS Choices, 2017).

What the Nursing Associate should be recording

There are many mantras in the field of health and social care, but one that you are bound to hear during your career is 'if it isn't written down, it never happened!'

Nevertheless, the documents or information required for each particular patient will depend on individual organizations. Organizational policies and procedures and departmental induction should prepare and support the nurse in this practice (RCN, 2017b). This may even vary from department to department, depending on the organization's policies and the ward or area the nurse works in, for example, if care pathways (discussed later) are in place. The consensus throughout the NHS, though, is that any records a person makes should contain first-hand knowledge only, as every practitioner will be accountable for their own entries.

Nurses have overall responsibility for coordinating and maintaining the patient's plan of care. Often, this is facilitated by models such as the Activities of Living (Roper et al., 2000). Broadly speaking, nurses should be recording any information about the patient that is clinically important. This information will

TABLE 7.1 Common Patient Documentation

Document	Description
Patient details page	E.g., Name, sex, age, address and phone number, marital status, next of kin, identifying data (e.g., hospital ID), admission date, diagnosis, admitting doctor/consultant, provisional date of discharge, dietary requirements
Medical history/current examination findings	Past and present complaints and illnesses, family history, current systemic examination of body system
Nursing process and care plan findings	Admission summary, a care plan which includes the patient's normal health status and the impact of their current illness on their activities of daily living. Tests already performed or pending, any referrals to the interprofessional team, dietary changes or restrictions, BMI, weight measurements, goals and evaluations of care
Progress notes	Nursing, physician/surgeon and other interprofessional (e.g. physiotherapist, dietician) follow-up plans or reviews
Applied nursing assessment tools	E.g., skin and pressure area assessments, risk assessments, mobility or moving and handling assessments
Laboratory and other results	Blood work, radiology reports, scan results
Consent forms	Surgical or other consent forms
Vital sign charts	Patient vital signs parameters
Medication charts	Record of drug administration: list of medications, routes, dosages, dates and times, signatures of persons administrating the medication
Discharge plan	Review of patient events and planned care following discharge from hospital/care facility
Predictive risk calculator (documentation)	Algorithm which calculates a specific, predictive risk according to the inputted selection of required data (e.g., height, weight and gender to determine healthy weight range – Body Mass Index)
Advance directives	'Living will'. A legal document in which a person specifies what actions should be taken for their health if they are no longer able to make decisions for themselves because of illness or incapacitation.
Do Not Resuscitate form	A legal form filled in either in hospital or the community. The document orders healthcare professionals to withhold from performing cardiopulmonary resuscitation on an individual patient.

normally be the result of the different phases of the nursing process. Each incident or entry should cover:

- a factual statement of a patient's status
- assessment information (e.g. vital signs)
- any prescribed monitoring interventions
- any communication between the nurse, the patient, the interprofessional team and the patient's family – this includes verbal and telephone conversations
- any interventions applied (e.g., patient education, treatments, counselling, etc.)
- expectations on outcomes and patient responses to treatments
- plans for follow-ups or discharge planning.

Best practice indicates that certain criteria are observed when completing documentation (Beach & Oates, 2014). Each specific episode of care should be dated and have a chronological time entry using the 24-hour clock. Entries should end with the writer's designation and surname, as well as their signature. Documentation errors must be corrected in accordance with organizational policy, although best practice indicates that no entries should be made between lines and no erasing of information should be made with correction products. If an error is made, it is suggested that the words or sentences are rectified by drawing a single line through them and writing 'mistake' over the entry, accompanied by the nurse's initials, time and date of the rectification. Further direction in record-keeping dos and don'ts are listed in Table 7.2.

REFLECTION 7.3

At work, take the opportunity to look at entries in a patient's notes to which you have authorized access. Consider the points made in Table 7.2.

Do the notes comply with the suggestions in the table? How could they be improved?

Documentation in the home setting

Those who provide care to people in their own homes must also adhere to the stringent guidelines associated with documentation talked about in this chapter. The legal and professional requirements discussed are just as significant when caring for people within their homes as when working in hospitals or clinics. The sharing of nursing or other health notes with patients or their families is a key element of care planning and involving them in this should be encouraged.

Healthcare providers have for many years routinely left notes in the patient's home, in part to enhance and maintain continuity of care, as well as to include the patient and other supporters of their health in the delivery of services. Ensuring that patient records are kept in the home also facilitates information-sharing between designated carers. This is especially important in the community setting, because healthcare workers often practise autonomously and there may be long periods between visits by different people involved in the delivery of care.

FACTORS THAT INFLUENCE POOR RECORD-KEEPING

Time constraints and workload are aspects that nurses cite when discussing substandard care. In their study, Ball et al. (2014) examined the issues surrounding 'care left undone', as reported by nurses. Forty-seven percent of participants complained of being unable to complete progress notes or updating of care plans by the end of their shifts. The study concludes that missed work impacts heavily on the quality and safety of the care environment and can potentially lead to poorer patient outcomes.

The intensification of patient documentation has also been cited as detracting from direct patient contact (Yee et al., 2012;

TABLE 7.2. Record-Keeping Dos and Don'ts (Adapted from Abbas, 2017)

Do	Don't
• Write legibly and simply. • Use black ink to write, where possible. • Avoid using pencil. Entries in pencil can be erased or fade with time. • Ensure good grammar, spelling and punctuation. • Sign and date your entries. • If it is your first entry, your name should clearly appear next to your signature so that later entries are traceable to you. • Your designation should be made clear. • Countersign any entries made by a student. • The 24-hour clock should be used to clarify entry times. • Your accounts should follow organizational guidance and policy in record-keeping. • You should check that any documentation you fill in matches the individual patient's detail (e.g., correct name, date of birth and hospital ID). • Your accounts should be objective. State facts and observations. • Document any discharge planning early on so that strategies or interventions can be planned in a timely manner. • Record a patient's verbal and non-verbal response if they have refused treatment. • Make sure your entry makes sense to anyone who may read it after. • Avoid abbreviations unless specifically approved in your organization's record-keeping policy. • Ensure that continuation sheets or multi-page documents are numbered and follow each other in order. • Ensure that patient records are stored securely, as per your organization's or department's policy, when they are not in use.	• Defer making entries until the end of your shift. You may forget to input important/relevant information if you are tired or in a hurry. • Make vague statements (e.g., comfortable, plan unchanged). These statements do not provide detail and cannot be considered evidence of care. • Mistakes in records should not be altered using correctional fluid. A line should be drawn over mistakes and initialled, timed and dated by the person who wrote it. • Leave spacing within document text. Other people may use this space to add information that is not written by you. Draw a line through any unused space in documents. • Complete or write records for somebody else. Other people are accountable for their actions and decisions. If you sign an entry, you are assuming accountability. • Destroy records. • Use inappropriate, slang or text speak language. • Falsify records in any manner.

Jardien-Baboo et al., 2016) Record-keeping is often perceived as being less important by nurses than hands-on interventions or face-to-face patient time. This may contribute to the general feeling among nurses that maintaining documentation is onerous, and explains to some extent the 'failures' in complying with documentation found in the literature.

ELECTRONIC HEALTH RECORDS (EHR)

Most EHR rely on the input of specific data, such as statistics or numerical values. There are many advantages in using EHR. For example, it facilitates the accessibility to medication and medical history from Primary Care sources when patients are admitted into hospital (Beach & Oates, 2014). However, because of the ease with which information can be transferred via email, this can pose increased risk of sharing patients' information with other parties unnecessarily and without a patient's express consent.

Data can also be collated for research much more easily, and privacy and confidentiality can be better managed, if only the necessary people are able to access patient files (Menachemi & Collum, 2011). Healthcare organizations and trusts have a duty to provide regulations and policies to ensure that patient- information is handled carefully (NHS Digital, 2015). Box 7.2 summarizes the main principles for employees to ensure that they comply with the set rules.

Studies also show that electronic prescribing improves safety through the reduction of errors (Radley et al., 2013) and may also diminish adverse drug reactions (Nuckols et al., 2014).

> ### BOX 7.2 Information Governance Alliance NHS Staff Responsibilities in Sharing Digital Information (NHS Digital, 2015)
>
> • Explore your organization's policy for information-sharing. Make sure you understand its regulations.
> • Explanations must be given to patients/clients about who their information is going to be shared with. Consent must be obtained before proceeding.
> • Confidential information must only be shared on a 'need to know' basis.
> • Do not share passwords or login information with any other person.
> • Log out of computers after you have finished using them.
> • Information stored on phones or other electronic devices must follow secure data protection organizational policies.
> • Electronic health records and other documentation should be tracked as per organizational policy to ensure that records are easily traced.
> • Ensure that you do not permit unauthorized viewing of information by leaving it open and unmonitored on computer screens.

Nevertheless, there are also significant potential limitations with maintaining computerized records. Healthcare workers need considerable education and training to learn new computerized systems and problems with internet connectivity may make notes irretrievable (Menachemi & Collum, 2011).

Another drawback could be the tendency to streamline electronic documentation to increase productivity. One of the most important roles of the nurse is to monitor for signs of decline in their patients (Douw et al., 2015). However, because the detection of patient problems in nursing does not only depend on tangible evidence, subtle signs of deterioration in patients picked up by non-calculable patient symptoms could be missed.

Vital sign charts, like the National Early Warning Score (NEWS 2, see Chapter 20) assign scores reliant on measurable data, such as the numerical values correlating to temperature and blood pressure. Action and escalation plans of treatment are triggered by the scores generated from the inputted numerical values. These charts are often managed electronically in hospital because remote access allows doctors and other legitimate health and social care staff who are not on the ward to view patient charts from other locations. Optional data, such as subjective symptoms from individual patients cannot be assessed. Decisions for treatments may only be based on the data seen via a screen, not as the result of a physical examination. On the other hand, if mistakes are made inputting statistical data, this could increase the risk of mismanagement treatment for a patient. Other outcome predictors, like risk calculators (e.g. cardiovascular or diabetes risk tests), also rely only on objective data.

It is vital, therefore, that when standardized charts are employed, additional supplemental information is available via progress notes or care plans to justify interventions. The documenting of concerns about patients requires a detailed rationale from healthcare workers and there should not be a sole dependence on electronic documentation, which may limit information.

CRITICAL AWARENESS

You are accountable for your record-keeping. Apply care and diligence when maintaining documentation.

❗ HOTSPOT

Remember that healthcare workers have a duty of care, even when writing. Ensure that nothing that you put down on record could be interpreted as being:
- insulting or abusive e.g., this smelly man
- prejudiced
- discriminatory in any way.

AUDITING AS A MEANS OF IMPROVING RECORD-KEEPING COMPLIANCE

The aim of clinical audits is to examine whether aspects of care are being provided in line with standards, and if standards are not being met, to see where improvements may be made (NHS England, 2017). In healthcare, this retrospective data is used to support change and open opportunities to educate and develop staff and practices. For example, if failures are persistently noted with one type of document, further investigation may indicate that the document is poorly designed or that personnel do not understand how to complete it properly.

Changes are always necessary in healthcare, but people often resist it because of fears that workload and pressure on an already overburdened system will increase (Sherman, 2011). However, auditing can help to overcome resistance, especially if professionals are involved in the gathering of data and the process of implementing the adjustments required to make improvements (Flottorp et al., 2010).

NURSING DOCUMENTATION

Care plans, bundles and pathways

Care plans are beneficial to both nurses and patients because they assist nurses in prioritizing a patient's needs and organizing how these can be attended to (Resar et al., 2012).

They are normally structured around the principles of holism, which takes into account a person's physical mental and social condition and spiritual influences in the treatment of illness. An example of this is the framework of care, Activities of Living, based on the Human Needs model by Roper, Logan and Tierney (1980). Attention, however, should be applied when using formatted, standardized plans as they may steer nurses away from developing person-centred care (Burt et al., 2014). Examples of substandard nursing notes that deviate from this are provided in Box 7.3.

When considering goal-setting, it is useful to use criteria-based principles, such as SMART, to help structure a plan (see Box 7.4)

The application of SMART fits nicely around the concepts of care planning:
- Who the plan is for (the patient and the nursing/ interprofessional team). (Specific)
- What the short-term and long-term goals are. (Specific)
- What measures are needed to determine that the goals have been reached. (Measurable)
- Realistic goals developed in partnership with the patient. (Agreed upon)
- What resources and people are required in the development of these goals (interventions, the patient, family, nurses and other professionals). (Realistic)
- How soon the plan will need to be re-evaluated. (Timely)

Care plans that are guided by the nursing process contribute to quality and safety in care. They direct the nurse in writing a

---

BOX 7.3 Examples of Substandard Nursing Progress Notes

1. 'Patient has had a comfortable day. S/B doctor, no changes.'
2. 'Patient appeared disorientated, but was no problem other than getting out of bed on his own.'
3. 'Refused medication. Doctor informed.'
4. 'Blood work requested for tomorrow.'
5. 'Wife spoken to today re prognosis. She seemed to understand the information given.'
6. 'Eating poorly. Referral made to Dietician.'

BOX 7.4 How SMART Can Be Used in the Structuring of a Plan

Specific	• Well defined
	• Clear to anyone who requires knowledge of the project
Measurable	• The goal must be obtainable and be able to be assessed
Agreed Upon	• Agreement must be reached with stakeholders on what the goals should be
Realistic	• Within the availability of resources, knowledge and time
Time-Based	• Enough time must be allocated to achieve the goal

precise record, and aid in the thinking and processing of information towards problem-solving.

Care bundles are relatively new to the field of healthcare, having only been introduced in the early 1990s. Described as a group of evidence-based interventions delivered consistently together in goal-directed therapy (Horner & Bellamy, 2012), bundles have been proved to achieve positive outcomes (Levy et al., 2010; Institute for Healthcare Improvement, 2017).

However, the definition implies that its elements should function as a package to prove most effective, deviating from person-centred care, which is at odds with the fundamental aim of nursing. For that reason, to fit in with nursing plans, care bundles are normally implemented within the framework of the nursing process. This enables the aspects of holistic and evidence-based care to be combined to improve patient outcomes. An example of a problem-oriented care plan using a tool (SOAPIER) is provided in Box 7.5.

Similarly to bundles, care pathways were first implemented by the NHS at the beginning of the 1990s. They allow for the standardization of interventions in patients who meet required criteria; for example, the application of prophylactic anti-embolic stockings during the perioperative period. The benefits of pathways are that they map out the care for patients with comparable conditions across the different health disciplines and organizations (Centre for Policy on Ageing, 2014). Yet, as with bundles, they can also present constraints in holistic care.

Like most standardized tools, bundles and pathways are most effective when the course of care or journey for the patient is predictable (Allen et al., 2009). Regrettably, while it is hoped that patients meet certain outcomes, this is almost impossible to guarantee. Thus, nurses should never be hesitant to question whether care needs to be adapted to fit an individual's needs, so that the patient's participation in their care is respected.

REFLECTION 7.4

Consider the six statements in Box 7.5 given as examples of substandard nursing progress notes.

What information do you think is missing that may provide better information about the different given situations?

Medication charts

Generally, medication records require similar information, but most organizations design or adapt their own medication documentation. This is because the information contained within them must comply with their policies. Nevertheless, medication policies should be clear about what nurses can and cannot record within these charts, and nurses should be assessed on this knowledge.

Medication charts include the patient's names and personal identifiers, as well as the following:
- Date of initial prescription of the drug
- The name of the drug being prescribed (in block letters). Best practice indicates that generic form of the drug name is used
- The pharmacokinetics properties and dose of the drug, e.g., 10 mg modified release

- The strength of the medication
- The route for administration
- If the drug must be given at a certain time, the 24-hour clock should be used to specify when
- 'When necessary' medications must specify use and have minimum and maximum doses stated and interval times highlighted, e.g., paracetamol 1 g, PO, no more than 4 g in 24 hours. Minimum interval 4 hours between doses
- Drugs must be accompanied by the clearly printed name of the prescriber, as well as a signature.

When nurses administer medication, their signatures ratify that they have performed the required safety checks and actions. It is therefore of paramount importance that the nurse has followed all the correct procedures identified within the document should the patient react adversely to a medication.

REFLECTION 7.5

Look at this list of commonly used abbreviations in healthcare. What do you think each one means?

Answers at the end of the chapter.

Acronym

CABG

DOA

FROM

NAD

Rx

Most organizations allow a selected number of abbreviations to be used within their setting. Usually, these are specified in their policy for documentation. Nevertheless, abbreviations should be used with caution as they could be misinterpreted or confused by other common word shortenings if documentation is transferred from one setting to another (RCN, 2014). To avoid errors or misunderstandings, it is therefore advisable to use full words when writing in free text.

CASE STUDY 7.2   Mr Kingsley – Abbreviations

Mr Kingsley is a 65-year-old man with moderately advanced dementia and type 2 diabetes. He is in hospital for intravenous antibiotics because of a urine infection. Additional to the antibiotics, he is also prescribed 35 units of Lantus insulin in the evening by his doctor.

This is documented as 'Lantus 35iu nocte' on his medication chart. Hospital policy indicates that no abbreviations must be used in medication charts to prevent errors.

The nurse who is administering his medication that evening is busy and is distracted while she is dealing with Mr Kingsley's medications. She decides that she will phone the doctor to rewrite his chart after her workload has eased, but misreads the abbreviation iu (international unit) for iv (intravenous). She proceeds to administer his medication through the cannula he has for antibiotics.

1. What is the policy in your organization about the use of abbreviations in documentation?
2. Who is at fault here? Explain and provide a priority order for your reasons. Discuss this with someone else. Are you in agreement about your evaluation of the situation?
3. What implications could this medication error have for Mr Kingsley?

BOX 7.5   SOAPIER: An Example of a Problem-Oriented Tool to Document Changes in a Patient's Condition

The following allows the nurse to implement a structured approach to identify patient problems and subsequently clarify a plan of care.

Subjective data: (e.g., How is the patient describing their symptoms?)

Objective data: (e.g., What do you see on assessment of the patient?)

Assessment (e.g., What are their vital signs?)

Plan (e.g., Will you be altering their current plan of care? Will you be phoning a doctor?)

Intervention (e.g., Have you implemented an intervention/treatment? What is it? What did you do?)

Evaluation (e.g., How did the patient respond to the treatment?)

Revision (e.g., When do you intend to review your patient/current care plan for effectiveness?)

Application of SOAPIER

Mr Jefferson, 19 years old, is on a surgical unit following an uncomplicated appendectomy 2 days ago. He has been recovering well and tolerating oral fluids for the last 10 hours. He has been mobilizing gently around his room, his pain has been well managed with regularly prescribed IV and PR paracetamol/anti-inflammatories (numerical pain score of 4, 1 hour ago from 6 prior to pain relief) but has not had his bowels open yet. He had decreased, but audible bowel sounds this morning and afternoon on examination. He used the call bell at 18.45 hrs to call a nurse. When the nurse attends to him, he can see that he looks pale, sweaty, grimacing and moaning and has vomited bilious content into his emesis bowl. When asked what is wrong, he explains that his abdominal pain score has increased to 8 and he feels nauseous and unwell. The nurse assesses and examines him and records the following in his progress report:

09.30 hrs Mr Jefferson has been seen by his surgeon (Mr Desmond) who is happy with his current progress. His IV Hartman's infusion can be discontinued if he is tolerating oral fluids after 6 hours. He can start with 100 mL of water every hour for 4 hours, and if tolerating well, he can drink clear fluids freely thereafter. Bowel sounds will require monitoring every 4 hours. At present, they are hypoactive. He can mobilize as much as he feels able. Vital signs: afebrile, radial pulse is 82 bpm and is regular, 15 BRpm, B/P 112/71 mmHg, SpO$_2$ 99% on air, AVPU: A, Pain score 3, PR Diclofenac due at 10.00 hrs. PLAN: Monitor pain, monitor bowel sounds 4 hourly, monitor fluid intake and output 4 hourly.

14.00 hrs Revision: Tolerating oral fluids well – current oral intake 400 mL. No nausea reported. Urine output presently 220 mL. BNO. Hypoactive bowel sounds. Pain score 2. Vital signs within acceptable limits.

17.20 hrs Revision: IV fluids discontinued. Cannula left in for the moment as remains on IV medications but it will need to be reassessed for purpose/removed tomorrow. On free oral fluids. C/O increased abdominal discomfort – Pain score 6. IV paracetamol 1 g given. Vital signs: radial pulse elevated at 101 bpm (regular). Possibly related to pain. PLAN: Will review approx. half an hour to see whether paracetamol has reduced pain and pulse.

17.35 hrs Revision: Observations improved following paracetamol. Pain score 4, pulse 94 bpm, temp 37.4°C. PLAN: Continue with plan from 09.30 hrs.

18.55 hrs **S**: Assistance call by Mr Jefferson. He feels unwell, has vomited 250 mL bilious content. Is C/O increased generalized abdominal pain, pain score 8.

O: Looks pale and sweaty, hands clammy but RUQ abdomen over wound area looks swollen and feels warm. Wound undressed looking slightly red but no severe signs of inflammation or infection.

A: Vital signs: Temp 38.6°C, B/P 97/53 mmHg, radial pulse 113 bpm (regular), RR 22 BRpm, SpO$_2$ 95% on air. AVPU: A. BNO. Bowel sounds absent. Intake approx. 1,700 mL; 980 mL oral, 400 mL IV Harts, 300 mL meds. Output 630 mL urine, 250 mL vomit (+820 mL). Possible intestinal obstruction or septic picture.

P: Continuous observations until reviewed by surgeon. Mr Desmond has been called and asked to come and assess patient in the next 10 minutes.

I: IV Ondansetron given for nausea and placed in bed on L side to improve pain/help nausea. Recommended on NPO until review by surgeon. Check x-match of blood available if needed for theatre.

19.15 hrs **E**: Reviewed by surgeon. For urgent U/S abdomen as possible obstruction of bowel. Blood work requested for FBC, U&Es, LFTs, CRP and blood cultures. Urine and sputum cultures requested and pending. IV fluids (Harts) recommenced, 1 L every 8 hours. Consideration to urinary catheterization will be given following blood results and progression of vital signs. OD staff advised re possible surgery. Plan will be updated following U/S. No further nausea or vomiting following Ondansetron. Vital signs: Temp 38.4°C, B/P 95/50 mmHg, radial pulse 123 bpm (regular), RR 20 BRpm, SpO$_2$ 94% on air (C/O humidified 24% O$_2$ via nasal cannula as per prescription). AVPU: A. Pain score 7.

19.35 R: U/S performed at bedside. Abscess seen forming under wound. C/O IV antibiotics and for drainage of abscess in OD in 1 hour. Continue with 15 minute observations. Temp 38.4°C, B/P 100/52 mmHg, radial pulse 116 bpm (regular), RR 20 BRpm, SpO$_2$ 97% on 24% O$_2$ via nasal cannula. AVPU: A. IV Morphine 4 mg given for pain as per prescription. Current Pain score 4.

Abbreviations used in the case study:

RR: Respiration Rate

bpm: beats per minute

BRpm: breaths per minute

B/P: Blood Pressure

SpO$_2$: saturation of oxygen via pulse oximetry

BNO: Bowels not opened

C/O: Complaint of pain

RUQ: Right upper quadrant

L: Left

NPO: Nil Per Os (nothing by mouth)

FBC: Full blood count (includes white count)

U&Es: Urea and electrolytes

LFTs: Liver function tests

CRP: C-reactive protein (levels increase during inflammation/infection)

Re: concerning/about

OD: Operating Department

IV: Intravenous

PR: Per rectum

AVPU: Alert, Verbal, Pain, Unresponsive

U/S: ultrasound

O$_2$: Oxygen

For further information on maintaining medication records, please see Chapter 17, Medicines Management.

AT THE GP SURGERY

Familiarity with the policies and procedures in your place of work is a must. This includes in general practices, which may have local or specific guidelines to ensure patient information is kept safe. How information relating to them may be used should be made clear to the people who employ their services.

Take a few minutes at work to observe colleagues using computers to read or pass on information to colleagues in other settings, such as hospitals.

Computers or any other smart/digital devices should never be left unattended with visible patient information on the monitors. Healthcare workers must be mindful to log out of shared computers once they have completed tasks to ensure no other person has access to their data.

Data protection also applies to swipe/access cards and passwords, which should never be shared with other people.

! HOTSPOT

Emails may not be attended to straightaway, so any urgent concerns or patient referrals must be communicated directly to the intended recipient.

CASE STUDY 7.3   Mr Olivetti – Confidentiality

Mr Olivetti is a new patient admitted during the night and allocated to you after you arrive for your early shift. He has been admitted for investigations as he is severely jaundiced. You are told by the nurse in charge that you are to get a bedside handover by the night nurse leaving her shift. He is in a bay with three other patients. As handover begins, you start to get increasingly uncomfortable at the manner in which your colleague is delivering her information. Although curtains are drawn around Mr Olivetti's bed, it is apparent that the other patients in the room can hear what is being said. Your colleague proceeds to provide data about the amount of alcohol Mr Olivetti is known to consume and explains that he is being observed for withdrawal.

As the handover continues, you become aware that Mr Olivetti looks upset and angry as other personal information about him is disclosed.
1. What are the issues with this bedside handover?
2. How could you overcome these issues, but still include the patient during handover?

COMMUNITIES OF CARE

Those in places of detention

Individuals who are detained may occasionally be required to attend healthcare services, such as hospital, not available within their secure setting environments. People may arrive from a number of places, including prison, the courts, immigration services and mental or learning disability centres.

These individuals are entitled to the same standards of care afforded to the general public, and they should be reassured that their information will be given the same consideration expected by anyone else.

Detained patients will return to secure settings where their care may need to be continued by healthcare professionals working in those settings. It is necessary for ease of transfer between facilities that any relevant information is communicated promptly. This is particularly important, for example, when the patient is returning with medication or instructions for follow-up care to safeguard continuity of care. The emphasis on effective communication between healthcare and detention centres cannot be underestimated (RCN, 2017c).

LOOKING BACK, FEEDING FORWARD

This chapter provides an overview of the main requirements relating to the professional and legal responsibilities of the nurse regarding documentation.

Effective communication, which includes good record-keeping, is the keystone of good healthcare (2017b). High standards in the maintenance of documentation are paramount to ensure safe quality care.

Professional and organizational guidelines and policies should be followed to promote the accuracy and consistency of written or electronic paperwork.

The implications of poor record-keeping should be made clear to nurses. Good record-keeping is a professional and legal requirement. Nurses are accountable for the care interventions that they implement and must be able to justify their decisions and actions.

ANSWERS TO REFLECTION 7.5

Acronym	Meaning
CABG	Coronary Artery Bypass Graft
	Consider how a patient might feel if they saw CABG written in their notes and did not know what it stands for.
DOA	Dead on Arrival **OR** Date of Admission
	Consider how this may impact follow-up information about a patient if the person confuses the abbreviations.
FROM	Full Range of Movement
NAD	No Abnormalities Detected
Rx	Prescription/treatment

REFERENCES

Abbas, A.D., 2017. Nursing Documentation. http://www.conursing.uobaghdad.edu.iq/uploads/others/d.ali%20d/Nursing%20Documentation.pdf.

Allen, D., Gillen, E., Rixon, L., 2009. Systematic review of the effectiveness of integrated care pathways: what works, for whom, in which circumstances? Int. J. Evid. Based Healthc. 7 (2), 61–74.

Ball, J.E., Murrells, T., Rafferty, A.M., et al., 2014. Care left undone during nursing shifts: associations with workload and perceived quality of care. BMJ Qual. Saf. 23, 116–125.

Beach, J., Oates, J., 2014. Maintaining best practice in record-keeping and documentation. Nurs. Stand. 28 (36), 45–50.

Burt, J., Rick, J., Blakeman, T., et al., 2014. Care plans and care planning in long term conditions: a conceptual model. Prim. Health Care Res. Dev. 15 (4), 342–354.

Caldicott, F., 1997. Report on the Review of Patient-Identifiable Information. http://webarchive.nationalarchives.gov.uk/20130124064947/http:/www.dh.gov.uk/prod_consum_dh/groups/dh_digitalassets/@dh/@en/documents/digitalasset/dh_4068404.pdf.

Caldicott, F., 2013. To share or not to share. The information governance review. Department of Health, London.

Centre for Policy on Ageing, 2014. The effectiveness of care pathways in health and social care. http://www.cpa.org.uk/information/reviews/CPA-Rapid-Review-Effectiveness-of-care-pathways.pdf.

Data Protection Act, 1998. https://www.gov.uk/data-protection/the-data-protection-act.

Douw, G., Schoonhoven, L., Holwerda, T., et al., 2015. Nurses' worry or concern and early recognition of deteriorating patients on general wards in acute care hospitals: a systematic review. https://ccforum.biomedcentral.com/articles/10.1186/s13054-015-0950-5.

Flottorp, S.A., Jamtvedt, G., Gibis, B., McKee, M., 2010. Using Audit and Feedback to Health Professionals to Improve the Quality and Safety of Health Care. World Health Organization, Geneva.

Horner, D.L., Bellamy, M.C., 2012. Care bundles in intensive care. Contin. Educ. Anaesth. Crit. Care Pain 12 (4), 199–202.

Human Rights Act, 1998. http://www.legislation.gov.uk/ukpga/1998/42/schedule/1/part/I/chapter/7.v.

Information Government Alliance, 2016. Records management Code of Practice for Health and Social Care. Information Government Alliance, NHS England. https://www.gov.uk/government/uploads/system/uploads/attachment_data/file/192572/2900774_InfoGovernance_accv2.pdf.

Institute for Healthcare Improvement, 2017. 10 IHI Innovations to Improve Health and Health Care. http://www.ihi.org/resources/Pages/Publications/10-IHI-Innovations-to-Improve-Health-and-Health-Care.aspx.

Jardien-Baboo, J., Van Rooyen, D., Ricks, E., et al., 2016. Perceptions of patient-centred care at public hospitals in Nelson Mandela Bay. http://www.sciencedirect.com/science/article/pii/S1025984816300114.

Levy, M.M., Dellinger, R.P., Townsend, S.R., et al., 2010. The Surviving Sepsis Campaign: results of an international guideline-based performance improvement program targeting severe sepsis. Intensive Care Med. 36, 222–223.

Menachemi, N., Collum, T.H., 2011. Benefits and drawbacks of electronic health record systems. https://www.ncbi.nlm.nih.gov/pmc/articles/PMC3270933/.

NHS Choices, 2017. Your health and care records. http://www.nhs.uk/NHSEngland/thenhs/records/healthrecords/Pages/overview.aspx.

NHS Digital, 2015. IG Guide for New Staff in Health and Social Care (leaflet). https://digital.nhs.uk/information-governance-alliance/resources/information-sharing-resources.

NHS England, 2017. Clinical Audit. https://www.england.nhs.uk/ourwork/qual-clin-lead/clinaudit/.

Nuckols, T.K., Smith-Spangler, C., Morton, S.C., et al., 2014. The effectiveness of computerized order entry at reducing preventable adverse drug events and medication errors in hospital settings: a systematic review and meta-analysis. Syst. Rev. 4 (3), 56.

Nursing and Midwifery Council (NMC), 2017a. Annual Fitness to Practise Report 2016–2017. London, NMC.

Nursing and Midwifery Council (NMC), 2017b. Record Keeping Guidance. http://www.advancedpractice.scot.nhs.uk/legal-and-ethics-guidance/documentation-and-record-keeping.aspx?tab=TabResources.

Nursing and Midwifery Council, 2018. The Code. Professional Standards of Practice and Behaviour for Nurses, Midwives and Nursing Associates. London: NMC. https://www.nmc.org.uk/standards/code/.

Radley, D.C., Wasserman, M.R., Olsho, L.E., et al., 2013. Reduction in medication errors in hospitals due to adoption of computerized provider order entry systems. J. Am. Med. Inform. Assoc. 20, 470–476.

Resar, R., Griffin, F.A., Haraden, C., et al., 2012. Using Care Bundles to Improve Health Care Quality. http://www.ihi.org/resources/Pages/IHIWhitePapers/UsingCareBundles.aspx.

Roper, N., Logan, W.W., Tierney, A.J., 1980. The Elements of Nursing. Churchill Livingstone.

Roper, N., Logan, W.W., Tierney, A.J., 2000. The Roper-Logan-Tierney Model of Nursing: Based on Activities of Living. Elsevier Health Sciences, Edinburgh.

Royal College of Nursing (RCN), 2014. Abbreviations and other short forms in patient/client records. London, RCN.

Royal College of Nursing (RCN), 2017a. Duty of Care. https://www.rcn.org.uk/get-help/rcn-advice/duty-of-care.

Royal College of Nursing (RCN), 2017b. Training: statutory and mandatory. https://www.rcn.org.uk/get-help/rcn-advice/training-statutory-and-mandatory.

Royal College of Nursing (RCN), 2017c. Supporting nursing staff caring for patients from places of detention. https://www.rcn.org.uk/professional-development/publications/pub-005856.

Sherman, R., 2011. Why is change so hard? http://www.emergingrnleader.com/why-is-change-so-hard/.

World Health Organization, 2007. Communication during patient handovers. 1, 3. Geneva, WHO.

Yee, T., Needleman, J., Pearson, M., et al., 2012. The influence of integrated electronic medical records and computerized nursing notes on nurses' time spent in documentation. Comput. Inform. Nurs. 30 (6), 287–292.

8

The 6Cs

Noleen P. Jones

OBJECTIVES

By the end of this chapter, the reader will be able to:

1. Comprehend what the core values of good care are through the 6Cs
2. Explore behaviours and attitudes that positively contribute to the quality of care
3. Discuss the principles of person-centred care
4. Identify problems within organizational cultures that could impede the delivery of care
5. Understand what dignified care means
6. Discuss how positive and negative interactions impact on the patient experience

KEY WORDS

Care	Courage	Support
Compassion	Commitment	Respect
Competence	Dignity	
Communication	Honesty	

CHAPTER AIM

The aim of this chapter is to enable the Nursing Associate (NA) to understand the concepts of care through an analysis of the 6Cs.

SELF TEST

1. Provide a definition for:
   Care
   Compassion
   Competence
   Communication
   Courage
   Commitment
2. What do you understand by values and beliefs?
3. Describe person-centred care.
4. How does patient-centred care differ from person-centred care?
5. Explain 'shared decision-making'.
6. Provide a definition for dignity.
7. What is empowerment?
8. Explain what 'values' and 'beliefs' are.
9. Provide examples of how a patient's values and beliefs may influence the delivery of care.
10. Consider how decision-making is affected if an individual is unable to make their own choices in healthcare.

INTRODUCTION

The provision of care has evolved enormously since the establishment of the first nursing school by Florence Nightingale more than 150 years ago. Nursing Associates (NAs) today need to be highly skilled as well as educated, and able to make decisions based on the needs of each individual patient. The many roles of the NA include supporting the role of the Registered Nurse in promoting patient comfort and well-being, the monitoring and assessing of interventions or care plans, providing patients and their families with education to manage medical conditions, and coordinating the process of care within multidisciplinary teamwork.

However, the NA's overall responsibility is to ensure that patients are looked after, and that they are treated safely and well within the healthcare system. Although this should always be the case, there is evidence to show that poor care exists (Health Service Ombudsman, 2011; Francis, 2013). Reports of sub-par care must be investigated in order for healthcare professionals to learn from them and improve future patient experiences, but we must all have a benchmark. This is why the 6Cs, explained and examined through this chapter, are so crucial as the reference point for all nursing processes. The 6Cs combine to ensure that the patient is at the centre of all that is done (see Fig. 8.1) The findings of the Francis Report (2013), which investigated incidents at the Mid Staffordshire Trust, will be used as the main examples to highlight unacceptable standards of care.

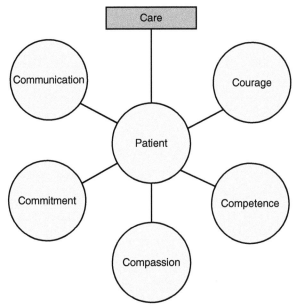

Fig. 8.1 Patient at the Centre of the 6Cs.

HOW WE CAN LEARN FROM POOR CARE

In November 2007, Julie Bailey set up the 'Cure the NHS' campaign group after her mother, Bella, died in November 2007 at Stafford Hospital. Julie described through the media how her mother had died in agony and terror, neglected by nurses during the final days of her life. She reported being horrified on her visits to the hospital, and that she observed that Bella's situation was not unique; other patients had endured similar suffering and mistreatment. Julie's campaign instigated a number of investigations which catalysed the Government and the Department of Health (DH) to act and make changes to the provision of care within the National Health Service (NHS).

Subsequent to Julie's whistle-blowing, more damaging stories emerged in the media from other patients and relatives cared for within the same trust. These included accounts of patients drinking from vases, and falling out of bed and being left on the floor, their cries overlooked. Service users claimed that untrained receptionists in Accident and Emergency were being asked to carry out the triaging of patients. Furthermore, visitors recounted that they were shocked by the hospital's squalid conditions, which they feared were increasing patients' chances of developing infections.

Prompted by these experiences, The Healthcare Commission (2009) conducted an investigation into the higher-than-average mortality rates for emergency admissions at two Mid Staffordshire Hospitals. The published results highlighted that the number of deaths were 27%–45% higher than would have been expected at a comparable NHS trust.

The continuing narratives in the press from service users and the report from the Healthcare Commission resulted in a public outcry, which forced a public investigation into the claims of neglect by the Mid Staffordshire Trust. The inquiry was headed by Robert Francis, QC, in 2010.

The failings identified by Robert Francis were published in 2013. The report stated how the healthcare system repeatedly disregarded the warning signs of poor care. Included were the harrowing stories of appalling and preventable suffering recounted by hundreds of people. The report concluded with 290 recommendations towards the improvement of care. The main ones are listed:

1. A list of clear, fundamental standards that every patient is entitled to expect.
2. The development of honest partnerships with patients, the public and healthcare professionals, which healthcare providers must comply with.
3. Non-compliance should not be accepted and any organization not able to fulfil their duties should be prevented from continuing a service that exposes patients to risk.
4. To cause death or serious harm to a patient by non-compliance without acceptable reasons for why fundamental standards were not achieved should be a criminal offence.
5. Training standards should ensure that qualified nurses are competent to deliver compassionate care to a consistent standard.
6. Healthcare assistants should be subject to mandatory regulation.

Consequently, the National Advisory Group on the Safety of Patients in England (2013) was charged with analysing the root of the problems brought to light by service users, as well as considering the recommendations made by Sir Robert Francis. Their task was to formulate an explicit action plan for the Government and the NHS to implement change and reduce the likelihood of similar incidents.

The DH also issued a response to assure the public that they were learning from the Francis Report. The publication, *Putting Patients First and Foremost* (2013), promised to instigate and deliver changes in the provision of care.

In what the DH defined a 'watershed moment', a historical event for the NHS, they pledged their five-point plan to:

1. Prevent problems
2. Detect problems quickly
3. Take action promptly
4. Ensure robust accountability
5. Ensure staff are trained and motivated

(DH, 2013a).

In the wake of the media reports of poor nursing, and just preceding the damning findings by Francis, nursing was already reacting to transform patient care. The call was put out to nurses from all fields by the Chief Nursing Officer for England, Jane Cummings, and the Director of Nursing for the Department of Health, Public Health England, Viv Bennett. They were asked to participate in the development of a new rolling approach to ensure high standards of care were consistently delivered. The strategy was to be based on identifying, improving and building on the core values that underpin nursing care. What emerged from this discussion was that certain principles of care must exist for patients to experience positive outcomes. The 6Cs, discussed in more depth later, were selected as the set of principles that would become the foundations of a shared purpose in nursing. How these applied to the refinement of care were laid out in the paper, *Compassion in Practice* (Cummings & Bennett, 2012).

> **❗ HOTSPOT**
>
> It is your duty of care to make known to your manager/supervisor any concerns you may have about below-standard care provided to patients.

Furthermore, six main points for action or areas for development were correspondingly decided within the document:

1. Helping people to stay independent, maximizing well-being and improving health
2. Working with people to provide a positive experience of care.
3. Delivering high-quality care.
4. Measuring the impact of care.
5. Building and strengthening leadership.
6. Ensuring the right staff, with the right skills in the right place. (Cummings & Bennett, 2012).

The strategy programme was to run over 3 years, during which time the detailed action plan would be deployed. Evaluation of the programme would be continuous and culminate in a review after 3 years. The paper, *Compassion for Practice. Evidencing the Impact* (2015) reflected on the observable achievements since the implementation of the nursing strategy. The evidence used to measure success and plan for further improvement consisted of examining samples of whether the action areas identified in *Compassion in Practice* (2012) had caused any positive impact. Staff experiences provided the backdrop for the discussion within this paper.

Overall, the strategy was deemed a success, with feedback from patients vindicating the action and indicating an improvement in care (Ipsos MORI, 2015). Nurses reported that they felt satisfied with their involvement in the transformation of care. Nevertheless, the review also cautioned that in order for the momentum to continue, the focus and drive for proactivity must be maintained. Achieving this is only possible through the engagement of staff, a positive work culture and the provision of tools to enable better conditions in the NHS.

> **REFLECTION 8.1**
>
> Think of an occasion that you have witnessed, been involved in or heard about involving the substandard care of a patient.
> 1. What factors may have influenced this?
> 2. How would you handle a similar episode today to prevent this from happening again?

CARE IN THE HOME SETTING

The Francis Report concentrated on the shortcomings within institution-based care, but the NA must also be cognisant of the standards of care provided in a community setting, such as a patient's home. High-quality standards must be maintained wherever care is provided, but it is especially important to remember that when offering care in a patient's home, the carer is a guest who has been invited in.

The role of the care worker is to help people to maximize their independence and well-being and, where possible, to improve health outcomes. In the home setting, this is often achieved with the partnership of family, friends and others employed to support patients.

Culture change must run through the veins of all healthcare settings, and this can only be accomplished through the consistent application of the 6Cs by all health and social care organizations (DH, 2013b).

EXAMINING THE 6CS

> **CRITICAL AWARENESS**
>
> Before going on to read about the 6Cs, you may find this video helps to put them into context.
> https://www.youtube.com/watch?v=jDeoQ5XT-sc

Care

Care can be a complex term to explain because it requires context when applied to nursing. Frequently, it is described as the intervention that the members of the nursing team must undertake to support a patient. For example, personal care refers to the interactions related to assisting individuals to bathe, dress or eat. Compassionate care is about treating patients respectfully and without prejudice. The presence of good quality care can also make the difference between life and death and conversely, as discussed in the introduction to this chapter, the absence of care can adversely affect patients psychologically, emotionally and physically in the short or long term.

> **❗ HOTSPOT**
>
> Prejudice and discrimination has no place in the healthcare setting. Care must be provided holistically and be focused on the health and well-being of the patient.

Nevertheless, while 'care' as a characteristic falls within a multifaceted continuum, it is clear that patients have every right to expect that all its aspects are delivered positively, competently and in a timely fashion.

This is why it is vital that patients' opinions and beliefs are included in the treatment choices offered. Patients should feel able to trust that their carers will provide and deliver safe, effective, high-quality care at every step of their journey. The development of a therapeutic relationship between the NA and patient is absolutely crucial because it allows the patient to explore their feelings and express what is important to them. The relationship is necessary as NAs must understand the people they are looking after so that their ideals, beliefs and needs become more easily recognizable.

Positive interactions with patients can only develop if the NA is self-aware. Getting to know their patients may be challenging, as their own values and beliefs may contrast significantly with their patients'. Reflection and evaluation of practices are considered critical parts of the nursing role. The NA must identify and confront weaknesses, such as impatience, before they lead to behaviour likely to provoke conflict. Introspection enables the nurse to analyse experiences at work and scrutinize how well care was given so that it can be improved if required (Oelofsen, 2012). The delivery of the entire package of care defines nursing, and it starts and ends with the ability to connect with people, whatever their background or circumstances.

Compassion

This is an emotion that extends from empathy. It is not just about being able to understand how another person is feeling but being compelled to help to alleviate distress. Compassion can also be an intelligent kindness, through which deliberate thought is employed to overcome or prevent suffering (Campling, 2015). In all aspects of nursing, compassion must be at the heart of every interaction. NAs must treat their patients as they would like to be attended to themselves – with courtesy and respect. Patient narratives reveal that they will especially remember how they felt when they were being looked after: whether the nursing staff were thoughtful and considerate of their choices, if they were treated as if they mattered, if their pain was managed quickly or if they had to wait long periods to be attended (Royal College of Nursing, 2017).

Patience is a prerequisite for compassionate care. It is never the patient's fault if the NA is busy, and yet sometimes, patients are apportioned the blame for making the job harder. If the NA starts feeling overwhelmed by the number of tasks they have to get through, they should take a step back and reprioritize their work. Spending time with patients is always more important. A supportive and caring departmental culture will permit this to happen. Looking after the sick and vulnerable should be considered a privilege because, although it can be hard, when it is done well, it is also one of the most satisfying and rewarding experiences a member of the nursing team can be part of.

Competence

Nurses and NAs must regularly revise their knowledge and skills to keep up to date with the latest practices. Attending courses relevant to their field or area of work, for example, will enhance or advance the nurse's ability to provide a good service (Nursing and Midwifery Council, 2018). Reading up on the latest practices ensures that clinical decision-making is supported by evidence-based research and strengthens the delivery of quality-assured care. Remember, any actions undertaken by the NA must always be justifiable and defendable.

> **! HOTSPOT**
>
> A key hallmark of any professional discipline is that practitioners update their understanding and knowledge. The NA can be called to account for their actions or omissions and will have to demonstrate that their practice is contemporary.

It is therefore of paramount importance for NAs to know the limits of their practice, and they must only undertake work that they feel confident and skilled in doing. It is also essential that they are aware of when to ask for help. Additionally, nursing staff need to regularly attend role appraisals and provide updated documents to revalidate their fitness to practice. Yearly appraisals are normally obligatory, but also useful as both practitioners and managers can clarify aims and develop action plans towards career and job progression. It is advised that NAs compile a portfolio to help them organize pertinent documentation and keep track of their achievements. Portfolios are also a reflective opportunity, as NAs can return to them for progress reports or to see if they are meeting their own expectations of themselves.

Compliance requirements are constantly being reviewed to ensure that all members of the nursing team meet the required standards. Nursing assessment of competence includes observing the execution of clinical skills, which gives an assessor an understanding of the individual's aptitude for a particular task. Clinical supervision in the workplace was implemented in the early 1990s (DH, 1993) with the primary purpose of ensuring that patients are cared for safely by competent and accountable practitioners. It complements self-development and the professional integrity required by the NMC. Competence and suitability for the role is assessed by peers through shared learning, discussions and mentoring, leading to motivation and assurances of a supportive professional environment in which everyone is valued for their contribution. The employer, for example the NHS, is responsible for supporting healthcare professionals to maximize their potential through personal and professional development.

Communication

Effective communication is the lynchpin of healthcare, as the exchange of information between the patient and multidisciplinary care team is central to the development of a therapeutic relationship and the setting of goals and outcomes. Communication is always a two-way process, and both the sender and receiver of the exchange must participate to ensure that the information being imparted is understood. Thus, active listening on the part of the NA is crucial to effective dialogue.

Channels of communication are affected by the environment and individual values, and are also influenced by situations and emotions (Kourkouta & Papathanasiou, 2014). Communication requires attentiveness during the information exchange and relies on the interpretation and understanding of the significance of verbal and non-verbal signals by all the parties involved. Every person has individual traits that inform their conduct in the process of communication. This will influence how they cooperate, or accept possible treatments, as well as how they will self-manage health.

The NA will need particular skill in communicating with the patient, especially when handling sensitive information. The Royal College of Physicians (2014) suggest that professionals who have contact with dying patients and their families should undertake mandatory communication skills training to be able to best support people at the end of life.

How the message is delivered is just as crucial as the content. Cultural sensitivity is a necessity in today's global, multicultural society. Information must be delivered so that, whatever their background, patients are able to understand what is being said. Translation may be required when English is not the patient's first language. Where possible, this should be both verbal and written.

An appropriate tone of voice and the use of patient-friendly language can enhance the exchange and relax patients who are feeling anxious (Bramhall, 2014).

Above all, thoughtfulness and kindness must be evident in the way the NA delivers a message. They must speak to patients courteously and respectfully. Essentially, communication allows the nurse to assess situations and learn about their patients' needs (Connolly, 2016). It is only then that they will be able to enrich their patients' self-esteem and help patients take control of their journey.

REFLECTION 8.2

1. Identify possible non-verbal signals of communication and explore what these may mean.
2. How may you elicit more information to confirm your visual interpretation?

Communication among colleagues should be kept professional, simple and precise. This includes written communication, which should be legible and traceable to the individual writer of the report. Moreover, all members of the nursing team require knowledge of the processes that assist the flow of communication within their organization. This includes understanding and upholding protocols and policies, referring patients to other members of the multidisciplinary team, consulting experts for advice and accessing and completing online or written documentation.

For more information on communication, please refer to Chapter 9.

Courage

Being courageous means having the strength to do what you think is right. The NA must be prepared to stand by what they believe, and maintain the values and standards expected by the profession. Nonetheless, having the mentality to confront fear or tension depends on the support received from outside forces, such as the climate of support in the workplace. If the organizational culture is closed to improvement because of a tendency to secrecy, healthcare professionals could be conflicted about reporting concerns because they may fear being victimized or ostracized.

A survey undertaken by the NHS in 2016 found that 30% of staff felt the culture in their workplace would not back whistleblowers. Results like these demonstrate that the pledge by the NHS of honesty and transparency is still a long way from being realized. Moreover, when nursing staff find themselves intimidated by colleagues, isolation or stress can make them feel demoralized and quickly lead to burnout or attrition. Bullying is a reality in the workplace, with 13%–18% of staff reporting harassment from either their managers or colleagues (NHS, 2016).

Leaders within an organization, however, have a duty to encourage, listen and act appropriately if concerns are presented to them. Nevertheless, NAs must remember that they are accountable and must 'Act without delay if…there is a risk to patient safety or public protection' (Nursing and Midwifery Council, 2018). Francis (2013) found that one of the main issues leading to the incidences at Mid Staffordshire that significantly impacted

on patient care was the power imbalance between professionals and service users. NAs must therefore challenge care that is lacking and advocate for those who cannot speak for themselves.

Direction is important in organizations and nursing staff usually lead the provision of care. Patients look to them for advocacy and safety when they are ill. They must speak up in their patients' best interests and the NHS has a moral obligation to provide backing to staff members who raise concerns on behalf of their patients (Francis, 2015).

Commitment

Commitment can be defined as a dedication or obligation to a cause. Inspired by leaders who can visualize and direct people along agreed pathways, commitment usually arises from a unified purpose. In nursing, this also involves a duty to uphold the professional code. The public rely on healthcare professionals to lead by example, even in their private lives. The NA therefore must look after their own health, as well as maintaining their conduct outside work so that they are effective role models and provide the best possible guidance for patients. Furthermore, they must be adaptable to change, thus accepting the responsibility of continuing to develop throughout their careers.

Commitment also means accepting that working in healthcare can be challenging. More often than not, there are often no straightforward solutions to problems. However, staff must develop, and have support to develop, coping mechanisms to prevent stress from inhibiting performance (Maben et al., 2012). Organizations and trusts may deliver this support through expressed acknowledgement when staff are under pressure; specific training, such as management or assertiveness courses; and rewards and incentives, such as pay rises or opportunities in career progression. The employer's duty includes looking after staff well-being and so they need to provide safe, accommodating and suitable conditions within the work environment.

PERSON-CENTRED CARE

Person-centred care is a phrase that is applied when considering a patient's individual healthcare needs.

Every single person is unique: their lives have been shaped by their own personalities, experiences and values or beliefs. This influences how they respond to problems or how they make choices, and it is why nurses must be able to adjust care according to an individual's wishes.

❗ HOTSPOT

NAs must demonstrate respect, not only to the patients and the families they provide care for, but also to other professionals and support workers.

There are many viewpoints on what NAs need to be aware of when applying person-centredness to the delivery of care. Fundamentally, the discussions revolve around getting to know the individual as well as possible. This can present complications in a number of ways, most of all because the person requiring care is not often given the choice of who is assigned to look after them in the healthcare setting, and an emotional connection is thought to be one of the most important aspects in developing a relationship through which people can reveal their innermost wishes.

This may seem like a huge problem, given the limited time period during which patients and NAs may be able to develop a relationship, let alone one that requires such depth. Furthermore, patients who are in ill health are naturally vulnerable and may also be overwhelmed or under pressure to make quick decisions.

The onus, therefore, falls on the NA to become perceptive and knowledgeable, to understand what characteristics make people distinctive, and to arm themselves with knowledge about different cultures and societies, as well as developing the skills to handle interactions with patients to effectively acquire information that helps them to understand each individual as well as they can.

CRITICAL AWARENESS

You must be reflective and introspective to prevent your own attitudes or beliefs from influencing patient choices.

Dignity

Dignity is an individual perception that is interpreted by each person in their own way, depending on their values, ideas or beliefs. The Royal College of Nursing (RCN) (2008) defines dignity as being 'concerned with how people feel, think and behave in relation to the worth or values of themselves and others', basic principles for achieving self-actualization or self-acceptance. Routes to self-actualization are diverse and are determined by many factors, such as confidence, age, economic status, culture and personal goals. Dignity is recognized as the most elementary of human rights (Human Dignity Trust, 2017), while the Social Care Institute for Excellence (2013) proposes that Dignity in Care is '…the kind of care, in any setting, which supports and promotes, and does not undermine, a person's self-respect, regardless of difference'.

How dignity is perceived by service users reflects the span and complexity of individual interpretation (Stratton, 2008; Patients Association, 2010). Subjective interpretations describe feelings of comfort, safety, being in control and having an opinion that is valued, while objective descriptions concern issues associated with physical presentation and behaviours. Unsurprisingly, the lack of consensus on what dignity is can result in poor care, especially if it means largely different things for nurses and patients.

What is uniformly agreed about dignity is that everyone should be treated with humanity, sensitivity and respect. This does not stop being true in situations where patients are incapable of explaining how they would like to be cared for. NAs must then draw on family or close friends who are more likely to have knowledge of individual's personal preferences. This, together with applied understanding of the patient's cultural and social background, will ensure that NAs can best advocate for their patient's wishes.

REFLECTION 8.3

Think of what aspects of dignity you might want to consider in these settings:
1. A ward for people recovering from facial surgeries, including the removal of tumours or the correction of trauma. Some of these patients might be experiencing surgery for the first time.
2. A family planning clinic.

Elderly care

The Francis Report has resulted in dignity becoming a principal concern in relation to the care provided for older and vulnerable people.

Older people in care report that they often feel excluded from decision-making, and that their experience and wisdom is seen as being of no value once they require help (Stratton, 2008). They are patronized and depersonalized. They become that 'little, old lady in bed 10 who needs her nappy changed'.

The ways in which dignity can be upheld include seemingly inconsequential things, like encouraging your elderly resident to select food from a menu, asking them how they would like to be addressed and handling hygiene tasks sensitively. It does not take much to show respect, and it can make the world of difference to somebody who may have contact only with carers or support workers for much of their time.

! HOTSPOT

Think about what kind of things may cause offence or make you feel vulnerable or unloved.

Knock before entering a patient's room and be mindful of offering the patient choices so that they will feel included in their care.

Privacy and confidentiality

Privacy and confidentiality are terms that are often used interchangeably to describe how protected information between professionals and their clients should be shared. Despite this, they do not necessarily have the same legitimacy in law.

Privacy is a right that entitles people to protect the information they share with somebody else from being passed on to a third party without their consent. Confidentiality is an ethical obligation, usually affirmed by a code of practice, such as the NMC or the RCN. It is pivotal to the preservation of trust between healthcare professionals and service users. For advice on confidentiality from the RCN, please go to: https://www.rcn.org.uk/get-help/rcn-advice/confidentiality.

The rules about privacy and confidentiality within healthcare do not always have clear boundaries. An individual's rights to object or veto the sharing of information between parties should, wherever possible, be respected. Yet, there may be circumstances where this presents a dilemma for the healthcare professional. For example, if a vulnerable patient informs a nurse that they have been harmed or if an individual imparts the intention to harm themselves or others, this will require discussion with other members of the care team in the patient's best interests (Caldicott, 2013).

All healthcare professionals should know how to protect patient data, but they also need to understand when this is not in the patient's best interests, and what situations warrant confidentiality breaches. Fortunately, there is guidance for NAs to turn to which will assist them in maintaining the code of confidentiality. The revised Caldicott Principles (2013) provide healthcare professionals with seven regulations that should be considered when the need to breaking confidentiality is being weighed.

CRITICAL AWARENESS

Honesty and trustworthiness are the building blocks of any relationship. The development of trust and the exchanging of information are essential to achieve shared goals.

REFLECTION 8.4

Read through the following scenario, then answer the questions below.

Mrs Victor, a 59-year-old, had changed address and joined a new GP surgery. She had been very happy with her previous GP, who knew her well, and had a good relationship with the nurses who worked there and understood her needs.

However, the first time Mrs Victor attended her appointment at the new surgery, she was a little shocked when the doctor was able to access the results of several tests via computer that she had thought available only to her previous doctor.

She was affronted that she had not been asked whether the availability of this information was acceptable to her and was a little alarmed about what else might be on there for anybody to read.

She leaves the consultation room without mentioning her concerns to the doctor. The practice nurse who had been present during Mrs Victor's appointment notices how upset she looks as she follows her out.

1. How could the nurse approach Mrs Victor to discover what may be wrong?
2. Do you think the sharing of Mrs Victor's information is in her best interests? If so, imagine a contrary point of view. Does your argument stand up to that?

Empathy

Simply put, empathy is the ability to understand and imagine another person's experience. Often referred to as 'putting yourself in someone else's shoes', an appreciation of the actions or reactions of others can convey support and understanding, allowing trust to develop between patients and healthcare professionals. For example, people who are ill may feel anxious, alone and misunderstood. Fears can be diminished when healthcare professionals demonstrate that they care about a person's concerns (Haslam, 2015). Empathy should, therefore, not only be an internal process. Healthcare professionals have a duty to manifest their support to patients, and this should be demonstrated through effective and positive nursing interactions and communication.

Nevertheless, it is necessary too for NAs to maintain professional objectivity in order to best advocate for their patients. Integrity is fundamental in the nurse–patient relationship, as this will lead to patient empowerment and encourage patients to take charge of their health needs. The NA must thus be able to set aside their own opinions so that these do not influence their perceptions of a patient's situation. This can be most challenging when the healthcare professional is asked to visualize themselves in a patient's shoes, because they may not see themselves acting or feeling in the same way.

Other barriers to empathy are time constraints, which limit patient contact, or anxiety on the part of the healthcare professional leading to emotional fatigue (Hardee & Platt, 2013). Patients may admit to feeling a nuisance when they ask a busy NA for help or complain that a NA seems distant and uninviting of interaction, making them feel undervalued. Empowerment of patients can only be achieved if the nursing team recognize the obstacles that can make patients feel excluded in their own care process. Reflection is a useful way to identify and tackle problems such as negative behaviours, which may result in adverse patient experiences.

CASE STUDY 8.1   Michael

Michael is a 32-year-old single man who has been admitted to your ward for an elective temporary ileostomy following some serious flare-ups of his ulcerative colitis. He has no other medical history. Michael is laughing and joking throughout the admission process, although it is clear that he is nervous. When you suggest that he may have questions for you at the end, he shrugs, looks uncomfortable and remains silent.

REFLECTION 8.5

Reflecting on Michael's situation in the case study, what skills would you need to engage or prompt your patient to explore any fears or anxieties he may have?

What questions may he have that he may find embarrassing or awkward to ask?

Empowerment

Healthcare professionals have a responsibility to help patients make the right choices for themselves about their health. Often, your role in these situations is to encourage patients to develop the confidence to question and inform themselves about their conditions. Once a patient has a good grasp of their problems, they are usually more able to see the options or pathways available to them, and through this participate in their care.

Studies have repeatedly shown that the patient's main worry when they are unwell is whether or not they are in safe hands (Rathert, 2011; Torpie, 2014; Mako et al., 2016). Providing a structured care plan tailored towards an individual must therefore treat the whole person, taking into account existing chronic problems which may not necessarily be impacting on their immediate health. Where there is continuous contact, for instance in a long-term care setting, the relationship between the NA and patient becomes much stronger. The NA is able to better advocate for patients they know well, particularly if they possess the knowledge and competencies to manage chronic conditions.

The essence of a good nurse or NA is the ability to inspire patients to take control over their well-being, and for this to happen, you must feel empowered yourself.

NAs must be assisted in developing the necessary skills to support patients, but also feel respected and supported in their work environments. To achieve the correct balance of autonomy and inclusiveness may seem like an impossibility for nurses in their workplace setting, especially in organizations that autocratically impose targets or restrictions. However, high-quality care can only be realized in environments in which the nurse feels satisfied, appreciated and able to take action within the scope of their abilities.

CASE STUDY 8.2 Mrs D'Angelo

Mrs D'Angelo is an 80-year-old widow who lives alone. She has been referred to a district nursing team because of a chronic leg ulcer. She has a past medical history of two myocardial infarctions in the last 11 years, which culminated in four coronary artery bypass grafts 2 years ago. She is also morbidly obese. Her last BMI measured at over 40 and this, together with her leg ulcer, makes it difficult for her to move around. She has type 2 diabetes, which she manages poorly, but blames her weight gain over the last few years on the venous leg ulcer that developed on the gaiter area of her left leg after bypass surgery. The ulcer causes her enormous discomfort and disrupts her 'life in general'. The ulcer has never fully healed since initiation, but it has been better at times. A quick visual assessment by the district nurse identifies that the ulcer is exposed and looking red and inflamed.

A read through previous notes makes the nurse aware that Mrs D'Angelo has previously been prescribed compression bandage therapy. Mrs D'Angelo's concordance with this therapy has been patchy. She does not keep the bandages on consistently as recommended by best practice because they are uncomfortable and bulky, restricting her mobility even further. Other issues that Mrs D'Angelo associates with her ulcer are pain and insomnia.

She has good support at home from her daughter, Anabella, who is a nurse and helps care for her. Anabella visits her daily and assists her with some chores.

Mrs D'Angelo has declined a referral before because she is fed up of 'seeing so many doctors who never listen to what I want, anyway'. From the nurse's conversations with her, it is clear that she has given up on the ulcer ever healing.

REFLECTION 8.6

1. Compression Bandaging is the gold standard treatment for leg ulcer management. What issues may be preventing Mrs D'Angelo's compliance with treatment?
2. What further knowledge do you need about Mrs D'Angelo to empower her towards making a decision about what is best for her?

LOOKING BACK, FEEDING FORWARD

The 6Cs are a values framework for nursing and their importance in delivering a good service for patients cannot be underestimated because patients should be the primary focus for all organizations involved in the transaction of care. Service users are entitled to positive experiences in healthcare, and nurses are the focal force in ensuring that this is possible.

Employing the 6Cs will assist nurses in their interactions and engagement with service users, as well as engendering a sustainable culture of considerate care.

Nonetheless, the need for compassion and vocation within healthcare must be a vision that does not just sit with nursing. It requires a whole systems approach which includes everyone who provides a service in the provision of care. Organizations have a duty to empower patients and staff towards making beneficial choices. This can only be possible if patients are able to participate in all the decisions that concern them.

REFERENCES

Bramhall, E., 2014. Effective communication skills in nursing practice. Nurs. Stand. 29 (14), 53–59.

Caldicott, F., 2013. To share or not to share. The information governance review. Department of Health, London.

Cummings, J., Bennett, V., 2012. Compassion in Practice: Nursing, Midwifery and Care Staff. Our Vision and Strategy. NHS Commissioning Board, Leeds.

Campling, P., 2015. Reforming the culture of healthcare: the case for intelligent kindness. BJPsych Bull 39 (1), 1–5.

Connolly, M., 2016. Listening skills 1: How to improve your listening skills. Nurs. Times 45 (46), 10–12.

Department of Health (DH), 1993. Vision for the Future. HMSO, London.

Department of Health (DH), 2013a. Patients First and Foremost. The Initial Government Response to the Report of The Mid Staffordshire NHS Foundation Trust Public Inquiry. https://www.gov.uk/government/uploads/system/uploads/attachment_data/file/170701/Patients_First_and_Foremost.pdf.

Department of Health (DH), 2013b. Compassion in Practice One Year On. https://www.england.nhs.uk/wp-content/uploads/2016/05/cip-one-year-on.pdf.

Francis, R., 2013. Report of the Mid Staffordshire NHS Foundation Trust Public Inquiry: executive summary. Stationery Office, London.

Francis, R., 2015. Freedom to Speak Up. http://webarchive.nationalarchives.gov.uk/20150218150343/https://freedomtospeakup.org.uk/wp-content/uploads/2014/07/F2SU_web.pdf.

Haslam, D., 2015. More than kindness. Journal of Compassionate Healthcare https://jcompassionatehc.biomedcentral.com/articles/10.1186/s40639-015-0015-2.

Hardee, J.T., Platt, F.W., 2013. Exploring and overcoming barriers to clinical empathic communication. http://www.tandfonline.com/doi/abs/10.1179/cih.2010.3.1.17.

Health Service Ombudsman, 2011. Care and Compassion? Report of the Health Service Ombudsman on Ten Investigations into NHS Care of Older People. Health Service, London.

Healthcare Commission, 2009. Investigation into Mid Staffordshire NHS Foundation Trust. http://www.nhshistory.net/midstaffs.pdf.

Human Dignity Trust, 2017. Human Dignity is The Basis of Fundamental Human Rights http://www.humandignitytrust.org/pages/OUR%20WORK/Why%20Human%20Dignity.

Ipsos MORI, 2015. Public Perceptions of the NHS and Social Care Survey. https://www.gov.uk/government/uploads/system/uploads/attachment_data/file/444783/NHS_tracker_acc.pdf.

Kirkup, B., 2015. The Report of the Morecambe Bay Investigation. https://www.gov.uk/government/uploads/system/uploads/attachment_data/file/408480/47487_MBI_Accessible_v0.1.pdf.

Kourkouta, L., Papathanasiou, I.V., 2014. Communication in Nursing Practice. https://www.ncbi.nlm.nih.gov/pmc/articles/PMC3990376/.

Maben, J., Peccei, R., Adams, M., et al., 2012. Exploring the relationship between patients' experiences of care and the influence of staff motivation, affect and wellbeing. Final Report. London. National Institute for Health Research Service Delivery and Health Programme.

Mako, T., Svanäng, P., Bjersa, K., 2016. Patients' perceptions of the meaning of good care in surgical care: a grounded theory study. https://bmcnurs.biomedcentral.com/articles/10.1186/s12912-016-0168-0.

National Advisory Group on the Safety of Patients in England, 2013. A Promise to Learn. A Commitment to Act: Improving the Safety of Patients in England. https://www.gov.uk/government/publications/berwick-review-into-patient-safety.

National Health Service, 2015. Compassion in Practice. Evidencing the impact. https://www.england.nhs.uk/wp-content/uploads/2016/05/cip-yr-3.pdf.

National Health Service, 2016. Briefing notes: issue highlighted by the 2016 NHS staff survey in England. http://www.nhsstaffsurveys.com/Caches/Files/20170306_ST16_National%20Briefing_v6.0.pdf.

Nursing and Midwifery Council, 2018. The Code. Professional Standards of Practice and Behaviour for Nurses, Midwives and Nursing Associates. London: NMC. https://www.nmc.org.uk/standards/code/.

Oelofsen, N., 2012. Using reflective practice in frontline nursing. Nurs. Times 108 (24), 22–24.

Oxford English Dictionary, 2017. Definition of dignity. https://en.oxforddictionaries.com/definition/dignity.

Patients Association, 2010. Listening to patients speaking up for a change. http://www.bgs.org.uk/pdf_cms/reference/patients_association_report.pdf.

Rathert, C., et al., 2011. Beyond service quality: the mediating role of patient safety perceptions in the patient experience-satisfaction relationship. Health Care Manage. Rev. 36 (4), 359–368.

Royal College of Nursing (RCN), 2008. Dignity. https://www.rcn.org.uk/professional-development/publications/pub-003298.

Royal College of Nursing (RCN), 2017. Patient Voices. Stories from the Royal College of Nursing quality improvement programme. http://www.patientvoices.org.uk/rcnqip.htm.

Royal College of Physicians, 2014. National Care of the Dying Audit for Hospitals, England. RCP, London.

Social Care Institute for Care, 2013. Dignity in Care. Overview of selected research: what dignity means. http://www.scie.org.uk/publications/guides/guide15/selectedresearch/whatdignitymeans.asp.

Stratton, D., 2008. Dignity in Healthcare. https://www.ageaction.ie/sites/default/files/dignity_in_healthcare.pdf.

Torpie, K., 2014. Customer service vs patient care. J Patient Exp 1 (2), 1–8.

9

Effective Communication Skills

Carrie Grainger

OBJECTIVES

By the end of the chapter the reader will be able to:

1. Understand the importance of effective communication in nursing care and therapeutic relationships
2. Examine the impacts of culture, values and power in communication exchange
3. Explore the impacts of verbal, non-verbal and proxemics in communication exchange
4. Recognize potential barriers to effective communication
5. Consider the challenges when engaging in difficult and challenging conversations
6. Appreciate the role of the Nursing Associate in effective communication with patients, families, colleagues and the wider healthcare team.

KEY WORDS

Culture

Values

Non-verbal

Verbal

Therapeutic

Intent

Power

Interpersonal

Mirroring

Proxemics

CHAPTER AIM

The aim of this chapter is to provide the reader with an understanding of the importance of effective communication skills in delivering care in a holistic, non-judgemental and compassionate manner.

SELF TEST

1. How might our culture and values influence how we communicate with others?
2. What is meant by active listening?
3. How might using OARS and SPIKES improve communication?
4. What skills might you employ to diffuse an emotional/ challenging situation with an upset relative?
5. What is meant by a 'therapeutic relationship'?
6. What cues might you use to demonstrate you were empathetic?
7. How and when might you adapt your communication style for different groups?
8. Describe how voice qualities might affect communication.
9. What are proxemics?
10. What potential barriers to communication might occur in healthcare and non-healthcare settings?

INTRODUCTION

In this chapter, the role of effective communication in nursing care is considered. The first part will explore the importance of effective communication, not only in building therapeutic relationships with patients and clients, but also in working collaboratively with a range of health and social care professionals. As healthcare is now delivered in a variety of settings, it is important for the Nursing Associate to build professional relationships with peers and colleagues to effectively and sensitively communicate with, and advocate for, the needs of their patients and families.

The second part of this chapter will examine technical and practical strategies that facilitate effective communication, including building a toolbox of approaches that can be utilized in practice. There will be a consideration of the challenges around engaging in more difficult conversations and how to identify potential barriers to communication.

WHY IS COMMUNICATION IMPORTANT?

Communication is a central component of human interaction, and the ability to communicate is learnt from an early age. Babies cannot speak, yet have the ability to communicate their needs to their parents through smiling, gurgling, laughing and crying, and their parents can respond appropriately to these needs by reading these communication cues (Barber, 2016). When working well, communication is a two-way process, a dance of reciprocity, an interactive dialogue, an expansive and immersive tool essential in building relationships.

Communication is fundamental to nursing practice and underpins every interaction within healthcare delivery. The Nursing and Midwifery Council (NMC) recognizes the importance of effective, culturally sensitive communication in the delivery of individualized care, which is responsive to the personal and health needs of service users and their families (NMC, 2018). Effective communication can help patients, service users, colleagues and peers feel valued, at ease and in control, which in turn can improve outcomes and experiences for service users and their families (Kourkouta and Papathanasiou, 2014; Clarke, 2015; Propp et al., 2010). Written communication is an effective way for health professionals to communicate with each other (Clarke, 2015).

The NHS constitution outlines seven key principles that govern the way the NHS operates, including values developed by and for patients, the public and NHS staff. This document recognizes the importance of seeing patients as *partners* in their care, rather than as passive recipients, meaning services reflect the needs and wants of service users and their families and highlight the importance of communication (DH, 2015). Communication is a key element in the Department of Health's report *Compassion in Practice* (2012) and makes up one of the '6Cs' of nursing, representing a core set of values that underpin compassionate practice.

The 6Cs of nursing are:
- Care
- Compassion
- Competence
- Communication
- Courage
- Commitment

See Chapter 8 for more information about the 6Cs.

> '*Communication is central to successful caring relationships and to effective team working. Listening is as important as what we say and do and essential for "no decision about me without me". Communication is the key to a good workplace with benefits for those in our care and staff alike.*' (DH, 2012).

In recent years, it has become more apparent how important effective communication in nursing and healthcare is. Documented failures in both health and social care settings have recognized the role of poor communication and interpersonal skills in contributing to substandard care (Francis, 2013; Berwick, 2013; Cavendish, 2013). Following an investigation and public inquiry into serious failings at Mid Staffordshire NHS Trust, The Francis Report (2013) made several recommendations, many of which were related to communication. These recommendations included identifying the role of a nurse as an 'essential point of communication' between the patient, patient's family

and the medical staff, particularly in hospital ward rounds, in order to be an effective advocate for patients (Francis, 2013; Entwistle, 2013a). The Francis Report also recommended the regulation of healthcare assistants. Skills for Care and Skills for Health (2013) were commissioned by the Government to produce a minimum training standard and code of conduct for healthcare assistants applicable in different care settings, which includes social care. As a minimum, it is advised that healthcare assistants receive training on what constitutes 'good communication', which would include identifying barriers to communication, and accessing support where appropriate, such as interpretation services and confidentiality (Francis, 2013; Skills for Care and Skills for Health, 2013; Entwistle, 2013b, 2013c).

THERAPEUTIC RELATIONSHIPS: COMMUNICATING THROUGH CARING

Interpersonal relationships are a central aspect of healthcare and the role of the Nursing Associate. In nursing, the development of therapeutic relationships is essential for the delivery of high quality, effective care (Reid Searl et al., 2014). Most time spent delivering nursing care will be through direct patient contact, involving communication exchanges (Munyisia, Yu & Hailey, 2011). Achieving and maintaining a good relationship with patients and their families can be transformative in care delivery and can have positive impacts for both the care giver and receiver (Stonehouse, 2016).

Nurse–patient relationships were originally explored through the work of Hildegarde Peplau, who was interested in their dynamics (Peplau, 1962). Peplau theorized about the importance of interpersonal relationships between nurses and their patients and developed her 'theory of interpersonal relations', which emphasized the need for *dynamic* rather than *passive* nurse-patient relationships. Key to this was the ability to effectively communicate. In essence, her theory acknowledged the creation of a shared experience, which resonates with the 6Cs and NHS constitution (DH, 2015).

A therapeutic relationship is seen as a professional, interactive relationship between a patient, their family and nurse, which is supportive in nature and aimed at facilitating change, such as a transition from ill health or distress to a desired state of health and well-being (Sharples, 2013). The required components for the development of a therapeutic relationship include:
- Trust
- Intimacy
- Respect
- Rapport
- Genuineness
- Empathy.

(Stonehouse, 2016).

A therapeutic relationship requires an acknowledgement of self-awareness, particularly around one's values and beliefs and a recognition of professional boundaries alongside proficient interpersonal skills, which include effective communication strategies, such as effective listening skills (Callwood, Cooke &

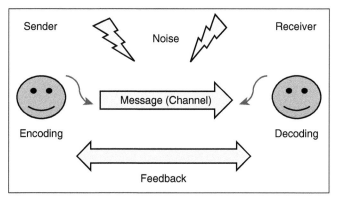

Fig. 9.1 The Process of Communication (Shannon & Weaver, 1948).

Allen, 2016; Sharples, 2013; McCabe & Timmons, 2013; Stonehouse, 2015; Tregoning, 2015).

Communication theory

The communication process, whether written, oral or non-verbally displayed, can at times only take seconds or minutes to occur. However, it is often fraught with potential breakdowns, misunderstandings and misinterpretations. For example, responding to an email from your boss who was enquiring as to whether you can work an extra shift in CAPS LOCK might be perceived as an angry response, yet, it might simply have been a mistake by the sender hitting the wrong computer keys. Barriers to communication can include language barriers, background noise and personal values. In order for communication to be effective and understood, much more time and effort needs to be afforded to it then we are often prepared or able to give.

THE COMMUNICATION PROCESS

Communication is a two-way interactive process for the exchange of information, and this exchange is in demonstrated in Fig. 9.1. For a message to be sent, the communication process requires a message, a sender and a receiver. The 'sender', also known as the 'communicator', is the person who initiates the message regardless of its form – the form might be verbal or non-verbal, conscious or unconscious. Once a message is sent, it needs to be received. The 'receiver', also known as the 'interpreter', is the person or persons to whom the message is sent. The 'message' itself relates to the particular content that is sent and received. The 'channel' or 'medium' refers to the means by which the message is sent, so this could be through the written word, such as email, or spoken voice, such as the telephone. The setting or environment in which the message is conveyed is referred to as the 'context' and can be an important factor for consideration by the Nursing Associate, such as finding a quiet, private place to deliver bad news. 'Feedback' relates to the success of communication from the receiver, often determining how well the message was understood. In the process of 'encoding' messages, the sender will use verbal and non-verbal cues to transfer a message that they feel the receiver will understand. 'Decoding' relates to how the message is

translated and interpreted by the receiver. Effective communication is only accomplished if the message is received in the way it was intended.

VERBAL AND NON-VERBAL COMMUNICATION

The content of messages contains both verbal and non-verbal communication. Verbal communication refers to the articulation of words, phrases and sentences that are actually spoken (Corcoran, 2013). Non-verbal communication refers to features of communication that relate not only to vocal *sounds*, such as prosodic elements (which refer to intonation and rhythm) and paralinguistic features (such as vocal expressions, for example, 'mmm'), but also those features that can be expressed through the body – through eye contact, posture, or gesture (Corcoran, 2013).

In the late 1960s and early 1970s, psychologist Albert Mehrabian famously explored the impacts of what is both said *and* done during communication exchanges (Mehrabian, 1971). His experiments looked at the relative importance people give to verbal and non-verbal communications in relation to the occurrence of inconsistent messages in conversations relating to likes and dislikes. He noted that non-verbal cues were often incongruent with verbal messages (meaning that what is said by the sender does not match their facial expression) and developed a formula of 7%–38%–55%. This is often referred to in communication texts, but also widely generalized to refer to all types of communications:

- 7% of meaning is in words that are spoken
- 38% of meaning is in the way it is said
- 55% of meaning is in facial expression.

Mehrabian's findings were rather more complex than this suggests as his formula related to how much of a message in regard to *feelings* is relayed in a specific way. He found that 7% of a message relating to feelings and attitude is relayed in the *words that are spoken*, 38% of a message pertaining to feelings and attitudes is paralinguistic, that is, relayed in the *ways* the words are spoken, and 55% of a message pertaining to feelings and attitudes is in the *facial expression*. This means that people tend to have more belief in the expression they see rather than the words spoken (Mehrabian, 1971). The interpretation of Mehrabian's findings is important in relation to communication in terms of understanding how messages are conveyed (in both the receiving and sending) and also in understanding differences in words and meanings and the impacts of body language.

Verbal communication

Verbal communication refers to the use of language to convey messages, and it is acknowledged that words can be used to promote the health, well-being and independence of individuals (Draper et al., 2013; Clarke, 2015). Language gives expression to values and is integral to the professional accountability of the nursing profession (Allen et al., 2007). Language and words also carry great power and have the ability to irreconcilably damage and undermine.

COMMUNITIES OF CARE
Care of Older People

The Commission on Dignity and Care for Older People Age UK, (2012) reported that the use of language by professionals in communicating with older people could have serious detrimental effects on self-confidence, skills and the ability to care for themselves and recommended that 'language that degenerates older people has no place in a caring society'.

Assumptions about potential hearing loss, the use of slower speech patterns, patronizing tones and the use of affectionate terms such as 'love' have long been adopted as ways of communicating with older people, reinforcing ageist stereotypes and can undermine independence and confidence.

Older people need to be shown respect and dignity, and should be treated as individuals, with specific needs.

! HOTSPOT

The way we use, understand and interpret language is often through the identities or roles we adopt, such as mother, father, doctor, nurse, which has implications in the way people respond to us and is influenced by our behaviours, beliefs, values and culture, including professional culture. How people view and interact with us is implicated by the roles we might assume at any one time. Culture, values and identity are reasons why language used by professionals can have such a powerful effect on the well-being of others. Inevitably, because of the type of work nursing involves, language may elicit authority or power over patients, but as we have seen in cases such as the Winterbourne View care home (where residents were subjected to horrific abuse at the hands of those who should have been caring for them), this is a dangerous position to adopt and negatively impacts on building relationships with patients and families and on quality of care.

It is important for the Nursing Associate to reflect on how culture, values and beliefs may influence how we behave and how others behave towards us, and develop strategies to minimize these effects, such as considering the type of language we use and how we speak to others.

REFLECTION 9.1

It is important to recognize that in most communication, verbal and non-verbal will be occurring simultaneously, conveying messages from a sender to a recipient. However, it is likely that the amount of attention afforded to each type of communication by the recipient will be dependent on different things. How might someone who has a hearing loss adopt different strategies to facilitate more effective communication?

Non-verbal communication

Non-verbal communication is the way in which messages are conveyed through a variety of physical means. These can include eye contact, facial expression, posture, the distance between sender and receiver (proxemics), movements and gestures (kinesics), affect, and touch (haptics). It is important to look at these in further detail to encourage the Nursing Associate to consider the implications of non-verbal messages when communicating with others, especially as these happen during communication interactions whether we are aware of it or not. It is also likely that non-verbal signals are affected by both personal and professional culture and by the health and condition of the patient.

Kinesics (movements and gestures)

Kinesics is concerned with non-verbal communication related to movement either through parts or the whole of the body. There are essentially five kinesics that are important to communication: emblems, regulators, illustrators, affect, and adapters (Roebuck, 2017).

An *emblem* is a hand movement or gesture that can be used to represent its verbal counterpart. For example, a 'V sign' for victory or peace or a 'thumbs up' sign implying something is good and 'thumbs down' implying something is bad. The OK symbol, used to express when someone is OK, is made when the forefinger and thumb connect to make an O shape. The remaining fingers are held upright. Emblems are often employed as a way of 'universally communicating'. The gesture we make to a waiter in a restaurant when we want to get our food bill is another example.

Although using emblems might be helpful in certain situations, for example if it is difficult to hear someone because of background noise, it is important to recognize the impact of culture. Whilst we live in a global world, emblems have a strong cultural component and therefore do not transcend the use of other forms of communication to convey understanding. Many emblems may have different meanings in different cultures and contexts, so cultural awareness is important as they have the potential to be misinterpreted. For example, the 'OK' emblem, popular in the UK, has different meanings in other countries where it can be seen as insulting.

Roebuck (2017) discusses the use of emblems by vulnerable groups in health and social care settings and acknowledges how some service users may make use of symbolic or gestured communication, such as Makaton, so it is important for practitioners to be attuned to this. Whilst it would be difficult for a Nursing Associate to be able to learn an entirely new language, learning the odd phrases or symbols would be helpful for someone working in that context. In a sense, it is a bit like visiting a foreign country; learning a few key phrases to help improve communication with local people is a good idea. In a working context, it can improve attentiveness to the needs of those the Nursing Associate is caring for. Failure to recognize key ways in which someone might be communicating may increase a patient's vulnerability and susceptibility to poor health and poor outcomes.

Illustrators, regulators and adapters

Illustrators have less of a cultural component and are natural movements used to illustrate what is being said (Roebuck, 2017). For example, when describing an object, you may point to it, or if describing a person who is tall, you might indicate their height through your hands. Illustrators can therefore be helpful to reinforce what you are saying. Although there is less cultural influence, there can still be differences in the way that some cultures might use these gestures, so it is important to be mindful of this when decoding them.

Regulators are the movements and signs that regulate, modulate and maintain the flow of speech during conversations, essentially the art of 'turn taking' in exchanges (Devito, 2013). Regulators are often used in giving and receiving feedback. This could be through the use of smiling or nodding your head when encouraging someone to continue talking or opening your mouth slightly when you wish to speak. Different cultures may use different regulators to demonstrate understanding, and it would be beneficial to consider that if someone does not pick up on your cues it is because they may be adhering to their own cultural norms, rather than simply ignoring yours (Roebuck, 2017).

Adapters are unconscious movements conveying messages about our needs. They are motivated by an inner drive, and are usually postural changes or movements made to make us feel more comfortable, such as scratching an itch or fidgeting (Devito, 2013). Most of the time these actions are performed unconsciously or at least at a low level of awareness.

> **⚠ HOTSPOT**
>
> There may be associated cultural and social norms that impact on our use of adapters; for example, some adapters could not be used in a public setting as it would be viewed as inappropriate. It is important to consider conditions or situations that might disinhibit patients and promote the use of inappropriate adapters and how you might respond to these. For example, think about how someone with dementia might use adapters.

Facial expression, affective display and eye contact

The face is like a projector and has a great capacity to communicate emotion, both consciously and unconsciously. The saying 'It's written all over your face' is often used to indicate that the expression on someone's face is representative of their true feelings. Charles Darwin was first to suggest a universality of some facial expressions focusing on the ability of the face to express distinct primary emotions, a theory further developed by Dr Paul Ekman in the 1970s (Darwin, 1872; Ekman, 1972). The expressions, responses to and understanding of happiness, surprise, anger, sadness, fear and disgust were seen to share commonality across cultures.

Micro expressions are facial expressions that occur fleetingly and are often involuntary and can expose true emotion. This makes decoding facial expressions a complex and imprecise business (Roebuck, 2017). It is important to acknowledge that whilst this indicates that facial expression can be universal, cultures may differ in terms of the acceptability of how these emotions are expressed (Roebuck, 2017). What we do know is that first impressions count and are an important component of healthcare, having a direct impact on how people view and utilize a service.

> **⚠ HOTSPOT**
>
> Smiling is good for you. The habitual act of smiling helps the mind move to a more positive state, and encourages positive thinking. Happiness triggers productivity and creativity. If you smile at someone, it is highly likely they will reciprocate with a smile, which is triggered by mirror neurons in the brain's cortex.
>
> Smiles are infectious, so infect someone today!

Affect

Affect refers to body or facial movements that display a certain emotional state (Devito, 2013; Roebuck, 2017). We have already considered the use of facial expressions to convey emotion, but the body is also a tool to display affect. There can sometimes be a disconnect with the face and the body conveying different messages and we can often be more concerned about what our face is doing rather than how the message is being conveyed through our bodies (Mehrabian, 1971; Ekman, 1972). A lack of affective display may well be perceived by someone as a lack of emotion but may actually relate to social or cultural norms. For example, two angry people may display their anger in differing ways, with one becoming aggressive, whilst the other remains quiet and passive.

Eye contact

Eye contact is considered an important non-verbal tool and provides humans with an innate form of communication. Eye contact is a way of making a connection with another individual, demonstrating focus and attention, and increases the receiver's status, so the message conveyed by the duration, direction and quality of eye contact can be really powerful (Roebuck, 2017). Eye avoidance or looking away might be adopted as a method to respect privacy, shut out distraction or increase concentration. Culture can influence comfort in eye contact, and it is also important to recognize this within patient groups.

> **CRITICAL AWARENESS**
>
> It is noted that there are differences in the length of normal gaze; for example, in people with mental illness, dementia, with a learning disability or on the autistic spectrum. This has the potential to be misinterpreted by nursing staff, perhaps as threat or lack of interest (Roebuck, 2017). The Nursing Associate needs to be mindful that assumptions like this can impact on the caring relationship and utilize adapters to counter them.

Proxemics

Proxemics is the study of space and how it is used, how it makes us feel more or less comfortable and how we arrange objects and ourselves in relation to the space around us (orientation). Proxemics was first theorized by the anthropologist Edward Hall (1966), following studies conducted on animal behaviour. Hall devised a model by which acceptable distances are used to achieve communication goals in different settings. In Hall's (1966) model, intimate distances (15–45 cm) are seen as those that occur when we engage in intimate contact, for example, when we hug another person, whisper something or touch somebody. A person distance is described as 45–120 cm; we tend to engage in this type of contact with family members or our close friends. Social distance (1.20–3.50 m) is demonstrated when we are communicating with those who are colleagues, usually with someone known fairly well to us, those we might feel more comfortable interacting with at a closer distance. In public distance (3.50–7.50 m) physical space is seen, for example, when we are in a lecture theatre or in a public speaking situation. Talking in front of a class full of students or giving a case study presentation whilst at work could be seen as public distance.

Hall surmised that these distances are deliberately chosen by individuals depending on the situation or context. Proxemic

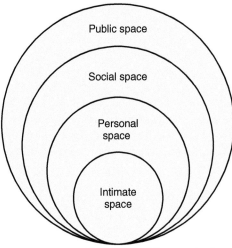

Fig. 9.2 Physical Distance and Communication.

behaviour tends to be learnt through the observation of others, usually within cultures and populations, rather than through explicit instruction, hence why there might be differences in acceptability of personal distance and physical contact within different cultures, especially in relation to intimacy (Hall, 1966) (Fig. 9.2). The physical distances between communicators are also dependent on the type of relationship they have. This is particularly important when considering the role of the Nursing Associate and the types of healthcare activities the Nursing Associate will engage in.

> **! HOTSPOT**
>
> Boundaries of personal space can be tested within cultural, social or vulnerable groups, such as those living with dementia, or a learning disability. For example, standing very close or far away may influence how we react to someone, if we or they feel threatened, so it is important to consider how we might react to and behave towards others. Think about your positioning when you are working with different patient groups.

Touch (haptics)

Touch is perhaps the most primal but complex way of communicating meaning, as it can communicate basic messages and responses in a powerful way, so is governed by cultural norms and values. Touch is a fundamental part of the nursing process and it is important to recognize different forms of touch that are adopted to communicate different messages or meanings. In social settings some touch is ritualistic, such as greeting by shaking hands. Other touch is task orientated, in order to carry out specific tasks and roles; however, this touch may well have an emotional impact to the receiver, especially if someone feels vulnerable (Roebuck, 2017). Touch is also used to convey or express positive emotion, such as affection, support, trust or emotional containment and is referred to as 'therapeutic caring touch' (Devito, 2013).

> **! HOTSPOT**
>
> Some touch is unwanted. This can be influenced by a number of factors including the age and gender of the people interacting, familiarity, role, occupation and personal comfort (Roebuck, 2017).

The use of and receipt of touch is complex, as we have already seen, and this can affect how people may utilize it within practice. Staff can be fearful of using touch in some circumstances, for instance with particular vulnerable groups, but it is also important to recognize the beneficial effects. Therefore touch should be responsive, appropriate and considerate to the needs and values of the patient, but we must ask permission.

LISTENING SKILLS AND THE ART OF CONVERSATION

As a Nursing Associate, perhaps the most important communication skill you will need to develop is that of listening. By effectively listening to people, the Nursing Associate will be able to enable patients and their families to talk about their experiences and associated feelings, and identify any needs and wants. During the Francis Inquiry (2013) it was noted that many families had not felt listened to or valued. A good listener will help people feel valued, appreciated, understood, recognized and respected. There are a number of features that demonstrate active listening is taking place. Good eye contact denotes attentiveness and focus on the patient. Body language is another equally important feature; displaying an open posture, arms unfolded, mirroring gestures and facing the patient indicates that the Nursing Associate is ready and interested to listen to what is being said (Scriven, 2010; Lynall, 2012; Roebuck, 2017).

Listening is an active process. A good listener needs to give the speaker full attention, making a conscious effort not only to listen to the words, but also to be aware of the feelings and meaning behind what is being said. Listening therefore involves tuning-in to and making note of both verbal and non-verbal cues to gain a real understanding of a situation. This is referred to as 'active listening' (Scriven, 2010). Devito (2013) notes that listening is a process made up of six elements:

1. Receiving (receiving the message)
2. Attending (paying attention to what is important – avoiding distractions, such as background noise)
3. Understanding (making sense of what is being said or shown through verbal and non-verbal cues)
4. Evaluating (what it means)
5. Responding (giving feedback – verbal or non-verbal)
6. Remembering.

Table 9.1 describes some key active listening skills.

A good listener will allow and encourage someone to talk without interruption, giving them the space to express their feelings or concerns and explore knowledge, attitudes and values. Active listening is about searching for meaning behind what is being said. This cannot be achieved if the listener is only hearing

TABLE 9.1   Some Key Active Listening Skills

Non-verbal listening skills	Meaning
Smiling	Smiling can be powerful in affirming messages being received and show that the listener is paying attention to what is said.
Eye contact	It is always helpful to look at the speaker, although too much eye contact can be intimidating, so looking away for short times or softening the gaze is helpful.
Posture	The attentive listener will have a tendency to lean forward or tilt or nod the head towards the speaker.
Mirroring	Adopting facial expressions or posture of the other person, i.e., sitting with legs crossed if the speaker is doing the same. Helpful to demonstrate empathy.
Distraction	Refraining from distractions like fidgeting, or looking at a phone or watch shows attentiveness.

Verbal listening skills	Meaning
Positive reinforcement	Can be helpful for encouraging speaker. 'Yes, I see…' 'Mmm' Can also be disingenuous if used too frequently and can distract from what is being said.
Remembering	Can demonstrate attentiveness, such as recalling parts of a conversation to ensure messages have been received and understood.
Questioning	Helpful to build clarity and reinforces interest in what the speaker may be saying.
Reflecting	Paraphrasing the speaker's words can be beneficial for clarity and understanding and reinforce messages.
Clarification	Using open-ended questions or reflection to expand on and gain more understanding.
Summarizing	Repeating what has been said in the speaker's own words. It also gives the speaker an opportunity to correct anything that has been misunderstood.

what is said rather than actively engaging in the process. Active listening is a skill that can be a challenge when practising it, but a gift when it is received.

REFLECTION 9.2

Skilful active listening is about being in the moment. It is very easy to get distracted when listening to someone else speak. You may find that your mind wanders to something that might be occupying your thoughts, or it may be that you become pre-occupied with planning how you might respond, or distracted by the knowledge that there are another six people on the ward you need to attend to before the morning ward round. The conversation may get you thinking about a similar experience you may have had, and the feelings it left you with. Think about a time when you have struggled to focus on a conversation with a friend. What factors contributed to your lack of attentiveness?

You will need to adopt strategies that can assist you in becoming a focused listener. There are many approaches that are helpful to learn which encourage active listening and meaningful conversations.

Helping and enabling people to talk

Have you ever been in a situation where you felt that you couldn't tell someone how you were feeling, or that you felt that someone wasn't interested in what you had to say? Sometimes starting a conversation can be the most difficult, and it might be especially difficult for those people who are in our care. People may feel powerless to speak in the context of healthcare because of situations and environments that are unfamiliar to them, such as being in a hospital ward, and the Nursing Associate needs to be able to make people feel at ease and valued and build rapport.

A welcoming approach is a good start, and it is important to acknowledge what makes patients feel valued and connected. Attentiveness is key here – do not be distracted or preoccupied by other tasks. Focus should be on the patient and good eye contact, positioning and orientation (proxemics) will help as it demonstrates that our focus is on the individual and they are the most important person to us at that moment (Rezende et al., 2015; Lynall, 2012).

To enable people to begin to talk, it can be useful to offer them a specific invitation to speak (Scriven, 2010). This requires the Nursing Associate to be attuned and attentive to both verbal and non-verbal cues. An example of an invitation could be as follows: 'Mahmood, you look rather worried about this examination today, are you?' or 'You don't seem to be yourself today, Rita, is there something on your mind?' or 'Hello, so what is it that can I help you with today?'. Inviting people to speak helps to demonstrate that you value what is important to them, facilitating rapport. It also helps establish a more collaborative approach to care.

Questioning skills

A key component of listening is understanding. An active listener needs to understand what is meant or being felt based on the patient's response. To facilitate understanding, and also help patients engage in conversation, the Nursing Associate needs to develop effective questioning skills. There are different types of questions that can be useful in different circumstances and contexts to facilitate understanding, namely open and closed, biased and multiple questions (Scriven, 2010).

Open questions

Open questions refer to questions that encourage dialogue. These are really high-value questions that initiate learning and enhance connections with others. Open questions can solicit the listener's thoughts and feelings, enriching the conversation by providing an opportunity to respond more fully, giving greater understanding of situations, behaviours, attitudes and values. They can encourage the responder to be much more reflective and revealing in their responses. Open questions can also demonstrate mindful curiosity and interest of the asker that, over time, facilitates development of reciprocal behaviour, which in turn enhances the relationship. Reciprocity, as we have already seen, is an important element in therapeutic relationships. There are some key words that are used to facilitate open questioning, such as 'how', 'what', 'feel' and 'think'. An example of an open question is 'What do you think about…?' or 'How did that make you feel?'

Closed questions

Closed questions are those that usually require short factual responses, such as a 'yes' or 'no' answer, usually confirmatory in nature. For example, 'Is that your address?' 'Can you reach that water jug?' Closed questions are less useful when encouraging dialogue or getting to know someone or getting them to talk in more detail.

Biased questions

Biased questions are those that are likely to indicate what the listener wants or expects to hear, and can be rather leading in nature (Scriven, 2010). An example of a biased question is 'You are feeling better today, aren't you?'. In this case, it is likely that the respondent will answer in a way that is expected of them, rather than say how they actually feel. This type of questioning can be rather disingenuous. It might be tempting, for example, to ask a biased question if the ward is full, the unit needs empty beds and staff need to make decisions about who to discharge home.

Multiple questions

Multiple questions are ones that contain more than one question and can be extremely confusing and overwhelming. A listener is unlikely to know which question to answer or indeed remember all the elements of the question. An example of a multiple question is 'Did you understand what the doctor told you? Would you like to talk with her again? Would you like me to go through it with you?' Asking questions in this way can be challenging for the responder, particularly in situations where there may already be some confusion or distress. It prohibits people thinking and processing information clearly. For example, questioning someone with dementia in this way would prove distressing, as their ability to process information is challenged by their cognitive decline (Hobson, 2012).

CRITICAL AWARENESS

Encouraging responses from patients should be seen as an art form as well as a skill. It should express humble enquiry or mindful curiosity as opposed to confrontation or prying. It is important to ask as opposed to tell: *telling* can disable people, whereas *asking* can empower them (it says, 'I am interested in you'). This can lead to an improvement in relationships. (Adapted from Schein, 2013; Dyche & Epstein, 2011.)

Response and feedback

Another component of effective listening is feedback and response. This can be useful for a number of reasons. Firstly, feedback can be helpful to check out understanding. For example, after instructing a patient on how to monitor their blood sugar, it would be important to make sure they understood what was said and done. Effective questioning will check what they remember and whether they have mastered the skill (Scriven, 2010). This is important, especially when there may be concerns over how much someone has understood. This needs to be done in an empathetic, sensitive manner, particularly as understanding could be compromised due to a variety of reasons, such as distress or anxiety, capacity to understand due to disability or impairment, or perhaps due to limited skills in language or comprehension. Feedback can also be helpful in facilitating dialogues or conversations. It is much easier to engage in conversation with someone when they are responsive and attentive to you.

Scriven (2010) highlights two key points to note about getting feedback. Firstly, it is the responsibility of the communicator, not the listener, to ensure that what has been communicated has be received and understood. Using sensitive questioning will demonstrate that it is your responsibility as the Nursing Associate to ensure that you have been understood by the patient.

CRITICAL AWARENESS

When the Nursing Associate asks questions such as, 'May I check to ensure that *I have addressed everything* – could you just go over what you have understood so far?', it places the emphasis on the Nursing Associate and their responsibility to be understood, rather than on the person listening.

You should try not to use statements or questions that indicate that you think what has been said and done has not been understood by the receiver, for example, '*I* do not think that *you* have fully understood me' or 'Have *you* learnt it yet – can *you* show me?' (Adapted from Scriven, 2010).

Secondly, in order to be sensitive and empathetic whilst checking out understanding, the type of questioning you use is important. Using open questions again facilitates a deeper comprehension and gives more opportunity for meaningful feedback. If you use closed questions to elicit feedback, the respondent might just answer 'yes' because they are too embarrassed to admit they do not understand, or are intimidated or scared and do not want to look foolish (Scriven, 2010).

Using OARS (Motivational Interviewing (MI))

There are some other communication tools that the Nursing Associate may find helpful in facilitating the art of therapeutic conversations to improve understanding and motivate change.

Motivational Interviewing (MI) is a person-centred approach to counselling developed to elicit personal motivations to facilitate change in health-related behaviours (Miller & Rollnick, 2012;

Droppa & Lee, 2014). It has its origins in addiction counselling, but some of its approaches and tools can be adopted and utilized effectively to develop communication skills and meaningful rapport, interactions and relationships with patients. Indeed, the spirit of MI is in the collaborative partnership that develops between patient and nurse. MI uses a basic communication style represented by the acronym OARS which stands for:

Open questions
Affirmations
Reflections
Summary
(Miller & Rollnick, 2012).

These four elements are described symbolically, guiding the patient through a dynamic interaction in a conversational partnership (Klonek & Kauffeld, 2015).

The benefits of adopting open questioning have already been addressed, but it is important to remember that this type of questioning encourages people to talk and allows for deeper thinking and elaboration of a topic

Affirmations refer to statements that recognize the patient's strengths and can be beneficial in building rapport as they promote positive feelings and increase self-esteem.

As a tool for effective communication, reflective listening is helpful for expressing empathy. By listening and reflecting back what is said to the patient, the Nursing Associate can demonstrate that they have an understanding and can see things from the perspective of the patient. It can also be useful to gain clarity.

> **! HOTSPOT**
>
> Reflection can be both simple and complex. It is important when reflecting to not just repeat verbatim what is said by the patient and therefore requires skill and effort to do well. Reflections should be statements that re-phrase the client's words and thoughts to establish clarity.

Summarizing is another type of reflecting and involves the nurse summarizing what has been talked about, and can be an effective way of moving the conversation on, shifting attention to the next issue and demonstrating that the client has been listened to and is valued (Miller & Rollnick, 2012). Table 9.2 gives some examples of each element and how OARS might be utilized in a conversation.

CASE STUDY 9.1   Conversation Using OARS (adapted from Widder, 2017)

The Nursing Associate has been seeing Jim for a number of days at his home and has been discussing his journey of giving up smoking. Look at how the Nursing Associate uses OARS to demonstrate empathy and understanding and to guide the conversation in a positive way.

Jim: I am constantly being told that I should give up smoking, and now the doctor and health visitor are telling me… but I've tried so many times, I know I need to but I just don't know how.

Nursing Associate: So, what I am hearing from you is you know you need to give up, but you know it will be hard and are wondering if all the effort to give up will be worth it? *(Reflective listening)*

Jim: Yes, I have tried before and it was a complete disaster!

Nursing Associate: So, your previous attempt was difficult… *(Reflection)* Can you tell me about that experience-what it was like for you giving up? *(Open question)*

Jim: Well, the first time I tried it was when my partner was pregnant with our first child. It didn't last long…the not smoking I mean…

Nursing Associate: That was a lovely thing to do for your child. *(Affirmation)* So, tell me about what was it that made you go back to smoking and what keeps you smoking? *(Getting the client's perspective)*

Jim: The baby was 6 months, and wasn't sleeping well…neither were we!

Nursing Associate: That must have been a difficult time for you as a new dad. *(Reflective listening)*

Jim: Yes, she was a poor sleeper for quite a while…

Nursing Associate: But you were able to keep on track for a few months *(Affirmation)* so what things did you do that you found that were helpful? *(Getting the client's perspective)*

Jim: My partner and I tried to quit together, although she has been better at it than me.

Nursing Associate: So, what are your thoughts about smoking now?

Jim: I would like to be smoke-free like my partner. We did set up a room in the house which is smoke free, when the baby was born. I think I might give it another go.

Nursing Associate: That's great, you made some important changes and it's good that you are willing to give it another try. *(Affirming)* So today we have talked about when you first tried quitting smoking – when you became a dad, and what made you return to smoking, and also your motivation to be smoke-free like your partner. *(Summarizing)*

TABLE 9.2   Some Examples of How OARS May Be Used

Open-ended questions	Affirmations	Reflections	Summaries
Nurse: 'You seem a bit worried about your discharge home. Can you tell me a little more about how its making you feel?'	**Nurse:** 'When you went home last time, you did really well keeping to the treatment plan we made.'	**Patient:** 'I am worried that I might not be able to care for myself at home-I'm scared' **Nurse:** 'So going home is something that is concerning you?'	**Nurse:** 'So today we have talked about how you have felt about being in hospital, what your main concerns are about going home, and your plans for when you get home.'

Motivational interviewing is a skilled process that requires time, training and practice; however, the use of OARS can certainly be beneficial in developing effective communication strategies that enhance therapeutic relationships.

BREAKING BAD NEWS – THE 'ART' OF A DIFFICULT CONVERSATION

Nursing Associates have an important role in providing information to patients and their families. In practice, there will be times where the Nursing Associate may have to engage in a more 'difficult' conversation. This is mostly related to communicating bad news, for example informing a patient about delays or discussing an issue relating to treatment or a patient's condition. Generally, communicating bad news relates to the imparting or receiving of knowledge or information that is either bad, sad or difficult (Fallowfield & Jenkins, 2004). If handled poorly, this communication can have significant ramifications for the patient experience and impact on the rapport between patient and Nursing Associate, ultimately affecting the relationship (Warnock, 2014; Baer & Weinstein, 2013). The way bad news is delivered is also an important factor in how it is received, understood and dealt with by the patient and their family (Royal College of Nursing (RCN), 2013).

It is important to acknowledge that there are many pitfalls when communicating about difficult topics, both in personal and professional situations.

Often, we tend to make assumptions about how people might respond and concern ourselves with about how we might make them feel: will they be angry, get distressed? These feelings make us hesitant about engaging in a difficult conversation altogether, which then leads to avoidance of the issue and a lack of resolution (Patton, Stone & Heen, 2010; Grimsley, 2010).

This can also be true within nursing practice. We may tend to make assumptions about what a patient and their family may want to know, how they feel about or what they understand about their condition. But there may be a risk that by trying to minimize the impact of giving bad news or exploring difficult topics, we actually miss opportunities to try to help the patient cope better and plan ahead (Baer & Weinstein, 2013).

There are, of course, cultural implications at play here too. There are often cultural preferences relating to how difficult information is managed, such as withholding information directly from the patient as a way of helping the patient cope with the situation or when families 'carry' the burden of information whilst the patient is shielded from it (Warnock, 2014). It is therefore important to ascertain the needs of both the patient and the family.

Often driving the avoidance behind tackling 'bad news' or 'difficult conversations' is the emotion behind it (Patton, Stone & Heen, 2010; Grimsley, 2010). It has been acknowledged that nurses can sometimes address emotional responses with fact rather than empathy, which may not be helpful to the patient (Baer & Weinstein, 2013). This is likely to be related to the associated fear that we have in the emotional responses of others reacting to bad news and how we then react to them. By developing skills and strategies in effective communication, the Nursing Associate can begin to feel more prepared to deal with more 'difficult conversations'.

As we have already acknowledged the way bad news is delivered is significant in improving patient outcomes and experiences and there are a number of frameworks and strategies that have been developed to support 'difficult conversations', such as SBAR (see Box 9.1) (see also chapter 7) and SPIKES (Warnock, 2014;

BOX 9.2 Breaking Bad News Using an ABCDE Easy Framework

The ABCDE mnemonic for breaking bad news:
Advance preparation
Build a therapeutic environment/relationship
Communicate well
Deal with patient and family reactions
Encourage and validate emotions

(RCN, 2013. Adapted from Rabow & McPhee, 1999.)

RCN, 2013). It can be helpful for the Nursing Associate to consider some of these frameworks alongside some of the communication strategies already discussed, such as active listening, open questioning and developing good rapport and relationships.

The RCN has developed a simple four-stage framework adapted for delivering bad news that takes elements of other frameworks and models (RCN 2013). The four elements relate to *preparation, communication, planning* and *follow up*. **Preparation** relates to considerations you make before the conversation, such as considering cultural issues, settings in which you might deliver the news, and rehearsing what you might say. **Communication** relates to issues such as building rapport, giving adequate time to the conversation, and the impact of body language, for instance eye contact and touch. It also includes exploring what is already known by the patient or family and checking understanding. **Planning** involves ensuring that the patient or family have an action plan, which might include clarifying the next steps, such as how to make contact again. **Follow up** relates to maintaining good relationships in cases of ongoing communication, and signposting for further support (RCN, 2013).

Breaking bad news can be helped by thinking of the easy framework outlined in Box 9.2.

The SPIKES communication tool, although originally developed for end of life care is also a useful tool to support the delivery of bad news (Baile et al., 2000; Baer & Weinstein, 2013; RCN, 2013). SPIKES is a mnemonic, which refers to:
Setting
Perception
Information (and invitation)
Knowledge
Empathy
Strategy and Summary.

Step 1: Setting

This relates to ensuring the setting is appropriate, so privacy is very important, with no interruptions from others, or indeed from the Nursing Associate when the patient or family is speaking. So being attentive to the patient and engaging active listening skills is paramount. Baile et al. (2000) acknowledge that those practitioners who sit down during difficult consultations tend to demonstrate more effectively to the patient that they are more attentive, have time and will not rush things. Alongside this, maintaining eye contact is an important way of establishing rapport and emotional connection.

Step 2: Perception

This relates to ascertaining the patient's understanding of what is happening, so asking open questions can be beneficial here. Helpful questions could be 'How much do you understand about what is happening here?' or 'What have you been told about why your operation has been postponed?'.

Step 3: Information

This step concerns providing information in a way that is responsive to the needs of the patient and their family, helping to avoid information overload. It is about using language that is familiar to the patient and delivering messages in small chunks rather than in one overwhelming message. It is important to remember that information will not be retained in highly stressful or anxious situations, so the pace should be led by the patient and their family.

Step 4: Knowledge

In its simplest term this refers to acknowledging that some of the information imparted might be difficult to hear, and so preparing the patient and their family for what might come next.

Step 5: Empathy

This step is about the Nursing Associate being responsive to the emotional needs of the patient and their family. The skill here is to observe, listen out for, name emotional responses and identify the source of the emotion. For instance, saying things like 'I can see this incident is making you angry,' or 'How is this making you feel?'. It is also about acknowledging that they may not want to talk about things now, so giving them space, or just being there with a quiet touch may be just as important as the words spoken.

Step 6: Strategy and summarizing

The last steps involve summarizing the information and giving the patient the chance to ask further questions and make a further plan. Patients will feel less anxious or unclear if there is a clear future plan about what will happen next, and this is relevant regardless of the situation. See Table 9.3 for a summary of the SPIKES model.

LOOKING BACK, FEEDING FORWARD

This chapter has introduced the Nursing Associate to some fundamental skills and knowledge required for effective communication. Communication is an art and a skill, much like the nursing profession. Whether or not it is performed well, it will be remembered and shape the experiences of service users and their families. Improving communication takes time, practice, persistence, courage and reflection.

Effective communication is paramount to building relationships and it is important to acknowledge and evaluate how your own attitudes, values and behaviours may be reflected in your professional role and how you provide and deliver care to others. It is important for the Nursing Associate to be responsible for effectively communicating to patients, and that the ways in which

TABLE 9.3   Summary of SPIKES Model (adapted from Baile et al., 2000)

Spike steps	Considerations
Setting (and setting up)	• Preparation • Arrange some privacy-use a private area/space in order to reduce interruptions • Involve significant others (family members if the patient prefers this) • Sitting down (with no barriers in between you such as a table or desk) • Make good eye contact • Manage time constraints and distractions-such as asking for mobiles to be on silent
Perception	• Giving an invitation to talk • Use open questions
Information	• Let the patient lead the pace of the conversation • Give time for questions
Knowledge	• Preparing the patient for bad news • Using language appropriate for patient-no jargon or technical terminology
Empathy	• Observe emotional responses such as crying • Acknowledge the emotion through questions or statements- *'I can see this is very upsetting'* or *'I can tell you were not expecting this'* • Use touch, silence or other responses to demonstrate empathy
Summary/Strategy	• Summarize the conversation to ensure understanding • Make a future plan to help reduce anxiety

you communicate will influence the success of that communication exchange and whether you have been understood.

An important feature of communication relates to self-awareness of values, culture, beliefs and attitudes. It is important the Nursing Associate be attuned to factors that may inhibit or become a barrier to effective communication, including settings, choice of language, non-verbal cues, such as body language and proximity, and to develop skills and tools to minimize the harmful effects of these barriers.

REFERENCES

Age, U.K., 2012. Delivering Dignity: Securing Dignity in Care for Older People in Hospital and Care Homes. Available at: http://www.ageuk.org.uk/Global/Delivering%20Dignity%20Report.pdf?dtrk=true.

Allen, S., Chapman, Y., O'Connor, M., Francis, K., 2007. The importance of language for nursing. Does it convey commonality of meaning and is it important to do so. Aust. J. Adv. Nurs. 24 (4), 47–51.

Baer, L., Weinstein, E., 2013. Improving oncology nurses' communication skills for difficult conversations. Clin. J. Oncol. Nurs. 17 (3), 45–51.

Baile, W.F., Buckman, R., Lenzi, R., et al., 2000. SPIKES – a six step protocol for delivering bad news: application to the patient with cancer. Oncologist 5, 302–311.

Barber, C., 2016. Communication, ethics and healthcare assistants. British Journal of Healthcare Assistants. 10 (7), 332–335.

Berwick, D., 2013. A promise to learn – a commitment to act: improving the safety of patients in England. London: DH. https://www.gov.uk/government/publications/berwick-review-into-patient-safety.

Callwood, A., Cooke, D., Allan, H., 2016. Value-based recruitment in Midwifery; do the values align to what women say is important to them. J. Adv. Nurs. https://www.researchgate.net/publication/303828183_Value-based_recruitment_in_midwifery_do_the_values_align_with_what_women_say_is_important_to_them.

Cavendish, C., 2013. The Cavendish Review: An Independent Review into Healthcare Assistants and Support Workers in the NHS and Social Care Settings, https://www.gov.uk/government/publications/review-of-healthcare-assistants-and-support-workers-in-nhs-and-social-care.

Clarke, P., 2015. Communication skills required when working with older people. Working Papers in the Health Sciences 1:12. https://www.southampton.ac.uk/assets/centresresearch/documents/wphs/PC%20Communication%20skills%20required%20when%20working2.pdf.

Corcoran, N., 2013. Theories and models. In: Corcoran, N. (Ed.), Communicating Health: Strategies for Health Promotion, second ed. Sage Publications, pp. 5–28, (Chapter 1).

Darwin, C., 1872. The Expression of the Emotions in Man and Animals. John Murray, London.

Davey, N., Cole, A., 2015. Safe Communication: Design, implement and measure: A guide to improving transfers of care and handover. https://www.england.nhs.uk/signuptosafety/wp-content/uploads/sites/16/2015/09/safe-comms-design-implmnt-meas.pdf.

Department of Health, 2015. The NHS Constitution: The NHS belongs to us all. London, DH. https://www.gov.uk/government/publications/the-nhs-constitution-for-england/the-nhs-constitution-for-england.

Department of Health and NHS Commissioning Board, 2012. Compassion in practice – nursing, midwifery and care staff – our vision and strategy. London, DH. https://www.england.nhs.uk/wp-content/uploads/2012/12/compassion-in-practice.pdf.

Devito, J., 2013. Interpersonal Communication, thirteenth ed. Pearson.

Draper, P., Wray, J., Burley, S., 2013. Exploring nurses' use of language with older people. Nurs. Older People 25 (9), 18–23.

Droppa, M., Lee, H., 2014. Motivational Interviewing: a journey to improve health. Nursing 44 (3), 40–50.

Dyche, L., Epstein, R., 2011. Curiosity and Medical Education. https://www.researchgate.net/profile/Ronald_Epstein/

publication/51199054_Curiosity_and_medical_education/links/02e7e53226d01dc2b1000000.pdf.

Ekman, P., 1972. Universals and cultural differences in facial expressions of emotions. In: Cole, J. (Ed.), Nebraska Symposium on Motivation. University of Nebraska Press, Lincoln, NB, pp. 207–282. https://1ammce38pkj41n8xkp1iocwe-wpengine.netdna-ssl.com/wp-content/uploads/2013/07/Universals-And-Cultural-Differences-In-Facial-Expressions-Of.pdf.

Entwistle, F., 2013a. How Nurses can lead from the front line. Nurs. Times 109 (12), 15.

Entwistle, F., 2013b. Mandatory registration for healthcare assistants. Nurs. Times 19 (10), 17.

Entwistle, F., 2013c. Minimum training standards for HCAs. Nurs. Times 19 (17), 17.

Fallowfield, L., Jenkins, V., 2004. Communicating sad, bad and difficult news in medicine. Lancet 36, 312–319.

Francis, R., (2013). Report of the Mid Staffordshire NHS Foundation Trust Public Inquiry. London, The Stationery Office. http://www.midstaffspublicinquiry.com/report.

Grimsley, A., 2010. Vital Conversations: A Practical Approach to Handling Difficult Conversations, Managing Conflict, Giving Feedback and Influencing Difficult People, first ed. Barnes-Holland Publishing.

Hall, E.T., 1966. The Hidden Dimension. Doubleday Anchor Books, NY.

Hobson, P., 2012. Communication: making sense of what people with dementia say. British Journal of Healthcare Assistants 6 (7), 334–337.

Klonek, F., Kauffeld, S., 2015. Providing engineers with OARS and EARS: effects of a skills based vocational training in Motivational Interviewing for engineers in higher education. Higher Education, Skills and Work Based Learning 5 (2), 117–134.

Kourkouta, L., Papathanasiou, I., 2014. Communication in nursing practice. Mater. Sociomed. 26 (1), 65–67. https://www.ncbi.nlm.nih.gov/pmc/articles/PMC3990376/.

Lynall, A., 2012. 'It takes two to tango!' – communication skills for getting the best out of a consultation. British Journal of Healthcare Assistants 6 (1), 32–34.

McCabe, C., Timmons, F., 2013. Communication Skills for Nursing Practice, second ed. Palgrave Macmillan, Basingstoke.

Mehrabian, A., 1971. Silent Messages: Implicit Communications of Emotions and Attitudes. Wadsworth Publishing Company, Belmont.

Miller, W., Rollnick, S., 2012. Motivational Interviewing; Helping People Change, third ed. Guildford Press.

Munyisia, E., Yu, P., Hailey, D., 2011. How nursing staff spend their time on activities in a nursing home: an observational study. J. Adv. Nurs. 67 (9), 1908–1917.

Nursing and Midwifery Council, 2018. The Code. Professional Standards of Practice and Behaviour for Nurses, Midwives and Nursing Associates. London: NMC. https://www.nmc.org.uk/standards/code/.

Patton, B., Stone, D., Heen, S., 2010. Difficult Conversations; How to Discuss What Matters Most. Penguin, London.

Peplau, H., 1962. Interpersonal techniques: the crux of psychiatric nursing. Am. J. Nurs. 62 (6), 49.

Propp, K.M., Apker, J., Zabava Ford, W., et al., 2010. Meeting the complex needs of the health care team: identification of nurse-team communication practices perceived to enhance patient outcomes. Qual. Health Res. 20 (1), 15–28.

Rabow, M.W., McPhee, S.J., 1999. Beyond breaking bad news: how to help patients who suffer. West. J. Med. 171, 260–263.

Reid Searl, K., McAllister, M., Dwyer, T., et al., 2014. Little people, big lessons: an innovative strategy to develop interpersonal skills in undergraduate nursing students. Nurse Educ. Today 1201–1206.

Rezende, R.C., Oliveira, R.M.P., Aruujo, S.T.P., et al., 2015. Body language in healthcare: a contribution to nursing communication. Rev. Bras. Enferm. 68 (3), 430–436. http://www.scielo.br/pdf/reben/v68n3/en_0034-7167-reben-68-03-0490.pdf.

Roebuck, A., 2017. Rethinking Communication in Health and Social Care. Palgrave Macmillan.

Royal College of Nursing, 2013. Breaking bad news: supporting parents when they are told of their child's diagnosis. London, RCN publication.

Schein, E., 2013. Humble Inquiry: The Art of Asking Instead of Telling. Berrett-Koehler Publishers.

Scriven, A., 2010. Promoting Health: A Practical Guide, sixth ed. Bailliere Tindall.

Shannon, C.E., Weaver, W., 1948. A mathematical theory of communication. The Bell System Technical Journal 27, July, October. 379–423, 623–656.

Sharples, N., 2013. Relationship, helping and communication skills. In: Brooker, C., Waugh, A. (Eds.), Foundations of Nursing Practice: Fundamentals of Nursing Care, second ed. Mosby Elsevier, London.

Skills for Care and Skills for Health, 2013. Code of conduct for Healthcare Support Workers and Adult Social Care Workers. http://www.skillsforcare.org.uk/Standards-legislation/Code-of-Conduct/Code-of-Conduct.aspx.

Stonehouse, D., 2015. Professionalism and what it means for you. British Journal of Healthcare Assistants 9 (9), 455–457.

Stonehouse, D., 2016. HCAs and APs building a therapeutic relationship. British Journal of Healthcare Assistants 10 (9), 460–463.

Tregoning, C., 2015. Communication skills and enhancing clinical practice through reflective learning: a case study. British Journal of Healthcare Assistants 9 (2), 66–69.

Warnock, C., 2014. Breaking bad news: issues relating to nursing practice. Nurs. Stand. 28 (45), 51–58.

Widder, R., 2017. Learning to use motivational interviewing effectively; modules. J. Contin. Educ. Nurs. 48 (7), 312–319.

10

Taking a Patient History and Physical Examination

Ian Peate

OBJECTIVES

By the end of the chapter the reader will be able to:

1. Understand the importance of communicating effectively in order to obtain a patient history and to carry out a physical examination
2. Be aware of the knowledge and skills needed to gather information and use the data in a meaningful manner
3. Describe the key components of history-taking
4. Discuss the various activities that need to be carried out in order to undertake a systematic physical examination
5. Understand the need for sensitivity when taking a patient history and undertaking a physical examination
6. Appreciate the role and function of the Nursing Associate (NA) during history-taking and physical examination

KEY WORDS

Therapeutic
Communication
Diagnosis
Prognosis

Syndrome
Respect
Signs
Symptoms

Cues
Lifestyle

CHAPTER AIMS

The chapter aims to introduce the reader to the key skills, knowledge and attitudes required to undertake a patient history and physical examination in a holistic, safe and sensitive manner.

SELF TEST

1. What is the basis of a true patient history?
2. What is said to be at the heart of good history-taking?
3. Describe therapeutic touch.
4. How might you facilitate establishing rapport with patients?
5. What is active listening?
6. Differentiate between signs and symptoms.
7. How might you display a non-judgemental attitude when taking a patient history?
8. How can you ensure that the patient is at the centre of all that is done?
9. As a Nursing Associate you must be aware of your own personal attitudes, values and ethical viewpoints; how do you ensure you do this when taking a patient history?
10. Distinguish between acute and chronic conditions.

INTRODUCTION

The skills needed to take a patient's history effectively and to undertake a physical examination competently require the Nursing Associate (NA) to use all of their senses to 'listen'. The patient must be given permission to tell you their story freely and they must never feel as if you are judging them or the lifestyle they have chosen. When asking questions, try to keep them as open as possible. Constantly check your understanding with the patient. Always keep an open mind and always ask yourself if you are making assumptions, and if so, be aware of this. It is essential that you are prepared to reconsider the causes of symptoms that you may have decided upon.

CRITICAL AWARENESS

You must demonstrate a commitment to patient-centred care, showing a non-judgmental attitude, promoting equality and respecting diversity.

The NA must have an understanding of anatomy, physiology and pathophysiology prior to commencing history-taking and physical examination.

SIGNS AND SYMPTOMS

Often the terms 'signs' and 'symptoms' are used interchangeably; however, there is a difference between the two. Any *objective* evidence of disease, such as a skin rash, for example, is a *sign*. *Subjective* data that the patient tells the NA about, such as fatigue or lower back pain, is a *symptom*; we only know about these symptoms if the patient tells us.

Symptoms are something that the patient feels or observes themselves that they regard as abnormal, such as pain, diarrhoea, vomiting or diminishing eyesight. Symptoms are discovered by taking a 'history'; this means questioning a person – having a dialogue between the NA and the patient. A headache or hallucinations can only be experienced by the person; they cannot be observed by others and are therefore symptoms.

Signs are physical or functional abnormalities that are obtained by undertaking a physical examination, such as tenderness, a wheeze heard when listening to the patient's chest (auscultation), a swelling felt by palpation. Taking a patient's blood pressure is a sign as this is an objective measurement.

A skin rash can be considered both a sign and a symptom: the rash is observable, therefore, it is a sign, but the patient may itch because of the rash and this is a symptom. Hypertension (high blood pressure) may be a sign and as a result of the hypertension the patient may have a headache – a symptom of the hypertension.

ACUTE AND CHRONIC CONDITIONS

To determine if a patient has an acute or a chronic condition the NA is required to obtain a full history from the patient. There are increasing numbers of people living with chronic (long-term) conditions in the UK. The number of people in England with one or more long-term condition is 15 million and this is projected to increase to around 18 million by 2025 (House of Commons Health Committee, 2014).

Chronic condition and acute condition are often considered to be at the opposite ends of the spectrum (see Fig. 10.1). Those with a chronic long-term condition may experience acute exacerbations of their illness and this can require admission to acute hospital services. Patients with chronic conditions may also experience acute conditions that are unrelated to their chronic condition. Distinguishing between acute and chronic conditions is important so that appropriate care plans are put in place to address individual care needs. This can only be achieved if the NA gathers the correct information when obtaining a patient history.

Acute conditions

These conditions are severe and sudden in onset; they usually have a relatively brief duration, such as fractured bone or an acute asthmatic attack. Acute conditions can be minor or serious and many people with an acute illness often present in general practice. Patients with these conditions requiring short-term medical or surgical management are often cared for in an acute hospital.

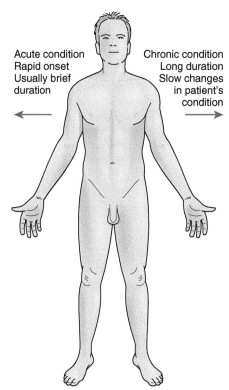

Fig. 10.1 The Acute–Chronic Continuum (Modified from Waugh & Grant, 2018).

Chronic conditions

Chronic conditions can be seen as a long-term developing syndrome, such as osteoporosis or chronic obstructive pulmonary disease (COPD). A disease is a collection of signs and symptoms that characterizes a particular condition. A syndrome is a combination of symptoms and/or signs that usually occur together, for example malabsorption syndrome. This syndrome consists of chronic diarrhoea with fatty stools and multiple nutritional deficiencies. A syndrome can produce a number of signs and symptoms.

In practice, the link between acute and chronic illness is not always obvious.

CASE STUDY 10.1   Mrs Rawal

Mrs Rawal, aged 86, is admitted to the surgical admissions unit. She has fallen at home and sustained a fracture of the mid shaft of her right femur and mid shaft right humerus. Mrs Rawal also has COPD and has a worsening cough, alongside an increase in volume of her respiratory secretions. Mrs Rawal also takes medication for depression.

REFLECTION 10.1

Consider Mrs Rawal in Case Study 10.1. She has a significant acute illness, as well as chronic illnesses. Now reflect on the following points:
- What is the acute illness?
- What are the chronic illnesses?
- Where does Mrs Rawal need to be nursed?
- What is the focus of care?
- How can you ensure Mrs Rawal is at the centre of all that is done?

AT THE GP SURGERY

Minor acute illnesses that present at the GP surgery include some of the commonest problems seen in general practice, for example, upper respiratory tract infections; ear, nose or throat infections; muscular skeletal conditions; or skin rashes.

Major acute illnesses may also present as an acute exacerbation (a worsening) of an underlying chronic illness, for example, myocardial infarction or diabetic coma, or the sudden onset of a previously undiagnosed condition, like epilepsy or stroke or an acute emotional or psychological problem.

CARE IN THE HOME SETTING

Chronic illness represents a significant challenge for the NHS. There is a growing trend to care for people with long-term conditions in community settings. To do this effectively requires a significant new way of thinking with regard to the way care is delivered, moving away from care delivered in a hospital setting, and towards a community-based, responsive, adaptable, flexible service. This involves far more than simply changing the location where care is delivered; it requires a significant whole-system change. Chronic disease management in the home setting provides the NA and other healthcare providers with opportunities for improvements in patient care and service quality as well as a reduction in costs.

DIAGNOSIS AND PROGNOSIS

The majority of diagnoses are made on history alone, recognizing patterns of symptoms (Snadden et al., 2013), with 5%–10% being made on examination, and the rest on investigation. A diagnosis occurs when the data the patient provides is translated into the name of the disease. Diagnosis can also have the effect of labelling people, as well as classifying their illness, and because of this can determine how a patient is treated. Taking histories and performing examinations in a competent and skilful manner is fundamental to clinical practice and effective diagnosis.

Diagnosis

Diagnosis is revealed in the patient's history, by listening to the patient's story. A good history is one that reveals the patient's ideas, concerns and expectations, as well as any associated diagnosis. Often it is the history alone that uncovers a diagnosis; sometimes, this is all that is required. A complete description will involve a knowledge of the causation (aetiology), as well as any anatomical and functional changes that are present. The NA gathers of all the relevant facts concerning the past and present history of the illness, along with the patient's condition as revealed by a full clinical examination.

Differential diagnosis

Differential diagnosis is the process of weighing the probability of one disease versus that of other diseases that could possibly account for a patient's illness. The differential diagnosis for depression can include a wide variety of medical disorders, for example:
- Central nervous system diseases (Parkinson's disease, dementia, multiple sclerosis, neoplastic lesions)
- Endocrine disorders (hyperthyroidism, hypothyroidism)
- Drug-related conditions (cocaine abuse, side effects of some CNS depressants)
- Infectious disease (mononucleosis)
- Sleep-related disorders.

Drake (2012) notes that a final differential diagnosis involves making 'best match' of the signs and symptoms aligned to the pathophysiological possibilities. He gives an example: backache and haematuria is a classic presentation of renal cell carcinoma in a middle aged or elderly patient; however, this diagnosis would be improbable in a 25-year-old.

Prognosis

Prognosis is a prediction of the chance of recovery or survival from a disease. A prognosis is based on statistics from studies on the general population of how a disease acts. Prognosis can vary for any single disease. For example, with lung cancer it depends on a number of factors, such as the stage of disease at diagnosis, the type of lung cancer and gender. Prognosis is different for every person. Important differences that affect prognosis include age, general health, the presence of co-existing medical conditions and the patient's ability to tolerate treatment.

COMMUNITIES OF CARE
Children

Children's ability to communicate is dependent on age and development. For example, the neonate's subtle signals may only be sensed by its mother, yet the teenager is usually able to communicate as an adult. From around 3 years of age, the child is capable of complex thought structures. The NA should never assume that the child's account will have any less credence than the adult's. The NA should introduce themselves to the child and ask how the child prefers to be addressed. Eye contact is reassuring for an older child but not for younger ones. Ensure you have toys available for the child throughout the consultation. If with their family, note how the child is interacting with parents, carers and siblings. Make sure you know what prompted the referral and what the parent or the carer thinks is wrong with the child.

CHAPERONE

Prior to undertaking a history and performing a physical examination, the patient should be offered a chaperone (an impartial observer). This applies even if the NA is the same gender as the patient. A chaperone is a third person who is usually of the same sex as the patient and usually a healthcare professional (Davey, 2014). The chaperone will be present during an examination and this must be provided irrespective of any organizational constraints or settings.

A relative or friend of the patient is not an impartial observer, and as such, would not normally be seen as a suitable chaperone. However, the NA should fulfil a reasonable request to have such a person present as well as a chaperone. The healthcare professional chaperone can act as advocate for the patient, providing an explanation of what will happen during the examination, as well as providing the patient with reasons why. The chaperone is well placed to assess the patient's understanding of what has been said to them, as well as providing a reassuring presence whilst the person is having the examination, safeguarding against any unnecessary discomfort, pain, humiliation or intimidation.

❗ HOTSPOT

Record any discussion about chaperones and the outcome in the patients' medical records or notes. If a chaperone is present, make a record of that fact and make a note of their identity. If the patient did not want a chaperone, record that the offer was made and declined.

INTERPRETERS

Interpretation is the oral transmission of meaning from one language to another. In face-to-face interpreting, the interpreter acts as a language transmitter between the health professional and the patient, aiding communication where a language barrier exists.

The use of a professional interpreter can help in taking a history and when performing an examination. The use of professional interpreters can also enhance the quality of care (Kaur, Oakley & Venn, 2014). Choosing an appropriate interpreter requires much thought. They need not only to be fluent in English and the identified other language, but in some cases also the same dialect as the patient. They must also be trained in specialist terminology and understand the health service; this can help to ensure accurate communication. Professional interpreters are trained in interpreting techniques, managing three-way communication and the interview process. There are many issues that a patient may be unwilling or unable to disclose in front of a partner, friend or family member; this should be acknowledged, respected and understood by the interpreter.

Using an independent professional interpreter will encourage a full, frank and honest discussion. Professional interpreters can encourage the patient to actively ask questions (active participation) ensuring they have a full understanding of their diagnosis and, if appropriate, the proposed course of treatment.

A family member, carer, friend or member of staff may act as interpreter; however, there a number of issues that should be given consideration. It may be hard for them to remain neutral because they are a relative or a fellow healthcare professional. Professional interpreters have no such conflict. Family members or friends may not have the same level of expertise in both languages or in specialist terminology. They are unlikely to have all the skills that professional interpreters are trained in. Their presence could have an impact on the patient's right to privacy and confidentiality; this may also deter the patient from expressing themselves fully and freely (Talley & O'Connor, 2014).

COMMUNITIES OF CARE

Deaf People

A qualified British Sign Language (BSL) interpreter should be used in any situation where complex and/or technical information needs to be communicated, such as in formal consultation with health and social care staff. Qualified and accredited interpreters minimize the risk of misunderstanding; they are also bound by a professional code of practice that addresses the issue of confidentiality. The patient, family member or friend who is deaf may request an interpreter, or when the healthcare provider becomes aware that the patient is deaf, an interpreter can be contracted.

Sign language interpreters are necessary in any situation where information is being exchanged and this requires effective communication. This will include, but is not limited to:

- Taking a patient's medical history
- Giving diagnoses
- Performing medical procedures
- Explaining treatment planning
- Explaining medicine prescription and regimen
- Providing patient education or counselling
- Describing discharge and follow up plans
- Admitting to emergency departments/urgent care.

Makaton is another type of communication system that may also be used.

HISTORY-TAKING

History-taking is a part of the consultation; it does not exist in isolation. This essential activity requires effective communication skills to gather information about the patient. It is the most important component of any clinical encounter. The ability to take a clinical history is central to developing and establishing an effective relationship with the patient. The process is about collaboration and consultation, as well ensuring a holistic approach.

Blainey (2014) suggests a systematic approach as used in several professions:
- Presenting complaint
- History of presenting complaint
- Past medical history
- Drug history
- Family history
- Social history
- Systems enquiry

A focused approach is required, and although the particular history-taking framework can differ between professional groups, the skills required for effective history-taking are shared by all healthcare professions.

Obtaining a patient history is more than the gathering of information. If it is carried out in an effective manner, it has the potential to reveal the nature and extent of the problem that the person is experiencing, the background to the problem and the impact the problem is having, as well as the patient's concerns, ideas and expectations. It is important, therefore, to have structure and order, in the form of a framework, to guide the process.

History-taking will ultimately rely on the NA's communication skills. When these are applied in the right way and in accordance with the context, it can result in a successful encounter for both patient and NA. Employing effective communication skills will enable the patient to tell the story of their illness and articulate their needs. When the patient is unable to provide their own history (the primary source), key information will need to be gathered from other sources (secondary sources), such as records, relatives, or other healthcare staff.

The reason for taking a history needs to be clear; for example, it may be that you are trying to make a diagnosis, or determine a patient's fitness for surgery. See Box 10.1 for some reasons why a patient's history may be taken.

The history reveals many things, including the patient's subjective experience of their condition and the impact this is having on their life. The physical examination and any investigations

BOX 10.1 Some Reasons Why a Patient History May Need to be Taken

- Establish the system(s) that are responsible for the symptom(s)
- Make a diagnosis
- Identify a differential diagnosis
- Gather data about the patient's health status
- Explain the cause(s) of the disease process
- Determine fitness to undergo an anaesthetic for surgery
- Understand the patient's individual circumstances, concerns, aspirations, expectations and beliefs

that follow will help to confirm or contest the differential diagnosis that has been made based on the history. In an acute illness or life-threatening situation, physical assessment skills will be paramount: recognizing and interpreting clinical signs will be a priority.

Taking a history

The NA needs to be fully prepared. If possible, review the patient's health records before seeing them. This may give some idea of their past medical history and provide some insight into the patient's presenting condition.

There are two aspects associated with the history:
1. Getting to know the patient and their medical background
2. Getting to know the condition – the presenting problem.

COMMUNITIES OF CARE

The Older Adult

Extra time should be scheduled into a consultation with a patient who is older. An older patent who is ill may be slower in their responses. They may also have a sensory impairment, such as hearing loss, or cognitive problems, such as dementia. They are also likely to have a longer health history than a younger person.

Environment

The choice of environment where the history-taking is to take place may already be set. For example, in a hospital setting it might be at the patient's bed where privacy is difficult as the only physical barrier between patients are curtains. You should also consider ambient noise. Explain to the patient if you are in a hospital setting that the conversation may be overheard and you are aware that they may not wish to give answers to sensitive questions.

The environment can also have an impact on undertaking a physical examination. You should always be sensitive to dignity and patient privacy.

History-taking and physical examination can be an exhausting experience for the patient. Prior to taking a history or undertaking a physical examination, it is essential to ask if the patient is able and willing to cooperate. It is essential that the patient's comfort is kept in mind throughout the process.

CRITICAL AWARENESS

Clear, sensitive and effective communication with the patient and their advocates is essential for a successful consultation.

Frameworks

The content of the history needed to arrive at a diagnosis in a health and social care setting will depend on:
- The presenting symptoms
- The patient's concerns
- The past medical, psychological and social history.

A general framework suggested for history-taking can be found in Box 10.2.

De Wit et al. (2017) provide a focused assessment framework that is traditionally used by staff who adopt a psychosocial or

BOX 10.2 A Suggested Framework for History-Taking

- Presenting complaint.
- History of presenting complaint, including investigations, treatment and referrals already arranged and provided.
- Past medical history: significant past diseases/illnesses, surgery, including complications, trauma.
- Drug history: now and past, prescribed and over-the-counter, allergies.
- Family history: especially parents, siblings and children.
- Social history: smoking, alcohol, drugs, accommodation and living arrangements, marital status, baseline functioning, occupation, pets and hobbies.
- Systems review: cardiovascular system, respiratory system, gastrointestinal system, nervous system, musculoskeletal system, genitourinary system.

TABLE 10.1 Aspects of the Focused Assessment (Adapted from de Wit et al., 2017)

Aspects of the framework	Description
Social assessment	• Patient identification, gender, age, occupation • Social support (family friends) • Mobility • Services accessed in the community (such as home help)
Physical assessment	• Reason for admission • Current health problems • Current consultations with other healthcare professionals, for example, therapists, doctors
Review of systems	• Head and neck • Chest • Abdominal • Genitourinary • Extremities and musculoskeletal systems
Psychological assessment	• Experience of depression, anxiety, other mental health concerns • Unusual memory problems • Difficulty with cognition
Current mediations	• Prescribed medication and reasons for taking them • Over-the-counter medications and reason for taking them

humanistic approach to history-taking. This is primarily aimed at identifying problems and needs (see Table 10.1).

Taking a history from a patient tests your communication skills and your understanding about what to ask. Specific questions will vary depending on the type of history you are taking; however, the general framework in Box 10.2 is a good basis to follow. Remember that you may need to gather a collateral history from a relative, friend or carer – for instance if you are with a child, or an adult who is unconscious.

The presenting complaint

As early as possible, identify the reason the patient is presenting. Was there a trigger? This is what the patient tells you is wrong. The presenting condition should be given briefly and as far as possible in the patient's own words. For example, 'water-work problems'. Note the duration of the presenting problem in hours, days, months or years – do not note 'since Monday'. If there is more than one presenting complaint, list in order of importance.

History of presenting complaint

You should gain as much information you can about the patient's specific complaint. If the presenting compliant is dysuria (difficulty in passing urine), for instance, use the mnemonic SOCRATES:

Site: Where exactly is the pain?

Onset: When did it start, was it constant/intermittent, gradual/sudden?

Character: What is the pain like, e.g., sharp, burning?

Radiation: Does it radiate/move anywhere?

Associations: Is there anything else associated with the pain, e.g., sweating, vomiting?

Time course: Does it follow any time pattern, how long does it last?

Exacerbating/relieving factors: Does anything make it better or worse?

Severity: How severe is the pain, (using a pain score, e.g., the 1–10 scale)?

Past medical history

Ask and gather information about the patient's other medical problems, if they have any. Ask about illnesses and determine dates, ask about childhood infections, any tropical infections, hypertension (high blood pressure), diabetes, tuberculosis (TB), jaundice and epilepsy – note if absent. Has the patient had any operations or injuries and if so, when. Are there any ongoing issues? Is their vaccination regimen up to date? For women, obtain an obstetric and menstrual history.

Drug history

Determine what medications the patient is taking: are they over-the-counter or prescribed? List medications accurately, find out about dosage and how often the patient is taking them, for example once-a-day, twice-a-day. What are they taking them for? At this point, it is a good idea to find out if the patient has any allergies or adverse drug reactions. Ask the patient about recreational drug use.

Family history

Gather information about the patient's family history, such as diabetes or cardiac history. Find out if there are any genetic conditions within the family, e.g., polycystic kidney disease. Are there any similar or serious illnesses in parents, grandparents, siblings? Note the age of family members who have died and cause of death.

Social history

This gives you the chance to find out more about the patient's background: is the patient employed, what work do they do? Enquire about smoking (current or ex-smoker – cigarettes, pipe, cigars), ask about alcohol, history of alcohol intake, how much consumed, when they drink, what type of alcohol. If not already asked, enquire if the patient uses any illegal substances, such as cannabis or cocaine. Where does the patient live, what kind of property, do they have to climb stairs? Who lives with the patient? Are they a carer for an elderly parent or a child?

The following LOST mnemonic can be used when gathering a social history:

Living situation: house/flat/nursing home, who is at home, dependants, carers, coping with activities of living

Occupation

Smoking and alcohol: cigarettes, cigars, pipe, how many, how often, calculate units of alcohol per week, recreational drug use

Travel: recent travel

APPLYING COMMUNICATION AND CONSULTATION SKILLS

Chapter 9 deals in depth with the important issue of effective communication. Remember that in patient-healthcare worker interactions, communication is both verbal and non-verbal. Your style, your posture, your physical position (distance) with regard to the patient and your body language all contribute to the outcome of the interaction. You should be relaxed and aim to radiate confidence with a smile and a greeting. The opening greeting should be given much consideration as this can encourage or inhibit rapport. Aim to have good eye contact, shake hands (the handshake can provide diagnostic clues; see Table 10.2) with the patient and show an active interest in them. This can help to create trust and encourage honest, open and effective communication.

You may need to offer an apology if the patient has been kept waiting. By doing this you are showing respect to the person. Try to avoid writing as the patient provides you with their story.

TABLE 10.2 The Handshake (Adapted from Douglas & Bevan, 2013)

Features	Potential diagnosis
Cold, sweaty hands	Anxiety
Cold, dry hands	Raynaud phenomenon (a condition that affects the blood supply to certain parts of the body – fingers and toes)
Hot, sweaty hands	Hyperthyroidism (overactive thyroid)
Large, fleshy, sweaty hands	Acromegaly (a condition in which the body produces too much growth hormone, leading to the excess growth of body tissues)
Dry, coarse skin	Regular exposure to water
	Manual occupation
	Hypothyroidism (underactive thyroid)
Delayed relaxation of grip	Myotonic dystrophy (an inherited genetic condition gradually causes muscles to weaken, leads to an increasing degree of disability)
Deformed hands/ fingers	Trauma
	Dupuytren contracture (condition affects the hands and fingers, causes one or more fingers to bend into the palm of the hand)
	Rheumatoid arthritis

If you do need to write things down, explain this to the patient, and state what sort of thing you are writing, in order for them to understand that you are still listening to them.

Be aware that patients vary in how they present; many of them will be anxious. This can manifest in a number of ways, for example:

- The quiet patient who may only provide monosyllabic answers (you may need use direct questioning)
- The patient who comes across as being over-confident
- The patient who is annoyed at having to wait for the appointment
- The patient who has been in the waiting room for a while, giving them time to mull over the worst or become angry
- The patient who requires much reassurance.

Listen fully and permit the patient to tell you the story that they have been storing up; use all of your senses to listen. This can be encouraged by active listening, demonstrating interest and being attentive to the patient. Provide the patient with an opportunity to tell you the narrative that they have prepared. By doing this you will have a better chance of understanding the patient's true perception of their experience of an illness, when it developed (the onset) and the importance to the patient of the symptoms they have (this provides you with their perspective).

Note and record each of the major symptoms in the order that the patient presents them to you. Then refer back to this initial picture and break down any further aspects of the history that you need. Some patients do not come readily prepared with a narrative of their illness, and in this situation, it is unavoidable to use questioning and clarification to 'draw out' the history. However, if your prompting sparks off a narrative, then try to hear it out if it seems to be relevant.

If appropriate, you should make full use of any communication aids available to you such as translators, sign language interpreters, picture boards and drawings done by the patient showing what and where the signs and symptoms are.

A good history-taking exercise is one where the patient has revealed their thoughts, concerns and expectations, as well as any associated diagnosis. You should not dominate the history-taking event with a list of questions that you want answered; listening is at the centre of good history-taking. The history is likely to be much less informative and less useful if you do not seek the patient's viewpoint. Respond to the patient's needs; for example, if the patient appears to be experiencing discomfort, is tired, or seems to be in pain, then acknowledge this and respond appropriately, you should not simply continue.

It takes practice to obtain a full and meaningful history, and the NA has to work hard to focus and concentrate on what is being said and what is not being said. The skills required to obtain the patient's true story can be learned; this goes beyond knowing what questions to ask.

Types of questions

Open-ended questions

These are the gold standard questions of historical enquiry. They do not suggest a 'right' answer – they give the patient a chance to express what is on their mind. The use of open-ended questioning is discussed further in Chapter 9.

Questions with options

It may be necessary on occasion to 'pin down' exactly what it is that a patient means by a particular statement. If this is the case, and you cannot obtain the information you are seeking through the use of open-ended questioning, then consider offering the patient some options to indicate what information it is that you need. For example, if a female patient complains of 'passing blood' and it is difficult to determine what it is she means, even after you have provided an opportunity to expand on the subject, ask: 'Is that in your water or your motions?' Caution must be used with this approach as there is a danger of getting the answer that you wanted as opposed to what it is the patient means (she might in this case be referring to the passing of blood vaginally).

Leading questions

A leading question is one that assumes the answer; for example, 'You didn't finish the course of antibiotics prescribed, did you?' As opposed to 'Did you finish the course of antibiotics prescribed?' In the first question an assumption is being made: that the patient did not finish the antibiotics and this leads the patient to give a specific answer. In the second example, no assumptions are made about whether or not the patient finished the antibiotics. This approach is more likely to yield a true response. It is easy to ask a leading question without being aware of it, and this is particularly so if we think we know what the answer will be. Leading questions presume knowledge about something that is not known and are inclined to lead the patient down a path that is framed by your own assumptions. It is preferable to ask an open question.

CASE STUDY 10.2   OLDCARTS

Karl Sanofi, 36 years old, is at the GP surgery. He is complaining of pain in his left foot. The pain started 2 weeks ago when he was at the beach. Karl describes this as a severe burning pain on the outside heel of this left foot. His pain is worse in the morning and when he walks barefoot. When he applies ice to his foot, his pain improves. Karl informs the NA that he has been taking paracetamol twice a day. The pain lasts for around 2 to 3 hours in the morning and after he is up and about walking it tends to subside.

Based on the history above, identify each of the characteristics that Karl describes using the mnemonic OLDCARTS

Onset
Location
Duration
Characteristics
Aggravating factors
Relieving factors
Timing
Severity

Adapted from Ball et al. (2015)

Recapping

Recapping or summarizing occurs after the history has been taken. It is beneficial to provide the patient with a run-down of what they have told you as far as you understand it. For example: 'So, Marcia, from what I understand you have been gaining weight, feeling sick and have had trouble when swallowing – particularly

OSCE 10.1

INSTRUCTIONS: Look at the following questions and provide the examiner with the answers in a more appropriate form.

You have 4 minutes to complete the exercise. You are marked out of 10. Only move on to the next station when told.

1. *And you have never experienced any kind of illness like this before?*
   Better expressed as:

/Mark

2. *There is no history of dementia in your family, is there?*
   Better expressed as:

/Mark

3. *Do you really think this is related to your headaches?*
   Better expressed as:

/Mark

4. *How much pain are you experiencing?*
   Better expressed as:

/Mark

5. *How often have you had unsafe sex?*
   Better expressed as:

/Mark

6. *How often do you smoke?*
   Better expressed as:

/Mark

7. *And you do not have diabetes or asthma?*
   Better expressed as:

/Mark

8. *What else are you concerned about?*
   Better expressed as:

/Mark

9. *You don't have any other problems, do you?*
   Better expressed as:

/Mark

10. *And you have no allergies?*
    Better expressed as:

/Mark

Marks out of ten:
/10

Suggested answers
1. Have you ever experienced anything like this before?
2. Is there any history of dementia in your family?
3. Why do you think this is related to your headaches?
4. Are you in any pain?
5. Have you ever had unsafe sex?
6. Do you smoke?
7. Do you have diabetes or asthma?
8. Are you concerned about anything else?
9. Do you have any other problems?
10. Are you allergic to anything?

---

late at night, and you feel that the whole situation is getting you down. Is that correct?'. If Marcia provides a nod of approval or she expresses agreement with the story, then you can be certain that you are getting what it is that Marcia wants to tell you. Equally, it gives her an opportunity to correct or add anything. Using this recapping technique can help avoid misinterpretation and incorrect assumptions, offering you a chance to correct those misunderstandings.

Concluding the history

End the history-taking session by asking the patient if there is anything they want to add, ask you or share with you. This can help you to provide further information if there is something that they have not understood and it may also uncover something that has been troubling them that has not yet been touched upon. It provides a chance to confirm that a shared understanding has been achieved between the NA and patient. You should always keep an open mind and check that you are not making assumptions. Check that what you think is wrong with the patient is what the patient thinks is what is wrong with them.

BOX 10.3 Ending the Consultation

- When the history-taking has been completed, inform the patient of this and that you have addressed everything that you need to.
- Ensure that the patient has nothing more to add.
- Recap the information and check it is complete and accurate.
- Provide an explanation of what will happen next.
- Thank the patient.

! HOTSPOT

It is important at the end of the consultation to let the patient know what will happen next.

See Box 10.3: Ending the consultation.

THE PHYSICAL EXAMINATION

The physical examination is a key part of a continuum that usually occurs after the history-taking of the present illness and

OSCE 10.2

INSTRUCTIONS: In this OSCE you are required to demonstrate that you are able to use a general framework in order to gain good marks. You are marked on your ability to explain to the examiner the various aspects of the history-taking, below.

Look at the framework and provide the examiner with the answers. You have 4 minutes to complete the exercise; you are marked out of 30. Only move on to the next station when told.

Introduce self

(Introduces self, gains consent, asks the patient's permission to take notes.)

Marks
/2

Present compliant

(Listens to what the patient says is wrong with them.)

Marks
/2

History of presenting complaint

(Gains as much information about the specific complaint.)
Uses the SOCRATES acronym.

S
O
C
R
A
T
E
S

Marks
/4

Past medical history

(Gathers information about the patient's other medical problems (if they have any).)

Marks
/2

Drug history

(Finds out what medications the patient is taking: dosage, frequency, reason for taking them. Identifies if the patient has any allergies.)

Marks
/2

Family history

(Gathers information about the patient's family history. Finds out if there are any genetic conditions within the family.)

Marks
/2

Social history

(Finds out more about the patient's background, also asks about smoking and alcohol. Asks the patient if they use any illegal substances. Also finds out who lives with the patient.)

Marks
/2

Review of systems

(Gathers a small amount of information regarding the other systems if not covered in history of presenting complaint. Is able to discuss the three main systems.)

Marks
/8

Summary of history

(Completes history, reviews what the patient has said. Repeats back the important points so patient can make any corrections, rectify any misunderstandings or errors.)

Marks
/2

Patient question feedback

(Determines if the patient has questions that they want to ask. Refers as necessary.)

Marks
/2

Ends consultation

(Thanks patient for their time and explains next steps.)

Marks
/2

Marks out of thirty:
/30

---

before the therapeutic outcome. The examination should proceed in an orderly fashion. Just like history-taking, the physical examination should adopt a directed systematic approach based on what has been obtained from the history itself (Donald et al., 2014). An overview of a routine approach will be discussed here. However, the examination process will be dictated by patient needs. It should be flexible, as some systems may need to be examined in more detail than others

As is the case with history-taking, the NA is required to exhibit exemplary communication skills in a physical examination. When the history is being taken, much information (clues) will be amassed regarding the patient, their education and their social background. There will also be physical signs to pick up on. Good technique includes using this information to inform the examination in order to yield a correct result.

Observation prior to the laying on of hands is essential. Florence Nightingale wrote that observation was the best skill that a nurse can possess – the same could be said of the NA: the first part of the physical examination is to observe.

Preparation and the optimal environment

The patient should be comfortable and warm and their dignity protected. Ensure that the patient is in a relaxed position, is wearing a gown if needed or draped correctly, avoid any unnecessary exposure. Seek permission prior to touching the patient. The examination surface should be at a height that is appropriate for the examiner; a step should be provide for the patient to get on to it. Light sources and curtains should be arranged in such a way they are suitable for the examination. Try to eliminate any distractions, such as mobile telephones, laptops, television sets, radios and other noise.

COMMUNITIES OF CARE
Children

Whenever possible, parents should always be present when children are examined.

A chaperone should be offered and the decision documented. Determine if a translator is required. Equipment required will be determined by patient needs.

! HOTSPOT

Collect all the equipment you need prior to commencing the examination.

Take vital signs and observe the patient. You can obtain valuable information from the facies (facial expression), skin colouration, gait, handshake and personal hygiene (this may be related to physical, psychological and social background). Document your initial observations. Evaluate the radial pulse, noting rate and rhythm. Measure brachial blood pressure. Measure height and weight. Inspect the patient's nails, skin and hair. Note the general appearance, body habitus (general constitution, physical build), distribution of hair, muscle mass, coordination, odours and breathing pattern.

An overview of the review of systems

The systems to be reviewed will be determined by the patient's needs. It is not always necessary or appropriate to review all systems. The NA may need to seek advice or be provided with instructions regarding the systems to be examined. This section of the chapter provides a brief overview of the following (see Fig. 10.2):
- Head and neck
- Lungs
- Cardiovascular
- Abdomen.

More detailed information regarding the various systems can be found in other textbooks as well by observing other health and social care practitioners at work.

Examination should always be carried out in a respectful and gentle manner. The NA will develop skills with practice enabling the identification of any deviations from normal. The following four components (skills) will need to be developed:
- Inspection
- Auscultation
- Palpation
- Percussion.

You must ensure that you record all findings as per local policy and procedure.

Inspection

Inspection requires visual examination; for example, when examining the abdomen, note should be made of the shape, the presence of any skin abnormalities, abdominal masses and the movement of the abdominal wall with respiration. Abnormalities that have been detected on inspection can provide clues to abnormal pathology; these can then be further investigated with auscultation, palpation and percussion if appropriate.

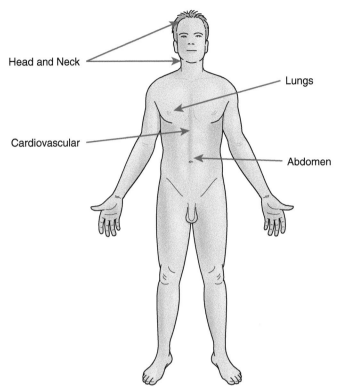

Fig. 10.2 Review of the Systems.

Auscultation

'Auscultation' is the term for using a stethoscope to listen to the sounds inside the body; for example, the heart, lungs and abdomen (gastrointestinal tract). The stethoscope is placed on bare skin, and the NA listens to the specific area of the body under examination. This test poses no risks or side effects.

Palpation

This concerns feeling; for example, placing the fingers over an artery to measure a person's pulse. The NA can palpate abnormalities with the pulse and plan care accordingly. Palpation of the abdominal wall can help to detect abdominal tenderness or the presence of abdominal masses (see Fig. 10.3). It is also possible for the liver and kidneys to be palpated.

Percussion

Percussion involves the skilled tapping of the fingers on various parts of the body, for example, the abdomen. Percussion is used to listen for sounds based on the organs or body parts underneath the skin. Hollow sounds are heard during percussion of body parts filled with air (for example, the lungs) and much duller sounds above an organ, such as the liver, or bodily fluids (for example, the urinary bladder) (see Fig. 10.4).

Head and neck

Examination of the head and neck includes assessment of:
- Head
- Eyes
- Ears

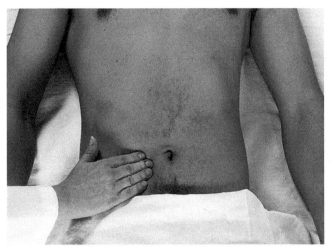

Fig. 10.3 Technique for Palpation (Williams, 2018) (From Potter, PA, Perry AG, Stockert P, & Hall A: Fundamentals of Nursing, eighth ed., Mosby, St Louis; 2014).

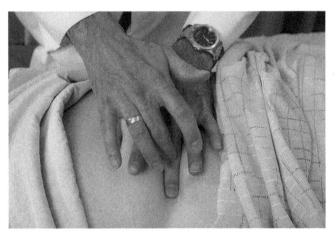

Fig. 10.4 Technique for Percussion (Williams, 2018).

- Nose
- Mouth
- Sinuses.

The face is inspected for symmetry, smile, frown and jaw movement which can provide information about nerve abnormalities. Head tilting towards one side may indicate hearing loss in that ear.

Opening the mouth provides the NA with a view of the patient's tonsils, dentition (decay, repair and bite), tongue and gums. Observe the lips for colour.

Inspect and examine the conjunctiva, sclera, cornea and iris of each eye. Test pupils for irregularity, accommodation and reaction using a pen torch. Evaluate visual fields and visual acuity as per your organization's policy.

Inspect and examine the ears, note the patient's responses to questions being asked, determine if a hearing aid is present. Examine the pinnae and periauricular tissues.

Inspect the nose externally, observe for skin colour, shape, symmetry. Note any deformity, inflammation, discharge, swelling or presence of bleeding. Examine the nares; if the person has a nasogastric tube in situ, inspect the nares for any signs of excoriation, inflammation or discharge. Use a pen torch to do the inspection; if needed stabilize the tube.

The head and face contain a number of sinuses; these are open cavities that communicate with the upper airway. The sinuses are inspected using palpation and percussion. Directly palpate and percuss the skin overlying the frontal and maxillary sinuses. If there is pain, this may suggest underlying inflammation.

Inspect and palpate the neck. Ask the patient to flex and hyperextend the neck, turning the head from side to side. This can detect any muscle weakness, strain and the range of movement. Lymph nodes are inspected with the patient tilting the head slightly; palpate the lymph nodes of the head and neck gently and note if the lymph nodes are enlarged, tender, inflamed or fixed as this may indicate local infection, systemic disease or neoplasm.

Lungs

Use inspection, palpation, percussion and auscultation. Alteration in respiratory function can be life threatening.

Observe the patient on first meeting for signs of cyanosis, breathlessness and mental state (does the patient appear confused). Shake hands and feel the temperature of the hands and fingers. Inspect the thorax for shape, deformity and asymmetry. Note the position of the spine, slope of the ribs and any changes during inspiration and expiration. Determine the rate, rhythm and depth of breathing.

Palpate the chest wall (posterior and anterior) on both sides, note any masses, pulsations or unusual movement and areas of localized tenderness. Observe for any signs of surgery (scars). Observe as the patient breathes – both sides of the thorax should expand equally during normal breathing. Percussion with the hand placed over specific aspects of the anterior, lateral and posterior chest wall allows the NA to hear any abnormalities as the patient breathes in and out. Percussion sounds can range from resonant to dull. Normal lung produces a resonant note.

Auscultation involves the use of a stethoscope to listen to breath sounds and the movement of air in and out of the lungs, comparing both sides. The patient should be relaxed breathing deeply through an open mouth. Sounds heard may include:
- Crackles (rales)
- Rhonchi (gurgling)
- Wheeze (this can inspiratory or expiratory)
- Pleural rub (a grating sound usually heard on inspiration).

Findings should be noted. Include the quality and amplitude of breath sounds.

CASE STUDY 10.3   Mr Riddle

Mr Clive Riddle is a 62-year-old gentleman living at home in a bungalow with his wife. Clive has not worked for 16 years. He receives disability living allowance. The community nurse was asked to visit Clive at home. He presented with a history of reduced mobility and was finding it difficult managing at home due to his increasing breathlessness. Medical history included COPD, sleep apnoea, obesity, hypertension and diabetes. Over the previous 12 months, he had been admitted to hospital twice as a result of unstable COPD, as well as the impact of co-morbid conditions. Clive is taking antibiotics for a chest infection.

Clive's wife expressed concern about his condition, and that he was so short of breath sometimes 'he can hardly speak'. The community nurse made the following observations on entering the patient's living room:
- Clive was sitting in a chair leaning over a table
- He was sleepy
- He was obese with a pendulous abdominal apron extending forward to his knees
- He was breathless
- He was pale and his lips were blue-tinged
- Clive was breathing through pursed lips.

A respiratory examination was performed; central cyanosis was present with rapid shallow breathing: 28 breaths per minute.

Chest expansion was symmetrical; chest percussion revealed a dull percussion note to mid zones on both sides. Decreased resonance was noted in lung bases.

Auscultation identified diminished breath sounds at the lung bases and upper lobe bronchial breathing. Muffled sounds were heard in lung bases on vocal resonance.

Findings from the physical examination and the history (provided by Clive, his wife and his medical notes), the sleepiness, tachypnoea, recurring exacerbation of COPD and chest infection, required an urgent response. There was a need for Clive to receive treatment in hospital, including oxygen, intravenous antibiotic therapy and further investigations. This was discussed with Clive so as to enable him to understand the diagnosis and for him to be a part of his care and management.

REFLECTION 10.2

It is clear that Mr Riddle is acutely ill and needs to be admitted to hospital.

Having obtained a history and performed a physical examination, can you think of any other examinations, investigations or tests that Mr Riddle may require?

Reflect on what these might be and consider how you would prepare Mr and Mrs Riddle prior to having the tests, investigations or examinations performed.

Cardiovascular

A careful and detailed clinical assessment is vital to assess the likely cause and severity of any symptoms, organize appropriate investigations and referrals and to assess the patient's individual risk of cardiovascular disease.

Observe the patient at first meeting and note their general appearance (anorexic, overweight, obese). Does the patient look unwell, anxious, distressed, breathless, cyanotic? Measure radial and brachial pulse noting rate and rhythm. Measure and record blood pressure. An electrocardiograph (ECG) may be required. Auscultation of the heart requires a skilled clinician to undertake this activity and to interpret findings.

Explain to the patient what is to be done. Sufficient clothing should be removed from the waist up, while at the same time protecting the patient's dignity. Try to ensure the environment is quiet when undertaking auscultation. Heart sounds (these may be normal or abnormal) are caused by turbulent blood flow and they include the sound of the closing heart valves. The bell of the stethoscope detects lower-frequency sounds, whilst the diaphragm is better for higher frequencies. The bell is usually used to listen to the mitral valve and the diaphragm at all other

sites. Auscultation is usually performed with the patient sitting up or reclined at about 45 degrees.

The stethoscope is used to listen to heart sounds. A normal heartbeat sounds like 'lub-dub', which are the sounds of the heart valves closing. If this 'lub-dub' sound changes, often with additional sounds being heard, this may indicate an abnormality. Listen for the first and second heart sounds. The first heart sound is the 'lub', which is also called 'S_1' and occurs when the tricuspid and mitral valves are snapping shut when systole begins. S_1 is at its loudest at the apex of the heart, over the tricuspid and mitral valves. The second heart sound, which is the 'dub' or S_2, happens when the aortic and pulmonary valves close at the beginning of diastole. S_2 therefore is heard best at the base of the heart.

Abdomen

It takes time to develop the skills require to undertake an examination of the abdomen. What is to be carried out and what is not to be carried out during the examination of the abdomen will be determined by the patient's needs and any instructions the NA has been given.

The patient should be prepared appropriately and adequately undressed (from mid chest to waist); leave the chest and legs covered. If needed, help to make the patient comfortable in a warm and private environment, lying with the head elevated a little and supported by a pillow. The arms should be placed alongside the body; this can help to relax the abdominal muscles. Explain the process and procedure and gain informed consent. The height of the bed or examination couch should allow a comfortable examination whilst you are standing upright. In a patient's home the bed may not be height adjustable. Assume the most comfortable position you can. This may require that you sit on a chair during the examination.

Observe the patient when you first meet them:
- Does the patient look unwell?
- Is there any pain apparent?
- Is the patient writhing or lying still?
- Are there any signs of jaundice?
- Is there evidence of dehydration?
- Are there any indications of weight loss or wasting?
- Leaning over the face to inspect respiration. At this point you can smell the patient's breath. Note any smell of alcohol.

Inspect the abdomen and note any distension, abdominal respiration, bruising, scars, presence of a stoma, herniae and any visible peristalsis. A mass may be evident.

Ensure hands are warm prior to palpating the abdomen. Place a pillow under the patient's knees; this can aid relaxation of abdominal musculature. If the patient is in pain, ask them to point to the site. When palpating the abdomen be alert to the response of the patient's abdominal muscles, observing their face for signs of discomfort.

Begin with light palpation, gaining the patient's confidence and helping to relax them, then perform deeper palpation. Use the flat of the hand with the fingers for deep palpation. Examine each region of the abdomen in turn, starting away from any site of pain. Observe for signs of localized guarding and rebound tenderness. Generalized 'board-like' rigidity and rebound tenderness can indicate an abnormality. In abdominal palpation, also examine the liver, spleen, gallbladder and kidneys for evidence of enlargement.

Percussion of the abdomen can be helpful in allowing the NA to determine if abdominal distension is because of tumours or collection of fluid or gas. Auscultation enables bowel sounds to be heard through a stethoscope.

> **❗ HOTSPOT**
>
> Absent bowel sounds or increased bowel sounds can indicate abnormality.

Undertaking a rectal examination is an important aspect of the abdominal examination (it is also an important part of the genitourinary examination). This is an intimate physical examination, which should be conducted in an appropriate manner to detect disease and to enhance patient comfort. Any findings must be recorded and reported.

LOOKING BACK, FEEDING FORWARD

This chapter has introduced the NA to the important activities of taking a patient history and undertaking a physical examination. Both of these activities require much skill, and the skills required have to be learned and honed over time. The NA is required to have an understanding of anatomy, physiology and pathophysiology if the history-taking and physical examination are to meet the needs of the patient.

A systematic approach is required to ensure that the examination and the taking of the history are thorough. There are several models that can be used to guide the NA – a body systems approach is one such model. The needs of the patient may dictate the model to be used.

There are four physical skills that have to be mastered when physically examining the patient – investigation, percussion, auscultation and palpation. When taking a history, the NA will need to communicate effectively using all of the senses to listen to the patient's story.

When the NA is able to take a patient's history and to undertake a physical examination in a confident manner, this will contribute to care that is patient-centred and holistic. Caring effectively for people requires knowledge acquired to be applied in an appropriate manner, and practical skills, attitudes and behaviours to be consistently displayed in a positive manner. The emphasis should always be on placing the patient at the centre of all that is done.

REFERENCES

Ball, J.W., Dains, J.E., Benedict, W.G., et al., 2015. Student Laboratory Manual for Seidel's Guide to Physical Examination, eighth ed. Elsevier, St Louis.

Blainey, S., 2014. Consultation and Clinical History Taking. In: Ransom, M., Abbott, H.Braithwaite, W. (Eds.), Clinical Examination Skills for Healthcare Professionals. M and K Publishing, Keswick, pp. 1–19. Chapter 1.

de Wit, S.C., Stromberg, H.K., Dallred, C., 2017. Medical-Surgical Nursing, Concepts and Practice, third ed. Elsevier, St Louis.

Davey, P., 2014. Medicine at a Glance, forth ed. Wiley, Oxford.

Donald, A., Stein, M., Scott-Hill, C., Chavda, S.J., 2014. The Hands On Guide to the Foundation Programme. Wiley, Oxford.

Douglas, G., Bevan, J., 2013. The General Examination. In: Douglas, G., Nicol, F.Robertson, C. (Eds.), Macleod's Clinical Examination, thirteenth ed. Elsevier, Edinburgh, pp. 41–62. Chapter 3.

Drake, W.M., 2012. General Patient Examination and Differential Diagnosis. In: Glynn, M., Drake, W. (Eds.), Hutchinson's Clinical Methods. An Integrated Approach to Clinical Practice, twenty third ed. Saunders, Edinburgh, pp. 15–30. Chapter 2.

House of Commons Health Committee, 2014. Managing the Care of People with Long-term Conditions. http://www.publications.parliament.uk/pa/cm201415/cmselect/cmhealth/401/401.pdf.

Kaur, R., Oakley, S., Venn, P., 2014. Using Face-to-Face Interpreters in Healthcare. Nurs. Times 110 (21), 20–21.

Snadden, D., Laing, R., Potts, R., et al., 2013. History Taking and General Examination. In: Douglas, G., Nicol, F.Robertson, C. (Eds.), Macleod's Clinical Examination, thirteenth ed. Elsevier, Edinburgh, pp. 5–39. Chapter 2.

Talley, N.J., O'Connor, S., 2014. Clinical Examination. A Systematic Guide to Physical Diagnosis, seventh ed. Livingston, Sydney Churchill.

Waugh, A., Grant, A., 2018. Ross and Wilson Anatomy and Physiology in Health and Illness, thirteenth ed. Elsevier, Edinburgh.

Williams, P., 2018. de Wit's Fundamental Concepts and Skills for Nursing, fifth ed. Elsevier, St Louis.

11

A Systematic Approach to Nursing Care

Ian Peate

OBJECTIVES

By the end of the chapter the reader will be able to:

1. Understand the concept of a systematic approach to nursing care
2. Discuss the various steps associated with a systematic approach to care
3. Relate a systemic approach to care provision
4. Identify ways in which a systematic approach to care can assist the Nursing Associate (NA) in problem solving
5. Recognize the need to plan care using a nursing model
6. Consider various types of care plans

KEY WORDS

Individual	Assessment	Systematic
Judgement	Patient-centred	Process
Communication	Competence	
Evidence-based	Nursing models	

CHAPTER AIM

This chapter aims to introduce the reader to a systematic approach to the provision of high-quality nursing care.

SELF TEST

1. How many stages are associated with a systematic approach to care?
2. What is the purpose of data collection?
3. What do you understand by a 'problem statement'?
4. How does the Nursing Associate formulate goals in relation to care giving?
5. What are the skills of assessment?
6. How might the Nursing Associate build a therapeutic nurse–patient relationship?
7. What resources might the Nursing Associate use to obtain a full patient history?
8. Why does the care provided to people have to be clearly communicated and documented?
9. Name three nursing models.
10. What do you understand by patient-centred care?

INTRODUCTION

The Nursing Associate (NA) is required to provide care that is safe, effective and based on the needs of the patient. Using a systematic approach to care enables the NA to do this. The nursing process was first conceived by Orlando (1961) and extensively used in the 1970s and 1980s in the USA where it originated, and then in the UK. It is said to be an organized, deliberate, systematic way to deliver nursing care and employs a step-by-step process to solve problems. The nursing process provides a way to implement caregiving and combines the art and the science of nursing. The NA focuses on the patient as an individual, identifies health-care needs and the strengths of the patient, establishes and delivers a plan of action to meet patient needs, and evaluates the outcomes of the plan and their actions. It is a circular process incorporating ongoing assessment, nursing diagnosis, planning, implementation and evaluation (see Fig. 11.1).

The NA is required to work within all aspects of the nursing process, offering high-quality, holistic, patient-centred care to individuals and providing support to the registered nurse in the assessment, planning and evaluation of care. Responsibility as primary assessor, planner and evaluator of care remains with the registered nurse (Health Education England (HEE), 2016).

The NA will develop an understanding of the nursing process and the rationale for each of the stages, which will help them appreciate the importance of the registered nurse's role as they undertake a holistic assessment prior to planning care, and the need for the NAs to employ their own skills of ongoing assessment and evaluation, and identifying when an individual requires their plan of care revisiting – this may be due to improvement, deviation or deterioration of needs (HEE, 2017).

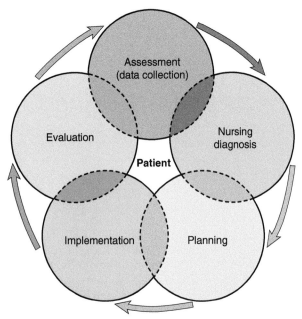

Fig. 11.1 The Cyclical Nature of the Nursing Process (Williams, 2018).

TABLE 11.1 A Comparison of the Scientific Method with the Nursing Process (Adapted from Williams, 2018)	
Step in scientific method	**Step in the nursing process**
Define the problem. Gather information	**Assessment (data collection)** Undertake a patient history, complete a physical assessment and gather results of any diagnostic tests. Use assessment tools
Analyse the information (data)	**Nursing diagnosis** Consider assessment database and tools and identify problems. Choose nursing diagnoses
Develop solutions. Make a decision	**Planning** Determine preferred outcomes. Select interventions to achieve those outcomes
Implement the decision	**Implementation** Implement chosen interventions
Evaluate the decision	**Evaluation** Assess the result of the interventions; decide if the outcomes have been accomplished; revise the care plan if outcomes are not being met. Interventions that are no longer needed should be stopped

The nursing process is akin to methods used to organize tasks that are part of daily life. In planning a week's holiday, for instance, the goal is to ensure each person going on holiday enjoys themselves. The assessment phase, or the collection of data, involves surveying the holiday destinations available that meet the budget. These data are then analysed to determine what destination meets needs and to plan the journey and the mode of transport. Implementation includes booking, packing a suitcase and going on the holiday. Evaluation is performed to determine whether the holiday was a success. Did those who went enjoy the destination? Was the time there long enough? Did they have enough spending money? Would they go to the same destination again? Would they go with same group of people? Was it value for money? This process is not a new way of thinking and doing, but here we are applying it to a nursing context.

CRITICAL AWARENESS

Imagine you were buying a new car for you, your partner and your family. Go through the process required to arrive at a decision. How did the process you went through reflect a systematic approach? Using systematic processes in everyday life is not new.

PROBLEM SOLVING

Nursing incorporates scientific knowledge and research methods. To solve problems, scientists use a consistent, logical method called the 'scientific method'. The scientist first defines the problem and then gathers information, analyses the information and develops solutions. The scientist makes a decision about which solution to use, implements the decision and then evaluates the outcome of the decision.

The nursing process has a number of characteristics similar to the scientific method. A comparison of the scientific method with the nursing process is outlined in Table 11.1.

Decisions are required to solve problems, and NAs make decisions as they go through each step of the nursing process. Effective decision-making is about selecting the best actions to meet a chosen goal and is part of the critical thinking process. Often the NA has to make decisions quickly, sometimes during emergencies. Another aspect of the role is to help patients make decisions, which may be during episodes of crisis. The NA problem-solves on a continual basis and critical thinking enhances the outcomes of the problem-solving process.

Decision-making is complex and often requires the choosing of an option from a range of options. Decisions can be influenced by:

- Conscious choice
- Rational thinking
- Personal factors
- Motivation to do something (for whatever reason).

Decisions made have consequences, and when caring for people this can be positive or negative. Emotions, feelings, moods and memories can impact on choices (Hertz, 2013).

REFLECTION 11.1

Think about a recent decision you have made and reflect on that decision:
- Why did the decision need to be made?
- What was it that led you to make that decision?
- What factors needed to be taken into account?
- What alternatives did you think about? Were any available?
- What was the outcome of the decision?

Chapter 13 may help you to reflect in an effective manner.

There are five steps associated with the problem-solving process:

1. Clearly define the problem.
2. Think about all potential alternative solutions to the problem.
3. Consider the possible outcomes for all alternatives.
4. Make a prediction of the likelihood of each outcome occurring.
5. Choose the alternative with the best opportunity to succeed, along with the least unwanted outcomes.

THE NURSING PROCESS

The five components of the nursing process are:

1. Assessment (data collection)
2. Nursing diagnosis
3. Planning
4. Implementation
5. Evaluation.

An overview of each component of the nursing process can be found in Table 11.2. The overall aim of this systematic, cyclical, dynamic process is to explore with the patient (when appropriate) the patient's health status, identify any actual or potential healthcare problems, determine desired outcomes (the goals of care intervention), deliver certain nursing interventions that will help to solve the problems and promote health, and evaluate care and ascertain if the outcomes have been achieved. Often, the components overlap as the NA is continually assessing and evaluating whether the effects of actions have resulted in the desired impact.

The formulation of a patient's care plan requires collaboration between the patient, NAs, registered nurses and other health and care team members. Patient input during the planning stage will result in greater success with the care plan and care coordination. The NA has a responsibility for the collection of data to assist with the assessment phase of the nursing process. The nursing process allows for constant alterations in the care plan as the patient's condition changes.

Critical thinking

Using critical thinking and the nursing process can help develop good clinical reasoning skills that result in solid, safe clinical judgements. What does this mean? In this context, 'critical' means requiring careful judgement and 'thinking' means to reason. Critical thinking is a purposeful, directed mental activity through which ideas are created and evaluated: thinking is expansive, data is analysed, problems are anticipated, experience is reflected upon, plans are constructed and desired outcomes determined. Critical thinking and clinical reasoning are required to problem-solve in a creative way and to produce new ideas and solutions. Critical thinking involves a variety of skills. To be able to think critically in nursing requires knowledge and skills, as well as appropriate attitudes, that are important for trainee Nursing Associates to acquire.

In complex and ever-changing healthcare environments, NAs have to be prepared to critically analyse large amounts of information (data). They do this so that they can weigh up the evidence supporting any arguments for and against particular care issues or procedures.

Nursing practice demands that NAs exhibit sound judgement and decision-making skills because critical thinking and clinical decision-making are key components of nursing practice. The NA's ability to recognize and respond to signs of a deteriorating patient in a timely manner is critical in ensuring positive patient outcomes (Purling & King, 2012).

The focus of the NA's clinical judgement is on quality evidence-based care delivery. As such, observational and reasoning skills will result in sound and reliable clinical judgements. Clinical judgement is critical to nursing; it can be complex, as the NA is required to use observation skills, identify relevant information and recognize the relationships among given elements through reasoning and assessment. These are all components of the nursing process. Clinical reasoning is the process by which NAs observe a patient's status, process the information, come to an understanding of the patient problem, plan and implement interventions and evaluate outcomes with reflection and learning from the process (Levett-Jones et al., 2010).

Assessment

This is the first stage of the nursing process and requires the NA to collect information about the patient. Assessment (just like all other aspects of the nursing process) is not a one-off

TABLE 11.2 Components of the Nursing Process	
Component	**Discussion**
Assessment (the collection of data)	Collecting, organizing, documenting and validating data regarding a patient's health status. Assessment data can be obtained from the patient, the family, a primary care worker, diagnostic tests and information about the patient from other health or care professionals, such as a dietician.
Nursing diagnosis	The process by which the assessment data are sorted and analysed, enabling actual and potential health problems to be identified. The factors contributing to the problems are considered and specific nursing diagnoses are chosen for the patient's care plan.
Planning	A series of steps by which the NA and the patient (where appropriate) set priorities and goals to eliminate or reduce the impact of the identified problems. The goals are specific expected outcomes. The NA and the patient work in partnership and choose specific interventions for each nursing diagnosis. The interventions assist the patient so that they meet the expected outcomes. The expected outcomes and nursing interventions are a part of the patient's nursing care plan.
Implementation	Implementing the nursing interventions is done in a systematic way. The NA carries out the interventions. How the patient responds to the care given is documented.
Evaluation	This requires the NA to assess the patient's response to the nursing care. The responses are compared with the expected outcomes to find out whether they have been achieved or not. The care plan is reassessed, and if required, changes are made.

activity; assessments are made initially (this provides a baseline) and continually throughout the delivery of patient care. The information gathered concerns the patient's psychological, physiological (biological), sociological and spiritual status. The information that is gathered during this stage will inform all other stages of the nursing process, and therefore the care the patient receives. Assessing needs is a complex and important activity.

There are many ways in which data (information) can be collected. Usually, a patient interview will be undertaken to determine the patient's health history and nursing care history. Information is also gathered about the patient's family health history as some conditions are genetic (Sorrentino & Remmert, 2017). A physical examination is undertaken along with general and specific observations that also provide assessment data. Patient interaction is heaviest during this phase as the NA encourages the person to tell their story. When the data is gathered it is documented according to local policy and procedure. The data may be documented electronically or by hand. Taking a patient history and undertaking physical examining is discussed in depth in Chapter 10, while Chapter 7 considers the important issue of documentation.

The purpose of assessment is to do the following:

- Validate a diagnosis
- Provide the basis for the delivery of effective care
- Assist with decision-making
- Offer holistic care
- Enable comparisons of the patient health status to be made (particularly during the evaluation stage of the nursing process).

The initial assessment, also known as the admission assessment, takes place when the patient first enters the healthcare facility; for example, when the practice nurse first meets the patient in the general practice. This assessment begins the therapeutic nurse–patient relationship.

AT THE GP SURGERY

Mrs Annie Sclara (known as 'Nonnie') is a 78-year-old lady who lives at home alone in a bungalow. She has come to see the practice nurse at the GP surgery for a repeat prescription for her hypertension medication, amlodipine. Nonnie has recently been taking some new 'pills' for her blood pressure. The practice nurse notices that Nonnie has a large haematoma to her left temple and asks Nonnie what happened. Nonnie tells her that she got up to make a cup of tea one afternoon after watching *Countdown* and she had a 'funny turn' tripped and hit her head on the side of the table. She informs the practice nurse that she is fine, she just had a bad head for a few days, but 'to be honest, I have not been feeling a hundred percent since the fall. I have been a bit giddy'.

Working with Nonnie, the practice nurse takes patient history and performs a physical examination using a range of equipment to observe and measure in order to complete a full assessment of needs.

The practice nurse's findings reveal that Annie is hypotensive; she has a blood pressure of 100/55 mm Hg (sitting) and 90/50 mm Hg (standing). The nurse arranges for Nonnie to be seen by the GP for a review of her anti-hypertensive medications.

Types of data

Data can be from a primary source (the patient) or a secondary source (others). Primary data is the most reliable as this comes directly from the patient. This is what the patient says the issues are, what the problems are and also how they manage them. The patient is often considered to be the most accurate reporter. The patient who is alert and orientated can provide information about the current condition, past condition and lifestyle issues.

Data that has been collected can be objective or subjective. Lappin (2018) notes that objective data can be related to the symptoms a patient may be experiencing, for example, tachycardia or pyrexia. Objective data are detectable by an observer and can be measured or tested against an agreed criterion or standard – they can be seen, smelt, felt or heard. For example, when a stethoscope is placed on the chest the NA may be able to hear an inspiratory or expiratory wheeze. Subjective data, on the other hand, is information that is personal to the patient and often focuses on the patient's experience. These are verbal statements the patient makes; for example, a feeling of nausea or a description of pain.

CRITICAL AWARENESS

Can you differentiate between objective and subjective data?

	Objective/subjective
Pain	
Hypertension	
Tiredness	
Cyanosis	
Dizziness	
I can hear voices telling me what to do	
Capillary nail refill	
Reports tripping over	
Atrial fibrillation	
I have been itching	
I am experiencing palpitations and am anxious all the time	
Anaemia	

NB Did you collect the information through communication with the patient (subjective) or is the information something you measured or observed (objective)?

Assessment tools

The data that is gathered during the assessment stage must be complete, factual and accurate. The NA should avoid jumping to any conclusions (assumptions) and should always attempt to be objective about any data gathered (measured). Assessment tools can help with this. Chapter 20 addresses data gathering and monitoring. When possible and appropriate, the patient should be involved in using the assessment tool. The choice of tool will depend on the clinical setting, although usually, the choice is related to the assessment of clinical variables with measurement of clinical interventions (Ward et al., 2014).

Using an assessment tool, for example the Malnutrition Universal Screening Tool (MUST), Mini Mental State Examination (MMSE), Alcohol Use Disorders Identification Test (AUDIT) or the Braden Scale, can assist the NA to make objective judgements that will impact on patient care. In Chapter 36 the Glasgow Coma Scale (GCS) is described. This is a neurological scale that aims to provide an objective and reliable way of recording the conscious state of a person for initial as well as subsequent assessment. A patient is assessed against the criteria of the scale, the resulting points giving a patient score.

CRITICAL AWARENESS

Whilst the use of assessment tools is helpful in making accurate measurements and providing a basis on which to provide care and evaluate care interventions, any assessment tool can only be as good as the person using it. The NA has to understand the reason why the tool is being used, its appropriateness, its limitations and above all how to use it. Failure to use the right tool for the right purpose and in the right way may result in harm to the patient.

COMMUNITIES OF CARE

Children

Providing effective pain management for children can be complex and challenging. All areas that treat and care for children should assess pain carefully and have a policy in place that addresses pain management. It is important that babies, children and young people have their pain recognized, assessed, treated and evaluated. For this to happen, those who work with children should be trained in assessing children's pain and use an appropriate assessment tool.

Healthcare professionals, such as the NA, are in the ideal position to assess children's pain, and they should also include the parents' and carers' views. The use of pain assessment tools can help to provide an organized standardized approach using a common language for written and visual observations.

Whenever possible, behavioural measurement of pain should be used along with self-reported and physiological signs. When self-reporting is not possible, interpretation of pain behaviours and decisions concerning treatment of pain require careful consideration of the context in which the pain behaviours are observed.

(Adapted from RCN, 2009)

The observations that the NA makes about a patient play a key part in assessment. The NA provides care, and as such, is able to observe and gather objective and subjective data (see Table 11.3).

Nursing diagnosis

Using the information gathered, the registered nurse makes the nursing diagnosis. Nursing diagnoses and medical diagnoses are not the same thing. A nursing diagnosis describes a healthcare condition that can be treated or alleviated by nursing measures or interventions. A doctor makes a medical diagnosis and identifies a disease; the condition is then treated by drugs, therapies and surgery to palliate, cure or heal.

Planning

The planning stage of the nursing process occurs when all the data have been gathered. It should be reiterated that assessment is not a one-off activity; it is continuous, occurring whenever the patient's condition dictates. Maslow's Hierarchy of Needs (see Critical Awareness box) can help when setting priorities.

CRITICAL AWARENESS

Maslow's Hierarchy of Needs theory maintains that a person does not meet a higher need until the needs of the current level have been satisfied.

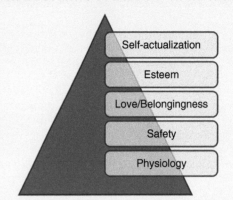

Self-actualization – e.g., realizing potential, personal growth, morality, spontaneity, creativity, accepting and acceptance.
Esteem – e.g., confidence, self-esteem, achievement, dignity, respect.
Love/Belongingness – e.g., love, friendship, affection, intimacy, trust, family.
Safety – e.g., security of body, environment, employment, resources, health, property, protection from the elements.
Physiological – e.g., air, food, warmth, rest, water, sex, sleep, other factors towards homeostasis.

(Adapted from Maslow, 1954)

A plan of action now needs to be developed; where possible this should be done with the patient. When there are multiple diagnoses, these have to be prioritized and plans of care written for each one. Priorities relate to the most important thing for the patient. Goals (aims, intents, ends) are set in this stage, and each problem is assigned a clear, measurable goal for the expected beneficial outcome (Barrett et al., 2012). The planning phase can also be extended to the prescribing of care phase. When goals have been set and priorities identified, then care has to be prescribed.

When goals are being set Barrett et al. (2012) suggest these four questions have to be answered:
• Who is meant to achieve the goal?
• What is it that they are meant to achieve?
• How are they meant to do it?
• When do they have to do it by?

As a reminder of what to include in a goal statement, the mnemonic PRODUCT may provide direction:

Patient-centred: Is the goal focused on the patient's needs?

Recordable: Are you able to document the progress towards the goal?

Observable: Can you evaluate progress?

Directive: Is the goal clear: who, what, where, when?

Understandable: Has the goal been written in an easy-to-read and comprehensible way?

Credible: Can the goal be realistically achieved by the patient?

Time frame: Does the goal state when it is meant to be achieved by?

Planning, therefore, is the process of developing a plan and establishing SMART goals (see Table 11.4). These are needed in

TABLE 11.3   The Skills of Assessment

Observation (using sight, smell, hearing, touch)	Objective data	Subjective data
You can see how the patient gets up from a chair, how they sit, lie and walk	You count pulse	The patient expresses to you their feeling of paranoia
You are able to observe the colour of a patient's skin; you can see if they are pale, flushed, cyanotic	You calculate Body Mass Index (BMI)	The patient tells you they feel as if they are going to vomit
You can see if the patient's limbs are oedematous (swollen); see if the abdomen is distended	You measure blood pressure	The patient relates to you that they feel they 'cannot go on any more'
You listen to the way a patient speaks (or does not), you listen to their breathing; through a stethoscope, you listen to chest sounds, and you take their blood pressure	You measure oxygen saturation	A patient tells you they feel pain when they pass urine
You touch the patient and determine if they are cold, clammy, sweating or if the skin is dry. You touch the patient to take their pulse	You measure a peak flow rate	
You use the sense of smell to tell if the patient's urine is malodorous; you can smell an infected wound and you can detect the smell of acetone on a person's breath		

TABLE 11.4   The Acronym SMART

S	Specific
M	Measurable
A	Attainable
R	Realistic/relevant
T	Time restricted

order to achieve a desired outcome, for example reducing pain or improving respiratory function.

SMART goals are developed to provide the patient (as well as those offering care and support) with a focused set of activities that are formulated (wherever possible with the patient) to improve their condition. The goals that have been set can be short-term or long-term and must focus on the individual outcome.

CRITICAL AWARENESS

Goals/aims and the specific activities that will help to achieve the healthcare goal will all contain the following:
- The date
- An action verb, such as 'monitor', 'instruct', 'auscultate', or something equally descriptive.
- Content – the where and the what of the activity; for example, 'applying antiembolic stockings on both legs from toe to top of the thigh'.
- A time element – defines how long or how often the nursing action will occur.
- Completed documentation, signature and designation of prescriber.
All goals should be SMART.

The prescription of care comes after the SMART goals have been set and nursing interventions selected. A nursing intervention does not have to be a doctor's order; they are actions taken by the nursing team to help the patient reach a goal – and so they are nursing actions. The prescription sets the direction; it is logically sequenced and clear about who, what, when and where needs to be done. The care prescription should be supported by the best available evidence – local guidance and protocols can be used to help with this. Attention needs to be paid

to the resources available, otherwise the prescription of care and the goals set will be unachievable and meaningless.

The goals set and care prescribed have to be documented. There are legal, ethical and professional issues associated with documentation (see Chapter 4 and Chapter 5).

Implementation

This stage follows on from the planning, goals setting and pre-scribing of care; it is the 'doing' stage of the nursing process. The NA excels at this stage, working from the care plan (the prescription) in the provision of high-quality, safe and effective nursing care.

How care is organized and delivered, and by whom, has an impact on goal attainment. The mode of delivery will depend on the specific care area. Care that is offered in a general practice will differ from that delivered in the intensive care unit – the philosophies of care will be different. The philosophy of care will dictate the model of care used, describing the role of, and the relationship between, the patient and the NA.

Delegation of care is an important issue. The NA has to be aware of the implication of delegating or receiving delegated activity incorrectly.

Care has to be provided in an individual and holistic manner. The plan of care should have taken into consideration any cultural issues, for example the provision of a place to pray or the choice of a vegan diet. Acknowledging and responding to the patient's psychological, physiological, sociological and spiritual needs demonstrates respect and positive regard and ensures that those you care for are your main concern.

REFLECTION 11.2

Reflect on the issues you would need to take into account when providing care for a patient admitted for hip replacement surgery. The patient is vegan.

Any aspects of care that have been delivered must be documented using local policy and procedure. This is also true of any element of care delivery that has been *omitted*, along with the reasons why.

REFLECTION 11.3

You are caring for Mr Saleh and he has refused his dose of clozapine. What actions do you take?

Evaluation

This is the final stage of the nursing process. In many respects the skills, knowledge and attitudes required for this stage are similar to assessment. Once the NA has implemented the prescription of care (the care plan), it is essential that the intended outcomes of care are evaluated to determine if they have been achieved – if the patient has progressed towards the achievement of the expected outcome. This echoes the fact that effective planning is essential if evaluation is to be successful. The planned outcomes are the measures by which the effectiveness of care interventions are evaluated. If there are no stated expectations of care (outcomes) during the planning stage, then it will not be possible to measure progress from the baseline; evaluation involves reassessment.

As in the assessment stage, the NA gathers data to check if there has been any progress in achieving the goals or targets set. Evaluation provides the opportunity to alert staff to any deterioration in the patient's health, as well as any progress that is being made. The patient, the NA, and, if appropriate, the patient's family should all be involved in the evaluation stage.

When the anticipated outcomes have not been achieved, the nursing process occurs again. Just as assessment is a complex process, so too is evaluation. Williams (2018) suggests that evaluation has a quality-assurance aspect associated with it as it can help to determine why some aspects of care worked and why others did not.

ASPIRE is an acronym that stands for:

Assess
Systematic nursing diagnosis
Plan
Implement
Recheck
Evaluate.

In this approach (Barrett et al., 2012), there are six stages. The additional stage is recheck, something that can often be overlooked. ASPIRE is also cyclical in nature.

MODELS OF NURSING

Nursing models incorporate fundamental concepts, values and beliefs about contemporary nursing. Any model is a conceptual framework or tool that is used to represent and understand a complex phenomenon or situation. Think of the London Underground map. This is a model; it represents a complex transport network and is used by people to navigate the underground system. It helps people understand how to get from A to B.

Nursing models have similarities with physical models. They are composed of different parts, and when brought together, they can guide the NA with regard to nursing and what it is about. The model provides the NA with an understanding of what nursing is and what those who nurse and care for people do. Models also provide direction to the NA about what the patient's needs may be.

There are a number of nursing models available, each having different perspectives concerning beliefs and values about people, health, the environment and nursing. However, whilst there are differences, there are also similarities. It would be inappropriate to have only one model of nursing as the people we offer care to are complex beings and will have different needs. For example, a model of care that focuses on the physical aspects of health might be inappropriate for those with mental health issues; a model that is child focused may be inappropriate for adults, and a model whose philosophy of care concentrates on musculoskeletal disorders might not be suitable for men with urological problems. Even in the same field of nursing there are different models that aim to address the needs and concerns of different patient groups. It is important that the right model is used for the right patient.

A brief overview of one commonly used model of nursing in a general care setting in the UK is described below.

Roper, Logan & Tierney: Activities of Living Model

This model provides a picture of nursing that sees the individual as a whole as opposed to parts of a whole. Three nurse theorists were responsible for the inception and development of the model. The model has undergone further developments, originally being called the Activities of Daily Living Model and now the Activities of Living Model (Roper, Logan & Tierney, 2000; Holland et al., 2008).

There are a number of components associated with this model (see Box 11.1). When these various components are considered together in order to help assess the unique needs of the individual, then patient-centred care can flourish. The NA needs to understand the component parts and how they can come together in order to consider the person holistically.

Individuality

Each person is an individual: each person is unique. There are many commonalities in how people perform their activities of living; however, there are also differences and this is what makes the person unique. This model emphasizes how the person should be at the centre of all stages of the problem-solving approach to care (the nursing process).

BOX 11.1   The Activities of Living

1. Maintaining a safe environment
2. Communicating
3. Breathing
4. Eating and drinking
5. Eliminating
6. Personal cleansing and dressing
7. Controlling body temperature
8. Mobilizing
9. Working and playing
10. Expressing sexuality
11. Sleeping
12. Dying

The twelve activities of living

Twelve activities of living were identified by Roper et al. (2000). Most of us carry out many of these activities on a daily basis (it is accepted that dying is not an activity that is performed on a daily basis, hence the need for the change in the name of the model from the Activities of Daily Living to the Activities of Living). Using the twelve activities as a guide to assessment can help the NA, along with the patient, when appropriate, address needs or identify where there may be a deficit in addressing needs.

The twelve activities should be thought of broadly; the NA should steer clear of thinking about them in a restrictive way – they are not a checklist or boxes that need to be filled. Thinking creatively can help to broaden your horizon and the patient's; each activity will impact on the others; they should not be considered in isolation.

CRITICAL AWARENESS

Respiratory insufficiency can impact on a number of aspects of a person's life. Think about the activity of breathing. A person with a breathing problem may have difficulty carrying out a number of other activities of living in an independent manner, such as (but not limited to):

* the ability to communicate
* the ability to maintain a safe environment
* being able to eat and drink
* being able to mobilize
* being able to attend to personal hygiene and dressing.

Whilst this is just one activity (breathing), note how it impacts in a number of other ways. This may require the NA to intervene in attempting to assist the patient with their unique needs.

REFLECTION 11.4

Consider Roper et al.'s twelve Activities of Living and then compare them to Maslow's Hierarchy of Needs. Can you see any similarity here?

Dependence–independence continuum

The purpose of nursing, according to Henderson (1960), is:

> *'To assist the individual, sick or well, in the performance of those activities contributing to health or its recovery (or to a peaceful death) that he would perform unaided if he had the necessary strength, will, or knowledge and to do this in such a way as to help him gain independence as rapidly as possible.'*

There are times when patients will depend on the NA to assist them with all of the twelve activities of living, for example, an unconscious patient. Others may be dependent on the NA for only some of the activities that they could do for themselves if they had the necessary strength, will or knowledge (Henderson, 1960). Yet others will need no assistance. The dependence–independence continuum enables the NA to identify where the patient is with regard to their degree of dependence and their ability to carry out the activities of living, aided or unaided.

Factors that contribute to dependence or independence are wide and varied. Barrett et al. (2012) group these under the following three headings:

* Maturity
* Social and economic circumstances
* Cultural background.

The life-span continuum

Another component of the Activities of Living Model is the life-span continuum, from conception to death. Roper et al. (2000) suggest that a person passes through a number of developmental stages:

1. Infancy (conception to 5 years)
2. Childhood (6–12 years)
3. Adolescence (13–18 years)
4. Early adulthood (19–30 years)
5. Middle years (31–45 years)
6. Late adulthood (46–65 years)
7. Old age (66 years and older)

Not all people will pass through these developmental stages; life might be cut short and the next developmental milestone may not be reached. The NA needs to give consideration to where a person is on the life-span continuum when assessing and planning needs as this will impact on the person's ability to undertake the activities of living.

The five influencing factors

The five influencing factors are key components in Roper et al.'s (2000) model (see Table 11.5). These factors can impact on how a person develops (the life-span continuum) and degree of dependence (the dependence–independence continuum). The influencing factors will all impact on the activities of living.

There are many positive aspects attributed to the Roper et al. (2000) model of nursing. It is used in a number of care settings throughout the UK. The model considers the physical and psychological aspects of the person's being set against the five influencing factors. It is not, however, the panacea for all ills that befall people requiring nursing. The model is limited in so far as it appears to focus very much on the biological aspects. However, the way the model is interpreted and used locally can help to negate this criticism. There is much potential for the model to help provide people with patient-centred, holistic care.

REFLECTION 11.5

Without looking back, can you list the twelve activities of living?

LOOKING BACK, FEEDING FORWARD

The nursing process provides the NA with ways to provide care that is systematic and patient-centred; it is the essential core of practice for the NA to deliver holistic care. The nursing process is a scientific method that is used to ensure the quality of patient care. This approach can be broken down into a number of separate steps or stages. The nursing process can be seen as a problem-solving approach to the identification and treatment of patient

TABLE 11.5   The Five Influencing Factors (Adapted from Roper et al., 2000)

Factor	Discussion
Biological	Biological factors, such as infection, genetics, diseases and disability can impact on a person's health.
Psychological	The person's emotions, personality, mood, levels of stress, anxiety and fear and cognitive functioning. Psychological factors must be given due consideration during the assessment and planning phases of the nursing process. This factor is just as important as the biological or physical factors.
Sociocultural	Issues such as cultural norms, religion, gender, values and spirituality. There are key issues that the NA must give due respect to when caring for people.
Environmental	The environment has an ability to enhance or negatively impact on a person's health and well-being. Where a person lives, the conditions of their housing, the neighbourhood and local, national and global environments are all important components that require consideration by the NA when providing care.
Politicoeconomic	How resources are managed and distributed by governments, social policies and practices and legislation all have the potential to impact both positively and negatively on how people enjoy good health.

problems. It provides a framework for the practice of nursing and the knowledge, decisions and actions that NAs bring to patient care.

This chapter has provided an overview of the nursing process and how it can be used in various care settings. The key message is that the patient must be at the centre of all that is done. Understanding the rationale for introducing a systematic, holistic, problem-solving approach to care delivery, in partnership with the patient (and if appropriate, the family), can help the NA respond in an effective way to the needs of the people they offer care and support to.

A model of care is required in order to make full and effective use of the nursing process – the nursing process and models of care go hand in hand. This chapter has looked at the Roper, Logan and Tierney Model of Care (Roper et al., 2000), but there are a number of other models of care available. The philosophy of care, the patient group and the care setting often dictates which model is to be used.

REFERENCES

Barrett, D., Wilson, B., Wollands, S., 2012. Care Planning. A Guide for Nurses, second ed. Pearson, Essex.

Health Education England, 2016. NA Curriculum Framework. https://www.hee.nhs.uk/sites/default/files/documents/Curriculum%20Framework%20Nursing%20Associate.pdf.

Henderson, V., 1960. Basic Principles of Nursing Care. International Council of Nurses, London.

Hertz, N., 2013. Eyes Wide Open: How to Make Decisions in a Confusing World. HarperCollins, London.

Holland, K., Jenkins, J., Solomon, J., Whittam, S., 2008. Applying the Roper-Logan-Tierney Model in Practice, second ed. Churchill Livingstone, Edinburgh.

Lappin, M., 2018. The Nursing Process. In: Peate, I., Wild, K. (Eds.), Nursing Care and Practice, Knowledge and Care. Wiley, Oxford, pp. 111–128. Chapter 6.

Levett-Jones, T., Hoffman, K., Dempsey, Y., et al., 2010. The 'Five Rights' of Clinical Reasoning: An Educational Model to Enhance Nursing Students' Ability to Identify and Manage Clinically 'At Risk' Patients. Nurse Educ. Today 30 (6), 515–520.

Maslow, A.H., 1954. Motivation and Personality. Harper and Row, New York.

Orlando, I.J., 1961. The Dynamic Nurse-Patient Relationship: Function, Process and Principles. Putnam, New York.

Purling, A., King, L., 2012. A Literature Review: Graduate Nurses' Preparedness for Recognising and Responding to the Deteriorating Patient. J. Clin. Nurs. 21 (23–24), 3451–3465.

Roper, N., Logan, W., Tierney, A., 2000. The Roper, Logan and Tierney Model of Nursing. Churchill Livingstone, Edinburgh.

Royal College of Nursing, 2009. The Recognition and Assessment of Acute Pain in Children. https://www.rcn.org.uk/professional-development/publications/pub-003542.

Sorrentino, S.A., Remmert, L.N., 2017. Mosby's Textbook for Nursing Assistants, ninth ed. Elsevier, St Louis.

Ward, V., Schorstein, R., Nightingale, P., et al., 2014. Assessment and Discharge. In: Dougherty, L., Lister, S. (Eds.), The Royal Marsden Manual of Clinical Nursing Procedures, ninth ed. Wiley., Oxford, pp. 9–47. Chapter 2.

Williams, P., 2018. De Wit's Fundamental Concepts and Skills for Nursing, fifth ed. Elsevier, St Louis.

12

Leading and Managing Care Provision

Ian Peate

OBJECTIVES

By the end of the chapter the reader will be able to:

1. Explain the principles underpinning leadership and management
2. Outline the role of the Nursing Associate (NA) as a member of a multidisciplinary team and the factors associated with teamworking
3. Understand the various aspects associated with collective leadership
4. Demonstrate an understanding of leadership styles
5. Understand issues associated with conflict in the workplace
6. Demonstrate an ability to prioritize workload and recognize where elements of care can safely be delegated to others

KEY WORDS

Self-awareness	Management	Workload
Safety	Teamworking	Role model
Communication	Delegation	
Leadership	Competence	

CHAPTER AIM

The aim of this chapter is to explain the principles and under-pinning frameworks that are associated with managing and leading care provision.

SELF TEST

1. List the traits associated with effective leaders and managers.
2. Why is it important for an effective leader to engage in self-awareness?
3. Explain the significance of working with others in teams to deliver and improve service provision.
4. What factors must be taken into account before delegating care provision or accepting delegated activities?
5. What does effective teamwork look and feel like?
6. How might the NA offer support and feedback to others they may work with?

INTRODUCTION

The Nursing Associate (NA) works as part of wider multidisci-plinary teams and plays a key role in securing high-quality care and excellent outcomes for patients. For people to be cared for effectively, the NA must have an understanding of the key issues that are associated with being a successful leader in order to offer care that is safe and results in positive care outcomes. The NA is required to understand the principles and competencies that accompany effective leadership and successful teamworking. As well as understanding leadership frameworks, there is also an essential requirement for the NA to be able to acknowledge and recognize their own personal qualities; these will include values, principles and assumptions as they lead and manage care. When these components are acknowledged and understood, the NA can develop strategies that will help them to adapt their personal behaviour as necessary. The first step towards managing care provision and leading is to be self-aware.

SELF-AWARENESS

Being self-aware means that you are conscious of your beliefs, values, qualities, strengths and limitations. It is an important attribute to have when managing and providing care. Self-awareness is vital for understanding and developing good inter-personal skills, as well as building therapeutic relationships with patients and their families. Through self-awareness, the NA is able to consciously learn about themselves and how they interact with other members of the multidisciplinary team. The NA needs to understand themselves before they can begin to understand the people they provide care for.

Self-awareness is concerned with learning how to better understand why it is you feel what you feel and why you are behaving in a particular way. Once this concept is understood there is an opportunity to change things about yourself, enabling you to create what it is that you want. It is difficult, if not impossible, to change and become self-accepting if you are unsure about who you are. Being clear about who you are and what you want can provide you with the confidence that is needed to make changes.

CASE STUDY 12.1 Kerry

Kerry, an NA working on a surgical ward, is helping a patient who has a newly formed stoma to change her bag. Kerry notices that there is a pus-like substance oozing from the stoma wound site and the surrounding skin looks inflamed.

Although Kerry is an experienced NA and competent at standard wound care, she is aware of the risks associated with wounds in the post-operative period, and as such, she knows that for her to treat this would be outside her sphere of competence. She is aware that the wound must be assessed by a registered nurse. Kerry informs the patient she wants another nurse to look at it and reports it to the registered nurse, who takes over the care of the patient's wound.

In this case study, Kerry has acted according to the protocols of her place of work and is able to justify her actions. She has been able to demonstrate her understanding of accountability and responsibility towards the patient.

CRITICAL AWARENESS

Think about describing yourself to another person. Do not mention anything about the external things in your life, for example, your friends, family, what you are studying, where you live and so on. Focus only on yourself, how you feel and behave; identify some of your strengths and weaknesses.

In this exercise, did you manage to explore your thoughts, feelings and behaviours?

Having a clear understanding of your thought and behaviour patterns can help you in understanding other people. This ability to empathize assists in forming and sustaining more effective personal and professional relationships.

The Johari Window

The Johari Window is a technique that can help people to better understand their relationship with themselves and others. It was created in 1955 by two psychologists Joseph Luft and Harry Ingham.

The Johari Window can be approached from many perspectives and provides four basic forms of the self:
1. The known self
2. The hidden self
3. The blind self
4. The unknown self.

The known self

This is what you and others see in you. This part is the part that you are able to discuss freely with others. For most of the time, you agree with this view that you and others have of you.

The hidden self

This is what you see in yourself, but others do not. In this part, you can hide things that are very private about yourself. This information is information that you do not want to be disclosed for the reason of protection. It might also be that you may be ashamed of these areas and that you feel a vulnerability about having your faults and weaknesses laid bare. This area of the window applies equally to those good qualities that you do not want exposed, maybe due to modesty.

The blind self

The blind self is what you do not see in yourself, but others see in you. You may consider yourself to be an open-minded person when, in reality, those people around you do not agree. This area also works the other way, for example, you might see yourself as an 'uninteresting, boring person'; however, other people might consider you very interesting and very bright. There may be times when those around you may not tell you what it is that they see as they may fear causing offence. This is the area that people sometimes detect when what you say and what you do, do not match. There may be times when body language reveals this mismatch.

The unknown self

This is the self that neither you nor others can see. In this aspect of the window, there could be good and bad things that you and others are unaware of. This might relate to unexploited talents and skills that are yet to be explored by you, your friends, co-workers or managers.

The Johari Window remains particularly relevant today where there is an emphasis on behaviour, empathy, cooperation, multidisciplinary group relationships and self-development. The Johari Window is like a window with four panes.

The panes of the window can be changed in size, reflecting the relevant proportions of each type of 'knowledge' of and about a particular person in a given group or team situation (see Case Study 12.2).

CASE STUDY 12.2 Kalifa

Kalifa was a newly qualified NA. She secured a position on the very busy regional burns unit in a tertiary care centre where she had never worked before. This was her first job as an NA.

Her new co-workers knew little about Kalifa; they had not worked with her previously. In this context, the unknown and hidden areas of the Johari Window will be larger and the open area will be small. As others do not know much about Kalifa, the blind spot also will be smaller (see Fig. 12.1).

As the team and Kalifa learn more about each other, and Kalifa also learns more about herself, the Johari Window will change shape.

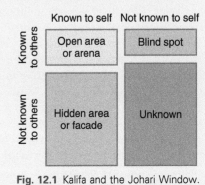

Fig. 12.1 Kalifa and the Johari Window.

REFLECTION 12.1 **Using the Johari Window**

Step one

Start in the open area of the Johari window (the known self). In this window, make some notes about yourself. Think about what your strengths and your weaknesses are. What it is about you that you are comfortable with and willing to share with others? Try to be honest and clear about what it is you know about yourself already.

Step two

Involve other people and ask them for feedback about yourself and be prepared to seriously consider their feedback. This does not mean that you have to act upon everything that has been said, but you should listen and think about it. Be sure to give the person who provided the feedback some acknowledgement or thanks for making the effort to share their thoughts with you. Depending on how confident you are, this can either be done as a group exercise or on a one-to-one basis. Providing feedback is a skill – some people are better at it than others. When you have received feedback, you should be respectful and listen and reflect on what has been said. It may be that when you have received the feedback you might want to explore it further and this can lead to discovery about yourself.

LEADING AND MANAGING

The role of the manager and/or leader is pivotal in any care environment. Leaders and managers have the skills to bring individuals and teams together aligned to organizational purpose and they also have the ability to ensure organizational infrastructure is embedded as patterns of behaviour among staff. They have to make the connection between the patient experience and the team's personal experience of work; they must get to know the team individually and be aware of their needs and their unique opportunity to contribute and to notice and respond to signs of need. This is a tall order for any leader or manager.

REFLECTION 12.2

Make a list of the attributes that you think a good leader should possess. Once you have formulated your list, do you think you have any of the skills to be a good leader?

The key leadership contribution of nursing staff is in ensuring and maintaining high standards and in delivering change. *Leading Change, Adding Value* (DH, 2016) sets out ambitions and commitments that demonstrate the leadership potential and role that nurses (including NAs) have and must enact. However, the whole workforce working together need to recognize the potential to manage the challenges that are being faced today that will shape the future, for those we offer care to, as well as for staff. All of us are leaders, and we have the potential to influence and lead improvement, whether delivering care and support in care homes, the independent and private sector or in NHS funded services. Leadership and management in any healthcare setting aims to maintain and improve patient care and is crucial to delivering change.

TABLE 12.1 **Comparison of Leadership and Management Attributes (Tomey, 2009)**

	Leadership	Management
Motto	Do the right things	Do things right
Challenge	Change	Continuity
Focus	Purpose	Structure and procedure
Time frame	Future	Present
Methods	Strategies	Schedules
Questions	Why?	Who, what, where, when, how?
Outcomes	Journeys	Destinations
Human	Potential	Performance

Leadership and management

Often the terms 'leadership' and 'management' are used interchangeably; however, although they are very closely connected, they do not have the same meaning. Wilcox (2014) suggests that a leader selects and assumes a role, whereas a manager is assigned or appointed to a role.

In Table 12.1 Tomey (2009) makes a comparison of leadership and management attributes.

One of the most cited definitions that delineates leadership and management comes from Kotter (1996). He states that management processes are concerned with planning, budgeting, organizing, staffing, controlling and problem-solving and that leadership processes involve establishing direction, aligning people, motivating and inspiring them. It is evident that leadership requires a significant number of management skills; however, it is more than just management, which might be briefly summarized as 'getting the job done' (King's Fund, 2011). It essentially involves organizing the human and technical resources that are required to ensure that the organization's goals are met. Leadership in the health and social care environment is required from the boardroom down to wherever hands-on care occurs. Table 12.2 provides an overview of contrasting facets of a leader and a manager, with advantages and disadvantages of each style.

Many leaders in their day-to-day work exhibit a number of traits that may relate to all of the styles exhibited in Table 12.2. In complex and varied organizations such as the health service, leaders may have to adapt their approach to the situation or context in which they find themselves.

Laissez faire

In this style of leadership very little supervision is exercised by the leader – a hands-off approach is preferred. Those who use this approach are referred to as 'passive avoidant type leaders' (Kibble and Chen, 2015). Such a leader prefers that people do what they need to do on their own; they may trust that those they are leading will be able to perform well and not need any guidance. This approach promotes independent thinking and encourages autonomy. However, it can also have several negative consequences.

- Important decisions will not be made on time
- Fewer changes happen in the workplace
- Quality improvements will only happen when the situation requires it.

TABLE 12.2 Leadership and Management Styles (Adapted from Burns, 2015)

Leadership style	Advantages/Strengths	Disadvantages/Weaknesses
Laissez-faire. These leaders exercise minimal influence and adopt a 'hands-off' approach (e.g., they often take a non-directive or inactive approach – leaving those who are following to decide upon the actions needed themselves).	Groups of fully autonomous and independent care workers working together can feel empowered to make decisions.	Outcome can often result in a lack of direction (disordered, frustrating, demoralizing and unproductive). This occurs mainly where there is tension or a clash of work ethic values among members of the team.
Autocratic/Authoritarian/Transactional. Top-down approach is evident here (controlling, directing, goal/target setting). Often the use of recognition and reward inducements to encourage motivation. Transactional leaders usually focus more on tasks (e.g., dominate and make decisions without allowing or considering the views of others).	In some situations, can be very efficient (e.g., cardiac arrest). Emphasis on the ability of leader/manager to monitor and correct others.	Has the potential to stifle creativity, may foster dependence, submissiveness and loss of individuality. There is little/limited collaboration and delegation. Shared values are not communicated and this may lead to discontent, hostility and even aggression among members of the group or followers.
Democratic. Leaders work with and guide rather than direct followers.	Increases job satisfaction for followers as they feel more motivated to become involved. Empowers followers.	Takes more time and effort to carry out effectively.
Transformational. Based on the notion that leaders motivate others to perform by encouraging a shared vision and altering their perception of reality (e.g., shares the decision-making and planning processes and also has responsibility for their implementation.)		

This style is often used by inexperienced leaders who are still learning, or by managers who are providing cover, waiting for someone to replace them. It could be suggested that a laissez-faire approach to leading is indeed (due to the absence of leadership) not leading at all.

Autocratic/authoritarian/transactional

In this approach, the leader calls all the shots. Decisions are made quickly without any kind of consultation with staff and all the power is focused at the top with everyone else passively following. Any team members who disagree with the autocratic leader and do not do as they are told are often punished to keep them in line. In this approach, knowledge is usually kept in the hands of the few to ensure it is kept with those in power. This is a good approach to use when fast action is necessary, such as a cardiac arrest or other emergency. However, when mistakes happen, it is usual for an authoritarian to make an example of others by chastising them in front of their peers. The blame is always on the individuals, regardless of the fault processes (Kibble & Chen, 2015).

Democratic

This style is the opposite of the authoritarian leadership style. The democratic leader encourages the team to speak up and take part in the decision-making process. An open communication approach is promoted, and all staff members should feel that their voices matter. With this approach, staff are encouraged to have more concern about the things that are going on in the organization with an understanding that they can influence situations if they act on them. Members of the team are given their own individual responsibilities and they assume accountability for reaching certain targets. When they receive feedback on their performance, this can permit them to adjust their approach if necessary. The emphasis is on improving the quality of the care and the systems and processes that will enable this, not on finding errors that may have been made by an individual team member.

BOX 12.1 Four Key Attributes Associated with Transformational Nurse Leaders (Adapted from Burns, 1978; Wong & Cummings, 2009)

1. The leader is seen as a role model, never requiring nursing staff to do something that they would not do.
2. They inspire motivation in their followers by having a strong vision about their work.
3. They are concerned about individuals and demonstrate real concern for their needs and feelings. They do this through mentoring and supporting individuals.
4. They challenge and develop the followers, encouraging them to be innovative and creative, as well as nurturing independent thinkers.

Transformational

Akin to democratic leadership is transformational leadership. In 1978, James McGregor Burns introduced the transformation leadership theory. It was described as leadership that occurs when the leader engages with followers in a way that raises their level of performance as well as their motivation. Transformational leaders encourage others to find meaning and value in their work, which can enable them to make significant contributions to the organization. Box 12.1 highlights four key attributes associated with transformational nurse leaders.

Transformational leadership contrasts with transactional leadership approaches where staff are driven in an authoritarian way as opposed to being led, so that 'followers' are worked on instead of worked with.

Table 12.3 provides an overview of leadership styles.

Collective leadership

Leadership often has an image of a single leader, a hero. With collective leadership, however, leadership is seen as a dynamic process of exchange between several people who are a part of a

TABLE 12.3   An Overview of Leadership Styles (Adapted from Wild, 2014)

Leadership Style	Traits	Influence
Laissez-faire	Permits others to make decisions Allows others to manage and control their own work Expects others to work autonomously and to ask for help if needed Adopts a 'hands-off' approach	Positive: works well in environments where the team is highly skilled, motivated and able to work independently Negative: in environments where the team is inexperienced the team may become demotivated, miss opportunities for development and can fall behind with deadlines
Authoritarian	Decision-maker Task-orientated High standards Planning and expecting others to follow In control, maintains power over others	Positive: when directions need to be clear and directed, e.g., in an emergency situation or when working with a novice Negative: can engender staff dependency, and can result in demotivation and may stifle creativity
Democratic	Team player Shares ideas Has mutual respect of others' ideas Delegates in order to develop others Interacts and seeks opinions	Positive: adopts a team approach, which can elicit more effective solutions. Respect from team members who feel developed Negative: in emergency situations where delay in decision-making might be seen as lack of competence
Bureaucratic	Obeys the rule book Is governed by policy and regulations Adheres to a close set of values and standards Is a strict disciplinarian	Positive: in situations where exact and precise ways of working are required, e.g., high-risk areas Negative: teams may feel indifferent, powerless and frustrated
Situational	Adapts style to manage specific situations Identifies the performance, competencies and commitment of others Flexible Recognizes the relationship between the leader's supportive and directive behaviour and the competence of followers Offers emotional support and is an effective communicator	Positive: allows for contingencies, and can be effective when providing support to newly registered NAs and students Negative: too much emphasis on leaders and not enough on group interaction

network of relationships that go beyond leader and follower. Collective leadership questions the traditional notions in which individuals become the source of leadership. This approach embraces the idea that many individuals within a system can lead, or that groups of people, structures and processes may use leadership in order to help move towards a shared goal.

Collective leadership is a leadership framework which is sometimes referred to as 'compassionate leadership' or 'distributed leadership' (NHS Improvement, 2017). According to West et al. (2015), a collective leadership culture is one that is characterized by shared leadership, where there is still a formal hierarchy, but the power flow is situationally dependent on who has the expertise at each moment. Such a culture is valuable, especially at team level. Collective leadership reflects the assumption that acts of leadership should come from anybody, not only from those who are in formal positions of authority.

If patients and service users in health and social care settings are to receive continually improving, high-quality, compassionate care, then a collective leadership approach is required. To ensure high-quality care it is important that all staff are engaged and committed. Each interaction that every member of staff has, every day, both with each other and the people they offer care to, will influence the extent to which the organization is able to provide high-quality and compassionate care. As well as engaging all members of staff in the organization, it is essential that patients and those who use services are also part of the leadership process.

The Department of Health and Health and Social Care (2017) in Northern Ireland noted that where there is a culture of

collective leadership it brings with it benefits for staff. It also leads to improved quality of care, results in a better experience for those who use services and delivers greater sustainability of those services. Fig. 12.2 provides an overview of the Department of Health and Health and Social Care (2017) Collective Leadership Strategy.

> **REFLECTION 12.3**
>
> What do you think may be the advantages and disadvantages of collective leadership?

TEAMWORKING

A team is a group of people, with each member of the team having different skills, who work together to accomplish a common goal. Teams, as opposed to individuals, can bring together the skills, experiences and disciplines that are required to offer care and support to the people who use services. Teamwork is the process of working together with a group of people to achieve a common goal.

Good teams do not just happen, they emerge over time. The basis for a team emerging is that everyone in the team understands, respects and values their own role, as well as the roles of other members. All team members have to be clear about:

- what they can and cannot do or the boundaries of their role
- the degree of freedom they have when making decisions

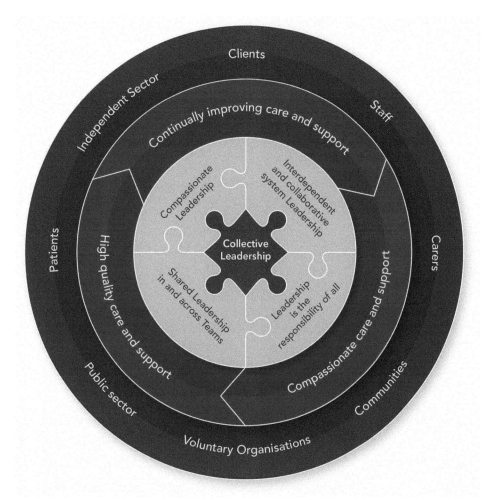

Fig. 12.2 Department of Health and Health and Social Care Collective Leadership Strategy (Department of Health and Health and Social Care, 2017).

- who they delegate activities to and who delegates activities to them
- how their function will be assessed, and what are the key things that they are expected to do
- where they can go for advice, support and supervision
- the boundaries to their freedom with regard to creativity and initiative
- how the team and team members will be supported to grow and develop.

Regardless of the leadership framework, unless there is effective teamwork in place, any strategy will be destined to fail. The NA and other healthcare staff have to work interdependently across professional boundaries, all aiming to provide high-quality and safe care for patients (Lyubovnikova & West, 2013).

Where multi-professional teams work together in an effective way, patient satisfaction is higher; healthcare delivery is more effective; there are increased levels of innovation in the delivery of new and improved ways of caring for patients; there are lower instances of staff stress, absenteeism and turnover; and there is more consistent communication with patients (West et al., 2015). D'Innocenzo et al. (2014) point out that leadership that ensures

effective team and inter-teamworking within and across organizational boundaries is key if NHS organizations will meet the challenges that they face.

From a historical perspective, the nursing team has always consisted of nurses, health visitors, students, support workers and associate practitioners with all of these staff delivering various elements of nursing care and each member of the team having a different level of responsibility and decision-making power. This team has grown, however, and become more complex over the years as new roles have been created, including the NA. In many settings, support workers are now providing a considerable amount of hands-on care. See Box 12.2 for the components of effective teamworking.

Many of the challenges in teamworking come about because people who are in the team are not clear about their role or function. Often, they do not fully understand what it is that they or other team members should be doing. When this happens, conflict is more likely to occur. It is essential when working as a team member that the NA is clear about their role and the roles of others. This approach has the potential to reduce tensions in the team.

CRITICAL AWARENESS

Working in a dynamic and constantly changing environment such as healthcare can be challenging. However, if you can develop the skills and attitudes that underpin effective teamworking, including understanding and valuing your role and the roles of other team members, knowing the team's objectives and playing a positive part in team meetings, you will come to recognize the many benefits that teamworking brings, not only to the quality of care patients receive, but also to the quality of the work experience.

Good teams:
- are creative in how they organize services
- make good decisions
- respond effectively to sudden changes
- provide high-quality services to patients.

MANAGING CONFLICT

Workplace conflict is a major source of stress for nurses. Conflict is often seen as a bad thing; however, it is a natural part of interactions with others. When conflict is addressed effectively it has the ability to improve interpersonal relationships (Balzer-Riley, 2017).

Conflict can be defined as a disagreement or struggle that happens when there is either a real or perceived threat or difference in the desires, thoughts, attitudes, feelings, or behaviours of two or more parties. It exists as a tension or struggle coming from mutually exclusive or opposing actions, thoughts, opinions or feelings. Conflict may be internal or external to an individual or a group. It can be positive as well as negative (Huber, 2017). It can be described as an expression of disagreement between at least two individuals and it frequently comes about as a difference of approach, opinion, intention or interpretation (Sullivan & Garland, 2013). Being able to manage conflict in a constructive and creative manner can be a challenge. Adopting a positive approach to conflict resolution can benefit patients as well as staff and it also gives support to the effective functioning of clinical teams.

Types of conflict

Finkelman and Kenner (2015) suggest there are three types of conflict:
1. Intrapersonal
2. Interpersonal
3. Intergroup

Intrapersonal conflict

This refers to personal unfulfilled needs and is associated with expectations and goals that result in tension, stress and disharmony within the individual (Huber 2017). It occurs when the person argues with themselves about something. For example, an NA may experience intrapersonal conflict in striving for a work–life balance.

Interpersonal conflict

This type of conflict occurs between two or more people who have differing values, goals or beliefs (Marquis & Huston, 2017). It might occur, for example, if an NA requests specific annual leave, but the nurse manager is unable to allocate these days off due to staff shortages. These types of conflict are not limited only to NAs. Patients can enter into an interpersonal conflict with an NA if they do not agree with an assessment or recommendation. Interpersonal conflict can be overt, for instance when it results in a person verbally making known a disagreement with someone else.

Relationship conflict concerns interpersonal incompatibilities, such as feelings of tension and friction. Here personal issues, feelings of dislike among group members and irritation, frustration and impatience may occur.

Task conflict is an awareness of differences in viewpoints and opinions about a group task. This is similar to relationship conflict; it relates more to and concerns conflict that emerges regarding ideas and differences of opinion about the task in hand. Task conflicts may be accompanied by lively discussions and personal excitement, but by definition, these are not constructive because of the intense negative interpersonal emotions that are often associated with relationship conflict.

Intergroup conflict

This type of conflict occurs between two or more groups of people, departments, or organizations (Marquis & Huston, 2017); it can also be known as interorganizational conflict. For example, an intergroup conflict might take place between the National Health Service and trade unions in relation to payment of staff and conditions of service.

Another example of intergroup conflict is when two or more departments in the same organization or department (unit) are competing for resources, particularly money, equipment and staff. Ongoing organizational conflicts can have a negative impact on staff and the department or unit, as constant competition for resources can create stress resulting in poor service provision.

Potential causes of conflict

As with other social processes, there are many reasons and conditions that can engender conflict. One analysis of conflict in the work environment (Almost, 2006) indicated that the precursors to conflict arise from the following factors:
- individual characteristics
- interpersonal factors
- organizational factors.

Individual characteristics include differing opinions and values, as well as demographic differences, which include gender and educational differences and generational (age) diversity. Interpersonal factors include lack of trust, feelings of injustice or disrespect and inadequate or poor communication. Organizational factors include interdependence and changes due to restructuring.

Huber (2017) suggests that a common condition that can lead to conflict is incompatible goals. The common goal in the provision of healthcare is to deliver safe, effective, quality care for patients; however, different disciplines may have different ideas on how best to provide this service, which may result in conflict.

Differences between beliefs and values can often cause conflict in the healthcare setting (Sullivan & Garland, 2013). An individual's beliefs and values develop from how they were socialized, their experiences and their personal set of beliefs.

Conflict can surface when individuals from different disciplines have roles and responsibilities that overlap. When there is lack of clarity associated with role and responsibility (which can happen to any member of the team), conflict is likely to arise.

In a health service where austerity has been the order of the day for a number of years, competition for resources is a common situation that leads to conflict (Finkelman & Kenner, 2015). With tight budgets, staff shortages and a lack of equipment, conflict is likely.

Sullivan & Garland (2013) suggest that the human behaviours that can cause conflict include:

- Blaming
- Accusing
- Insulting
- Using hostile language
- Making assumptions.

Impact of conflict

Whilst conflict includes positive and negative effects, Almost (2006) has noted that there is more empirical evidence for negative outcomes than for positive outcomes. The main effects of conflict are:

- individual effects
- interpersonal relationships
- organizational effects.

Individual effects can include job stress, job dissatisfaction, absenteeism, intent to leave, increased grievances, psychosomatic complaints and negative emotions. Organizational effects include reduced coordination and collaboration at work and reduced productivity. Interpersonal relationships included positive and negative outcomes. The positive outcomes are stronger relationships and team cohesiveness, whereas negative outcomes include negative perceptions of others, hostility and avoidance.

Functional (positive) outcomes include improved group performance, better quality of decision making, encouragement of creativity and innovation, generation of interest and curiosity, provision of a way to problem-solve and the creation of an environment for self-evaluation and change. However, dysfunctional (negative) outcomes include the development of discontent, a reduction in group effectiveness, interrupted communication, diminished group cohesiveness and in-fighting among members of the group, which then distorts the focus of the group on its goals (Robbins & Judge, 2015).

Managing conflict

There is no one single best method to manage conflict. The situation itself, the urgency associated with any decision that needs to be made, organizational culture, the power and status of those involved, the importance of the issue, the time that is available and the maturity of the individuals involved in the conflict are factors that will influence the strategy that is chosen (Marquis & Huston, 2017). The way conflict is managed will also depend on the style and strategy chosen by the manager.

It is essential to take action as soon as there is any sign of conflict surfacing so if there are bad feelings, these will not linger and intensify. In a group situation, the best place to clear the air is in a group meeting. Here, issues can be defined and strategies worked out for managing the points of disagreement.

To work effectively as part of a team, NAs must establish positive respectful relationships. Positive working relationships are the result of good communication, mutual acceptance and understanding, use of persuasion – as opposed to coercion – and a balance of reason and emotion. The active management of conflict is a key part of building positive collegial relationships. Those who work together to manage conflict in an effective way will help to promote a working environment that creates positive outcomes for both patients and healthcare staff.

Colleagues should address conflict directly as opposed to avoiding it, focusing on the behaviours that led to the conflict rather than personally on a colleague. Validate any assumptions that are being made through open dialogue with colleagues instead of acting on misperceptions or suppositions. The NA should collaborate with colleagues to identify the underlying cause of the conflict. In some instances, a neutral party (such as a professional mediator) may be necessary (College of Nurses of Ontario, 2017).

Conflict is more than just a disagreement. When ignored, a conflict will continue to fester. We will all respond to conflict based on what our perceptions of the situation are. Conflict has the potential to trigger strong emotions, but conflict should also be seen as an opportunity for growth.

MANAGING CHANGE

Change management is complex and is driven by a number of factors and can have an impact on patients, staff and organizations. How change is managed is key to its successful implementation and just like conflict, often change is seen as negative, yet can also have positive ramifications (Jones & Bennett, 2012).

Reasons for change

There are many reasons for change, and in any organization there are many factors that will drive change. Reasons for change may occur at three levels (see Table 12.4).

Identifying where changes are coming from is important so that their worth or applicability can be evaluated and their rationale communicated to others. One aspect of change that has had an impact on the public and healthcare professionals over recent years in England is the transformation of urgent and emergency care services (see Table 12.5).

TABLE 12.4 Levels of Change (Adapted from Jones & Bennett, 2012)

Level	Example
The micro level	Occurs where changes may originate from the client, the unit or the department
The meso level	Includes the health and/or social care organization and the community
The macro level	Is affected by national or international (i.e., World Health Organization, European Union) policy

TABLE 12.5 Levels of Change Related to Urgent and Emergency Care Services (Adapted from Jones & Bennett, 2012)

Level	Example
The micro level	This can include public/community dissatisfaction or complaints and/or staff complaints
The meso level	The drivers here may include key performance indicators concerning waiting times for those requiring urgent or emergency services and/or community/public dissatisfaction
The macro level	National policy in the form of guidance from the DH regarding transformation of urgent and emergency care (DH, 2015)

Force field analysis is a tool that can help to identify and evaluate the forces for and against a change. Lewin's force field analysis tool (Lewin, 1947) is one such approach.

REFLECTION 12.4

Think of a change in your place of work that you would like to instigate. Using the force field analysis, what are the drivers and barriers to the change initiative you have thought about? How might you address the imbalance? How can you turn the barriers into drivers? Who might provide you with help to turn this around?

In order for any proposed change to be effective, the forces driving the change have to be stronger than the forces resisting it. The resistant forces could be centred on the availability of physical and human resources and finance. They are often centred on the psychological responses of those involved in and affected by the change. Often the most visible symbol of change is a physical change. Important changes to agreed working practices are accompanied by social and psychological changes (Jones & Barnett, 2012).

A leader has to try to understand what is underpinning a person's resistance to change. Those reasons may be manifold, but could include the following:

- An unwillingness to give up something that the individual values
- A lack of understanding and appreciation of the change and its consequences
- A lack of belief in the change with regard to its benefits for the organization (perceived or actual)
- A low tolerance of change.

Once aware of the resisting forces, it is often possible to minimize them through discussing and addressing the salient points with the key players.

DELEGATION

Delegation can be defined as directing another to carry out work or perform a duty. It is about empowering one person to act on behalf of another. Over the last decade the task of delegation has changed, as have health and social care teams. The nursing team is now made up of a range of different people all bringing with them different skills and levels of competence.

CASE STUDY 12.3 Shona

Shona, a healthcare assistant, is working on a busy medical ward. She has undertaken a patient's nutritional assessment using the Malnutrition Universal Screening Tool (MUST). Shona has been assessed during a training session on nutritional assessment at the hospital as competent to carry out this assessment.

This aspect of Shona's role forms a part of her job description (this is a responsibility). As part of his NA role, Freddie has delegated this activity to Shona. He is fully aware of Shona's level of competence and what her responsibilities are.

Freddie remains professionally responsible for appropriate delegation and Shona is accountable for her actions (although not currently regulated).

The principles of delegation have been discussed in Chapter 6, and Chapter 4 addresses the important issue of duty of care. All those who provide health and social services are accountable to the criminal and civil courts to ensure that the activities they carry out conform to legal requirements. Furthermore, employees are accountable to their employer as they adhere to the terms and conditions in their contract of employment. All registered practitioners are also accountable to regulatory bodies in terms of standards of practice and patient care.

For the NA to be accountable for their decision to delegate tasks and duties to others, they must:

- Only delegate tasks and duties that are within the other person's scope of competence, ensuring that the person fully understands the instructions
- Make sure that everyone they delegate tasks to is sufficiently supervised and supported in order for them to provide safe and compassionate care
- Confirm that the outcome of any task that has been delegated meets the required standard.

(Royal College of Nursing (RCN), 2017)

Table 12.6 provides a delegation checklist; if you can answer yes to all of the questions in the checklist, then delegation is appropriate. If you are unable to answer yes, then it is inappropriate to delegate the task, as it would not be in the best interests of the patient.

LOOKING BACK, FEEDING FORWARD

Managing care provision is complex, and in the health and social care field, no two days are ever the same. The NA is required to

TABLE 12.6 The Delegation Checklist (Adapted from RCN, 2017)

Item	Check
Is delegation in the patient's best interests?	
Have you considered the clinical risk that may be involved in delegating?	
Do you have authority to delegate the work, as well as the appropriate clinical knowledge?	
Does the person being delegated to have the skills and knowledge needed to carry out the activity, including communication and interpersonal skills, and are they also considered clinically competent?	
Does the health care assistant have the capacity to take on additional work?	
Are you able to provide support and supervision and check that the outcome of the delegation meets the required standard?	

manage care that is safe and compassionate, and in order to do this they need to develop their leadership and management skills. This chapter has provided some insight into the complexities of management and leadership.

The role and function of the NA is set to grow and develop. There will be much need for current and future NAs to develop their clinical and management skills. The key aim has to be to ensure that care delivered at all times and in all situations is safe, with the patient at the centre of all that is done.

REFERENCES

Almost, J., 2005. Conflict within nursing work environments: concept analysis. J. Adv. Nurs. 53 (4), 444–453.

Balzer-Riley, J., 2017. Communication in Nursing, eighth ed. Mosby, St Louis.

Burns, D., 2015. Leadership and management. In: Burns, D. (Ed.), Foundations of Adult Nursing. Sage, London, pp. 205–242, (Chapter 8).

Burns, J.M., 1978. Leadership. Harper and Row Publishers, New York.

College of Nurses of Ontario, 2017. Conflict Prevention and Management https://www.cno.org/globalassets/docs/prac/47004_conflict_prev.pdf.

Department of Health (DH), 2015. Safer, Faster, Better: Good Practice in Delivering Urgent and Emergency Care. A Guide for Local Health and Social Care Communities. https://www.england.nhs.uk/wp-content/uploads/2015/06/trans-uec.pdf.

Department of Health (DH), 2016. Leading Change, Adding Value https://www.england.nhs.uk/wp-content/uploads/2016/05/nursing-framework.pdf.

Department of Health and Health and Social Care, 2017. HSC Collective Leadership Strategy https://www.health-ni.gov.uk/sites/default/files/publications/health/hsc-collective-leadership-strategy.pdf.

D'Innocenzo, L., Mathieu, J.E., Kukenberger, M.R., 2014. A meta-analysis of different forms of shared leadership – team performance relations. Journal of Management. doi:10.1177/0149206314525205.

Finkelman, A., Kenner, C., 2015. Leadership and Management for Nurses: Core Competencies for Quality Care, third ed. Pearson, New Jersey.

Huber, D.L., 2017. Leadership. Nursing Care Management, sixth ed. Saunders, Philadelphia.

Jones, L., Bennett, C.L., 2012. Leadership in Health and Social Care. An Introduction for Emerging Leaders. Lantern Publishing, Banbury.

Kibble, M.R., Chen, H., 2015. Leadership in Surgery. Springer International, New York.

King's Fund, 2011. The Future of Leadership and Management in the NHS. No More Heroes. King's Fund, London.

Kotter, J.P., 1996. Leading Change. Harvard Business School Press, Boston.

Lewin, K., 1947. Frontiers in group dynamics: concept, method and reality in social science; social equilibria and social change. Human Relations 1, 5–41.

Luft, J., Ingham, H., 1955.. The Johari Window, A Graphic Model of Interpersonal Awareness. Proceedings of the Western Training Laboratory in Group Development. Los Angeles, UCLA.

Lyubovnikova, J., West, M.A., 2013. Why teamwork matters: enabling health care team effectiveness for the delivery of high quality patient care. In: Salas, E., Tannembaum, S.I., Cohen, D., Latham, G. (Eds.), Developing and Enhancing Teamwork in Organizations. Jossey Bass., San Francisco, pp. 331–372.

Marquis, B.L., Huston, C.J., 2017. Leadership Roles and Management Functions in Nursing: Theory and Application, ninth ed. Wolters, Philadelphia.

NHS Improvement, 2017. Culture and Leadership Programme. Phase 2. https://improvement.nhs.uk/uploads/documents/01-NHS104-Phase_2_Toolkit_060717_FINAL.pdf.

Peate, I., 2016. The Essential Guide to Becoming a Staff Nurse. Wiley, Oxford.

Robbins, S.P., Judge, T.A., 2015. Essentials of Organizational Behavior, thirteenth ed. Pearson, New Jersey.

Royal College of Nursing (RCN), 2017. Accountability and Delegation: A Guide for the Nursing Team. https://www.rcn.org.uk/professional-development/publications/pub-006465.

Salas, E., Diaz-Granados, D., Klein, C., et al., 2009. Does team training improve team performance? A meta-analysis. Hum. Factors 50 (6), 903–933.

Sullivan, J., Garland, G., 2013. Practical Leadership and Management in Healthcare for Nurses and Allied Health Professionals. Pearson, London.

Tomey, A.M., 2009. Guide to Nursing Management and Leadership, sixth ed. Elsevier, St Louis.

West, M., Armit, K., Loewenthal, L., et al., 2015. Leadership and Leadership Development in Health Care: The Evidence Base. King's Fund, London.

Wilcox, J.W., 2014. Challenges of nursing management and leadership. In: Zerwekh, J., Zerwekh-Garneau, A. (Eds.), Nursing Today. Transition and Trends. Elsevier, St Louis, pp. 194–221, (Chapter 10).

Wild, K., 2014. The professional nurse and contemporary practice. In: Peate, I., Wild, K.Nair, M. (Eds.), Nursing Practice, Knowledge and Care. Wiley, Oxford, pp. 25–49, (Chapter 2).

Wong, C.A., Cummings, G.G., 2009. The relationship between nursing leadership and patient outcomes: a systematic review. J. Nurs. Manag. 15, 508–521.

Reflective Practice

Jacqueline Chang

OBJECTIVES

By the end of this chapter the reader will be able to:
1. Understand the importance of reflective practice in healthcare
2. Be able to identify key literature that supports reflective practice
3. Understand some of the commonly used reflective models
4. Know how to use different models of reflection to aid reflective practice
5. Understand the practicalities of reflective practice
6. Feel confident to include reflection in their practice both clinically and academically

KEY WORDS

Academic writing
Candour
Formal reflection
Literature

Reflective blog
Reflective practice
Reflective models
Revalidation

Safeguarding
The 6Cs

CHAPTER AIM

This chapter will look at the art of reflection. It will explain why the Nursing Associate (NA) and other healthcare professionals should reflect upon their practice. It will then describe some common reflection models and provide exercises to help the reflector identify which models they work with best. It will explain the different types of formal reflection and highlight some of the challenges of reflection.

SELF TEST

1. What do you understand by the term 'reflection'?
2. How often should a healthcare professional reflect on their practice?
3. What should a healthcare practitioner reflect upon?
4. How long should a reflection take?
5. What guidelines emphasize the importance of reflective practice?
6. What reflective models have you heard of?
7. What different formats of reflection are there?
8. What do you think the benefits of reflective practice are?
9. Which of the 6Cs relate to reflective practice?
10. Why do you think some people don't use reflection to evaluate their practice?

INTRODUCTION

Reflection, other than the throwing back of light or heat, is defined by the Oxford English Dictionary as 'serious thought or consideration' (2017). For healthcare, this is further interpreted as giving serious thought to our practice and that of our peers. Reflection is not a new concept. It was written about in 1933 by John Dewey, who described it as a process that is both deliberate and active. He stated that it involves 'careful consideration of any belief or supposed form of knowledge in the light of the grounds that support it, and further conclusions to which it leads' (Dewey, 1933).

Reflection is something that everybody does. We all think about the care we have delivered and how we have reacted in certain situations. However, we do not always look deeply enough to really assess our own practice. By seriously considering our own practice we can identify deficits, develop and improve what we do and learn from others.

THE IMPORTANCE OF REFLECTION IN HEALTHCARE

There are some aspects of guidance from the Nursing and Midwifery Council (NMC) and the Department of Health that highlight the importance of reflective practice. These are the

6Cs, The Code, NMC Revalidation, the Professional Duty of Candour and the Francis Report. Their relationship to reflective practice is summarized here.

The Francis Report (2013)

The Mid Staffordshire Enquiry of 2013 highlighted the importance of healthcare practitioners assessing their own practice and the practice of their peers. The report investigated mistreatment and poor care delivery and made recommendations for all healthcare providers about how this should be prevented in the future. Among the many problems that Sir Robert Francis found, the negative culture traits in that specific Trust included defensiveness and a lack of openness to criticism. In order to prevent this happening again, he recommended creating a culture of openness, transparency and candour. This is intrinsically linked to reflection because in reflecting on the care we deliver, we are able to self-regulate and maintain our professional standards.

The Code (2018)

Nursing Associates will be regulated by the NMC and they will work under The Code (2015). This is the same professional code that First level Registered Nurses work under, and it states that in order to practise effectively, a registered healthcare professional should be able to 'reflect and act on any feedback you receive to improve your practice' (Nursing and Midwifery Council, 2018a).

Revalidation (2017)

In order to validate their nursing registration with the NMC all registered nurses have to demonstrate effective reflection of practice through five written reflections, which are then discussed via peer conversation (NMC, 2017a).

NAs are also going to be validated by the NMC, and the NMC Standards of Proficiency for Nursing Associates (2018b) states what is expected of them. One of the standards is that NAs will be accountable for their practice and within that, they must be able to 'acknowledge and articulate the demands of professional practice and demonstrate how to recognize signs of vulnerability in themselves or their colleagues and the action required to minimise risks to health' (NMC, 2018b). In standard number 4, working in teams, the NA must 'understand ways in which they can improve their own personal performance and the quality of care they provide' and also, they must 'contribute to team reflection activities to promote improvements in practice and services'. In standard number 6, the NA must 'demonstrate an understanding of their own role and contribution, and the issues which require management by themselves and others, when involved in the care of a person who is undergoing a transition of care between professionals, setting and services'. In order to do all of these things, the NA must have an understanding of reflection and be comfortable with looking critically at their own practice.

Duty of Candour (2016)

One of the recommendations of the Francis report (2013) was for healthcare practitioners to be honest and open about making mistakes. This led to the publication of the Professional Duty of Candour in 2016. This duty tells healthcare workers to be open and honest when something happens that could, or does, affect their care in a negative way (NMC/General Medical Council, 2015; NMC, 2017b). The duty tells healthcare professionals to report any incidents or near misses to their line managers for follow up. Being a reflective practitioner is an essential element of candour. By reflecting on practice, healthcare professionals can see where errors have occurred and what could have been prevented. If healthcare professionals are not reflective, they are unable to identify any areas that may require development.

The 6Cs (2012)

Compassion in Practice was published by the Department of Health in 2012. This policy was released following public consultation to reflect the needs of the healthcare workforce. The Compassion in Practice policy is underpinned by 'the 6Cs', which are discussed here and in more detail in Chapter 8.

The 6Cs are identified values that should always be considered when delivering care. The report itself acknowledges that these are not new ideas, but this policy formalizes them. Box 13.1 provides an overview of the 6Cs.

BOX 13.1 The 6Cs (DH, 2012)

Care

Care is our core business and that of our organizations. The care we deliver helps the individual person and improves the health of the whole community. Caring defines us and our work. People receiving care expect it to be right for them, consistently, throughout every stage of their life.

Compassion

Compassion is how care is given through relationships based on empathy, respect and dignity – it can also be described as intelligent kindness and is central to how people perceive their care.

Competence

Competence means all those in caring roles must have the ability to understand an individual's health and social needs and the expertise, clinical and technical knowledge to deliver effective care and treatments based on research and evidence.

Communication

Communication is central to successful caring relationships and to effective team working. Listening is as important as what we say and do, and essential for 'no decision about me without me'. Communication is the key to a good workplace and benefits those in our care and staff alike.

Courage

Courage enables us to do the right thing for the people we care for, to speak up when we have concerns and to have the personal strength and vision to innovate and to embrace new ways of working.

Commitment

A commitment to our patients and populations is a cornerstone of what we do. We need to build on our commitment to improve the care and experience of our patients, to take action to make this vision and strategy a reality for all and meet the health, care and support challenges ahead.

Contains public sector information licensed under the Open Government Licence v3.0.

The relevance of the 6Cs to reflection is quite simple. By reflecting on our practice, we are maintaining all six of the Cs. We reflect about the care we give, or the care we have seen being given, to try to ensure that the best possible care is being delivered. The process of reflecting on our practice will enable us to look at the compassion we express through our care. Reflection asks us to consider other points of view, which promotes empathy and understanding. Reflection will encourage competence as it examines the care we are giving, and through using literature, helps us to ensure we are competent in our care delivery. Communication is a vital element of reflection, whether you are reflecting verbally or in a written format. It takes courage to be able to criticize your own practice and the practice of your colleagues. Reflection also shows commitment to your job. Reflection can only help your practice, and to want to do that, you must be committed to your work.

MODELS TO AID REFLECTION

There are many models to help professionals reflect, and some are considered here. The benefit of using a model is that it provides structure for the reflection. Without a model, it is easy to describe what has happened, how you felt and how you feel now, but the models make the reflector probe deeper into the event and along with the literature, support actions and feelings.

All reflective cycles have the same basic criteria of describing the event, analyzing the event and considering what to do with the information gathered from the analysis. Some cycles are relatively simple, whereas others offer a lot more guidance. All of the cycles are good reflection tools and every reflector should find the tool that they like to use the most. At times, you will be told which one to use for academic work, but when conducting your own reflections, you can choose whichever cycle you prefer.

Reflection in action/reflection on action

In 1983 Schön described reflections as having two different timescales as described in Table 13.1.

Reflection in action is spontaneous. Adaptations to care need to be made in the moment to provide safer or more appropriate care and therefore a formal model is not appropriate for these situations. However, after the event, it would be appropriate to reflect on action to help your personal development and learn from the situation you have just experienced.

TABLE 13.1 Reflection in Action, Reflection on Action (Schön, 1983)	
Stage 1: Reflection in action	This is when you are able to reflect on behaviour and feelings during an episode of care and can change actions at that point.
Stage 2: Reflection on action	This involves looking back at an interaction and evaluating behaviour and opinions after the event has occurred.

The following reflective models focus on ways to reflect on action.

Kolb's Learning Cycle

This was published in 1984 and is a useful model for nurses and other healthcare providers to use. It consists of four stages that are integrated and cyclical in nature.

Stage 1: Concrete experiences

Asks the reflector to describe what actually happened (the experience).

Stage 2: Reflective observation

Asks the reflector to think about that experience. This is easier for some people than for others and guidance may be needed for this. It requires the reflector to reflect and review.

Stage 3: Abstract conceptualization

Having thought about the experience the reflector should consider how a different outcome might have occurred by acting in a different way. This is about creating a hypothesis.

Stage 4: Active experimentation

The process of testing out the hypothesis that arose from stage 3.

Gibbs' Reflective Cycle

This was published in 1998 (see Fig. 13.1) and consists of six stages.

Stage 1: Description

Describe what happened. This section should be quite short.

Stage 2: Feelings

The reflector should think about how they felt during the episode. It is sometimes worth considering how you feel about it once some time has passed.

Stage 3: Evaluation

Consider what was good and what was bad about the episode.

Stage 4: Analysis

This is the main element of this cycle. The reflector should consider how they felt, the positive and negative points

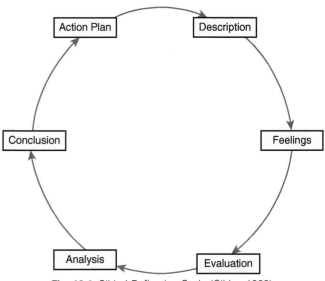

Fig. 13.1 Gibbs' Reflective Cycle (Gibbs, 1988).

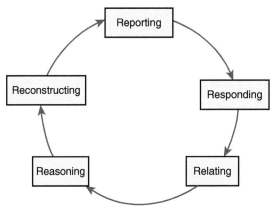

Fig. 13.2 Bain's Framework (Bain et al., 2002).

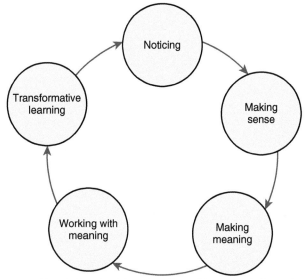

Fig. 13.3 Moon's Levels of Learning (From Moon, 1999. Reproduced with permission from Taylor & Francis Books UK).

and what sense can be made of this. When writing essays, this is the stage that requires most of the literature support where you can really look at what affected the situation at the time.

Stage 5: Conclusion

This is a short stage which allows the reflector to pull the different elements together.

Stage 6: Action plan

This final stage asks the reflector to describe what they would do should the situation occur again.

Bain's Framework (5Rs)

This was published in 1999 (see Fig. 13.2) and has five stages.

Stage 1: Reporting

The reflector describes the episode that occurred.

Stage 2: Responding

The reflector describes how they felt during the episode and consider why that was.

Stage 3: Relating

Explains what happened and looks at areas that could have been managed better.

Stage 4: Reasoning

Uses literature to demonstrate a greater understanding of the episode.

Stage 5: Reconstructing.

The reflector states what they would do should the same or a similar situation arise again.

Moon's Levels of Learning

This was published in 1999 (see Fig. 13.3) and consists of five stages.

Stage 1: Noticing

This is when the reflector notices that an event is interesting or important and wants to reflect on it.

Stage 2: Making sense

The reflector needs to understand why they noticed this episode and begin to try to understand it better.

Stage 3: Making meaning

The reflector begins to understand the issues by asking questions and linking thoughts together.

Stage 4: Working with meaning

This is the stage that utilizes literature in order for the reflector to link their own ideas and learn from other experiences.

Stage 5: Transformative learning

Utilizing the literature read and ideas formed, the reflector can decide how they would act should a similar situation occur again.

Johns' model for structured reflection

This was published in 2000 and is structured differently from the other frameworks. It has two sections and each section has cue questions; these are outlined in Table 13.2.

How to decide which model to use

The models are all similar with the same goal, but it is important to find the one that you like best. Consider which of the five models described you think is structured best for you. When you work with each model, consider which probing questions you can relate to the most and which do not seem comfortable to you.

CHALLENGES OF REFLECTION

The main challenge of reflection is knowing where to emphasize the discussion and analysis. It is easy to describe the event, and often too much time is spent on this. The core element of reflection is the analysis/conceptualization/reasoning/working with meaning section. This is where the learning and development is explained. This section uses the art of reflection and the literature to support the development of the reflector. It is also the most challenging part of the reflective cycle, but it is the most important one for improving practice.

TABLE 13.2 Johns' Model for Structure Development (Johns, 2000)

Stage 1: Looking in	• Find some time and a quiet space to be able to focus on yourself.
	• Pay close attention to your emotions and your feelings and thoughts and write these down with honesty.
Stage 2: Looking out	• Describe the event.
	• Identify significant issues.
	• Consider different elements of the event, including what you were trying to achieve, why you responded the way you did, what the consequences were, how others were feeling and how you knew others were feeling that way.
	• Explain why you felt the way that you felt.
	• Consider whether you acted in the best way possible for the best reasons.
	• Look at what factors influenced your behaviour and what knowledge affected your actions.
	• Reflect on the event and relate it to other experiences, considering how it could have been managed better. What, if anything, would have been different had you acted differently? How do you feel now and how could you react in the future?

When to reflect on practice

Arguably, healthcare professionals reflect in action constantly; it is just not formalized. Because the work is with members of the public, practice has to constantly be adapted to suit the person receiving care. However, there is a difference between subconscious reflection and formalized reflection. The question of when it is appropriate to formally reflect is an interesting one. During an academic course you will be instructed to find an incident and reflect upon it. But Francis (2013) asks that all healthcare professionals reflect on their practice regularly to self-monitor their work. Finding an episode to reflect on may seem daunting at first, but it is likely that each shift will provide at least one episode that is suitable for reflection. It may be an encounter with a patient, a relative, or a staff member. It needs to be something that stood out to you and that you feel you could learn from. It is helpful to formally reflect after there has been time to feel less emotionally charged about the event to enable looking at the episode from a perspective different from your instinctive one.

Reflection does not only have to be carried out on negative episodes. We learn from positive experiences also. There is no perfect episode to reflect upon. The episode simply needs to be one that could be used to either consolidate good practice or identify how to improve practice.

How to reflect on practice

The essential element of reflection is finding the time to sit and think about the episode. This can be challenging to find, but it is important. There is no specific time that a reflective episode should be allocated. Reflection can be verbal with a peer or manager soon after the event, or it can be more

formalized by taking some time at the end of the shift in a quiet place to write a short reflection using a model that is suitable. To fully reflect, some literature support is required, but that might not be manageable for every reflection that is done, although it is best practice and it would be advisable to find time perhaps later, to look at literature surrounding the topic.

TYPES OF FORMAL REFLECTION

There are three types of formal reflection:
• The first is a personal reflection. This is where you sit somewhere quiet and take the time to think about a certain episode and reflect upon it with the goal of learning and growing as a practitioner. The reflection is personal, and the development is personal.
• The second type of reflection is facilitated reflection. This is called clinical supervision in some areas and this is an oral reflection where you work through an episode with someone listening and offering pointers to aid your reflection. The reflection and the growth is still personal, but the process is aided by another person. The facilitator has an obligation to keep all discussions from these sessions confidential.
• The third type of reflection is group reflection. Some clinical areas support group supervision where a group of healthcare workers meet to reflect upon episodes of care. This might be after a particularly distressing incident where people need support, or an unsafe incident where lessons need to be learnt. These reflective groups should be confidential, and there has to be trust within the room that everything said will remain confidential.

❗ HOTSPOT

When something happens during a work day that you want to reflect upon later, jot down some key words about how you are feeling in that moment as you might not remember later. Be honest with how you are feeling; you will work through these emotions later.

You might want to use a concept map or a list depending on what method you prefer.

❗ HOTSPOT

When doing a personal informal reflection, it is not essential to use literature. However, when writing a reflection for an academic piece of work, it is imperative to use literature to analyze the episode to be able to support any ideas or action plans you make.

CRITICAL AWARENESS

As well as using literature to support your thoughts you must be mindful of the use of emotive language in academic work. It is important to express how you are feeling but consider the language you are using and make sure it is non-judgemental and appropriate for academic work.

CRITICAL AWARENESS

Important Note!

Whilst it has been stated that any facilitated reflection needs to be kept confidential, it is also essential that all details of the patient involved are kept confidential too. Think about what is being written down and whether these details are necessary to facilitate your learning.

REFLECTION 13.1

- Think back on your day today. Did any particular event stand out to you? An interaction with someone or a conversation perhaps? Why does this event stick out? What has made it significant for you today? Did it go well? Could it have gone better? How?
- Consider your last clinical shift. Was there something that stands out for you? An interaction with a patient perhaps, or with a relative or a member of staff?
- If someone asks you to tell one story from your work, what would that story be? Why would you choose that story in particular? What makes it special for you?

CARE IN THE HOME SETTING

You are on a community placement and go to visit a patient with a Staff Nurse to administer his daily insulin. Once there, the patient informs you that he requires personal care as he has been incontinent of urine. The Staff Nurse politely informs him that she is unable to do that as she was only coming to give him his insulin and she has other patients to see. You feel that this was the wrong thing to do, but you do not say anything and you leave with the Staff Nurse. Later you do discuss this with the Staff Nurse who maintains she was too busy to provide personal care and also that personal care is the job of the carers, not the community nurses.

Use Gibbs' Reflective Cycle to reflect upon this episode.

Description – As above.

Feelings – I felt guilty towards the patient for not doing something that is really important to maintain his dignity and his skin integrity. I felt angry towards the Staff Nurse, but I also felt unable to challenge her due to being a trainee NA.

Evaluation – From my perspective this was a largely negative experience for the patient and for me. The patient did not have his needs dealt with and the risk of causing skin deterioration from this is high. It is also unfair to leave someone in dirty clothing when they want to get changed.

Analysis – I was concerned that refusing to provide this care was negligent of us. As healthcare professionals, we have a duty of care and I do not feel we met that duty by leaving the patient in soiled clothing.

Conclusion – I feel we did not meet our duty of care and we neglected our patient's needs. I should have been able to stand up for the patient and express my concerns.

Action Plan – If I were in the situation again, I would challenge the nurse politely and state that I feel we need to provide this personal care to prevent skin deterioration. If the Staff Nurse still refused to provide the care, I would document it and discuss it with the larger team.

Reflect on the scenarios given in Case Studies 13.1 and 13.2 and Reflection 13.2. Another example of a short reflective account is provided in the Communities of Care box at the end of the chapter.

CASE STUDY 13.1

You are working in your place of employment on a very busy acute medical ward and you are therefore counted in the staff numbers on the ward (this particular ward often experiences staff shortages). You find out that there is an opportunity to watch a liver biopsy and you have asked if it would be OK for you to observe it. You would be off the ward for approximately 30 minutes as this is being done in the medical investigations department.

The nurse in charge tells you that you cannot go as you are needed to care for the patients. You feel this is unfair because, although you are not supernumerary, you are still a trainee NA and you should be allowed to develop whilst at work.

Reflect on this case study. The response below uses Bain's framework for reflection.

Reporting – *As above.*

Responding – I felt angry with the nurse in charge as I felt I was disadvantaged due to being in my home work environment. Had I been on placement, I would have been allowed to go. Thirty minutes is not a long time to be off the ward and I had done all the jobs that I had been allocated for that time. I did not feel that leaving the ward for 30 minutes would cause a big problem for care delivery and I felt the nurse in charge was not recognizing my status as a trainee, even when I am in my home environment.

Relating – Retrospectively, I can see the viewpoint of the nurse in charge. Her main responsibility is for the safety of the patients. There needs to be a certain number of healthcare workers on the ward at all times in case an incident occurs and even though I had finished my tasks, more that I could have helped with might have arisen and it was impossible to predict this. There were other members of the team struggling with their workload that day and I did need to help them to meet patient needs.

Reasoning – I did not appreciate the staff-patient ratio required on wards at all times. By leaving for 30 minutes, I would have left the ward short-staffed, which could have been viewed as dangerous. Also, if I was allowed to go and develop, there is no reason why other members of staff couldn't request to go and observe procedures at any time. We all have a right and need to develop whether we are on a course or not as it enhances our practice delivery. If everyone left whenever they wanted to, the ward could be left in an unsafe situation affecting patient safety.

Reconstructing – Were an opportunity to arise again, I would look at the ward situation and consider the workload of the entire unit, not just me. If I felt that everyone was up to date with their work, then I would ask to be excused. Otherwise I would not and I will make sure I take full advantages of all opportunities when supernumerary in placement.

REFLECTION 13.2

You have worked very hard on a 1500-word essay and are pleased with the product that you handed in. However, you are very disappointed with the mark that you received. All of your colleagues tell you not to worry about it as it was a pass, but you are angry. You demand the work be re-marked, but the teaching team refuse. You want to make a formal complaint about the mark given.

Reflect on this scenario using Johns' Model for Structured Reflection to assess the situation.

CASE STUDY 13.2

You are working a weekend shift and during this shift you find two of your colleagues are having a heated discussion. This escalates to an argument and their behaviour soon becomes very unprofessional and is bordering on violent. You step in to separate them and manage to calm the situation down. Afterwards, the ward sister asks to see you and commends you for your courage and behaviour.

Reflect upon this positive outcome using Kolb's Learning Cycle to aid your work. You may have identified different feelings and themes. Your analysis may be different from the response shown here. Reflection is personal and subjective. These responses are to act as an example.

Concrete experiences – *As above.*

Reflective observation – Looking back, I am not sure if intervening without knowing what was really happening was the best action to take. However, instinctively I did not know what else to do. For two healthcare professionals to be arguing so expressively while in the workplace was shocking for me to witness, and I am sure all of the patients and their families were shocked too. I felt it was unprofessional and embarrassing and would have a knock-on effect for care provision due to a loss of trust in the professional attitude of the staff.

Abstract conceptualization – There were other members of staff on the ward who did not intervene. I am not sure why, but I think they felt it wasn't their business or they didn't want to make things worse. I had not considered that by intervening the arguing parties might become angry and violent with me. Retrospectively, that could have happened, and I put myself in a vulnerable position.

Active experimentation – If this situation arose again, I would again intervene and try to calm down the situation. I am pleased with how I reacted and maintain it was the correct course of action.

Not everybody reflects on their practice

Reflection is clearly important and will help develop all healthcare professionals. Formal written reflection is a particularly important development tool. However, despite this, a lot of healthcare professionals do not participate in reflective practice. There are many reasons for this, including the following:

- Reflection is hard. To be able to make sense of a situation when you are emotionally involved is a challenge. To consider the situation from another point of view is not something that a lot people are willing to do.
- As healthcare professionals we work long hours and we are tired. To then take time to reflect on a situation can feel like too much work once the shift has finished.
- Some healthcare professionals do not see the value of reflection because they feel their practice is appropriate and that they do not need to reassess how they do things.
- The need to use literature to help develop can seem like an onerous task for an already busy healthcare worker. However, without literature the reflection is simply a personal blog with no evidence-based development. Without the up-to-date knowledge, the reflection is not affective, and therefore it is not done.

However, despite these reasons, reflection is an essential skill for the healthcare professional and it helps you work within the 6Cs. If you can take the time to regularly reflect, your practice will be consistently improved and this will impact on care delivery.

CRITICAL AWARENESS

Your personal reflection may have an impact on your workplace. If you identify unsafe practice, you have an obligation to report this under safeguarding laws. For this, it would be advisable to contact your union representative for support. There are many resources on the Nursing and Midwifery Council website to help guide you through your responsibilities if you think a vulnerable person needs safeguarding.

COMMUNITIES OF CARE

Mental Health

You are on a mental health placement and you develop a good working relationship with one specific service user. Your mentor asks to see you one shift and informs you that your relationship with the service user is inappropriate and unprofessional. You feel this is unfair as the service user is opening up to you and communicating well with you.

Example of reflection on this situation using Moon's Levels of Learning.

Noticing – As above.

Making sense – I was both hurt and offended by the mentor's comments. I felt my professional integrity was being questioned and my personal morals. However, as I spoke with other people about the situation I started to understand that it wasn't just about an inappropriate relationship, it was also about how I was being perceived by other service users and other staff members.

Making meaning – Looking back, I understand that I was spending too much time with one particular patient, and although the relationship was not inappropriate, my conduct was, and I can now see how it might have been perceived that way. I should deliver my care evenly to as many service users as I can and not spend consistently more time with one particular patient. By spending more time with one patient, I was making myself vulnerable for complaints from other patients and vulnerable for the one specific service user to say untrue things about me.

Working with meaning – Documentation is essential in healthcare because, whilst the patients in our care are vulnerable, so are we, the healthcare workers. If conversations are not documented, there is no way to prove what was discussed. Also, all conversations with a service user should be discussed with the wider team as well. I am an inexperienced member of the team and there may be verbal cues that I am not picking up. By discussing the interactions with the wider team, it is easier to ensure the health needs are met.

Transformative learning – I have learnt it is important to be transparent in relationships with service users and to document all interactions to ensure that I am not put in a vulnerable position again.

LOOKING BACK, FEEDING FORWARD

This chapter has explained the importance of reflective practice and identified the documents where it is stipulated. Some common reflective models have been provided and explained, with examples. The management of reflection in practice has been discussed.

Reflective practice is an essential tool of the healthcare professional and one that needs to be perfected as early in a career as possible. This will enhance learning and career prospects.

REFERENCES

Bain, J.D., Ballantyne, R., Mills, C., Lester, N.C., 2002. Reflecting on Practice: Student Teachers' Perspectives. Post Pressed, Flaxton, Qld.

Department of Health (DH), 2012. Compassion in Practice. Nursing, Midwifery and Care Staff. Our Vision Our Strategy. https://www.england.nhs.uk/wp-content/uploads/2012/12/compassion-in-practice.pdf.

Dewey, J., 1933. How We Think: A Restatement of the Relation of Reflective Thinking to the Educative Process, revised edition. Heath, Boston, p. 1910.

Francis, R., 2013. Report of the Mid Staffordshire NHS Foundation Trust Public Inquiry Executive Summary. TSO, London.

Gibbs, G., 1988. Learning by Doing: A Guide to Teaching and Learning Methods. Oxford Further Education Unit, Oxford.

Johns, C., 2000. Becoming a Reflective Practitioner: a Reflective and Holistic Approach to Clinical Nursing, Practice Development and Clinical Supervision. Blackwell Science, Oxford.

Kolb, D., 1984. Experiential Learning: Experience as the Source of Learning and Development. Prentice Hall, Englewood Cliffs (N.J.), Prentice Hall.

Moon, J., 1999. Reflection in Learning and Professional Development: Theory and practice. Routledge-Falmer, Abingdon.

Nursing and Midwifery Council, 2015. The Code: Professional standards of practice and behaviour for nurses and midwives.

London, Nursing and Midwifery Council. https://www.nmc.org.uk/standards/code/.

Nursing and Midwifery Council, 2017a. Revalidation. London, Nursing and Midwifery Council. http://revalidation.nmc.org.uk/.

Nursing and Midwifery Council, 2017b. Safeguarding Standards. London, Nursing and Midwifery Council. https://www.nmc.org.uk/standards/safeguarding/.

Nursing and Midwifery Council, 2017. Standards of Proficiency for Nursing Associates (working draft). London, Nursing and Midwifery Council. https://www.nmc.org.uk/standards/nursing-associates/developing-standards-and-requirements/.

Nursing and Midwifery Council, 2018a. The Code. Professional Standards of Practice and Behaviour for Nurses, Midwives and Nursing Associates. London: NMC. https://www.nmc.org.uk/standards/code/.

Nursing and Midwifery Council, 2018b. Standards of Proficiency for Nursing Associates. London: NMC. https://www.nmc.org.uk/globalassets/sitedocuments/education-standards/nursing-associates-proficiency-standards.pdf.

Nursing and Midwifery Council/General Medical Council, 2015. Openness and Honesty When Things Go Wrong. The Professional Duty of Candour. London, Nursing and Midwifery Council. https://www.nmc.org.uk/standards/guidance/the-professional-duty-of-candour/.

Schön, D., 1983. The Reflective Practitioner: How Professionals Think in Action. Temple Smith, London.

14

Evidence-Based Practice

Janine Archer, Louise Bowden

CHAPTER AIM

The chapter aims to introduce the reader to the importance of developing the key knowledge, skills and attitudes to support the use of best evidence to underpin the Nursing Associate's clinical practice.

SELF TEST

1. What do you understand by the term 'evidence-based practice'?
2. Why is evidence-based nursing practice important?
3. What are the three key parts that make up evidence-based nursing practice?
4. Describe the different sections of PICO.
5. Name an electronic database relevant to your practice.
6. What type of evidence is considered the gold standard?
7. Name two reasons why patients might not voice their preferences.
8. What are the three elements of clinical expertise?
9. How does 'best evidence' influence patient care?
10. What is the role of the Nursing Associate in evidence-based nursing practice?

INTRODUCTION

Nursing is a challenging yet rewarding discipline. Public and professional expectations are that members of the nursing profession deliver high-quality care supported by evidence-based practice (EBP). This can be achieved by developing and supporting patient-centred approaches to care using the most current evidence. Many of the tasks that nurses carry out are underpinned by best evidence, and it is important that Nursing Associates (NAs) have the necessary knowledge, skills and attitudes to engage in evidence-based practice to meet expectations and deliver high-quality care.

> **CRITICAL AWARENESS**
>
> You will need to demonstrate a commitment to evidence-based practice by developing the required knowledge, skills and attitudes to engage with best evidence to deliver high-quality care.

WHAT IS EVIDENCE-BASED PRACTICE?

EBP in healthcare is not new, with one of the first references to it appearing over 25 years ago. Over time there has been a growing

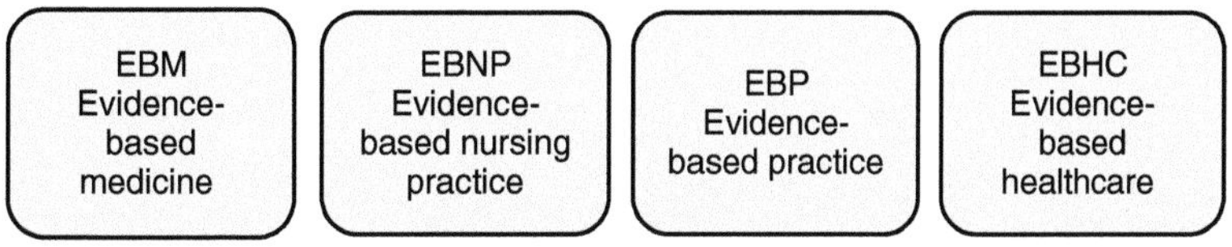

Fig. 14.1 Some Terms Used in the Literature.

interest to develop EBP and it is probably useful to note some of the key terms you will likely come across in the literature (see Fig. 14.1).

As this text relates to the role of the NA within the nursing profession, the rest of this chapter, where appropriate, will adopt the term 'evidence-based nursing practice' (EBNP).

A historical example of EBNP dates to Florence Nightingale, who was interested in mortality rates and causes of death during the Crimean War. She collected information and identified that more soldiers were dying of disease rather than battle wounds, highlighting an urgent need for hygiene standards to improve in military hospitals. She changed the hospital routines, improved hygiene and saved many lives with her determination and hard work. This historical example demonstrates how information can be collected and used to change nursing practice and improve patient outcomes.

COMMUNITIES OF CARE

Mental Health Nursing

From 1935 until 1974 a range of chemical and electrical experiments were carried out on homosexual men in psychiatric institutions. Named 'aversion therapy' this was intended to deter homosexuality, which at the time was considered a criminal act. The treatments offered were barbaric and included attaching electrodes to genitalia and sending electric shocks whilst the person looked at pictures of naked people of the same sex. When pictures of the opposite sex were shown no electric shock was administered. The 'patient' was given the ability to change the picture and therefore avoid the electric shock. Despite there being a belief that it worked, there is no evidence to support this claim. Homosexuality is no longer considered an illness that can be 'cured' and was decriminalized in 1967 and declassified as mental disorder in 1973.

Back in 1999, the Department of Health in their 'Making a Difference' report stated that practice needs to be evidence-based and identified that the nursing profession needed better access to high-quality research and training in appraisal skills to translate research findings into practice.

REFLECTION 14.1

Do you think the view of the Department of Health was right?
 How well has it been achieved? Can you think of any barriers that may have limited the implementation of evidence-based nursing practice?
 Is it relevant for NAs today? Considering your own training, how does the curriculum prepare you to deliver evidence-based nursing practice? What more might you need to learn?

There is no one agreed definition of EBP in the literature. One of the earliest and best recognized definitions of evidence-based medicine is: 'the conscientious, explicit and judicious use of current best evidence in making decisions about the care of individual patients' (Sackett et al., 1996). Other early definitions of EBP, include: 'Making decisions about groups of patients and/or populations and basing such decisions on a careful appraisal of the best evidence available' (Gray, 1997) and 'A combination of clinical expertise and best available evidence, together with patient preferences to inform decision making' (Fleming & Cullum, 1997).

As EBP evolved, Polit and Beck in 2008 defined EBP as 'The use of best clinical evidence in making patient care decisions' and continued by saying 'such evidence typically comes from research conducted by nurses and other health care professionals'. This definition highlights the importance of research in EBP and recognizes the benefits of drawing on a wide range of research, not solely that conducted by nurses. However, it has limitations. Systematic research is the best quality research, but is not always available; nursing care, and particularly mental health nursing, remains under-researched. As EBP continued to evolve, Polit and Beck revised their definition in 2016 to: 'Using the best evidence (as well as clinical judgement and patient preferences) in making patient care decisions, and "best evidence" typically comes from research conducted by nurses and other healthcare professionals.' This revised definition recognizes the importance of clinical judgement and patient preferences alongside the use of best evidence.

Whilst there is no single agreed definition of EBP/EBNP, the NMC (2018) states that NAs, 'use their knowledge and experience to make evidence based decisions and solve problems' and 'take into account the personal situation, characteristics, preferences and wishes of people, their families and carers when providing care'.

Although definitions of EBP/EBNP vary, ultimately all share the same common principle: 'Doing the right thing in the right way for the right patient at the right time' (Royal College of Nursing, 1996).

CRITICAL AWARENESS

Consider why patient preferences are important in evidence-based nursing practice.
 What opportunities and challenges does this raise for NAs?

As healthcare evolves and the demands on the nursing profession increase, EBNP is an increasingly important factor in improving the patient experience and challenges the common attitude of 'but we've always done it this way'.

It is important to note that clinical practice that is evidence-based might not always be best practice; for example, research trials often exclude certain patient groups, such as those who drink alcohol excessively, have suicidal thoughts or comorbidities. Thus, in addition to the evidence base, we also need to take into account other important issues, such as patient preference and clinical expertise.

The three key parts of EBNP are identified in the definition by Polit and Beck (2016) as (1) evidence base; (2) patient preference; and (3) clinical expertise. All three of these are required to identify the 'best evidence' to inform EBNP. Each of these three key parts will be discussed in more detail later in the chapter.

WHY IS EVIDENCE-BASED NURSING PRACTICE IMPORTANT?

EBNP is important for NAs and is implicit in many of the Department of Health's (DH) documents including the *NHS Plan* (DH, 2000) and the Darzi report (DH, 2008). More recently, the *Five Year Forward View* (National Health Service (NHS) England, 2014) calls for greater use of evidence-based approaches within nursing practice. One of the key themes in Health Education England's (HEE) *Shape of Caring Review* (2015) focuses on supporting and enabling research, innovation and evidence-based practice within the nursing profession. Specifically, the Nursing and Midwifery Council's (NMC) 2018 standards of proficiency for NAs clearly states that nursing associates will provide evidence-based patient-centred care. So EBNP is important because the Department of Health and Regulators of the NA role tell us we must provide it.

EBNP is also important because evidence can be used to support current practice, to defend what we do and why we do it. The demand for EBNP is fuelled by the increasing professional and public demand for accountability in safety and quality improvement in nursing practice. The Francis Inquiry (DH, 2010) provides a harrowing account of how inadequate nursing care can result in poor patient outcomes and provides the impetus for us all to provide high-quality, compassionate, patient-centred nursing care based on the best evidence.

We have identified that EBNP is not a new phenomenon; however, it is also important to recognize that there are many areas of nursing that continue to lack high-quality research. Therefore, it is important that NAs should also be involved in developing nursing practice and we can do this by being involved in audit and research, listening to our patients and broadening our expertise.

The nursing profession is also constantly evolving. Youngblut and Brooten (2001) recognized that when evidence is used to 'define best practices rather than to support existing practices, nursing care keeps pace with the latest technological advances and takes advantage of new knowledge developments'. Thus, not only is it important that we know that our current practice is evidence-based, but we also need to ensure we remain updated so that our practice evolves with developing evidence.

After looking at the following case study and reflecting on your own clinical examples we will explore the three key stages of EBNP: evidence base, patient preference and clinical expertise.

CASE STUDY 14.1 Evidence-Based Practice

Mr Jones is an 86-year-old man with chronic obstructive pulmonary disease (COPD) who has been admitted to the medical ward from a local care home. The NA on shift sees that Mr Jones has not eaten his dinner or drunk any of his water.

- The NA is aware that COPD is a progressive lung disease caused by chronic inflammation and damage to the respiratory system, which is making it difficult for Mr Jones to breathe, which in turn may be making him anxious. (NICE, 2010)
- The NA knows malnutrition and dehydration are both causes and consequences of illness and both have significant impacts on health outcomes. (NHS England, 2015)
- The NA is aware that neglect of fundamental nursing care was a major concern raised in the Francis Inquiry. (DH, 2010)
- The NA approaches Mr Jones and sits at his level as she is aware non-verbal communication is important in building a rapport and reducing anxiety. (Bach & Grant, 2015)
- Concerned that he looks thin and pale, the NA asks Mr Jones why he has not eaten or drunk anything, being aware that there are various causes and consequences of malnutrition in COPD which will need to be investigated. (Malnutrition Pathway, 2016)
- After checking that there are no medical issues, the NA gains consent from Mr Jones to help him with his diet and gently encourages him to eat and drink small amounts. (DH, 2009)
- The NA then checks the medical notes to see if Mr Jones's BMI has been calculated and asks about weight loss, as recommended by NICE (2006).
- Using the Malnutrition Universal Screening Tool (MUST) flowchart as guidance, the NA reports the findings to the registered nurse and suggests Mr Jones is put on a care plan so his dietary and fluid intake is observed, encouraged and recorded as per Trust policy. (NICE, 2006)
- The NA documents the discussion in the nursing notes and asks the healthcare assistant to encourage oral nutritional supplements as per NICE guidelines (NICE, 2006) and detailed in the care plan. Intake is documented in the nursing notes.
- The NA liaises with the dietician for advice, discusses the care plan with Mr Jones and the care home staff present and informs the medical team.
- The NA is aware they have worked within their scope of practice according to the NMC's draft standards of proficiency for NAs (2017).

PART A: EVIDENCE BASE

Nursing care is very complex and can be extremely challenging at times. Traditionally, the qualified nurse makes the clinical decisions and allocates tasks to the healthcare assistant, who carries out the tasks as requested. Therefore, using an evidence base to underpin clinical practice is likely to be a new experience for many NAs. Nursing Associates can break up this part of EBNP into three steps:
1. Identifying questions about clinical practice.
2. Finding the evidence to answer the questions.
3. Assessing the quality of the evidence.

Step 1: identifying questions about clinical practice

We can sometimes get stuck in a rut of doing things because 'we've always done it this way'. Without an enquiring mind, ineffective nursing practice would continue, and patient outcomes

BOX 14.1 Identifying a Question About Clinical Practice

Think of an everyday task you do (e.g., turn a patient, help a patient mobilize), then ask yourself:
* What evidence is there to support what I am doing?
* What does the patient/carer think about what I am doing?
* Does what I am doing have the desired patient outcome?
* Is this the best option for this individual patient? What are the other options?
* Am I following national/local policy/guidance?
* Do the registered nurses do the same things? If not, why not?

BOX 14.2 Examples of Broad Questions

What are sexually transmitted diseases?
How can you stop smoking?
What is diabetes?
How do you prevent pressure sores?
Do antidepressants work?

would not improve. It is only because of an enquiring mind that the barbaric treatment of homosexuals, mentioned earlier in this chapter, ceases to be implemented in clinical practice today.

Identifying questions about clinical practice can be challenging and sometimes feel daunting with thoughts ranging from 'I feel overwhelmed by the number of questions I have' to 'I can't think of anything'.

To start to identify questions about clinical practice you can do the following:
* Listen to your patients (preferences).
* Think about the care you provide (reflection and clinical expertise).
* Talk with colleagues (clinical expertise).
* Examine trust/local priorities (evidence base).
* Identify agendas of national policy/guidance (evidence base).

Box 14.1 provides some example questions you could ask yourself to help you identify a clinical question about your practice.

Often questions arise in clinical practice without us having to think too hard, for instance 'Why does the patient continue to smoke cigarettes following a myocardial infarction (heart attack)?' or 'Why is this wound not improving?' The role of the NA in providing EBNP in situations like this is to identify and examine the available evidence by asking 'Why do people smoke? Why does this patient continue to smoke? Are there biological, psychological, social and/or cultural factors that might be relevant? What is the risk to health if they continue to smoke? What interventions work and are they available? How might I help the patient to make an informed decision about whether to continue smoking or to try to quit?'

We can sometimes feel overwhelmed by the many different questions that we could ask about clinical practice. If we were to continually question everything, then nothing would get done, but without an inquisitive mind nothing would change either. It is important here to narrow down or prioritize the questions by considering if the question is about the following:
* High risk, e.g., falls, managing suicidal patients.
* High volume, e.g., things that occur frequently that will depend on the area in which you work and could include things such as catheter care, fluid intake.
* High benefit, e.g., has a significant impact on patient outcomes, such as pain management, infection control.
* Something that you are passionate about!

Identifying a good clinical question involves identifying a broad topic/area of interest (see Box 14.2 for some examples), then narrowing it down.

If you start to identify the evidence based only on broad questions, then you would be inundated with an enormous amount of information, much of which is likely to be irrelevant for the patients you are caring for. Therefore, broad questions need to be refined. Making your questions specific will focus your inquiry and is important when identifying and examining the evidence for narrowing down your search and making the evidence you find more relevant for your patient group.

A well-crafted clinical question is very important. A commonly used mnemonic in evidenced-based practice is PICO (Richardson et al., 1995):

P = patient or problem
I = intervention or issue of interest or exposure to something
C = comparison
O = outcomes.

Asking a PICO question increases the likelihood that the best and most relevant evidence will be found efficiently.

Note that not all questions have all four components, and when identifying the components of PICO, it is important to create brief, specific responses.

For (P) think about the people you are interested in: children, adults, the elderly? Are they a specific population (hospitalized, community)? Do they have a specific health condition (dementia, diabetes, and so on)?

For (I) consider which interventions or issues you are interested in (e.g., exercise, hand washing, music therapy); what you want to do for the patient (e.g., administer a drug, request a test); and what factors might influence the prognosis of the patient (e.g., age or comorbidities).

For (C) identify the main alternative with which to compare the intervention. Are you trying to decide if a particular bandage is better than another or if meal supplements are more effective than a normal diet? Your clinical question may not always have a specific comparison.

For (O) ask what you can hope to achieve, measure, improve or affect. What are you trying to do for the patient: Relieve or eliminate the symptoms? Reduce the number of adverse events? Improve test scores?

Areas to consider and examples from the four fields of nursing practice can be found in Table 14.1.

In wording your clinical question, you can move the different stages around and broaden a particular aspect. For example: What are the benefits of using e-cigarettes over ordinary cigarettes in adult patients with COPD? Here we have listed the outcome first and made it less specific (it no longer just focuses solely on lung function). Sometimes it makes sense to reword the question. Take the learning disability example 'Is autism in boys rather

TABLE 14.1   The Four Stages to Identifying Specific Questions

	1	2	3	4
	Patient or problem	Intervention or issue of interest	Comparison (if relevant)	Outcomes
	Ask:	Ask:	Ask:	Ask:
	'How would I describe my patient/s?'	'Which intervention am I interested in?' 'What do I want to do for the patient?' 'What factors might influence the prognosis of the patient?'	'What is the main alternative to compare with the intervention?'	'What are we hoping to achieve/measure?' 'What outcome could this intervention improve/affect?' 'What are we trying to do for the patient?'
Example: Mental health	In adults with psychosis...	is cognitive behaviour therapy more effective than...	antipsychotics...	in reducing hallucinations and delusions?
Example: Children and young people	In children experiencing pain...	is analgesia more effective than...	play therapy...	in reducing their pain score?
Example: Adult	Are adult smokers with chronic obstructive pulmonary disease (COPD)...	who use e- cigarettes...	compared to those who use tobacco cigarettes...	more likely to experience improved lung function?
Example: Learning disability	Is autism...	in boys...	rather than girls...	more prevalent?

BOX 14.3   Examples of Specific Questions

- What are the most effective smoking cessation interventions available for adults with COPD?
- Which wound dressing is most appropriate for a third degree burn to a child's arm?
- Do special observations reduce the incidence of self-harm on a female acute mental health admission ward?
- Does having the flu vaccination reduce hospital admissions for pneumonia in older people?

than girls more prevalent?' This would be better written as 'Is autism more prevalent in boys or girls?'

An alternative mnemonic is PICOT where T is the time it takes for the intervention to achieve the outcome(s).

Box 14.3 shows some more examples of clinical practice questions relevant for NAs.

REFLECTION 14.2

Identify the components of PICO in the examples of specific questions in Box 14.2. Remember they might not all have all four components.

CASE STUDY 14.2

James Owen is a 30-year-old man who has been admitted to A&E on a Saturday evening with 'a racing heart, feeling shaky and vomiting'. He has refused to cooperate with the qualified nurse's assessment and is becoming increasingly angry.

REFLECTION 14.3

Based on the information provided in the Case Study, identify two clinical questions that an NA might ask. Use PICO to guide you.

Step 2: finding the evidence to answer the questions

Once a specific clinical question has been posed following step 1, the next step is to find the evidence to answer the question.

Access to the internet means that we have lots of information available to us at the touch of a button. This can be really useful when trying to explore a clinical practice question as it means you can access information in a quick and efficient manner, often without the need to leave your area of work. On the other hand, it can also bring challenges by overloading us with information.

To help us not to feel overloaded, this step can be broken down as follows:

1) Identify the key words. Key words help you stay on focus whilst searching.
2) Identify where to look. It is important to use credible sources of information.
3) Identify who can help. There are a variety of resources and people available to help.

The first thing to do involves using the PICO question to identify key terms. To take our examples from Table 14.1, the adult example of a specific clinical question was: 'Are adult smokers with chronic obstructive pulmonary disease (COPD) who use e-cigarettes, compared to those who continue to smoke tobacco cigarettes, more likely to experience improved lung function?'

The key words here would be:

- adults
- smokers
- chronic obstructive pulmonary disease (COPD)
- e-cigarettes
- cigarettes
- improved
- lung function.

REFLECTION 14.4

Identify the key words in the following specific question:
  In adults with psychosis, is cognitive behaviour therapy more effective than antipsychotics in reducing hallucinations and delusions?

Once key words have been identified, it is also important to consider any other similar terms that may have been used in the literature to describe the same/similar thing, for instance, community and clinic. This will ensure your search captures the relevant literature. In the previous example, you would not just include the term 'psychosis' in your search as the more specific term 'schizophrenia' is sometimes used. By not including both terms your search might miss some highly relevant evidence. Other examples from the earlier example include: improved/increased/better, adults/patients and COPD/chronic obstructive pulmonary disease/lung disease. You also need to consider other ways of spelling a word, for example 'behaviour' is spelt 'behavior' in the USA, where a lot of research is generated.

Secondly, finding the best evidence to answer the question involves considering where to look.

You could choose to spend the day at the library searching all the volumes of *Nursing Times* but that would be exhausting and be a very narrow search. You could spend the week there and also search the *Nursing Standard*, but this would be very tiring and your search likely to be subject to many human errors and omissions.

You could put your question into an internet search engine, but as the information supplied could be from any source and is not filtered in any way, that might bring up random pieces of unreliable information.

Another option would be to use an academic search engine that only searches through scholarly literature and is therefore more reliable than a regular search engine. You can find such a resource by typing 'academic search engine' into your usual search engine.

An important issue to consider when looking for the *best* evidence is to consider how credible the evidence is. We will discuss how to appraise the quality of the evidence later in the chapter, but we also need to consider where we get the information from. Taking the standard search engine Google versus the academic version Google Scholar as an example, which do you think will produce the most credible results?

REFLECTION 14.5

Copy and paste the question: 'Are adult smokers with chronic obstructive pulmonary disease (COPD) who use e-cigarettes, compared to those who continue to smoke tobacco cigarettes, more likely to experience improved lung function?' firstly into Google, and then into Google Scholar.
• What do you notice about the information you are provided with?
• How many results does each one give you?
• How credible are the sources of information?
• Can you filter the results further?

A more effective and efficient way to find the best evidence is to use an electronic database search to find the information you need. However, this will require some training and support from someone experienced in using electronic databases, such as a librarian or online training package (see Stage 3).

You will also need to identify the databases you use because databases specialize in single subject areas. For example, there are nursing databases, education databases and business databases. The key here is to pick a database that matches the subject matter of your chosen topic. CINAHL, for instance, is the main database for nursing and allied health professionals, whereas PsycINFO is commonly used in mental health. However, if you were interested in a question related to mental health nursing, you would probably use both CINAHL and PsycINFO (among others).

If you are going to use electronic databases to conduct your searches, then you will also need to consider using Boolean operators. When searching electronic databases, you can use Boolean operators to either narrow or broaden your searches. The three Boolean operators are AND, OR and NOT and they connect the different key terms you will use in your search strategy (see Box 14.4).

In addition to Boolean operators, you will need to consider using truncation and/or wild cards that are relevant to different electronic databases. For example, using the * symbol as truncation in certain databases; for example, 'depress*' rather than 'depression' will expand your search to include not only the term 'depression', but also 'depressive' and 'depressed'. Wildcards are symbols used to represent different letters either at the end of a word or within a word, for instance where you know other countries have a different spelling. Thus 'speciali#es' will pick up both 'specialises' and 'specializes' (American spelling).

Using electronic databases for the first time can be a challenge, so it is always advisable to seek training, online resources or support. This links to the third stage, identifying key people or resources available to help you, in this case with your search strategy. If you are registered with an educational establishment

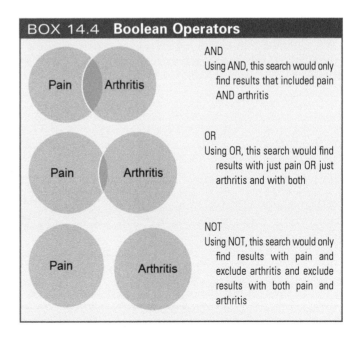

BOX 14.4 **Boolean Operators**

AND
Using AND, this search would only find results that included pain AND arthritis

OR
Using OR, this search would find results with just pain OR just arthritis and with both

NOT
Using NOT, this search would only find results with pain and exclude arthritis and exclude results with both pain and arthritis

such as a university or college or if you are employed by an organization with access to a library, speak to the librarian; they usually have lots of resources and expertise to help you with your searches. The library may also provide online resources and training. It is important that you do start the work yourself, so follow stages 1 and 2 and then you should be able to go to the librarian with an outline plan of your search strategy.

Step 3: assessing the quality of the evidence

We have already noted that EBNP requires clinical expertise, evidence base and patient preferences. The 'best available evidence' is determined by the quality of the evidence available and it is essential for NAs to be able to evaluate the strength of the evidence so they can determine how appropriate it is. One method of doing this is to be familiar with the 'hierarchy of evidence' (see Fig. 14.2).

At the top of the hierarchy of evidence are systematic reviews. These summarize the results of carefully designed healthcare studies (e.g., randomized controlled trials (RCTs)) and provide high-quality evidence on the effectiveness of healthcare interventions. Such systematic reviews often underpin the development of clinical guidelines on a specific healthcare topic, such as those issued by NICE (National Institute for Health and Care Excellence), as discussed later in the chapter.

Often considered the gold standard of evidence, 'Cochrane' systematic reviews are placed at the top of the pyramid. These systematic reviews are subject to additional scrutiny and have to follow strict guidelines laid out by the Cochrane Collaboration. There are many Cochrane reviews on a variety of healthcare topics.

A Cochrane systematic review includes a comprehensive search of the literature and then uses appropriate methods to collate the information from a number of RCTs. This then produces a summary of all the RCTs covering a particular topic, so the evidence tends to be more reliable. Other high-quality evidence that summarizes multiple research reports includes non-Cochrane systematic reviews and meta-analyses, evidence guidelines and evidence summaries.

REFLECTION 14.6
Accessing Cochrane Reviews

Using a search engine, look for the Cochrane Library.
    See if you can locate a review by one of the authors of this chapter on depression and anxiety.
    Read the abstract and plain language summary.
    How many RCTs were included in this review?
    Now see if you can find a Cochrane review on a topic related to your current practice area.
    Read the abstract and plain language summary.
    How many RCTs are included in that review?
    Can you see how these systematic reviews collate evidence from a number of other sources? This increases the number of people studied (sample size), which can lead to more meaningful results.

The next layer of the hierarchy, RCTs, are generally accepted as the most reliable evidence of whether a treatment is effective and are conducted using a clear and transparent process (methodology). In RCTs, patients/subjects are randomized into two or more groups. Randomized means that the people being studied

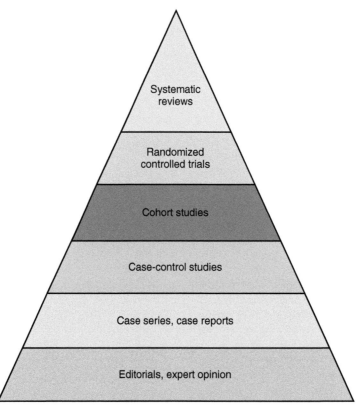

Fig. 14.2 The Hierarchy of Evidence.

(sample) are put into groups in a random way so that the researcher has no say in who goes into which group. The groups are used to compare a particular issue, for instance comparing a specific drug with a placebo (medication that appears real, but has no effect, like a sugar pill) or an intervention with people on a waiting list. One of these groups is the intervention group and one is the comparison group or 'control' group. For example, the intervention group receives a specific cancer drug and the other group (the control) get a placebo tablet with no active ingredients. Another example in people with type 2 diabetes might be that the intervention group receives an evidence-based web-based self-management programme, whereas the control group gets access to only a simple information website. Depending on what outcomes the researchers are interested in, by comparing the groups they might be able to say how one of the interventions is better than the other. RCTs are usually published in respected academic journals, such as the *British Journal of Nursing* and the *Journal of Community Nursing*, and are subject to independent peer-review.

The next few layers of the hierarchy include cohort and case control studies. Cohort studies begin with a group of people (a cohort) free of disease. These subjects are then grouped by whether they are exposed to a potential cause of disease. They are then followed over time to see if the development of new cases of the disease (or other outcome) differs between the groups. A case-control study begins with the selection of subjects with a disease (cases) and compares with subjects without the disease (control). The controls are people who would have been 'cases' if they had developed the disease (so they were people at risk of getting the disease). These studies tend to be considered 'good' even though they do not use randomization to allocate the subjects to the groups. The information collected is decided before it occurs (prospective), and although not randomized, the groups tend to be similar. Cohort studies are useful to examine the cause of disease because you follow people from exposure to the occurrence of the disease. Case control studies are especially useful for rare diseases, as you select the cases yourself.

Then there are case series and case reports, which are considered 'poor' studies with a non-randomized control group. Data are gathered after the event (retrospectively) and the groups are poorly matched. These types of studies describe the issues of interest rather than analysing the data. Case reports tend to focus on one individual, whereas case series are a group of patients who usually share one or more thing in common, such as disease, treatment, or side effect.

Finally, editorials and expert opinion make up the lowest level of the hierarchy. This includes studies with no control group, anecdotal evidence and testimonial.

However, not all research is conducted to a high standard and there are tools available to assess (or appraise) the quality of systematic reviews and individual studies, such as RCTs, cohort or case-control studies.

Critical appraisal, defined by Duffy (2005) as 'an objective, structured approach that results in a better understanding of a study's strengths and weaknesses', is a structured approach that allows the NA to identify evidence that comes from rigorous, reliable, unbiased and methodologically appropriate research.

A commonly used appraisal tool is the Critical Appraisal Skills Programme (CASP). This is a set of eight critical appraisal tools designed to be used when reading research. For different types of research, they ask a series of questions and require the appraiser to make judgements based on the information provided in the research. Once all questions have been attempted, the appraiser makes an overall judgement of the paper based on the responses to the questions. To access these resources, type 'Critical Appraisal Skills Programme' into your search engine.

Learning to use appraisal tools is beyond the scope of this chapter, but there will be people in your organization who can help. Contact your organization's Research and Development team or the university's library services.

Although systematic reviews and RCTs are considered the gold standard of evidence, that does not mean that the evidence at lower levels of the hierarchy is not important; in fact, many of the clinically relevant RCTs have developed from ideas conceived in clinical practice. It is, however, imperative wherever possible to use evidence of the highest quality to inform practice.

Despite it being important for all members of the nursing profession to have skills in accessing and appraising the best evidence, often they are too busy and do not have the time or the skills to continuously identify, appraise and make clinical sense of new research. Thankfully, there are resources available to NAs, and the other health and social care professionals, that have already assessed and summarized available evidence.

Evidence summaries are useful but the NAs, like registered nurses, need to be aware of where they are accessing the evidence from to ensure it is from a credible source. There are many different sources that summarize information, but there is a risk that the meaning and results of the original source of evidence has been misrepresented. Therefore the NA must always access information from a credible source. For example, if you want to find out information on 'what is the best treatment for type 2 diabetes' you could go to Wikipedia, but anyone, including non-healthcare professionals, can post on there, so the information may not be credible. You could go to a leading national charity for diabetes, and although they may conduct their own research, they tend to report the evidence from research conducted by other people. This information again could be misrepresented and may not be credible. You could try NHS Choices which has been certified as a producer of reliable health and social care information by The Information Standard, a certification scheme for health and social care information established by the Department of Health. NHS Choices can be a good starting point, especially on a topic you are not familiar with. However, NHS Choices is aimed at patients and the general public and may not contain all the information you require.

In the UK, one of the more credible bodies that informs evidence-based practice, by developing clinical guidelines, is the National Institute for Health and Care Excellence (NICE). NICE sets guidelines based on proven research, often from all levels of the evidence hierarchy, that has been subject to scrutiny. The overarching aim of NICE is to improve health and social care through evidence-based guidance. Therefore, this is a really useful place for the NA to find evidence summaries and evidence guidelines. Focused on clinically relevant topics, NICE searches the literature, assesses the quality of the evidence and then makes clinical recommendations based on the best available evidence, which can range from expert opinion through to Cochrane reviews. You can browse the website by topics including conditions and diseases, health protection, lifestyle and well-being, population groups, service delivery, organisation and staffing and finally settings.

NICE also has 'NICE Evidence,' an online search engine that identifies relevant clinical, public health and social care guidance. This was set up in 2009 as part of Lord Darzi's strategy for the future of the NHS, as mentioned earlier in this chapter. There is also access to resources purchased on behalf of the NHS, including the Healthcare Databases Advance Search (HDAS), which is a collaboration between NICE and Health Education England (HEE) and enables access to a range of health-related databases and professional journals.

Another useful resource for NAs is the Joanna Briggs Institute, which promotes evidence-based practice through systematic reviews and resources designed to enable healthcare professionals to access, assess and utilize high-quality evidence.

This section has focused on identifying, accessing and assessing the evidence base, but, as previously identified, this alone does not guarantee EBNP. The next two parts of this chapter will focus on the other two important aspects of EBNP: patient preferences and clinical expertise.

PART B: PATIENT PREFERENCE

The NMC (2018) state that NAs should work in partnership with patients to provide EBNP. For this to occur, firstly NAs need to engage with patients and families so that they are active participants in their own care (Gluyas, 2015). The philosophy of person-centred care is to facilitate participation as an understanding of values and preferences and can empower patients to be involved in their own care (Manley & Marriot, 2011).

Understanding patient preferences should not just be seen as an information gathering exercise; it is about 'getting to know the patient'. The development of a therapeutic relationship with patients and families can help to elicit patient preferences. The basis of a therapeutic relationship is rapport with the patient and family and the establishment of trust between them and the NA. The therapeutic relationship is a two-way process that also allows the NA to share information and knowledge with the patient about their care and treatment process (Price, 2017; Manley & Marriot, 2011).

Nursing associates are required to develop and maintain therapeutic relationships with patients and families to provide person-centred care that reflects patient preferences (NMC, 2018; HEE, 2016). In your role as an NA, you are well placed to take the time to determine what is important to the patient and their family. This should occur as a conversation where you can elicit patient preferences and enable them to participate in their care by helping them understand information on their health and treatment options (Gluyas, 2015).

There are, however, barriers to patients sharing their preferences with healthcare professionals, including NAs. Health professionals caring for patients from black, Asian and minority ethnic (BAME) groups need to understand how they access information in order to share their perception of care (Innes, MacPherson & McCabe, 2006). Taylor and colleagues (2013) state that cultural differences, such as differing attitudes and health beliefs, can impede active participation in care planning. The NMC (2018) states that NAs should demonstrate an understanding of different cultures, which you should have developed during your foundation degree education (HEE, 2016).

Patients can still adopt a passive role in their care despite literature to support their participation. This can be due to many reasons, such as feeling overwhelmed by their environment or being anxious about their health or treatment (Gluyas & Morrison, 2013). Gluyas (2015) also notes that healthcare professionals can lack the necessary skills to engage with patients, impeding participation as there is a lack of relationship to elicit their preferences. Your foundation degree should have provided you with fundamental skills in patient engagement, which you can develop in clinical practice (HEE, 2016).

Health literacy describes the patient's ability to understand information about health and to use it to make decisions. Factors that can influence a patient's health literacy include their age, education, mental health status and ethnic background (Wachter, 2012). Larson and colleagues (2011) have noted the added factor of the quality of the relationship between patient and healthcare professional. Therefore, as an NA providing evidence-based care, it is not enough to elicit patient preferences; there is also the need to ensure that the health information patients receive is understood and used by the patients and families (Gluyas, 2015).

REFLECTION 14.9

Thinking of your own clinical practice:

Have there been times when patients you are caring for have been passive in stating their preferences? Why do you think this was? Could you have done more to enable the patient to have more of an active part in their care decisions?

PART C: CLINICAL EXPERTISE

Clinical expertise is developed from experience, knowledge and clinical skills (Fig. 14.3). Haynes, Devereaux and Guyatt (2002) acknowledged that traditionally, clinical expertise was credited to medics. However, nurses and other healthcare professionals, such as physiotherapists or speech and language therapists, can also develop clinical expertise. Clinical expertise informs decision-making, judgement and EBNP. All healthcare professionals from novice level to expert (Benner, 1982) can develop clinical expertise through theoretical knowledge and the skills gained in clinical practice.

It is important to recognize that clinical expertise differs from clinical preference. According to Haynes, Devereaux and Guyatt (2002), a healthcare professional's individual preferences often have an influence on their actions, which may lead to variation in patient management based simply on the person providing the care. Clinical expertise is underpinned by theoretical

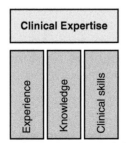

Fig. 14.3 The Three Component Parts of 'Clinical Expertise'.

and practical knowledge, whereas the same can not always be said for a healthcare professional's individual preference. For example, when taking a capillary blood sample for full blood count (FBC) investigation, nurses traditionally used Vaseline to maintain the formation of the blood droplet for collecting the sample in the specimen bottle. Despite evidence suggesting this practice could derange the blood result, some nurses continue to use Vaseline as it is their favoured method based on their clinical preference.

The NMC (2018) states that NAs will use their knowledge and experience to make evidence-based decisions about patient care and solve any arising problems. Although there is some opinion that a lack of guidance on how to do this at the bedside hinders the process, other literature supports the use of evidence-based decision-making (Thompson et al., 2004). Health Education England (2016) designed a curriculum where NAs qualify with sufficient underpinning knowledge for the delivery of care; this includes an understanding of evidence-based practice and clinical decision-making. This theoretical knowledge gained from academia, together with clinical knowledge and experience, informs your clinical expertise. Clinical knowledge is developed by linking theory to practice, by applying your academic knowledge to clinical experience. An example of this would be establishing an understanding of the pathophysiology of a disease through the experience of caring for a patient with that disease.

The NMC (2018) state that NAs must possess communication skills to deliver effective care and provide information using a wide range of strategies. Your role at the bedside puts you at the forefront of patient care where you will learn to talk to patients, developing a therapeutic relationship to allow patients to discuss their concerns or feelings about their treatment or diagnosis. What you have learnt about good communication will inform your experience and clinical knowledge to enable you to explain procedures and investigations and provide updates to the patient.

AT THE GP SURGERY

While working in a GP surgery, you are asked to obtain blood samples from 6-year-old Amina, who has presented with a fever and been diagnosed with an ear infection. The GP has provided advice on using anti-pyretic medicine for fever associated distress.

Amina's mother asks you about the blood tests and shares her concerns about the advice given on only administering anti-pyretic medication if Amina is distressed.

As a Nursing Associate, you have developed clinical expertise in communication and can explain what the blood tests are and understand Amina's mother's concern. You are able to explain the advice given, but without the evidence you are unable to provide the rationale for it.

Clinical expertise on its own without best evidence or patient choice is not evidence-based practice. Clinical expertise allows the application of evidence to a patient or clinical situation and helps to inform clinical decision-making. Evidence should never be used alone to make a decision or as a solution to a problem. Clinical expertise is needed to determine if the evidence can be applied to the patient and if it is appropriate to do so.

As a Nursing Associate, your clinical expertise will allow you to evaluate whether the best evidence available is appropriate and applicable to your patient.

Using 'best evidence' to inform clinical decision-making and patient care

This chapter has already explored the importance of EBNP, highlighting three key components: the evidence base, patient preferences and clinical expertise. The NA will demonstrate EBNP through clinical decision-making, which is integral to clinical practice and underpinned by these three elements. Clinical decision-making may be undertaken by an individual or a team of healthcare professionals from the same discipline or across various disciplines.

Examples of clinical decision-making in everyday practice include the decisions taken about the order of patients taken for emergency surgery or the prioritization of care for a group of patients.

> ### REFLECTION 14.10
> Thinking about your last shift:
> * What clinical decisions were made?
> * Who made these decisions?
> * What do you think informed the decision-making?

Evidence-based decision-making involves actively using the evidence base alongside patient preference and clinical expertise to inform clinical decision-making, taking into account the resources required. The process of clinical decision-making can result in choosing from a list of options with the patient. In evidence-based decision-making, these options are informed by an evaluation of all the 'best evidence', including the evidence base, patient preferences and clinical expertise (Thompson et al., 2004).

As an NA supporting the registered nurse, you will participate in clinical decision-making in everyday practice, although you may not realize the full extent of your role within decision-making. The NMC (2018) state that NAs should encourage shared decision-making to support patients in managing their own care. An example of this may be encouraging a patient to mobilize so that they can regain their independence after surgery. However, there are decisions that are outside an NA's remit, such as making specialist referrals and altering a plan of care (HEE, 2016). An example of this may be that, after the use of a nutritional screening tool, a patient needs a referral to a dietician and and be commenced on a fluid balance/diet chart. Although you would not make this decision autonomously, working within your role you would support the registered nurse. Your role would be as an advocate for the patient ensuring they are informed of the decision in order to empower them to become partners in the process (NMC, 2018; HEE, 2016).

> ### REFLECTION 14.11
> Think of some examples of decisions you have made within clinical practice.
> * Have you made them autonomously?
> * What has been your role within the multi-disciplinary team when a decision needs to be made about a patient?
> * Did you work in partnership with the patient and include them in the decision-making process?
> * Did you ensure the patient's preference was heard within that shared decision-making process?

Making the right decision relies on finding the right solution from whichever source is appropriate using the best evidence.

Reviewing EBNP

Simply because we practice EBNP does not necessarily mean that we provide the best care possible. EBNP is a continuous process, and once implemented, the NA will review the care provided and identify any areas for improvement. In collaboration with the registered nurse, changes may then be made to the patient's plan for care.

LOOKING BACK, FEEDING FORWARD

This chapter has explored the issue of evidence-based nursing practice and the role of the NA. It has broken EBNP into three key parts. Part A, the evidence base, included an introduction to the different stages, including (1) identifying questions about clinical practice, (2) finding the evidence and (3) assessing the quality of the evidence. Parts B, patient preference, and C, clinical expertise, complete the key ingredients that form 'best evidence' upon which to base clinical decision-making and patient care. The role of the NA in implementing EBNP was explored and how the NA will need to utilize available resources to support embedding EBNP into their current and future clinical practice.

Nursing Associates need to engage with evidence-based nursing practice owing to the increasing complexity of healthcare because the Department of Health dictates that care should be based on the best evidence, because we need to comply with NMC standards and codes of conduct, and because we need to make informed clinical decisions and be part of an effective multidisciplinary care team.

REFERENCES

Bach, S., Grant, A., 2015. Communication and Interpersonal Skills in Nursing, third ed. Sage, London.

Benner, P., 1982. From novice to expert. Am. J. Nurs. 82 (3), 402–407.

Casey, A., 1988. A partnership with child and family. Sr Nurse 8 (4), 8–9.

Coyne, I., Hallstrom, I., Soderback, M., 2016. Reframing the focus from a family centred to a child centred care approach for children's healthcare. J. Child Health Care 20 (4), 494–502.

Department of Health, 1999. Making a Difference. Stationery Office., London. http://webarchive.nationalarchives.gov.uk/20120524072447/http://www.dh.gov.uk/prod_consum_dh/groups/dh_digitalassets/@dh/@en/documents/digitalasset/dh_4074704.pdf.

Department of Health, 2000. The NHS Plan. A Plan for Investment. A Plan for Reform. Stationery Office., London. http://1nj5ms2lli5hdggbe3mm7ms5.wpengine.netdna-cdn.com/files/2010/03/pnsuk1.pdf.

Department of Health, 2008. High Quality Care for All: NHS Next Stage Review Final Report. Stationery Office., London. https://www.gov.uk/government/uploads/system/uploads/attachment_data/file/228836/7432.pdf.

Department of Health, 2009. Reference Guide to Consent for Examination or Treatment, Second ed. Stationery Office., London. https://www.gov.uk/government/uploads/system/uploads/attachment_data/file/138296/dh_103653__1_.pdf.

Department of Health, 2010. Independent Inquiry Into Care Provided by Mid Staffordshire NHS Foundation Trust January 2005–March 2009. Chaired by Robert Francis QC. Stationery Office, London.

Duffy, J.R., 2005. Critically appraising quantitative research. Nurs. Health Sci. 7 (4), 281–283. https://doi.org/10.1111/j.1442-2018.2005.00248.x.

Fleming, K., Cullum, N., 1997. Doing the right thing. Nurs. Stand. 12, 28–30.

Gluyas, H., Morrison, P., 2013. Patient Safety: An Essential Guide. Palgrave, London.

Gluyas, H., 2015. Patient centred care: improving healthcare outcomes. Nurs. Stand. 30 (4), 50–57.

Gray, J.A.M., 1997. Evidence-Based Health Care: How to Make Health Policy and Management Decisions. Churchill Livingstone, New York.

Haynes, B.R., Devereaux, P.J., Guyatt, G.H., 2002. Clinical expertise in the era of evidence-based medicine and patient choice. Evid. Based Med. 7, 36–38. doi:10.1136/ebm.7.2.36.

Health Education England, 2015. Raising the Bar: Shape of Caring: A Review of the Future Education and Training of Registered Nurses and Care Assistants. Health Education England, London. http://hee.nhs.uk/wp-content/blogs.dir/321/files/2015/03/2348-Shape-of-caring-review-FINAL.pdf.

Health Education England, 2016. Nursing Associate Curriculum Framework. Health Education England, London.

Innes, A., Macpherson, S., McCabe, L., 2006. Promoting Person-Centred Care at the Front Line. Joseph Rowntree Foundation, York.

Larsson, I., Sahlsten, M., Segesten, K., Plos, K., 2011. Patients' perceptions of barriers for participation in nursing care. Scand. J. Caring Sci. 25 (3), 575–582.

Malnutrition Pathway, 2016. Managing Malnutrition in COPD. http://www.malnutritionpathway.co.uk/files/uploads/Managing_Malnutrition_in_COPD_document_-_final.pdf.

Manley, K., Marriot, S., 2011. Person-centred care: principle of nursing practice D. Nurs. Stand. 25 (31), 35–37.

NHS England, 2014. NHS Five Year Forward View. NHS England, London. www.england.nhs.uk/ourwork/futurenhs/.

NHS England, 2015. Guidance – Commissioning Excellent Nutrition and Hydration. NHS England, London. https://www.england.nhs.uk/wp-content/uploads/2015/10/nut-hyd-guid.pdf.

NICE, 2006. Nutrition support for adults: oral nutrition support, enteral tube feeding and parenteral nutrition. Clinical Guideline 32. https://www.nice.org.uk/guidance/cg32.

NICE, 2010. Chronic obstructive pulmonary disease in over 16s: diagnosis and management. Clinical guideline 101. https://www.nice.org.uk/guidance/cg101.

Nursing and Midwifery Council, 2018. Standards of Proficiency for Nursing Associates. London: NMC. https://www.nmc.org.uk/globalassets/sitedocuments/education-standards/nursing-associates-proficiency-standards.pdf.

Polit, D.F., Beck, C.T., 2008. Nursing Research: Generating and Assessing Evidence for Nursing Practice, eighth ed. Wolters Kluwer, Philadelphia, PA. ISBN 9780781794688.

Polit, D.F., Beck, C.T., 2016. Nursing Research: Generating and Assessing Evidence for Nursing Practice, tenth ed. Wolters Kluwer, Philadelphia, PA. ISBN 9781496308924.

Price, B., 2017. Developing patient rapport, trust and therapeutic relationships. Nurs. Stand. 31 (50), 52–61.

Richardson, W.S., Wilson, M.C., Nishikawa, J., Hayward, R.S.A., 1995. The well-built clinical question: a key to evidence-based decisions. ACP J. Club 123, A12–A13. doi:10.7326/ACPJC-1995-123-3-A12.

Royal College of Nursing, 1996. Clinical Effectiveness. RCN, London.

Sackett, D.L., Rosenberg, W.M.C., Muir Gray, J.A., et al., 1996. Evidence based medicine: what it is and what it isn't. Br. Med. J. 312, 71–72. doi: https://doi.org/10.1136/bmj.312.7023.71.

Taylor, S., Nicolle, C., Maguire, M., 2013. Cross-cultural communication barriers in healthcare. Nurs. Stand. 27 (31), 35–43.

Thompson, C., Cullum, N., McCaughan, D., et al., 2004. Nurses, information use, and clinical decision making – the real world potential for evidence-based decisions in nursing. Evid. Based Nurs. 7 (3), 68–72.

Wachter, R., 2012. Understanding Patient Safety, second ed. McGraw-Hill, San Francisco CA.

Youngblut, J.M., Brooten, D., 2001. Evidence-based nursing practice: why is it important? AACN Clin. Issues 12 (4), 468–476.

15

Health Education and Promotion

Carmel Blackie

OBJECTIVES

By the end of the chapter the reader will be able to:
1. Discuss the complex issue of health
2. Understand the concepts of health education and health promotion
3. Describe a number of approaches to health promotion
4. Appreciate the role and function of the Nursing Associate (NA) in including episodes of health education and health

promotion within care delivery and therapeutic communication
5. Describe strategies that can be used locally and nationally to help improve the health of the nation
6. Identify the challenges that may be encountered when implementing health promotion and health education strategies

KEY WORDS

Health	Locus of control	Public health
Education	Prevention	Equity and equality
Promotion	Belief	Diversity
Empowerment	Models	

CHAPTER AIM

The chapter aims to introduce the reader to the key skills, knowledge and attitudes required to provide health promotion within the context of a therapeutic relationship.

SELF TEST

1. What is health?
2. Can you differentiate between health promotion and health education?
3. What are the three main areas of knowledge required for effective health education and health promotion?
4. Why are health promotion and health education necessary?
5. What is meant by the concept of locus of control?
6. What is empowerment?
7. How does public health relate to health promotion and health education?
8. Should a person who refuses to take health advice offered to them be penalized in terms of their care?
9. There are five main approaches to health promotion; what are these?

10. How can you ensure a commitment to diversity and equality when offering health promotion and health education?

INTRODUCTION

Health promotion and health education are core elements within the role of the Nursing Associate (NA); in fact, all healthcare professionals are responsible for offering advice and guidance to enable the people to whom they offer care to make effective choices related to their health and well-being (Soni & Bailey, 2013). All clinical contact with people receiving healthcare is an opportunity for health promotion and health education. This is offered within the context of a therapeutic relationship designed to empower the person to take as much control of their own situation as they are able to. All engagement between a professional healthcare provider and the person using the service has a therapeutic element, and it is not casual. Health promotion and health education are complex and intertwined elements; there are a number of definitions and a variety of models and approaches to health promotion and health education. Unfortunately, there is no universal agreement as to which approach or model is the best to use. Healthcare itself is complex, as are people, and in practice, a variety of models and approaches are used.

It is essential that the NA understands the concepts of health promotion and health education to be able to work appropriately with the people they serve. The NA must understand the definitions of health education and health promotion; be aware of a variety of approaches and be able to offer individualized advice, recognizing the person's individuality and self-determination.

Health promotion is the overarching strategic activity that has the intention to improve health for populations. It is linked to public health and uses a public-health approach based upon epidemiological data to determine which areas and topics to target. The emphasis within the public health agenda, and therefore the priorities for health promotion, alter to meet the identified need. Some of the priorities within health promotion help to shape society; in this way healthcare professionals carrying out health promotion initiatives can be seen as agents of social change and could be regarded as carrying out government agendas. The ethical element within health promotion practice is important. For instance, parenting advice to new parents is designed to optimize the outcome for the child and the family, and in so doing, help the child to achieve their potential. Initiatives in relation to this, such as Sure Start, have been shown to reduce disadvantage and the issues associated with it, such as underachievement in education. The ethical principles important to consider here are beneficence: actively seeking to do good, and non-malfeasance: actively seeking to do no harm. These ethical principles are opposite sides of the same coin.

Health promotion is about the prevention of harm; this can relate to disease or to harms caused by social disadvantage. Measurement of the effectiveness of initiatives can be problematic: if a thing is prevented, how is it measured? Some health promotion initiatives take time to realize; this can mean that several generations pass by before an outcome is seen. An example of this is the health of a newborn child, which relates to its mother's health at conception and also its maternal grandmother's health when the infant's mother was in utero (Rillamas-Sun, Harlow & Randolph, 2014). All the ova that the mother will produce are created in utero. Thus, the infant's health is a three-generational project. Health advice to young women in 2018 will have an effect on their grandchildren's health outcomes. When thought about seriously, this is an awesome responsibility.

Reflection is an important part of all practice and particularly so in relation to health promotion. For instance, is the advice appropriate for the person? How does it affect their ability to be independent? A useful model to help the practitioner to decide whether they are engaging in an appropriate activity is to use a model of reflection – any will do. What is important is always asking the same questions: What was my aim? What did I do? What were the outcomes for the client, for myself and for others involved? What other actions could I have taken? What would the consequences of these alternative actions be? After reflecting the practitioner could use Carper's (1978) *Ways of Knowing in Nursing* to further explore why they have acted as they did and what knowledge they need to develop further. In this way the practitioner can develop an action plan for their own development moving forward. It is this which makes a lifelong learner and safe practitioner. Johns' (1995) *Model of Guided Reflection* uses this approach, and is regarded as an excellent tool (see Chapter 14 for a discussion of other reflective models). The domains of knowledge for practice identified by Carper (1978) help the individual to analyse what knowledge they require to develop their skills and knowledge in the future (Box 15.1). It is an aid to action planning for our ongoing learning and is invaluable for that reason. Reflection without planning is only reminiscence and does not move practice on.

In considering health promotion, it is also important to consider two further elements or domains of practice: unknowing and sociopolitical knowledge (Box 15.2). These were identified by Christopher Johns (1995), and relate to the context of practice. This is something that is changing within the National Health Service (NHS). The King's Fund illustrates this very well in two videos created in 2013 at the start of the reform implementation and updated in 2017.

BOX 15.1 Carper's Ways of Knowing (Carper, 1978)

Carper split the knowledge required for nursing into four domains or areas. Each domain influences the way in which practice is delivered.
1. Empirical Knowledge
   Guidelines and theory that can be applied to practice.
2. Personal Knowledge
   You as an individual, you the person delivering the care; the culture and belief system that forms you, your preferences and biases.
3. Moral and Ethical Knowledge
   The rights and wrongs within the situation and ethics. The two cardinal principles here are beneficence, actively seeking to do good, and non-malfeasance, actively seeking to do no harm.
4. Aesthetic Knowledge
   The art of delivering care to the person cared for. It fuses the knowledge required with the person who has eliminated their own biases and preferences and acts with professional integrity, seeking to do good and to do no harm and, in doing so, is therapeutically present in the moment for the person cared for. It is the beauty of practice.

BOX 15.2 Unknowing and Sociopolitical Knowledge (Johns, 1995)

Unknowing

Relates to the practitioner's understanding that they do not know the client to the full at the outset and must learn about them in partnership. This is fundamental to good health promotion practice. After all, tailoring information to the person requires insight into their lives and needs.

Sociopolitical knowledge

Relates to understanding society and the context within which practice is executed. This is mission critical within health promotion activity because so much of it relates to the wider public health and societal agenda of government. Awareness of this is critical to ethical and appropriate practice.

Health education is the activity related to delivering care to people and translates the health promotion agenda into practical advice and projects. It concentrates on the work that clinicians carry out with individual people. This can be a person, a family group or a small community of people with the same condition. For instance, an NA could advise a person with type 2 diabetes about their health and how diet and exercise relate to their well-being. The NA could also give health education advice to the person's family/partner related to shopping, cooking and family meals and maintaining a healthy weight. The NA could also give guidance to a group of people with type 2 diabetes as part of a structured programme, such as the DESMOND programme (https://www.desmond-project.org.uk/), which is designed to enable people living with diabetes to better understand their condition and to make realistic and healthy choices about the way in which they conduct their lives.

Nursing Associates are part of the NHS workforce, and keeping the workforce healthy is a public health agenda issue (Soni & Bailey, 2013). An example of an NHS Trust endeavouring to keep their workforce healthy and effective can be seen in the following example from The NHS's Role in the Public's Health. A Report from the NHS Future Forum (Soni & Bailey, 2013):

'The Walton Centre NHS Foundation Trust, a specialist neuroscience trust, employs roughly 950 staff. The Trust developed a local strategy for improving staff health and well-being, 'Work Well the Walton Way'. They asked staff how they wanted support with issues like obesity, smoking, physical exercise and staff engagement, and fed their views into an action plan. This led to initiatives on the ground including virtual health and well-being champions in every ward and department, onsite zumba, table tennis and Pilates, an in-house weight management course, a cycle scheme, a running club and staff counselling. The trust has maintained communications and engagement with staff throughout, holding regular staff summits with the executive team so that the staff have an opportunity to feedback and ask questions. Since introducing the strategy, the trust has seen staff sickness fall from over 7% in January 2010 to less than 4% now. Staff feedback has been positive, and staff survey results have shown more positive attitudes to health and well-being and job satisfaction.'

When offering health promotion and health education, it is important to be aware of models of health promotion practice. These can be split into three areas for ease of discussion: descriptive, prescriptive and process. It is important to remember that these models are often interlinked and used together in the practice setting.

1. Descriptive models: e.g., Downie (1991); Beattie's Model (1991). Descriptive models describe the activities within health promotion and health education. They consider the relationships between these and the impact upon health promotion and health education of the organizations and aspects of society within which they are delivered. This is an important aspect of the usefulness of the model as inequalities in health, and within society generally, are important determinants of health and life outcomes. An example of this is the social class gradient in educational achievement. Education directly affects the length of life of an individual (Feinstein et al., 2006). This unfairness has an impact upon the stability and coherence of society.

2. Prescriptive models: e.g., programmes derived from government policy in response to health data. These models are concerned with enabling people to change their behaviour and are practical in their approach.

3. A process approach: e.g., Prochaska & DiClementi (1983). This uses learning theory to create ways to deliver health promotion messages and links to understanding the person. Another example is Motivational Interviewing (MI).

UNDERSTANDING THE CONCEPT OF HEALTH

Understanding the meaning behind a term that we take for granted in everyday language is of critical importance for clinicians delivering health promotion and health education.

The World Health Organization (WHO) (1946) defined the concept of health as: 'a state of complete physical, mental and social well-being and not just the absence of disease or infirmity.'

This definition attempts to include the determinants of health and elements within a healthy life. It is moving away from a medical model of health, which is the absence of disease, to a concept that is more holistic and incorporates social aspects of life, including family support, work and inclusion within a social network with physical and mental aspects. This definition of health is very broad and has been criticized as being unobtainable. It also excludes those who have any form of disability. For example, a short-sighted person would potentially not count as being healthy within this definition. This is ludicrous, and in fact the definition makes it hard for the health service and healthcare professionals to achieve these goals.

In 1984, the WHO later refined its definition to include some explanation of the concepts and issues:

'The extent to which an individual or group is able, on the one hand, to realise aspirations and satisfy needs: and on the other hand, to change or cope with the environment. Health is, therefore, seen as a resource for everyday living, not an object of living: it is a positive concept emphasising social and personal resources, as well as physical capacities.'

This definition is also broad and addresses the person's ability to function, to contribute to society and to achieve their dreams. It is inclusive and allows forms of physical or mental challenges to be included. For example, people who compete in the Invictus Games or Paralympics are entirely healthy in the 1984 definition; in the 1946 definition of health, they are not.

Since its creation in 1946, the definition of health by the WHO has been criticized for its emphasis on wholeness, and to an extent, perfection. Even in the adapted version, there would be some groups who would fall outside of its remit.

As technology in medical care increases and people are living longer with conditions that in past generations would have cut their lives short, it is important to redefine what is meant by health. The way in which health is defined underpins policy decisions made by government and so affects practice. Huber et al. (2011) puts this case very forcefully when he argues that the time is right to introduce a 21st-century approach to defining health that is linked to the ability to be adaptable and self-managing, regardless of a person's situation and the physical, intellectual, social and emotional issues that they face on the course of their life's journey. Huber et al. (2011) propose this because of the rise in long-term conditions within populations that leave people living longer, but with functional problems/morbidity. As populations age, the pattern of disease changes and so the advice offered, and the health service and professionals' response to changing needs must adapt.

For clinicians, including NAs, practising within the current context of care, it is important to adopt a wide and inclusive definition. In the contemporary context, as Huber et al. (2011) argue, being healthy also means being able to cope with stress and to have a flexible approach to life and the challenges that may arise. For instance, the stress of unemployment, threats of terrorism and financial issues, can all weigh heavily upon a person in contemporary Britain.

Accesses to healthcare and to good healthcare advice affects health, but healthcare services are not the only important factor. The following issues are just as important in achieving good health:

- where a person lives
- the surrounding environment
- genetics
- income
- education
- relationships with friends and family.

These can be summarized as:

- The social and economic environment: including how wealthy a family or community is
- The physical environment: including parasites that exist in an area, or pollution levels
- The person's characteristics and behaviours: including the genes that a person is born with and their lifestyle choices.

To be healthy, and to remain so, it is important for people to be active and to be engaged within society (The New Economics Foundation, 2008). To this end, people should do the following:

- Connect with others at each stage of life: i.e., children need friends and groups as do adults.
- Be active regardless of age or ability and take an interest in social pursuits. Examples of this can be sports or volunteering.
- Take notice of the environment and engage with the seasons and nature. Live part of life outdoors.
- Continue to learn throughout life. For instance, learning new skills and taking on challenges, however small.
- Contribute something to others so as not to feel in receipt of help all the time. This raises self-esteem and is good for mental health.

REFLECTION 15.1

Consider ways in which the NA could encourage people at various stages of life to become more engaged within their local community, regardless of ability and situation.

It is clear that some of the issues that affect people's health are broader than the health service itself can deal with and therefore beyond the remit of a clinician, or of one professional group to improve alone. Teamworking across disciplines is essential, as is working in partnership with people and communities. The WHO advocates an approach to offering health promotion that targets people at different life stages (Kuruvilla et al., 2018). This means that the health advice given to a young mother would be individual and different from the information provided for her when she is in the menopause phase of her life. A life-stage approach to health is a useful model to use because it is practical and logical (Pickin & St Ledger, 1997). It is important, too, that the health professional seeks to influence policies which affect health. For example, supporting a community to lobby its member of parliament for safe play areas is using political pressure to achieve a goal. NAs and other health professionals engaging with communities to achieve policy change must be above party politics. It is 'politics with a small p' that is relevant here. Like the monarch, health professionals in the practice context are above party politics.

REFLECTION 15.2

Make a list of the things that mean good health to you. Ask another person (someone older or younger than yourself) what it means to them. Compare and contrast the lists. Are there any similarities to your list? What are the differences?

In his seminal work *Pedagogy of the Oppressed*, published first in 1968, Paolo Freire suggests that if a person is empowered to take charge of their own health through health promotion and health education, then the skills and confidence that they learn can be used in other areas of their life, as individuals, within families and within a community and nation. In this way, the empowerment of people is a means to peaceful revolution. Freire was writing in the context of a turbulent South America in the 1970s; in the democracy of contemporary Britain it would be a goal to achieve greater equity for all.

What do we mean by inequity and inequality? The terms are used often interchangeably but are actually quite distinct. This information taken from *Global Health Europe* (2009) explains the situation well:

'Inequity and inequality: these terms are sometimes confused, but are not interchangeable, inequity refers to unfair, avoidable differences arising from poor governance, corruption or cultural exclusion while inequality simply refers to the uneven distribution of health or health resources as a result of genetic or other factors or the lack of resources.'

Essentially, people in Western democratic societies, such as the UK where there is a National Health Service free at the point of delivery, have access to health services to meet their needs. To get this, they must be in the system; some are not, and these people are usually those with greatest need, as Tudor Hart (1971) in *The Inverse Care Law* describes. Once within the system, services are available to meet need without reference to gender, ethnicity or religion. Sometimes the services do not operate as fast as a person would like, but that is another matter.

There are essentially four factors that affect health, death and disease:
1. Inadequacies in the provision of healthcare
2. Lifestyle and behavioural factors and choices
3. Environmental factors, such as pollution
4. Biophysical characteristics, such as genetics.

Individuals have their own autonomy and self-efficacy within the system, and some people have more personal resources available to them than others. This includes the level of individual socio-economic status and educational background, social networks and social class. To ensure health equity, extra resources, which can be financial or legislative, are required to aid the disadvantaged. The approach of government to this challenge varies according to the political party in power.

REFLECTION 15.3

How do you think being unemployed could impact negatively on a person's health and well-being?

Some important principles to understand when offering health promotion and health education are locus of control and self-efficacy.

Locus of control

Locus of control, in the context here as it relates to health, was defined by a psychologist called Julian Rotter in the 1950s as part of a theory of social learning and was published in 1966. It refers to the extent to which people believe that they have control over events in their lives. A health locus of control can be internal to a person or external to them. It links to a person's belief as to whether their health is influenced and controlled by their own behaviours and personal choices, that is, internal to them and under their control, or whether their health is affected only by outside agency and so is external to them and is outside of their control. Where a person's locus of control is sited determines whether they are active or passive as participants in their care. This is an important concept to keep in mind in relation to health promotion as it will determine the way that advice is offered and received. These outside agencies can include karma, luck, random chance, inescapable fate or influential people, such as healthcare professionals. Research has shown that, where a person has an internal locus of control, they have better physical and mental health and are more proactive in seeking out ways in which to be healthy. An external locus of control leads to poorer physical and mental well-being and people are less proactive in seeking out health information. People with an external locus of control often see the health professional as powerful and so are likely to follow advice, for example in relation to taking medication, but the downside of this compliance is that they are more likely to feel disabled or to have more pain.

Self-efficacy

Self-efficacy was identified by Albert Bandura in 1977. It relates to a person's ability to take charge of their situation and to be active or passive within what is happening. It links to locus of

control and it is a psychological adaptation to the situation that the person finds themselves in. A person with high self-efficacy and confidence will expend a lot of effort in achieving their goals and is likely to succeed. A person with low self-efficacy is likely to expend less and to give up.

Examples of this in relation to health promotion can be seen in people who are trying to stop smoking or who are trying to lose weight.

AT THE GP SURGERY

The NA and other clinicians working within the general practice setting have a unique opportunity to offer a range of health promotion and health education initiatives. These include weight management, smoking cessation, healthy eating and the importance of exercise. This advice and input is given within the context of a consultation.

Health summary

So, it is important to be aware that health includes physical, mental and social well-being; it is a resource for living a full life.
- Health is not only the absence of disease, but also includes resilience, which is the ability to recover from adversity and illness and to bounce back.
- Good health is affected by genetics, the environment, social relationships, education, income and location.
- Making healthy choices regarding diet and exercise, early managing of risk factors, screening for diseases and developing and utilizing coping mechanisms improve a person's health and well-being.
- Health is achieved across generations and we are linked to the past and the future.
- Health can be defined as physical, mental and social well-being, and as a resource for living a full life.

CASE STUDY 15.1   Sarah

Sarah Arthur is 36 years old. She is obese, with a BMI of 40. She has a 2-year-old daughter who weighs 4.30 kg. Sarah had gestational diabetes. She sees her GP because she is tired and lethargic and, after a fasting blood sugar test, the GP diagnoses Sarah as having pre-diabetes. The NA is asked to support Sara through a programme of advice as to how she can reduce her weight and so minimize her risk of developing type 2 diabetes.

The NA uses Motivational Interviewing techniques to encourage Sarah to identify her goals and priorities, and following this, Sarah is introduced to the 8-week blood sugar diet (Mosley, 2017). She follows this and is seen weekly by the NA so that the NA can offer support. The NA continues to use Motivational Interviewing techniques to ensure that Sarah remains focused and is on track to achieve her realistic goals. At the end of the 8-week period, Sarah has lost 4 kg. She does not feel as tired and, although she is still significantly overweight, her weight loss has given her the confidence to start to walk regularly with a local group of young mothers.

HEALTH PROMOTION IN THE HOME SETTING

There is a growing trend to care for people with long-term conditions in community settings. Health promotion and health education opportunities are embedded within episodes of care at home. For instance, the NA can offer advice and support to carers looking after people with dementia or frail people at home.

This can include advice about keeping themselves as well and as stress free as possible. Health visitors who work with children and families at home channel all their effort into health promotion through the surveillance programmes offered to all children and families under the Healthy Child Programme started in 2009. This is a 0–19 service shared between midwives, health visitors, school nurses and the skill mixed teams who work with them.

Earlier in the chapter, the difference between health promotion and health education was mentioned. It is important to understand this in more detail. Health promotion was first coined as a term related to public health practice in 1974; this was as part of a health bill in Canada. There was emphasis then on redefining healthcare provision, much as there is now within the UK, where rebalancing of the health services is moving the system away from cure and treatment to prevention (Health and Social Care Act 2012). The emphasis within the current NHS is on service design and long-term conditions and within this, public health and health promotion are key elements.

Health education is a tailored approach offered to individuals, families and small groups. Its aim is to provide information that then enables people to make informed choices about their lives and so to change their behaviour for the good. Paolo Freire (2017 [1968]) saw this as a means to peaceful revolution; to create a just society all it takes is to empower people to take charge of their health and the rest follows. The skills people develop carry on into other aspects of their lives. The World Health Organisation in 2018 defines health education as 'any combination of learning experiences designed to help individuals and communities improve their health by increasing their knowledge or influencing their attitudes'. This can be found on the WHO website at http://www.who.int/topics/health_ednucation/en/.

Some of the approaches to health promotion can be described as follows:

Medical approach

The aim of a medical approach to health promotion is to reduce premature death and the morbidity associated with this. This is important because the burden of cost to the NHS in relation to caring for people who are compromised by avoidable conditions is high. There is also a cost to society in the wider sense as, if people of working age are not able to work because of ill health, this reduces national productivity and tax revenues. This means that the money available to the NHS is reduced. A medical approach to health promotion uses scientific methods and data collection to both define the problem and to determine ways to address the problem. An example is targeting a population for screening, such as for bowel cancer, breast cancer, cervical cytology, high cholesterol and obesity. It is led by experts and tends to require participants to accept the service.

Behaviour change approach

The aims of a behaviour change approach are to encourage individuals to change behaviours that carry risk and to adopt others that encourage healthy outcomes. This can only happen if the person subject to the approach is motivated to change, that is, they can see the benefit to themselves and will adopt new ways of thinking and behaving. This approach is used within many health campaigns. It depends upon the development of a

therapeutic relationship between the subject and their clinician. It is a partnership approach to effecting change to optimize their health and well-being. There is a danger within this approach of implying that the people targeted are somehow to blame for their situation. Behaviour-change approaches to health promotion outlined by NICE in 2007 can be found here: https://www.nice.org.uk/guidance/ph6/chapter/2-Considerations.

They added to this in 2014 with an individual guide to behaviour change in health promotion: http://www.makingeverycontactcount.co.uk/media/1020/01_nice-behaviour-change-individual-approaches.pdf

> **REFLECTION 15.4**
>
> Think about a smoking cessation programme (if possible attend one if you are able to on clinical placement). What are the key motivational factors people may have for wanting to reduce or give up smoking? How might the NA help to motivate people?

Educational approaches

Educational approaches aim to give people the knowledge and skills that they need to be able to effect changes in their lives that will then lead to greater health and well-being. Embedded within the approach is an understanding of learning theory and psychological approaches to learning. There are three main areas within this approach:

1. Cognitive: relates to information and how this is understood.
2. Affective: relates to how people feel and their emotions.
3. Behavioural: relates to the skills required for a particular task. The delivery of programmes within this tradition is led by the teacher/expert. However, participation is encouraged and role play is often used if it is within a group setting. This allows participants to identify their own emotions, attitudes and beliefs and compare these to others.

Empowerment approach

An empowerment approach (Tengland, 2007) to offering health promotion aims to enable a person to get in touch with the issues important to them. It has at its core respect for the person as an individual and it aims to be holistic in its approach. It aims to inspire confidence and to promote self-efficacy. This fits well with the approach to redefining health advocated by Huber mentioned earlier. There are two distinct elements within an empowerment approach to health promotion and health education: individual empowerment and community empowerment. It is relational in its approach and invests control in the subjects. Examples of this approach are used within contexts to encourage alcohol reduction, smoking cessation and weight loss.

Legislative approach

This final approach tries to achieve social change through legislation. Government policy introduces controls in society that affect people's ability to make the choices that impact on their lives. For instance, taxing confectionery makes it more expensive, thus aiming to reduce the amount of sugary food that people buy and eat. This in turn reduces obesity and consequently the amount of type 2 diabetes within the population. This in its turn reduces the burden of disease upon the individual and the burden upon society in terms of healthcare provision and associated health and social care costs. Within this model, factors known as determinants of health, such as education and economic status, gender, class, culture and so forth, are important. The focus is on changing the structures of society and influencing policy. This is a top-down approach that clinicians can influence. Examples can be seen in the Health Child Programme and in legislation such as the banning of smoking in public places.

PREVENTION OF ILL HEALTH AND DISEASE

Prevention of ill health and disease had traditionally been thought of as three elements:

- **Primary prevention** is the prevention of the onset of disease. Examples of this approach are the child immunization programme and the child surveillance programme, which monitors growth and development, among other things.
- **Secondary prevention** seeks to prevent existing ill health from worsening and becoming chronic. Examples of this are smoking cessation for people with lung disease or cancers.
- **Tertiary prevention** is concerned with supporting people who have long-term and intractable conditions. An example of this is diabetes education offered through the DESMOND programme cited earlier.

Downie (1991) expanded the three levels of prevention to four. These are similar to the three elements, but they challenge them too (see Table 15.1).

NATIONAL PRIORITIES FOR HEALTH PROMOTION AND HEALTH EDUCATION

There is a growing recognition that communities and individuals hold the key to their own health and well-being, and that a public health approach to enabling and empowering individuals

is critical to the NHS using resources most efficiently as we go into the future. The burden of disease to the individual and to society is very large and, in an age of limited financial resources, it is important for governments to create ways in which people can act in their own best interest, in partnership with health providers, to achieve a healthy society. An innovative approach to creating a health community can be seen in the New NHS Alliance initiative, which is a movement of people and organizations committed to building a sustainable, community-based health service. It has created a partnership with ITN Productions to create health education programmes. See what you think. Is this helpful to your practice?

http://www.nhsalliance.org/nhs-alliance-tv/communities-of-care/

In addition, the Government has established an agency to tackle health inequality. Health promotion is an important element of this (Box 15.3).

TABLE 15.1   Three Levels of Prevention (Downie, 1991)

Level of prevention	Description
Prevention of the onset of the disease.	Prevention at the earliest stage through aiming to work to reduce risk.
Prevention of the progression of the disease once it is established, but not identified within the person.	This relies upon screening. A good example of this is the cervical cytology programme offered by general practitioners and screening for bowel cancer offered to people over age 60 years.
Prevention of avoidable complications.	This relies upon follow up and good management. Client education is always an important element here.
Prevention of recurrence of the condition/disease.	This relies upon keeping the person healthy.

BOX 15.3   Government Aims in Supporting Health Improvement

The UK Government, via the NHS and partners, aims to support health improvement and says of itself that it will:

Improve health
We work with local government and the NHS to protect and improve health and well-being and to help people make healthier choices. We work to reduce health inequalities so the poorest and most poorly benefit most.

Empower the public
We work with partners to inform, educate, and empower people and communities, especially those in greatest need. We help people to take more control of their health and the things that affect their health.

Build a committed workforce
We work across the system to develop a robust public health workforce that is knowledgeable, capable and effective at improving health, promoting wellness and tackling health inequalities.

Use the evidence
We champion science and look to put research into practice – we always call on the best available evidence when advising, developing and implementing high-impact strategies to improve health outcomes.

Tackle health inequalities
We build partnerships and engage a wide range of stakeholders to help address health inequalities and influence the factors that affect the public's health.

Address public health priorities
PHE [Public Health England] is prioritising its efforts to achieve meaningful and measurable results quickly in a few key areas of public health, which we can tackle effectively and with known strategies. By setting out clear strategies and targets, and by working with public health partners, we can reduce health inequalities and lessen the overall burden of these diseases and conditions.

Well-being and mental health
Mental illness accounts for 23% of all ill health in England and affects more than one in four of the population at any time. Good mental health is linked to good physical health, education, employment and reduced crime and antisocial behaviour. We aim to expand access to services, improve the public uptake of promotion and prevention programs, and prioritise measures that have the greatest public impact. PHE will work with the NHS, local authorities and other partners to help more people have good mental health, improve the physical health and well-being of those with mental illness and ensure few people as possible suffer avoidable harm.

BOX 15.3 Government Aims in Supporting Health Improvement (Continued)

Diet, obesity and physical exercise

Poor diet, obesity and lack of exercise are all major causes of cardiovascular disease (CVD) and cancer. Poor diet accounts for one third of deaths from cancer and CVD. Lack of exercise increases the risk of CVD, and colorectal and breast cancers. Obesity increases the risk of type 2 diabetes, hypertension and colorectal cancer in men. We are making progress in these areas by supporting national and local initiatives to give people healthy choices that are easy and affordable. This includes improving the food in schools, hospitals and workplaces; reducing salt in processed and restaurant food; and improving opportunities for safe physical activity.

Smoking

Smoking accounts for 20% of new cases of cancer. Every year, tobacco causes nearly 1 in 5 deaths in England. For each death, 20 more people develop tobacco-related illnesses. Effective interventions include cessation programmes, tax increases, smoke-free policies, media campaigns and advertising restrictions.

Alcohol and drugs

Alcohol and drugs are cross-government issues. The costs of drug and alcohol misuse are similar to smoking and obesity but come more from crime. Drug-related crime is mainly acquisitive while alcohol-related crime is mainly violence and social disorder. Our first goal here is to prevent risky behavior and to help people stop misusing these substances.

HIV and sexual health

More than 100,000 people in the UK were living with HIV/AIDS by the end of 2012. Over half of those living with HIV in the UK were diagnosed late and this means their outcome may not be as positive as if their infection was diagnosed at an earlier stage.

Around half a million new sexually transmitted infections (STIs) were diagnosed in 2011 (a 2% rise from 2010). Among those most affected are young men and women, men who have sex with men and ethnic minority groups. The key things we can do to tackle this increase include; screening people for HIV/STI infections, early treatment, notifying partners so they can be tested, social marketing campaigns, providing access to condoms and promoting their use, and policies to address stigma and discrimination.

Life-course perspectives

PHE will focus its health improvement efforts on the life course, which means combining prevention and early intervention to support people as they pass through life's major transitions. This has 5 key benefits. It:
* promotes an holistic approach that sees the individual's total health and well-being needs
* encourages an asset-based approach that understands risk factors and the importance of the family as a protective factor

* focuses on outcomes and draws from the evidence base
* concentrates on prevention and early intervention, which includes reducing health inequalities and preventable mortality
* views public health as one agency for improving health and well-being outcomes.

Expert advisors will help PHE to develop, implement and monitor public and personal health and well-being across the five key stages of life. They will also help PHE to promote the value and effectiveness of this approach to our partners and stakeholders.

Healthy infants, children and youth

Focus on improving health and outcomes for mothers and infants, children, teens and young adults.

Healthy adults and older adults

Help all people and especially those at risk from health inequalities, to live a long and healthy life.

Healthy people in healthy places

Ensure the places where people live, work, learn and play protect and promote their health, especially for those at greater risk of health inequalities.

Healthcare public health

Support sound decision-making and policy changes within the NHS that deliver, evaluate and improve effective clinical preventive services that drive public health.

Health in all policies

Inform and support the Department of Health and other government partners in sound decision-making and policy changes at all levels to deliver and evaluate programs and to address the social factors that affect health.

National programmes
* Alcohol and drugs
* Cancer screening
* Dental public health
* UK National Screening Committee and other screening programs
* National health marketing campaigns
* NHS Health Check
* Nutrition and healthy food
* Offender health
* Public mental health
* Tobacco
* Sexual health
* Well-being and mental health

Contains public sector information licensed under the Open Government Licence v3.0.

LOOKING BACK, FEEDING FORWARD

Health promotion and health education are important and critical elements within the reforming NHS. Empowering the public to take charge of their own health is important for the personal well-being of individuals, as well as for managing resources for health effectively and efficiently.

The NA must understand that there are various approaches to delivering health promotion and health education and be aware that each encounter with a client is an opportunity for therapeutic engagement and a chance to change. The NA has to make each contact count.

Health is a complex construct. It has many aspects – some subjective and others objective. Health policy is influenced by the Government's agenda. Health and the uptake of healthcare are affected by culture, a person's religious beliefs, their age, gender, social class, socio-economic status, educational attainment and life experiences. In order for the NA to be an effective practitioner and work to empower people, it is important to understand health and the issues that impact upon it, such as the determinants of health and health inequity and inequality. It is also important to understand that it will never be possible to achieve exactly the same outcome for everyone, despite best efforts. This means that NAs and other health professionals and governments work to eliminate inequality wherever possible, and that this is the goal we aspire to. Understanding why inequality and inequity exist is important in tackling the issues inherent within them. Ultimately, improving health and well-being requires individuals to take charge of their own lives and health. Health professionals' input is key to assisting with this process. It will take many generations, but it is a worthwhile and humane goal. In this, the NA recognizes individual personhood and the value of each person, regardless of who they are.

REFERENCES

Aked, J. et al., 2008. Five ways to wellbeing. The New Economics Foundation. http://b.3cdn.net/nefoundation/8984c5089d5c2285ee_t4m6bhqq5.pdf.

Beattie, A., et al., 1991. Knowledge and control in health promotion: a test case for social policy and social theory. The Sociology of the Health Service. Routledge, New York.

Carper, B.A., 1978. Fundamental patterns of knowing in nursing. ANS 1 (1), 13–24.

Downie, R.S., 1991. The new medicine and the old ethics (book review). Sociol. Health Illness 13, 564–565.

Feinstein, L. et al., 2006. Measuring the effects of education on health and civic engagement. Proceedings of the Copenhagen Symposium. OECD, Paris.

Freire, P., 2017. [1968]. Pedagogy of the Oppressed. Harmondsworth, Penguin Modern Classics.

Global Health Europe. (2009) A Joint Project between Maastricht University, Graduate Institute Geneva, Global Health Program, Inequity and Inequality in Health. www.globalhealtheurope.org/index.php/resources/glossary/values/197-inequity-and-inequality-in-health.html.

Health and Social Care Act 2012. http://www.legislation.gov.ukpga/2012/7/contents/enacted.

Healthy Child Programme, 2009. https://www.gov.uk/government/publications/healthy-child-programme-5-to-19-years-old.

Huber, M., et al., 2011. How should we define health? BMJ 343, doi:10.1136/bmj.d4163.

Johns, C., 1995. The value of reflective practice for nursing. J. Clin. Nurs. 4, 23–30.

Kuruvilla, S., et al., 2018. A life-course approach to health; Synergy with sustainable development goals. Bull. World Health Org. 96, 42–50. doi:10.2471/BLT.17.198358.

Marmot Review. (2011) https://www.local.gov.uk/marmot-review-report-fair-society-healthy-lives.

Miller, W.R., Rollnick, S., 1991. Motivational Interviewing: Preparing People to Change Addictive Behavior. Guilford Press, New York.

Mosley, M., 2015. The 8-Week Blood Sugar Diet: Lose Weight Fast and Reprogramme Your Body for Life. Short Books Ltd, London.

Pickin, C., St Ledger, S., 1993, 1997. Assessing Health Needs Using The Life Cycle Framework. Open University Press, Buckingham.

Prochaska, J., DiClemente, C., 1983. Stages and processes of self-change in smoking: toward an integrative model of change. J. Consult. Clin. Psychol. 5, 390–395.

Prochaska, J.O., DiClemente, C.C., Norcross, J.C., 1992. In search of how people change: Applications to the addictive behaviors. Am. Psychol. 47, 1102–1114. PMID: 1329589.

Rillamas-Sun, E., Harlow, S.D., Randolph, J.F., 2014. Grandmothers' smoking in pregnancy and grandchildren's birth weight: comparisons by grandmother birth cohort. Matern. Child Health J. 18 (7), 1691–1698. doi:10.1007/s10995-013-1411-x.

Rotter, J.B., 1966. Generalized expectancies for internal versus external control of reinforcement. Psycholo. Monogr. 80, 1–28.

Soni, A., Bailey, V., 2013. The NHS's role in the public's health. A report from the NHS Future Forum. 1st ed. [ebook].

Tengland, P.A., 2007. Empowerment: a goal or a means for health promotion? Med. Health Care Philos. 10, 197–207.

The Kings Fund, 2013. An Alternative Guide to the NHS in England. 27 June. https://youtu.be/8CSp6HsQVtw.

The Kings Fund, 2017. How Does the NHS in England Work? An Alternative Guide. 6 October. https://www.kingsfund.org.uk/audio-video/how-does-nhs-in-england-work.

Tudor Hart, J., 1971. The Inverse Care Law. The Lancet. 297 (7696), 405–412.

Twist, J., 2011. Work Well the Walton Way. http://www.nhsemployers.org/case-studies-and-resources/2011/10/work-well-the-walton-way.

World Health Organizaton, 1946. Preamble to the Constitution of the World Health Organization as adopted by the International Health Conference, New York, 19–22 June 1946; signed on 22 July 1946 by the representatives of 61 States (Official Records of the World Health Organization, no. 2, p. 100) and entered into force on 7 April 1948.

World Health Organization, n.d. http://www.who.int/topics/health_promotion/en/, http://www.who.int/topics/health_education/en/.

World Health Organization, Health and Welfare Canada & Canadian Public Health Association, 1986. Ottawa Charter for Health Promotion: An International Conference on Health Promotion— the Move Towards a New Public Health, Nov. 17–21, Ottawa. World Health Organization, Geneva, Switzerland.

16

Infection Prevention and Control

Sandra Netto

OBJECTIVES

By the end of the chapter the reader will be able to:

1. Describe the different types of microbes that cause infections
2. Understand the path of infection and how microbes can be transmitted
3. Recognize the importance of using standard precautions and apply this to all patients with the aim of reducing healthcare-associated infections
4. Appreciate the role of the Nursing Associate in applying infection prevention and control principles in healthcare

KEY WORDS

Infection
Prevention
Control
Transmission

Precaution
Handwashing
Microorganisms
Bacteria

Viruses
Pathogens

CHAPTER AIM

This chapter aims to familiarize the Nursing Associate (NA) with the chain of infection and infection transmission. Through acquiring the knowledge and skills, the NA will be able to apply the standard principles of infection prevention and control to reduce healthcare-associated infections.

SELF TEST

1. List the signs and symptoms of infection.
2. What is meant by the chain of infection?
3. What role does the nurse play in preventing infection?
4. What are the 5 moments for hand hygiene?
5. What do you understand by personal protective equipment?
6. How should sharps be disposed of safely?
7. In the case of needle stick injury, what does your local policy and procedure require you to do?
8. How do you safely dispose of contaminated laundry according to policy and procedure?
9. What are body fluids?
10. What are blood-borne viruses?

INTRODUCTION

Healthcare-associated infections (HAI) have become a significant threat to patient safety over the last 20 years, causing considerable morbidity and mortality to patients and imposing a financial burden on healthcare trusts in terms of the economic consequences when dealing with these infections. The increase in technological advances with treatments and interventions in healthcare, coupled with the increasing rise in multi-resistant strains of disease-causing organisms, has led to both government and the public becoming more aware of the risks associated with healthcare interventions and the healthcare environment.

The English National Point Prevalence Survey (Health Protection Agency, 2012) identified that 6.4% of inpatients in acute care hospitals in 2011 acquired a healthcare-associated infection. The six most common types of healthcare-associated infections were pneumonia and other respiratory infections (22.8%), urinary tract infections (16.2%), surgical site infections (15.7%), clinical sepsis (10.5%), gastrointestinal infections (8.8%) and bloodstream infections (7.3%) (Fig. 16.1).

This chapter will concentrate on measures to reduce the risk of transmission in the healthcare setting, with the aim of protecting patients, visitors and staff from acquiring a healthcare-associated infection. It is not possible in a chapter of this size to address all issues associated with infection, prevention and control. The Nursing Associate (NA) is advised to delve deeper into the subject area, accessing other texts that focus on infection prevention and control. The NA should always adhere to local policy and procedure to guide their practice and ensure patient care is safe, effective and evidence-based.

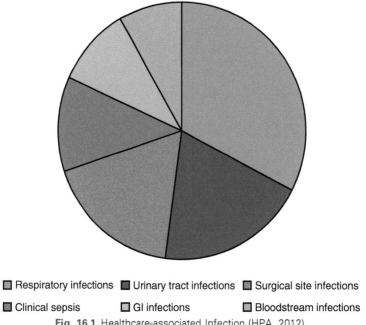

☐ Respiratory infections ■ Urinary tract infections ■ Surgical site infections

■ Clinical sepsis ☐ GI infections ■ Bloodstream infections

Fig. 16.1 Healthcare-associated Infection (HPA, 2012).

The NA, as a member of the multidisciplinary team, is a key player in the fight against infection and in ensuring that processes and procedures are in place to reduce risk and prevent infection.

MICROORGANISMS (MICROBES)

Microorganisms (also known as microbes) are small living organisms that can only be seen with a microscope. Microbes are everywhere – in the air, soil, water and food. They also colonize our body – in the nose, mouth, respiratory tract, stomach and intestine. The surface of the body (skin) is also densely populated with microorganisms; these are known as commensals and cause no harm. They are referred to as the 'normal flora' of the body. The following are types of microbe:

- Bacteria – single-celled organisms that multiply rapidly. Bacteria have three basic shapes, round, rod shaped and curved or spiral, and can be seen in pairs, chains or clusters. They are also classified by their need for oxygen. Aerobic bacteria need oxygen to grow and anaerobic bacteria thrive without oxygen.
- Viruses – an assemblage of particles of nucleic acids, RNA or DNA, with a protein outer layer or membranous envelope. Viruses need a host cell to multiply – they cannot replicate alone.
- Fungi – a diverse group of organisms including yeasts, moulds and mushrooms. Some species cause disease in humans, such as ringworm and oral and vaginal candida, but fungi can cause more serious infection in the immunocompromised patient. They need a warm, moist environment to survive.
- Protozoa – single-celled animals that divide in two. They have complicated life cycles and most are aquatic. Some are animal parasites.

- Rickettsia – small bacteria that cannot grow outside the cells of their host. They are found in vectors, such as fleas, lice and ticks, and are transmitted via the bite of the vector animal.
- Prions – protein particles that do not have nucleic acids and are not destroyed by the same methods as bacteria and viruses. They can cause degenerative neurological disease, such as Creutzfeldt-Jakob disease (CJD), the human form of mad cow disease.
- Helminths – parasitic worms, such as pinworms (common in children), tapeworms or roundworms.

INFECTION

An infection is the process whereby microbes invade the body and multiply causing tissue damage at the site of infection, and in the worst case, the death of the host. Microbes capable of causing disease are called pathogens. Some pathogens can produce harmful toxins or endotoxins that cause disease in people. However, the body also hosts non-pathogenic microbes (normal flora), which sit in or on the body and prevent harmful pathogens from colonizing or multiplying. Infection can manifest both physically and physiologically, and the signs of infection can be either localized to one area – such as the site of invasion – or throughout the whole body, this is called 'systemic spread'. The path of infection is as follows:

- Entry: pathogen enters the host.
- Attachment: pathogen attaches to tissues in the body and enters them.
- Multiplication: once inside the host and having the right environment to grow and survive, the pathogen will begin to multiply. This can be local at the site of entering or may

BOX 16.1 Some Signs and Symptoms of Infection

- Pyrexia (high temperature)
- Chills, muscle aches
- Tiredness and loss of energy (lethargy)
- Nausea, vomiting, diarrhoea
- Discharge or pus from infected area
- Redness, swelling, heat and loss of function at site
- Loss of appetite

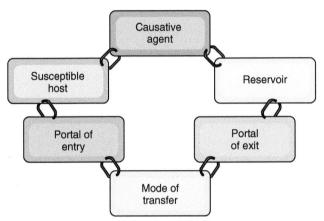

Fig. 16.2 The Chain of Infection.

spread into the bloodstream or other body sites. Signs of infection may begin to show at this stage.

- Evasion of the host defences: the pathogen will try to avoid the host's immune system which is there to defend the host.
- Damage to tissues/host: damage from infection may be severe enough to cause lasting damage to tissues and, in some cases, death of the host.

Signs of infection

The signs of infection are due to the inflammatory response by the body's immune system (see Chapter 27) with the aim to localize the infection and limit the spread. See Box 16.1 for some signs and symptoms of infection.

COMMUNITIES OF CARE

The Older Person

It must be noted that the immune system changes with aging and older people are more susceptible to infections. The signs of infection may not be as pronounced, as there may not be pyrexia, or signs of redness or swelling. However, this group may be more confused and agitated.

The chain of infection

The chain of infection (Fig. 16.2) is where microbes can be passed from one person or contaminated article to another person,

for them to then become infected. There are several requirements needed for this to happen:

- A pathogenic microbe
- A reservoir where microbes can survive (people, food, articles)
- An exit point (body fluids, respiratory secretions)
- A route of transmission (direct contact, airborne, contaminated article)
- A suitable place of entry (respiratory tract, broken skin, gut)
- A susceptible host (immunocompromised, non-immune).

Microbial reservoirs

Microbial reservoirs are where microbes live and grow. People, animals, plants, soil, food and water are all common reservoirs, but microbes can also contaminate articles and lie in the environment for several months. Microbes need water and nourishment to grow and most grow best at body temperature. Some need oxygen, but some survive and grow without this.

Portal of exit

This is where the pathogenic microbe finds a way to leave its current host and move to another. There are several ways this can be done:

- Via the respiratory tract: by coughing, sneezing and respiratory secretions, e.g., measles, influenza, *Mycobacterium tuberculosis*.
- Via the gastrointestinal tract: by diarrhoea, vomiting, microbes in faeces, e.g., Norovirus, *Clostridium difficile*, *Salmonella typhi*.
- Via the skin and mucous membranes: through open or exuding wounds, e.g., methicillin-resistant *Staphylococcus aureus* (MRSA), sexually transmitted infections.
- Via blood and body fluids: through an open wound or piercing of the skin or mucous membranes, e.g., human immunodeficiency virus (HIV), hepatitis B, hepatitis C.

Routes of microbial transmission

There are several ways that microbes can transfer from one person to another. To be able to transmit infection, a pathogen must have an entry point and an exit point and can use a range of different mechanisms to find a new host. Some pathogens have the ability to spread more easily than others and this makes them more infectious or contagious. However, microbes cannot spread by themselves, and spread will be as a result of direct or indirect contact. Establishing the source and route of transmission is therefore important so that the appropriate infection control measures can be put in place.

- Direct contact: Microbes are spread by direct contact with body fluids or on the surfaces of an infected person. Examples are: sexually transmitted infections (*Chlamydia trachomatis*), via kissing (Epstein-Barr virus), from mother to child in utero (rubella) or piercing of the skin with a contaminated article from the environment (tetanus).
- Indirect contact: Microbes are transmitted indirectly through contaminated people, animals or inanimate objects in the environment. They spread via vehicles such as hands,

equipment, contaminated food/water or infective particles in the air.

- Airborne: Microbes travel either via droplets, which are heavy particles burdened with microbes but do not travel very far (less than 1 metre), or by a fine spray where particles are very small and light but stay suspended in the air for a long time and can travel more than 1 metre.
- Vectors: Insects or animals that can indirectly transmit microbes; note, however, this is not a usual mode of transmission for infection in a healthcare setting.

Portal of entry

Microbes can enter the body by several ways where they can multiply and cause infection or sit in the host without causing harm.

- The respiratory tract by inhaling in the microbes.
- The gastrointestinal tract by ingestion and absorption.
- The urinary tract by direct or indirect contact with an infected person or contaminated article or equipment.
- The bloodstream through openings in the skin, contaminated needles or vectors. such as mosquitoes.
- The skin through cuts, grazes or cannula sites.

A susceptible host

A susceptible host can be anyone. However, people admitted into a healthcare setting may be more vulnerable. Some people are more at risk than others of acquiring an infection:

- Older adults – may have poor nutrition, chronic illness, poor mobility and frail skin integrity and more frequent visits to hospital.
- Very young children – immature immune system.
- Immunosuppressed patients – such as those receiving treatments that will suppress the immune system, e.g., chemotherapy, steroid therapy.
- Chronic illness – chronic diseases, such as diabetes and HIV, can cause people to become more prone to infection due to an impaired immune system.
- Indwelling devices – cannulas, urinary catheters, feeding tubes and prosthetic implants all provide access for microbes to enter the body and colonize, so can be a focus for infection.

Healthcare-associated infection

This term applies to any person developing an infection due to treatment or being cared for in a healthcare setting. This can be in hospital (secondary/tertiary care), in a GP clinic or home setting (primary care) or in a nursing home. Healthcare associated infections (HAIs) can be caused by the patient's own normal flora (for example *E. coli* in the gut passes into the urinary tract due to poor personal hygiene) or can be passed indirectly by healthcare workers on their hands as a result of poor hand hygiene or from the environment due to poor disinfection and sterilization of equipment or cleaning of the hospital environment.

CARE IN THE HOME SETTING

Care is now being delivered in a wide range of community settings, such as residential homes, patients' own homes and nursing homes. This poses a challenge for carers as sometimes infection control policies in the healthcare setting may be unsuitable for use in the community and may need adapting. However, it is important that all staff caring for patients in the community apply the principles of infection prevention and control by using standard precautions when delivering care.

Challenges faced in the community:

Hand hygiene

In patients' homes, hand hygiene facilities may not be ideal; therefore staff are encouraged to:

- carry alcohol hand rub/gel or antibacterial hand wipes
- only use soap from a pump dispenser, not a bar of soap
- dry hands with paper towels or a clean towel
- adhere to hand hygiene techniques.

Patient environment at home

The main aim of hygiene in the home is to target those places where pathogenic microbes may reside and have the potential to cause infection, such as bathrooms and kitchens.

Normal cleaning, such as vacuuming, damp dusting and cleaning surfaces are generally enough in the home; however, tact maybe needed when advising cleaning methods as carers/patients may feel the house is clean enough already and not see this as important.

Disposing of clinical waste

The healthcare trust has the primary responsibility for the disposing of any healthcare waste in the patient's home. Staff must ensure that the patient/carer recognizes the procedure for disposing of clinical waste at home.

- **Non-hazardous waste** – should be double bagged and disposed of in household waste with owner's permission. This includes small dressings, sanitary towels and incontinence pads.
- **Hazardous waste (infectious, sharps, etc.)** – households where hazardous waste is generated should have an approved clinical bin/sharps bin (rigid, leak proof and sealed) in the house and arrangements with the waste contractor must be made by the community staff for collection and disposal.

Home loans equipment:

- Patient equipment must be deemed safe to handle before being sent for repair or returned into storage.
- Soiled items of equipment should be cleaned with warm water and detergent.
- When selecting beds, chairs and mattresses for patients, ensure items are easy-clean and made of an impermeable material.
- Gloves should be used when handling soiled or contaminated equipment.
- Hand hygiene must be performed after removal of gloves.

BREAKING THE CHAIN OF INFECTION

It is important for the NA and other healthcare professionals to recognize the requirements within the chain for an infection to be transmitted. Interrupting one of the links makes it harder for microbes to spread.

Cross transmission of infection can be halted at any point in the chain of infection. The implementation of standard precautions helps facilitate the breaking of the chain. These precautions are there to protect the NA as much as the patient and should be used for every patient contact.

Standard precautions include the following:
- Hand hygiene
- Use of personal protective equipment (PPE)
- Respiratory and cough etiquette
- Transmission-based precautions
- Patient placement and assessment of infection risk
- Safe handling of linen
- Safe handling of clinical waste (including sharps management)
- Occupational safety
- Management of blood and body spills
- Decontamination of medical and patient equipment
- Environmental cleaning
- Using single-use or sterile equipment and Aseptic Non Touch Technique (ANTT®) when performing procedures

Hand hygiene

The most common vehicle for transmitting infection in healthcare settings is via the hands of healthcare workers (WHO, 2009a; Loveday et al., 2014). Hands are colonized with two types of flora: resident flora, which are found on the uppermost surface of the skin and are mostly of low pathogenicity and normal flora to the body, and transient flora, which are microbes picked up by the hands from contaminated surfaces, such as patients, other people and the environment. Pittet et al., (1999) demonstrated that pathogens are more likely to be picked up when handling moist, heavily contaminated substances, such as body fluids, as these microbes are readily transferred from one person to another or to any object touched. Transient carriage can include a vast range of multi-resistant bacteria, such as MRSA, *Acinetobacter* and other gram-negative bacteria, which, if transferred to a susceptible site, such as a cannula or open wound, can cause life-threatening infections and may consequently result in an HAI.

Hand hygiene is the most effective way to reduce the number of microbes on the hands, thus minimizing the risk of transferring them from person to person or from one object to another. The aim of hand washing is to remove the transient microbes picked up via patient care or in the patient environment.

When to wash your hands

Patients are placed at risk when the healthcare worker has contaminated hands. The World Health Organization (WHO) has developed a framework called the 'Five Moments of Hand Hygiene' where a moment is deemed an actual risk of when a pathogen can be transmitted from a person or contaminated surface by the NA's hands (Fig. 16.3). Therefore the timing of when to perform hand hygiene is crucial. The five stages are:

1. Before patient contact
2. Before a procedure
3. After a procedure or handling body fluids
4. After patient contact and removal of gloves
5. After contact with the patient environment.

Other indications for hand hygiene are:
- Before and after handling food and drink
- After handling clinical waste and laundry
- After removing gloves
- After using the toilet
- Before leaving the clinical area.

Hand decontamination is the process that either physically removes dirt, blood or body fluids from the hands by hand washing, or destroys and removes microbes on the hands with alcohol hand rub or antimicrobial hand wash.

What hand decontamination method to use

There are various ways to decontaminate the hands, such as by using liquid soap and water, alcohol-based hand rub (ABHR) or antiseptic/antimicrobial agents such as chlorhexidine 4% or povidone/iodine solution. Extensive research has shown that there is no evidence to suggest that one method of hand decontamination agent is more effective than another (Loveday et al., 2014). Choosing an agent for decontaminating the hands must depend on the NA undertaking an assessment of what episode of care is to be carried out, the availability of resources at the point of care and personal preference of the available products.

Soap and water. Effective hand washing with liquid soap and water will remove transient microbes and render the hands socially clean. This level of decontamination is sufficient for most episodes in clinical care and social interaction.

Alcohol-based hand rub (ABHR). This will also remove transient microbes and render the hands socially clean. ABHRs have also been shown to reduce the amount of resident flora on the hands, making them an effective agent for most episodes in clinical care and social contact. However, they are not effective against viruses, such as norovirus, or spore-forming microbes, such as *C. difficile*, where soap and water need to be used. They are also not a good agent to use if the hands are visibly soiled.

Liquid soap preparation containing antibacterial/microbial agent. These agents remove both transient and resident flora from the hands and some will have a lasting effect. This level of decontamination will be used when episodes of care require prolonged reduction of microbes on the hands, such as when performing invasive procedures, surgery or in some outbreak situations.

Hand hygiene technique

Hand hygiene involves both the liquid preparation used and the process used to decontaminate the hands. The wearing of jewellery and false/acrylic nails has been identified as being the cause of some outbreaks in the healthcare environment, as microbes can get trapped under rings or nails/nail beds and are not easily removed by hand washing. Therefore, before effective hand decontamination can take place, all jewellery must be removed from the hands and wrists before entering the clinical area and nails should be short and free from nail polish and nail art. Long sleeves that cover the wrist also affect good hand decontamination and

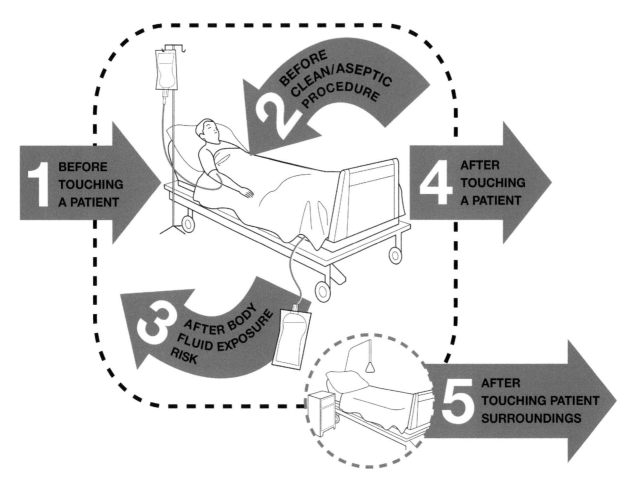

1	BEFORE TOUCHING A PATIENT	WHEN?	Clean your hands before touching a patient when approaching him/her.
		WHY?	To protect the patient against harmful germs carried on your hands.
2	BEFORE CLEAN/ ASEPTIC PROCEDURE	WHEN?	Clean your hands immediately before performing a clean/aseptic procedure.
		WHY?	To protect the patient against harmful germs, including the patient's own, from entering his/her body.
3	AFTER BODY FLUID EXPOSURE RISK	WHEN?	Clean your hands immediately after an exposure risk to body fluids (and after glove removal).
		WHY?	To protect yourself and the health-care environment from harmful patient germs.
4	AFTER TOUCHING A PATIENT	WHEN?	Clean your hands after touching a patient and her/his immediate surroundings, when leaving the patient's side.
		WHY?	To protect yourself and the health-care environment from harmful patient germs.
5	AFTER TOUCHING PATIENT SURROUNDINGS	WHEN?	Clean your hands after touching any object or furniture in the patient's immediate surroundings, when leaving – even if the patient has not been touched.
		WHY?	To protect yourself and the health-care environment from harmful patient germs.

Fig. 16.3 A Guide to the 5 Moments for Hand Hygiene (WHO, 2009b).

must be removed. Most healthcare organizations include the 'bare below the elbow' recommendation as part of their uniform policy.

Hands should be washed properly to ensure that all microbes are removed. However, in a study undertaken many years ago, Taylor (1978) noted that nurses frequently missed areas of the hands when washing (Fig. 16.4). Hands should be washed in a systematic way to ensure all areas of the hands and wrists are covered.

Handwashing technique

Hand washing should be done in three stages:

1. Preparation – wetting the hands and applying the appropriate hand hygiene solution.

2. Washing – a six-stage technique is recommended (Ayliffe et al., 1978) to ensure the solution comes into contact with all areas of the hands and wrists. This should be done for at least 20 seconds.

3. Drying – hands should be dried thoroughly with a dabbing method to ensure no residue of moisture is left.

Fig. 16.5 outlines the correct method for washing hands with soap and water.

When using an ABHR, the solution must still come into contact with all of the hand and wrist and the same hand washing technique must be used. The hands must be rubbed until the liquid has evaporated.

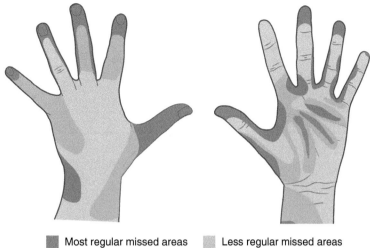

■ Most regular missed areas   ▨ Less regular missed areas

Fig. 16.4 The Seminal Work of Taylor (1978): Missed Areas of Handwashing.

Care of the skin

Frequent handwashing, especially with antibacterial/microbial solutions, can damage the skin and alter the normal flora of the hands. Poor hand hygiene technique, where the hands are not dried thoroughly, or using antimicrobial preparations when not needed, can lead to dry chapped skin. Sore hands can also lead to increased colonization of microbes on the skin, which in turn can increase the risk of transmission. Therefore, the use of an emollient hand cream to moisturize the skin regularly should be encouraged and be available in all clinical areas.

CRITICAL AWARENESS

Little research has been done into the role that carers and patients have in transmitting infection in the healthcare setting, especially in outbreak situations. Therefore, it is just as important to educate both patients and carers in effective hand washing and inform them of the hand-hygiene facilities available to them in the healthcare setting.

Personal protective equipment (PPE)

Many excretions and secretions from the patient harbour pathogenic microbes and are a source of infection that can then be transmitted to others. Protective clothing, such as gloves, aprons, goggles and masks, should be worn if it is anticipated that the NA may be in contact with such substances, thus helping to reduce the risk of transmission. Selection of the appropriate PPE requires the NA assessing the patient and the care activity that is to take place.

Gloves

Gloves are an important element of PPE and are used every day as part of clinical care. There are several types of gloves available:

- Medical examination gloves – for use in clinical care to prevent contamination with blood, body fluids or pathogenic microbes. These can be non-sterile or sterile, depending on the task.
- Surgical gloves – sterile gloves used by the NA during surgery or for other invasive procedures.

The NA should wear gloves for any activity involving blood, body fluids or exposure to mucous membrane and must be discarded (using local policy and procedure) after each patient contact/procedure, or if heavily soiled. The choice of glove should always be based on an assessment of risk to what should be suitable for the task and materials being handled (Fig. 16.6).

Although gloves offer protection for staff and reduce the risk of hand contamination, they do not eliminate the risk completely. Gloves may be torn and, if not removed correctly, the hands can become contaminated; therefore it is important to learn how to remove gloves without contaminating the hands. Hand hygiene must always be performed after removing gloves (Fig. 16.7).

CRITICAL AWARENESS

Latex Allergy

Latex gloves are made from natural rubber. Sensitivity can develop after repeated exposure to latex. Limiting the use of latex may prevent allergic reactions in staff.

Allergic reactions can manifest in several ways:
- Contact dermatitis – the most common symptoms are dry, itchy irritated skin most often on the hands
- Allergic contact dermatitis – normally happens 24–96 hours after use and looks like a rash all over hands
- Latex allergy (immediate hypersensitivity) – within minutes of use. Symptoms can vary from skin redness, hives and itching to wheezing, coughing or difficulty in breathing.

Staff should therefore also have access to non-latex gloves, such as nitrile, vinyl or polymer gloves. If latex gloves are used, then powder free ones should be available.

Aprons and gowns

Aprons should be used by all staff if there is a risk of contaminating the uniform with sprays or splashes of blood or body fluids, either from close patient contact or from handling equipment or materials soiled with such. In most cases, plastic disposable aprons provide adequate protection and must be single-use and discarded as clinical waste after each procedure and between patients.

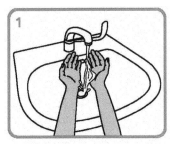

Wet hands
with water

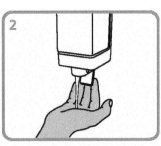

Apply enough soap
to cover all
hand surfaces

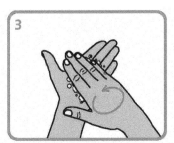

Rub hands palm
to palm

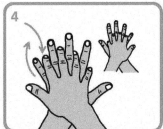

Rub back of each hand
with palm of other hand
with fingers interlaced

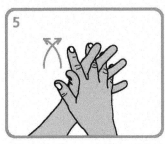

Rub palm to palm with
fingers interlaced

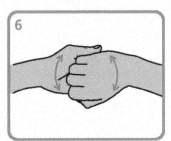

Rub with back of fingers
to opposing palms with
fingers interlocked

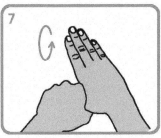

Rub each thumb clasped
in opposite hand using a
rotational movement

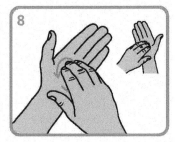

Rub tips of fingers in
opposite palm in a
circular motion

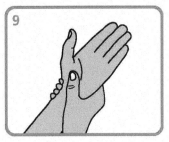

Rub each wrist with
opposite hand

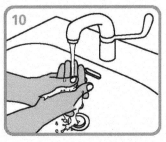

Rinse hands
with water

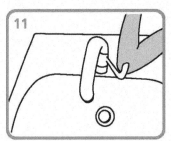

Use elbow to
turn off tap

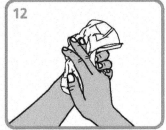

Dry thoroughly with
a single-use towel

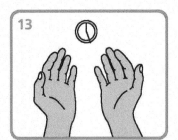

Hand washing should take
15–30 seconds

Fig. 16.5 Handwashing Technique Using Soap and Water (World Health Organization, 2009c).

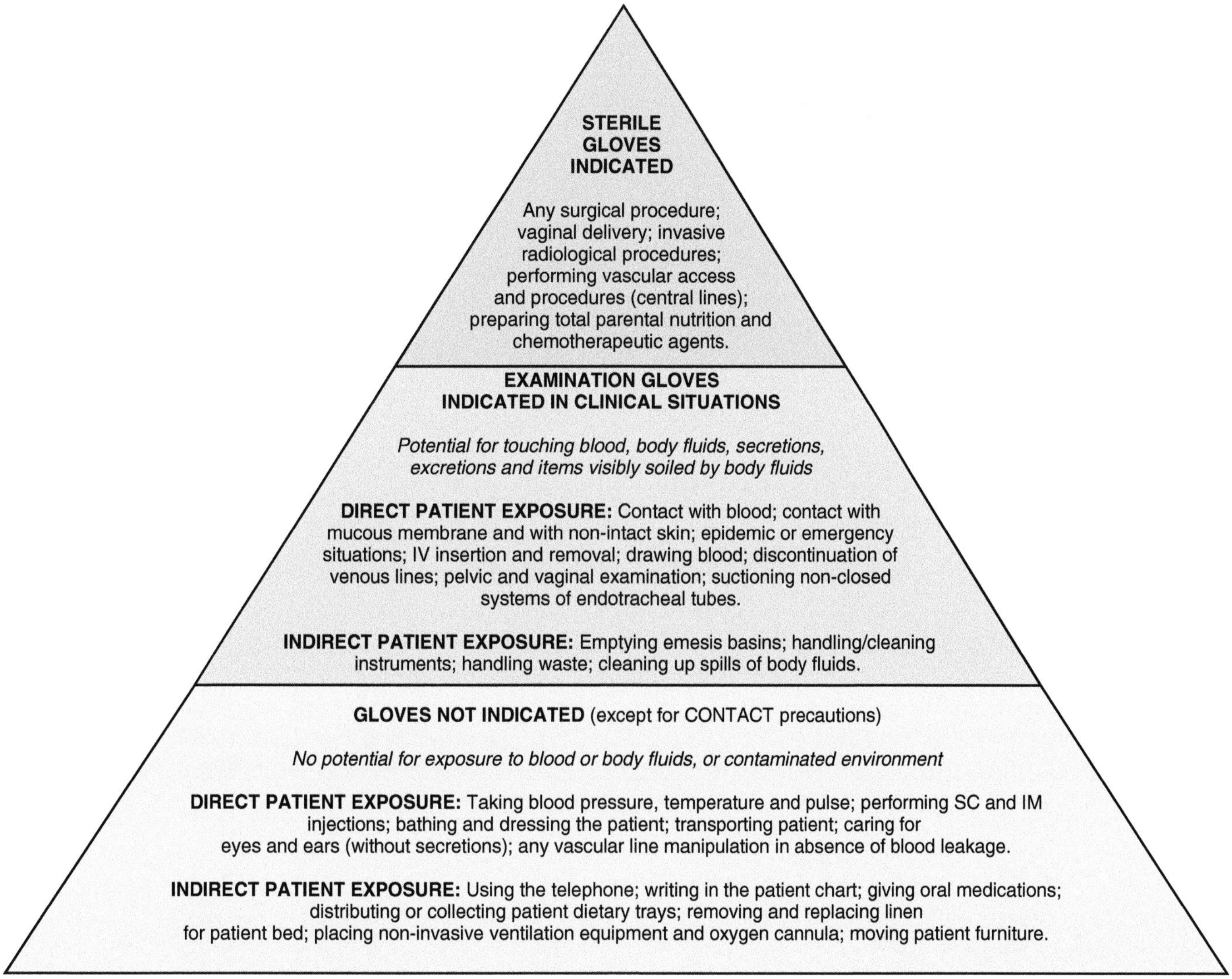

STERILE GLOVES INDICATED

Any surgical procedure; vaginal delivery; invasive radiological procedures; performing vascular access and procedures (central lines); preparing total parental nutrition and chemotherapeutic agents.

EXAMINATION GLOVES INDICATED IN CLINICAL SITUATIONS

Potential for touching blood, body fluids, secretions, excretions and items visibly soiled by body fluids

DIRECT PATIENT EXPOSURE: Contact with blood; contact with mucous membrane and with non-intact skin; epidemic or emergency situations; IV insertion and removal; drawing blood; discontinuation of venous lines; pelvic and vaginal examination; suctioning non-closed systems of endotracheal tubes.

INDIRECT PATIENT EXPOSURE: Emptying emesis basins; handling/cleaning instruments; handling waste; cleaning up spills of body fluids.

GLOVES NOT INDICATED (except for CONTACT precautions)

No potential for exposure to blood or body fluids, or contaminated environment

DIRECT PATIENT EXPOSURE: Taking blood pressure, temperature and pulse; performing SC and IM injections; bathing and dressing the patient; transporting patient; caring for eyes and ears (without secretions); any vascular line manipulation in absence of blood leakage.

INDIRECT PATIENT EXPOSURE: Using the telephone; writing in the patient chart; giving oral medications; distributing or collecting patient dietary trays; removing and replacing linen for patient bed; placing non-invasive ventilation equipment and oxygen cannula; moving patient furniture.

Fig. 16.6 The Glove Pyramid (WHO, 2009d).

Gowns or suits should only be used if there is a possibility of extensive splashing of blood or body fluids. They should be fluid repellent and should protect all areas of the body from contamination. All soiled gowns/suits should be removed promptly and carefully so as not to contaminate the wearer and be discarded in clinical waste. Hand hygiene must be performed after removal of aprons, gowns and suits.

Facial protection

Facial protection must be worn when carrying out any activity where there is a risk of blood or body fluid spray or splash. Goggles and masks must be used together to provide adequate protection of the mucous membranes of the eyes, nose and mouth.

Eye protection. Goggles provide adequate protection from splashes to the eyes but are seldom used by healthcare workers. A face shield or goggles and a fluid-resistant surgical mask should be worn by staff when performing aerosol generating procedures or if there is a risk of an eye/mouth splash. Ordinary corrective glasses must not be used as a substitute for eye protection – goggles or a face shield must be worn over the top.

Eye protection must be removed or changed:
- when soiled with blood or body fluids
- in accordance with manufacturer's advice
- at the end of the procedure
- when leaving the clinical area.

Face masks

These are used to protect staff from blood/body fluid splashes, and for protection against respiratory droplets and airborne infectious agents. They are also used to prevent droplets from the nose and mouth of staff reaching the patient when performing invasive procedures, such as central venous catheter (CVC) insertion. There are different categories of face masks and it depends on the task to be undertaken and the risk of exposure to infectious agents, which mask to use.

Surgical masks. These can be used as a barrier to protect the nose and mouth from blood and body fluid splashes but are not effective in filtering respiratory particles. They do not prevent small droplets from being inhaled around the side of mask as there is no adequate seal between the mask and the wearer.

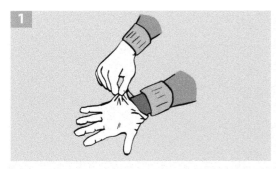

With both hands gloved, grasp the outside
of one glove at the top of your wrist, being careful
not to touch your bare skin.

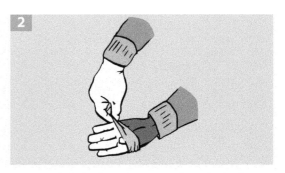

Peel off the first glove, away from the body,
from the wrists to the tips of the fingers.
As you do so, turn the glove inside out.

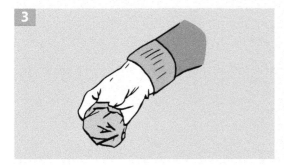

Grasp the glove that has just been removed in
the hand that still has a glove on.

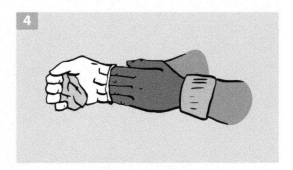

With your bare hand, take off the second
glove by putting your fingers inside the
top of the glove, near the wrist.

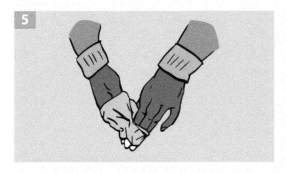

The second glove is turned inside out
whilst angling it away from the body.
The first glove is now inside the second.

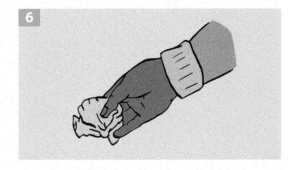

Dispose of the gloves safely. Do not reuse the gloves.

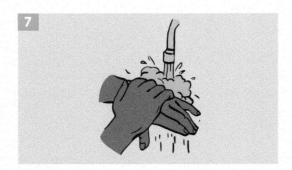

Clean your hands immediately after removing gloves
and before touching any objects or surfaces.

Fig. 16.7 Safely Removing Gloves. How to protect yourself with step-by-step glove removal.

Therefore specialized respiratory equipment with filters may be needed in nursing patients infected with a respiratory pathogen. Surgical masks should be fluid resistant and close fitting to avoid exhaled air escaping from the sides of the mask. Surgical masks should be changed:

- if the integrity of the mask is compromised – such as soiled with blood/body fluids, or a build up of moisture from an extended period of use
- in line with manufacturer's guidance
- at the end of the procedure.

Respiratory protective equipment (RPE). Respiratory masks (FFP3) are designed to prevent infectious droplets from being inhaled into the respiratory tract or coming into contact with the mucous membranes of the nose and mouth. They should be used when caring for patients infected with certain respiratory pathogens, such as multi-resistant pulmonary tuberculosis,

pandemic influenza and severe acute respiratory syndrome (SARS). FFP3 masks should be:

- worn prior to entering the room of a patient with a suspected airborne infection
- well-fitting to provide a close seal around the nose and mouth. A fit check test should be performed before entering the room. Staff with facial hair may not have as close a fit as those who are clean shaven. In this case staff must not enter the room.
- used in line with manufacturer's guidance.
- untouched once in place.
- properly fitted. If the mask does not fit properly then staff should not enter the room.

See Fig. 16.8 how to fit a respiratory mask correctly.

Some staff may be uncomfortable with the FFP3 mask as they may feel that they cannot breathe. Most masks have a valve

How to put on and fit check an **FFP3 RESPIRATOR**

Follow these five steps to fit your respirator correctly

Tip: It may be helpful to look in the mirror when fitting your respirator

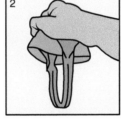
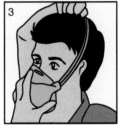
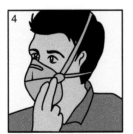

1. Hold the respirator in one hand and separate the edges to fully open it with the other hand. Bend the nose wire (where present) at the top of the respirator to form a gentle curve.

2. Turn the respirator upside down to expose the two headbands, and then separate them using your index finger and thumb. Hold the headbands with your index finger and thumb and cup the respirator under your chin.

3. Position the upper headband on the crown of your head, above the ears, not over them. Position the lower strap at the back of your head below your ears.

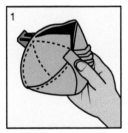
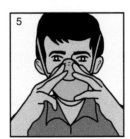

4. Ensure that the respirator is flat against your cheeks.

5. Mould the nosepiece across the bridge of your nose by firmly pressing down with your fingers until you have a good facial fit. If a good fit cannot be achieved, do not proceed.

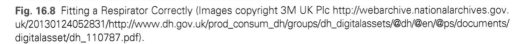

Fig. 16.8 Fitting a Respirator Correctly (Images copyright 3M UK Plc http://webarchive.nationalarchives.gov.uk/20130124052831/http://www.dh.gov.uk/prod_consum_dh/groups/dh_digitalassets/@dh/@en/@ps/documents/digitalasset/dh_110787.pdf).

to allow for easy breathing; however, if the person becomes anxious about their breathing, they should leave the room immediately and only then remove the mask as directed.

Removal of the mask should occur:
- after task or procedure has finished
- if visibly soiled with blood/body fluids
- after leaving the patient area
- after the removal of gloves, aprons and goggles.

The mask should be discarded as clinical waste and the wearer should wash their hands after removal.

> ### ⚠ HOTSPOT
>
> Patients with infections should wear a surgical face mask when being moved to another area. Surgical face masks will prevent infectious droplets being transmitted into the air. FFP3 masks should not be used with patients as there is no filtration of air in the mask. All staff escorting patients with infections must use FFP3 masks when the patient is being transferred.

Removing PPE

To avoid the risk of self-contamination by staff when removing PPE, a set sequence of removal is recommended:
1. gloves
2. aprons
3. eye protection (when worn)
4. mask (when worn).

See Fig. 16.9 for a guide to removing PPE. All PPE should be discarded as clinical waste and hand hygiene must be performed.

Cough etiquette

Part of standard precautions is the implementation of the infection control measure of cough etiquette. Infected persons with respiratory symptoms should be advised on how to prevent the spread of respiratory infection.

HOW TO SAFELY REMOVE PERSONAL PROTECTIVE EQUIPMENT (PPE) EXAMPLE 1

There are a variety of ways to safely remove PPE without contaminating your clothing, skin, or mucous membranes with potentially infectious materials. Here is one example. **Remove all PPE before exiting the patient room** except a respirator, if worn. Remove the respirator **after** leaving the patient room and closing the door. Remove PPE in the following sequence:

1. GLOVES
- Outside of gloves are contaminated!
- If your hands get contaminated during glove removal, immediately wash your hands or use an alcohol-based hand sanitizer
- Using a gloved hand, grasp the palm area of the other gloved hand and peel off first glove
- Hold removed glove in gloved hand
- Slide fingers of ungloved hand under remaining glove at wrist and peel off second glove over first glove
- Discard gloves in a waste container

2. GOGGLES OR FACE SHIELD
- Outside of goggles or face shield are contaminated!
- If your hands get contaminated during goggle or face shield removal, immediately wash your hands or use an alcohol-based hand sanitizer
- Remove goggles or face shield from the back by lifting head band or ear pieces
- If the item is reusable, place in designated receptacle for reprocessing. Otherwise, discard in a waste container

3. GOWN
- Gown front and sleeves are contaminated!
- If your hands get contaminated during gown removal, immediately wash your hands or use an alcohol-based hand sanitizer
- Unfasten gown ties, taking care that sleeves don't contact your body when reaching for ties
- Pull gown away from neck and shoulders, touching inside of gown only
- Turn gown inside out
- Fold or roll into a bundle and discard in a waste container

4. MASK OR RESPIRATOR
- Front of mask/respirator is contaminated — DO NOT TOUCH!
- If your hands get contaminated during mask/respirator removal, immediately wash your hands or use an alcohol-based hand sanitizer
- Grasp bottom ties or elastics of the mask/respirator, then the ones at the top, and remove without touching the front
- Discard in a waste container

5. WASH HANDS OR USE AN ALCOHOL-BASED HAND SANITIZER IMMEDIATELY AFTER REMOVING ALL PPE
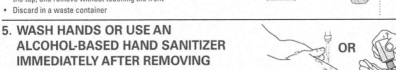
OR

PERFORM HAND HYGIENE BETWEEN STEPS IF HANDS BECOME CONTAMINATED AND IMMEDIATELY AFTER REMOVING ALL PPE

Fig. 16.9 How to Remove PPE (Reproduced with permission from the Centers for Disease Control and Prevention).

HOW TO SAFELY REMOVE PERSONAL PROTECTIVE EQUIPMENT (PPE) EXAMPLE 2

Here is another way to safely remove PPE without contaminating your clothing, skin, or mucous membranes with potentially infectious materials. **Remove all PPE before exiting the patient room** except a respirator, if worn. Remove the respirator **after** leaving the patient room and closing the door. Remove PPE in the following sequence:

1. GOWN AND GLOVES

- Gown front and sleeves and the outside of gloves are contaminated!
- If your hands get contaminated during gown or glove removal, immediately wash your hands or use an alcohol-based hand sanitizer
- Grasp the gown in the front and pull away from your body so that the ties break, touching outside of gown only with gloved hands
- While removing the gown, fold or roll the gown inside-out into a bundle
- As you are removing the gown, peel off your gloves at the same time, only touching the inside of the gloves and gown with your bare hands. Place the gown and gloves into a waste container

2. GOGGLES OR FACE SHIELD

- Outside of goggles or face shield are contaminated!
- If your hands get contaminated during goggle or face shield removal, immediately wash your hands or use an alcohol-based hand sanitizer
- Remove goggles or face shield from the back by lifting head band and without touching the front of the goggles or face shield
- If the item is reusable, place in designated receptacle for reprocessing. Otherwise, discard in a waste container

3. MASK OR RESPIRATOR

- Front of mask/respirator is contaminated — DO NOT TOUCH!
- If your hands get contaminated during mask/respirator removal, immediately wash your hands or use an alcohol-based hand sanitizer
- Grasp bottom ties or elastics of the mask/respirator, then the ones at the top, and remove without touching the front
- Discard in a waste container

4. WASH HANDS OR USE AN ALCOHOL-BASED HAND SANITIZER IMMEDIATELY AFTER REMOVING ALL PPE

OR

PERFORM HAND HYGIENE BETWEEN STEPS IF HANDS BECOME CONTAMINATED AND IMMEDIATELY AFTER REMOVING ALL PPE

Fig. 16.9, cont'd

This includes:

- Covering the nose and mouth with a tissue when coughing or sneezing
- If no tissue is available, covering the nose and mouth with the crux of the elbow when coughing or sneezing rather than the hands
- Disposal of used tissues directly into the waste bin, not leaving them lying around
- Wash hands afterwards.

Transmission-based precautions

Using standard precautions alone may not be enough to prevent cross transmission of infections to patients in the healthcare setting. Additional precautions may need to be considered when caring for patients:

- With symptoms of an infection
- Who may be incubating an infection, but have no symptoms
- Who are colonized with multi-resistant or pathogenic microbes which can then be passed on.

Transmission based precautions are additional methods and are categorized according to the method of transmission.

Contact precautions

Contact is the most common means by which infections are spread. These precautions are used to prevent and control infections spread by direct or indirect contact with the patient, equipment or the immediate patient environment (see Box 16.2).

Droplet precautions. Used to prevent and control infections from the respiratory tract via droplets that do not travel very

BOX 16.2   Contact Precautions

- Patient should be placed in a single room and explain the rationale.
- Use of PPE – gloves and apron.
- Limit movement of patient to other areas – unless necessary.
- Use single-use items or dedicated patient equipment where possible.
- Clean and disinfect patient equipment after use if needed for other patients.
- Ensure daily cleaning and disinfection of patient's room – focusing on hand touch areas and immediate patient environment.
- Perform hand hygiene.

BOX 16.3   Droplet Precautions

- Place patient in a single room and explain the rationale.
- Use PPE – gloves, apron and mask (see PPE).
- Teach patient cough etiquette.
- Limit movement of patient to other areas – unless necessary, place surgical mask on patient if moved to prevent droplet spread.
- Use single-use items or dedicated patient equipment where possible.
- Clean and disinfect patient equipment after use if needed for other patients.
- Ensure daily cleaning and disinfection of patient's room – focusing on hand touch areas and immediate patient environment.
- Perform hand hygiene.

BOX 16.4   Airborne Precautions

- Place patient in single room, with door closed to prevent spread. In the case of multi-resistant TB, negative pressure air flow room should be sought.
- Use PPE – gloves, aprons with long sleeve and FFP3 respiratory mask ensuring fit test is done.
- Teach patient cough etiquette.
- Restrict susceptible staff (i.e., non-immune staff to measles or chickenpox, pregnant women) entering room and caring for patient.
- Limit movement of patient to other areas unless necessary. Place surgical mask on patient.
- Use single-use items or dedicated patient equipment where possible.
- Clean and disinfect patient equipment after use if needed for other patients.
- Ensure daily cleaning and disinfection of patient's room – focusing on hand touch areas and immediate patient environment.
- Perform hand hygiene.

CRITICAL AWARENESS

Patient Placement/Accommodation

It is imperative that an assessment of the patient is made when they enter the healthcare area to determine if there is any risk of infection transmission. Those patients who have experienced:

- diarrhoea, vomiting, fever, respiratory symptoms or unexplained rash
- a history of testing positive for a multidrug-resistant microbe (such as methicillin-resistant *Staphylococcus aureus* (MRSA), extended spectrum beta-lactamase (ESBL), Carbapenemase producing *enterobacteriaceae* (CPE)
- hospitalization abroad in last 12 months

have to be isolated in a single room along with the appropriate precautions in place awaiting investigation or screening. Patients have to stay in isolation until their symptoms have cleared and they are no longer thought to be an infection risk.

Cohorting of patients

Patients may be placed together when:

- there are several cases of the same infection
- no single rooms are available
- it is more appropriate to cohort patients.

It is a requirement that those patients who are cohorted be placed at least 1 metre apart. Consideration should be given to assigning a dedicated team to cohorted patients as an added infection control measure as this can reduce the risk of cross infection.

(Adapted from CDC, 2007)

Protective isolation

This is used to create a safe environment for patients who are more susceptible to infections because of a compromised immune system. These patients' immune systems can be compromised in many ways:

- through treatments – such as chemotherapy, steroid therapy
- blood disorders – such as neutropenia (low white blood cell count), pancytopenia (deficiency in all blood cell types)
- organ transplant, bone marrow or stem cell transplant
- blood cancers
- burns – where the skin is compromised
- immune disorders – such as HIV.

The decision to implement protective isolation should be made by the patient's consultant and the nurse in charge of the area. An explanation underpinning the reason why there is a need for protective isolation should be given to the patient and, if appropriate, the family.

The following patient placement and precautions are needed:

- single room with en-suite facilities and the door closed
- hand hygiene – following the WHO 5 moments for hand hygiene (see Fig. 16.3)
- PPE – depending on the task to be performed
- minimal staff caring for patient – staff with respiratory infections, oral/facial herpes or with any other signs or infections must not care for the patient
- restricted visitors – children under the age of 10 must not be allowed, and visitors with signs of infection must be excluded
- flowers/plants are a reservoir for bacteria and must be avoided
- good personal hygiene must be encouraged to prevent self-infection from resident flora

far (less than 1 metre) but can penetrate the mucosal surface of persons (see Box 16.3).

Airborne precautions. Used to prevent and control respiratory infections that spread via aerosol transmission and can be inhaled into the lungs or contaminate the mucosal surfaces of others (e.g., measles, chickenpox, tuberculosis (TB)) (see Box 16.4).

Notices should be placed on the doors of rooms with contact, droplet or airborne precautions in place as they act as an aide memoire to staff on entering.

TABLE 16.1 Categories of Linen

Type of linen	Description
Clean linen	Freshly laundered linen ready for use
Used linen	Used but not contaminated with blood or body fluids
Infectious linen	Linen used by a person known or suspected to be infectious or contaminated with blood or body fluids, such as faeces

TABLE 16.2 Types of Waste (WHO, 2014)

Type of waste	Example
Healthcare waste	Any waste produced by healthcare activities, such as articles contaminated with blood or body fluids, waste from isolation rooms or human tissue or body parts, cultures and culture plates from pathology.
Special (hazardous) waste	Waste that contains hazardous substances, such as medications (which are pharmaceutical waste), chemotherapy treatments (which are cytotoxic), and x-ray diagnostic or therapeutic materials (which are radioactive waste).
General waste	Recyclable, such as glass, paper, plastic and cardboard, and waste that cannot be recycled.

- regular assessment of immune system – performing daily full blood counts to assess white cell count.

In some instances, specialized rooms with positive pressure ventilation may be used depending on the level of immunosuppression; these rooms must not be used for isolating patients with respiratory/droplet infections.

Safe handling of linen

Linen in the healthcare setting is divided into several categories: these are outlined in Table 16.1.

Clean linen

- Hospital linen must be washed for at least 10 minutes at 65°C.
- Linen should be stored in a clean designated area, preferably in a closed cupboard or a designated trolley that is covered to prevent contamination.
- Clean linen that is ripped or torn is unfit for use and returned to laundry.

Used linen

- Ensure laundry skip at point of use.
- When removing bed/trolley linen – ensure gloves and apron are worn.
- Do not rinse, shake or sort linen or re-handle once bagged.
- Do not place used linen on the floor.
- Be careful not to place inappropriate items, such as incontinence sheets, dentures or jewellery, in the laundry bag along with linen.
- Laundry bags must not be overfull and must be sealed with cord.

Infectious linen

- Linen should be removed and placed into water soluble or alginate bags and sealed, before placing in the laundry bag. This enables minimal handling by staff as the linen will not need to be removed from the bags because they dissolve in the wash.
- All laundry bags should be labelled and dated and placed in a designated area for collection.

> **! HOTSPOT**
>
> When handling used or infectious linen, gloves and aprons should be used at all times and clean linen should never be placed alongside used linen. Hand hygiene must be performed after removal of gloves.

Safe handling of clinical waste

Of all the waste that healthcare settings generate, it is estimated that 85% is considered general, non-hazardous waste, which can be disposed of as domestic waste. The remaining 15% is thought to be infectious, toxic or radioactive waste, which is hazardous to the public and needs to be disposed of as clinical waste (WHO, 2014).

The Health Technical Memorandum (HTM) 07-01 on the Safe Handling of Healthcare Waste (DH, 2013b) provides guidance to all those involved in the management of healthcare waste. This includes waste classification, segregation, storage, packaging, transport, treatment and disposal. Types of waste are described in Table 16.2.

Management of clinical waste

Healthcare waste needs to be segregated according to the level of hazard to the public. Guidance follows the HTM 07-01 (DH, 2013b) and is as follows:

- Non-hazardous, general waste – normally goes to landfill and can be put in black refuse bags and placed in designated domestic waste bins or recycling bins situated in the clinical area.
- Healthcare waste – which is high risk and hazardous, should be placed in designated bins which are made of hard plastic and can be sealed tight to prevent leakage. Thick colour-coded plastic bags may also be used in some healthcare organizations – this waste may be coloured according to hazard and maybe be autoclaved or either incinerated or sent to landfill.
- Special (hazardous) waste – this tends to be chemical waste and will need to be disposed of in the designated bins or bags with special arrangements made for transportation and disposal.

When handling clinical waste, the NA must:

- ensure PPE, such as gloves and aprons, are worn; waste collectors should be provided with heavy duty gloves
- ensure waste is disposed of at the point of use
- be trained on local policy for handling and disposing of clinical waste
- ensure bins or bags are well sealed and labelled with the clinical area

- ensure bins or bags are only two-thirds filled, not heavy or overflowing; bags must not be ripped or torn
- ensure bins and bags are placed in the designated collection point for disposal
- perform hand hygiene after removal of gloves.

Disposal of sharps

A sharp is defined as a needle, blade or any other sharp medical instrument capable of cutting or piercing the skin (Health and Safety Executive, 2013). A sharps or percutaneous injury is an incident that involves the sharp piercing the skin.

In healthcare, the safe handling and disposal of sharps is part of clinical waste management and is there to protect staff, patients and visitors from acquiring a blood-borne pathogen through an injury.

The estimated risk of acquiring a blood-borne virus through percutaneous injury is:

- hepatitis B, 1:3
- hepatitis C, 1:30
- HIV, 1:300

Health Protection Agency (2012).

The following are infection control measures to prevent sharps injury:

- Used sharps should be handled as little as possible and discarded by the person who used it – **YOU USE IT, YOU BIN IT**
- Needles should not be re-sheathed, bent or disassembled after use
- Sharps should be discarded immediately at the point of use in designated sharps box
- Place sharps boxes at waist height and closed when not in use
- Do not over fill, close when fill line is reached
- Discard after 3 months if not filled.

Sharps boxes:

- must conform to UN3291/BS EN ISO 32907:2012
- be yellow with wording such as 'Danger, for sharps use only', 'For incineration' and have a biohazard sticker
- be made of hard plastic – resistant to penetration – and should not leak
- should have a handle with a closing device and must remain closed when not in use
- have a locking mechanism that, once locked, cannot be re-opened
- located as close as possible to the point of use.

See Fig. 16.10 illustrates a commonly used type of sharps box.

Occupational exposure and sharps injury management

Occupational exposure to blood-borne viruses (BBV) can be percutaneous (piercing of the skin) or mucocutaneous (exposure to the mucous membranes of the eye, nose and mouth). The following first aid actions should be taken immediately following any occupational exposure:

For sharps/percutaneous injury:

- Do not suck puncture site.
- Encourage active bleeding by gently squeezing the puncture site.

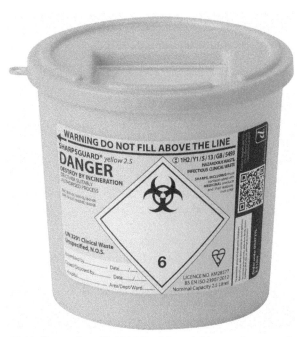

Fig. 16.10 Sharps Box (© 2018 Daniels – A Mauser Company http://www.daniels.co.uk).

- Wash area well with soap and water: do not scrub area or use antimicrobial solutions.
- Cover with a waterproof plaster.
- Report incident to line manager.

For mucocutaneous exposure:

- Exposed mucous membranes of the eyes should be irrigated thoroughly with water.
- Irrigation with water should be done before and after removal of contact lens if used.
- Mouth should be rinsed with water, which should be spat out, not swallowed.
- Report incident to line manager.

Staff immunization and post-exposure prophylaxis (PEP)

Any vaccine preventable disease that can be spread from person to person poses a risk to both healthcare workers and patients (DH, 2013a). Nursing Associates have a duty of care towards their patients and all measures should be taken to protect them from communicable disease.

Immunization will:

- protect staff and their families from infections acquired in work
- protect patients, including vulnerable patients who have not responded to or cannot have immunization
- protect other healthcare workers.

The main aim is to ensure that all staff that have regular and direct contact with patients are immunized. The level of immunization needed will depend on the exposure risk.

Routine immunization of healthcare workers

- All staff should be up to date with routine immunizations, such as tetanus, diphtheria, polio and MMR.

- Hepatitis B vaccine – should be given to staff in direct contact with blood and blood-stained body fluids, and those at risk of being bitten or deliberately injured by patients.
- BCG vaccine – should be given to staff who have close contact with infectious patients or who work with patients who are immune-compromised.
- Varicella vaccine – staff who have direct patient contact and who have not had or are unaware of having had chickenpox or herpes zoster infection should be tested and vaccinated for varicella if not immune.
- Influenza vaccine – annual vaccination for influenza is recommended for all clinical staff to help reduce the transmission of influenza to vulnerable patients.

! HOTSPOT

Staff who have a significant exposure to blood or blood-stained body fluids where the source patient is known to be, or found to be, positive for a blood-borne infection should report all incidents promptly to their line manager so that a risk assessment of the exposure can be made and post exposure prophylaxis given if required.

Management of blood and body fluid spills

Body fluids are any fluids produced by the body, including the following:
- Blood
- Urine
- Faeces
- Tears
- Saliva
- Breast milk
- Amniotic fluid
- Cerebrospinal fluid
- Pleural fluid
- Peritoneal fluid
- Vomit
- Bile
- Digestive juices
- Pus

Any body fluids can have the potential to transmit infection, although those containing blood are more hazardous. Spills must be contained and decontaminated immediately, using appropriate PPE (gloves, apron and facial protection if needed). Local policy and procedure must be followed at all times. Staff responsible for clearing spills must be trained to do so.

Management of spills:
- Put on PPE
- Close area where spill occurred
- Place absorbent pads/towels on spill to soak up excess fluid
- Place absorbent pads/towels in clinical waste bins
- Clean with sodium hypochlorite solution 1:10,000 dilution
- Discard PPE as clinical waste
- Ensure area is cleaned and dried

Urine spills should not be treated with sodium hypochlorite or any chlorine solution, as this will release a chlorine gas. Larger spills should be treated with absorbent granules and scooped up once solidified. Spill kits should be accessible in areas where

BOX 16.5 The Decontamination Process

- Cleaning: the removal of visible dirt and matter from objects and surfaces, normally done manually or mechanically by washer disinfectors or ultrasonic cleansers using detergents or enzymatic products.
- Disinfection: a process using physical and chemical agents that eliminates many pathogenic organisms from objects and surfaces. However, bacterial spores and viruses may survive this. Moist heat or liquid chemicals are the most common methods used.
- Sterilization: total eradication of all infective organisms from the surface of objects. Can be carried out by various methods, such as steam, dry heat, liquid sterilizing agents and gases. The choice of which level of decontamination needs to be used depends on the risk of infection to the patient. The risk level is normally categorized as High, Intermediate or Low.

larger spills are more likely to occur, such as accident and emergency and operating theatres (Rutala & Weber, 2008).

Post-exposure management

Additional measures may be required following an exposure incident to an infected person, contaminated instrument or a pathogen. Further advice on management should be sought from an occupational health doctor or consultant microbiologist.

Decontamination of patient and medical equipment

Patient equipment can be contaminated with blood and body fluids, which may harbour infectious microbes. Therefore, decontamination of patient equipment is essential to prevent the spread of infection and minimize the risk of patients acquiring HAI. Decontamination means the removal of unwanted material from the surface area to reduce the level of infection. The decontamination process can be done in three ways (see Box 16.5).

Categories of risk

1. High risk
   - In close contact with a break in the skin or mucous membranes
   - Items introduced into sterile body areas
   Recommendation: Sterilization
2. Intermediate risk
   - In contact with mucous membranes
   - Contaminated with virulent or transmissible organisms
   - Prior to use on immunocompromised patients
   Recommendation: Sterilization or disinfection
3. Low risk
   - In contact with healthy skin
   - Not in contact with the patient
   Recommendation: Cleaning and disinfection

Care equipment classification

Single-use – these are items that are used once then discarded and must never be re-used, even with the same patient. Single-use items normally carry a symbol (Fig. 16.11)

Needles and syringes are single-use items and should never be used more than once. Medications from a single-use vial or intravenous fluid bags must never be used between multiple patients.

Fig. 16.11 Single-use Symbol

Single-patient-use – equipment or items that can be used again on the same patient.

Reusable invasive equipment – equipment, such as instruments that are used once, then cleaned and sent for sterilization.

Reusable non-invasive equipment – such as commodes, blood pressure cuffs, bed mattresses, wheelchairs and patient trolleys are to be cleaned:

- between patient use
- after blood or body fluid contamination
- at regular intervals if not in use
- before sending for inspection, servicing or repair.

After cleaning, equipment should be rinsed and dried, and stored clean and dry.

CRITICAL AWARENESS

When storing items that have been disinfected or sterilized, it is important to ensure that recontamination does not occur.

Therefore, sterile items should be stored:

- at the point of use – treatment areas, clinical rooms, operating theatres
- in a clean dedicated area and not used for other purposes
- in a way as to enable a good rotation of stock
- on shelves that are easy to clean and have free movement of air around the items
- above floor level, away from direct sunlight and in a cool, dry environment.

Before use, sterile items should be checked to ensure packaging is intact, with no evidence of contamination, and perishable items have not expired.

Environmental cleaning

A clean environment plays an important part in the reduction of HAI in the healthcare setting. Routine cleaning is an important aspect of ensuring a dust-free environment and a reduction in the level of microbial contamination that sits in dust. A cluttered environment hinders cleaning and traps dust.

Within the care environment, the sites closest to the patient, 'the patient zone', and surfaces frequently touched by staff and visitors, have been identified as having the highest level of microbial contamination. Therefore, environmental cleaning should focus more on these areas:

- Patient zone – bed rails, bed table, chair, call bell, locker, bed linen and any medical equipment, such as infusion pumps and tubing close to the bed.
- Frequently touched areas by staff and visitors – door handles, taps, television monitors, telephones.

Cleaning of the care environment

For routine cleaning – a fresh solution of neutral pH detergent with hot water should be used. Cleaning solution should be changed when dirty and prior to moving to a new location. Cleaning of sanitary areas, for example, toilets, sinks, baths, taps and bathroom fixtures, should be with a disinfectant or combined detergent/disinfectant product. All fixtures should be rinsed and dried after using disinfectant. Patient isolation rooms or cohort rooms require enhanced cleaning, which must be done daily using a combined detergent/disinfectant solution.

However, 'hand touch' areas that are more frequently touched, such as door/toilet handles, lockers and tables and commodes, will need to be decontaminated more frequently, especially in cases of diarrhoea.

Terminal decontamination should be done when the isolation/cohort room has been vacated if the patient has been transferred, has left or is no longer considered infectious.

- Remove all items from the room.
- Dispose of all waste and disposable items as clinical waste.
- Bag bed linen and manage as infectious linen.
- Change curtains.
- The room must be cleaned from the highest to the lowest point using a detergent/disinfectant solution which contains 1,000 ppm available chlorine.
- All reusable equipment must be decontaminated on removal from room
- Cleaning equipment must be disposed of or decontaminated after use.

Colour coding of cleaning equipment

All reusable cleaning equipment should be colour-coded in accordance with the National Patient Safety Agency (NPSA) colour coding hospital cleaning materials and equipment (NPSA, 2007) directive.

Cleaning equipment should only be used in the area indicated by its colour. Colour coded areas are:

RED – bathrooms, washrooms, showers, toilets, sinks and bathroom floors

BLUE – public areas such as wards, departments, offices and other public areas

GREEN – ward kitchen areas and patient food service areas in ward area

YELLOW – isolation areas

It should be noted that:

- Only cleaning products supplied by the healthcare organization should be used.
- All ward and treatment areas should be de-cluttered regularly to enable cleaning.
- Cleaning solutions should be diluted in accordance with manufacturer's instructions.
- All staff should use PPE (single-use gloves) when handling cleaning solution.
- Hands must be washed after removal of gloves.
- All staff should have access to cleaning products and materials in the ward area.
- Cleaning materials should be rinsed and dried upright and in a designated area.
- Single-use cleaning materials do not need to be colour-coded and must be discarded after use.
- Everyone has a responsibility to keep the clinical area clutter free and clean.

Asepsis

Asepsis means 'free from pathogenic organisms' (Merriam-Webster, 2010). Asepsis needs to be maintained by NAs and other staff when performing medical, surgical or invasive procedures that compromise the body's natural defence mechanisms and can lead to the introduction of microbes into the body.

Aseptic technique is a generic term describing the practice and process involved in protecting patients from infection during any type of invasive procedure. It aims to prevent transmitting microbes to vulnerable sites of the patient by ensuring all sterilized parts of devices in contact with or inserted into susceptible body sites are not contaminated during the procedure. Aseptic technique is used in all clinical and care settings from and including surgical procedures performed in dedicated operating theatres to ward and community settings when inserting medical devices, maintaining indwelling devices and dressing open wounds.

Aseptic Non Touch Technique (ANTT®)

ANTT® is a specific type of aseptic technique with a unique theory and practice framework (NICE, 2012).

Originated by Rowley et al. (2010), The ANTT Clinical Practice Framework is now used extensively by healthcare organizations internationally to help improve aseptic practice in healthcare and community settings through standardized practice. This is done in two ways:

- By providing a clear and precise set of rules and theory to teach aseptic technique safely and efficiently
- Setting clear ANTT guidelines for clinical procedures which are often done in hospital or in the community, thus enabling staff to perform aseptic procedures in a consistent manner.
- ANTT is based on the 10 key principles outlined in Box 16.6.
  Key-Parts and Key-Sites. A Key-Site is any portal of entry into the patient including breaches of skin integrity, such as a wound, and involves any site where devices are inserted. Key-Parts are aseptic parts of the procedure or equipment that will have direct contact with either another Key-Part or a Key-Site of the patient (Rowley et al., 2001).

⚠ HOTSPOT

If Key-Parts become contaminated during the procedure, then this could provide a direct route for transmission of infection to the patient. Key-Parts on the patient, for example, intravenous ports, hubs and lumens, are critical, and it is therefore important that effective cleaning is undertaken. It is recommended that chlorhexidine 2% with 70% alcohol impregnated wipes are used.

(Adapted from Loveday et al., 2014)

Standard-ANTT or Surgical-ANTT

The types of ANTT for any given procedure is selected according to the complexity of maintaining of asepsis for any given procedure. This is risk assessed by the NA.

Standard-ANTT. This typically incorporates procedures which are technically simple, take less than 20 minutes to do and involves smaller Key-Sites and Key-Parts (such as intravenous therapy or peripheral cannulation). Standard-ANTT includes:

- a main General Aseptic Field (e.g., a procedure tray) and Micro Critical Aseptic Fields (e.g., sterilized caps or the inside of equipment packaging)
- non-sterile gloves – relies on a non-touch technique to protect Key-Parts
- hand hygiene – an essential component of ANTT

In Standard-ANTT, if Key-Parts or Key-Sites cannot be managed with a non-touch technique, then sterile gloves and hand hygiene with antimicrobial solution must be used.

BOX 16.6 The Foundation Principles and Safeguards of ANTT

The ANTT Clinical Practice Framework provides practitioners and healthcare organizations with a robustly defined and reproducible process by which to teach and apply safe aseptic technique.

Clinical practice
Principle 1
Asepsis is the aim for all invasive clinical procedures, including the maintenance and use of invasive clinical devices (*'For surgery to community care'*)

Principle 2
Asepsis is achieved by 'Key-Part and Key-Site Protection'; Protecting Key-Parts and Key-Sites from microorganisms transferred from the healthcare worker and the immediate environment

Principle 3
ANTT needs to be efficient as well as safe; therefore Surgical-ANTT is used for complicated procedures and Standard-ANTT for uncomplicated procedures

Principle 4
The need for Surgical or Standard-ANTT is determined by ANTT risk assessment that is based on the technical difficulty of achieving asepsis

Safeguard 1
Basic Infective Precautions
Basic infective precautions such as environmental controls, hand cleaning and disinfecting medical devices, significantly reduce the risk of contaminating Key-Parts and Key-Sites

Safeguard 2
Identification of Key-Parts and Key-Sites
Key-Parts are the critical parts of the procedure equipment that, if contaminated, are most likely to cause infection. Key-Sites are open wounds and medical device access sites

Safeguard 3
Non Touch Technique
Non Touch Technique is a critical skill that protects Key-Parts and Key-Sites from the healthcare worker and the procedure environment. It is essential in Standard-ANTT and desirable in Surgical-ANTT

Safeguard 4
Aseptic Field Management
Aseptic Fields protect Key-Parts and Key-Sites from the immediate procedure environment. Surgical and Standard-ANTT require different aseptic field management

Clinical and organizational management
Principle 5
Aseptic practice should be standardized

Principle 6
Safe aseptic technique is reliant upon effective healthcare worker training and environments and equipment that are fit for purpose

(Copyright © 2016 Aseptic Non Touch Technique (ANTT®) www.antt.org enquiries@antt.org).

Surgical-ANTT. This should be used when procedures are technically more complex, take longer than 20 minutes to perform and involve larger Key-Sites or Key-Parts (e.g., the insertion of a CVC line or surgery in theatre). Surgical-ANTT includes:

- a main Critical Aseptic Field (a sterilized drape)
- sterile gloves and barrier precautions, such as gowning
- surgical hand scrub with antimicrobial solution
- relying on non-touch technique where practical to do so.

OUTBREAK MANAGEMENT

Public Health England (2014) has defined an outbreak as:

- two or more people experiencing similar illness and are linked in time or place
- a greater than expected rate of infection compared with the usual background rate for the time and place where outbreak has occurred
- a single case of a rare disease such as diphtheria, botulism, rabies, polio
- a suspected, anticipated or actual event involving microbial or chemical contamination of food or water.

Outbreaks can occur anywhere but become more of a threat if in hospital or care home as there is the likelihood of faster spread due to crowding and the presence of more-vulnerable people. Outbreaks can disrupt service delivery to the patients and can lead to the closure of wards and staff absence and prove costly for healthcare trusts. Therefore, prompt identification and management of outbreaks are essential.

Identifying the start

The NA must be aware at all times of any increase in illness in patients or staff in their clinical area. The period of increased incidence (PII) is where there is an unexpected increase in the number of cases of infectious illness at one time. Depending on the type of organism causing the symptoms, outbreaks can start in many ways. For example, a norovirus outbreak may start with several cases developing symptoms all at once, whereas an outbreak of Salmonella may be characterized by two or three cases spread over several days.

Action taken in a period of increased incidence

- Isolate or cohort patients and instigate barrier precautions – use of gloves, aprons and masks if needed.
- Ensure specimens from symptomatic cases are collected: if diarrhoea – stool specimens must be tested for norovirus, bacterial culture and *C. difficile.*
- Clinically assess each case as the patient may have underlying pathology causing symptoms.
- Inform the infection prevention and control team and alert the domestic services manager as more supplies and increased cleaning in clinical area may be required.
- Keep a record of all cases, including date of onset, symptoms reported, food history, medication history and specimens collected for surveillance purposes.

Box 16.7 provides information on outbreak control measures.

BOX 16.7   Outbreak Control Measures (Norovirus Working Party, 2012)

Ward
- Close affected bay(s) to admissions and transfers.
- Keep doors to single-occupancy room(s) and bay(s) closed.
- Place signage on the door(s) informing all visitors of the closed status and restricting visits to essential staff and essential social visitors only.
- Place patients within the ward for the optimal safety of all patients.
- Prepare for reopening by planning the earliest date for a terminal clean.

Healthcare workers (HCWs)
- Ensure all staff are aware of the norovirus situation and how norovirus is transmitted.
- Ensure all staff are aware of the work exclusion policy and the need to go off duty at first symptoms.
- Allocate staff to duties in either affected or non-affected areas of the ward but not both unless unavoidable (e.g., therapists).

Patient and relative information
- Provide all affected patients and visitors with information on the outbreak and the control measures they should adopt.
- Advise visitors of the personal risk and how they might reduce this risk.

Continuous monitoring and communications
- Maintain an up-to-date record of all patients and staff with symptoms.
- Monitor all affected patients for signs of dehydration and correct as necessary.
- Maintain a regular briefing to the organizational management, public health organizations and media office.

Personal protective equipment (PPE)
- Use gloves and apron to prevent personal contamination with faeces or vomitus.
- Consider use of face protection with a mask only if there is a risk of droplets or aerosols.

Hand hygiene
- Use liquid soap and warm water as per WHO 5 moments.
- Encourage and assist patients with hand hygiene.

Environment
- Remove exposed foods, e.g., fruit bowls, and prohibit eating and drinking by staff within clinical areas.
- Intensify cleaning ensuring affected areas are cleaned and disinfected. Toilets used by affected patients must be included.
- Decontaminate frequently touched surfaces with detergent and disinfectant containing 1000 ppm available chlorine.*

Equipment
- Use single-patient use equipment wherever possible.
- Decontaminate all other equipment immediately after use.

Linen
- Whilst clinical area is closed, discard linen from the closed area in a water soluble (alginate) bag and then a secondary bag.

Spillages
- Wearing PPE, decontaminate all faecal and vomit spillages.
- Remove spillages with paper towels, and then decontaminate the area with an agent containing 1000 ppm available chlorine.*
- Discard all waste as healthcare waste. Remove PPE and wash hands with liquid soap and warm water.

*Guidelines for management of Norovirus outbreaks in acute, community and social care settings (Norovirus Working Party, 2012).

Environmental decontamination in an outbreak

Effective cleaning and removal of organic matter should be done before disinfection in the clinical area. Disinfection should be carried out using 0.1% sodium hypochlorite (1000 ppm available chlorine). Staff should wear PPE (gloves and aprons) and follow standard precautions.

Box 16.8 provides advice concerning environmental decontamination during an outbreak.

The infection prevention and control committee will consider when an outbreak is over as factors such as a small number of cases having persistent symptoms can make this difficult to determine. However, once the outbreak is declared over, all staff should remain vigilant in case there is a re-emergence of symptoms.

Further points to consider
Visitors

- Visitors who have symptoms should not visit until clear of symptoms for 48 hours.
- Visitors who are not infected should be given leaflets and discouraged from visiting during the outbreak.
- Non-essential visitors should not be allowed to enter whilst outbreak precautions are in place.
- Visiting will be at the discretion of the nurse in charge. All visitors allowed to enter must use standard precautions (gloves, apron and handwashing).

Staff

- Staff who are symptomatic should be excluded from work until clear of symptoms for 48 hours.
- Staff working in affected areas should not be sent to other wards in the same shift but may work in another area if free of symptoms.

BOX 16.8 Environmental Decontamination During an Outbreak (Norovirus Working Party, 2012)

- Increase frequency of cleaning using dedicated domestic staff where possible and avoiding transfer of domestic staff to other areas.
- Clean from unaffected to affected areas, and within affected areas from least likely-contaminated areas to most highly contaminated areas.
- Use disposable cleaning materials including mops and cloths.
- Where reusable microfibre cloths suitable for use with chlorine releasing disinfectants are in use, the system must be supported by a robust laundry service and adherence to manufacturer's instructions.
- Dedicate reusable cleaning equipment to affected areas and thoroughly decontaminate between uses e.g., mop handles and buckets.
- After cleaning, disinfect with 0.1% sodium hypochlorite (1000 ppm available chlorine).
- Pay particular attention to frequently touched surface, such as bed tables, door handles, toilet flush handles and taps.
- Cleaning staff and other staff who undertake cleaning tasks should follow standard infection control precautions and wear appropriate personal protective equipment (PPE) including disposable gloves and apron.
- National and local colour coding for PPE and cleaning equipment should be adhered to, to avoid cross contamination.

LOOKING BACK, FEEDING FORWARD

It is not possible in a chapter of this size to discuss all the issues associated with infection prevention and control. The NA has a key role to play in ensuring patients are safe and that care delivered is effective. Healthcare-associated infections can develop either as a direct result of healthcare intervention (e.g., medical or surgical treatment) or from being in contact with a healthcare setting.

This chapter has identified that healthcare-associated infections can arise across a wide range of clinical conditions and have the potential to affect people of all ages. Infection can exacerbate existing or underlying conditions, they may cause a delay in recovery and can impact negatively on a person's health and well-being. Healthcare-associated infections may occur in people who are otherwise healthy, particularly if invasive procedures or devices are being used. The NA, other healthcare workers, family members and carers may also be at risk of acquiring infections when they offer care to people. There are a number of factors that can increase the risk of acquiring an infection. However, when the NA utilizes high standards of infection prevention and control in their practice, including providing clean environments, this can minimize risk.

REFERENCES

Association for Safe Aseptic Practice, 2017. ANTT. http://antt.org/ANTT_Site/home.html.
Ayliffe, G.A.J., Babb, J.R., Quoraishi, A.H., et al., 1978. A test for hygienic hand disinfection. J. Clin. Pathol. 31, 923.
Centre for Disease Control and Prevention, 2007. Guideline for Isolation Precautions: Preventing Transmission of Infectious Agents in the Healthcare Setting. https://www.cdc.gov/infectioncontrol/guidelines/isolation/index.html.
Department of Health (DH), 2013a. Immunisation against infectious disease. https://www.gov.uk/government/immunisation of healthcare-and-laboratory-staff-the-green-book-chapter 12.
Department of Health (DH), 2013b. Health Technical Memorandum 07-01: Safe management of healthcare waste. https://www.gov.uk/government/uploads/system/uploads/attachment_data/file/167976/HTM_07-01_Final.pdf.
Gibraltar Health Authority, 2016. Infectious Disease Outbreaks in Hospital Policy. http://ghanet/wp-content/uploads/2016/04/IC-0127-Infectious-Disease-Outbreaks-in-Hospital-Policy.pdf.
Health Protection Agency, 2008. Eye of the Needle: United Kingdom surveillance of significant occupational exposure to bloodborne viruses in healthcare workers. https://www.his.org.uk/files/1513/7085/4781/1_Eye_of_the_needle_2012_accessible.pdf.
Health Protection Agency, 2012. English National Point Prevalence Survey on Healthcare associated infections and Antimicrobial Use, 2011. http://webarchive.nationalarchives.gov.uk/20140714095446/http://www.hpa.org.uk/webc/HPAwebFile/HPAweb_C/1317134304594.
Health Protection Scotland, 2015. National Infection Prevention and Control Manual. http://www.nipcm.hps.scot.nhs.uk/chapter-1-standard-infection-control-precautions-sicps/.
Health and Safety Executive, 2013. Health and Safety (Sharp Instruments in Healthcare) Regulations 2013. Guidance for employers and employees – Health Services information sheet 7. http://apps.who.int/iris/bitstream/10665/85349/1/9789241548564_eng.pdf?ua=1.

Loveday, H.P., et al., 2014. Epic 3: National Evidence-Based Guidelines for Preventing Healthcare-Associated Infections in NHS Hospitals in England. https://www.his.org.uk/files/3113/8693/4808/epic3_National_Evidence-Based_Guidelines_for_Preventing_HCAI_in_NHSE.pdf.

Merriam-Webster, 2010. Merriam-Webster Online Dictionary: Aseptic. https://www.merriam-webster.com/dictionary/aseptic.

NICE, 2012. Infection prevention and control of healthcare associated infections in primary and community care. National Institute for Health and Clinical Excellence clinical guideline [CG139]. https://guidance.nice.org.uk/CG139/Guidance/pdf/English.

National Patient Safety Agency, 2007. The National Specifications for Cleanliness in the NHS: Guidance on setting and measuring performance outcomes in primary, medical and dental premises. http://www.nrls.npsa.nhs.uk/EasySiteWeb/getresource.axd?AssetID=75245%20.

Norovirus Working Party, 2012. Guidelines for the management of norovirus outbreaks in acute and community health and social care settings. https://www.gov.uk/government/uploads/system/uploads/attachment_data/file/322943/Guidance_for_managing_norovirus_outbreaks_in_healthcare_settings.pdf.

Pittet, D., et al., 1999. Bacterial contamination of the hands of hospital staff during routine care. Arch. Intern. Med. 159, 821–826.

Public Health England, 2014. Communicable Disease Outbreak Management Operational Guidance. https://www.gov.uk/government/uploads/system/uploads/attachment_data/file/343723/12_8_2014_CD_Outbreak_Guidance_REandCT_2__2_.pdf.

Rowley, S., 2001. Aseptic Non Touch Technique. Nursing Times. Infect. Control Suppl. 97 (7), V1–V111.

Rowley, S., Clare, S., Maqueen, S., Molyneux, R., 2010. ANTT v2: An updated practice framework for aseptic technique. Br. J. Nur.

19 (5), S5–S11. https://www.researchgate.net/profile/Simon_Clare/publication/42542104_ANTT_v2_An_updated_practice_framework_for_aseptic_technique/links/004635256ad6e1bacb000000/ANTT-v2-An-updated-practice-framework-for-aseptic-technique.pdf.

Rutala, W.A., Weber, D.J., 2008. Healthcare Infection Control Practices Advisory Committee (HICPAC). Guideline for Disinfection and Sterilisation in Healthcare Facilities. Centre for Disease Control and Prevention. https://www.his.org.uk/files/1513/7085/4781/1_Eye_of_the_needle_2012_accessible.pdf.

Taylor, L., 1978. An evaluation of handwashing techniques. Nurs. Times 74, 108–110.

World Health Organization, 2009a. WHO guidelines on Hand Hygiene in Healthcare: First Global Patient Safety Challenge, Cleaner Care is Safer Care. http://apps.who.int/iris/bitstream/10665/44102/1/9789241597906_eng.pdf.

World Health Organization, 2009b. Your Five Moments for Hand Hygiene. http://www.who.int/gpsc/5may/Your_5_Moments_For_Hand_Hygiene_Poster.pdf?ua=1.

World Health Organization, 2009c. WHO Guidelines on Hand Hygiene in Health Care: A Summary. http://www.who.int/gpsc/5may/tools/who_guidelines-handhygiene_summary.pdf.

World Health Organization, 2009d. Glove Use Information Leaflet. https://www.google.com/url?sa=i&rct=j&q=&esrc=s&source=images&cd=&cad=rja&uact=8&ved=0ahUKEwj_-unhpZ3XAhXKNxQKHZPMDvkQjRwIBw&url=https%3A%2F%2Fwww.slideshare.net%2Fsarahammam%2Fppe-46464803&psig=AOvVaw2z2yYdJgitZxwTlDEVMpAr&ust=1509622921927881.

World Health Organization, 2014. Safe management of wastes from health-care activities. http://apps.who.int/iris/bitstream/10665/85349/1/9789241548564_eng.pdf?ua=1.

17

Medicines Management

Paul Deslandes, Ben Pitcher and Simon Young

OBJECTIVES

By the end of the chapter the reader will be able to:
1. Define the term 'medicines management' and appreciate its use in healthcare practice
2. Acknowledge the importance of a patient-centred approach to medicines management
3. Describe the key underpinning pharmacology relevant to medicines management
4. Apply pharmacological principles to the therapeutic use of medicines
5. Acknowledge the role of regulatory and advisory bodies in ensuring the safe, efficacious and cost-effective use of medicines
6. Appreciate the role the Nursing Associate (NA) has and their accountability in the use of medicines in healthcare practice

KEY WORDS

Medicines
Pharmacology
Pharmacokinetics
Pharmacodynamics

Pharmacotherapeutics
Dosing
Administration
Concordance/compliance/adherence

Adverse drug reaction
Accountability

CHAPTER AIM

This chapter aims to introduce the reader to the key knowledge required to approach safe and effective medicines management.

SELF TEST

1. What is medicines management?
2. What are the four aspects of pharmacokinetics?
3. List three mechanisms through which drugs exert a therapeutic effect.
4. Find three examples of medicines having a local effect.
5. Find three examples of medicines having a systemic effect.
6. Is polypharmacy a good or bad approach to managing medicines?
7. How does managing medicines vary during different stages of life?
8. What are the 5 Rs?
9. What are the three legal categories of medicines?
10. What is the importance of pharmacovigilance and incident reporting in safely managing medicines?

INTRODUCTION

Medications are the most commonly used therapeutic intervention in modern healthcare. Medicines provide a safe and effective means by which many signs, symptoms and even entire disease processes can be managed. In 2016, 1104 million items of medication were dispensed by community pharmacies in England (NHS Digital, 2017). Statistics suggest that half of the adult population in the UK take prescribed medication. The Nursing Associate (NA) will therefore have a role in appropriately managing these medicines and maximizing the benefits of their use for patients.

Consider the availability of medicines to the general public and how easy medicines are to obtain in pharmacies and shops. This suggests that some medicines are safe enough for people to manage without always needing healthcare intervention. Many medicines are only available on prescription because they require intervention and input from a healthcare professional (prescriber and the wider healthcare team) to ensure their safe use. Examples include powerful cancer chemotherapy drugs, antibiotics and the more potent pain killers (analgesics). However, medicines that can be purchased from shops and other retail outlets 'over the counter' (e.g., paracetamol), are not free of side effects and can cause problems if used incorrectly. Taking medicines is therefore a matter of weighing up the benefits of using the medication versus the risks posed from side effects and other adverse events. Not all patients will gain the same benefit from using a medication and some will suffer particular side effects, whilst others will not. The effectiveness of a medicine will differ from person to person due to biological variability.

CRITICAL AWARENESS

The term 'medicines optimization' is used in healthcare; it describes a patient-focused approach to getting the best outcomes from the money and time invested in medicines-use. It defines a holistic approach; an increasing engagement with patient-centred professionalism and increased partnership between clinical professionals and patients to maximize the benefits and the choices made when using medications.

Medicines management can be defined as a system of processes and behaviours that determines how medicines are used by healthcare professionals and patients. As with medicines optimization, effective medicines management puts primary focus on the needs of the patient, thus improving the delivery of care and better informing the decision-making of the individuals. The aim is to improve adherence to a given regimen and to improve patient outcomes.

There are strategies that can be used to improve adherence to medication regimens. Educating patients about their medication, that is the risks and benefits and how they will present, is important. Increasingly, it is acknowledged that there is a strong behavioural element associated with medicines-use and the NA can have a role to play in assisting the patient in making their optimal choice.

CASE STUDY 17.1   Mr Simons

Mr Simons is a 46-year-old man who has been diagnosed with high blood pressure (hypertension). He has been prescribed ramipril (a medicine commonly used in the management of hypertension) to lower his blood pressure and reduce his risk of more serious cardiovascular disease. He has developed an irritating dry cough (a fairly common side effect with this medicine) and wants to stop taking the medication. He wasn't feeling ill when he was diagnosed with high blood pressure, is fed up with having to remember to take his medicines and the side effect is troublesome when he is trying to sleep.

After reading the chapter, consider the knowledge and skills you could use to help Mr Simons.

PHARMACOLOGY

If you are involved in the administration of medicines, it is important to have an understanding of how they work. If you understand how the medicine works, it can help you understand and even predict side effects and drug interactions.

The study of the way in which drugs interact with the human body is called clinical pharmacology. Clinical pharmacology is in turn divided into two categories: pharmacokinetics and pharmacodynamics (Young & Pitcher, 2015).

Pharmacokinetics

Pharmacokinetics considers how a drug enters the body, how it moves around the body, how the body tries to deactivate the drug and how it eventually leaves the body. These principles are usually discussed in terms of absorption, distribution, metabolism and elimination (often shortened to ADME).

Absorption

Absorption considers how the drug enters the body. There are a variety of ways in which this can be achieved, termed *routes of administration*. Different routes of administration will allow entry of the drug at different speeds and to different extents. The proportion of the administered drug that reaches the bloodstream from a given route is termed the *bioavailability*. Intravenous administration directly into the blood results in 100% bioavailability, whereas other routes, such as *oral*, may result in lower bioavailability. Therefore, giving a drug intravenously can have a much larger effect than giving the same amount orally.

Distribution

Distribution considers how the drug moves around the body and into and out of different tissues. Some drugs can cross cell membranes easily, allowing them to move into tissues quickly. Other drugs do not, slowing their entry into tissues and even preventing them from entering certain tissues, such as the brain.

Metabolism

The body will try to destroy a drug as if it were a poison. Many different enzymes are used to convert a drug into an inactive metabolite, which is easy to remove from the body. The majority of drug metabolism takes place in the liver, although other tissues (e.g., the kidney) also have the capacity to metabolize drugs. Many factors, such as other medicines, certain foods, smoking or damage to the liver, can influence the rate and extent of drug metabolism.

Elimination

Drugs need to be eliminated from the body. The major route for drug elimination is via the kidneys, although drugs are also eliminated in faeces, sweat and breath. If a patient's kidneys are not functioning properly, their ability to eliminate drugs from the body may be diminished. This change in pharmacokinetics can require an adjustment of dose. When discussing a drug's rate of elimination, it is often talked about in terms of half-life. A half-life is the time taken for the amount of drug in a system to reduce by half.

Pharmacodynamics

Pharmacodynamics considers how the drug actually works. This usually relates to the stimulation or inhibition of an existing control mechanism within the body. For example, opioid analgesics are able to suppress pain because they stimulate pain control mechanisms that exist naturally in the body.

BOX 17.1 Examples of Blocking and Stimulating Receptors

Adrenaline has effects throughout the body. By binding to receptors on the heart, it makes your heart rate and blood pressure go up. By binding to receptors in your lungs, it causes the airways to dilate.

Stimulating a receptor
Medicines such as salbutamol bind to and stimulate certain receptors (called beta-2 receptors) in the lung. This causes the airway to open up, which is known as bronchodilation (and makes breathing easier).

Blocking a receptor
Medicines such as atenolol bind to and block certain receptors (called beta-1 receptors) on the heart. This prevents adrenaline from binding to these receptors and therefore reduces heart rate and blood pressure.

BOX 17.2 Example of Enzyme Inhibition

When our tissues experience a noxious stimulus (damage or irritant), it uses a group of enzymes called cyclooxygenases to produce chemical messengers that cause inflammation. Drugs, such as aspirin and ibuprofen, inhibit the cyclooxygenase enzymes and thereby reduce the production of the chemical messengers, decreasing inflammation.

BOX 17.3 Examples of Transport Proteins

The sodium glucose transport protein SGLT2 is found in the kidney and is responsible for the reabsorption of glucose from the filtered urine back into the body. The drug dapagliflozin blocks this transporter and therefore prevents glucose from being reabsorbed, causing it to be lost from the body. This is useful in diabetes because it helps to maintain the patient's blood sugar at an appropriate level.

Serotonin selective reuptake inhibitors (SSRIs)
The serotonin transport protein is found in nerve cell membranes and is responsible for returning the neurotransmitter serotonin back into the nerve cell (neurone) following its release. Fluoxetine and paroxetine are SSRIs. They block the serotonin transport protein, resulting in increased levels of serotonin, resulting in a subsequent elevation of mood (antidepressant effect).

Receptors

The body uses chemical messengers to control and sustain physiological processes, such as blood pressure, body temperature and heart rate. These messengers include neurotransmitters (which facilitate communication between neurones or from neurones directly onto target organs) and hormones released into the bloodstream from glands. For these chemicals to have an effect, the target cells must have a receptor. These receptors make excellent targets for drugs. Many drugs either stimulate or block receptors and thereby either stimulate or block the associated physiological processes. See Box 17.1 for an example of stimulating and blocking receptors.

Enzymes

Enzymes are molecules that help to facilitate chemical reactions. Enzymes are often discussed in the context of digestion or drug metabolism. However, they play a role in a huge number of chemical reactions throughout the body. As enzymes are involved in facilitating various processes and producing chemical messengers, if a drug inhibits an enzyme it will block that process or production of the molecule (Box 17.2).

Transport proteins

The function of the cell membrane is to regulate the movement of water and electrolytes into and out of the cell. Membrane spanning proteins are used to 'pump' molecules into or out of the cell. Using a drug to alter the activity of these transport proteins influences the movement of molecules, affecting the functioning of the cell in question (Box 17.3).

Pharmacotherapeutics

Pharmacotherapeutics is a term used to describe the way in which medicines are used for the treatment, prevention and diagnosis of illnesses in clinical practice. Pharmacotherapeutics relies in part upon knowledge of pharmacokinetic and pharmacodynamic principles and involves the application of these to the management of individual patients.

Routes of administration

Before any medicine can have an effect, it must successfully reach its site of action in the body. Medicines can be administered using a number of different routes, although not all of them are appropriate for all medicines. Some routes result in distribution of the medicine throughout the body, where it can affect many tissues (a systemic effect). Others result in the medicine having a local action at the site of administration. Systemic administration allows the medicine to reach a target within the body which may not be readily accessible and where a local route would therefore be impractical.

The most commonly encountered route of systemic administration (particularly in the UK) is oral (swallowing the medicine via the mouth), sometimes termed enteral administration. After being swallowed, the medicine is subsequently absorbed from the gastrointestinal tract, typically from the small intestine, from where it passes through the liver before reaching the blood stream. Rectal administration also results in absorption from the gastrointestinal tract. Other routes resulting in a systemic effect of the drug can include via veins, muscle and subcutaneous tissue following injection, and, in some cases, via the skin and lung. Compared to the oral route, these have the advantage of avoiding first-pass metabolism in the liver.

Local administration, such as to the vagina or the eye, may be used to treat conditions of these tissues whilst limiting the amount of drug entering the systemic circulation. Administration to the skin or lung may result in a local or systemic effect depending upon the medicine and its formulation. Box 17.4 provides examples of systemic routes of administration and Box 17.5 highlights some local routes of administration.

BOX 17.4   Some Examples of Systemic Routes of Administration

Oral (e.g., amoxicillin capsules)
Rectal (e.g., paracetamol suppositories)
Lung (e.g., inhaled anaesthetics)
Veins (intravenous injection) (e.g., ceftriaxone)
Muscle (intramuscular injection) (e.g., Risperdal Consta®)
Subcutaneous injection (e.g., insulin glargine)
Sublingual (under the tongue) (e.g., glyceryl trinitrate spray)
Skin (transdermal) (e.g., fentanyl patches)

BOX 17.5   Examples of Local Routes of Administration

Skin (topical) (e.g., hydrocortisone cream)
Lung (e.g., salbutamol inhaler)
Subcutaneous injection (e.g., lidocaine)
Vaginal (e.g., clotrimazole cream)
Eye (e.g., timolol eye drops)

Each route of administration has its advantages and disadvantages. Oral administration is usually convenient for the patient. However, the medicine will be exposed to stomach acid and enzymes that may alter it chemically and render it less effective. This means that some drugs cannot be given orally and must be given by an alternative route, such as via injection. A good example is insulin, which, due to its protein structure, will be broken down by digestive enzymes and therefore must be given by an alternative route. Medicines administered via the gastrointestinal tract also typically undergo some degree of first-pass metabolism in either the intestinal wall, the liver or a combination of both. This may reduce the amount of medicine that is delivered to the body (bioavailability) and forms a possible basis for drug interactions. Any medication administered via the gastrointestinal tract will be distributed widely in the body and will be able to act in the target tissue, as well as in other tissues, which may result in adverse effects (e.g., constipation caused by opioids).

Local administration usually has the advantage of reducing adverse effects associated with the medicine as it remains in, and acts on, the target tissue. However, even when using a local route of administration, there may be some absorption of the medicine into the body resulting in a degree of systemic effect (e.g., timolol eye drops causing narrowing of the airways, making breathing more difficult).

The choice of route may form part of the discussion between the prescriber and patient when deciding upon the best treatment option for a particular illness. In some cases, the route of administration will be determined by the physiological state of the patient. For example, if someone is unconscious, the oral route will typically be impractical and other routes (such as intravenous or rectal) will need to be considered.

Medicine formulation

The formulation of a medicine refers to the physical form in which it is produced for administration to the patient. Different routes of administration require different formulations to allow safe and effective delivery of the medicine.

Medicines administered orally are typically formulated as tablets, capsules or liquids. Of these, liquid formulations are perhaps the most straightforward; the drug is carried in a liquid vehicle and is exposed to the stomach and duodenum before absorption from the small intestine. Tablet and capsule formulations may also expose the drug to the stomach, and result in absorption from the small intestine. However, they can also be designed to protect the drug from the stomach contents. These are usually termed enteric coated (E/C) or gastro-protective tablets or capsules and represent a useful way of delivering drugs that are affected by the acidic conditions of the stomach, for example, proton pump inhibitors, or which may have an irritant effect.

Tablets and capsules can also be designed to release the drug gradually over time to delay absorption from the small intestine; these are termed modified or extended release (M/R or X/L) formulations. This approach is useful for prolonging the duration of action of drugs with short half-lives (e.g., lithium, venlafaxine) to allow once or twice a day dosing.

Typically, injections may be formulated as either solutions (where the drug is dissolved in a liquid) or suspensions (when the drug will not dissolve). Injections for intravenous, intrathecal (into the spinal canal) or intravitreal (into the eye) use are typically solutions that have a rapid effect following administration. Those for intramuscular or subcutaneous use may be solutions designed to exert acute effects but can also be suspensions of less soluble drug particles. Injectable suspensions may be useful where a prolonged effect of the medicine is required, such as with certain types of insulin and long-acting antipsychotic injections (e.g., paliperidone palmitate). The gentle shaking of the vial to ensure even distribution of the drug particles is important prior to the administration of a suspension. The sterility of injections is very important due to the potential risk of infection for the patient. Therefore, injections must be handled in a way that minimizes the risk of microbial contamination.

Medicines applied to the skin may be in the form of creams or ointments where a local effect is required (e.g., topical steroids in the treatment of atopic eczema). However, the skin can also be used as a route for systemic administration, with an increasing number of medicines administered across the skin (transdermally). Some examples include rivastigmine used in dementia, rotigotine for Parkinson disease, fentanyl for the management of pain and, of course, nicotine as an aid to smoking cessation. These are all formulated as adhesive patches that contain a reservoir of the medicine, which is gradually released through the skin over time.

Medicine dosing

The dosing of a medicine involves consideration of both the frequency (how often the medicine should be given) and the quantity that should be given. The aim is to maintain the concentration of the drug within its therapeutic range.

The pharmacokinetics of the drug, its formulation and route of delivery all determine the frequency of dosing. Drugs with a short half-life tend to require more frequent dosing (unless formulated as modified release preparations), whereas those with a longer half-life can be given less frequently. Medicines administered orally as modified release preparations, transdermally in patches, intramuscularly by long-acting injection and subcutaneously as implants, are generally given less frequently than other formulations. The pharmacodynamic effect of the medicine may also be a factor in determining its frequency of dosing. Some medicines, such as vaccines, which have a prolonged effect on the immune system, are given at intervals of months or years.

To improve patient adherence, it is usually preferable to dose medicines less frequently (for example on a daily rather than four times per day basis). As a result, medicines with a short half-life requiring multiple daily doses, are often superseded by longer-acting medicines with similar pharmacodynamic properties (an example is the diabetes medicine gliclazide, which is more commonly used than the shorter acting tolbutamide). The frequency of dosing can also be an important consideration for children attending school or nursery, where administration during school hours may be difficult.

The quantity of dose to be given is strongly influenced by elements of the drug's pharmacodynamic properties. Drugs that have a stronger effect at their site of action typically require a smaller dose than those with a weaker effect (e.g., 30 mg of morphine will have approximately equivalent effects to 240 mg of codeine). However, pharmacokinetic factors will also influence the final dose. The extent to which the drug is absorbed if given orally, distributed to its site of action, metabolized and eliminated from the body are all important factors to consider. A medicine's pharmacokinetics are also relevant when adjusting the dose for patients with hepatic or renal impairment, or when managing drug interactions.

Adverse drug reactions (ADRs)

ADRs (sometimes referred to as side effects) are unwanted and/or harmful reactions that occur after taking a medication (or after a medicine has been administered). For a reaction to be deemed an ADR, it must have been caused by the medicine, or suspected to have been caused by the medicine.

CRITICAL AWARENESS

Adverse Drug Reaction (ADR)

'An appreciably harmful or unpleasant reaction, resulting from an intervention related to the use of a medicinal product, which predicts hazard from future administration and warrants prevention or specific treatment, or alteration of dosage regimen, or withdrawal of the product'.

Reprinted with permission from Elsevier (Edwards, I.R, & Aronson, J.K. (2000) Adverse drug reactions: definitions, diagnosis, and management. Lancet 356:1255–1259).

ADRs are a cause of both ill health and death, and the recognition and management of ADRs are an important part of the NA role. The NA should become familiar with medicines that are commonly used in their area of practice and become aware of their associated ADRs. This is an important facet of medicines

TABLE 17.1 Some Examples of Important ADRs

Medication	Significant ADR
Penicillin based antibiotics	Allergic reaction and anaphylaxis
Opioid analgesics	Constipation and respiratory depression
NSAIDs	Gastrointestinal irritation and bleeding
Antihistamines	Drowsiness

management; many patients will suffer ADRs and, as a consequence, discontinue their treatment. Effective management of ADRs is necessary to ensure patient safety and optimize outcomes. Children, older adults and the critically unwell are more susceptible to ADRs. Other factors increasing the chance of the patient suffering ADRs include chronic disease states such as diabetes and polypharmacy (NICE, 2017). Table 17.1 outlines examples of some important ADRs.

Drug interactions

A drug interaction is a situation in which a medication (e.g., Medication A) influences the activity of another medication(s) (e.g., Medication B) taken by the same patient. Medication A can increase, decrease or even produce a new effect of Medication B if the two medications interact and this may result in the patient experiencing an ADR. If Medication A is causing an increase in the effect of Medication B, the NA may spot an increase in the ADRs associated with Medication B and/or an increase in the therapeutic effect of Medication B. If Medication B is an anti-hypertensive drug (a drug that lowers blood pressure), its effect is enhanced and the patient's blood pressure readings will be somewhat lower than expected (a sign associated with the interaction) and the patient may describe feeling faint or light-headed (a symptom associated with the interaction).

Drug interactions occur in the human body. In contrast, drug incompatibilities, another term often used in managing medicines, occur in IV infusion containers, infusion lines and syringes. Drug interactions are a result of two or more medicines influencing each other in biological systems; drug incompatibilities occur as chemical reactions in the environment in which medicines are delivered to the body. In addition to medications interacting with each other, food, smoking and environmental chemicals can interact. Interactions are important as they can cause illness, worsen illness or, in extreme cases, cause death. Many medicines can be used safely in combination and prescribers and pharmacists are educated to use these combinations or spot where drug interactions might occur. Older adults and the critically unwell are particularly susceptible to drug interactions due the incidence of polypharmacy in these groups.

Medicines and the older person

Managing medicines in older people requires some key considerations related to the physiological process of ageing. Whilst it is incorrect to generalize that managing medicines is more complex in the elderly, there are important changes associated with ageing that define some of the ways medicines are best used.

Ageing usually results in a decline in kidney (renal) function. As renal function declines, the ability to eliminate/excrete some drugs changes. This may require dosage adjustments in older patients. Other physiological changes, such as a reduced ability to balance, can mean that ADRs such as light-headedness and dizziness may be more pronounced in the older patient. The increased sensitivity could make an individual more likely to fall and expose them to greater risk from using that medication. As humans age, they are more likely to develop chronic diseases, such as diabetes, Parkinson disease and cancer. In addition to the increased likelihood of developing these diseases, the likelihood of having more than one chronic condition increases with age. Those with chronic diseases and multiple chronic diseases tend to be more significantly affected by ADRs and more likely to be affected by drug interactions (especially as the number of medications they take increases).

Other aspects of ageing, such as declining eyesight and hearing issues, memory problems and decreased dexterity, can also affect adherence to medication regimens. Simple issues, such as opening medication bottles and cartons, reading medicines labels, listening to and following verbal instructions, are issues to be carefully taken into account when the NA manages medicines for the older patient.

Managing medicines in other specialist groups

Managing medicines in children has many considerations that parallel those in the older patient. At the various stages of development, children mature anatomically and physiologically, consequently influencing the response to medicines. As children age from birth to 12 years of age, the pharmacokinetic processes (ADME) change and mature. This means that medicine starting doses, dosing intervals and maximum doses vary from those in adults and must often be calculated on an individual basis.

Medicines management during pregnancy and breast-feeding is complex and requires careful consideration of the risks and benefits both to the mother and to the foetus (or in the case of breastfeeding, to the child). The use of established medicines with greater evidence to support safety may be preferable to the use of newer medicines where evidence may be less readily available. It is generally advisable to seek specialist advice when using medicines in pregnancy and during breastfeeding. Local medicines information centres, the UK Teratology Information Service and the UK Drugs in Lactation Advisory Service can provide such advice.

Medicines in hepatic and renal impairment

A patient's hepatic (liver) and renal (kidney) function can have a significant impact on the dosing requirements of many commonly used medicines. Similarly, many medicines have adverse effects on the liver and kidney, which may impact the functioning of these organs.

The liver metabolizes a large proportion of medicines, and hepatic impairment can directly reduce metabolism, leading to drug accumulation and toxic effects. Estimation of the ability of the liver to metabolize drugs is difficult as liver function tests are not always a reliable guide; however, dose reductions (either as amount of drug or frequency of dosing) may be necessary.

Patients with hepatic impairment may have associated physiological changes that influence medicines management. These include the risk of hepatic encephalopathy (a brain disorder associated with advanced liver disease) being increased by the use of sedative medicines and those causing constipation, and changes in the production of substances that facilitate blood clotting (clotting factors) that can alter the effectiveness of medicines used to stop the blood from clotting (anticoagulants). The use of shorter-acting medicines (to avoid accumulation) and those that do not undergo hepatic metabolism or elimination, may be preferred.

Changes in renal function can have a significant effect on plasma levels and dosing requirements of medicines. This is particularly important for medicines such as digoxin and lithium, where toxicity may result from increased plasma levels, and doses should be reduced accordingly. However, dosage adjustment is necessary for many medicines when they are used in patients with renal impairment. The kidney must excrete certain medicines for them to exert their therapeutic effect (e.g., nitrofurantoin). Therefore, these may not be effective in patients with renal impairment and alternatives will need to be considered. A number of medicines can worsen renal function (e.g., ACE inhibitors and NSAIDs) and should be avoided in patients with existing renal impairment. When these medicines are prescribed for any patient, renal function should be regularly monitored for signs of deterioration.

LEGAL ASPECTS OF MEDICINES MANAGEMENT

Human Medicines Regulations 2012 (HMR)

Medicines and the way they are used have the capacity to prevent, treat and cure disease. In contrast, if medicines are misused, they have great capacity to do real harm. The powerful nature of medicines mean that it is necessary to have systems in place to ensure they are used correctly and all transactions associated with medicines have corresponding legislation and regulation to govern their use.

The way in which medicines are handled by the NA in their day-to-day activities is governed by a legal framework: the Human Medicines Regulations 2012 (HMR). (http://www.legislation.gov.uk/uksi/2012/1916/contents/made). The NA is required to adhere to any local policies or procedures that may be in place. The law as it is set out in the HMR also governs and guides regulators like the General Medical Council, the Nursing and Midwifery Council, the General Pharmaceutical Council and the Health and Care Professions Council, who protect the public by ensuring their registrants use medicines safely and legally.

The HMR are a comprehensive set of laws that deal with the way medicines transactions occur in the UK. The HMR provide a legal definition of a medicinal product, which is then used to define how those medicines are transacted. The regulations cover important areas in the day to day working life of the NA. The HMR define what is, or is not, a medicine; this influences what can be bought over the counter and when a prescription is needed to obtain a medicine. The law also guides the governance that oversees the way medicines are handled in the workplace, for example, policies by which medicines are administered, how transactions are recorded, and what medicines that usually need a prescription might be administered in emergency medical situations. The HMR also defines who is entitled to prescribe medicines in the UK and which advisory bodies will guide the evidence supporting the use of medicines. Prescribing was traditionally the role of the doctor, the dentist or vet. Currently, midwives, nurses, pharmacists and physiotherapists (as well as certain other healthcare professionals) can also become prescribers.

Other issues covered by the HMR include how medicines are imported or exported to the UK and the rules by which medicines can be advertised.

CLASSIFICATION OF MEDICINES

The HMR directly or indirectly define three categories of medicine in the UK.

Prescription only medicines (POM)

These are medicines with the strictest level of control. As the name suggests, the prescription is key for legalizing many transactions involving these medicines. These medicines cannot be bought or sold without a prescription or other valid documentation. The law dictates the nature of the prescription, and how it should be written and verified to make any transactions involving POMs legal. The regulations governing POMs also guide their storage in pharmacies and hospitals (but not in patients' homes). The majority of medicines encountered by the NA as part of their everyday work will be POM.

> **! HOTSPOT**
>
> Controlled drugs (CDs) are a sub category of POM. These medicines are liable to misuse. There are additional rules and restrictions on their use, including procedures for storage, recording and verifying administration and their disposal. The Misuse of Drugs Act 1971 defines many categories of controlled drugs and the degrees of control exercised over their use and handling in healthcare settings.

Supplying POMs for emergency situations

In certain circumstances, the HMR allows POMs to be supplied without them being prescribed. This is typically in anticipation of the need to treat emergencies, such as opioid overdose with naloxone.

Pharmacy medicines (P)

This category of medicines can only be sold by a pharmacist, or under the supervision of a pharmacist, on a registered pharmacy premises. Some POMs are available as P medicines but have greater restrictions on their use compared with when they are prescribed.

General sales list (GSL) medicines

This category of medicines has the lowest level of control over their use. They can be sold and supplied from a range of retail outlets (and vending machines) without any healthcare professional oversight or control. The medicines must be sold in their original manufacturer's packing and supplied with their patient information leaflet (PIL). Medicines in the P and GSL categories are often referred to as 'over the counter' medicines (OTC) as they can be bought over the counter rather than being obtained by consultation with a prescriber. A subcategory of GSL medicines exists, termed PO medicines, which can only be sold from pharmacy premises.

MONITORING THE SAFETY OF MEDICINES

The importance of establishing the safety of medicines was brought into focus by the adverse effects associated with the use of thalidomide in pregnant women in the 1960s. This ultimately led to the introduction of the 1968 Medicines Act and the introduction of more robust systems to monitor adverse effects of medicines used in clinical practice (pharmacovigilance). In the UK, the Medicines and Healthcare products Regulatory Agency (MHRA) is responsible for pharmacovigilance. The Yellow Card system forms the basis for reporting adverse drug reactions when a medicine is being used in practice (MHRA, 2017). This is particularly important for new medicines and those where there are safety concerns. This is denoted using a black triangle symbol in any literature relating to the product, such as the Summary of Product Characteristics (SPC).

> **REFLECTION 17.1 What Information Can the NA Gather from the SPC?**
>
> Mr Simons (see Case Study 17.1) has an irritating dry cough when taking ramipril. Have a look at the SPC for ramipril and see what information you can find to support Mr Simons and his concerns about the side effect.
>
> You can search for the SPC for ramipril at the following link: http://www.medicines.org.uk

PERSONAL ACCOUNTABILITY

Medicines administration

The 5 Rs

Medicines are powerful tools. It is essential that the NA undertakes reasonable checks to ensure they are giving the right medicines to the right patients. To assist with this, a systematic approach to medicines administration has been developed, known as the 5 Rs or Five Rights of Drug Administration (see Jones, 2009). The 5 Rs are:
- Right Patient
- Right Time
- Right Drug
- Right Dose
- Right Route.

Right patient. It is essential that before administering a medicine you ensure that you are administering it to the right patient. This involves verifying the patient's identity by checking their name, address and date of birth, both with the patient and on the chart or medication label. Please remember that a patient may not always be able to answer questions (an unconscious patient) or may not be able to answer them accurately (a patient with severe dementia). In such cases, checking the patient's identification bracelet can help confirm their identity.

Right time. The timing of the medicine administration must be correct. Medicine administration usually spaces the dosing of drugs evenly throughout the day. This is intended to prevent unwanted gaps in therapy and ensure stable levels of the drug within the body. Giving medicine doses too close together could result in overdose, and giving them too far apart can result in a failure of therapy and return of symptoms.

Right drug/medicine. Checking that you have the correct medicine seems like the most obvious thing to do. However, there are a number of potential pitfalls that can lead to the wrong medicine being administered (e.g., two different medicines with very similar names or packaging). It is important that the medicine is correct, that it is the correct formulation and, in some cases, the correct brand. Some medicines, such as modified release preparations, must be given as the same brand, as the rate of release of the drug can vary.

Right dose. In the majority of cases, a medicine will have a standard dose. In these cases, checking you have the correct dose can be relatively straightforward (e.g., checking the prescribed dose against that found in the BNF). However, for some medicines the dose is calculated according to specific variables, such as the patient's age, weight, seriousness of the condition or a specific biochemical marker. There are also instances where a drug dose may be altered to account for a patient's other illnesses, such as renal failure.

Once you have confirmed that that you have the right dose, it may be necessary to calculate how this dose will be administered. This may involve determining how many tablets or how much liquid will be required to provide the required dose. When undertaking these calculations, it is important for you to check the strength of the preparation you are using. A typical dose of ibuprofen is 400 mg. This will require two 200 mg tablets or one 400 mg tablet. Incorrectly identifying the strength of the tablets or liquid can result in accidental overdose.

REFLECTION 17.2 Right Dose

Mr Simons (see Case Study 17.1) is taking ramipril 7.5 mg once a day. Have a look at the BNF and see what combinations of strength and formulation of ramipril could be given to Mr Simons.

Right route. It must be confirmed that the medicine is given via the correct route. This is important as the dose and onset of action can vary between routes. There may also be specific reasons why a particular route was avoided.

The Five Rights should form the basis of checks for administration of medicines in all settings. It is important to remember, however, that these checks only verify that the medicine being administered is what has been written on the chart. You must also consider the possibility that the drug was written in error. You should addionally ask yourself the following questions;

- Has the patient been prescribed a standard dose when their condition (e.g. renal failure) requires a non-standard dose?
- Is this patient allergic to this medicine?
- Will this medicine interact with any other treatments that the patient is receiving?
- Does the patient's condition mean that it is unsuitable or unsafe to give this medicine at this time?

If the answer to any of these questions is yes, the direction to administer the medicine should be checked with a senior member of staff or, ideally, with the prescriber.

Consent

Before engaging in any form of interaction with a patient, it is essential to gain consent. A patient must give permission for you to wash, dress or feed them, or to administer medication. Our patients should always have the right to refuse care, even if we feel the care is in their best interest. Failure to gain consent means that any care you give, no matter how well-intentioned, is essentially a form of assault.

When obtaining consent, it is important to ensure that the consent is 'informed'. This means that for a patient to give permission for a drug to be administered, they should be informed about what it is and why they are being given it. Any notable side effects or potential risks should be explained so that a patient can make an honest judgement as to whether they wish to give consent. Issues can sometimes arise if a patient is unable to fully understand what the treatment is for. This can occur if a patient is very young, has an altered state of consciousness or is mentally unwell.

Mental capacity

Mental capacity describes the ability of a person to make informed decisions about what they do and how they are treated. This may apply to all aspects of life choices, including whether to consent to medical treatment. If a person is deemed to have capacity to make a decision, then that decision must be respected even if, in the case of medical treatment, a healthcare professional may not consider it to be the best course of action. In the UK, the Mental Capacity Act 2005 outlines the process to follow when someone's capacity is in doubt and allows for someone to make plans should they lose the capacity to make certain decisions in the future. The Act describes how a person's mental capacity is assessed. The two-stage process initially identifies whether a person is likely to have an impairment in brain function (e.g., through a medical condition), and then determines whether this has an impact on their decision-making ability. To make an informed decision, a person must be able to understand relevant information relating to a given decision, retain that information and use it to consider the options to come to a decision, and be able to express that decision. It is important to note that a person's mental capacity may fluctuate over time; therefore, an assessment of their ability to make a given decision may need to be made on separate occasions. Similarly, a person may have the capacity to make certain decisions, but not other more complex ones. Where a person lacks capacity, the choice to proceed or not must be made by whoever needs the decision (e.g., the nurse or NA administering a medicine), taking into account factors such as the person's previous views and beliefs. The decision must be made in the person's best interest. The Act makes provision for a person to nominate a trusted person to take decisions on their behalf (Lasting Power of Attorney) in the event that they lose capacity in the future.

REFLECTION 17.3 Mental Capacity and the NA

Mr Simons (see Case Study 17.1) has been admitted to hospital for closer monitoring of his hypertension. During the medicines administration 'round,' he tells you that he doesn't want to take his ramipril. He clearly understands the reason the ramipril has been prescribed and the potential consequences of not taking it.

Do you have the right to insist he takes his ramipril?

Covert administration

Covert administration describes the circumstances in which a drug is administered to a patient without their knowledge, typically by hiding it in food. This is a complex area, which on the surface seems to breach the requirement to gain consent for any medication that you give. The difficulty comes with patients who are unable to fully understand what they are refusing. This may be due to issues such as confusion or a reduced level of consciousness. In these circumstances, it may be viewed in the patient's best interest to covertly administer the medication. However, whilst it is acknowledged that this is sometimes necessary, it should not be undertaken lightly. The decision to administer drugs covertly should not be made by a single practitioner in isolation. It should be discussed with other members of the multi-disciplinary team and the patient's family. Any decision to do this should be outlined clearly in the patient's notes and it should be reviewed regularly.

REFLECTION 17.4. Covert Administration

Whilst in hospital Mr Simons is still refusing his ramipril. One of your colleagues suggests that because he might suffer harm if he does not take his ramipril, it could be given covertly in his food.

Consider how you would approach this scenario.

Dealing with controlled drugs

Controlled drugs (CDs) have a significant potential to be misused and the risk of harm from their misuse can be substantial. The classification of a medicine as a CD places additional requirements on the healthcare professional with regard to their use. The Misuse of Drugs Act 1971, and its associated regulations, outline the legal framework governing the use of CDs. The National Institute for Health and Care Excellence (NICE) guideline *Controlled Drugs: Safe Use and Management* [NG46] (www.nice.org.uk/guidance/ng46) outlines what 'systems and processes' should be in place for managing CDs in all healthcare environments (except care homes).

There are issues considered in the guideline that will directly affect the practice of the NA:
- Record keeping required by organizations when handling CDs
- Risk assessment in the use of CDs
- Processes for reporting incidents involving CDs to monitor patterns of misuse and potential criminal activity
- Processes and requirements by which CDs are prescribed, obtained and supplied
- Processes for safe administration, handling and disposal of CDs.

The issues that most affect the everyday activity of the NA will centre on obtaining controlled drugs for use in the clinical environment, their storage and handing, their administration and their safe disposal.

REFLECTION 17.5

Visit the NICE website at the web address:
https://www.nice.org.uk/guidance/ng46

Review the recommended procedures that NICE suggests and compare them with some of your areas of practice where CDs are handled.

Do the procedures in use follow the guidelines precisely and, if not, what are the differences? Do colleagues ask questions or analyse the suitability of administering the controlled drug in the way NICE suggests or do they have their own way of checking the administration is safe and correct and making the appropriate records?

You will notice some variance in the exact practice from clinical area to clinical area, but you will hopefully see some consistency of practice around the guideline.

Patient Group Directions (PGDs)

A Patient Group Direction (PGD) is a set of written instructions that facilitates the supply or administration of medicines to patients, usually in planned circumstances. PGDs are used in many contexts in healthcare, for instance in vaccination clinics and in sexual health clinics, to ensure a patient has access to medication without the need for a prescription or undergoing the comprehensive consultation that is required before a prescription is written.

PGDs are usually fairly substantial documents that are put together by a multi-disciplinary team, such as senior doctors, pharmacists and nurses. Essentially, the team who put the PGD together are outlining the circumstances in which a healthcare professional can supply a medicine without a prescription or intervention. A range of healthcare professionals use them in various aspects of their practice; for instance, paramedics, pharmacists, midwives and dieticians.

PGDs contain important information that carefully defines the parameters of the medicines supply related to the PGD. The PGD will only be used in a given area of business, such as a Hospital Trust, Clinical Commissioning Board or Health Board. Each PGD will have a start and end date within which it is to be used, a description of the medicines that can be administered or supplied, the class of healthcare professional who can supply the medicines, the conditions/situations in which the PGD applies and, most importantly, inclusion and exclusion criteria, dosages (and associated side effects, cautions and warnings) and further details, such as the procedure for 'following up' the patient and where the patient needs to go for further advice. PGDs cannot be used to supply certain medicines, such as those that do not have marketing authorizations, abortifacients and certain controlled drugs.

Procedures for safe use of medicines
Record keeping
Information relating to the use of medicines for a patient typically does not fall to a single practitioner, but to a team. This highlights the importance of accurate and contemporaneous record keeping.

To ensure that everyone involved in the patient's care is aware of what medicine has or has not been given to a patient, records *must* be kept. The most common form of medicines record keeping is the patient 'medication chart'. This is a list of medicines prescribed for a patient with instructions of when they should be given. In a ward setting, this is commonly kept at the end of a patient's bed. A record should be kept of any medicine that is given, identifying who administered it. If the medicine is to be given when needed, rather than at specific intervals, a record of the time of the administration must also be recorded. This is necessary to prevent accidental overdosing of the patient. Should a patient be unable to take the medicine, or choose not to take it, a record that the administration was attempted but not completed should be made. Some medication charts use codes to identify why the medicine was not given. It may also be necessary to record additional information about why the medicine was not administered in the patient's notes. Some medicines (such as those given intravenously or those given to children) may require a second person to check that everything is correct prior to administration. In these instances, a record of who double-checked the medicine must also be kept.

Records should be made promptly after the medicine was administered and should be clear, legible and, if written on paper, should be written in indelible ink. Many care environments are utilizing more computerized means of recording interventions. These require the same information to be recorded, using the practitioner's log-in identification as proof of who administered in place of a signature. At all times, the NA must adhere to local policy and procedure.

Storage
Medicines should be stored in a secure location. In a patient's home, the patient can choose how the medicine is stored, but it is still recommended that it be stored in a secure place where other people (children in particular) cannot get into it. In a hospital environment, a patient's own medicines will typically be kept in a locked cabinet by their bed. The ward stock of medicines will typically be kept in locked cupboards or on a locked 'drug trolley'. These have traditionally been locked with a key; however, more modern computer control storage units can be accessed using a password or security card.

Expiry dates
The concept of expiry dates on food is widely known; expiry dates on medicines are similar. After a period, medicines lose their effectiveness and sterile products lose their sterility, thus rendering them unsafe to use. It is essential that before a medicine is administered, it is checked to make sure that it (and all the equipment used for administration) is within the expiry date. Multi-dose containers (e.g., insulin vials) contain more than a single dose of the medicine. When using these, it is prudent to note when the container was first accessed, as the contents may become unusable after a specific period.

Refrigerated storage
In much the same way that some foods must kept chilled to prevent them from spoiling, so too should some medicines. Most care settings where medicines are stored will have a fridge specifically set aside for this (which may also need to be lockable). In patients' own homes, their own fridge will be used. Typically, medicines that require refrigerated storage should be kept at a temperature between 2°C and 8°C; they should not be allowed to freeze.

Disposal
There are circumstances where medicines either go out of date or are no longer needed. Practitioners should be careful when considering how they dispose of unwanted medicines. Medicines should not be disposed of in domestic waste bins, flushed down toilets or washed down the sink. Unused medicines should be disposed of using suitable equipment or, if appropriate, returned to a pharmacy for safe disposal. Local policy and procedure will dictate how medicines are to be disposed of.

Prescribing/administration errors
The prescribing and administration of medicines is a process undertaken by humans, and as such, is subject to the potential for human error. It is because of this potential for error that a range of checking mechanisms is undertaken to ensure that, if there is a mistake, it is identified before it reaches the patient.

If you identify that an error has occurred in the prescribing or the administration of a medicine, then you must report it to a senior member of staff. An error must be reported whether it was made by yourself or by another practitioner, even if it did not reach the patient or cause any harm. NAs have a duty of candour; this means that they have a responsibility to be honest about and report any error they encounter, even if this has consequences for the practitioner involved, the work area or organization. All healthcare settings will have formal mechanisms for the recording and reporting of errors or patient incidents. To improve patient safety and facilitate future learning, it is important that these procedures be completed with as much information as possible.

LOOKING BACK, FEEDING FORWARD

This chapter has provided the reader with insight and understanding concerning medicines management with a discussion of the important factors that can impinge on this activity. In order to provide care that is safe and therapeutic, the NA must master the principles that underpin safe and effective administration and optimisation of medicines ensuring that local policy and procedure is adhered to.

Demonstrating an understanding of how medicines are managed safely ensures the NA is practicing within their sphere of competence demonstrating that the patient is central to all that is done. The ability to understand and the importance of being able to recognise the effects of medicines, allergies, drug sensitivities, side effects as well as adverse reactions have been addressed in this chapter.

REFERENCES

Edwards, I.R., Aronson, J.K., 2000. Adverse drug reactions: definitions, diagnosis, and management. Lancet 356, 1255–1259.

Jones, S.W., 2009. Reducing medication administration errors in nursing practice. Nurs. Stand. 23 (50), 40–46.

Medicines and Healthcare Products Regulatory Agency, 2017. Yellow Card. Available at: https://yellowcard.mhra.gov.uk/.

National Institute for health and Care Excellence (NICE), 2017. KTT18 Multimorbidity and polypharmacy.

NHS Digital, 2017. Prescriptions Dispensed in the Community, Statistics for England – 2006–2016. https://digital.nhs.uk/catalogue/PUB30014.

Young, R.S., Pitcher, B., 2015. Medicines Management for Nurses at a Glance. Wiley-Blackwell, London.

SUGGESTED READING

Dougherty, L., Lister, S.E. (Eds.), 2015. The Royal Marsden Manual of Clinical Nursing Procedures, ninth ed., professional edition. West Sussex, Chichester; John Wiley & Sons Inc, Hoboken, NJ.

Royal College of Nursing. Consent. https://www.rcn.org.uk/get-help/rcn-advice/consent.

Moving and Handling

Hamish MacGregor

OBJECTIVES

By the end of the chapter the reader will able to:

1. Understand the law in relation to moving and handling and apply it to practice
2. Understand the importance of good back care and the promotion of good musculoskeletal health
3. Understand the risk assessment process and how it applies to good patient handling
4. Apply the safe principles of moving and handling in the patient setting
5. Be aware of the importance of safer moving and handling in relation to both staff safety and good patient care
6. Be able to deliver (after suitable and sufficient face-to-face practical moving and handling training) some safer handling techniques within a hospital or community setting

KEY WORDS

Safety	Principles	Load
Hazard	Legislation	Equipment
Risk	Responsibilities	
Assessment	Supervision	

CHAPTER AIM

The chapter aims to provide the reader with the necessary knowledge and skills needed to deliver safe and effective moving and handling in a variety of healthcare settings.

SELF TEST

1. Name three pieces of legislation relating to moving and handling.
2. How often should a hoist be inspected and checked by a competent person?
3. State three things you may need to know about the handler when carrying out a risk assessment.
4. Name three assessment factors to be considered that relate to the environment.
5. How many vertebrae are there in the human spine?
6. State three things necessary to maintain a healthy back.
7. Describe a stable mobile base.
8. State four things you would check about a hoist before using it.
9. State four areas you would assess about the patient before standing them.
10. What is the maximum load that can be moved at waist height in ideal conditions by a woman?

INTRODUCTION

The carrying out of effective patient moving and handling requires the Nursing Associate (NA) to use all their observation skills to ensure a suitable and sufficient risk assessment before they start. Once an assessment has been made, the NA must use the practical skills they have developed in practice and in the simulation room to ensure the handling technique used is safe for both the patient and the handler(s). The patient must be treated with dignity and compassion at all times. The handling technique used must be fully explained to the patient and carried out so that it maximizes independence and minimizes discomfort.

LEGAL ASPECTS

Moving and handling is underpinned by legislation and there are a number of laws, regulations and guidance that the NA must adhere to. These legal aspects are interspaced throughout this chapter. The NA must also ensure they and adhering to local policy and procedure at all times.

Health and Safety at Work Act 1974 (HASAWA)

The NA needs to know about the legal aspects related to moving and handling. The HASAWA places responsibility on both employers and employees. As a trainee NA, you need to be aware of the responsibilities of the employee. As a qualified NA, you need to be aware of the responsibilities for both the employer and employees, as the definition of an employer is anyone who manages or supervises anyone else. Therefore, as an NA you will, at times, be responsible for the supervision of students and healthcare assistants.

Broadly speaking, the responsibilities of the employer are as follows:

- Provide equipment that is safe, with a safe system of work in place to back this up.
- Ensure safety in connection with the use, storage and transport of loads (a load in this context could be defined as a person) and substances hazardous to health.
- Provide information, instruction, training and supervision. This will include moving and handling training. It needs to be emphasized that, when on clinical placement, you must ensure that you are receiving adequate supervision in relation to patient handling, and if it is not sufficient, you need to communicate this to your link lecturer from the university (or the person responsible for your training).
- Maintain a safe working environment. Remember as a trainee NA, your environment can be a hospital, a day centre, a nursing home or a patient's home, and all these areas need to be deemed safe by your clinical supervisor.
- Provide a written health and safety policy statement. This will be two-fold, one from the university and one from the managers of the organization that you are on clinical placement with.

As an employee you are required to do the following:

- Take reasonable care of your own health and that of your colleagues. This includes not only your acts, but your omissions, i.e., not only things that you do that can put you, your colleagues or your patient at risk, but also the things that you may fail to do to reduce risk to all.
- Not recklessly or intentionally interfere or misuse anything provided for health and safety.
- Be willing to receive training provided by your employer. This means that if the training is provided and you have been given the time and opportunity to attend, then you must do this.

> **⚠ HOTSPOT**
>
> Prior to moving or handing people or other loads the NA must undertake appropriate training. The employer is responsible for providing this training.

Management of Health and Safety at Work Regulations 1999

These regulations require employers to carry out risk assessments on tasks considered hazardous in the workplace. These assessments must be done by a competent person. A competent person is someone with the necessary ability, knowledge and skills to carry out risk assessments. This could be you if you have received suitable and sufficient training. More information on risk assessment is provided later in this chapter.

For assessments to be carried out, hazards need to be identified. A hazard is something with the potential to cause harm. An example from patient handling would be a dependent patient who is not able to move themselves from bed to chair.

A risk is defined as the chance of something causing harm. The risk of harm here would be the NA sustaining a back injury by physically moving the patient from bed to chair without assistance or the aid of moving and handling equipment.

Regulations ask for the risk to be 'reduced as far as is reasonably practicable'. An example in this respect would be a patient being provided with a hoist and sling to move them from bed to chair. The hoist and sling would need to be assessed as suitable for this patient, be properly maintained and in good working order and the handlers using the hoist would have to be trained and deemed competent to operate the hoist.

Manual Handling Operations Regulations (1992) as amended 2002 (MHOR, 1992)

Like the Health and Safety at Work Act (HASAWA), these regulations also put responsibilities onto both employers and employees. The employer has a duty to do the following:

- Avoid the need for manual handling tasks so far as it is reasonably practicable to do so. In relation to patients, this will usually mean the patient being encouraged to do as much for themselves as possible. This will not only reduce the risk of a musculoskeletal injury for the handler, but also increase patient independence, promote dignity and potentially reduce the length of patient stay if in hospital.
- Assess all moving and handling tasks where there is a perceived risk. This is covered in a more general way by the health and safety legislation. The MHOR (1992) is applying the assessment process specifically to moving and handling.
- Reduce the risk of injury to the lowest level reasonably practicable. This is both for the patient and the handler. It is important to note that the regulations use the word 'reduce', not 'remove'. This is vital as it recognizes that all patient handling has some level of risk; even when it has been reduced, there is still some residual risk as it is not possible to eliminate risk completely.
- Review all assessments as changes occur and/or at regular scheduled intervals. In relation to patient handling, it is important to have regular review dates as it provides a forum to assess the patient whose condition does not change dramatically over time, for example the longer-stay patient in a nursing home. In the case of the acute hospital patient, their condition can change very rapidly (e.g., pre and post-operatively), therefore continuous assessment of their handling needs is essential.

The employee has a duty to:

- Follow appropriate systems provided for handling of loads (and patients) by the employer. If you as the NA do not agree with this system of work, you can refuse to carry out this handling task if you deem it unsafe. This of course will be based on a suitable and sufficient risk assessment carried out by you. You are also supported by the HASAWA as it defines that you as an employee 'take reasonable care of your own health and that of your colleagues'.

- Report accidents and near misses. You should ensure that you are familiar with the accident/incident reporting procedure of the organization you are working in. In addition, you should report any near misses. An example of a near miss would be if a patient nearly fell from the edge of the bed as it was not low enough for them to reach the floor with their feet. This could highlight that there was a fault with the bed or that the patient was short in stature and needed an extra low bed. The reporting of these incidents as a near miss might prevent an accident happening in the future.

> **! HOTSPOT**
>
> If the NA does not agree with any systems of work related to moving and handling, or deems it unsafe, they can refuse to carry out a handling task.

Lifting Operations and Lifting Equipment Regulations 1998 (LOLER)

These regulations require the following:
- Lifting equipment should have adequate strength and stability for its proposed use.
- Risk from positioning and installing lifting equipment should be minimized as far as is reasonably possible.
- Equipment has to be marked indicating its safe working load.
- Equipment that lifts people must be examined by a competent person at 6-monthly intervals.

As this applies to equipment whose primary function is to lift people, it would be reasonable to use the example of a patient hoist. It is important that the correct hoist is used for the correct patient in the correct environment. For example, a patient in their own home may have a ceiling tracking hoist as opposed to a mobile hoist as it would:

1. Take up less space than a mobile hoist.
2. Be easier for the handler to move in the domestic environment.
3. Be operable by one person rather than two, which may be more suitable in a patient's home environment.

To continue with the example of hoists, regulations also require that a hoist is serviced every 6 months and then inspected in the next 6 months after the first year of being put in service. The handler must therefore look for a label on the hoist that tells them when the hoist was last serviced and checked and when it is next due. This should always be at 6-monthly intervals. Do not, under any circumstances, use a hoist that is out of date as, if there is an accident to a patient, you, or a colleague, then it would be your responsibility, not the employer's, because you as the handler had not checked if the hoist was compliant with the regulations.

In addition, the hoist and the sling must be marked with a Safe Working Load (SWL). Therefore, the handler should determine an accurate weight of the patient before putting them in the hoist and sling.

Provision and Use of Work Equipment Regulations 1998 (PUWER)

These regulations state that:
- Equipment is used for operations that it is designed for. Therefore, it is not acceptable to use a bed sheet to move a patient as it is not designed for this purpose. An appropriate slide sheet that has been assessed as suitable for the patient would be a safe system of work that would comply with the regulations to move the patient.
- Equipment is maintained efficiently, and a maintenance log is kept up to date. Before using equipment, check the maintenance schedule if in doubt.

> **! HOTSPOT**
>
> It is absolutely unacceptable for the NA to use a bed sheet to move a patient.

This link http://www.hse.gov.uk/pubns/hsis4.pdf from the Health and Safety Executive gives a list of moving and handling equipment used in health and social care and indicates whether LOLER or PUWER applies.

Reporting of Injuries, Diseases and Dangerous Occurrences Regulations 2013 (RIDDOR)

- RIDDOR places responsibilities on employers to report injuries deemed 'reportable' under the Regulations. Part 4 of the regulation is the one that is most commonly applied in relation to back or other musculoskeletal injuries that can happen to patient handlers.

Over-seven-day incapacitation of a worker

Accidents must be reported directly to the Health and Safety Executive where they result in an employee or self-employed person being away from work, or unable to perform their normal work duties, for more than 7 consecutive days as the result of their injury. This 7-day period does not include the day of the accident, but does include weekends and rest days. The report must be made within 15 days of the accident.

Over-three-day incapacitation

Accidents must be recorded in the organization's incident reporting system, but not reported where they result in a worker being incapacitated for more than 3 consecutive days. The employer must keep an accident book under the Social Security (Claims and Payments) Regulations 1979, and, having recorded the incident in the accident book, will have fulfilled their obligations under the regulations.

Human Rights Act 1998

It may seem that it is unusual that this Act applies to moving and handling, but there are two articles from the Act that can apply (Table 18.1).

TABLE 18.1   The Human Rights Act and Its Application to Moving and Handling

Article	Description
Article 3: Prohibition of Torture (Ref 7)	Patients who have not had a handling technique carried out correctly could be regarded as having care that is inhuman and degrading. An example of this may be when a hoist sling is incorrectly fitted causing the patient pain, fear and anxiety.
Article 8: Right to respect for home, private and social life (Ref 8)	It is important that when moving and handling patients, you are respectful, listen to their fears and approach them with an open mind using your professional knowledge and skills. Remember, if in doubt, seek advice.

RISK ASSESSMENT

Risk assessment is an integral part of all good moving and handling. Although the MHOR clearly sets out the risk assessment process associated with moving and handling, it is essential to demystify this and take a common-sense approach to both patient and load handling. The process of risk assessment in general is something that we all carry out in our day to day lives. For example, when we cross the road, particularly at a crossing without waiting for the 'green man', this involves complex risk assessment skills to work out if we can get across the road before the oncoming vehicle hits us. This expertise can be translated into the skills necessary to carry out effective moving and handling assessments.

There are a number of component parts of a moving and handling risk assessment.

Task

- Can you apply the key safe principles of moving and handling? (See later section on 'Safe Principles of Moving and Handling'.) This is often a good, quick checklist to carry out before attempting a handling task. For example, if you are unable to adopt a stable mobile base, it may be because there is not enough room for you to have your feet apart and it may be necessary to move a bed, a chair or a bedside locker before you attempt the handling task.
- Be aware of adopting static postures, e.g., leaning over a low bed for a prolonged period.
- Minimize the amount of twisting from the waist. If you move your feet in the direction you are moving, you can reduce twisting by about 80%.
- Ensure there are sufficient breaks in the prolonged handling task.

Individual capability of the handler(s)

Does the handling task involve any of the following?
- Require a certain level of fitness? We all have different levels of fitness that affect our ability to move objects and people.
- Require levels of knowledge, skill and competence? All handling tasks require levels of knowledge before you can attempt them. In addition, there needs to be a development of skill

and competence before these tasks can be carried out safely. The quality, length, content and frequency of training can affect all of this.
- Require specialist training?
- Present a risk to those with pre-existing health problems? This can be both short-term and longer-term injuries.
- Present a risk to pregnant staff? All pregnant staff must have a suitable and sufficient risk assessment carried out by their manager while working and pregnant (MHSW, 1999: Regulation 16).

Load or person

When assessing a load, consider the following factors:
- Weight
- Size and shape
- Difficulty to hold; e.g., does it have handholds?
- Uneven weight distribution
- Potentially harmful; e.g., hot or have sharp edges.

When assessing a person, we need to apply some of these criteria, specifically weight, size, shape and distribution of weight. For example, legs can be heavy, particularly when a person has impaired movement in the lower limbs. In addition, other factors we will need to consider are:
- The patient's level of understanding. If the patient cannot understand, either due to a language or cognitive problem, then they are unlikely to be able to cooperate or follow instructions.
- The patient's motivation. A patient may have the ability to carry out certain activities, but if they are unwilling to do this, for whatever reason, then this can affect the amount of input necessary from the handler and may necessitate further assessment.
- Medical condition that may affect handling. Many conditions, such as stroke or Parkinson disease, will require specialist knowledge and skill before the patient is moved.
- The patient's level of consciousness.
- Attachments, such as intravenous lines or catheters. These may impede the patient's movement and require additional staff to manage them during patient transfer.
- The patient's level of pain and how well this is being controlled. A patient who is in pain will not be able to maximize their movement potential.

Environment

Factors that can be considered with regard to the environment include the following:
- Is there enough space? If not, then more space needs to be created. If this is not possible, a full ergonomic assessment may be needed to maximize the space.
- Are there any obstacles that could be moved to create more space?
- Is the flooring safe, e.g., is it dry and hazard free?
- Are there stairs to be negotiated?
- Is there enough light?
- Is the temperature comfortable to work in? Temperatures too high or too low can cause problems for both patients and handlers.

Equipment

Factors for consideration include the following:
- Is it fit for the task?
- Is it in good working order?
- Has it been serviced and checked in accordance with current regulations?
- Has an SWL been identified?
- Do people need specialized training to operate the equipment?

Other influencing factors

These include the following:
- Compromised staffing levels
- Levels of stress and other psychosocial factors
- Pressures at work and/or at home affecting handlers
- Organizational climate and culture.

STRUCTURE AND FUNCTION OF THE SPINE

The spine is one of the strongest structures of the body and it gives us a great range of movement. It starts at the atlas at the base of the skull and finishes at the coccyx, the base of the spine. The main functions of the spine are to support the body's weight and to protect the spinal cord. It is important to understand the basic anatomy of the spine to understand how you can protect it when you are carrying out moving and handling tasks. In this link you can see how the biopsychosocial view of back pain has implications on how we apply lifting techniques:

http://www.pain-ed.com/blog/2017/07/05/does-the-biopsychosocial-view-of-back-pain-have-implications-on-how-we-teach-lifting-technique/

The vertebrae

There are 33 vertebrae that make up the spine and these are divided into four areas (Fig. 18.1).
1. The Cervical Spine
    This consists of seven vertebrae from the base of the skull to the beginning of the thoracic spine. The cervical spine allows a great deal of movement, letting the head, neck and shoulders move in multiple directions.
2. The Thoracic Spine
    This consists of 12 vertebrae from the cervical spine to the lumbar spine. This area has less movement as the ribs are attached to the vertebrae here.
3. The Lumbar Spine
    This area has the five largest vertebrae. It takes the full weight of the upper body and, like the cervical spine, has a full range of movement.
4. The Sacrum and Coccyx:
    This consists of nine separate vertebrae which are fused to form two bones. Five of these vertebrae form the sacrum and four form the coccyx.

The intervertebral discs

These act as shock absorbers between the vertebrae. There are 6 in the cervical spine, 12 in the thoracic spine and 5 in the

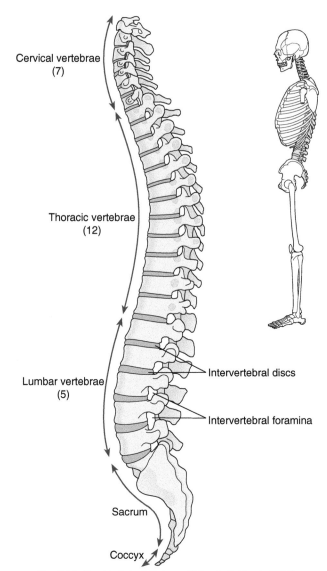

Fig. 18.1 The Vertebral Column (Waugh & Grant, 2018).

lumbar spine. Additionally, they act as a spacer between the vertebrae and allow movement between the vertebrae.

The disc has two layers; the outer part is called the annulus and the inner part is the nucleus. The outer part is made up of 16–20 C-shaped rings that are laid out in opposite directions and give the disc strength. The nucleus is the central core of the disc and is made of a soft gelatinous material. Problems occur with the discs when they are unevenly loaded; this most commonly occurs when there is a combination of forward and side bending. In extreme cases, the nucleus can push through the outside wall causing the disc to bulge. This is incorrectly called a slipped disc but is in fact a prolapsed or herniated disc (Fig. 18.2). The discs are attached to the vertebrae above and below by ligaments.

The facet joints

These work like hinges and are located at the back of the vertebra. Their role is to allow the spine a good range of movement when

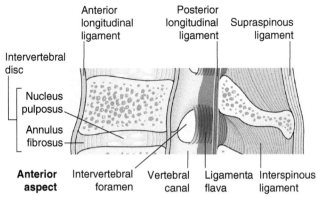

Fig. 18.2 Section of the Vertebral Column Showing the Ligaments, Intervertebral Discs and Intervertebral Foramina (Waugh & Grant, 2018).

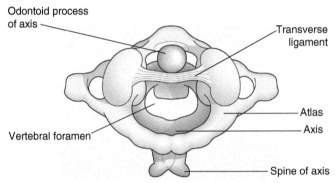

Fig. 18.3 The Upper Cervical Vertebrae (Waugh & Grant, 2018).

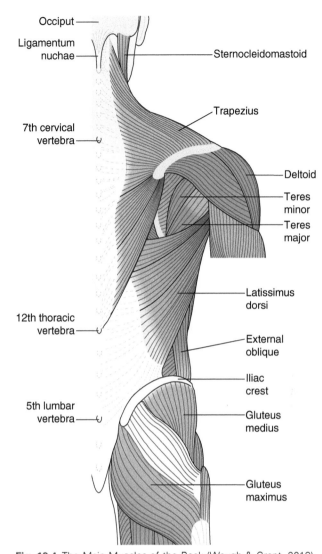

Fig. 18.4 The Main Muscles of the Back (Waugh & Grant, 2018).

bending and twisting. They also give the spine stability. About 25% of our body weight rests on the facet joints.

Muscles and ligaments

The ligaments are made of fibrous connecting tissue and these connect the vertebrae. Back pain can be a symptom of the ligaments being overstretched or, in some cases, torn. This is particularly true in lower back pain (Fig. 18.3).

The muscles of the back are divided into two groups. The extrinsic muscles deal with movement of the upper extremities and the shoulders. The intrinsic muscles deal with the movement of the vertebral column and assist in maintaining posture. Injury to the intrinsic muscles can occur when poor moving and handling techniques have been carried out, particularly over a period of time. It is for this reason that we need to bend at the hips and knees, not the lower back, when lifting objects from a low level (Fig. 18.4).

Looking after your back

As an NA it essential to look after your back.

- The best way to prevent/manage back problems is to do some form of regular exercise and maintain a healthy lifestyle. Many different forms of exercise help back pain – it is most important to choose an activity that you enjoy, and that is convenient for you. Exercise will help strengthen the back muscles.
- Try to minimize bending and twisting at the same time.

- Bend at the hips and knees, not the back, whenever possible.
- Hold loads close to your body (see later section on 'Safe principles of handling').
- Carry loads in a rucksack with the straps over both shoulders.
- Be posturally aware. Avoid slouching in a chair or over a desk or walking with shoulders hunched.
- Use a chair that supports you in a good posture. Feet flat on the floor, lower limbs at ninety degrees. Keep changing your posture.
- Lose any excess weight.
- Have a mattress that suits your height, weight, age and sleeping position.

(http://www.nhs.uk/Livewell/Backpain/Pages/Topbacktips.aspx)

Working at computers and laptops

Part of your studying will involve the use of computers and possibly laptops or tablets. There is evidence to suggest that adopting poor postures when at a workstation can be a contributory factor to cumulative back pain. To minimize this, here are a few tips that might help.

Chairs and desks:

- It is important that you can sit in an upright position at a desk.
- Your chair should be adjusted to allow you to sit with your hips and knees at approximately 90 degrees.
- Your feet should be flat on the floor. If this is not possible you will need a footstool.
- Your back should be upright (in line and your head held upright).
- Your screen should be adjusted to allow your eyes to be in line with the top third of the screen.
- Your elbows should be at 90 degrees and your hands relaxed in front of your keyboard.
- If you use a mouse a lot, try and use your short-cut keys as much as possible, e.g., F7 = spell check. You should have a mouse mat with a wrist support, this will keep your wrist and hand in a more neutral position.
- You should not spend more than 20 to 30 minutes at your computer before getting up to change your posture.

Use of laptop stands, external keyboards and mouse:

- Laptops and tablets can be made safer by using laptop or tablet stands in association with an external keyboard and mouse. This will allow the user to mimic sitting at a desktop, and therefore allow them to adopt a better posture.

Carrying laptops:

- Carrying laptops over one shoulder puts the body out of alignment and, with prolonged use, can cause cumulative back pain. It is better to carry a laptop in a rucksack designed for the purpose, ideally with wheels, as this will allow it to be wheeled as well as carried.

Further information on setting up a workstation is available on http://backcare.org.uk/wp-content/uploads/2015/02/Setting-up-your-Workstation-Factsheet.pdf, plus more information at www.backcare.org.uk.

SAFE PRINCIPLES OF MOVING AND HANDLING

This can act as a checklist when assessing a patient or a load before a move.

Avoid the handling task

The first thing we need to think of is whether we can avoid this handling task. This may prove difficult in relation to load handling but can be a positive action in relation to patient handling. If we can encourage the patient to do as much as possible for themselves, this will assist in their rehabilitation, increase self-esteem, promote dignity and, if they are in hospital, may reduce their hospital stay. To promote this, it is necessary to have honed your risk assessment skills to help you decide when it is practicable to encourage or allow the patient to move independently or what level of intervention they will need from the handler. Remember as well as your nursing colleagues, there are others in the multidisciplinary team who will be able to help, such as physiotherapists and occupational therapists.

Keep your spine in line

This relates to keeping your spine in neutral position without bending, stretching or twisting. It is important to remember that your spine is one of the strongest parts of your body and responds well to movement, but excessive bending and twisting may lead to cumulative back pain.

Hold loads close

Keep a load as close to you as possible as when you move it away from you, the effort required will make it seem heavier. This can feel as much as five times heavier when the load is at arms' length. In relation to patient handling, this principle also applies. Here you will have to apply your assessment skills to the patient as it is necessary to consider dignity and privacy, the patient's personal choice and their cognitive state.

Stable mobile base

This is the position of your feet that you adopt when carrying out a handling task. Your feet should be about shoulder width apart and your knees soft and flexible. You should be in a walk stance position (Fig. 18.5). This will allow you to transfer your weight from one leg to the other using the major muscle groups of your thighs and buttocks.

Controversial techniques

During your practical moving and handling training you will be taught some safe moving and handling techniques. You may see some techniques that are not acceptable when you are on

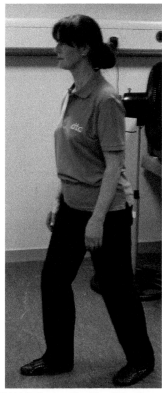

Fig. 18.5 Walk Stance Position (MacGregor, 2016).

placement. These are called controversial techniques as they should not be used except in very exceptional circumstances, such as a fire. An example of this is a drag lift, where the patient is lifted up the bed or chair under the arms. This is unsafe for the patient and can cause pain, subluxation of the shoulder, nerve damage and even fractures in the frail elderly. If you see this, or any other controversial technique happening, speak to a member of the team, your link lecturer or the moving and handling adviser.

Common pieces of moving and handling equipment

Please note this is not an exhaustive list and these are just some examples of common moving and handling aids you will see on clinical placement. Like with all equipment, you must ensure that you have had suitable and sufficient training beforehand and that you are competent to use the equipment. You can injure yourself and/or the patient by incorrect use of any of the equipment detailed here.

> **❗ HOTSPOT**
>
> Never take chances with any piece of equipment. If in doubt do not use.

Beds

These may not be immediately apparent as moving and handling equipment, and technically they are not, but many patient handling techniques can be made simpler for the handler and safer for the patient if there is a bed that is appropriate to that patient's needs.

The most common example is an electric profiling bed. This has the benefit of raising and lowering to allow easier egress and access for the patient. It also has a back rest that can be raised and lowered, and a knee break, which will stop the patient from sliding down the bed. This is beneficial as it helps maintain the patient's independence and therefore promotes dignity. It also reduces the amount of patient handling. There are many types of these beds with different controls and options. It is vital that you familiarize yourself with the beds in your clinical area and ensure that you know how to operate them safely.

There is also a range of specialist beds that can help with patients who have more complex moving and handling issues. Some examples of these follow.

Low-level beds

These lower to the floor, often to a height of 12 cm (Fig. 18.6). They can be helpful for patients of a short stature who are unable to get into and out of a normal height bed, thus impeding their ability to mobilize independently. These beds are also useful for patients who are at risk of falling out of bed or climbing over side rails.

Bariatric beds

These are for larger patients who need a larger bed in order to safely meet their care needs. The Aurum Bariatric Bed (Fig. 18.7).

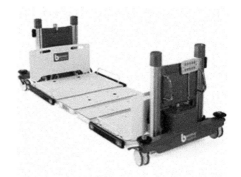

Fig. 18.6 The Deprimo Floor-Level Bed (Reproduced with permission from Benmor Medical UK).

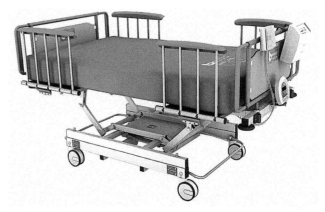

Fig. 18.7 Bariatric Bed (Reproduced with permission from Benmor Medical UK).

is an example of this and has a safe working load of 490 kg and a maximum patient weight of 440 kg. The bed has a width expandable mattress platform which expands from 920 mm (36") to 1220 mm (48"). This is important, as the size and shape of a bariatric patient can present as much of a challenge as weight in providing compassionate and dignified care to these patients.

Hoists

These are designed to assist or move a patient from bed to chair, for example. These work in conjunction with a sling that will support the patient. You must have training and be competent in the use of the hoist and sling before using them. There are certain legal requirements you must comply with before using the hoist and the sling, such as ensuring that the patient is within the safe working load of both the hoist and sling and that the equipment has been checked/serviced by a competent person in the past 6 months (see earlier section on Lifting Operations and Lifting Equipment Regulations in Legal Aspects).

> **❗ HOTSPOT**
>
> Before using any piece of equipment, you must always ensure you know how to use it.

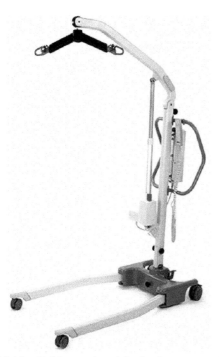

Fig. 18.8 Mobile Hoist: used mainly in the community (Joerns Healthcare UK).

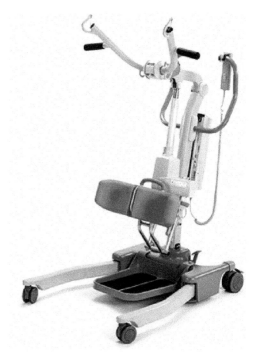

Fig. 18.9 Compact Standing Hoist (Joerns Healthcare UK) (Photo: Guldmann A/S).

There are many types of hoists that you will see in practice. Here are just a few common examples.

Mobile passive hoists. These are sometimes referred to as full body hoists. They will take the full weight of the patient and are moved by the handlers. These come with varying safe working loads ranging from small community hoists (typical SWL 150–200 kg; Fig. 18.8) to hospital hoists (typical SWL 190 kg–227 kg) to bariatric hoists up to 320 kg.

Standing hoists. These assist the patient into a standing position from sitting either as a therapeutic handling technique or to assist the patient in personal care. These can be small and compact for use in the community (Fig. 18.9) or larger and multifunctional for a hospital or rehabilitation facility (Fig. 18.10).

Ceiling tracking and gantry hoists. These are often seen in residential facilities or in people's homes. They are fixed in place either to the ceiling or on a gantry system that is place over the patient's bed and chair/wheelchair/commode (Figs 18.11 and 18.12). These can be used by one handler after a comprehensive risk assessment has been carried out and the handler has sufficient knowledge and skills to operate the hoist safely.

Slings

There are a wide range of slings available that are designed to meet the handling needs of the most complex patient.

Slings are attached to the hoist either by a loop system (Fig. 18.13) or a clip system (Fig. 18.14).

These are NOT interchangeable and loop slings can only be used with hoists with a spreader bar that takes loop slings

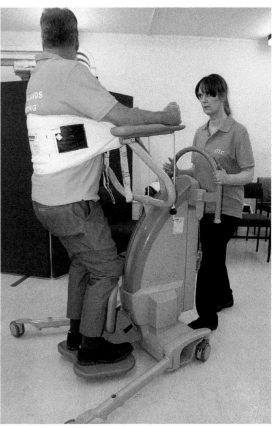

Fig. 18.10 Larger Acute Hospital Standing Hoist.

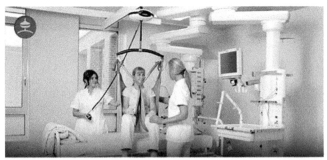

Fig. 18.11 Ceiling Tracking Hoist (Winncare Nordic, Taarnborgvej 12C, 4220 Korsoer, Denmark +45 70 27 37 20. http://winncare.com).

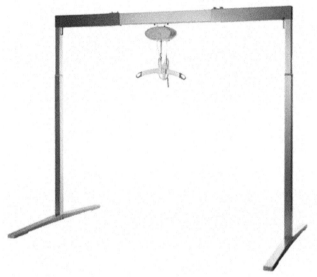

Fig. 18.12 Gantry Hoist (Photo: Guldmann A/S).

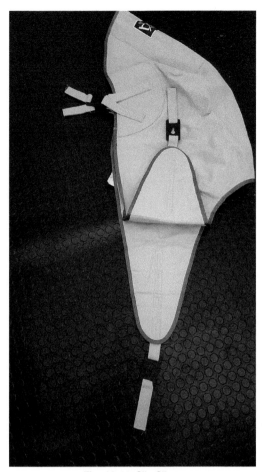

Fig. 18.14 Clip Sling.

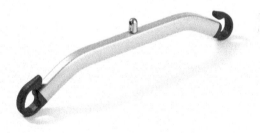

Fig. 18.15 Loop Sling Spreader Bar (Etac R82, Unit D4A, Coombswood Business Park East, Coombswood Way, Halesowen, West Midlands, B62 8BH, 0121 561 2222. enquiries@etac.uk.R82.com www.etac.com/uk).

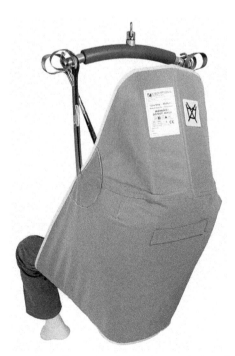

Fig. 18.13 Loop Sling (Reproduced with the permission of Cromptons Healthcare by MIP, MIP (UK) Ltd. http://www.cromptons.co.uk).

(Fig. 18.15) and clip slings can only be used with hoists that have a spreader bar that can accommodate clips (Fig. 18.16).

The other broad categories of slings are disposable slings, largely used in hospitals for infection control purposes. These are thrown away when the sling is soiled, or the patient is discharged. The other type of sling is washable and is more commonly used in the community. These must be washed in accordance with the manufacturer's instructions, which will be attached to the sling. Failure to do this can severely damage the sling and make it unsafe for use.

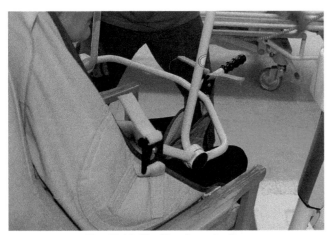

Fig. 18.16 Clip Sling Spreader Bar.

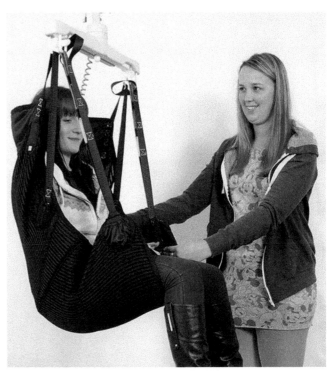

Fig. 18.17 In-situ or All-day Sling (Care and Independence).

Specialist slings

There are a large number of specialist slings available. The most important thing is not to attempt to use a sling that you are unfamiliar with. Examples of specialist slings would be all day or in-situ slings (Fig. 18.17).

Unlike conventional slings, these are designed to be left under the patient for lengthy periods of time, as they do not have ridges and allow the air to flow around the patient. Another more common specialist sling is an amputee sling. These are designed for patients who have a thigh or above knee amputation and can be used for single or double amputees.

Non-mechanical standing and raising aids

These are pieces of equipment that assist the patient to stand but require the patient to have some ability to cooperate. They must have some strength in their legs and arms to enable them to use the equipment. An example of these is the rota stand (Fig. 18.18), which can pivot a patient from a bed to a chair.

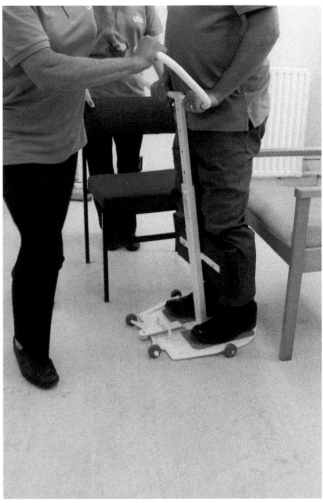

Fig. 18.18 Rota Stand.

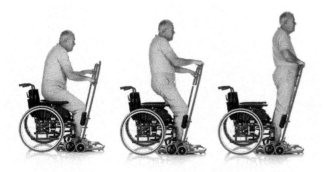

Fig. 18.19 Romedic Re-turn (Handicare UK).

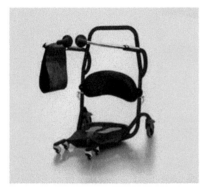

Fig. 18.20 Cricket II (from the Helping Hand Company).

This must not be used to move a patient from A to B; it is purely a pivot transfer. A more sophisticated version of this is a Re-turn (Fig. 18.19). This not only turns, but allows the patient to be moved a short distance.

There are also non-mechanical standing and raising aids that are designed to transport the patient from one area to another, for example from chair to toilet. Examples of these are the Sara Stedy and the Cricket (Fig. 18.20).

Slide sheets

There are broadly two different types of slide sheets.
- Roller or tubular slide sheets. These are made in a continuous roll.
- Flat slide sheets. These are used in pairs and one is placed on top of the other.

The purpose of these slide sheets is to move the patient up and down the bed or side to side in bed or to turn the patient on their side. They are placed under the patient and provide a low friction surface that enables the patient to be easily moved without causing any damage to their skin.

It is essential that you have face-to-face moving and handling training to use this type of equipment in order to use the slide sheets effectively without causing damage to the patient, yourself or your colleagues.

PRACTICAL MOVING AND HANDLING TECHNIQUES

These, plus some others, will all be covered in your practical moving and handling session during your course. This section is to act as a reminder for you and cannot replace face-to-face training where your practice can be assessed, and feedback given.

Load handling, pushing and pulling

You should always assess the load to be moved, a box for example, before moving it (see earlier section on Risk Assessment). Do not lift something that is too heavy. The Manual Handling Operations Regulations 1992 gives guidance on the maximum loads that men and women can lift before a risk assessment is necessary. This looks at the position of the load in relation to the handler (Fig. 18.21).

When pushing something, for example a bed or a wheelchair, keep as close to the object as possible. If it is a bed, ensure it is the correct height that enables you to maintain an upright posture. All hospital beds have a free-wheel and steer option which allows you to control the bed efficiently; make sure you know how to use this. It is preferable to push rather than pull.

Assisting a patient from a chair into a standing position

Firstly, an assessment has to be carried out with the patient to determine if it is safe to stand the patient from the chair. This could either be with verbal instructions, assistance of one or two handlers or using equipment, such as a standing hoist.

The assessment of the patient should always include:
- The strength in their legs, which will include range of movement.
- The strength of their arms. This is necessary to ensure that they can push themselves up from the chair.
- That they have some core strength and balance. This can often be assessed when asking the patient if they can move to the front of the chair in preparation to stand.
- The patient's cognitive state, e.g., can they understand and follow instructions.
- That their level of pain has been assessed and appropriate analgesia given before the technique is instituted.

The following example covers standing a patient up from the chair with two handlers. Only proceed once the assessment has been carried out and it is deemed safe. That is, that the patient's consent has been obtained and they are ready to move, and you and your colleague are competent to carry out this technique.

The handlers should stand either side of the patient's chair, facing the same way as the patient with their inside leg back and their outside leg forward in a walk stance position. Their arms next to the patient should be crossed at the patient's back, with their hands just above the belt line; the handlers' outer hands should be in front of the patient's shoulders. (Figs 18.22 and 18.23).

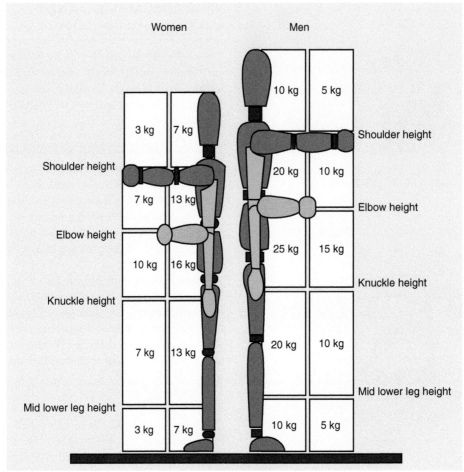

Fig. 18.21 Numerical Guidance. (Manual Handling Operations Regulations 1992).

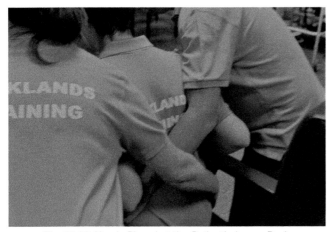

Fig. 18.22 Hands Placed at the Patient's Lower Back.

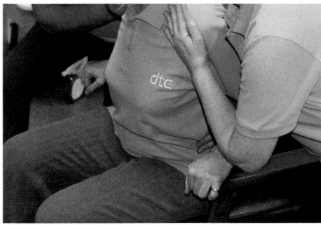

Fig. 18.23 Hands Placed at the Front of the Patient's Shoulders.

The handlers should adopt a walk stance position either side of the patient's chair and, using a weight transfer technique, *assist* the patient to stand. At the same time, the patient should be encouraged to push up with their arms, move their head forward until their 'nose is over their toes' and push up with their legs. Instructions, such as 'Ready, Steady, Stand' will help the handlers and the patient to be coordinated.

Once the patient has stood up, then it is important that the handler moves close to their side and offers them their hand in a 'palm to palm grip' with thumbs tucked in (Fig. 18.24).

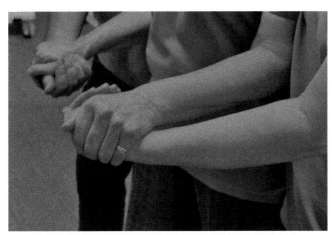

Fig. 18.24 Handhold with Patient with Thumbs Tucked In.

Alternatively, the patient may be handed a walking frame. This must only be done when the patient has stood safely. They must not use the walking frame as a standing aid.

If you are then walking the patient, carry out a few checks, such as asking them to take a few steps on the spot before they set off.

Moving a person in bed

As an NA, moving patients in bed is one of the most common patient-handling manoeuvres you will carry out. Here are a few key points that you should adhere to prior to the moving the patient.

- Carry out an on-the-spot risk assessment to ascertain the patient's ability.
- Ensure that the bed is at a correct height so that you can avoid overstretching.
- If working with another handler who is at the opposite side of the bed, ensure that you only work on your side of the bed, i.e., work within the 50% rule. Do not stretch over to the other side of the bed unless it is absolutely essential.
- If you require equipment, ensure that it is at hand, in good working order, checked according to any relevant legislation, e.g., LOLER, and ensure that you are competent to use it.

Use of a mobile passive hoist

The most common type of hoist in use is the mobile passive hoist. You will need comprehensive face-to-face training before you can use a hoist. In all but the most exceptional circumstances, there must always be two people to operate a mobile passive hoist.

Principles of the safe use of a mobile passive hoist and sling:

1. Check the risk assessment/handling plan if you are unfamiliar with the patient.
2. Assess the patient prior to using the hoist. Is the handling plan still valid?
3. Always select the appropriate hoist, sling and attachments for the task in hand.
4. Check the sling.
   a. Is it clean and in good condition?
   b. Has it been checked in the past 6 months by a competent person?
   c. Is there any loose stitching?
   d. If it is a sling with loop attachments, are the straps frayed?
   e. If the sling is a type with plastic clips, are there any cracks in the plastic?
   f. Can you read the label with the SWL and other information on it?
   g. If the sling is disposable, is it still fit for purpose?

If there is a problem with any of the <u>above</u>, then the sling must not be used.

5. Check the hoist.
   a. When was it last serviced/checked?
      Under the Lifting Operations and Lifting Equipment Regulations (LOLER, 1998), hoists must be serviced every year and checked every 6 months by a competent person.
   b. Has the battery been fully charged?
      To ensure that this happens there should be a protocol/procedure outlining a system that guarantees that the batteries always remain charged.
   c. Are the wheels moving freely?
   d. Is the emergency lower working correctly?
   e. Does the emergency stop work?
6. Check the lifting capacity of the hoist. Does it match the weight of the patient? *If there is any discrepancy, do not use the hoist and seek advice.*
7. Explain the lift to the patient and any assisting handlers.
8. Prepare the handling area. A great deal of room is necessary to operate a mobile hoist. If you are unfamiliar with the patient and/or hoist, practise the manoeuvre prior to lifting the patient, to ensure that there is sufficient space.
9. Insert the sling ensuring that the patient is in the centre of the sling; make sure that the sling is correctly positioned and free of creases. You will normally need a second person to assist you in carrying out this task.
10. If you have difficulty in inserting the sling you may have to use slide sheets to help you. Are you competent to do this?
11. Check your posture.
12. Attach the hoist to the sling correctly. If in doubt, ask advice.
13. Explain the procedure to the patient again. Reassure them.
14. Ensure that the brakes are OFF. Raise the patient up from the bed, chair or floor until the sling is taut and check that the loops/clips are in place and have not slipped off. Once you have checked this raise and transfer the patient smoothly and efficiently. Another handler must be available to prevent the sling from swinging or moving unduly.
15. Do not raise the patient higher than is necessary.
16. When pushing the hoist, be aware of your posture and avoid twisting. If you have to turn the hoist, it may be easier to move it from the side. Are you competent to carry out this procedure?
17. Push the hoist the shortest possible distance and remember a hoist *is not for transporting patients from A to B*. Use a wheelchair to move someone rather than the hoist.
18. Minimize the amount of time that the patient is in the sling. Comfort is of prime consideration.

19. Ensure that the patient is correctly positioned in the new location to prevent further moving and handling when the sling has been removed.
20. Remove the sling carefully to avoid damaging the patient's skin. Check their skin. Check your posture.
21. Pack away all equipment safely.
22. If the hoist is not being used immediately afterwards, does it need to go on charge?
23. Do not use a hoist that you are unfamiliar with; if in doubt, seek advice.

NB. This is *general* guidance on the use of a mobile hoist. Each manoeuvre is different and will need a suitable and sufficient assessment before hoisting is carried out.

REFLECTION 18.1

Where in the organization where you are working would you find the protocols and procedures that are related the various pieces of manual handing equipment?

WORKING WITH BARIATRIC (PLUS SIZE) PATIENTS

There are an increasing number of patients who are deemed to be bariatric. It is generally accepted that a bariatric (plus size) patient is one who weighs over 159 kg (25 stone) or has a body mass index (BMI) of 30+ (Newcastle Hospitals NHS Trust, Moving and Handling of the Bariatric (Plus Size) Patient, 2015).

When working with a bariatric patient, it is often necessary to access specialist moving and handling equipment that has a higher SWL than conventional equipment. Examples include beds, chairs, commodes, hoists and slings. If these are not immediately available, there are a number of specialist bariatric equipment companies who will hire out equipment and can usually deliver in a number of hours. The equipment does take up more space and therefore part of your risk assessment is to ensure that the environment is suitable. For example, in a hospital environment, it may be necessary to use two bed spaces.

For more information, see the case study on assessing a bariatric patient in MacGregor, 2016.

MOVING AND HANDLING IN THE COMMUNITY

Moving and handling in the community presents its own challenges. The main differences are outlined here.
- If you are working in a patient's home, then you will need to negotiate with them and their family with regard to the use of equipment, the number of handlers or any other care handling needs that might affect the way that they want their home to be organized. However, this is your place of work and it is important to have systems that do not put you or the patient at risk. There is also the Health and Safety at Work

Act to consider. This states that you are responsible for your own health and safety and that of your colleagues.
- You could, as a qualified NA, be providing single-handed care. This will involve you working on your own and using more specialized moving and handling equipment. Therefore, you will need to have the competence to use these pieces of equipment. In addition, you will need to be aware of the lone worker policies and protocols of your employing organization.
- Some procedures in the community, such as leg ulcer dressings, whether carried out in the patient's home or in a community clinic, can present a number of postural challenges for the NA due to working at a low level. It is important that this is rigorously assessed by a competent person in order that the risk is reduced to the lowest reasonably practicable level. This may involve making a number of changes in a patient's home, and if this is not an acceptable option for the patient, then they may have to attend a community clinic to have their leg ulcers dressed. In a clinic there should be a more ergonomically designed environment with more space and variable-height couches.

REFLECTION 18.2

Think about your own home. How might you feel if you had to have specialist moving and handling equipment installed? Do you think this might have an impact on how you might enjoy a 'homely' environment? How might you help to promote 'normality' in the home setting?

COMMUNITIES OF CARE
Working with the Elderly

This group of patients tends to have the most complex handling issues. One aspect that may have to be addressed is if the patient has some degree of dementia. This may present itself in a behavioural way, for instance, if the patient is out of their usual environment, they may be fearful, anxious and disorientated. You will need to assess these patients carefully and determine if equipment, such as a hoist, causes too much anxiety for the patient. If this is the case, it may be necessary to introduce another system of handling.

COMMUNITIES OF CARE
Working with Children

It may not seem immediately apparent that children can present challenges with regard to moving and handling, but the following need to be considered:
- Children can be defined in health and social care as up to 16 years of age. In the case of children with complex needs, this may go up to 19 years of age. This means that you can be working with large young adults.
- Many children who require moving and handling have complex needs, such as those with cerebral palsy, muscular dystrophy or a number of other deteriorating or life-limiting conditions. These children need the handler to have a high level of skill in moving and handling to meet their needs in a safe and dignified way, at the same time acknowledging the needs of not only them, but of their parents and siblings.

CASE STUDY 18.1 Community

Mrs Smith is 90 years old. She is physically very frail and arthritic and her mobility is poor. She is looked after by her 94-year-old husband, who is finding it increasingly difficult to manage but does not want to have home carers coming into the house as it will invade their privacy.

The biggest problem is when Mrs Smith gets up in the morning as she is very short in stature and, with her arthritis, this is a long and painful process for both her and her husband.

Name two things, short-term, that might help make this moving and handling task better for both of them.

Possible answers:

1. A low-level bed may enable Mrs Smith to get out of bed more easily as her feet would more easily reach the floor.
2. Having Mrs Smith's analgesia and anti-inflammatory medication reviewed may help not only in type and dosage, but also in timing (e.g., half an hour before getting up).

CASE STUDY 18.2 Residential Home

Mr Sawatzky is 79 years old and has been a resident of the home for 2 years. His mobility fluctuates, and he is a keen to maintain as much of his independence as possible.

You have been asked to ensure that you take him for a short walk at least twice in the course of the morning. You do not know him too well so you want to assess his mobility before you take him for a walk.

What five areas would you want to assess before standing Mr Sawatzky up to walk?

Possible answers:

1. The strength in his legs, including the range of movement
2. The strength in his arms
3. His core strength when sitting at the front of the chair
4. His cognitive state, e.g., can he understand and follow instructions?
5. His level of pain, if any, and if it is sufficiently well controlled before he goes for a walk

For further reading on this topic see Ruszala and Alexander (2015).

LOOKING BACK, FEEDING FORWARD

Patients who the NA offers care to often have very complex and varying needs. The role of the NA is to respond to those needs in an effective manner whilst ensuring compassion and dignity.

No one should routinely manually lift patients. There are other methods available for manual handling, including hoists, sliding aids, electric profiling beds and other specialized equipment. Patient manual handling should only continue in those instances that do not involve lifting most or all a patient's weight. This chapter has provided insight into some of the specialized equipment that the NA is likely to use in hospital and community settings.

The Health and Safety Executive, the body responsible for the encouragement, regulation and enforcement of workplace health, safety and welfare, advise a balanced approach to managing the risks from patient handling. There are a number regulations and laws in place to ensure the safety not only of these we offer care to, but also to those who provide that care. Employers are legally obliged to provide a safe working environment for their staff. This chapter has gone some way to providing an overview of the most important laws and regulations that impact on safe moving and handing.

An emphasis has been put on the importance of ensuring an assessment of needs is carried out and, where appropriate, an assessment of risk is undertaken and documented in the patient's individual handling plan. This is usually found in the nursing assessment and care plan documentation. The safety of the patient is paramount and they are indeed at the heart of all that is done. As part of their multi-faceted role, the NA must ensure that they are also safe, as well as ensuring the safety of those they work with and care for.

REFERENCES

Alexander, P., Johnson, C., 2011. Moving and Handling of Children. National Back Exchange, Towcester.

MacGregor, H., 2016. Moving and Handling Patients at a Glance. Wiley Blackwell.

Ruszala, S., Alexander, P., 2015. Moving and Handling in the Community and Residential Care. National Back Exchange, Towcester.

Waugh, A., Grant, A., 2018. Ross and Wilson Anatomy and Physiology in Health and Illness, thirteenth ed. Elsevier, Edinburgh.

Regulations, Guidance and Resources

Backcare

www.backcare.org.uk.

Health and Safety at Work Act 1974.

www.hse.gov.uk/legisation/hswa.htm.

Human Rights Act 1998 Article 3.

https://www.equalityhumanrights.com/en/human-rights-act/article-3-freedom-torture-and-inhuman-or-degrading-treatment.

Human Rights Act 1998 Article 8.

https://www.equalityhumanrights.com/en/human-rights-act/article-8-respect-your-private-and-family-life.

LOLER.

http://www.hse.gov.uk/work-equipment-machinery/loler.htm.

Management of Health and Safety at Work Regulations (MHSW) 1999.

Manual Handling Operations Regulations (MHOR), 1992. L23 (4th Edition, 2016). HSE, London.

http://www.legislation.gov.uk/uksi/1999/3242/contents/made.

Manual Handling Operations Regulations 1992 (as amended).
    L23. 2002.
www.hse.gov.uk/pubns/books/123.htm.
PUWER.
http://www.hse.gov.uk/work-equipment-machinery/puwer.htm.
RIDDOR 2013.
http://www.hse.gov.uk/pubns/indg453.pdf.

The Social Security (Claims and Payments) Regulations 1979.
http://www.legislation.gov.uk/uksi/1979/628/contents/made.
Newcastle Hospitals NHS Trust, 2015. Moving and Handling of the
    Bariatric (Plus Size) Patient.
www.newcastle-hospitals.org.uk/
    MovingandHandlingoftheBariatricPatient201507.pdf.

First Aid

Sigurd Haveland

OBJECTIVES

By the end of this chapter the reader will be able to:
1. Have an awareness of the ethics relevant to the first aider, as well as the relevant guidelines associated with first aid
2. Assess an incident by applying principles of scene safety
3. Describe the DR<C>ABCDE framework
4. Understand the structured primary and secondary survey approach
5. Recognize and administer first aid to those in need
6. Appreciate the principles behind effective CPR and rescue breaths

KEY WORDS

Airway	Resuscitation	Preservation
Assessment	Safety	Prevention
Ventilation	Consent	
Circulation	Skills	

CHAPTER AIM

The aim of this chapter is to provide the reader with an understanding of the principles underpinning first aid procedures.

SELF TEST

1. What is the chain of survival?
2. List the 4 Ps.
3. Why is scene safety and a 360-degree appraisal important?
4. What is the 'Golden Hour'?
5. What is the AVPU scale?
6. How would you recognize peripheral cyanosis?
7. What steps should be taken if you witness an acid attack?
8. What is a 'rescue breath'?
9. Name the types/classifications of wounds.
10. Where (location) do most burn accidents happen?

INTRODUCTION

It is not possible in a chapter of this size to address every aspect of first aid. Instead, it aims to provide the reader with insight and understanding of the key/salient issues that need to be given consideration when providing care as a first aider. Further understanding can be gained by accessing both human and material resources.

There is no legal duty for the Nursing Associate (NA) to volunteer help in an emergency situation. The legal duty of care normally only arises when a practitioner has assumed some responsibility for the care of the person concerned. As a result of this, if an NA is at a road traffic accident, they do not have a legal duty of care to offer aid to any person who is injured in the accident (Royal College of Nursing, 2017). Many people incorrectly believe that NAs and nurses have first aid training that would help the injured person; however, this is not always the case.

Every year many people could have been saved from death due to injuries and illnesses if adequate and timely assistance had been provided. For the chain of survival to work, it is essential that the first link, the witness of an accident, engages and activates the chain of survival. It must be remembered that even a child, when equipped with simple first aid skills and a degree of self-confidence, has the potential to be this first link and save a life.

The chain of survival

Maximizing the chances of surviving a cardiac arrest requires following a sequence:
1. Immediate recognition of cardiac arrest and calling for help.
2. Prompt initiation of cardiopulmonary resuscitation.
3. Performing defibrillation as soon as possible.
4. Optimal post resuscitation care.

Relevant guidelines

- Resuscitation Council (UK) (2015)
- European Resuscitation Council (ERC) (2015)

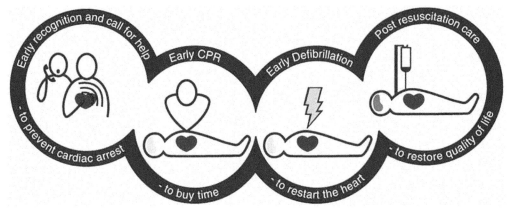

Fig. 19.1 Chain of Survival (Reproduced with the kind permission of the Resuscitation Council (UK). https://www.resus.org.uk/resuscitation-guidelines/adultbasic-life-support-and-automated-external-defibrillation/).

TABLE 19.1	Forms of Consent
Types of consent	**Description**
Expressed consent	On informing, either verbally or by writing, the casualty of your intentions and reasoning, they clearly understand and express consent (permission to treat)
Implied consent	If the casualty is unconscious or lacks mental capacity (alert, orientated and coherent) to give consent, you can assume they would ask for assistance and give consent, so you may start treatment
If the casualty cannot verbally communicate or write due to a language barrier or deafness, they may also imply consent or non-consent by expressions of body language and/or other nonverbal cues.	

- International Liaison Committee on Resuscitation (ILCOR) (2015)
- International Federation of Red Cross and Red Crescent Societies (2016).

Although in its most basic form, first aid can be perceived as merely the initial assistance given to a casualty, its intervention must not be underestimated, since in serious injuries or illnesses, it can mitigate long-term disabilities and reverse a process that might have resulted in a fatal outcome. Elementary first aid has four goals or '4 Ps':

- **Preserve life** – stopping the progression of illness or injury, which left untreated, may result in death
- **Prevent** – further illness or injury form deteriorating and minimize future disability
- **Promote recovery** – try to assist the casualty's healing mechanisms
- **Protect the unconscious** – position and, if necessary move the unconscious casualty to prevent aspiration, hypo/hyperthermia or other environmental injuries.

AT THE SCENE

Approaching and sizing up the scene

Sizing up the scene or knowing what is going on around you is often termed 'situational awareness'. This requires a 360-degree appraisal to avoid any surprise and is summed using the acronym **SCENE:**

- **S** – Safety: perform a dynamic risk assessment; are there any dangers now or any that could develop during the progression of the incident?
- **C** – Cause: including mechanism of injury. Compare and contrast events leading to the incident with your casualty's findings, if conscious and coherent.
- **E** – Environment: consider access and egress for others who may need to come to assist. Consider climatic conditions and time of day.
- **N** – Number: is there more than one casualty?
- **E** – Extra resources required: make a prompt decision whether the situation requires additional resources: ambulance, fire, police and/or coastguard.

Scene safety must include minimizing the risk of infection to the first aider, as well as to the casualty, by considering body-substance isolation. Minimum personal protective equipment may include a pair of clinical gloves and a facemask used as a barrier for mouth-to-mouth ventilation (see Chapter 16 for infection control).

The term 'Golden Hour' is a fundamental aspect of situational awareness and serves as a time guide for those attending a time-critical casualty with significant injury, prompting clinicians, as well as first aiders, that ideally this casualty should be in the operating theatre within the hour.

Consent

As a first aider, you must not assume that a casualty who needs help actually wants it. Before caring for a casualty, you must ask for and receive permission, or using the medical term, consent. If the casualty is able to think clearly and make a decision and declines consent, even a touch could qualify as physical assault or battery.

Consent comes in two forms expressed (informed) and implied (Table 19.1).

The first aider should not start treatment if an adult, who is coherent and able to decide, refuses the offer of treatment. The first aider only has the casualty's consent to treat them for a condition that affects their immediate health and should not provide any treatment that falls outside of their competency or skill-set.

The UK Resuscitation Council updates its guidelines every 5 years. Its last update was published in 2015. The European Resuscitation Council (ERC) and the International Liaison Committee on Resuscitation (ILCOR) also publish guidelines based on worldwide expert consensus of best practice from international evidence-based reviews. The ERC published guidelines specific for first aid for the first time in 2015.

Approaching the casualty
The primary survey
The primary survey makes reference to a structured approach for the initial management of an injured person. Its purpose is to systematically identify and then treat within the skill-set of the first aider any immediately or potentially life-threatening condition.

The DR<C>ABCDE framework reminds the first aider, as well as other pre-hospital care professionals, how to conduct an approach in a systematic manner. The acronym stands for:
- **D** – Danger – Apply SCENE
- **R** – Response
- **<C>** – catastrophic haemorrhage or bleeding (the rational for prioritizing <C> over A is that shock from blood volume loss secondary to uncontrolled severe bleeding is the most common shock scenario seen in pre-hospital practice and death from severe blood loss can occur in less than 5 minutes)
- **A** – Airway (with cervical spine control)
- **B** – Breathing
- **C** – Circulation
- **D** – Disability (related to consciousness)
  - o Consider Alert, Voice, Pain, Unresponsive (AVPU)
  - o Assess pupil size and reaction to light
  - o Unusual posturing
  - o Assess tone arms and legs
  - o Blood sugar – if suspected to be low or able to measure with equipment
- **E** – Exposure (secondary survey, discussed later in this chapter)

At the end of the primary survey, the patient should be in a stable condition, only baseline observations should have been performed.

> ⚠ **HOTSPOT**
>
> Treat and reassess at each stage of <C>ABCDE – do not move to next stage unless satisfied.

Response
The AVPU scale
The AVPU scale is a simple assessment tool to swiftly quantify and record a person's level of consciousness. It is also an indication of when to call the emergency medical services; if the person is not alert, this option should be considered.

The acronym refers to four possible situations: Alert, responsive to Voice, responsive to Pain and Unresponsive (Table 19.2).

Airway
Airway management is best performed applying a stepwise approach. A basic manoeuvre may be all that is required to enable adequate oxygenation and ventilation.

TABLE 19.2   AVPU: Looking at Each Level Closer

A Alert	The patient is fully awake and has normal motor power for that patient. However, the patient may not necessarily be fully coherent or orientated. Alertness can be further examined by noting the patient's orientation to Time, Person, Place and Events.
V Voice	The patient is prompted to respond by voice stimuli. This can be in subtle forms, such as purposeful movement, any purposeful sound (a moan, a grunt), a purposeful eye movement or motor movement, such as moving a limb or finger.
P Pain	The patient only responds to pain stimuli. Recognized sites for physical stimulation are applying pressure to the fingertips, pinching the trapezius, applying pressure to the supraorbital notch. Note: a paraplegic patient will not be able to feel any stimuli below the neck.
U Unresponsive	The patient not responding to voice or pain stimuli can be considered as unconscious.

> **CRITICAL AWARENESS**
>
> Current literature tells us that basic airway manoeuvres are often poorly performed or neglected. It must be reiterated that the basic and most simple things normally are the interventions with the greatest impact on the casualty's outcome.

Airway patency poses a fundamental question: is air flowing in and out of the lungs, hence is the casualty ventilating and oxygenating adequately? The quickest method of checking a patent airway is by talking to the casualty. A speaking patient with a normal sounding voice tells us their airway is patent and there are no obstructions. Simultaneously, eliciting a verbal response to a verbal stimulus also assesses the casualty's mentation or responsiveness.

The unresponsive casualty
Opening the airway of the unresponsive casualty
This requires the first aider to either employ the head-tilt/chin-lift manoeuvre or the jaw-thrust manoeuvre. The jaw-thrust manoeuvre is chiefly employed, but not limited to, managing a casualty with a high index of suspicion for a cervical spine injury.

> ⚠ **HOTSPOT**
>
> A patent with a cervical spine (neck) injury is vulnerable to spinal cord damage leading to permanent impairment of motor and sensory functions. If the respiratory muscles are affected, the patient may die.

If a patient is suspected of having a cervical spine injury and a jaw-thrust airway manoeuvre is required, the quickest way to protect the cervical spine is for someone to hold the patient's head and neck in a neutral position (without flex or extension) while another assesses <C> ABC.

To perform the head-tilt/chin-lift manoeuvre, approach the patient from the side and place the palm of one hand on the patient's forehead. Then push down gently, rolling the patient's head towards the top. Then, using the fingers of your free hand lightly lift the chin, which pulls soft tissue from the back of the upper airway, particularly the tongue (Fig. 19.2).

The jaw thrust requires more force to execute. The first aider should do the following:

1. Approach the supine casualty from behind the head, so that the provider is facing down the body. Kneel and place each hand with thumbs pointing up on either side of the casualty's face.
2. Steadily support the head in the neutral position (aligning the head, neck and spine). The thumbs or the thenars are then placed on the casualty's cheekbone, allowing the thumbs to act as pivot points so that the index and middle finger levers the jawbone from the angles of the mandible.
3. Taking care to not to tilt the neck, the provider gently pulls and draws up anteriorly (without extending neck), displacing jaw, lifting tongue and improving airway patency (Fig. 19.3).

> **! HOTSPOT**
>
> The term agonal gasps, also known as agonal breathing is associated with spasmodic, simultaneous movements of the diaphragm and muscles in the jaw, which a fish trying to breath out of water and is characterized by irregular, shallow, abrupt gasps. This phenomenon is commonly seen during a medical emergency, such as cardiac arrest, when the respiratory centre begins to be deprived of oxygen-rich blood. During the first minutes after a cardiac arrest up to 40% of victims, manifest agonal gasps. Remember this is NOT considered normal breathing and therefore it is an indication to commence cardiorespiratory resuscitation. https://www.resus.org.uk/resuscitation-guidelines/adult-basic-life-support-and-automated-external-defibrillation/.

Checking for breathing

Following the head-tilt/chin-lift, determining whether there is breathing should not take more than 10 seconds and is easily done by following a stepwise approach:

- Look
- Listen
- Feel.

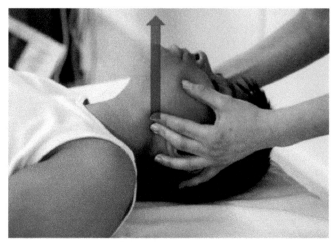

Fig. 19.3 Jaw-thrust.

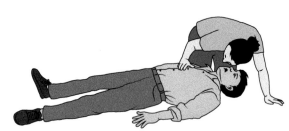

Fig. 19.4 Looking at and feeling the chest simultaneously can detect if there is any chest movement.

Checking for breathing is best done by leaning over the casualty with your cheek above the casualty's mouth, looking down at the chest with one hand on the chest

- **Look** – for foreign bodies in the mouth and remove obvious objects, dentures, lose teeth), scan for obvious deformities, swelling, burns or trauma to the mouth, face or front of the neck.
- **Listen** – for stridor, gurgling or snoring. The patient with an altered level of consciousness or unconscious gurgling indicates secretions or fluid (e.g., vomit) in the upper airway. Snoring indicates partial obstruction, normally as a result of the pharynx becoming partially obstructed due to loss of tone of the tongue or by the soft palate.
- **Feel** – with your cheeks for air movement in and out of mouth and with one hand for chest expansion, symmetry of chest wall and the respiratory pattern.

See Fig. 19.4.

If the casualty is breathing or starts to breathe following airway positioning, then the casualty should be placed in the recovery position and monitored until help arrives.

When assisting a casualty who has an altered level of consciousness or an unconscious casualty who is supine and you lack airway management equipment (such as suction) and/or specialized techniques (such as airway adjuncts) to manage the airway, neither the head-tilt/chin-lift nor the jaw thrust (or a combination of these) will prevent fluids or solids (blood, secretions, vomitus) from obstructing the airway. In this case, the casualty should be moved into the recovery position, also known as the safe airway position, drainage position, left lateral recumbent or the three-quarter prone.

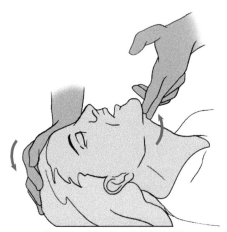

Fig. 19.2 The Head-tilt/Chin-lift.

Any patient experiencing an altered level of consciousness or unconscious needs to be moved into the recovery position.

Moving the casualty

To move the casualty from a supine position to the recovery position:
- Kneel at casualty's waist level.
- Grasp casualty's nearest hand and place the arm at right angles to the casualty's body.
- Lift the casualty's furthest leg from behind knee, until the foot is flat on floor.
- Using the casualty's same knee as lever, pull and flip the casualty onto their side.
- Place the casualty's head against their opposite side's hand, palms down against casualty's cheek.
- Ensure airway is patent by adjusting head using an adapted head-tilt/chin-lift.

Breathing

Breathing has two main functions:
1. To deliver, via the process of inhalation, air rich in oxygen to functional units of the lungs (alveoli) where gaseous exchange occurs and oxygen is diffused into the blood.
2. To remove carbon dioxide, a by-product of internal respiration, from the blood into the alveoli to be exhaled into the atmosphere.

Quick breathing assessment

A first aider should be observant of the following signs when assessing the efficiency of breathing:
- Is breathing too fast (higher than 29 breaths per minute) or too slow (lower than 9 breaths per minute)?
- Are breaths too shallow or deep?
- Are breath sounds absent or diminished?
- Are there any abnormal sounds, such as grunting, snoring, wheezing or stridor?
- Is there nasal flaring, use of respiratory accessory muscles or pursed lips?
- Is the patient in a tripod position or refusing to lie down?
- Is the patient cyanotic or listless?

Observe chest movement for equal rise and fall. No movement or asymmetry (one side of the chest rises while the other is still), may indicate poor ventilation in that lung or no inspiration at all. If the chest is sucked-in and the abdomen moves out during attempted inspiration (see-saw movement), this may indicate an airway obstruction.

Remember that determining someone is not breathing should not take more than 10 seconds.

Ventilation and oxygenation

Ventilation and oxygenation are separate but linked physiological processes and very important concepts to understand to adequately manage a casualty in respiratory distress or arrest.

Ventilation

This is the mechanical process of moving air in and out of the lungs for gaseous exchange. Assessment by a first aider requires rigorous vigilance of clinical signs to qualitatively determine adequate ventilation.

The casualty's respiratory rate can be used to evaluate the adequacy of ventilation. A respiratory rate below 9 respirations per minute is defined as hypoventilation. A respiratory rate above 29 is defined as hyperventilation and may lead to blowing out excessive volumes of carbon dioxide. Breathing outside these boundaries for prolonged periods can result in hypoxia (low levels of oxygen) and will also affect blood homeostasis.

Oxygenation

This is the process of oxygen diffusing across the alveoli into the blood and being taken up by a haemoglobin molecule. This in turn transports oxygen to all cells of the body.

Signs and symptoms of hypoxia

- Confusion
- Fast heart rate
- Rapid breathing
- Shortness of breath
- Sweating
- Restlessness
- Headache
- Dizziness, light-headedness and/or fainting spells
- Lack of coordination
- Visual disturbances
- Peripheral or central cyanosis
- A sense of euphoria.

Airway positioning

This requires optimizing ventilation and oxygenation by positioning the casualty's airway. Having a fundamental understanding of where the airway axes lie for the optimal patent airway will provide the first aider with an important tool when managing ventilations (Fig. 19.5).

The chin of the unconscious supine casualty often drops forward, resulting in soft tissues of upper airway (particularly the tongue) collapsing or falling backwards and obstructing the airway. Basic airway manoeuvres are best practised with a focus on optimizing head position with the head tilt/chin-lift and/or the two-handed jaw thrust. These manoeuvres will open most airways with no further action needed.

Circulation

In the context of first aid, circulation refers to recognizing signs of hypoxia and physiological shock, managing bleeding,

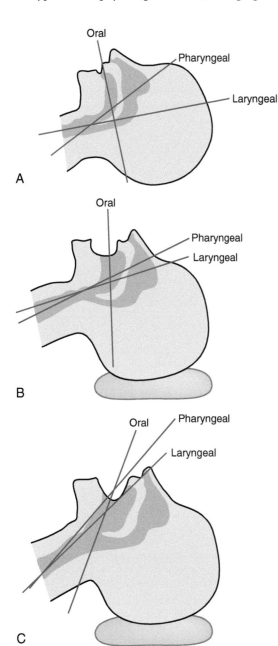

Fig. 19.5 Airway Axis. (A) The three axes of the airway with the head in a neutral position. (B) The three axes with the head in the 'sniffing' position. (C) The three axes after extending the head.

being able to locate palpable pulses and assisting circulation of blood.

Perfusion

In physiology, the process of perfusion is the process of oxygenated blood being delivered to cells and tissue.

Bleeding type

Arterial bleeding – this bleed is driven by direct pressure from the heart. Initially, under full pressure, the blood will pulsate and spurt with the heartbeat. As blood volume inside the body drops, a concomitant drop in pressure will result and bleeding will change from spurting to oozing. The blood will be bright red as it is well oxygenated.

Venous bleeding – a venous bleed has less pressure than an arterial bleed; the blood tends to gush or flow out. The blood will be dark red as it is poorly oxygenated.

Capillary bleeding – the bleed is limited to small blood vessels. It oozes out and generally leads to minor blood loss.

If the first aider observes any signs of severe or catastrophic bleeding <C> this must take priority over ABC.

> **! HOTSPOT**
>
> Serious venous bleeding must be considered almost as dangerous as serious arterial bleeding.

HAEMORRHAGING

Haemorrhaging is blood leaking from the vascular system. It can be:
- **External** (blood escaping from blood capillaries, veins and or arteries outside the body, through natural orifices – mouth, nose, ears, vagina, penis, anus – or through wounds).
- **Internal** (blood escaping from blood capillaries, veins and/ or arteries inside the body).

External blood loss: It is not always easy to assess the extent of blood volume lost since blood present on the ground is surface dependant. For instance, compare a patient who is on a marble floor against one on sandy ground.

Internal blood loss: Bleeding inside the body, for instance into a body cavity. It is concealed and thus not visible. Body cavities include:
- The chest or intrathoracic cavity
- The abdomen or intraabdominal cavity
- The pelvis
- Long bones (or the thigh where the femur is located).

Recognizing external bleeding
- Bleeding from an injury or a body opening, such as the mouth, nose or anus
- Vomiting blood

Recognizing internal bleeding
- Bruising
- A tender or swollen abdomen
- Shortened, swollen and deformed limbs (especially thighs).

- Cold, clammy skin
- Thirst
- Fractures
- Shock, indicated by a rapid, weak pulse, pallor, sweating, rapid breathing and decreased alertness

Body cavities

Knowledge of major body cavities is important to help the first aider appreciate potential spaces where internal blood loss may pool in trauma.

The skull

The skull or cranium, although a cavity, can be considered a vault since it has no potential to become a space where significant volumes of blood may collect leading to a concomitant decrease in blood volume. Traumatic brain injuries are beyond the scope of this chapter; suffice to mention that this type of injury complicates the dynamics of intracranial pressures, which may lead to fatal consequences.

The thorax

This is a bony case between the neck and the abdomen, enclosed by the clavicles, sternum, vertebrae and ribs and protecting vital organs, including the lungs and heart, and major vessels, and provides an anchorage for the respiratory muscles. Some important anatomical landmarks include the xiphoid process, the angle of Louis and the suprasternal notch.

The abdomen

The portion of the body that extends from the diaphragm to the pelvis. The abdomen embraces organs such as the stomach, intestines, spleen and urinary bladder.

The pelvis

The pelvic region is the area between the abdomen and the lower extremities, or legs. Its shape is imparted by a sturdy ring of bones, which also confers protection on the delicate organs of the abdominopelvic cavity.

Long bone

Another potential space for the accumulation of blood is the upper arm and upper leg when there is a femur shaft facture.

Nose bleed (epistaxis)

Epistaxis refers to blood flowing from one or both nostrils. Common courses include picking the nose, flying at high altitude, high blood pressure and strenuously blowing the nose. Any of these actions may rupture tiny blood vessels inside the nostrils.

Management of epistaxis

- Apply firm pressure, elevation and rest.
- The casualty needs to sit down with their head well forward and above heart level to ensure an effective airway and the continuation of breathing.
- Encourage the patient to apply firm pressure on the entire soft part of the nose releasing every 10 minutes (a swimming nose clip can be used instead of fingers).

- Most nosebleeds are minor and subside within a few minutes.
- Reassure.

If bleeding has stopped, then advise the person not to cough or sniff or blow their nose for a few hours as this may disrupt or dislodge the blood clot and bleeding may reoccur. If the nose bleed is related to a head injury or if bleeding continues after 30 minutes despite the above management, call emergency medical services.

Haemorrhagic/circulatory shock

Shock is a complex group of physiological abnormalities, which may be caused from a variety of illnesses and injuries. It is a life-threatening situation where the body does not have enough blood flow, leading to cells and tissue receiving inadequate supply of oxygen. If not recognized, understood and managed, circulatory shock can lead to multiple organ failure, including the brain, heart, liver and kidneys.

A first aider without equipment may be able to detect the signs and symptoms of stages 1 and 2 of shock:

Stage 1

Compensatory shock (also called compensated, or non-progressive shock): the body detects low perfusion and a number of compensatory mechanisms are activated. The person will not show significant outward signs and symptoms, although heart rate may increase, and extremities may be cool.

Stage 2

Decompensated shock (also called decompensated or progressive shock): compensatory mechanisms begin to fail and become incapable of maintaining adequate perfusion. The brain, which also relies on oxygen for is function, exhibits this by confusion, incoherence and disorientation.

Stage 3

Irreversible shock: constant low perfusion leads to a systematic shut down of vital organs and cell death. Its end point is death.

Shock

Shock is caused by three major dysfunctions occurring within the body:

- Cardiogenic shock: related to dysfunctions associated with the heart (for example, heart attack).
- Hypovolaemic shock: dysfunctions leading to a low total circulatory volume of blood (for example, severe blood loss).
- Septic shock: related to an overwhelming infection, generally through bacteria and their secretion of toxic chemicals (e.g., abdominal, lung or urinary infections).

Physiological shock is not to be confused with emotional shock.

Signs and symptoms of shock

- Mental status or behaviour – due to low perfusion to the brain: a progressive alteration in will be observed, including, but not limited to, altered level of consciousness apathy, restlessness, combativeness and agitation.

- Pulse – fast or very slow (more than 120 beats per minute or less than 40 beats per minute).
- Respiratory rate – high, above 29 breaths per minute.
- Skin – pale, clammy, cool, ashen skin, mottled skin.
- Other – nausea, vomiting, fainting enlarged pupils.

If shock is trauma related, do not forget the possibility of blunt trauma and potential internal bleeding into a body cavity/space.

Treatment for shock

If you suspect shock, or are in doubt, call emergency medical services.
- DR<C>ABCDE.
- If patient is not breathing after opening the airway, call for help and commence CPR.
- If patient is breathing and unconscious, turn them to recovery position and try to establish obvious cause.
- If breathing and conscious and following a secondary survey, consider laying casualty on their back and elevating their legs and feet slightly above heart level. If the casualty begins to vomit or bleed from the mouth turn them to recovery position.
- If you suspect an allergic reaction, follow steps under anaphylactic shock covered later in this chapter.
- Unless there are hazards, do not move patient.
- Keep patient warm and loosen any tight-fitting clothing.
- Reassure.

TRAUMA

Types of wounds

Laceration

This refers to an injury caused by tearing of the skin. If high forces are involved, this injury can incur damage to other tissues, including muscle, ligament, tendon, bone, blood vessels and nerves.

Abrasion

An injury caused by scraping against a rough surface. Although commonly a superficial injury with minor consequences, if extensive, these can be very painful and vulnerable to infection.

Avulsion

Also called degloving, avulsion refers to a partial or complete removal of the skin commonly following a violent accident where there are moving parts, which can also tear tissue beneath.

Puncture

A wound that pierces and penetrates the skin. The depth of penetration and damage to underlying tissues and organs depends on the length and penetration of the instrument that caused the puncture.

Contusion

This is a wound where the skin may be injured, but unbroken, and vessels beneath have been ruptured from a blunt-instrument blow.

Treating wounds

With all open wounds, there is a risk of infection, so wash your hands and use gloves (if you have any) to help prevent any infection passing between you and the casualty. If the wound is covered by the casualty's clothing, consider removing clothes as necessary to uncover the wound (do not forget to respect patient's dignity). If an object is protruding from the wound, do not to pull in out as it may be mitigating further bleeding by acting as a stopper. Management should include stabilizing the object and applying pressure around it using hands, dressing and/or clothing.

BURNS

CRITICAL AWARENESS

- The majority of burn accidents occur in the home.
- Burn accident statistics suggest that around three-quarters of all burn injuries in children are avoidable.
- In the European Union, burns and scalds are the fourth leading cause of injury death to children. Children under 5 years old experience the highest death rates.
- Young children in particular are more vulnerable to burn-related injury and death because their skin is thinner than adults' and they can experience serious deeper burns more quickly.
- It is thought that up to 1,900 injuries per year in the EU and approximately 40 fatalities per year are caused by children finding and playing with lighters.
- The leading cause of burn injury for children is scalding. Infants and the elderly are at the greatest risk of burn injury from scalding.
- In older adults, smoking and open flames are the key cause of burn injury.
- The risk of injury and death relative to exposure means that fireworks are one of the highest risk consumer products available.
- The way the body responds to severe burns may include a positive feedback inflammatory response and derangement of the coagulation cascade; this can be more damaging and life-threatening than the burn itself.

(European Child Safety Alliance, 2013; Glas, 2016; Nielsen, 2017).

This type of injury occurs when heat energy from external sources, is transferred to the skin and other tissues, raising its temperature and resulting in tissue damage and/or cell death. Thermal energy can be transferred by:
- Conduction
- Convection
- Radiation.

Types of burn

Different types of injury caused by heat energy:
- Thermal burn
- Chemical burn
- Radiation burn
- Electrical burn
- Electromagnetic energy burn.

Thermal burns

These occur when external heat sources that raise the temperature of the skin and tissues result in cell death or charring. Examples of heat sources include, for example, hot metals, scalding liquids, steam and flames.

Temperature

- Studies (e.g., Dewhirst et al., 2003) show surface temperatures of 44°C do not produce burns unless exposure time exceeds 6 hours.
- Between 44°C and 51°C the rate of epidermal necrosis approximately doubles with each degree of temperature increase.
- Water at 49°C takes ~10 minutes to cause significant burn injury.
- Water at 60°C causes a burn within 3 seconds.
- At ≥70°C, exposure time required to cause transepidermal necrosis is less than 1 second.

Contact time and temperature of source determines the depth of burn. Scalds with boiling water have shorter exposure time as water flows rapidly off skin, whilst hot fat, oil and other liquids that cling, continue to release energy into skin, causing considerably deeper and more serious burns.

Chemical burns

These are caused by strong acids, alkalis, detergents or solvents coming into contact with the skin and/or eyes. When dealing with chemical burns you should note the following:

- The nature of chemical
- Alkalis cause deep, penetrating burns
- Topical absorption by phenols and hydrofluoric acid cause poisoning and must be irrigated with copious amounts of water for a minimum of 20 minutes, ideally until definitive care is available

> **! HOTSPOT**
>
> Irrigation with water is effective up to 3 hours after injury.

Electrical burns

These are burns caused from electrical current. Depending on the power, there may be an entry and exit wound. Generally, the extent of damage is impossible to assess at time of injury.

Electromagnetic energy burns

These are caused by prolonged exposure to ultraviolet rays of the sun, or other sources of electromagnetic radiation, such as x-rays or nuclear radiation.

Classification of burn depth

Table 19.3 provides a classification of burn depth.

Assessing and estimating depth of burns may be challenging. Call for medical assistance if you suspect deep partial thickness or full thickness burns.

Management of burns
DR<C>ABCDE

- Stop the burning process as soon as possible.
- Remove casualty from heat source.
- Determine time of burn.
- Remove any clothing or jewellery near the burnt area of skin, including babies' nappies.
- Do not try to remove anything that is stuck to burnt skin, as this may cause further damage.
- Time taken to commence cool water irrigation and removal of clothing has a significant impact.
- Cool the burn with cool running water for at least 20 minutes, ideally until definitive care arrives. If burns are extensive and thus the area being cooled down is large, be vigilant as hypothermia could ensue and shock, if present, may worsen.
- Keep casualty warm. Use a blanket or layers of clothing away from burn area to prevent hypothermia.
- Avoid using ice or refrigerated water, which can cause further vasoconstriction and tissue damage.
- Do not apply creams, lotions, sprays or greasy substances, such as butter or toothpaste.
- Cover the burn loosely with cling film. If cling film is not available, use a clean, dry dressing or non-fluffy material. Do not wrap the burn tightly because swelling may lead to further injury.
- Sit the casualty upright as much as possible if the face or eyes are burnt. Avoid lying casualty down for long periods to help reduce swelling.

The upper airway is very susceptible to swelling and therefore obstruction following exposure to heat. Airway status may deteriorate rapidly. Cues of inhalation injury may be subtle and not appear in the first 24 hours. Indications of inhalation injury include the following:

- Face and/or neck burns
- Singed eyebrows
- Singed nasal hair and around the nose
- Carbon particles seen in sputum.

TABLE 19.3	**Classification of Burn Depth**		
Depth	**Cause**	**Appearance**	**Sensation**
Superficial	Sun, flash, minor scald	Dry, minor blisters, erythema, brisk capillary return	Painful
Superficial partial thickness (superficial dermal)	Scald	Moist, reddened with broken blisters, brisk capillary return	Painful
Deep partial thickness (deep dermal)	Scald, minor flame contact	Moist white slough, red mottled, sluggish capillary return	Painful to air and temperature / Painless
Full thickness	Flame, severe scald or flame contact	Dry, charred whitish. Absent capillary return	Painless (as sensory nerves together with other tissues have been damaged)

Another indication is if the casualty was involved in an explosion incident resulting in burns to head and torso.

When irrigating eyes, ensure fluid runs away from the non-affected eye.

Indications of when to call emergency medical services

- Large or deep burns that are bigger than the affected person's hand
- Burns of any size that cause white or charred skin
- Burns on the face, hands, arms, feet, legs or genitals with blisters
- All chemical and electrical burns
- Casualty is pregnant
- Casualty is over the age of 60 years or under the age of 5 years
- Medical condition, such as heart, lung or liver disease, or diabetes
- Casualty has a weakened immune system: HIV/AIDS, chemotherapy/cancer
- Casualty is in shock

If someone has breathed in smoke or fumes, some symptoms may be delayed. These include:

- Coughing
- Hoarseness
- Sore throat
- Difficulty breathing.

If in any doubt, call the emergency medical services

> **⚠ HOTSPOT**
>
> Avoid leaving a patient on their back if they are bleeding from the nose or mouth as it may obstruct the airway and complicate breathing. In they are conscious, lean them forward; if unconscious, flip them into the recovery position.

Acid attacks

Make sure you know what to do if you witness an acid attack. St John Ambulance (2017) suggest:

1. Make sure that the area around the casualty is safe. Wear gloves, preventing you coming into contact with the chemical. If the chemical is in powder form, it can be brushed off of the skin.
2. Flood the burn with water for a minimum of 20 minutes to disperse the chemical and stop the burning. Ensure the water does not collect underneath the casualty.
3. Gently remove any contaminated clothing while flooding the injury.
4. Arrange to send the casualty to hospital. Monitor vital signs, such as breathing, pulse and level of response.

Acid attack – chemical burn to the eye

1. Hold the casualty's affected eye under gently running cold water for at least 10 minutes. Irrigate the eyelid thoroughly both inside and out.
2. Ensure that contaminated water does not splash the uninjured eye.
3. Ask the casualty to hold a clean, non-fluffy pad over the injured eye.

4. Arrange to send the casualty to hospital.
5. Do not allow the casualty to touch the injured eye.
6. Do not forcibly remove a contact lens.

CARDIOPULMONARY RESUSCITATION (CPR)

The casualty who is unresponsive, unconscious and not breathing is normally in cardiac arrest and requires cardiopulmonary resuscitation (CPR).

Follow SCENE and the DR<C>AB approach.
Airway – open the airway employing an appropriate manoeuvre.
Breathing – if the patient is not breathing commence CPR.

Performing chest compressions

Place the heel of one hand on the sternum (centre of the patient's chest). Place your other hand on top of your first hand and interlock your fingers. Position yourself with your shoulders above your hands. Using your body weight (not just your arms), press straight down by 5–6 cm on their chest. It is said that 50 kg of weight is required to adequately compress an adult chest.

Try to perform chest compressions at a rate of 100–120 chest compressions a minute. It is critical to allow the chest to recoil completely between compressions.

If you have been trained in CPR, including ventilations or rescue breaths, and feel confident using your skills, you should give chest compressions with rescue breaths. If either untrained or unwilling to perform rescue breaths, the first aider should deliver continuous uninterrupted chest compressions at a rate of 100–120 per minute. This is known as compressions-only CPR.

However, health professionals are expected to conduct CPR in a targeted manner that is age group specific and includes ventilations.

> **⚠ HOTSPOT**
>
> Adults CPR: Compress to a depth of 5–6 cm, at a rate of 100– 20 per/minute and a ventilation to compression ratio of 2 ventilations to 30 compressions.

Performing CPR with ventilations

Following 30 compressions as instructed above, gently provide head-tilt and chin-lift, pinch the patient's nose, seal your mouth over the patient's mouth and blow steadily over 1 second. Repeat twice every 30 compressions while checking for chest rise. Aim to spend approximately 1 second inflating the lungs providing sufficient volume to ensure the chest visibly rises. Ventilations are given at a rate of 10–12 per minute or 1 approximately every 5 to 6 seconds. All efforts should be made to minimize interruption between ventilations and compressions.

To protect against body fluids, vomitus and cross-infection, it is recommended the first aider use a face seal or if equipped with a bag-valve-mask and competent in this skill, this should be used.

The ratio of chest compressions to ventilations is 30:2 for adults.

If there is evidence suggesting the cardiac arrest was through a lack of oxygen (apnoeic cardiac arrest; e.g., drowning, strangulation or suffocation), then the first aider should provide 5 ventilations before compressions. Following this, the ratio of 2 ventilations to 30 compressions is continued. Once CPR is commenced, it must be continued until:

- Emergency Medical Service arrive on scene
- There is Return of Spontaneous Circulation (ROSC). There are obvious signs of life such as breathing, coughing, movement, a palpable pulse or a measurable blood pressure.
- You are physically exhausted.

Automated external defibrillator (AED)

The AED is a device that delivers an electric shock to the heart when it is in cardiac arrest. Some facts about the AED:

- AEDs can be used on children over 1 year of age and adults.
- Using an AED before an ambulance arrives can double someone's chances of survival.
- Defibrillation within 3–5 minutes of collapse can produce survival rates as high as 50%–70%.
- Each minute of delay to defibrillation reduces the probability of survival to hospital discharge by 10%.
- Defibrillation on a wet surface is safe providing the rescuer is not in contact with the patient. If necessary, dry the patient's skin for good pad contact.
- Defibrillation of a patient on a metal surface is safe, providing the first aider is not in direct contact with the patient.
- Defibrillation in an aircraft or helicopter is safe because the metal surface in contact with the patient ensures that any leakage current is conducted away from the first aider.

If the first aider is alone and cardiac arrest is established and an AED is at hand, defibrillation takes precedence over airway, breathing or compressions.

Warning

Make sure no one is touching the patient during shock delivery, including you. Remember your situational awareness and perform a 360-degree assessment before pressing the shock button to avoid accidental injury to yourself or others.

Secondary survey or detailed assessment

This assessment is only performed after the first aider has completely assessed and managed any life-threatening problems identified in the primary survey (<C> ABC). As with the primary survey, it is also conducted using a structured approach.

 HOTSPOT

In approaching the patient do not forget to acquire consent and be attentive to the patient's dignity.

The approach

- First identify yourself.
- If appropriate, ask the patient to describe the history of the chief complaint.
- Seek information from bystanders, relatives or carers.

- Using a systematic head-toe approach, check the patient for any other possible injuries or illnesses. Do not forget to scan all over the body, including groin and back, and remember to note any rash.
- Assess body temperature.
- If possible, all information should be jotted down and handed over to medical emergency services on their arrival. At the end of the secondary survey history, relevant signs and symptoms should be noted.
- In trauma, the secondary survey may be a focused rapid systematic examination of the entire body completed within minutes to identify any bleeds and fractures and, if appropriate, sprains and strains.
- Cover patient with items of clothing or a blanket if at hand.
- Consider patient's dignity.

BROKEN BONES, DISLOCATIONS, SPRAINS AND STRAINS

- A fracture is a break or crack in the continuity of a bone.
- A dislocation is the displacement of one or more bones from their joint.
- A sprain occurs when ligament/s supporting a joint become overstretched and/or torn.
- A strain follows when fibres of a muscle or tendon are overstretched and/or torn.

Appropriate first aid for any of the above injuries aims to reduce pain and mitigate shock and the prospect of long-term complications.

Fractures and dislocations

Generally, a fracture is not life-threatening and may be concealed under the skin; a closed fracture. However, if the shattered bone/s severs or traps a nerve or blood vessel (complicated closed fracture), it may lead to neurological deficits or internal bleeding with a concomitant loss of motor function, sensations or circulatory volume. If blood loss pools into a large body cavity or a cavity with capacity to significantly expand (see earlier under Shock), the injury may become life-threatening.

Similarly, an open fracture can severe or trap nerves or blood vessels (complicated open fracture) and can also lead to neurological deficits or external bleeding with a concomitant loss of motor function, sensations or circulatory volume. In an open fracture, damaged blood vessels can lead to external bleeding; if severe and not adequately controlled, the injury will also become life-threatening. Therefore, if catastrophic bleeding is suspected either internally or observed externally, prompt management using adequate equipment needs to be employed to avoid exsanguination (blood loss to a degree sufficient to cause death). In both cases, the patient will also need to be treated for physiological shock.

It should be noted that the term 'open fracture' is not limited to injuries where bone is protruding from the skin. An open fracture also includes an injury where there is no protruding bone, where a fracture is suspected, and the skin has been broken around the site. This is because this opening can provide a passage for microorganisms to cause bone infection or osteomyelitis.

Signs and symptoms related to fractures

- Pain
- Loss of power
- Rapid swelling
- Tenderness
- Guarding
- Bruising
- Deformity – 'it does not look right' (Singletary et al., 2015)
- Irregularity – lumps, bumps, depressions, extended skin or stepping (particularly palpable when gently feeling along the vertebrae of the casualty, and may indicate dislocations and/or fractures)
- Exposed bone fragments
- Locked joint
- Limited range of motion
- Movement, but with unnatural direction – false motion
- When comparing and contrasting with the other limb it may look shorter, twisted or bent
- Crepitus – grinding sound or feeling when bones rub against each other
- Shock.

CRITICAL AWARENESS

Singletary et al. (2015) did not find any evidence supporting or opposing the first aider from straightening or gently realigning a suspected angulated long bone fracture before splinting, even in the presence of neurovascular compromise. Generally speaking, ILCOR (2015) suggests first aid providers should not move or try to straighten an injured extremity. However, if emergency services or definitive care is expected to be protracted, the first aider should, in an attempt to safeguard the patient, consider moving the injured limb or patient with prior splinting based on training, and setting to mitigate pain, prevent further injury and to facilitate safe transportation.

Signs and symptoms of dislocation

- Pain
- Marked deformity
- Swelling
- Pain aggravated by movement
- Tenderness on palpation
- Locked joint
- Numbness or impaired circulation to the limb or digit.

! HOTSPOT

- A fractured clavicle (collarbone) should be suspected if the affected side presents as a protrusion (these are the broken bones under the skin) and swelling in the middle of the collarbone, with very limited range of motion.
- An anterior dislocation of the shoulder should be suspected if there is an anterior prominence of the shoulder, the arm is anteriorly rotated, there is inability to move the arm, severe pain and a sensation of a 'dead arm'.

The approach

- Size up the scene – apply situational awareness to help you in decision-making throughout attendance and a 360-degree assessment to avoid any surprises.
- Obtain consent (informed/implied).
- Assess level of consciousness (AVPU).
- Undertake a primary survey (<C>ABCDE). If there is catastrophic bleeding, it requires immediate control.
- Secondary survey – use a rapid, focused trauma/physical assessment using a structured approach, for example DCAP-PBTLS (deformities, contusions, abrasions, punctures/penetrations, burns, tenderness, lacerations and swelling).

Once the first aider has established where the fracture, dislocation, sprain or strain is located, keep it simple by following three steps:

1. Assessment
2. Pain Management
3. Treatment.

Assessment

Differentiating between a fracture, dislocation, or connective tissue injury (sprain or strain) can be very difficult. If in any doubt, treat as for a fracture. Remember, trying to force a fracture or a dislocation back into its normal anatomy can cause further damage. Nevertheless, assessing the injury, as part of a holistic approach, may reveal crucial information that may impact management and will set a point of reference to determine any improvement or deterioration, including pain. To assess, follow a structured approach, for example: circulation, sensation and motor function (CSM).

Circulation, sensation and motor function
The approach

When managing a fracture, dislocation, sprain or strain, the first aider should establish a benchmark. Therefore, prior to and following any treatment, it is paramount to assess CSM. This physical assessment may reveal underlying neurological or vascular damage. Note, if you do observe any deterioration or loss in CSM during or following treatment (except following the application of a tourniquet), you may have to review treatment, which may include releasing applied bandages. Remember, any deterioration, including changes in CSM or AVPU, should be noted, together with time of occurrence.

How to apply CSM

The first aider should expose the area, making sure the patient has granted consent and their dignity is considered. Look and feel further along the limb (distal) to where the injury is (hands/fingers, feet/toes) and check circulation (blood flow) and the integrity of nerves, respectively. Then motor power and disability (pain and range of motion) can be assessed by looking at and feeling for the following:

Colour
- Are both extremities the same colour?
- Does it look purplish, pale or pink? (consider also palms of hands and soles of feet)

Sensation
- Touch the opposing extremities. Does the patient feel equal sensation?
- Is there any tingling or numbness?
- Is there a feeling of pins and needles?

Movement
- Can the patient move the limb freely?
- Does movement lead to pain?

Pain management

Pain management is a fundamental human right and, although pain may not be perceived as life-threatening, it has a direct physiological impact on respiratory rate, pulse rate and blood pressure. Moreover, addressing pain will not only mitigate detrimental physiological changes, it will also assist the first aider in managing the patient as they will be more willing to cooperate.

Pain management can be addressed by using a medication and/or a non-medication approach. As with CSM, it is important to establish a benchmark to enable the detection of trends of improvement or deterioration (refer to Box 19.1).

PQRST – a tool for pain

The first aider can consider pain by using PQRST.
- **P** – Provokes: What causes pain? What makes it better? What makes it worse?
- **Q** – Quality: Does it feel sharp, dull, stabbing, burning or crushing? Is it intermittent or constant?
- **R** – Radiate: Where did the pain start? Does it move? Does it spread to another location?
- **S** – Severity: Use the 1–10 pain scale (Box 19.1).
- **T** – Time: At what time did it start? How long has it lasted?

Treatment

Following pain management, the main objective of the physical treatment is to keep movement to a feasible minimum as movement will exacerbate pain and affect blood clotting and healing mechanisms. So, treatment will be influenced by the following:
- Does the patient need to be moved?
- Can the patient support the injured limb?
- Is there still much pain?
- Does the patient need to be transferred to require definitive treatment? How long will this take?

> **! HOTSPOT**
>
> Be practical. Sometimes less is more.

When managing closed fractures, as well as sprains and strains, the first aider should follow a structured approach such as PRICE to assist in decision making:
- **P** – Protect (unless it is totally necessary—for example, removing from hazards or having to turn the unconscious patient into the recovery position to protect the airway—do not move the patient).
- **R** – Rest the injury (advise the patient not to use or move the injured limb). Sling an arm or immobilize an injured leg by strapping it to the uninjured leg. Reassure.
- **I** – Ice (apply a wrapped ice pack to the injured area). Cold therapy can be applied for 15–20 minutes every 2–3 hours.
- **C** – Apply a supportive bandage to provide comfortable compression to the affected area to manage swelling.
- **E** – Elevate – allowing gravity to reduce swelling.

You should call emergency medical services if:
- The presenting injury is an open fracture.
- You have a high index of suspicion for a spinal, pelvic or head injury.
- If, during your CSM assessment, you observe loss of feeling, loss of movement, loss of sensation and/or limb is presenting marked changes in colour.
- The patient is showing signs of an altered conscious level.
- The patient is showing signs of physiological shock (see Signs and Symptoms of Shock).
- You are in any doubt.

MEDICAL EMERGENCIES

It is not possible in a chapter of this size to address all medical emergencies. The reader is advised to seek further information from other valid sources, such as St John's Ambulance Brigade (Austin et al., 2014).

Anaphylaxis

The immune system is key to protecting the body. But sometimes the system reacts to non-hazardous substances (allergens) producing immunoglobulin E (IgE) antibodies. This reaction is common and affects one in four people in the United Kingdom (Patient UK, 2017). Generally, such allergic reactions are mild, self-limiting, local in nature and non-life-threatening. However, at times the system reacts inappropriately, and a hypersensitive immune cascade leads to a systemic allergic response, known as anaphylaxis. This detrimental response releases immunological agents into the blood system, and when severe, anaphylactic shock may ensue and become a life-threatening condition. This escalation can happen within minutes or be delayed and not express symptoms for hours. The most common triggers responsible for an anaphylactic reaction are shown in Table 19.4.

> **BOX 19.1 Pain Scale**
>
> **Pain score range**
>
> | | |
> |---|---|
> | 0 | no pain |
> | 1–3 | pain increases to mild |
> | 4–6 | pain increases to moderate |
> | 7–10 | severe pain increases to imaginable or worst pain ever |

TABLE 19.4 Common Triggers Responsible for an Anaphylactic Reaction

Triggers	Example
Food	Peanuts, tree nuts, shellfish, cow's milk, soy, eggs, wheat
Insect bites or stings	Bee, wasp, ant
Medication	Antibiotics, ibuprofen, aspirin, penicillin
Latex	Rubber gloves, balloons, condoms, bottle teats
Exercise	Early signs include flushing and fatigue

Signs and symptoms

Different parts of the body can be affected simultaneously during a severe allergic reaction; however, the timeframe for signs and symptoms to develop varies depending on the cause. The first aider must be observant for the following signs and symptoms that may indicate anaphylaxis.

Airway
- Difficulty speaking, shortness of breath, persistent coughing, hoarseness, wheezing and/or other types of noisy breathing, swelling or tightness of throat and/or tongue severe asthma.

Skin
- Generalized flushing of the skin.
- Rash.
- Hives or welts anywhere on the body.

Gastrointestinal
- Abdominal pain, nausea and vomiting.

Cardiovascular and general disabilities
- Alterations in heart rate.
- Sudden onset of weakness, altered level of consciousness, dizziness, faintness, collapse, unconsciousness.
- Pale and floppy (particularly in children)
- During an anaphylactic shock, there is a lowering of blood pressure.

Mood
- Sense of impending doom.

Signs and symptoms of a mild to moderate reaction (it should be noted that these may precede anaphylaxis):
- Vomiting.
- Swelling of the lips, face, eyes.
- Tingling sensation in and around the mouth.
- Red raised itchy skin.
- Abdominal pain.
- Difficulty speaking or hoarse voice.

The signs and symptoms noted may be apparent or the casualty may develop a full anaphylactic reaction without these preceding signs.

Management of anaphylactic shock

Those individuals who are at risk of experiencing anaphylaxis are prescribed adrenaline autoinjectors and generally carry these with them (e.g., EpiPen®, AnaPen®).

COMMUNITIES OF CARE

Children

New legislation in the UK that came into force from 1 October 2017 enables emergency adrenaline autoinjectors to be available in schools (these are similar to the arrangement in place for asthma inhalers). A website for parents, pupils and school staff explains how to comply with the new arrangements.

The update to the law permits school staff to use autoinjectors to administer a dose of adrenaline of to a child who has previously been identified as at risk of a severe allergic reaction (anaphylaxis), but who does not have their device with them. It could also be used if the child's autoinjector is broken or out of date, or if a second dose is needed.

Managing the conscious anaphylactic patient

Follow DRABCD.
- Help patient to sit or lie in a position that assists breathing.
- As soon as anaphylaxis is suspected or manifesting, it is paramount that adrenaline is administered without delay.
- Call for an emergency medical services and remember to mention anaphylaxis; this will make the response more focused.
- Keep person in a lying (with legs elevated) or sitting position if composed.
- Monitor and record pulse, and quality and rate of breathing.
- If, after 5 minutes, the person is not responding to the first dose of adrenaline, a further dose may be administered.
- Adequately dispose of autoinjectors by handing them over to the ambulance crew.

If the person is unable to self-administer, you should assist or take over. EpiPen®, AnaPen® are adrenaline-based autoinjectors that work swiftly by relaxing smooth bronchial muscles and improving breathing, constricting dilated blood vessels, stimulating the heartbeat and reversing swelling around the face, mouth and lips.

! HOTSPOT
Remember, act immediately. Do not delay treatment.

Managing the unconscious anaphylactic patient

Follow DRABCDE.

If at hand, immediately administer the adrenaline autoinjector (EpiPen®, AnaPen®).

Heart attack (myocardial infarction)

A heart attack develops when a coronary artery (heart's own blood supply) is suddenly obstructed, for example, by a clot. If the obstruction affects a large area of the heart muscle and is left untreated, it will lead to a cardiac arrest.

Signs and symptoms

Consider the four Ps:
- Pain – a continuous uncomfortable pressure, fullness or squeezing pain in the centre of the chest, which may radiate to the jaw, neck, arms and occasionally upper abdomen. But note it can also have no symptoms, particularly in diabetic patients. Many people have warning signs hours, days or weeks in advance.
- Pale skin.
- Pulse (is it rapid, weak or absent?).
- Perspiration/sweating.

Other presentations
- Shortness of breath.
- Light-headedness, dizziness, fainting and/or nausea.

Managing the conscious suspected heart attack
- Assist patient to move into comfortable position, for example, on the floor leaning against wall, with knees bent and head and shoulders supported.

- Ask if they have any angina medication, for example, aspirin or glycerol trinitrate (GTN) spray.
- If yes, assist administration. If pain persists after five minutes following administration, suggest second dose or they take a second dose of GTN.
- If still in pain after another five minutes, or the pain returns, presume it is a heart attack and call emergency medical services.
- If they have no medication, and the pain does not go away after resting, call emergency medical services.
- Be aware the patient may develop shock.
- Keep checking their breathing, pulse and level of consciousness (AVPU).
- If they lose responsiveness at any point, follow ABCDE. You may need to do CPR.

Diabetic emergency

Hypoglycaemia is a term used to describe low glucose (sugar) levels. Generally speaking this condition is normally associated with known diabetic patients who have mismanaged their diabetic drug/s and blood glucose levels have fallen below a critical level (<4.0 mm/L). If left untreated the person will continue to deteriorate and eventually go into a diabetic coma, which is a life-threatening condition.

Recognition

- Mental status or behaviour – altered level of consciousness (AVPU), confused, irrational behaviour
- Weakness, hunger, tremors
- Pulse – fast
- Respiratory rate – high, above 29 breaths per minute
- Skin – pale, clammy, cool

Look out for a medical warning bracelet or necklace and medication, such as an insulin pen or blood glucose testing kit.

Management of the hypoglycaemic patient

The aim is to raise the patient's blood sugar (glucose) level as quickly as possible.

- Keep the person safe and, if necessary, obtain medical assistance.
- Advise patient to sit or lie down.
- If conscious, ask patient if they are diabetic and inform them they may be experiencing a hypoglycaemic episode.
- If the patient is conscious and able to follow commands, ask if they are carrying glucose tablets or gel. If not, you need to provide something sweet (preferably liquid/gel). This will instigate a glycaemic effect, raising blood sugar quickly. Remember, diet beverages do not have any sugar and need to be avoided.
- If the patient's conscious level is compromised, for example, only responds to pain stimuli in the AVPU scale, avoid giving solids and be cautious if using liquids since there is a high probability of choking and aspiration as the patient may not be able to maintain their airway. You should call emergency medical services.
- Provide reassurance.
- If the patient responds positively to the administration of glucose tablets and is alert, orientated and fully coherent, ask

if they would like you to call emergency medical services. If not, advise them to visit their health-practitioner despite fully recovery.

Management of the unconscious hypoglycaemic patient

- If breathing, place in the recovery position, call emergency medical services and monitor.
- If not breathing, follow ABC approach and be ready to commence CPR.

Asthma

An asthma attack is the sudden constriction of the smooth-muscle bands surrounding the bronchioles (bronchospasm). Additionally, there is inflammation of the bronchioles' mucus lining and more and thicker mucus is produced, leading to airway obstruction. Attacks are triggered by allergy-causing substances, respiratory viruses, colds and environmental triggers.

Common asthma triggers

A trigger is anything that irritates the airways and sets off asthma symptoms.

- Colds and flu
- Emotions
- Exercise
- Food
- Female hormones
- House dust mites
- Indoor environment
- Moulds and fungi
- Pollen
- Pollution
- Recreational drugs
- Sex
- Smoking and second-hand smoke
- Stress and anxiety
- Weather

Recognition

If you think someone is having an asthma attack, these are the seven key signs to look for:

1. Difficulty breathing or speaking
2. Breathing may get faster
3. Coughing
4. Tight chest
5. Noisy wheezy breathing
6. Grey-blue tinge to lips or nailbed (cyanosis)
7. Anxiety and distress.

Asthma management

- Allow patient to assume most comfortable position.
- Reassure patient and help them to control their breathing by advising to breathe slowly and deeply.
- If patient is having difficulty speaking, encourage them not to speak.
- If patient has a reliever inhaler, help the patient to use it straight away – one or two puffs immediately. If this does not improve condition, it may be a severe attack. Get them

to take one or two puffs of their inhaler every 2 minutes, until they have had 10 puffs.

- If patient continues to worsen or is becoming exhausted, or if it is their first attack, call emergency medical services and monitor.
- Anticipate patient may become unresponsive. If this occurs, open airway, check breathing, prepare to treat someone who has become unresponsive.
- Reassure.

Psychological first aid

Studies of human behaviour in victims of trauma have recognized the emotional distress that these patients suffer as psychological pain, which is as incapacitating as physical pain, but not as overt. Psychological first aid is an evidence-based approach to address emotional distress experienced by patients following exposure to a traumatic event. This is achieved by helping the patient tap into their own inherent resilience and empowers them to use the necessary coping skills to revert to a healthy state of mind. To read more, refer to the World Health Organization webpage on this subject (WHO, 2011).

LOOKING BACK, FEEDING FORWARD

The chapter has introduced the reader to some aspects of first aid. It is not possible to address all issues that the first aider may encounter. The aim of the chapter was to provide the reader with an awareness of the first aider's role and responsibility. The fundamental issues have been described and discussed and the NA is required to understand the principles underpinning first aid procedures and basic life support. They will need to develop their skills so that they are able to perform these activities safely and effectively.

The chapter has focused on the administration of basic first aid; however, there is also a need for the NA to be able to administer basic mental health first aid. Many organizations offer staff the opportunity to participate in first aid courses (physical and mental health), often a part of the induction period.

The NA must be aware that each situation is different and they are expected to use their professional judgement in each instance. If an NA has first aid training and can assist, then there is an expectation they will provide support in line with their knowledge and skill. If the NA is not experienced with the situation, then they should use their professional judgement to assist as much as they can; however, they have to acknowledge their limitations.

REFERENCES

Austin, M., Crawford, R., Armstrong, V.J., 2014. First Aid Manual: The Authorised Manual of St John's Ambulance, St Andrews First Aid and the British Red Cross, tenth ed. Dorling Kindersley, London.

Dewhirst, M., Viglianti, B., Lora-Michiels, L., Hoopes, P., 2003. Thermal dose Requirement for Tissue Effect: Experimental and Clinical Findings. https://www.ncbi.nlm.nih.gov/pmc/articles/PMC4188373/.

European Child Safety Alliance, 2013. Child Product safety Guide. http://ulsafetysmart.com/files/content/report/ProductSafetyGuideFINAL.pdf.

European Resuscitation Council, 2015. European Resuscitation Council Guidelines. https://cprguidelines.eu.

Glas, G., Levi, M., Schultz, M., 2016. Coagulopathy and its management in patients with severe burns. https://onlinelibrary.wiley.com/doi/pdf/10.1111/jth.13283.

International Liaison Committee on Resuscitation, 2015. 2015 Consensus. http://www.ilcor.org/consensus-2015/costr-2015-documents/.

International Federation of Red Cross and Red Crescent Societies, 2016. International First Aid and Resuscitation Guidelines 2016. http://www.ifrc.org/Global/Publications/Health/First-Aid-2016-Guidelines_EN.pdf.

Nielsen, C., Duethman, N., Howard, J., et al., 2017. Burns: Pathophysiology of Systemic Complications and Current Management. https://www.ncbi.nlm.nih.gov/pmc/articles/PMC5214064/pdf/bcr-38-e469.pdf.

Patient UK, 2017. Allergies. https://patient.info/health/allergies.

Resuscitation Council UK, 2015. Resuscitation Guidelines. https://www.resus.org.uk/resuscitation-guidelines/.

Singletary, E.M., Charlton, N.P., Epstein, J.L., et al., 2015. *Part 15*: first aid: 2015 American Heart Association and American Red Cross guidelines update for first aid. Circulation 132 (2), S574–S589.

St John Ambulance, 2017. First Aid for Acid Attacks. http://www.sja.org.uk/sja/what-we-do/latest-news/first-aid-for-acid-attacks.aspx.

World Health Organization, 2011. Psychological First Aid Guide for Field Workers. http://apps.who.int/iris/bitstream/10665/44615/1/9789241548205_eng.pdf.

20

Data Gathering and Patient Monitoring

Laura Park, Jaden Allan, Barry Hill

OBJECTIVES

By the end of the chapter, the reader will be able to:

1. Discuss skills and data gathering techniques including observation, interviewing, physical and mental health examination, and measurement
2. Describe patient data collecting, interpreting, utilizing, monitoring accurately and reporting information

concerning the health and well-being of the person receiving care
3. Demonstrate an understanding of appropriate use of technology
4. Describe the National Early Warning Score (NEWS) 2 and appropriate communication and handover techniques

KEY WORDS

- Communication
- Handover
- Vital signs
- Assessment

- Data
- Interpretation
- Decision-making
- Critical thinking

- Physical
- Outcomes

CHAPTER AIM

The aim of this chapter is to increase the reader's awareness and understanding of the role of data gathering and monitoring in the provision of safe and knowledgeable nursing care.

SELF TEST

1. What do you understand by open and closed questioning?
2. What does the acronym SBAR mean?
3. What is the National Early Warning Score?
4. List five commonly used physiological measurements.
5. What is said to be the fifth vital sign?
6. Differentiate between objective and subjective data.
7. What senses may be used in the data gathering process?
8. What is the Glasgow Coma Scale?
9. Why is it important to make known any deviations in patients' vital signs?
10. What is the number for cardiac arrest in the area where you are currently working?

INTRODUCTION

The care you give today will reflect on the profession tomorrow. This is important to remember when interacting with anyone in your Nursing Associate (NA) role.

> ### REFLECTION 20.1
>
> Think of a time when you received good service from someone that you have interacted with, such as a shopkeeper or interview panel member. If they were polite and courteous, your experience would have been positive, thus you associate the service you received with the establishment they worked in; it is the same in the NHS.

If you deliver high-quality personable care, a positive experience should occur. When you collect data from a person, you are requiring that individual to share their information with you; sometimes this information is sensitive or personal. To promote sharing and disclosure you are expected to maintain appropriate therapeutic relationships with those you care for and work with (Nursing and Midwifery Council (NMC), 2018b).

Communication is the process of sending and receiving information and barriers can disrupt this communication (World Health Organization (WHO), 2007; Arnold & Boggs, 2016). This is addressed later in this chapter. Chapter 9 addresses effective communication in detail. In 2013, Kate Gardner started the #Hellomynameis campaign (https://hellomynameis.org.uk/). This simply requests you to introduce yourself when you first meet a patient or carer. Thinking of the earlier example in Reflection 20.1, there would have been some form of introduction or welcome in that scenario. When you collect patient data, always remember the initial contact will define the relationship you have and can affect the results you obtain.

BOX 20.1   The ABCDE Approach

A: Airway – Is the airway clear; is the patient speaking? (Sound: Such as wheezing).

B: Breathing – Is the patient struggling to breathe? (Sight: Does the patient look in distress? Count the rate, rhythm and depth of respiration).

C: Circulation – Does the patient have a pulse? Is it a fast heart rate (tachycardia)? (Feel: The patient pulse rate, rhythm and amplitude (strength)).

D: Disability – Does the patient have pre-existing conditions, such as asthma?

E: Exposure/Examination – Look at the patient and you may need to expose areas to examine for injury (maintaining patient dignity always).

Reproduced with the kind permission of the Resuscitation Council (UK) 2015. https://www.resus.org.uk/resuscitation-guidelines/abcde-approach/

BOX 20.2   Fundamental Assessment Using the Senses

LOOK – Look at the patient, are there any signs of physiological or psychological change different from what you might expect? This may be a change in colour, such as a pale or flushed face. Does the patient look distressed or anxious?

LISTEN – Can you hear the patient breathing or an unusual sound? (Remember, at rest most of us cannot be heard when breathing; listen to a friend or relative when you are sitting next to them.)

FEEL – With consent, feel the patient's pulse. Is the patient hot to the touch?

SIGHT – As with 'LOOK' earlier, use your sight to note any unexpected changes in the patient's normal physiology and behaviour.

SOUND – Are there any unexpected sounds, such as a wheeze? Is the wheeze on inspiration or expiration? This could aid the diagnosis of respiratory issues.

SMELL – Is there an unusual odour coming from the patient's breath or their wound? This could suggest several conditions or infections.

CRITICAL AWARENESS

If you were ill, consider how you would like to be greeted by someone in hospital, the GP surgery or your own home. What information would you like to know about them and their role in your care?

CRITICAL AWARENESS

Take some time to observe a patient you are providing care to and note their airway; is there any difficulty? You can look to see if they are using the accessory muscles such as the shoulders and if they are breathing deeply (think of yourself after strenuous exercise). Listen, as someone with an increased respiration rate will often be breathing heavily.

Therapeutic relationships

Therapeutic relationships in healthcare, are relationships established between healthcare professionals and patients. The aim is to promote engagement between patient and professional to create a beneficial and trusting partnership. Therapeutic relationships usually include education, patient support, guidance and sometimes safeguarding, among others. The King's Fund (2017) believes that a good-quality therapeutic relationship improves both patient satisfaction and professional fulfilment, saves time and increases compliance with prescribed medication. However, they continue to recognize that the subtle and intangible elements that underpin a strong therapeutic relationship are difficult to define and to measure.

COLLECTING DATA AND INFORMATION

Assessment

Patients are at the heart of all we do. To care for someone, we must understand what is going on or what concerns them; thus, we must collect information that will allow us to provide the evidence-based care they need.

Collecting data about health and well-being can be complex, and when someone is critically ill, such as in intensive care, it is inevitably technology focused. However, the fundamental collection of data can be as simple as the alphabet: ABCDE (Resuscitation Council (UK), 2015) is a reminder of the order of observations to make with a new patient (Box 20.1). Following this initial assessment, we consider the senses used daily (look, listen and feel, and sight, sound and smell). You can undertake a fundamental assessment anywhere at any time (Box 20.2).

Mental health

In addition to the ABCDE structured assessment used for effective patient assessment and monitoring, it is important to recognize patients who have mental health needs, such as emotional and psychosocial requirements. These must not be discredited, as to provide true holistic and person-centred care NAs must acknowledge that people with mental health needs may also present with physical health problems.

According to the Royal College of Psychiatrists, people with mental disorders and disabilities have a higher risk of poor physical health and premature mortality than the general population. Those people who are detained under the Mental Health Act are at a significantly higher risk of death due to sudden and long-term health complications, intoxication and self-inflicted violence (SIV) (such as self-harming). According to the Care Quality Commission's (CQC) Mental Health Act Annual Report 2014/15, 227 (CQC, 2016) quality of care was being questioned by healthcare professionals, with questions being raised to the CQC specifically regarding the death of people detained in hospital.

In January 2017, the National Institute for Health and Care Excellence (NICE) published *Improving the physical health of people with serious mental illness: A quality improvement approach* (NICE, 2017a). Eight years after the Royal College of Psychiatrists' *Physical Health in Mental Health* report in 2009, NICE continued to observe that people with serious mental illness (SMI), such as schizophrenia or bipolar disorder, die earlier than the rest of the population due to preventable disease. This remains an intractable problem.

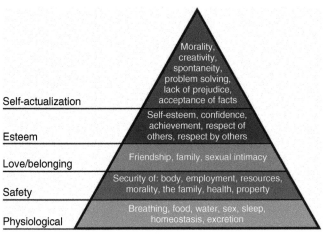

Fig. 20.1 Maslow's Hierarchy of Needs (1943)

BOX 20.4 Priority Problems

First level priority problems: Life-threatening immediate problems, such as respiratory arrest.
Second level priority problems: Urgent intervention required to reduce or halt deterioration, such as falling oxygen saturation.
Third level priority problems: Life-limiting issues that will affect the patient but are non-urgent in nature. These can include long-term conditions such as chronic obstructive pulmonary disease (COPD); continence assessment.
Collaborative problems: This includes multi-agency involvement to ensure the most effective care package is delivered.

Data collection

Jarvis (2016) and Dougherty & Lister (2015) highlight several assessments that include a total health and background assessment, such as those undertaken in a pre-admission clinic. This involves a focused or problem-based data collection approach around specific concerns, such as a patient presenting with a rash. In follow-up assessments, data collection is concerned with the checking of progress of a treatment, such as diabetic medication. One area of data collection for assessment that most trainees and staff are apprehensive about at the start of their careers is emergency data collection when rapid deterioration is occurring, or when a critically ill patient needs a rapid accurate assessment so that evidence-based care can then be provided. Health Education England (HEE, 2017) highlight the need for NAs to be able to carry out basic health monitoring.

Intentional rounding (IR)

IR has now been adopted into UK practice to direct nurses to intentionally check on patients frequently (usually hourly) in acute care settings. The purpose of these rounds is to monitor patients' needs, such as those required in Maslow's Hierarchy of needs (1943) (Fig. 20.1): does the patient require analgesia (pain control), support with walking, assistance to get to the bathroom or have specific nutrition and hydration requirements?

Harm-free care

One significant measure used by some NHS care providers in the delivery of harm-free care is the NHS Safety Thermometer (Box 20.3). This allows teams to measure harm and the proportion of patients that are 'harm free' during their working day, for example at shift handover or during ward rounds (Harm-FreeCare.org, 2017). The report *Delivering the NHS Safety Thermometer CQUIN 2013/14* (NHS Safety Thermometer, 2017), stipulates the following specific areas of patient monitoring focus:
• Falls
• Venous thrombus emboli (VTE)
• Catheters and urinary tract infections (UTIs)
• Pressure ulcers (PUs).

When monitoring patients, Jarvis (2016) provides a list of priority problems (Box 20.4).

Informed consent

As an NA, you will be collecting data to support care, evaluation of treatment and enhance the decision-making process by an appropriate member of staff (NMC, 2018b). You must ensure you obtain accurate data, which can sometimes be difficult if patients are aware they are being observed. It is important as a NA that you always ensure you have informed consent from your patient, explaining procedures thoroughly so that consent is given. This also applies to any data collection. Patients have a right to non-disclosure and may not want to participate or build a therapeutic relationship with an NA. Being open, transparent, and seeking permission for any procedure is a professional and legal requirement (NMC, 2018b). If a patient is unwilling to allow you to take vital signs, especially if you have concerns or the patient is deteriorating, please actively seek support from your mentor.

! HOTSPOT
Changing Normality

Ask a peer if you can count their respiration rate. Ask them to breath 'normally'. Observe if they change their respiration or become self-aware after your request.

When you inform someone you are going to observe them, they may change their actual behaviour, such as respiration in this example. For respiration counting, you may wish to observe from a vantage point (not directly in front of the patient). This ensures the patient does not change their current pattern. Some healthcare staff may say they are repeating a pulse count and then count respirations using peripheral vision.

Vital signs

Vital signs are clinical measurements (usually referred to as patient observations) that indicate the status of the body's organ function. Vital signs are measured by healthcare professionals to assess physical health parameters. These are a reliable indicator (especially when being compared to the patients' baseline observations) of deteriorating or improving health. Measuring vital signs allows a graph of data to be plotted onto a National Early Warning Score (NEWS) 2 observation chart (Fig. 20.2), to allow a trend to be seen by the practitioner. By using a NEWS2 chart, the patient's early warning score can also be calculated. It is important to note that a patient's vital signs change with age, weight, gender and disease. Vital signs can be measured in both secondary care (hospital) and primary care (community) settings.

There are opposing views on what exact parameters vital signs are categorized as, and which ones should be considered as vital. The newest and most contemporary evidence in the UK comes from the Royal College of Physicians in 2017a. The RCP does not necessarily refer to the patients' observations as vital signs; however, they do advocate six key observations to effectively calculate the NEWS, emphasizing these as vital components and key signs:

1. Respiratory rate (RR)
2. Oxygen saturations (O_2 sats)
3. Body temperature (BT)
4. Systolic blood pressure (SBP)
5. Pulse rate (heart rate)
6. Level of consciousness (LOC)

Respiratory rate (RR)

The respiratory rate is measured by observing the chest rise (from inspiration) and fall (from expiration) and should be counted as one breath every time both happen. The RR must be counted over a full minute if it is to be as accurate as possible. The normal respiratory rate of adults is 12–20 breaths per minute (BTS, 2017; RCP, 2017b). A respiratory rate less than 12 breaths per minute is termed bradypnoea, 12–20 is normal, more than 20 is tachypnoea. Breathing too slowly (bradypnoea) may encourage carbon dioxide to accumulate and change the pH of the blood, leading to changes in your patient's consciousness level. Breathing too fast (tachypnoea) may eventually lead to too much carbon dioxide being expelled from the blood. The patient will eventually collapse, and may stop breathing if they do not have enough carbon dioxide as this triggers and initiates breathing. Therefore, in line with your ABCDE assessment and systematic approach, any respiratory concerns must be raised immediately to your mentor or a senior clinical person, nurse, outreach team or doctor. The RR is a vitally important indicator of deterioration and statistically the observation that is most frequently missed (Smith et al., 2011).

Oxygen saturations

Oxygen saturations are measured using pulse oximetry: a red-light beam passes from the device into the cell tissue (usually the fingernail bed, but can be the earlobe), and measures the estimated oxygen amount in the red blood cells. This is completely non-invasive and is only an estimate. In a respiratory emergency, a more accurate reading would be gained from an arterial blood gas (ABG). Normal oxygen saturation is 94%–98% on room air for healthy adults, or 88%–92% in patients with chronic airway or lung diseases (BTS, 2017). 'Hypoxia' is the term used for low oxygen saturation and can be an indicator that the patient requires oxygen. The BTS publishes guidelines for the use of oxygen (BTS, 2017).

Body temperature

Body temperature can be measured orally, rectally, under the armpit (axillary), by ear, or by skin. Body temperature being or becoming abnormal can indicate a problem. Normothermia is between 35°C and 37°C. Fever (pyrexia) is a high temperature (more than 37°C). A body temperature between 37°C and 37.9°C is known as low grade pyrexia. A temperature of more than 38°C requires blood cultures (sepsis guidelines). Hypothermia is a low body temperature (less than 35°C).

Systolic blood pressure

Systolic blood pressure (SBP) is the top number of a recorded blood pressure and diastolic blood pressure (DBP) is the bottom number. For example 120/80 is a systolic BP of 120 and a diastolic BP of 80. The systolic blood pressure represents the pressure created when the heart beats (contracts). When the heart contacts, it pushes blood through the arteries within the body system. The diastolic blood pressure indicates the pressure in the arteries when the heart rests between beats. An easy way to remember this is when the heart stops, it is called diastole. Therefore, when the heart is not contracting, and is resting, this is the diastolic pressure. An SBP below 90 is recognized as hypotension (low blood pressure), 90–139 is normotension (normal blood pressure), and above 140 is hypertension (high blood pressure) (British National Formulary (BNF), 2017).

Pulse rate (heart rate)

The pulse rate is heart beats per minute (bpm). A low heart rate is considered less than 60 bpm (this is termed bradycardia (slow heart)), a normal pulse rate is considered 60–99 bpm, and a fast heart rate is considered more than 100 bpm and is termed tachycardia (fast heart). Taking the pulse rate is important as it allows the clinician to feel the pulse itself. Does it feel weak, or is it bounding and strong? This can give an indication of the overall blood pressure and the rhythm of the heart at a very early stage. When feeling the pulse, note if the hands are cold, are the peripheries cool to touch. This may indicate poor heart function or low blood pressure.

Level of Consciousness (LOC)

Consciousness. One of the fundamental observations that requires assessment is whether the patient is alert and aware or

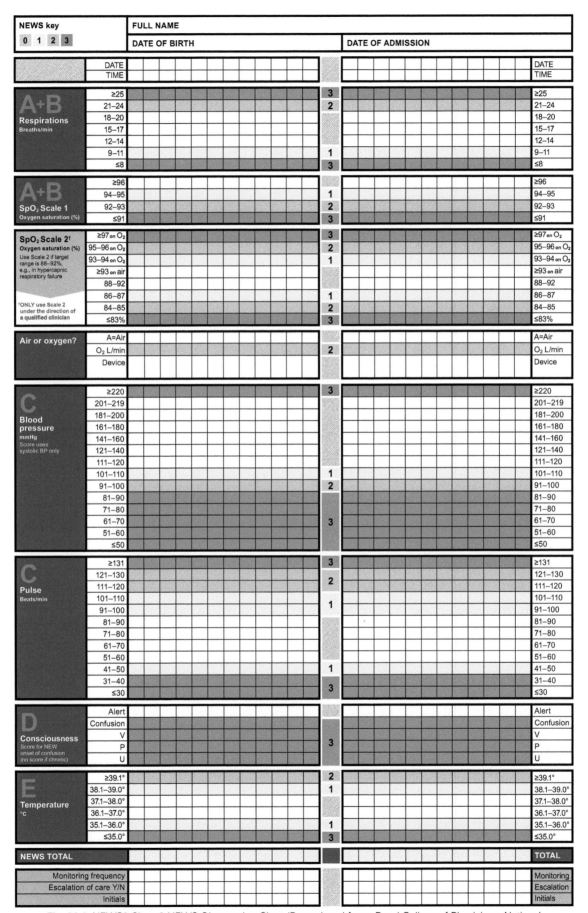

Fig. 20.2 NEWS2 Chart 3 NEWS Observation Chart (Reproduced from: Royal College of Physicians. National Early Warning Score (NEWS) 2: Standardising the assessment of acute-illness severity in the NHS. Updated report of a working party. London: RCP, 2017).

BOX 20.5   The AVPU Scale (McNarry & Goldhill, 2004)

A – Alert. Is the person fully aware and responding to you or others?

V – Voice. Will the person become aware when you use verbal commands or requests? (Consider the level they rouse to.)

P – Pain. Will the person only rouse when appropriate painful stimuli is used? (Ensure you are aware of appropriate stimuli and have had appropriate training before attempting any stimuli.)

U – Unresponsive. The person will not respond to any of the previous actions.

TABLE 20.1   AVPU and Relation to the GCS (Kelly et al., 2004)

AVPU	Relation to GCS and score
Alert	15
Voice	13
Pain	8
Unresponsive	3

BOX 20.6   Sepsis in Adults (UK Sepsis Trust, 2017)

According to The UK Sepsis Trust, the signs of sepsis in adults include:

Slurred speech or confusion
Extreme shivering or muscle pain
Passing no urine (in a day)
Severe breathlessness
It feels like you are going to die
Skin mottled or discoloured

BOX 20.7   Sepsis in Children (UK Sepsis Trust, 2017)

If a child is unwell with either a fever or very low temperature (or has had a fever in the last 24 hours), ask: could it be sepsis?

Any child who:
- is breathing very fast
- has a 'fit' or convulsion
- looks mottled, bluish, or pale
- has a rash that does not fade when you press it
- is very lethargic or difficult to wake
- feels abnormally cold to touch

Might have sepsis. Call 999 and ask: could it be sepsis?

Any child under 5 who:
- is not feeding
- is vomiting repeatedly
- has not had a wee or wet nappy for 12 hours

---

unconscious. This can be done immediately on approaching the patient and can start the assessment process and aid in prioritizing care (Schwitz, 2018). When collecting data on consciousness level, there are two main tools that can be used: Alert, Voice, Pain, Unresponsive (AVPU) and the Glasgow Coma Scale (GCS).

AVPU (McNarry & Goldhill, 2004) is a fundamental process that immediately assesses a person's consciousness level. Box 20.5 outlines the various stages that can be used to check if a patient is conscious. The NEWS2 chart will produce a score of 3 if the patient is only responding to Voice, Pain or is Unresponsive (RCP, 2017a).

It should be noted that misinterpretation can occur; a sleeping patient could be presumed unconscious during their afternoon snooze! Always consider the full context and patient-care requirement.

Glasgow Coma Scale (GCS) (www.glasgowcomascale.org) is based on a scoring system that provides an indication of the person's level of consciousness. This tool is commonly used in emergency care, high dependency and intensive therapy units. The scoring system can guide intervention and care. A declining score would suggest deterioration and risk to respiratory function. Kelly et al. (2004) suggest that the GCS score can relate to the AVPU (Table 20.1).

It should be acknowledged that alcohol-intoxication can be a barrier to assessment.

Collecting data concerning vital observations should be done following the correct procedures and steps, as well as adhering to local policies and procedures (DeWit, 2018; Dougherty & Lister, 2015). It is also essential you have a fundamental knowledge of anatomy and physiology (see Waugh and Grant, 2018) as this helps develop your understanding of any abnormal data. Data collected can be affected by conscious observation and 'white coat syndrome' where patients become nervous during data collection, such as blood pressure measurement (Blood Pressure UK, 2017). To ensure that monitoring is effective, specific data

is required for the recognition of a patient's early deterioration when using NEWS2. NICE (2007) and Resuscitation Council (UK) (2015) recognizes the importance of collecting data to identify deterioration at an early stage. All data must be documented on the appropriate record, such as a NEWS2 chart or electronic record and local policies and procedures must be followed.

INTERPRETING AND UTILIZING DATA

The NA provides essential support to the patient's care team (NMC, 2018b). The data gathered will assist in planning care delivered by the appropriate healthcare professional. To do this, you will be required to interpret the data and assessment you have undertaken and report this accordingly (Institute for Apprenticeships, 2017; NMC, 2018b). There are many tools and frameworks available to support interpretation of data and to assist in care planning (Department of Health (DH), 2010a, 2010b; DH, 2012; DH, 2016; National Health Service Improvement, no date). Conditions such as sepsis (see Glossary and Boxes 20.6 and 20.7) and pressure area risk are annually reviewed, and standards published. There is a variety of tools for assessment that all healthcare personnel can utilize (NICE, 2017b; Healthcare Improvement Scotland, 2009). It is essential that you use these tools in conjunction with your developing ability to make decisions. Use your professional judgement when applying these tools and other cues to interpret the data and act accordingly (Dougherty & Lister, 2015; Brooker & Nicol, 2011).

NEW score	Frequency of monitoring	Clinical response
0	Minimum 12 hourly	• Continue routine NEWS monitoring
Total 1–4	Minimum 4–6 hourly	• Inform registered nurse, who must assess the patient • Registered nurse decides whether increased frequency of monitoring and/or escalation of care is required
3 in single parameter	Minimum 1 hourly	• Registered nurse to inform medical team caring for the patient, who will review and decide whether escalation of care is necessary
Total 5 or more Urgent response threshold	Minimum 1 hourly	• Registered nurse to immediately inform the medical team caring for the patient • Registered nurse to request urgent assessment by a clinician or team with core competencies in the care of acutely ill patients • Provide clinical care in an environment with monitoring facilities
Total 7 or more Emergency response threshold	Continuous monitoring of vital signs	• Registered nurse to immediately inform the medical team caring for the patient – this should be at least at specialist registrar level • Emergency assessment by a team with critical care competencies, including practitioner(s) with advanced airway management skills • Consider transfer of care to a level 2 or 3 clinical care facility, ie higher-dependency unit or ICU • Clinical care in an environment with monitoring facilities

Fig. 20.3 NEWS2 Chart 4 Clinical Response to the NEWS Trigger Thresholds. (Reproduced from: Royal College of Physicians. National Early Warning Score (NEWS) 2: Standardising the assessment of acute-illness severity in the NHS. Updated report of a working party. London: RCP, 2017).

CASE STUDY 20.1 Pamela

You are allocated to look after Pamela, a 35-year-old female patient, following abdominal surgery. During the afternoon, you notice that Pamela's behaviour has changed. She has become less conversational and is also less interactive with you. She only appears to rouse to voice and appears pale and has a grey appearance.

Questions to Consider:
• What are Pamela's overall observations (vital signs) telling you?
• When were they last recorded?
• Has anything happened that could have caused a change in behaviour?
• Is there a concerning trend in her observations?
• Are the recorded observations moving towards the trigger points on the NEWS2 chart?

REFLECTION 20.3

In Case Study 20.1, the information indicates a change in Pamela's behaviour and physical presentation.
  What should you do next and with whom should you raise your concerns?

Using the assessment and data to guide the care requirements of the patient in a timely manner is highlighted by NICE (2007) and DH (2010a). This prevents deterioration and enhances recovery while promoting evidence-based care. This is done by using tools such as NEWS2 (RCP, 2017a) and can give direction on how often a review should occur, or the appropriate action to be taken Fig. 20.3.

It is the responsibility of the NA to raise and report any concerns and actions, as appropriate, and to follow local and national guidelines and policies to reduce the risk, or harm to those to whom you offer care (NMC, 2018a; Institute of Apprenticeships, 2017; Health Education England (HEE), 2017).

HANDOVER AND COMMUNICATION TECHNIQUES

Effective communication plays a central role within healthcare and the nursing profession. Contemporary nursing practice in the UK utilizes the well established 6Cs theory developed by the Chief Nursing Officer of NHS England, Jane Cummings (NHS England, 2016). The 6Cs are the value base for *Leading Change, Adding Value; a framework for nursing, midwifery and care staff*. These values are one of the great legacies created through 'Compassion in Practice', a 3-year strategy that concluded in March 2016. The 6Cs are:

1. Care
2. Compassion
3. Competence
4. Communication
5. Courage
6. Commitment.

See Chapter 8 for more information about the 6Cs.

The 6Cs are embedded into everything that nursing, midwifery and care staff do. We now need to bring the same focus to measuring the outcomes, experiences and use of resources involved in our work. In this way, we will be able to demonstrate an extra dimension to our value. *Leading Change, Adding Value* is a framework that nursing, midwifery and care staff can use to do this. It can be used by everyone, whatever their role, wherever they work.

Communication

Communication's position within the 6Cs affirms its fundamental role in patient safety and successful teamwork (NHS England, 2016). Additionally, the principles of the fundamentals of care (such as use of the 6Cs), are suggested throughout the NMC's Code and its inclusion as a national benchmarker echoes its importance within contemporary nursing practice (DH, 2010a; NMC, 2018a). However, although communication is widely acknowledged as an essential skill to possess, ineffective communication remains linked to errors within clinical practice (Frain, 2018). With healthcare teams encompassing interprofessional working (IPW) and a multi-disciplinary team (MDT) approach, team structure is more complex than ever. Consequently, developing NAs and healthcare professionals (HPCs), and ensuring they possess the skills to effectively communicate, is as vital as ever (Cracknell & Cooper, 2018). Chapter 9 address the essential use of effective communication.

Communication in its simplest form involves a sender and a receiver who interact to exchange verbal and non-verbal information (Bach & Grant, 2011). Communication in healthcare, however, is not always that simple. Barriers to communication can disrupt or interfere with messages being sent or received, which can lead to adverse effects for patients (Ballantyne, 2017). Having a level of insight into the potential communication barriers and knowledge of communication strategies and tools appropriate to the situation, can help NAs, nurses and healthcare professionals to be effective communicators (Elcock & Shapcott, 2015).

Communication tools and barriers
Communication tools

> **REFLECTION 20.4**
>
> Take some time to think about barriers to communications and make a list of some of the potential causes for ineffective communication within a healthcare setting.

An NA must be self-aware of how they communicate and the importance of effective communication, especially in large, complex healthcare environments. The absence of a standardized communication tool when sharing information has been found to be a contributor to ineffective communication (WHO, 2007). Handovers are specifically identified as high-risk for patient safety because it is the point where critical clinical information about patients is passed between healthcare professionals (Ballantyne, 2017). Consistently using a structured communication tool is seen to improve the quality of handovers, as the tool allows nurses and other professionals to organize and structure their thoughts (Renz et al., 2013). Additionally, taking a structured approach to clinical conversations, such as handovers, ensures critical information is both delivered on the one hand and heard on the other (Ballantyne, 2017). Additionally, structured communication tools can bridge the gap between the different communication styles that are often found among different professional groups (Achrekar et al., 2016). A number of different communication tools and frameworks can be used to assist healthcare professionals in conveying information. However, globally, the Situation, Background, Assessment and Recommendation (SBAR) handover tool has gained popularity across healthcare, military and aviation settings, who highly recommend its use to reduce communication barriers and to promote patient safety (WHO, 2007).

SBAR communication tool

Kaiser Permanente, a rapid-response team based in Colorado, USA, introduced the SBAR tool to aid patient safety (Achrekar et al., 2016). The tool aims to assist nurses and other professionals with structuring and standardizing their communication when handing over information about deteriorating patients (Dougherty & Lister, 2015). The SBAR tool does this by providing a structured method to prepare for communication. The SBAR tool is broken down into four sections, with each section having its own set of structured questions. This format reduces ineffective communication because it is easy to follow, the structured design enables the sharing of information to be focused, factual, clear and without repetition. The tool additionally helps prompt the receiver about what information to expect next (NHS Institute Innovation and Improvement, 2010).

Table 20.2 shows an example of the tool and the structured questions asked within each of the four sections.

What follows are some pointers to take into consideration for each section of the SBAR handover tool.

- Situation

Firstly, you need to say who you are. (Tip: make sure you say your full name, multiple professionals working in your area may

TABLE 20.2 SBAR Communication Tool

S	Situation	• I am (insert name/ profession) on (insert ward/ clinical environment) • I am calling about (insert patient name) who is (insert patient age) • The reason I am calling is because they have a NEWS of (insert score) or I am calling because I am concerned that ... (e.g., their pulse is (insert pulse), BP is (insert BP), they are in pain, they are short of breath)
B	Background	• (Insert patient's name) was admitted on (insert admission date) with (insert admission rationale e.g., chest infection) • They have been commenced on ... (insert medication name if appropriate) or they are currently taking ... • They are normally fit and well • During this admission they have had ... (e.g., operation, procedure, investigation)
A	Assessment	• Their last set of observations taken at (insert date and time) were ... (e.g., BP 90/40, pulse 120 bpm, respiratory rate 24 breaths per minute) • The patient's normal condition is ... (e.g., alert, pain free) • They are now ... (e.g., drowsy, confused) • I think the problem is ... or • I am not sure what the problem is, but (insert patient's name) is deteriorating
R	Recommendations	• I need you to come and review the patient within the next ... (give time allocation) • Is there anything I can do in the meantime ... (e.g., repeat observation)

have the same or a similar first name e.g. Laura, Lauren, Lorna. This will reduce any potential confusion later on, so say Laura Nkoma.)

Next you need to state your profession (nurse, NA, trainee NA, student nurse, sister) and where you are based. (Tip: you must state the department and/or the ward number/name.)

Finally, you need to state who you are concerned about (Tip: use the person's full name and age) and why you are concerned. (Tip: be specific, e.g., I am concerned because Mr Vlas is now short of breath.)

• Background

Here you need to give information about the patient, such as the reason for admission; their diagnosis; if they have recently undergone any investigations/procedures; medication that they are taking; and laboratory results. (Tip: ensure the information is relevant to the current situation. For instance, it may only be necessary to name the medication(s) that have just been commenced or medications linked to the current situation.)

Additionally, you need to give background information, such as past medical history. (Tip: remember to only give information that is significant, for example, surgeries that happened 20 years ago may not be significant to the patient's current condition.)

• Assessment

At this point, state the patient's vital signs (observations). (Tip: include the set of observations that were documented before the patient's change in condition, as well as their latest set of observations.)

You should also state the patient's normal condition and how they are now – for example, the patient is normally alert and is now only responsive to pain.

What you think the problem is. (Tip: do not feel pressured to give an answer if you do not know what is wrong with the patient, simply say that you are not sure what the problem is, but the patient is deteriorating.)

• Recommendation

Inform the receiver of the handover what you need/want – for instance, to review the patient in the next 15 minutes.

Finally, ask if there are any recommendations for what you should do, such as repeat observations. (Tip: if a recommendation is given, ensure you repeat the request back to the receiver.)

CASE STUDY 20.2A

Read the case study below and identify what information you would include and where it would go if using the SBAR framework. With the help of Table 20.2, construct your handover.

Hanna Fernandez is a 68-year-old woman who was admitted yesterday on ward 26 with a urinary tract infection (UTI). Hanna is currently on 200 mg of trimethoprim twice a day. Hanna is normally fit and well, fully independent, and lives with her husband in a two-storey home.

Hanna is currently on 4-hourly observations. Her last set of observations were:
• Blood Pressure: 115/78 mm Hg
• Pulse: 76 beats per minute
• Respiratory Rate: 12 breaths per minute
• Temperature: 36.6°C
• Oxygen saturation: 100% oxygen: none in situ (on Room Air 0.21%)
• NEWS = 0

Hanna's observations now are:
• Blood Pressure: 89/52 mm Hg
• Pulse: 111 beats per minute
• Respiratory Rate: 21 breaths per minute
• Temperature: 37.6°C
• Oxygen saturation: 94% oxygen: none in situ (on Room Air 0.21%)
• NEWS = 8

Hanna informs you that she now has pain in her abdomen. When talking to Hanna, you notice she appears confused.

REFLECTION 20.5

Look at the words below and think about how they can potentially be barriers to effective communication.
• Misunderstandings/misinterpretations
• Communication with a speaker whose first language is not English
• Accents
• Terminology/language
• Noises
• Distractions
• Poor telephone connections
• Time

CASE STUDY 20.2B

Read the case study below and identify what information you would include and where it would go if using the SBAR framework.

Yellow – situation
Red – Background
Green – Assessment

Hanna Fernandez is a 68-year-old female who was admitted yesterday onto ward 26 with a urinary tract infection (UTI). Hanna is currently on 200 mg of trimethoprim twice a day. Hanna is normally fit and well, fully independent, and lives with her husband in a two-storey home.

Hanna is currently on 4-hourly observations. Her last set of observations were:

Blood Pressure: 115/78 mm Hg
Pulse: 76 beats per minute
Respiratory Rate: 12 breaths per minute
Temperature: 36.6°C
Oxygen saturation: 100%
NEWS = 0

Hanna's observations now are:
Blood Pressure: 89/52 mm Hg
Pulse: 111 beats per minute
Respiratory Rate: 21 breaths per minute
Temperature: 37.6°C
Oxygen saturation: 94%
NEWS = 8

Hanna informs you that she now has pain in her abdomen. When talking to Hanna you notice she appears confused.

TABLE 20.3   SBAR Responses in Relation to the Case Study

S	Situation	• I am Laura Nkoma and I am a nurse on ward 26 • I am calling about Hanna Fernandez who is a 68- year-old female • The reason I am calling is because she has a NEWS of 9 or • I am calling because I am concerned that Hanna is now in pain, appears confused and her NEWS has gone from 0 to 8
B	Background	• Hanna was admitted on (yesterday's date) with a UTI • She has been commenced on trimethoprim 200 mg twice a day • Hanna is normally fit and well
A	Assessment	• Her last set of observations taken 4 hours ago (insert time) were: BP 115/78, pulse 76, respiratory rate 16, temperature 36.6 and oxygen saturations 100% resulting in an NEWS of 0 • Hanna's observations now are: BP 89/52, pulse 111, respiratory rate 21, temperature 37.6 and oxygen saturations 94% resulting in an NEWS of 9 • Hanna was previously not in pain • She is now complaining of pain in her abdomen and appears confused • I am not sure what the problem is but Hanna is deteriorating
R.	Recommendation	• I need you to come and review Hanna ASAP • Is there anything I can do in the meantime?

Table 20.3 shows the responses to SBAR in Case Studies 20.2a and 20.2b.

Early warning scores

The Department of Health (2000) first introduced the early warning score system in its critical care recommendations. Early Warning Score (EWS) tools, or track and trigger systems such as the National Early Warning Score (NEWS) 2 and Paediatric Early Warning Score (PEWS), are tools used by NAs, nurses and other healthcare professionals to assist in monitoring a patient's health status, in particular, those patients who are critically ill or who are at risk of deteriorating (Bilben et al., 2016). NICE (2007) published clinical guidelines on recognizing and responding to the acutely ill adult and recommends the implementation of early warning tools. Early recognition of the acutely ill patient means clinical decisions about their care can be made promptly (Foley, 2015).

National Early Warning Scores (NEWS)

The Royal College of Physicians (2017a) NEWS2 tool works using numerical data that NAs collect when carrying out physiological measurements on adults (vital observations) (Fig. 20.4). Each physiological measurement, for instance, blood pressure (BP), has allocated parameters, and each parameter has an attached score that ranges from 0–3. Once all physiological measurements have been recorded, their allocated scores are aggregated to calculate the NEWS (NICE, 2007). This score indicates a patient's clinical risk. Fig. 20.5 illustrates the RCP's NEWS2 4-stage threshold trigger system. The four trigger stages follow a colour code system low (grey), low-medium (yellow), medium (amber) and high (red); each stage in the trigger system has a clinical response for healthcare staff to follow (RCP, 2017c, 2017e).

Score of 0–4 (Grey) – This trigger calls for a ward-based response.
Score of 3 in any Individual Parameter (Yellow) – This trigger calls for an urgent ward-based response.
Score of 5–6 (Amber) – This is a key threshold that triggers a response for an urgent clinical review.
Score of 7 or more (Red) – This trigger requires an emergency clinical review.

To correctly and effectively monitor your patients' vital signs, and to calculate their NEWS accurately, the following physiological measurements should be recorded:
• Blood Pressure (BP) (Systolic)
• Respiratory Rate (RR)
• Pulse (heart rate)
• Temperature
• Air or oxygen
• Oxygen saturation – SpO$_2$ scale 1 (%)
• Oxygen saturation – SpO$_2$ scale 2 (%) **(Scale 2 should only be used if the target saturation range is 88%–92% and used under the direction of qualified clinicians)**
• Consciousness level
(RCP, 2017b, d).

The use of the NEWS2 tool in clinical practice has been shown to help NAs and nurses recognize deteriorating patients (Foley, 2015). However, there is currently no system that can be used across all departments and areas of care (Kyriacos, Jelsma & Jordan,

Physiological parameter	Score						
	3	2	1	0	1	2	3
Respiration rate (per minute)	≤8		9–11	12–20		21–24	≥25
SpO₂ Scale 1(%)	≤91	92–93	94–95	≥96			
SpO₂ Scale 2(%)	≤83	84–85	86–87	88–92 ≥93 on air	93–94 on oxygen	95–96 on oxygen	≥97 on oxygen
Air or oxygen?		Oxygen		Air			
Systolic blood pressure (mmHg)	≤90	91–100	101–110	111–219			≥220
Pulse (per minute)	≤40		41–50	51–90	91–110	111–130	≥131
Consciousness				Alert			CVPU
Temperature (°C)	≤35.0		35.1–36.0	36.1–38.0	38.1–39.0	≥39.1	

Fig. 20.4 NEWS2 Chart 1 The NEWS Scoring System. (Reproduced from: Royal College of Physicians. National Early Warning Score (NEWS) 2: Standardising the assessment of acute-illness severity in the NHS. Updated report of a working party. London: RCP, 2017).

NEW score	Clinical risk	Response
Aggregate score 0–4	Low	Ward-based response
Red score Score of 3 in any individual parameter	Low–medium	Urgent ward-based response*
Aggregate score 5–6	Medium	Key threshold for urgent response*
Aggregate score 7 or more	High	Urgent or emergency response**

* Response by a clinician or team with competence in the assessment and treatment of acutely ill patients and in recognising when the escalation of care to a critical care team is appropriate.
**The response team must also include staff with critical care skills, including airway management.

Fig. 20.5 NEWS2 Chart 2 NEWS Thresholds and Triggers (Reproduced from: Royal College of Physicians, 2017a. National Early Warning Score (NEWS) 2: Standardising the assessment of acute-illness severity in the NHS. Updated report of a working party. London: RCP).

2011). Therefore, NAs and other healthcare professionals need to have an awareness of alternative scoring systems and if any modifications have been made. Other physiological measurements that could potentially be included as part of the NEWS calculation are:
- Urine output (minimum urine output is 0.5 mL/kg per hour)
- Blood glucose reading (<4 mmols = hypoglycaemia; 4–9 mmols = normal; >10 mmols = hyperglycaemia)
- Pain assessment (NICE, 2007).

NEWS and the role of the Nursing Associate

The National Confidential Enquiry into Patient Outcome and Death (NCEPOD) (2015) notes that even though the use of the EWS tools are seen to reduce delays in diagnosing patients, not all healthcare professionals are using the scoring tools to identify deteriorating patients.

Nurses and NAs are responsible and accountable for reporting patients' NEWS (Foley, 2015). It is therefore important that they can accurately measure observations, interpret each of the physiological measurements, and adhere to their practice area's EWS system because inaccuracies can lead to incorrect scores, which can result in inappropriate clinical interventions (Higgins et al., 2008). It is recommended that NEWS2 should be used as a clinical assessment tool in conjunction with competent clinical judgement (RCP, 2017a).

CRITICAL AWARENESS

Using the NEWS2 tool (see Fig. 20.3) calculate the scores from the sets of observations below.

Observation set one:
Blood pressure: 118/70
Respiratory rate: 12
Temperature: 38.0
Pulse: 112
Oxygen saturations: 92%
Oxygen: Yes
Level of consciousness: Alert
NEWS =

Observations set two:
Blood pressure: 100/68
Respiratory rate: 20
Temperature: 37.2
Pulse: 117
Oxygen saturations: 96%
Oxygen: No
Level of consciousness: Alert
NEWS =

Observation set three:
Blood pressure: 85/52
Respiratory rate: 24
Temperature: 38.0
Pulse: 120
Oxygen saturations: 90%
Oxygen: Yes
Level of consciousness: Voice
NEWS =

Observations set four:
Blood pressure: 80/48
Respiratory rate: 11
Temperature: 37.2
Pulse: 48
Oxygen saturations: 92%
Oxygen: No
Level of consciousness: Pain
NEWS =

CRITICAL AWARENESS

Using the NEWS2 chart (see Fig. 20.4) identify the clinical risk from the sets of observations below.

Observation set one:
Blood pressure: 118/70
Respiratory rate: 12
Temperature: 38.0
Pulse: 112
Oxygen saturations: 92%
Oxygen: Yes
Level of consciousness: Alert
NEWS = 6

Observations set two:
Blood pressure: 100/68
Respiratory rate: 20
Temperature: 37.2
Pulse: 117
Oxygen saturations: 96%
Oxygen: No
Level of consciousness: Alert
NEWS = 4

Observation set three:
Blood pressure: 85/52
Respiratory rate: 24
Temperature: 38.0
Pulse: 120
Oxygen saturations: 90%
Oxygen: Yes
Level of consciousness: Voice
NEWS = 15

Observation set four:
Blood pressure: 80/48
Respiratory rate: 11
Temperature: 37.2
Pulse: 48
Oxygen saturations: 92%
Oxygen: No
Level of consciousness: Pain
NEWS = 10

Clinical risk:
Set one = medium
Set two = low
Set three = high
Set four = high

REFERENCES

Achrekar, M., Murthy, V., Kanan, S., et al., 2016. Introduction of Situation, Background, Assessment, Recommendation into Nursing Practice: A Prospective Study. Asia Pac. J. Oncol. Nurs. 3 (1), 45–50.

Arnold, E.C., Boggs, K.U., 2016. Interpersonal Relationships. Professional Communication, seventh ed. Elsevier, Missouri.

Bach, S., Grant, A., 2011. Communication & Interpersonal Skills in Nursing, second ed. Learning Matters, Exeter.

Ballantyne, H., 2017. Undertaking Effective Handovers in the Healthcare Setting. Nurs. Stand. 31 (45), 53–62.

Bilben, B., Grandal, L., Sovik, S., 2016. National early warning score (NEWS) as an emergency department predictor of disease severity and 90-day survival in the acutely dyspneic patient – a prospective observational study. Scand. J. Trauma Resusc. Emerg. Med. 24 (1), 80.

Blood Pressure UK, 2017. White Coat Hypertension. http://www.bloodpressureuk.org/BloodPressureandyou/Medicaltests/Whitecoateffect.

British National Formulary (BNF), 2017. British National Formulary. https://www.bnf.org/.

British Thoracic Society (BTS), 2017. Oxygen Guidelines. https://www.brit-thoracic.org.uk/document-library/clinical-information/oxygen/2017-emergency-oxygen-guideline/bts-guideline-for-oxygen-use-in-adults-in-healthcare-and-emergency-settings/.

Brooker, C., Nicol, M., 2011. Alexander's Nursing Practice, fourth ed. Churchill Livingston, Elsevier, London.

Care Quality Commission, 2016. Monitoring the Mental Health Act in 2015/2016. http://www.cqc.org.uk/sites/default/files/20161122_mhareport1516_web.pdf.

Cracknell, A., Cooper, N., 2018. Communication in Clinical Teams. In: Cooper, N., Frain, J. (Eds.), ABC of Clinical Communication. John Wiley & Sons Ltd, Chichester, West Sussex, pp. 29–34.

Department of Health (DH), 2000. Comprehensive Critical Care, a review of adult critical care services. http://webarchive.nationalarchives.gov.uk/20121014090959/http://www.dh.gov.uk/prod_consum_dh/groups/dh_digitalassets/@dh/@en/documents/digitalasset/dh_4082872.pdf.

Department of Health (DH), 2010a. Essence of Care 2010. https://www.gov.uk/government/publications/essence-of-care-2010.

Department of Health (DH), 2010b. How to use Essence of Care. https://www.gov.uk/government/uploads/system/uploads/attachment_data/file/216690/dh_119970.pdf.

Department of Health (DH), 2012. National framework for NHS continuing healthcare and NHS funded nursing care. https://www.gov.uk/government/publications/national-framework-for-nhs-continuing-healthcare-and-nhs-funded-nursing-care.

Department of Health (DH), 2013. NHS Outcomes Framework 2014/2015. https://www.gov.uk/government/uploads/system/uploads/attachment_data/file/256456/NHS_outcomes.pdf.

Department of Health (DH), 2016. NHS Outcomes Framework 2016 to 2017. https://www.gov.uk/government/publications/nhs-outcomes-framework-2016-to-2017.

Dougherty, L., Lister, S. (Eds.), 2015. The Royal Marsden Manual of Clinical Nursing procedures, ninth ed. John Wiley & sons, Ltd, Chichester, West Sussex.

Elcock, K., Shapcott, J., 2015. Core communication skills. In: Delves-Yates, C. (Ed.), Essentials of Nursing Practice. SAGE Publications Ltd, London, pp. 211–222.

Foley, V., 2015. Clinical Measurement. In: Delves-Yates, C. (Ed.), Essentials of Nursing Practice. SAGE Publications Ltd, London, pp. 349–378.

Frain, J., 2018. Why Clinical Communication Matters. In: Cooper, N., Frain, J. (Eds.), ABC of Clinical Communication. Chichester. John Wiley & Sons Ltd, West Sussex, pp. 1–6.

HarmFreeCare.org, 2017. Harm Free Care. http://harmfreecare.org/measurement/nhs-safety-thermometer/.

Health Education England (HEE), 2017. Nursing Associate Curriculum Framework. https://www.hee.nhs.uk/our-work/developing-our-workforce/nursing/nursing-associate-new-support-role-nursing.

Healthcare Improvement Scotland, 2009. Adapted Waterlow pressure area risk assessment chart. http://www.healthcareimprovementscotland.org/our_work/patient_safety/tissue_viability_resources/waterlow_risk_assessment_chart.aspx.

Higgins, Y., Maries-Tillott, C., Quinton, S., Richmond, J., 2008. Promoting Patient Safety using an Early Warning Scoring System. Nurs. Stand. 22 (44), 35–40.

Institute for Apprenticeships, 2017. Apprenticeship standard: nursing associate. https://www.gov.uk/government/publications/apprenticeship-standard-nursing-associate.

Jarvis, C., 2016. Physical assessment and health assessment, seventh ed. Elsevier, Missouri.

Kelly, C.A., Upex, A., Bateman, D.N., 2004. Comparison of consciousness level assessment in the poisoned patient using the Alert/Verbal/Painful/Unresponsive scale and Glasgow Coma Scale. Ann. Emerg. Med. 44 (2), 108–113.

King's Fund, 2017. The Therapeutic Relationship. https://www.kingsfund.org.uk/projects/gp-inquiry/therapeutic-relationship.

Kyriacos, U., Jelsma, J., Jordan, S., 2011. Monitoring vital signs using early warning scoring systems: a review of the literature. J. Nurs. Manag. 19 (3), 311–330.

Maslow, A.H., 1943. A theory of human motivation. Psychol. Rev. 50 (4), 370.

McNarry, A.F., Goldhill, D.R., 2004. Simple bedside assessment of level of consciousness: comparison of two simple assessment scales with the Glasgow Coma Scale. Anaesthesia 59 (1), 34–37.

National Confidential Enquiry into Patient Outcome and Death (NCEPOD), 2015. Sepsis patients at risk of death or long-term complications suffer critical delays in identifying and treating their condition, latest NCEPOD report says. http://www.ncepod.org.uk/2015report2/downloads/PressRelease.pdf.

National Health Service Improvement, no date. Improvement Hub. https://improvement.nhs.uk/improvement-hub/.

National Institute for Health and Care Excellence (NICE), 2007. Acutely ill adults in hospital: recognizing and responding to deterioration. https://www.nice.org.uk/guidance/cg50.

National Institute for Health and Care Excellence (NICE), 2017a. Improving the physical health of people with serious mental illness: A quality improvement approach. https://www.nice.org.uk/sharedlearning/improving-the-physical-health-of-people-with-serious-mental-illness-a-quality-improvement-approach.

National Institute for Health and Care Excellence (NICE), 2017b. Sepsis. Quality Standard [QS161]. https://www.nice.org.uk/guidance/qs161.

NHS, 2017. Safety Thermometer. https://www.safetythermometer.nhs.uk/index.php?option=com_content&view=article&id=2&Itemid=106.

NHS England, 2016. Leading Change, Adding Value, A framework for nursing, midwifery and care staff. https://www.england.nhs.uk/wp-content/uploads/2016/05/nursing-framework.pdf.

NHS Institute for Innovation and Improvement, 2010. The Handbook of Quality and Service Improvement Tools. http://webarchive.nationalarchives.gov.uk/20160805122939/http://www.nhsiq.nhs.uk/media/2760650/the_handbook_of_quality_and_service_improvement_tools_2010.pdf.

Nursing and Midwifery Council, 2018a. The Code. Professional Standards of Practice and Behaviour for Nurses, Midwives and Nursing Associates. https://www.nmc.org.uk/standards/code/.

Nursing and Midwifery Council, 2018b. Standards of Proficiency for Nursing Associates. London: NMC. https://www.nmc.org.uk/globalassets/sitedocuments/education-standards/nursing-associates-proficiency-standards.pdf.

Renz, S.M., Boltz, M.P., Wagner, L.M., et al., 2013. Examining the feasibility and utility of an SBAR protocol in long-term care. Geriatr. Nurs. (Minneap) 34 (4), 295–301.

Resuscitation Council (UK), 2015. The ABCDE approach. https://www.resus.org.uk/resuscitation-guidelines/abcde-approach/.

Royal College of Physicians, 2017a. National Early Warning Score (NEWS) 2: Standardising the assessment of acute-illness severity in the NHS. Updated report of a working party. RCP, London. https://www.rcplondon.ac.uk/projects/outputs/national-early-warning-score-news-2.

Royal College of Physicians, 2017b. National Early Warning Score (NEWS) 2: Standardising the assessment of acute-illness severity in the NHS [Chart 1 The NEWS scoring system]. https://www.rcplondon.ac.uk/projects/outputs/national-early-warning-score-news-2.

Royal College of Physicians, 2017c. National Early Warning Score (NEWS) 2: Standardising the assessment of acute-illness severity in the NHS [Chart 2 NEWS thresholds and triggers]. https://www.rcplondon.ac.uk/projects/outputs/national-early-warning-score-news-2.

Royal College of Physicians, 2017d. National Early Warning Score (NEWS) 2: Standardising the assessment of acute-illness severity in the NHS [Chart 3 NEWS Observation chart]. https://www.rcp.london.ac.uk/projects/outputs/national-early-warning-score-news-2.

Royal College of Physicians, 2017e. National Early Warning Score (NEWS) 2: Standardising the assessment of acute-illness severity in the NHS [Chart 4 Clinical response to NEWS trigger thresholds]. https://www.rcplondon.ac.uk/projects/outputs/national-early-warning-score-news-2.

Schmitz, S.M., 2018. Assessing health status. In: Williams, P. (Ed.), DeWit's Fundamental Concepts and Skills for Nursing, fifth ed. Elsevier., Missouri, pp. 375–396.

Smith, I., Mackay, J., Fahrid, N., Krucheck, D., 2011. Respiratory rate measurement: A comparison of methods. Br. J. Healthcare Assistants 5 (1), 18–23. http://respir8.com/Clinical%20Studies%20-%20Full%20Study.pdf.

The UK Sepsis Trust, 2017. What is sepsis? https://sepsistrust.org/what-is-sepsis/.

Waugh, A., Grant, A. (Eds.), 2018. Ross & Wilson's Anatomy and Physiology in Health and Illness, thirteenth ed. Elsevier, London.

World Health Organization, 2007. Communicating during patient hand-overs. http://www.who.int/patientsafety/solutions/patientsafety/PS-Solution3.pdf.

FURTHER READING

Hurley, K.F., 2011. OSCE and Clinical Skills Handbook, second ed. Elsevier, Toronto.

Liou, S., Chang, C., Tsai, H., Cheng, C., 2013. The effects of a deliberate practice program on nursing students' perception of clinical competence. Nurse Educ. Today 33, 358–363.

Platt, A., Tuffnell, C., Bradley, G., et al. (2011) Mapping of the International Nursing Association for Clinical Simulation and Learning (INACSL) (2011 to the simulation sessions for adult nursing students undertaking the 'Making it Real' Curriculum, Northumbria University. *Unpublished Report*, Northumbria University: UK. https://www.inacsl.org/i4a/pages/index.cfm?pageID=3407.

Unsworth, J., Melling, A., Allan, J., et al., 2014. Assessing human factors during simulation: The development and preliminary validation of the rescue assessment tool. J. Nurs. Educ. Pract. 4 (5), 52–63.

21

Breaking Bad News

Rosi Castle

OBJECTIVES

By the end of the chapter, the reader will be able to:

- Understand how bad news is defined in the literature and reflect on own experiences of receiving bad news
- Identify the barriers for staff and patients/relatives that may exist in the giving of bad news
- Examine the recipients lived experience of receiving the bad news and possible consequences
- Identify the various protocols and skills suggested in the literature
- Explore how bad news can be shared with patients/relatives with compassion and sensitivity
- Explore different clinical contexts in which breaking bad news can take place with an example in practice

KEY WORDS

Bad news

Effective communication

Barriers and strategies

Patient-centred care

Disclosure

Shared decision-making

Patient empowerment

Loss and grief

Emotional work

Self-awareness

CHAPTER AIM

The aim of this chapter is to help the reader understand and explore the issues relating to breaking bad news to patients, relatives or significant others and to encourage the reader to reflect on their own experience of being the bearer of bad news and how their practice may change in the light of reading this chapter.

SELF TEST

1. What do you understand by the term 'standard procedures'?
2. In what situations might you be required to break bad news to a person?
3. Describe the term 'trauma'.
4. What is the difference between empathy and sympathy?
5. From a personal perspective, what might be some of the barriers you may face when breaking bad news?
6. Discuss 'open' and 'closed' awareness.
7. Define grief and discuss how it may manifest.
8. Palliative care means what?
9. What are the overarching principles associated with hospice care?
10. What does the acronym in the BRAKES model mean?

INTRODUCTION

In this chapter we will look at the factors that need to be considered when breaking bad news and the suggested guidelines published on how to break bad news. We will examine how bad news is defined and interpreted by the patient or the Nursing Associate (NA), doctor or other health and social care staff.

There is now a realization that protocols alone may not give the healthcare worker enough guidance in breaking bad news. Warnock's work published in 2010 demonstrates that, rather than being a single episode, the experience of receiving bad news from the patient's perspective is more of a process or journey. Disclosure of bad news may involve the education of the patient, their family and significant others. A person's individual ability to cope will need to be identified to enable the patient to deal with the news and enable the provision of interventions to maximize those coping skills. There are many situations, therefore, where the healthcare professional may feel undermined or unprepared for the situation that they find themselves in when encountering a patient with challenging questions or when having to inform that patient of news that may be interpreted as bad. NAs and registered nurses are often left with the aftermath of bad news following a doctor's consultation. The NA can be seen as the practical manager of events following bad news, as well as the interpreter of medical information.

NAs are encouraged to understand that a patient-focused approach is good practice and therefore understanding how a patient may respond to news is part of the communication process (see Chapter 9 for a detailed discussion of the communication process). Empathy and compassionate care are emphasized, reminding the NA and other care staff to deliver care that embodies these values.

The Nursing and Midwifery Council (2018) states that one of the objectives for the NA was to be able to demonstrate proficiency in the ways in which individuals can contribute to their own health and well-being and be able to reflect on the importance of encouraging and empowering people to share in and shape decisions about their treatment and care. It is important, therefore, to understand the role that the NA can play in supporting patients, relatives and loved ones when these difficult situations arise. There is already a framework to ensure patient-centred care, called the 6Cs (see Chapter 8). The 6Cs are viewed as the principles that form the foundation of the *Compassion in Practice* national nursing strategy published in 2012.

Incorporating the 6Cs into practice can be challenging, and this is no different when breaking bad news (Box 21.1). If you are already in a position where you have delivered significant news or have other relevant experiences in your private life, does this reflect in your practice now?

> **! HOTSPOT**
>
> Care that embodies compassion and empathy is care that is respectful and will go some way to acknowledging the unique and individual needs of people.

> **! HOTSPOT**
>
> Always be aware of the 6Cs when communicating bad news.

However, there are also barriers to this that may have resonance with the NA themselves:
- Do I have enough knowledge?
- Will I be able to answer all their questions?

> **BOX 21.1 The 6Cs Related to Breaking Bad News**
>
> **The 6Cs**
>
> CARE – how you plan the encounter and are sensitive to the patient's/relatives' needs.
>
> COMPASSION – how you demonstrate empathy towards the patient/relative in this situation, being aware of the need to take time. See Gorniewicz, et al. (2017) 'In my view one categorical imperative, never be faster than your patient.'
>
> COMMUNICATION – be compassionate but truthful: 'No decision about me without me.' Making sure that the patient is given the opportunity to make autonomous decisions.
>
> COURAGE – to be able to face the patient/relatives with the truth.
>
> COMMITMENT – to continue with the encounter and to follow up to ensure clarity.
>
> COMPETENCE – to provide the necessary knowledge, skills and attributes to provide the information required by the recipients.

- What will I do if the patient does not respond favourably, or does not believe what I am saying?
- Do I have time to respond to their emotional feelings?
- Should I involve the relative?

> **! HOTSPOT**
>
> Breaking bad news is an intervention that must be managed with thought and knowledge if it is to be 'successful' for all concerned.

The way bad news is communicated can make a difference to patient outcomes (Porensky & Carpenter, 2016). In this chapter, some of these issues are explored to inform and support the NA's practice in the clinical area.

> **! HOTSPOT**
>
> The way in which the NA breaks bad news can have an impact on patient outcomes.

> **REFLECTION 21.1**
>
> - What do you consider to be bad news?
> - What does bad news mean to you?
> - Reflect on your own experiences of receiving bad news.
> - What was important to you about this experience and how has it changed the way you give bad news?

DEFINITION OF 'BAD NEWS'

Buckman (1984) defines bad news as: 'Any information likely to alter drastically a patient's view of his or her future'. Some writers describe this as significant bad news. What does bad news mean for a patient? This may come down to interpretation. For example, having a urinary catheter inserted could be bad news to a patient who feels that would be a violation of their body or who has experienced a painful or uncomfortable procedure previously. It could therefore be argued that bad news is in the eye of the beholder and therefore is self-defining (Dean & Willis, 2016). Consider Mr Singh in Case Study 21.1.

> **CASE STUDY 21.1 Mr Singh**
>
> Mr Singh is a 77-year-old gentleman admitted to hospital following several episodes of breathlessness, fatigue and fluid retention. Mr Singh lives at home with his wife on the eighth floor of an inner-city tower block. They have two daughters who live locally.
>
> Normally, he is an active person who walks his dog twice a day. He has had a hip replacement in the last 5 years with good recovery and outcomes.
>
> Investigations and a patient history undertaken previously at the health centre include a 12-lead ECG, systemic observations, chest x-ray, cardiac echocardiogram and full blood count.
>
> He has been diagnosed with left ventricular heart failure, possibly due to an earlier undetected myocardial infection. Mr Singh is told that he is required to be admitted to hospital where he will undergo further tests and he is given his diagnosis by the doctor on the ward round. The NA is asked to stay with the patient to answer any further questions that he may have. Mrs Singh and their daughters are due to visit later that evening.

REFLECTION 21.2

You are the NA caring for Mr Singh. Write down your possible feelings related to Mr Singh's care. What are the issues that come into your mind?

Breaking bad news: challenges for the patient and the NA

Historically in the medical hierarchical system, knowledge, and therefore power, emanated from the physician. The patient was entirely in the hands of the doctor and this paternalistic approach allowed the patient some freedom from information – the medical model of health (Jones, 1994). Glaser and Strauss (1965) identified this as 'closed awareness': the physician would decide what the patient should know.

However, with the advent of the patient as a consumer and patient-centred care, information about the patient is said to be the patient's property, and rather than simply accepting care provision, the patient can actively question the care they receive (Chowdhry, 2010). Healthcare professionals must therefore communicate their findings to the patient as 'open awareness'. Research in patients with cancer, for example, has found that patients generally prefer to know their diagnosis (Fallowfield et al., 2002). The literature carried out with patients who have cancer argues that non-disclosure can damage the health status of the recipient, either short- or long-term and therefore breaking bad news is not simply a communication task but should be seen in the wider context of health promotion, providing patients with the time to discuss their emotions and feelings (Corner, 1993). In other words, the way in which the news is broken can frame the patient's view of their situation, influencing their treatment compliance and health behaviour. Framing is a manner of communication, which can influence how information is conveyed by supporting some interpretations and downplaying others (Rodriguez et al., 2008) to either focus on the positive – the chance of a cure, or the negative – the chance of a relapse.

The concept of mind/body dualism can help us understand how psychological stress may affect the immune system, for example, and the health status of the recipient (Selye, 1976) if told bad news. Others will argue that not having any information can also cause stress and health consequences (Lowden, 1998). Along with the communication of any life-changing news, therefore, the necessary social support mechanisms are required to avoid the patient experiencing 'social death' preceding biological death (Field & James, 1993), where the patient feels isolated as others around them prepare for their loss. At this point it is important that the patient's ongoing palliative or other needs are met (Nicol, 2015). With regard to Mr Singh in Case Study 21.1, knowledge of the illness trajectory is not clear and there is a possibility that the acute exacerbations of the disease could indicate the patient's deteriorating condition (Wilmot, 2015; Brake & Jones, 2017). Watson et al. (2009) suggest that encouraging the patient to ask questions is a way of determining the timing of the disclosure and detail of information required and maintains hope for the patient.

Another important aspect of the communication process is the effectiveness of communication among the healthcare team (Wittenberg-Lyles et al., 2013). This may be more evident when there are differences in opinion between patients, relatives and care providers (Prouty et al., 2014). Tuffrey-Wijne (2013) found this disparity in her research with patients with learning difficulties who had cancer. Caregivers felt it was better for the patients not to know, to protect them from anxiety – which Tuffrey-Wijne found to be based on the carers' 'world view' rather than on any assessment of the individual. Since the Mental Capacity Act (2005), every attempt to involve the patient in decision-making, using the appropriate level of knowledge, is required by law.

Building a rapport with patients allows the NA to assess psychological needs (Taylor, 2016). Part of the role of the NA is to educate patients and support them from the beginning of the patient journey to the end of treatment (Benner, 1984) and provide information about diagnosis and illness trajectory.

It has already been noted that the recipient of bad news is not always supported once the initial conversation has ended, and this is where the NA will often be asked to follow up the patient's concerns. Arber and Gallagher (2003), for example, argue that models of communication for breaking bad news, such as the SPIKES protocol (Setting, Perception, Invitation, Knowledge, Emotion, Summary), and the guidelines on how to use the model, do not refer to emotional support. The focus is more on the *manner* of breaking bad news (and therefore on the professional) rather than on the person receiving that news (Arber & Gallagher 2003; Duke & Bailey, 2008). Farrell (1999) argued Buckman's (1992) protocol depends on formulas to give bad news resulting in the loss of the human element of how that news may be interpreted or understood.

In fact, back in 1991, Finlay and Dallimore (1991) had explored how parents felt the news of the death of their child had been managed. The results from this retrospective study seemed to suggest that there was greater satisfaction from those parents who had received the news from a police officer, who showed empathy and warmth and appeared upset, rather than those who had received the news from a nurse or doctor. Barriers to communication therefore also need to be examined.

REFLECTION 21.3

Back to Mr Singh in Case Study 21.1 who has been diagnosed with heart failure.

You, as the NA, have been asked to speak with the patient to answer any questions that he may have. He is visibly upset after the ward round has left.

What are your immediate concerns when responding to this patient? Discuss with your colleagues how you may go about this. Can you anticipate his reaction?

John Diamond said in his book about his initial diagnosis of cancer: 'any response to the news of one's own imminent death is a legitimate one' (Diamond, 1999). Therefore, there is certainly an element of the unknown when we are put in this situation, and there lies the first anxiety for the healthcare professional: the patient's reaction to the news and how to manage it. Later on in his book, Diamond talks about the spiritual responsibility for a disease once it has been diagnosed (Diamond, 1999), having to behave as a personal hero that wants to survive enough to get through in the end and 'the implied corollary that those who die are somehow lacking in moral fibre and the will to live'.

Therefore, being there for the patient and having difficult conversations that may clarify, or indeed confirm, their worst fears, is part of being caring and compassionate. For John Diamond, the loss of his voice (he was a broadcaster) was bad news enough, without the added fear of losing his life. Responding to the patient's emotions is said to be one of the most difficult challenges when breaking bad news. The patient may be experiencing elements of the grief response, such as disbelief/silence, crying, denial or even anger (Baile et al., 2000).

Cultural nuances may also need to be considered depending on the health belief system that the patient has been socialized in, and relevance to care across cultures remains under-researched (Baile et al., 2000; Buckman, 2005). Guidance for breaking bad news may also need to reflect cultural differences (Rollins & Hauck, 2015).

However, in her qualitative study of a London Hospice looking at the relations between the representation of professional practice and ethnic and cultural difference in palliative care work, Gunaratnam (2001) found what she called 'insecure practice' affecting intercultural work. A nurse in her study commented:

'I was thinking why it is so frightening and I think it is about communication, particularly around death. In our own culture it is difficult even when there are already agreed concepts and understanding around death, but when you are dealing with people from another culture you are adding another layer...You don't know if you are using the right words and even if you speak the same language the depth of understanding of the other persons culture is very shallow on one side ...in the context of dying we often have to reach out to people and take risks, and I think I might be more reluctant to do that with people from a different culture' (page 177).

The issue that Gunaratnam (2001) stresses later on in the chapter is that emphasis on this one aspect of a person's identity may mean that we culturalize instead of individualize the patient and consequently their care. This may also form a further barrier to the communication process.

As with Mr Singh (Case Study 21.1), many people are diagnosed with long-term conditions that may not have a predictable trajectory, which adds more complexity to how the news is broken and the surety of the information. Cremin (2016) emphasizes the need for shared decision-making so that patients can express their preferences, contributing to the concept of patient-centred care.

Becker et al. (2015) state in their discussion of breaking bad news for physicians that knowledge of the truth can free patients to actively participate in their medical care and can free physicians from sticking simply to the medical facts and allow a patient-centred approach.

REFLECTION 21.4

With regard to Mr Singh in Case Study 21.1, how can the NA and others create an atmosphere for him that is open and truthful?
Discuss this with your colleagues.

Models of breaking bad news

As mentioned earlier, the most commonly cited guideline for breaking bad news is the SPIKES protocol (Baile et al., 2000). This has been adapted in this chapter for the NA who is unlikely to give primary diagnosis/prognosis, but who will, however, be attempting to deal with the aftermath of that news with the patient (Box 21.2).

The SPIKES protocol could also be used for relatives who have experienced a sudden or expected loss.

AT THE GP SURGERY

Practice nurses also have to break bad news, and the NA may be required to assist with this. Often patients visiting the general practice are given results of tests or investigations that have been carried out at the surgery or in another healthcare establishment, such as hospital.

Patients may receive the results of biopsies, scans and blood tests – such as a positive result to a HIV test. Baile's (2000) SPIKES model can be employed to help when the result of the test is to be given to the patient.

Buckman's protocol (1992) adds some useful suggestions regarding giving bad news over the telephone (discussed later in the chapter) and how much information relatives may require to feel that their loved one was cared for until death. This was based on his own experiences in the clinical environment as a doctor. The death of a relative can be a traumatic time. Receiving clear, understandable information from a knowledgeable member of staff who is not afraid to speak of the death in an empathetic manner is essential (Reid et al., 2011; Fallowfield & Jenkins, 2004; Jurkovich et al., 2000; Wright, 1996). This protocol can provide the NA with a structured approach to communicating with relatives, for instance in the example below dealing with breaking bad news about a death.

Buckman's six-step protocol for breaking bad news (1992):

Step 1 Get the physical context of the conversation correct. Whenever possible, the NA should try not to break the news over the telephone. Some forward planning may be required, if possible, to avoid difficult conversations over the telephone. Always ensure that you check in the care plan whether the patient's relatives have asked to be involved and be there when the patient is dying.

Step 2 Assess how much the relatives already know about the patient's situation. The NA may know this already if they have been communicating with the family or have identified one or two key people to contact with information. This information should be in the patient's care plan.

Step 3 Find out how much the relatives want to know. It will be enough for some to simply know that their loved one is dead; however, others may wish to know more detail about what led up to the person's death. The more advanced planning and knowledge that the NA has about the patient and their family, then the easier it will be to anticipate their responses. Anecdotally, in my own experience it is the healthcare assistant, or another NA, or the hands-on nurse, who will have a closer relationship with the relatives and may provide useful information to the NA who may be managing the situation.

BOX 21.2 The SPIKES Model (Baile et al., 2000)

- **Step 1 – Setting up**

Choose an area that is private, either a separate room or a closed-off area that appears non-clinical. It may be that, if the patient is mobile or can use a wheelchair, you take them off the ward.

Make sure that you will not be disturbed during the meeting (Lomas et al., 2004; DH, 2010).

Involve others – If there are significant others who the patient feels should be involved in the discussion, then include them as well. If it is a large family, you may advise one or two key people among the relatives to be there.

Sit down with the patient – are they comfortable and open to talking with you at that precise moment? Use the communication strategy SOLER: sit Squarely, Open posture, Lean forward, Eye contact, Relaxed body language (Egan, 1975; Arthur, 1999).

It may be appropriate to include gentle reassurance by touch of the shoulder or holding hands. In Case Study 21.1, the patient has already been told some news that has visibly affected him. Radziewicz & Baile (2001) believe that touching may be supportive.

- **Step 2 – Assessing the patient's perception**

Before you tell, ask. Using open-ended questions establishes the patient's understanding (in this case of heart failure).

'What do you know about this condition and what did the doctor tell you?'

- **Step 3 Obtaining the patient's invitation**

Try to gauge how much information the patient wants. It may be that discussing the tests already carried out, such as the ECG and echocardiogram may need explaining. This may be enough at this stage. Whilst a majority of patients express a desire for full information about their diagnosis, prognosis and details of their illness, some patients may not be ready, so gentle questioning of what they would like to know is essential.

For example:

Did the doctor explain what heart failure is? Do you have any questions regarding their explanation? Are there particular issues that you would like to discuss?

This then leads in to Step 4.

- **Step 4 Giving knowledge and information to the patient**

If further explanation is requested, you need to frame your explanation according to the patient's current understanding; this is again the confirmation of the bad news that may have been said before. Check that they do not want anyone else with them and if they do, delay further discussion until that is possible. Otherwise say something like:

'Unfortunately following the tests that have been carried out the doctor has diagnosed that your heart is not pumping enough blood around the body – we are not sure why at this stage, but that is why you are experiencing breathlessness. For example, you said that going for a walk with your dog has become more difficult and that your legs have become swollen.'

In the above narrative the NA is not using medical jargon and is relating it to the patient's own lived experience of the condition. The NA is being open with the patient to avoid misunderstanding, but also trying to avoid being too blunt or excessively informative at this stage. As the patient requests more information, careful disclosure can occur.

If the patient asks about his prognosis, only answer this if you have all the facts and have checked with the physician. The patient may have looked up the condition himself on the internet and been frightened by what he has read.

- **Step 5 – Addressing the patient's emotions**

Explore with the patient what his understanding of the prognosis is and suggest a further meeting with the doctor once all the tests are completed.

- **Step 6 – Strategy and summary**

The emphasis should be on providing a summary of how the symptoms can be relieved so that that his quality of life can be improved and so exploring with him what is important in his life at this stage. What information the patient would like the family to be aware of and when that could be arranged would also be discussed.

From this you can correct misinformation and explain the bad news in a way that the patient will understand. Try to establish if the patient is being realistic about what you have said. Are they responding in an overly optimistic way or, conversely, displaying a pessimistic viewpoint?

Step 4 Provide information. When possible, this should include a diagnosis, the treatment the person received before death, and an offer of support.

The NA should explain medical jargon and measure out information in smaller doses to help the relatives take in or understand what is being said.

CRITICAL AWARENESS

The use of words such as 'passed on', 'passed away', 'passed' or 'lost' should be avoided as they may be misunderstood. The current view is that 'died' or 'dead' is more concrete and unequivocal (Harrahill, 1997).

Step 5 Respond to relatives' feelings. This step requires the NA to use good listening skills, as well as to have an awareness of non-verbal communication. The importance of responding to relatives' feelings was emphasized by Harrahill (2005) who noted that staff must ensure relatives have all their questions answered. It is also suggested that relatives are provided with contact details for the hospital, ensuring they can contact staff if any questions arise later (Harrahill, 2005).

Step 6 Prepare the relatives. Inform them of what might be expected of them after they have left the deceased; this includes offering advice on practical matters associated with the death. Time spent with the relatives following the breaking of bad news should not be rushed. Offering tea is a symbolic way of communicating to the relatives that they have some space and time to reflect on what has happened and take on board what the subsequent events may be. The room should be made available for them to stay for as long as they need to compose themselves (Lomas et al., 2004). Jurkovich et al. (2000) found that 19% of study participants described the attention given to the location of their conversation as poor. The study also found that 56% of participants felt the location of the conversation was of medium or high importance.

This is more difficult if the patient dies at night when, as the author experienced, even being given the opportunity to help lay their relative out (the provision of last offices) or just sit with the deceased, may not be encouraged. According to Wright (1996), relatives may feel they no longer have total ownership of their loved one once in hospital. They feel they must be granted permission to do things, such as view the body, hold their hand, or

> ### BOX 21.3 The BREAKS Protocol (Data from Narayanan et al., 2010)
>
> Background – setting the scene
> Rapport – getting the patient's narrative. Explore understanding
> Exploring – getting permission to give more information
> Announce – giving slow warning. Avoid bluntness
> Kindling – responding to emotion
> Summarize – paraphrasing what has been said and concerns of the patient.
> Documentation and ongoing plan discussed.

> ### BOX 21.4 Resources for Explaining to People with Intellectual Difficulties (Adapted from Tuffrey-Wijne, 2013)
>
> - Make an assessment of the patient's ability to understand, asking for support from family, support staff and colleagues in intellectual disability services if in doubt.
> - Use short, simple explanations and pictures (such as those in the 'Books Beyond Words'* series).
> - Avoid collusion with carers who may be over-protective.
> - Support the carers and give them all the information.
> - Create opportunities for the patient to ask questions and answer them truthfully.
>   Useful books include:
> *Am I going to die?* by S. Hollins and Tuffrey-Wijne, I. (2009).
> *Getting on with cancer* by Donaghey (2002) This tells the story of a woman who is diagnosed with cancer and then has surgery, radiotherapy and chemotherapy. Available from www.rcpsych.ac.uk/publications.

*'Books Beyond Words' is a series of picture books that has been developed to make communicating easier for people with learning difficulties.

speak to the deceased. The death of a relative is a traumatic time. Family members must receive clear, understandable information from a knowledgeable member of staff who is not afraid to speak of the death in an empathetic manner (Fallowfield & Jenkins, 2004; Jurkovich et al., 2000; Reid et al., 2011; Wright, 1996).

If families are not present at the time of death, they may feel guilty that their relative died 'alone' and they were unable to say goodbye (Wright, 1996). This highlights the need for NAs to encourage family members to spend as much time as they wish with the deceased, allowing them to say final goodbyes, which will help to promote normal grieving processes (Cooke, 2000). This is also stressed by Brown (2016), ensuring that relatives do not feel marginalized or uninvolved is vital as this could have negative effects for bereavement (Brown 2016).

Offering guidance on collecting the death certificate and registering the death can be explored with the relatives and usually there is a leaflet designed for this purpose that can be provided. This is helpful because information will not necessarily be understood or processed by the relatives at this time.

Another, more recent, model devised by Narayan et al. in 2010, is outlined in Box 21.3. It is represented by the acronym BREAKS: Background, Rapport, Exploring, Announce, Kindling, Summarize. It includes the important events following the breaking of bad news and acknowledges the emotional aspects of the encounter and how the communicator of the bad news should record concerns of the recipients and document this for follow up.

Telephone communication

The fear of many healthcare professionals, including NAs, is when a relative rings unexpectedly and wants information, or when the NA must ring a relative to give bad news. What to say in this situation will depend on a number of factors:

- Is this the significant relative that the NA has been communicating with? If not, who are they and how much information should be disclosed?
- Is the relative at home or somewhere relatively safe to receive bad news? It's important to check, especially if ringing or responding to a mobile number.
- Make sure they are not driving, and if they are, advise them to move to a safe space. Requesting that the relative be accompanied by someone is also be advised.

If the person has died, what should the NA disclose? Ethically, the Code (Nursing and Midwifery Council, 2018a) requires that those who provide care are open and truthful with patients and relatives,

as far as the law allows, and provide the information they want or need to know about their relative's healthcare and ongoing treatment sensitively and in a way they can understand. However, if the relative or patient is alone, or the NA feels they are vulnerable, Kendrick (1997) suggests that avoiding the truth in this situation can be ethically justified as staff are trying to prevent harm and want to make sure the situation is right for them to hear the bad news. Again, it will depend on the situation, such as how far the relative lives from the hospital. The important issue here is that staff do not imply that someone is alive when they are not, and if asked directly should respond truthfully (Buckman, 1992). If they do not do this, they may lose the trust of the patient's family when they find out that the time of death was before they were contacted. Guidance has since been developed to ensure that the conversation takes place as soon as possible.

Breaking bad news to patients with intellectual difficulties

Tuffrey-Wijne (2013) suggests ways of explaining bad news to patients with intellectual difficulties. As stated in the Mental Capacity Act 2005, an appropriate level of information is required by law (Tuffrey-Wijne, 2013). Every attempt should be made to invite the patient into the decision-making progress, or if this is not possible, then the process should be openly discussed and documented. Clarity among staff as to what has been disclosed and the reasons for withholding any information should be made explicit.

It is important to acknowledge the sadness that the person feels rather than trying to cheer the person up. The patient's understanding will depend on their cognitive capacity, and their experience (for example, of cancer in the family) as to how much they are told and in what format. Their understanding will also depend on their ability to comprehend the concept of time and the future (Box 21.4).

COMMUNITIES OF CARE

Learning Disabilities

Generally, there are few picture books that are available for adults and adolescents who are unable to read or who may have difficulty with reading. There are fewer books still that provide information about and address emotional issues, such as death and dying. *When somebody dies* is a book produced by Books Beyond Words. It explains the issues associated with death and dying in an appropriate and sensitive manner that people with intellectual and communication difficulties can more easily understand.

The stories in this text are told through colour pictures that include mime and body language, to communicate simple yet explicit messages. These help the 'readers' to manage their emotions and the events that may be associated with bereavement.

Telling the whole story in pictures can help people to prepare for an event or to deal with something that has already happened. 'Readers' are able to associate the pictures with their own experiences and they are not distracted or confused by any accompanying text. The pictures share information, show procedures and illustrate emotions that are relevant to death, dying and bereavement.

At the back of each book, there is support information provided as text. A suggested storyline provides one interpretation of what is taking place.

Emotional barriers related to breaking bad news

Parkes (1996) talks about the cost of commitment. When an emotional response is required from the person breaking bad news, the professional may feel committed and involved in that news and its consequences. To avoid this emotional attachment, some professionals develop strategies in which they remain detached and avoid any situation where an emotional response may occur, and thus the 'emotional labour' – the term used for this part of a nurse's work – involved (Smith, 2012). To remain objective and, some would argue, professional, by avoidance of any situation in which an emotional response may be likely, the NA will avoid a situation or a conversation with the patient or relatives. Emotional work as described by Sorensen and Ledema (2009) can lead to distress and imbalance in the relationship between the patient and the nurse.

There may also be feelings of anxiety if the NA has experienced a similar situation in their own life or if there are shared meanings related to the death, such as cultural identity or identification with the relatives, which can lead to a more personalized response (Penson & Fischer, 2002).

Being able to get closure when an encounter such as this is over can only be managed if the NA is supported, and if there is recognition of the trauma that can be involved. Reflection of the encounter and discussion with an agreed person is helpful. Breaking bad news guidance should include reference to care and support of the healthcare professional (Arber & Gallagher, 2003; Bousquet et al., 2015).

REFLECTION 21.5

Do you reflect on difficult conversations/encounters in order to reach closure? Discuss this with your colleagues.

Patient reactions

Being aware of the possible patient reactions and considering how to cope with this to support the patient is challenging. These are some typical responses.

- Why me?
- I don't understand it – I feel so well. It must be a mistake! – **Denial**
- What I have I done to deserve this? It isn't fair! – **Anger**
- How can I/they live longer? What can I do to achieve this? – **Bargaining**
- What's the point of treatment I'm a 'goner'. – **Depression**
- I will just have to live for today. – **Acceptance**

Kubler-Ross (1969) originally described these stages of loss when trying to understand the emotional reactions to the experiences of dying. The individual may move from denial of death to acceptance.

REFLECTION 21.6

- Denial
- Anger
- Bargaining
- Depression
- Acceptance

Think of personal examples of these coping mechanisms in your own everyday life – how do they fit with you? For example, if you are told you have failed an exam – how do you react?

These stages were originally viewed and presented in a linear fashion that the patient would go through ending in acceptance. However, Kubler-Ross (2009) has since agreed that these stages are interchangeable, and a person can oscillate between them depending on their mood and the circumstances they find themselves in. In addition, bargaining may not be a possibility for a relative when a patient dies. The stages also do not take into account cultural and individual ways of coping. Brown (2016) considered this approach to be reductionist and unhelpful as it rejects the person's ability to be empowered and utilize their own coping strategies. In other words, these ways of understanding a person's response may be helpful in trying to identify at what stage of the grief cycle the patient/relative is at and how best to help them (Brown, 2016); however, there is no set rule as to how someone should respond, and we should respect every individual's right to use a coping system that helps them at the time. There is no script explaining how one would feel in this situation, or how to understand, for example, what it is like to suddenly be put on 'death row'.

What studies seem to imply is that no news is good news and that uncertainty can increase suffering. A better understanding of the situation allows the patient some control over their care and the decisions that they need to make. It comes down to the basic tenet of caring that is patient-centred (Van Mossel et al., 2011).

Heaven et al. (2003) identified two elements to the act of breaking bad news: facilitation of the disclosure – so knowing the patient when possible, and positive responsiveness to what is disclosed. Becker et al. (2015) added that for patients, finding out the truth about their illness forces them to confront existential fears, such as:

- What will happen to me?
- Will I know when I am dying?
- What will it be like?
- Is there another place?

Becker et al. 2015 give an analogy of a physician bearing bad news as being that they must hold out the truth like a jacket, ready to help the patient put it on when they are ready.

It is also important to find out about, or make reference to, an integrated care plan with regard to whether the patient has a faith and whether they would like to discuss this further with a spiritual person who is available to come and talk. Such an approach could be adopted successfully by the NA.

It is important to remember that supportive care from day one is essential (NICE, 2004). Think about Mr Singh in Case Study 21.1 with a diagnosis of heart failure, and accompanying him on the journey, informing him of the issues as they arise and when he is ready to receive them. Involving his family when he feels it is appropriate would also be necessary. Addressing his quality of life and allowing him hope would all be part of the journey. However, simply focusing on hope may deny his need to talk about his dying and eventual death.

As mentioned earlier, protocols such as SPIKES give confidence to the news-breaker as to how to manage this intervention. However, the patient's experience is more difficult to define or manage (Arber & Gallagher, 2003; Fallowfield & Jenkins, 2004). In fact, Gardner (2016) says using 'formulaic' communication strategies may obscure the real issues.

It is therefore important to keep an open mind and to use these protocols in the service of creating and enhancing a communication intervention which, although it may be painful for the recipient, will allow them the choices to decide their own journey – its direction and speed.

REFLECTION 21.7

Reflect back on your own experiences of giving or receiving bad news now that you have read this chapter.

What are the communication skills and strategies you feel you have or you need to develop to support your patients, but at the same time take care of your professional and emotional self?

LOOKING BACK, FEEDING FORWARD

The NA is expected to be able to demonstrate proficiency when engaging in difficult conversations. This includes the ability to break bad news and to support those who may be feeling vulnerable or in distress, demonstrating conveying compassion and sensitivity, as well using appropriate communication strategies. This chapter has provided some insight as to how the NA may, when using the 6Cs, provide care that is sensitive and empathetic.

There are several models, frameworks and protocols that can be used in helping to decide the best approach, although it has to be acknowledged that there is no one best approach. The way bad news is broken is often context-dependent and the NA must be aware of this. Previous personal experiences may impact on how the news is delivered and the way the recipients react when being given bad news. Understanding the key issues that have been addressed in this chapter can help to offer care that is appropriate and timely.

REFERENCES

Ahmadi, A., Heydari, N., 2010. Is there a proper method of truth telling? J. Med. Ethics Hist. Med. 3 (2), 16–28.

Arber, A., Gallagher, A., 2003. Breaking Bad news revisited: the push for negotiated disclosure and changing practice implications. Int. J. Palliat. Nurs. 9, 166–172.

Arthur, D., 1999. Assessing nursing students' basic communication and interviewing skills; the development and testing of a rating scale. J. Adv. Nurs. 29 (3), 658–665.

Baghdari, N., Rad, M., Sabzevari, M.T., 2017. Effects of SPIKES-based Education by Role Playing and Multimedia Approaches on Breaking Bad News Skills in Midwifery Students (a comparison). Acta facultatis Medicae Naissensis 34 (2), 137–146.

Baile, W.F., Buckman, R., Lenzi, R., et al., 2000. SPIKES – a six-step protocol for delivering bad news; application to the patient with cancer. Oncologist 5 (4), 302–311.

Becker, G., Jors, K., Block, S., 2015. Discovering the truth beyond the truth. J. Pain Symptom Manage. 49 (3), 646–649.

Benner, P., 1984. From Novice to Expert. Excellence and Power in Clinical Nursing practice. Addison-Wesley, Menlo Parl. CA. In Taylor, S. (2016) The Psychological and psychosocial effects of head and neck cancer. Cancer Nurs. Pract. 15 (9), 33–37.

Bennett, V., Cummings, J., 2012. Compassion in Practice: Nursing, Midwifery and Care Staff, Our Vision and Strategy. DH and NHS Commissioning Board, London.

Bouquet, G., Ori, M., Winterton, S., et al., 2015. Breaking bad news in oncology; a metasynthesis. J. Clin. Oncol. 33 (22), 2437–2443.

Brake, R., Jones, I.D., 2017. Chronic heart failure part 1; pathophysiology, signs and symptoms. Nurs. Stand. 31 (19), 54–60.

Brown, M., 2016. Palliative Care in Nursing and Healthcare. Sage.

Bousquet, G., Orn, M., Winterton, S., et al., 2015. Breaking bad news in oncology: a metasynthesis. J. Clin. Oncol. 33 (22), 2237–2443.

Buckman, R., 1992. How to Break Bad News: A Guide for Healthcare Professionals. John Hopkins University Press, Baltimore, MD.

Buckman, R.A., 2005. Breaking bad news: the SPIKES strategy. Commun. Oncol. Mar/Apr, 138–141.

Buglass, E., 2010. Grief and bereavement theories. Nurs. Stand. 24 (41), 44–47.

Buckman, R., 1984. Breaking Bad News; why is it still so difficult? Br. Med. J. (Clin. Res. Ed.) 288, 1597–1599.

Chowdry, S., 2010. Exploring the concept of empathy in nursing; can it lead to abuse of patient trust? Nurs. Times 106 (42), 22–25.

Cooke, H., 2000. When Someone Dies. Butterworth-Heinemann, Oxford.

Corner, J., 1993. The impact of nurses' encounters with cancer on their attitudes. J. Clin. Nurs. 2 (6), 363–372.

Cremin, M., 2016. Encouraging shared decision making on treating men who have prostate cancer. Cancer Nurs. Pract. 15 (6), 32–36.

Cromwell, J., Goodrich, J., 2009. Exploring how to enable compassionate care in hospital to improve patient experience. Nurs. Times 105 (15), 14–21.

Dean, A., Willis, S., 2016. The use of Protocol in breaking bad news: evidence and ethos. In: J. Palliat. Nurs. 22 (6), 265–271.

Department of Health, 2010. Independent Enquiry into Care Provided by Mid Staffordshire NHS Foundation Trust. January 2005–March 2009, Vol 1.

Diamond, J., 1999. Because Cowards Get Cancer Too. Vermillion, London.

Donaghey, V., 2002. Getting on With Cancer. Gaskell/St Georges Hospital Medical School, London.

Duke, S., Bailey, C., 2008. Chapter 7. In: Payne, S., Seymour, J., Ingleton, C. (Eds.), Palliative Care Nursing – Principles and Evidence for Practice, second ed. OU press McGraw-Hill Education.

Egan, G., 1975. The Skilled Helper; a Client Centred Approach. Wadsworth Publishing Co Inc.

Fallowfield, L., Jenkins, V., 2004. Communicating sad, bad and difficult news in medicine. Lancet 363, 312–319.

Fallowfield, L., Jenkins, V., Farewell, V., et al., 2002. Efficacy of Cancer research UK communications skill model. Lancet 359 (9307), 650–656.

Farrell, M., 1999. The challenge of breaking bad news. Intensive Crit. Care Nurs. 15 (2), 101–110.

Field, D., James, N., 1993. Where and how people die. In: Clark, D. (Ed.), The Future for Palliative Care: Issues of Policy and Practice. Open University Press, Buckingham, pp. 6–29.

Finlay, I., Dallimore, D., 1991. Your child is dead. Br. Med. J. 302 (6791), 1524–1525.

Gardner, C., 2016. Medicine's uncanny valley; the problem of standardising communication. Lancet 386 (9998), 1032–1033.

Glaser, B., Strauss, A., 1965. Awareness of Dying. Aldine, Chicago.

Gorniewicz, J., Floyd, M., Krishnan, K., et al., 2017. Breaking bad news to patients with cancer: a randomised control trial of a brief communications skills training module incorporating the stories and preferences of actual patients. Patient Educ. Couns. 100, 655–666.

Gunaratnam, Y., 2001. Chapter 7: 177. In: Culley, L., Dyson, S. (Eds.), Ethnicity and Nursing Practice. Palgrave, Basingstoke.

Harrahill, M., 1997. Giving bad news compassionately – a two-hour medical school educational programme. J. Emerg. Nurs. 23 (5), 496–498.

Harrahill, M., 2005. Giving bad news gracefully. J. Emerg. Nurs. 31 (3), 312–314.

Heaven, C., Maguire, P., Green, C., 2003. A patient centred approach to defining and assessing interviewing competency. Epidemiol. Psichiatr. Soc. 12, 86–91.

Herth, K.A., 1990. Fostering hope in terminally ill people. J. Adv. Nurs. 15, 1250–1259.

Hollins, S., Tuffrey-Wijne, I., 2009. Am I Going to Die? Books beyond Words series. Royal College of Psychiatrists Publication, London.

Jenkins, V., Fallowfield, L., Saul, J., 2001. Information needs of patients with cancer; results from a large study in in the UK cancer centres. Br. J. Cancer 84, 48–51.

Jones, L., 1994. The Social Context of Health and Health Work. Macmillan.

Jurkovich, G., Pierce, M.D., Becky, R.N., 2000. Giving bad news; the family perspective. J. Trauma Acute Care Surg. 48 (5), 865–873.

Kendrick, K., 1997. Sudden death; walking into a minefield. Emergency Nurse 5 (1), 17–19.

Kubler-Ross, E., 1969. On Death and Dying. The Macmillan Company, New York.

Kubler-Ross, E., 2009. On Death and Dying; What the Dying Have to Teach Doctors, Nurses, Clergy and Their Own Family, fortieth anniversary ed. Routledge, Abingdon.

Lomas, D., Timmins, J., Harley, B., Mates, A., 2004. The development of best practice in breaking bad news to patients. Nurs. Times 100 (15), 28–30.

Lowden, B., 1998. The health consequences of disclosing bad news. Eur. J. Oncol. Nurs. 2 (4), 225–230.

Martins, R.G., Carvalho, I.P., 2013. Breaking bad news; patient preferences and health locus of control. Patient Education and Counselling 92, 67–73.

May, C., 1993. Disclosure of terminal prognoses in a general hospital; the nurse's view. J. Adv. Nurs. 18, 1362–1368.

McQueen, A., 2000. Nurse–patient relationships and partnership in hospital care. J. Clin. Nurs. 9 (5), 723–731.

Mishelmovich, N., Arber, A., Odelius, A., 2016. Breaking significant news: the experience of clinical nurse specialists in cancer and palliative care. Eur. J. Oncol. Nurs. 21, 153–159.

Narayanan, V., Bista, B., Koshy, C., 2010. 'BREAKS' Protocol for breaking bad news. Indian J. Palliat.Care 16 (92), 61–65.

National Institute for Health and Clinical Excellence (NICE), 2004. Improving Supportive and palliative Care for Adults with Cancer. https://www.nice.org.uk/guidance/csg4.

National Institute for Health and Care Excellence (NICE), 2015. Care of dying adults in the last days of life. https://www.nice.org.uk/guidance/ng31.

Nicol, J., 2015. Nursing Adults With Long Term Conditions, second ed. Sage.

Nursing and Midwifery Council, 2018a. The Code. Professional Standards of Practice and Behaviour for Nurses, Midwives and Nursing Associates. NMC., London. https://www.nmc.org.uk/standards/code/.

Nursing and Midwifery Council, 2018b. Standards of Proficiency for Nursing Associates. NMC., London. https://www.nmc.org.uk/globalassets/sitedocuments/education-standards/nursing-associates-proficiency-standards.pdf.

Parkes, C.M., 1996. Studies of Grief in Adult Life, third ed. Routledge, London.

Penson, P., Fischer, R., 2002. Palliative Care for People with Cancer, third ed. Arnold Publications, London.

Porensky, E.K., Carpenter, B.D., 2016. Breaking bad news; effects of forecasting diagnosis and framing prognosis. Patient Educ. Couns. 99, 68–76.

Prouty, C., Mazor, K.M., Greene, S.M., et al., 2014. Providers' perceptions of communication breakdowns in cancer care. J. Gen. Intern. Med. 29 (8), 112–113.

Radziewicz, R., Baile, W.F., 2001. Communication skills; breaking bad news in the clinical setting. Oncol. Nurs. Forum 28 (6), 951–953.

Reid, M., McDowell, J., Hoskins, R., 2011. Breaking bad news of death to relatives. Nurs. Times 107, 12–15.

Rodriguez, K.L., Gambino, F.J., Butow, P.N., et al., 2008. 'It's going to shorten your life': framing of oncologist–patient communication about prognosis. Psychooncology 17, 219–225.

Rollins, L.K., Hauck, F.R., 2015. Delivering breaking news in the context of culture; a patient centred approach. J. Clin. Outcomes Manag. 22 (1), 21–26.

Selye, H., 1976. Stress without distress. In: Serban, G. (Ed.), Psychopathology of Human Adaptation. Springer Book Archive, pp. 137–146.

Smith, P., 2012. The Emotional Labour of Nursing Revisited. Can Nurses Still Care? Palgrave Macmillan, Basingstoke.

Sorensen, R., Ledema, R., 2009. Emotional labour; clinicians' attitudes to death and dying. J. Health Organ. Manag. 23, 5–22.

Taylor, S., 2016. The psychological and psychosocial effects of head and neck cancer. Cancer Nursing Pract. 15 (9), 33–37.

Tudiver, F., Lang, F., 2017. Breaking bad news to patients with cancer; a randomised control trial of a brief communication skills training module incorporating the stories and preferences of actual patients. Patient Educ. Couns. 100, 655–666.

Tuffrey-Wijne, I., 2013. A new model for breaking bad news to people with intellectual disabilities. Palliat. Med. 27 (1), 5–12.

Van Mossel, C., Alford, M., Watson, H., 2011. Challenges of patient centred care practice or rhetoric? Nurs. Inq. 18, 278–289.

Warnock, C., Tod, A., Foster, J., Soveny, C., 2010. Breaking bad news in patient clinical settings; role of the nurse. J. Adv. Nurs. 66 (7), 1543–1555.

Warnock, C., 2014. Breaking bad news; issues relating to nursing practice. Nurs. Stand. 28 (45), 51–58.

Warnock, C., Buchanan, J., Tod, A.M., 2017. The difficulties experienced by nurses and healthcare staff involved in the process of breaking bad news. J. Adv. Nurs. 73 (7), 1632–1645.

Watson, M., Lucas, C., Hoy, A., et al., 2009. Oxford Handbook of Palliative Care, second ed. Oxford University Press, Oxford.

Wilmot, J., 2015. Palliative care of non-malignant conditions. In: Nicol, J. (Ed.), Nursing Adults With Long Term Conditions, second ed. Sage, London.

Wittenberg-Lyles, E., Goldsmith, J., Ferrell, B., 2013. Oncology nurse communication barriers to patient-centred care. Clin. J. Oncol. Nurs. 7 (2), 152–158.

Wright, B., 1996. Sudden Death: a Research Base for Practice. Churchill Livingstone, New York, NY.

22

Essay Writing

Shirley Sardeña

OBJECTIVES

By the end of this chapter the reader will be able to:
1. Deconstruct an essay question
2. Search for information resources to answer an essay question
3. Understand how to take notes and read papers analytically
4. Structure an essay plan
5. Discuss standard essay format
6. Understand the importance of drafts and checking work
7. Avoid plagiarism
8. Reference correctly

KEY WORDS

Assignment	Format	Rubric
Assessment	Proofreading	Critical analysis
Information	Plagiarism	
Structure	Regulations	

CHAPTER AIM

The aim of this chapter is to provide information on the skills you will need to write an essay.

SELF TEST

1. Name the key three key components of an essay.
2. What is Boolean logic?
3. List three reliable search engines.
4. What are the benefits of using an academic search engine?
5. Explain what a mind map is.
6. What does the acronym KISS stand for?
7. How would you describe a seminal text?
8. Why is it important to proofread your work?
9. What do you understand by the term 'plagiarism'?
10. How can you avoid plagiarism?

INTRODUCTION

Essay writing is a required skill for any academic course. Even in a practical course such as nursing, essay writing is used as an assessment tool. There will be other types of assessment during your course, for example, multiple choice questions, examinations and vivas. Chapter 3 provides hints and tips with regard to study as 'learning to learn', but this chapter focuses on the writing of an essay as part of a course assignment strategy.

THE PURPOSE OF ESSAY WRITING

While many student nurses (and students in general) do not like writing essays, there are many positives associated with this style of assessment. Essay writing allows you to demonstrate your knowledge of a subject. Unlike in an exam, you are able to prepare, plan and explore a subject area at your own pace (albeit within the timeframe of the assessment period). You are allowed, and expected, to use others' work to write an essay (correctly referenced – but more on that later) and to do so without having to memorize it, as you would in an exam.

> **! HOTSPOT**
>
> When you get your hand-in date, work out how many weeks you have to produce your essay. Set yourself a completion date one or two weeks before the actual date. This will allow you some 'extra time' if you get delayed. Time management is essential.

Another positive aspect of writing an essay is that you will have to carry out research. The process of researching allows you to extensively read around and think about the subject. So often, we learn at such a pace that we do not have the opportunity to pause and look at a subject in more depth, and really imbed that knowledge into our memory. In 10 years' time you will you probably still remember the essays you wrote while studying, but you will not necessarily recall exam questions.

Finally, writing is a skill, and being given the opportunity to write essays will allow you to learn and hone these skills. In an era of abbreviations, hash tags and emojis, the ability to express yourself through the written word is a valuable skill not only for your studies, but also for your employability.

Data from Health Education England (2017)

As with all skills, the more you practise the better you become. Some students will have a natural writing ability, whilst others will need to work harder to develop their writing skills. However, these are basic skills that can be learnt and will benefit all students.

I have an essay to write – What do I do?

Imagine the scenario: you attend a class and are told that assessment for the module will be a 2,500-word essay. The first thing to do is not to panic. Many students have fears and anxieties when faced with writing an essay for the first time. Fig. 22.1 shows some common responses.

There is no need to panic when faced with writing an essay. An organized approach should be adopted. You need to:
- understand the question
- know what you need to write about to answer the question
- know where to find the information you need
- know how to present your writing in academic essay format.

Understanding the question

Normally, an essay question will be set and the lecturer will explain what you are expected to write about. It is critical that you understand the question and what is being asked. Many institutions will use a rubric to help guide students. A rubric in its simplest form is a set of instructions, quite often in the form of a table. By studying this you will have a better understanding of what is required for you to complete your assignment. Some students do not recognize the value of a rubric, often only referring to it at the end, however it is strongly recommended that you use it as a guide throughout your assignment. Often students will provide an answer to what they 'think' the question is and not actually what is being asked. No matter how well written the essay, if it does not fulfil the requirements of the question, it will be wrong.

The easiest method to use to ensure you understand the question is to *deconstruct* it, that is, break it down into small sections. Let us use the example of this question:

Discuss how communication is used to improve patient care for the elderly.

The first step is to highlight the words that are the most important the essay title, then look at each of these words in turn and think about what they mean in the context of the question. Table 22.1 breaks down the above question.

Different essays will ask you different questions. Table 22.2 helps you understand the meaning behind some of the words commonly used.

After examining the question in this way, you should be able to put the question into your own words and have an idea how to answer it. For your own personal use, provide a little more information regarding what you will be writing about. For example:

'Discuss – write about the most important aspects of communication specifically focusing on communication with the elderly. Then discuss how communication with the elderly can be improved to ensure better patient care'.

You should now have a solid understanding of what is being asked of you and what you are expected to write your essay on. The next step is to design an essay plan.

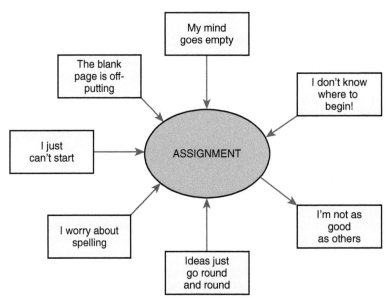

Fig. 22.1 Some Common Responses to Essay Writing.

TABLE 22.1 Examples of Meaning in Context

What does discuss mean?	Discuss means to identify important aspects of the subject and consider arguments for and against
What is communication?	You will need to provide a definition of 'communication' in the essay and then discuss how it is used with patients
How does the question use the word 'Improve'?	Highlight how communication may not be being used, or used well, and then show how it could be used better (improve) to benefit patients
What is patient care?	Explain what patient care is – work into the text the importance and the need for improvement
What limits does the word 'elderly' in the question place on your essay?	You have been provided with a specific demographic to consider, the 'elderly', so you should not be writing about any other group of people. You therefore need to think about, and include, the specific needs of this group

TABLE 22.2. Key Words Used in Assignment Criteria

Define	Give the exact meaning of ...
Discuss	Give important aspects and consider arguments for and against
Analyse	Examine in close detail and identify the important points
Compare	Show how two things are *similar*
Contrast	Show how two things are *different*
Evaluate	Give the usefulness (strengths and weaknesses, pros and cons)
Describe	Give the main features of something
Explain	Give a reason for something happening
Relate	Show connections between two or more things
Account for	Explain why something happens
Valid	Addresses the concept e.g., an assessment tool that measures what it was intended to measure
Reliable	Stable and consistent e.g., an assessment tool that always gives results that are error free and without bias
Component	An essential part that contributes to the whole

! HOTSPOT

When you are set an essay, make sure you ask the following:
• When is the hand-in date?
• How many tutorials on it can you have?
• Are there any specific requirements for presentations, e.g. format, font, line spacing?

THE ESSAY PLAN

It is essential to spend time at the beginning creating a good essay plan. Some students prefer to start reading and then think about how their essay will develop; however, if you have a good essay plan to start with, there are some distinct advantages:

• You will have a clearer idea of what information you need to find to support your arguments for your essay.
• You will stay more focused on the topic – and less likely to deviate from the essay title.
• Ultimately, it will save you time as you will be researching with a clear purpose.

In order to create a good essay plan, you need to understand the structure of an essay. Normally an essay is written in three parts:
1. The introduction
2. Main body
3. Conclusion.

Thinking of an essay in these three parts makes it far more manageable.

THE INTRODUCTION

The introduction provides a brief outline of the topic and what you plan to focus on. Make your introduction almost a guide for yourself for what you are going to write about. If we use the same essay question, *Discuss how communication is used to improve patient care for the elderly*, An example of an introduction could be the following:

'This essay will look at communication with the elderly and how communication can be used to improve patient care. Firstly, communication will be defined and discussed in relation to the specific needs of the elderly. It will address how communication is a vital skill in nursing and how it can be used to improve patient care by helping form therapeutic relationships with patients. Finally, the essay will conclude by summarizing its findings.'

As a draft introduction, this provides you with all the information you need to get started. You know from this introduction what will make up the main body of your assignment and how your conclusion will be written.

The main body of your assignment will be the largest part of your essay. It will be where you discuss the main issues. In this case, all the areas you have mentioned in your introduction will make up the main body.

Essays tend to follow the format of an argument, so, for example, you could write:

'The idea of using verbal communication with the elderly was thought to be of more importance than non-verbal skills (MadeUpFact, 2012). However, MadeUpFact (2016) states that this is not the case and that non-verbal skills are more important with the elderly due to some of their senses being impaired, i.e., sight and hearing.'

It is important to keep the idea of two sides of an argument in mind when looking for information, otherwise you could easily discard information that could be useful for your essay.

For this essay, and based on the introduction, these would be the areas you might look for information on:
• Communication
• Elderly and communication
• Importance of communication

- Nurses
- Therapeutic relationship benefits
- Restrictions that limit nurses' ability for effective communication: e.g., time, staff shortages, not knowing enough about patients due to poor hand-over
- Improvements
- Use of SOLER (Squarely, Open, Lean, Eye contact and Relaxed) (Egan, 2007).

After writing your introduction and starting to think about what you are going to research, you need to know how to find the information.

Finding useful resources

In the past, students could quite honestly claim to not be able to find adequate information. Before the internet, it was hugely time consuming to manually search indexes and databases to find the location of information in libraries. It was then even more time consuming to locate the material in the library stacks, search the books for the relevant information, and then queue at the photocopier to make copies. Many days of study were lost trying to locate suitable material, and quite often, after all that effort, you would just end up with information you were able find rather that what you actually needed.

The information age

The advent of the 'information age' has changed all this – we are used to finding information on the internet and receiving instant results. It has made searching for information much simpler and more comprehensive. However, as with most gains in life, there are also negatives – the main one being information overload.

To help with this we will now look at:
- Useful resources
- Building a search strategy
- Resources not to use.

The internet is your friend!!

The internet has made looking for information so much easier and quicker not only for everyday life, such as booking tickets, hotels and so on, but also for students.

> ### REFLECTION 22.1
>
> Reflect on how you use the internet to search for a hotel, or to book a holiday, or do online shopping. How did you do this? What skills did you have to use when doing this? Do you think some of those skills are transferable when searching for information for your studies?

Databases, electronic journals, eBooks and useful webpages

There are many online resources that your institution will make available to you. You may have access to Internurse.com and ScienceDirect.com, which are databases that hold journals. They are easy to navigate and will provide you with useful journal articles.

There are also many useful study skills webpages that various universities have made available via the internet. Look at The Open University study skills website: 'Skills for Open University study' which is an excellent resource and covers all aspects of study skills. (http://www2.open.ac.uk/students/skillsforstudy/).

Most databases will have a search box – similar to a search engine (see later), where you enter your search terms in the same way. Some will also have an advanced search where you can finely tune your investigation.

It is worthwhile familiarizing yourself both with what your institution has available and with databases. The great thing about electronic databases is that you can 'mess about' with them as much as you like while you are learning, and they will not break. At worse you will need to reboot your PC, so allow for time in your planning to familiarize yourself with resources.

Building a search strategy

If you are starting to search on an initial idea for your essay, your preferred internet search engine is a reasonable place to start.

To use a search engine, you only need to type your search terms in the box. Search engines are intuitive, so they will auto-correct any spelling mistakes (databases do not have this facility, so if your search result returns '0', check your spelling) and you do not have to be too careful.

You can also use Boolean logic to include and exclude things from your search strategy (Table 22.3).

Fig. 22.2 explains further how Boolean logic is used.

More often than not you are going to just search using the toolbar, but it can be useful to know these short cuts.

Some search en gines put the scholarly articles at the top and then the rest of the information they have found follows in order of relevance. Some of these links may lead you to information that is passworded, such as via Athens, a portal that manages access to certain databases. You may or may not have access to these, depending on where you are studying or working.

> ### ❗ HOTSPOT
> ### *Key Words*
>
> Understanding the keywords you need to use for your searches will speed up the process. It is always a good idea to jot down some key words before you start. Use the title to guide you and the subject you wish to write about to think of key words. Once you have started searching, when you find an article that is relevant use the key words provided on that article to lead you to others.

TABLE 22.3 Boolean Logic

AND	To link search terms together, e.g., dementia AND communication would search for both these terms
OR	To search for either/or. This is useful if you know that a subject can be referred to in two ways e.g., Non-verbal communication OR body language would search for either/or these terms
NOT	To exclude terms you would use NOT, e.g., communication NOT body language would search *only* for communication and *not* body language
*	Truncation can be used when there is more than one ending for a word and you want to search all of them, e.g., age* will retrieve age, aged and ageing

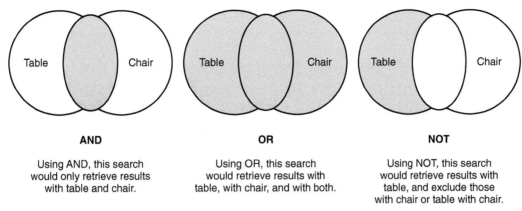

Fig. 22.2 Boolean Logic.

Search engines can also act as a portal to other databases. For example, you will probably want to use the National Institute for Health and Care Excellence (NICE); the Scottish Intercollegiate Guidelines Network (SIGN); Clinical Guidelines; Department of Health reports, and so forth to aide your learning. Looking for these types of documents may be far easier from a search engine than the actual direct website. So, for example, if looking for NICE Clinical Guidelines for Dementia, you could put 'Clinical Nice Guidelines Dementia' into the main toolbar.

There are also a number of academic search engines (eg. Google Scholar, WorldWideScience, Microsoft Academic, ResearchGate etc.) that are specifically aimed at researchers and students. They allow you to restrict the search using various parameters.

For instance, you can be given the option to select the years and introduce a custom date range. This is important as you will only really want to use material that is up to date. Most academic institutions may recommend that you do not use material older than 5 years; however, this will sometimes extend to 10 years. Obviously, there will be some material that is much older and still relevant. These are called 'seminal pieces of work'. An example of this would be the work done by Michael Argyle in the 1980s on body language. As his work is considered a 'seminal' piece, you would be able to use it and reference it. If in doubt whether or not a piece is seminal, take advice from your lecturers.

When you have located information you want to use, you should print off articles, webpages, etc., that are of interest. This is preferable to just saving to external drives, such as USB sticks, as this makes it harder to locate the reference or remember why you wanted it. You also cannot make notes as easily. When it comes to referencing, it is much harder if you do not have a physical copy.

Resources not to use

There are many sites and information resources available when you use the internet. Not all of them, however, are useful, and not all provide valid information. Blogs, for example, in general give accounts of people's personal experience and therefore are not of relevance to students and should not be used. Some sites are seen as the internet's encyclopaedias (and they do indeed store information on pretty much everything), but they may lack validity. These internet encyclopaedias can have information on their pages altered by any members of the public. Because

of this, their resource validity is questionable and therefore they should not be used. Again, if you are unclear which sites are suitable and which are not, speak to your lecturer.

CRITICAL AWARENESS

You need to be aware that not all information carries the same *validity* – that is the believability and credibility of what has been written.

The more you study and carry out research, the more you will see that certain authors and publishers are recognized for providing reliable information. In very simple terms, if you read an article in a tabloid newspaper on how eating 20 tomatoes a day will cure cancer written by a journalist who does not refer to any study, you will (should) automatically question the validity of what you are reading!! However, if you read an article on a trusted website that states the same and quotes a reputable source, you would be more inclined to believe it is true.

You are recognizing that there are more reliable sources available than tabloid newspapers and that some sources contain more reliable information than others. Be aware of the source of information and ask the questions: Where was this published? Who wrote it? What did they use as a source of reference? Asking these questions will help you assess the validity of information sources.

Critical analysis

You will be asked to 'critically analyse' the evidence you find. While this sounds very daunting, it is not as complicated as it first appears.

You are probably already using your own initiative to decide what evidence is good and what is not. For example, if you read an article in your local newspaper about diabetes, while it may give you information that is useful and written from a patient's perspective, it would not carry the same authority as a piece from Diabetes UK. You have probably critically analysed the work without realizing it. In its simplest form, critical analysis is looking at all the information that tells you whether something is a good or bad piece of work.

Here are some questions you could use to analyse a piece of work:

- Who wrote the piece? How qualified are they to write on the subject? Have they written on the subject before?
- Have you seen the author cited by others?
- How old is the piece?

- What kind of publication is it in? Is it from a peer reviewed journal, an international publication or local journal, a newspaper, etc.?
- Who was it written for? Students, health and social care practitioners, the general public?
- Did you understand it? Was it well written and logically presented?
- Could you see any contradictions with the argument?
- Does it only cover part of the argument (for example, does it only look at one section of the demographic, such as adults)?
- How does the article/evidence add to the overall argument?

When you look at any evidence you need to 'critically analyse' it to ascertain whether it is of value and whether it can be used in your assignment. Asking the previous questions of any piece of evidence will help you judge whether it is good material to use.

How to take notes and read actively

It is worth taking a moment to give you a few hints on how to read and take notes for the purpose of study. Taking notes in everyday life is very different from how you take notes when studying. You have probably jotted down a few reminders to yourself on a Post-it Note, maybe even taken notes during GCSEs and A levels, but it is very unlikely that anyone will have taught you how to take notes. Note-taking is almost considered an intuitive skill! It is not – it is a skill that can be learnt, and the better your note-taking skills, the better your ability to learn. Whilst there are study skills books that focus on this, here are a few pointers to get you started. Whatever you choose to use, note-taking involves the following:

- Writing down the main points.
- Summarizing/condensing those points.
- Remembering why you are making the notes: keep in mind the learning outcomes you are hoping your notes will help you achieve.
- Remembering what your assignment is about and what you are writing about.
- Understanding your notes.

> ### REFLECTION 22.2
>
> Think back on a time when you have been required to take notes and to read actively. This might have been while you were at school, at college or even while at work. How did you manage note-taking then?

Index/note cards

The classic way of taking notes has been on index cards. It forces you to condense the information for it to fit on the card. The most common way to use them is one card for each quotation or piece of information. You can then use the back of the card to store the reference details.

As each card holds one piece of information, it is easy to lay them out and order them to see how you will use the information in your essay and how you can flow between one point and another. Using index/note cards to revise for exams is particularly useful as you can use a rubber band to hold them all together in subjects and use them to study from.

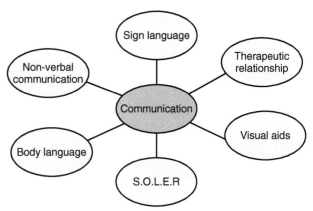

Fig. 22.3 An Example of a Mind Map for 'Communication'.

Mind mapping

If you are the sort of person who receives information better visually, mind mapping may be useful for you when taking notes. Mind mapping is placing an idea in the centre of a page and then breaking that concept down into smaller parts using lines branching out from the centre.

There are free mind mapping tools available on the internet that you may find useful. Also, the book *How to mind map* by Buzan (2002) is well worth looking at. An example of a mind map for communication can be found in Fig. 22.3.

Note taking

Note taking by hand is probably the most preferred method. The advantages are that as you write more slowly than you type, it gives your brain more time to absorb the information. Also, by having physical notes, you can arrange them in front of you and this can help you organize your information better. Physical notes also allow you to further organize the text by using, for example, highlighters and markers.

Digital note-taking

One advantage of taking digital notes is that they are easy to read, no matter how bad your handwriting! You can use your laptop or tablet to organize your notes into an order that works for you without having to re-type them. Apps such as Evernote, and One Note, among others, make it easy to jot down ideas while reading or listening to a lecture and store them on your device or on the cloud.

Whatever method you choose to use, key points to remember are:

- Use your own words – the process of reading, understanding and using your own words to record the information will help it become imbedded.
- If using a quote verbatim, make sure you reference the source.
- Keep it simple. The acronym KISS – **K**eep **I**t **S**hort and **S**imple – is useful to keep in your mind when making notes.
- Use symbols and abbreviation.
- Keep a note of references.
- Make sure you understand the notes you have made.
- Keep copies – if using hardcopy, take photocopies; if using electronic notes, back up to the cloud or another external source.

> **! HOTSPOT**
>
> When typing up your work on the computer, make sure you save on a regular basis. Keep more than one copy, for instance saving on two USB sticks, or saving to a separate drive. This could be your institution's drive if you are allowed to do so.

Reading actively

We all read; whether it is a novel, a newspaper or a webpage, the activity of reading is common to us all. But when we read, we often do it passively. For instance, when reading a fiction novel, it is usually for pleasure and to follow the story. There may be no need to refer to the story again other than to say it was a 'fantastic read' so we make no active attempt to engage further with the information. When you read for study, it is an active process – you are reading with the purpose of understanding and evaluating what you have read.

Many students will just read and re-read in the hope they will understand by some process of repetition. Unfortunately, this is not the case. You need to engage with the text by keeping in mind the purpose you are reading for. An example would be thinking about your essay question, or the specific point you are trying to make in your essay, while reading and looking for material to support it.

The following tips may help you engage with the material:

- Underline or highlight key words (if it is your own book or a photocopy).
- Make notes in the margins – summarize points, ask questions of the text, note where you think you can use it in your essay. This takes the highlighting stage a bit further. If you have a substantial amount to write, use sticky notes.
- Use your critical analysis skills – question the text: Who wrote it? Why? When? Who is the audience for the piece? Does it corroborate your other reading on the same subject?
- Look for signposts within the text. Words such as 'most importantly', 'in contrast', 'research shows…'

Reading for studying is an active process and should feel very different from how you read outside of studying.

The library

Hopefully, your institution will have a library (sometimes referred to as 'learning resource centres' or 'information hubs') that you can use. As part of your induction to the course, you should have the opportunity to attend a library induction. When we think of libraries we all automatically think of rows of books on shelves, but libraries nowadays offer so much more and can assist students in many ways.

As well as books, libraries offer electronic resources, such as online journals, eBooks and databases, and they will almost certainly have terminals where you can access the internet and printing facilities. They will also offer places to study that are quiet and where you can meet other students and peers.

The librarian will be able to recommend resources and generally steer you in the right direction to find what you need. They may offer tuition in carrying out literature searches and searching databases. Library services can often help with study skills and

may well offer classes in writing and referencing, among other skills. With all the activities you have to do when starting a new course, it can be hard to find the time to familiarize yourself with the library. However, it is well worth making the effort, and ultimately it will save you time.

MAIN BODY OF THE ESSAY

So now that you have found the articles, webpages and information that you want to use, it is time to focus on the main body of the essay. This is where you present the information you have gathered (answering the essay question) in a logical and clear manner, supporting the overall argument or idea of your essay.

The main body is structured in paragraphs. Ideally each paragraph should address one or two points that are discussed and analysed in detail, rather than many details that are only dealt with superficially.

As guidance:

- Paragraphs contain one or two main arguments.
- Outline the main idea(s) in the first sentence/s.
- Develop that sentence by using evidence to support. Examples of evidence could be data, facts, statistics and quotations. These you will have gathered from your reading.
- Explain in detail how the evidence supports your point.
- Finish the paragraph with the most important part of the overall argument or the point that you are trying to convey.
- A good paragraph will allow the reader to read the first and last sentence and understand the main idea of that paragraph.

Once you have managed to master one paragraph, you have to write another, and another… and then connect them to make sure they flow. As explained, paragraphs are used to present different arguments, so the order of the paragraphs is important to keep the 'thread' running throughout the essay. The essay should be set out in a logical way so that the reader can easily follow the argument/point you are trying to make.

You do not need to reiterate what was said in the previous paragraph to establish flow between your paragraphs. Rather, your first sentence should introduce the new topic/change of focus that this paragraph will be about.

An example of an essay that shows very easily the transition from one paragraph to another and the flow between all the paragraphs is provided below:

Example essay

As our society gets wealthier, are we doomed to become ever more unhappy? Discuss in the light of the Richard Layard article.

Over the past fifty years our society has become substantially richer and, because of this, we enjoy better health and a better quality of life. Many people own cars, refrigerators, DVDs and mobile phones and go on foreign holidays. But does this mean we are a happier society? Not according to Richard Layard. In this essay, I will consider his evidence for this view and his suggestions as to why this is the case.

Layard looked at various surveys taken in the USA, Japan, continental Europe and Britain for evidence of changes in happiness levels over this period. He reports that on average rich people are happier than poorer. But that, over the years, the proportions happy at different income levels have stayed about the same. In other words, in spite of the huge growth in average incomes, levels of happiness have not increased.

Layard also notes evidence of rising levels of depression. He quotes studies of depression among women in their thirties, published in 1982 and 2000, which show a rise from 16% to 29% in clinically diagnosed depression. (Layard, 2003, p 25). However, such figures should be treated with caution, since as a society we are now much more aware of depression and there is less stigma attached to admitting to it. This could be why reports of depression have increased, rather than any genuine increase in levels of depression.

It is particularly surprising to see reports of rising depression among young women, as their pay and job opportunities have improved. However, though women can now do the same jobs as men, with the same demands and responsibilities, they still get less pay. Layard suggests that women have become more unhappy at this unfairness because they are now more likely to include men in their reference groups.

It seems increasingly that the more other people have, the more we want. We do not seem to be happy with the fact that we have a free NHS. Instead, because a rich man can afford private healthcare we want the same. Consequently, rising incomes will never bring greater happiness. We will simply want more. Indeed, as we become increasingly aware of what other people have and as the gap between rich and poor grows ever wider, we seem likely to become increasingly unhappy with what we don't have. So it seems that, as we surround ourselves with more material wealth than would have seemed possible fifty years ago, we can only look ahead to becoming increasingly unhappy.

(417 words)

References

Layard, R. (2003) *The Secrets of Happiness*, New Statesman, 3 March 2003.

The Good Study Guide (2017) Lewis's essay improved.

Available at: www.goodstudyguide.co.uk (Last accessed 12 August 2017)

CONCLUSION

So, you are at the end of the essay. Hopefully you are feeling elated, but often the reality is that you are at the stage where you want to hand it in and you have no energy left. It is important that you preserve a little bit of energy to write a good conclusion. Remember this will be the last part that the assessor will read before assigning your mark.

Let us look at what a conclusion should do:

- Summarize the main points/arguments/findings in the essay.
- Link with the introduction.
- Predict future trends, suggest wider implications, outline need for further research.

Greetham (2013) explains that 'the most useful thing you can do in a conclusion is to tighten your essay up into a cohesive piece of work by picking up the theme you raised in your introduction, reflecting on it in the light of what you've discussed since' (p. 221).

As you can see, the idea of linking back to the introduction and then writing the conclusion is a common method. An example of this would be a conclusion that starts:

'As stated in the introduction the importance of communication in nursing has been discussed. It has shown that … (here you would list your main arguments) support communication as vital tool.'

Conclusions do not include any new evidence and therefore do not have any references. Conclusions are very much reflective pieces and as such should be written in a reflective manner.

Once you have written your essay, go through it and read it. Think specifically about whether the order which the essay is laid out is how you had originally wanted it and whether it would be easier to follow the argument if you moved paragraphs around. Do not forget, this is a draft, so you are still able to make changes to produce the best essay that you can.

DRAFTS AND PROOFREADING

At this point, you should have a draft of your essay. It is at this stage when you should start to relax. If you have planned your time well, hopefully you should be able to give yourself a day or two off from essay writing. This is important as sometimes, once you have got to the draft stage, you need to let it 'go cold' and then come back to it and start proofreading and finalizing. The reason for this gap is because quite often, when you have just written a piece of work, you are so familiar with it, if you check it straight away you read what you *think* is there rather than what is *actually* there. It is a strange phenomenon, but it happens!!!

So, after giving yourself a break, reread your essay. Do this actively, engaging with your essay, and do the following:

- Check for spelling and grammar mistakes.
- Check that your essay flows in a logical fashion. Move paragraphs around to make it flow better.
- Remove any repetition. Could you express yourself more concisely? Remove any waffling!
- Have you answered the question?
- Have you fulfilled what you said you would do in the introduction?
- Check your references.
- Is it in the correct format (you may have to present your work in a certain format, font, line spacing).
- Read it aloud.
- Ask a friend to read it.

> **❗ HOTSPOT**
>
> Read your work aloud. When you do this, it is easier to hear whether it flows. You will be able to hear which parts make sense and which parts need further clarification. While it may feel strange – it is a method that works.

Proofreading can take some time, so it is best not to leave it to the last minute. Allow yourself time to go through your essay in a methodical manner to ensure that you have time to make any changes that are necessary.

> **! HOTSPOT**
>
> It is very important you proofread your work, or ask someone to read your work for you. They do not need to know anything about nursing, they are just checking that it makes sense and that the grammar and spelling are correct.

REFERENCING AND BIBLIOGRAPHY

Throughout your research for your essay, you were asked to keep notes of where you have taken information from. This is because you have to use others' work to build your essay, but you must credit the authors whose work you have used. This is academic referencing.

You will almost certainly be introduced to referencing by your lecturers, and many libraries run informal sessions that teach referencing. Most academic institutions use the Harvard referencing system; basically, this is a standardized format for presenting the details about the pieces of work you have used.

Within your essay, when you refer to the work of others (for both books and journals), cite the authors and the date of their work. An example would be:

Smith (2016) explains that communication is a vital tool...

Or

Communication is a vital tool (Smith, 2016)...

This would be the same for websites, but using the website details as the author, for example:

Diabetes UK (2016) explores the subject of diabetes....

At the end of your essay, you must provide a detailed list of all the references used in it. This list gives the complete reference details, not just the author and year that appears in the essay citation.

Table 22.4 provides a brief guide for the most common types of resources used: a book, a journal and a website, and shows which details you need to have from each of these resources to be able to reference them in your list.

You will see that in the examples given that the title of the book or webpage appears in italics. For a journal article, the title is not italicized, but the journal name appears in italics. This is the Harvard system, but you will need to check with your own

institution what system they prefer and any slight changes they may have adopted from the standard form.

You may also be required to include a bibliography. This lists the resources you have read and that have informed you, but that you have not actually referenced within your essay. This is presented in the same way as a reference list.

> **! HOTSPOT**
>
> ***Thinking Time***
>
> You need to allow yourself time to think about your essay, what you want to write about, what you have already written, and how you can make it sound better. Students are often in 'doing' mode and sometimes you need to just stop and think about *what* you are doing. Some people like to think when they are jogging, washing up, walking the dog, and so on. Sometimes you need to stop writing and distract yourself with another activity and wait for that light-bulb moment!

Note about plagiarism

It is very important that you reference the work that you have used. You should never try and pass off someone else's work as your own. By correctly referencing, you avoid plagiarism; however, if you are in any doubt, speak to your lecturers.

LOOKING BACK, FEEDING FORWARD

You should now feel confident in the following:

- Understanding essay titles
- Carrying out literature searches
- Essay structure and format
- Referencing your work.

You should also be able to understand how to critically analyse your resources and select appropriate material. You can now take effective notes and read actively, which are skills that will help you throughout your study. After writing your essay, you will be able to check your work and compile a reference list to ensure that you avoid plagiarism.

This chapter has aimed to give you a brief guide to studying. However, there are far more in-depth books that you may also want to look at. Details of further resources are provided at the end of the chapter. As you progress through the course, your ability to carry out research and write essays will improve. Persevere, and by the end of the course you will have all of these skills finely tuned.

REFERENCES

Buzan, T., 2002. How to Mind Map. Thorson, London.

Egan, G., 2007. The Skilled Helper, ninth ed. Cengage, Belmont.

Good Study Guide, 2017. Lewis's essay improved. www.goodstudyguide.co.uk.

Greetham, B., 2013. How to Write Better Essays, third ed. Palgrave, Basingstoke.

Health Education England, 2017. Nursing Associate Curriculum Framework. https://www.hee.nhs.uk/sites/default/files/documents/Curriculum%20Framework%20Nursing%20Associate.pdf.

TABLE 22.4	Referencing
Item	**Details required**
Book	Author, Year, Title, edition (if not the first edition), place of publication and publisher.
	e.g. Buzan, T. (2002) *How to mind map.* London, Thorsons.
Website	Name of Website, Year, Title of the exact website page you are looking at, www.address, date you accessed
	Diabetes UK (2016) *Type 2 Diabetes.* Available at: https://www.diabetes.org.uk/Type-2-diabetes (Last accessed 5 June 2018)
Journal	Author, Year, Title of article, Title of journal, volume, issue, page numbers
	Smith, S. (2015) How to write an essay. *Education Daily.* 15,11: 12–20.

23

Nutrition

Rachel Wood

OBJECTIVES

By the end of the chapter the reader will be able to:

1. Understand the meaning of a healthy diet and how clinical conditions may affect this
2. Assess nutritional status, including malnutrition
3. Understand the relationship between the correct nutritional intake and a variety of clinical conditions
4. Outline the care required by a patient in need of nutritional support, including food fortification, enteral tube feeding and parenteral nutrition
5. Describe some common conditions and needs associated with nutrition and diet and how this may differ dependent on the type of patient, such as the elderly, and those from different cultures
6. Review the role of the Nursing Associate (NA) in promoting health and well-being

KEY WORDS

Malnutrition	Food fortification	Anaemia
Diabetes	Nutritional assessment	Coeliac disease
Nutrition support	MUST score	
Nasogastric feeding	Obesity	

CHAPTER AIM

This aim of this chapter is to provide the reader with an understanding of the skills and knowledge concerning nutrition to ensure all patients, including those with a variety of clinical conditions, are provided with safe, effective and compassionate care with regard to the correct nutritional input.

SELF-TEST

1. How would you describe a healthy diet?
2. What are the key macronutrients that form the basis of a healthy diet?
3. What is nutritional screening?
4. What does malnutrition mean?
5. Discuss nutrition support.
6. Name five conditions where adapting the diet can improve health and well-being.
7. What is iron-deficiency anaemia and how would you assess for it?
8. Define coeliac disease.
9. Define diabetes mellitus.
10. What dietary changes would you suggest to an adult recently diagnosed with diabetes?

INTRODUCTION

Food is essential to keep your body healthy, functioning and alive. Without sufficient nutrition, the body cannot function efficiently. All of the individual nutrients have an important role to play in improving outcomes for patients. Being able to assess how an individual's diet can be adapted is an essential aspect of the role of the Nursing Associate (NA).

A healthy diet must:

- provide the correct amount of energy in the form of calories, protein, fat and vitamins and minerals to maintain normal physiological functions and permit growth and development.

- protect the body against future conditions and the risk of disease.

ENERGY NEEDS

Energy is necessary for all basic physiological functions of the body, cell function and active transport pumps, but most importantly breathing, digestion and excretion. The brain is the most energy-demanding organ, but any activity we do requires energy – even sleeping. Infants, children and pregnant women require extra energy for growth as well as basic function.

Energy is provided from the macronutrients in our food (carbohydrate/fat/protein) that are broken down to smaller and more easily absorbed components, digested and absorbed. Some energy will be used straight away and some of it stored. If more energy is consumed than is required, excess gets stored. If not enough energy is consumed, the body utilizes its own stores to assist bodily functions. This is the basic concept of energy balance. Factors that influence basal metabolic rate (BMR) are body weight, gender, age and disease. Disease and its treatment can affect BMR, particularly if it has any influence on the thyroid gland as thyroid hormones play a key part in metabolism. Fever, trauma and stress can all increase energy expenditure short term, as can certain drugs, for example, caffeine, nicotine and amphetamines. Undernutrition can reduce BMR, as can some antidepressants and beta blockers.

Energy balance

$$\text{Energy intake} = \text{Energy output (BMR} +$$
$$\text{diet-induced thermogenesis} +$$
$$\text{physical activity)}$$

Energy intake derives from the food that is eaten. Hunger, appetite, mood, social and environmental factors can all contribute to the types and volume of food that is ingested. See Table 23.1 for the energy conversion factors used in the UK.

Table 23.1 shows that fat and alcohol are the most energy-dense foods and therefore, when weight loss is required, these are the two most important things to focus on when trying to reduce calorie intake.

Diet-induced thermogenesis is when the body processes the food eaten. This is the digestion, absorption, transporting and storing of food and nutrients and requires about 10% of the energy from the food eaten. Physical activity accounts for the rest of the calories the body burns up during the day and is by far the biggest variable that can influence weight gain and loss.

TABLE 23.1 Energy Conversion Factors Used in Current UK Composition Tables	
	Calories/g
Protein	4
Fat	9
Carbohydrate	3.75
Alcohol	7

When an individual is in energy balance, their weight and body composition remain constant; what they eat and the activity they do is stable and in equilibrium. If an individual is gaining too much weight, reducing their calorie intake and increasing their activity levels will shift the balance. Likewise, for individuals who are very underweight, increasing their calorie intake with energy-dense foods (fat) and reducing how much exercise they do will also shift the energy balance.

PROTEIN, FAT AND CARBOHYDRATES

Protein

Amino acids are the very simple building blocks of all proteins. There are many different proteins that are made up of the same 20 amino acids, but in different sequences and numbers. The proteins we eat can be broken down by the body and rebuilt into new amino acids or new protein structures. Eight amino acids are 'essential' amino acids, meaning the body cannot make them and they need to be provided in the diet. Proteins are digested by various peptidase enzymes and broken down into peptides and then amino acids before the body can use them for cell growth, repair, protein synthesis (including enzyme formation) and homeostasis. Dietary sources of protein can be animal or plant based.

Fat

Fat is an important component of living cells as essential fatty acids are required for cell walls and membrane structures. Fats are insoluble in water and greasy in texture. They consist of triglycerides (95% of fats we consume), phospholipids and cholesterol and fat-soluble vitamins. Fatty acids are combined with glycerol to make triglycerides and these can be easily broken down and resynthesized. The type of fatty acid determines the fat's physical characteristics and can be split up into the following:

- Saturated fatty acids
- Monounsaturated fatty acids
- Polyunsaturated fatty acids.

As with the essential amino acids, the essential fatty acids, linoleic and alpha linoleic fatty acids, need to be provided in the diet as the body is unable to make them itself. These essential fatty acids are vital as they act as metabolic regulators, as well as having many other benefits on the body's homeostasis.

Fat is broken down by lipase enzyme, but due to it being water insoluble, it has to be emulsified by bile salts from the liver first to allow the enzyme to work. Fats are then transported around the body as lipoproteins, which aid absorption.

Fat has many diverse functions in the body, including metabolic, storage and structural. Excess fat intake is stored in adipose tissue, which is an important energy reserve and insulates and protects the body.

UK recommendations are that fats should average 30% of nutritional intake, but actual intake remains over 40% (Whitton et al., 2011). Fats increase the palatability of the diet but can contribute to over-consumption of energy. Fats and oils, followed by meat and meat products, represent the highest percentage of fat intake in the diet.

TABLE 23.2   Vitamin and Minerals

Nutrient	Main function	Dietary sources
*Vitamin A	Growth, vision, antioxidant, normal cell growth and reproduction. High doses can be toxic in pregnancy	Liver, fortified margarines and fat spreads, dairy products, oily fish, eggs
*Vitamin D	Maintain calcium and phosphate levels for bone formation	Oily fish, meat, eggs, dairy
*Vitamin E	Antioxidant	Vegetable oils
*Vitamin K	Essential for blood clotting	Dark green leafy vegetables, vegetable oils
Thiamine	Release and utilization of energy from food	Fortified breakfast cereals, pork, nuts, pulses, yeast
Riboflavin (B2)	Normal growth, helps maintain integrity of eyes, skin, nervous system	Fortified cereals, yeast, liver and offal, green leafy vegetables, eggs
Niacin	Important in metabolism of fat	Meat, fish, fortified cereals, wholegrains, yeast extracts
Vitamin B6	Important in protein metabolism	Fortified cereals, wholegrains, meat, bananas, nuts and pulses
Folate	Synthesis of DNA/RNA and crucial role in cell division	Liver, yeast extract, green leafy vegetables, fortified cereals
Vitamin B12	Cofactor for enzymes involved in amino acid metabolism	Dairy, meat and fish
Vitamin C	Antioxidant, assists iron absorption	Citrus fruits, berries, strawberries, green vegetables
Calcium	Create and maintain skeletal structures	Dairy, fish containing soft bones, green leafy vegetables
Iron	Oxygen carrier in haemoglobin and myoglobin in muscles	Red meat, liver, fortified breakfast cereals, poultry and fish, green leafy vegetables, dried fruit
Zinc	Required for normal function of many metabolic pathways	Red meat, fish, dairy, poultry, eggs
Copper	Component of important enzymes	Shellfish, liver, nuts and cocoa
Selenium	Antioxidant defence, immune function and thyroid hormone metabolism	Fish, offal, nuts and eggs
Iodine	Forms part of the thyroid hormones, protein synthesis	Marine fish, shellfish, sea salt, seaweed, dairy

(*fat soluble vitamins)

! HOTSPOT

If fat is undigested, it will appear in the faeces. This produces a very waxy, (often pale in colour) foul-smelling stool that floats and is difficult to flush away. This is called steatorrhoea. Unabsorbed fats also remove other fat-soluble components, for example vitamins, and chronic steatorrhoea can be linked with specific vitamin deficiency.

Causes:
- Pancreatic insufficiency
- Gallstones
- Defects to small intestine leading to malabsorption.

TABLE 23.3   Eight Tips for Healthier Choices (FSA, 2005)

1. Base meals on starchy foods, such as wholegrain bread, potatoes, rice or pasta
2. Eat lots of fruit and vegetables
3. Have at least two portions of fish per week and include one of oily fish
4. Cut down on saturated fat and sugar
5. Try to eat less salt; adults should have less than 6 g salt per day
6. Drink plenty of water and other fluids
7. Get active and try to be a healthy weight
8. Don't skip breakfast
   And remember to enjoy your food!

Carbohydrates

Carbohydrates are found in plant and animal sources and are the cheapest energy source in the world. They should comprise 50% of energy intake, mainly of complex carbohydrates and sugars from milk and fruit. Non-milk extrinsic sugars should comprise no more than 10%.

Excessive intake of sugars can be detrimental for teeth and are linked to obesity and diabetes. Starches are much more desirable in the diet as they are broken down slowly in the body and often contain other nutrients and particularly fibre. See Table 23.2 for an overview of minerals and vitamins.

EATING A BALANCED DIET

Each individual has their own energy requirements based on their weight, height, body mass index (BMI) and activity levels. They also have specific requirements for each individual nutrient, and if these are not met on a regular basis, it can lead to deficiencies. The Food Standards Agency produced eight tips for Healthier Choices (FSA, 2005) (Table 23.3) but found it was very difficult for the general public to interpret. This led to a nationwide teaching guide *The balance of good health* (HEA, 2014). In July 2014, Public Health England reviewed this based on changing healthy eating messages and renamed it *The Eatwell Plate*, which was relaunched in 2016 (see Fig. 23.1).

The concept of the Eatwell Guide

The Eatwell Plate was updated to the Eatwell Guide in 2016 and was designed with the intention to change people's perception that meals should be centred on one food group, such as just protein foods, and to encourage a healthy balance of all of the food groups that is flexible and has variety, including fluids. Table 23.4 highlights the different food groups and the principal nutrients provided.

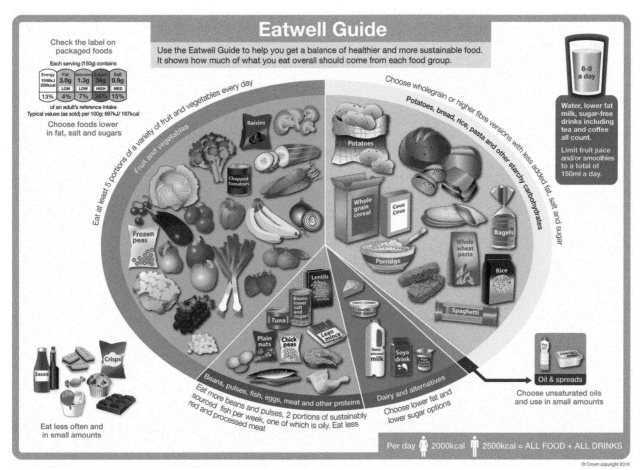

Fig. 23.1 The Eatwell Guide (PHE, 2016) (Crown copyright. Public Health England in association with the Welsh government, Food Standards Scotland and the Food Standards Agency in Northern Ireland).

COMPASSIONATE CARE

Nutrition and its association with an individual's health can be a very sensitive issue to address. Many chronic health conditions can be improved by changes to the diet, nutritional intake and lifestyle, for example, obesity, diabetes, coronary heart disease, Crohn's disease, coeliac disease and cystic fibrosis. Making healthier food choices can be difficult and requires support from family, friends and health professionals.

The NA needs to be able to offer care to people with malnutrition and identify appropriate methods of nutrition support within the community and in hospital settings. They must show empathy and understanding wherever possible, and also take into account their patients' wishes and views on treatment plans.

The NA must employ an open and non-judgmental attitude to those they care for, maintaining confidentiality at all times. The role of the NA is to offer support and reassurance; there is no place in a contemporary healthcare system for judgmental attitudes. Rassool (2015) points out how important it is to have an understanding of spiritual and cultural values when offering care; this applies to all aspects of care provision. The NA must be aware of the need to promote modesty and privacy. When

doing this, they are going some way to providing culturally competent care that ensures that the patient is at the centre of all that is done. Table 23.5 outlines the Essence of Care Benchmark for Privacy and Dignity (DH, 2015).

NUTRITIONAL ASSESSMENT

Nutritional assessment determines the extent to which an individual's nutritional needs are being met over a period of time. This can be relevant for assessing malnutrition within the hospital and also obesity within the community.

Early identification of those who are nutritionally depleted, or are at risk of becoming nutritionally depleted, is key to ensuring that timely and effective treatment plans are put into place. Nutritional screening tools can be quick and simple to use by nursing or medical staff on the first contact with the patient and will highlight the need for further nutritional assessment and intervention.

Factors in assessing nutritional status
Clinical

Acute or chronic illness, injury, trauma or surgery will all affect an individual's nutritional intake. During a stress response or

TABLE 23.4 The Different Food Groups and Principal Nutrients Provided

Food group	Foods included	Amount to be consumed	Principal nutrients provided
Bread, cereals and potatoes	Bread, breakfast cereals, oats, chapattis, pasta, rice, potatoes (choose wholegrain where possible)	1/3 of total volume of food eaten/day	• Carbohydrate as a source of energy • Fibre to help with bowel health • B vitamins • Calcium and iron
Fruits and vegetables	All types of fruit and vegetables i.e., fresh/frozen/tinned/dried/juice	1/3 of total volume of food eaten/day. Aim for at least 5 portions per day, limit juice to no more than 150 mL/day	• Vitamin C • Carotenes and other antioxidants • Folates • Fibre (soluble fibre) • Potassium
Milk/dairy products and alternatives	Milk Cheese Yoghurt Fromage frais Crème fraiche Soya	1/6 of the total food volume eaten/day 2–3 servings per day (e.g., 200 mL) glass of milk, 1 small yoghurt or 40 g of cheese	• Calcium • Protein • Fat soluble vitamins (A and D) • Riboflavin
Meat, fish and alternatives	Meat Poultry Offal Fish, meat and fish products Eggs Liver and kidney Pulses (beans and lentils) Nuts	1/6 of total food intake/day 2 servings per day Choose lean cuts of meat where possible and avoid frying. Aim for 2 portions of fish per week, at least one oily	• Protein • Iron • B vitamins • Zinc • Magnesium
Oils and spreads	Choose unsaturated oils and spread and eat in small amounts	Too much fat especially saturated fat in the diet can lead to high cholesterol and increase your risk of heart disease	• All types of fat are very high in energy; therefore use sparingly
Foods high in fat and sugar	Chocolate, cakes, biscuits, crisps, ice cream, butter, sugary drinks	These are not needed in the diet and should be eaten less often and in smaller amounts	
Fluid	Water, low-fat milk, low-sugar or sugar-free drinks including tea and coffee	6–8 glasses per day	• To keep your body well hydrated

TABLE 23.5 Benchmarks for Respect and Dignity (DH, 2015)

Factor	Best practice
Attitudes and behaviours	People and carers feel that they matter all of the time
Personal world and personal identity	Patients experience care in an environment that actively encompasses individual values, beliefs and personal relationships
Personal boundaries and space	People's personal space is protected by staff
Communication	People and carers experience communication with staff that respects their individuality
Privacy – confidentiality	People experience care that maintains their confidentiality
Privacy, dignity and modesty	People's care ensures their privacy and dignity and protects their modesty
Privacy – private area	People and carers can access an area that safely provides privacy

period of illness or following surgery, the body has increased nutritional requirements and to aid its recovery. This, coupled with increased losses and/or impaired absorption, can be challenging for a person who is unwell (Table 23.6).

Physical

Simple, holistic observations of a patient can be extremely useful in providing an indication of their nutritional status.

- Appearance – do they look thin/underweight/overweight? Look for signs of loose fitting clothing, dentures, or rings that could indicate recent weight loss. Assess their complexion: do they look pale, emaciated or is there any sign of hair loss that could indicate poor nutrition and vitamin deficiencies? Sunken eyes, dry mouth and fragile skin can all be signs of dehydration.
- Mobility – assess for signs of muscle wasting or poor mobility and weakness, which could indicate they might find buying, preparing and eating food more challenging.
- Mood – monitor for any signs of confusion, which can be a deteriorating clinical condition, or dehydration, particularly within the elderly population. Low mood, lethargy and poor concentration can be features of undernutrition.

TABLE 23.6   Effects of Illness, Injury and Surgery on Nutritional Status

Increased nutritional requirements	Increased nutritional losses	Impaired nutrient ingestion, digestion and/or absorption
Due to	Due to	Due to
• The metabolic response to trauma or surgery	• Vomiting	• Lack of appetite
• The metabolic costs of repairing tissue damage e.g., wounds, bedsores	• Diarrhoea	• Effects of other treatments on gastrointestinal tract e.g., radiotherapy
• Sepsis/infection	• Renal excretion	• Loss of absorptive surfaces e.g., resection of bowel, coeliac
• Involuntary activity e.g., tremors, spasms	• Surgical drains	disease, Crohn's disease
• Certain chronic conditions e.g., cystic fibrosis, burns	• Bleeding	• Swallowing difficulties or breathlessness on their ability to eat
	• Wound/fistula exudate and burns	• Difficulty self-feeding/chewing/maintaining food in their mouth

TABLE 23.7   Dietary Aspects to Explore with Patients

1. Current food and fluid intake – meal patterns and timings
2. Likes and dislikes
3. Changes to appetite and intake – and time period
4. Any other factors/clinical conditions affecting their food and fluid intake
   • Do dentures fit correctly, or have they lost them?
   • Do they need adapted cutlery due to arthritis?
   • Is swallowing challenging and do they need a texture modified diet (soft/pureed)?

TABLE 23.8   WHO Classification of Body Mass Index in Adults kg/m² (WHO, 1998)

Category	Caucasian population
Severely underweight	less than18.5
Underweight	18.5–20
Healthy/desirable	20–25
Overweight	25–30
Obese	30–40
Morbidly Obese	greater than 40

• Breathlessness – this can make it much more challenging for a person to eat, as well as prepare food; it can also be a sign of anaemia.

• Pressure sores/poor wound healing – this can be an indication of poor nutritional intake with inadequate calories and protein for the body to heal, as well as poor mobility.

• Oedema – this is linked with low albumin levels. It can reflect heart failure and prolonged protein deficiency in the diet.

It is really important if you have initial concerns about a patient's nutritional intake to explore their social circumstances and find out if they are aware of any 'unintentional' weight loss. For example, do they need any extra support in the community, do they have the cooking facilities and skills to cook? Often, there can be simple solutions that, with some guidance and support, can facilitate a better diet (Table 23.7).

Anthropometrics

Body weight as a single measurement is not helpful in assessing nutritional status. It can be useful if there are a series of weight records over a period of time to assess changes in body weight and a person's risk of malnutrition, but it does not indicate any changes in body composition or muscle wasting.

NICE (2006) uses weight loss as a guide to consider nutrition support if:

• there has been unintentional weight loss of more than 10% over a 3–6-month period

• BMI is less than 20 kg/m² AND there has been unintentional weight loss of more than 5% over 3–6 months.

The WHO classification of body mass index is given in Table 23.8.

OSCE 23.1   Body Mass Index

Instructions

In this OSCE you are required to accurately calculate the BMI for a patient.

Mr Syad Ayaz is a 68-year-old gentleman. He is 5 feet 7 inches tall and weighs 15 stone 12 pounds. What is his BMI?

You have to demonstrate that you are able to use the agreed formula for the accurate calculation in order to pass the assessment. You are marked on your ability to explain to the examiner the various aspects of the assessment.

Look at the patient details below and provide the correct answers using the criteria listed. All criteria have to be achieved to pass.

Criteria	Competent	Not competent
1 Provides a brief explanation to patient and informed consent gained Demonstrates the ability to perform effective hand decontamination		
2 Records the patient's height in metres using the stadiometer, accurately		
3 Accurately records the patient's weight in kilograms		
4 Calculates the patient's body mass index Weight in kg Height in m²		
5 Accurately documents height, weight and BMI		
6 Demonstrates and maintains a safe posture throughout and ensures the safety and comfort of the patient		
7 Demonstrates the ability to perform effective hand decontamination		

BMI =

MALNUTRITION

Malnutrition can be defined as: 'a state in which a deficiency or excess of energy, protein and other nutrients causes measurable adverse effects on tissue, body functions and clinical outcome' (Elia, 2000).

Malnutrition can mean both under and over-nutrition, and also an imbalance of micronutrients. It can widely be rectified with nutrition intervention (i.e., nutritional support). It is a common problem that can be extremely costly and can often be left unrecognized and untreated. Between 10% and 60% of adults that are admitted to hospital are at risk of malnutrition when screened using MUST (Malnutrition Universal Screening Tool) which is a recognized screening tool used in most hospitals. Likewise, malnutrition is just as much a problem in infants and children and now there is also much more recognition about screening infants and children on admission to hospital.

Those at risk of developing malnutrition:

• Young children
• The elderly
• Patients with chronic health conditions, e.g., malignancy, respiratory, gastrointestinal problems or renal disease
• Patients with multiple comorbidities
• Individuals undergoing complex surgery, transplantation or treatment for burns.

Malnutrition affects physical and psychological health and well-being; it can impact on recovery, increase mortality and further complications, and can increase hospital stay.

Signs and symptoms

Malnutrition occurs when the nutritional intake does not meet the nutritional needs of the body – the basic concept of energy balance. Malnutrition can occur for three main reasons:

1. Decreased dietary intake
2. Increased nutritional requirements
3. Inability to absorb or use the nutrients appropriately.

Higher rates of malnutrition are also seen in more deprived areas where there is an increase in poverty. Malnutrition can be related to the food not being available, not being easy enough to eat or of sufficient quality, or because intake is reduced due to disease-related factors, despite food availability. Disease is the most common cause of malnutrition in the UK. Fig. 23.2 provides an overview of malnutrition.

Consequences of malnutrition

• Poor wound healing, pressure sores.
• Reduced immune function, prolonged infections and risk of sepsis.
• Muscle wasting and muscle weakness. This can affect breathing and cardiac function, as well cause poor mobility.
• A change in gastrointestinal function that affects absorption and digestion of food.
• Apathy, lethargy and depression.
• Poor libido, fertility problems, poor pregnancy outcomes.

Diagnosis

Detecting malnutrition is a key concern for the NHS; it has costly effects on health outcomes, hospital stays and NHS resources, but it can also be treated. Screening is a procedure that those who have first contact with patients should undertake. It is a multidisciplinary responsibility and easily detects malnourishment or those at risk of malnutrition so that action plans for monitoring and treatment can be put in place.

'MUST' was developed by the Malnutrition Advisory Group, a standing committee of BAPEN (originally the British Association of Parenteral and Enteral Nutrition) and has been regularly reviewed since its launch in 2003, (Elia et al., 2003). It is endorsed by many government agencies, as well as the Royal College of Nursing (RCN). It is the most commonly used screening tool for adults in the UK.

MUST has been developed for use in the following:

• All adults including the elderly, the sick/healthy, free-living individuals
• Hospital wards
• Outpatient clinics
• General practice
• Community settings
• Public health

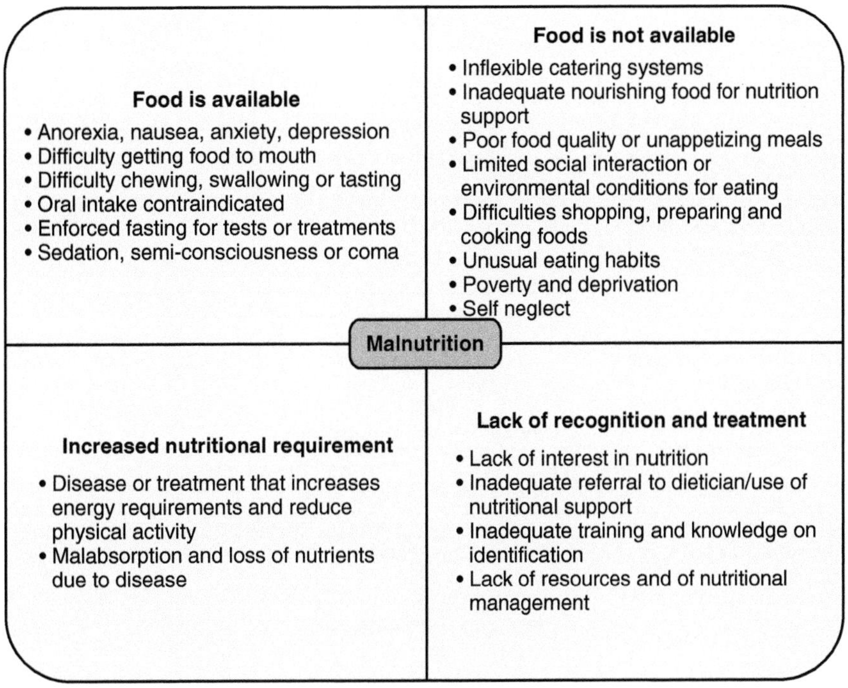

Food is available
- Anorexia, nausea, anxiety, depression
- Difficulty getting food to mouth
- Difficulty chewing, swallowing or tasting
- Oral intake contraindicated
- Enforced fasting for tests or treatments
- Sedation, semi-consciousness or coma

Food is not available
- Inflexible catering systems
- Inadequate nourishing food for nutrition support
- Poor food quality or unappetizing meals
- Limited social interaction or environmental conditions for eating
- Difficulties shopping, preparing and cooking foods
- Unusual eating habits
- Poverty and deprivation
- Self neglect

Malnutrition

Increased nutritional requirement
- Disease or treatment that increases energy requirements and reduce physical activity
- Malabsorption and loss of nutrients due to disease

Lack of recognition and treatment
- Lack of interest in nutrition
- Inadequate referral to dietician/use of nutritional support
- Inadequate training and knowledge on identification
- Lack of resources and of nutritional management

Fig. 23.2 Malnutrition.

MUST is a five-step screening tool; it has been validated and includes management guidelines (Fig. 23.3).

It is important to check what local screening tools and management guidelines are implemented wherever you are working. The NICE *Guideline for Nutrition Support in Adults* highlights the importance of screening and following the care quality standards for all patients seen within hospital or the community (NICE, 2012a). It relies on all care professionals having the correct training and competencies to deliver and provide safe, high-quality nutrition support. Table 23.9 outlines the five NICE quality standards for nutrition support.

! HOTSPOT

It is the responsibility of health and social care professionals, including the NA, to ensure they nutritionally screen people in their care. People admitted to hospital, attending an outpatient clinic for the first time, or having care in a community setting, should be offered checks for their risk of malnutrition using an accurate and reliable tool.

Care and treatment

Nutritional treatment of malnutrition is often termed 'nutrition support'. There are several steps to nutrition support and the type of intervention may depend on whether the individual is safe to eat and drink orally, whether they are acutely or chronically unwell, and for how long intervention may be required.

TABLE 23.9 NICE Quality Standards for Nutrition Support (NICE, 2012a)

Statement 1	People in care settings are screened for the risk of malnutrition using a validated screening tool.
Statement 2	People who are malnourished or at risk of malnutrition have a management care plan that aims to meet their nutritional requirements.
Statement 3	All people who are screened for the risk of malnutrition have their screening results and nutrition support goals documented and communicated in writing within and between settings.
Statement 4	People managing their own artificial nutrition support and/or their carers are trained to manage their nutrition delivery system and monitor their well-being.
Statement 5	People receiving nutrition support are offered a review of the indications, route, risks, benefits and goals of nutrition support at planned intervals.

Dietary fortification and modification

The aims of dietary fortification and modification are as follows:
- To increase the frequency of food and fluid intake, for example, little and often with eating, small meals and additional nourishing snacks in between meals (sandwich/yoghurt/biscuits/cheese and crackers) and encourage nourishing drinks (milky drinks, build-up drinks, hot chocolate).
- To increase the energy and nutrient content of foods and fluids already consumed. Energy-dense foods can be useful to increase calorie, protein and fat intake without increasing

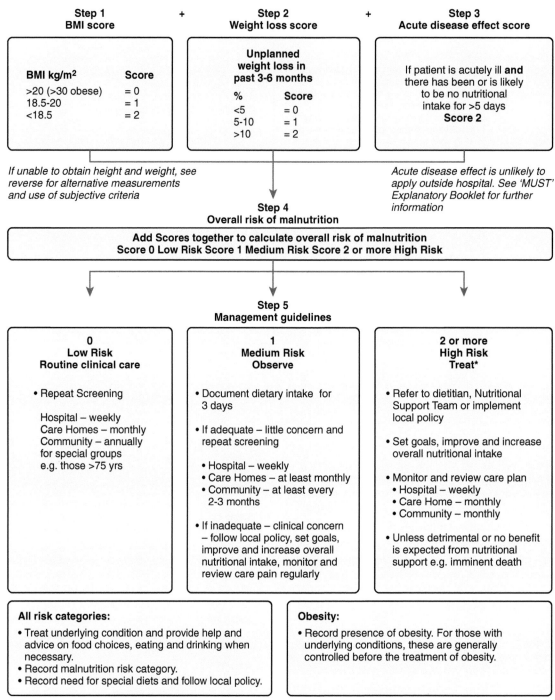

Step 1 BMI score	+	Step 2 Weight loss score	+	Step 3 Acute disease effect score

Step 1
BMI score

BMI kg/m²	Score
>20 (>30 obese)	= 0
18.5-20	= 1
<18.5	= 2

Step 2
Weight loss score

Unplanned weight loss in past 3-6 months

%	Score
<5	= 0
5-10	= 1
>10	= 2

Step 3
Acute disease effect score

If patient is acutely ill **and** there has been or is likely to be no nutritional intake for >5 days
Score 2

If unable to obtain height and weight, see reverse for alternative measurements and use of subjective criteria

Acute disease effect is unlikely to apply outside hospital. See 'MUST' Explanatory Booklet for further information

Step 4
Overall risk of malnutrition

Add Scores together to calculate overall risk of malnutrition
Score 0 Low Risk Score 1 Medium Risk Score 2 or more High Risk

Step 5
Management guidelines

0
Low Risk
Routine clinical care

• Repeat Screening

Hospital – weekly
Care Homes – monthly
Community – annually
for special groups
e.g. those >75 yrs

1
Medium Risk
Observe

• Document dietary intake for 3 days

• If adequate – little concern and repeat screening

• Hospital – weekly
• Care Homes – at least monthly
• Community – at least every 2-3 months

• If inadequate – clinical concern – follow local policy, set goals, improve and increase overall nutritional intake, monitor and review care pain regularly

2 or more
High Risk
Treat*

• Refer to dietitian, Nutritional Support Team or implement local policy

• Set goals, improve and increase overall nutritional intake

• Monitor and review care plan
• Hospital – weekly
• Care Home – monthly
• Community – monthly

• Unless detrimental or no benefit is expected from nutritional support e.g. imminent death

All risk categories:
• Treat underlying condition and provide help and advice on food choices, eating and drinking when necessary.
• Record malnutrition risk category.
• Record need for special diets and follow local policy.

Obesity:
• Record presence of obesity. For those with underlying conditions, these are generally controlled before the treatment of obesity.

Re-assess subjects identified at risk as they move through care settings

Fig. 23.3 MUST Screening Tool (Reproduced with permission from BAPEN).

the quantity of food eaten. Dairy products are really helpful for this method, for example adding extra butter/cream/cheese to mashed potato, full fat yoghurts or cream with fruit, creamy milk-based puddings.

Oral nutritional supplements

These are nutritional drinks that come in a variety of flavours but are predominantly milk-based and provide additional calories, protein, fat and micronutrients. They are to be used in addition to the diet not as a replacement. Nutritional supplements, such as Fortisips or Ensure, plus milkshake drinks, must be prescribed for disease-related malnutrition as well as for a variety of other conditions. However, because of the high costs to the NHS, their use should be monitored and ideally should only be considered when dietary measures alone have not been sufficient.

Enteral feeding

Enteral feeding is indicated when oral nutrition is insufficient or unsafe (NICE, 2012b) and most commonly used for the following conditions:

- Stroke/dysphagia/neuromuscular conditions
- Unconscious/sedated (critical care)
- Physiological anorexia
- Gastrointestinal obstruction (head and neck conditions)
- Increased need for extra calories/protein, i.e., pre/post-surgery or stress on the body (infection)
- Psychological problems.

Feeding enterally is far superior to parenteral nutrition and carries much less risk (Heyland et al., 2003). It helps maintain gut function and structure and is physiologically much more beneficial.

Enteral feeding can be delivered directly into the stomach (gastric) using a nasogastric tube or gastrostomy or beyond the stomach (post pyloric), directly into the jejunum, which is the middle section of the small intestine, via nasojejunal, gastrojejunostomy or jejunostomy (Fig. 23.4).

Nasogastric feeding is most commonly used in hospitals to provide short-term nutrition support, that is, up to 4 weeks. A fine-bore tube is used for feeding (6–9 FG (French gauge)), usually with an integral guide wire (Stylet) and is inserted transnasally into the stomach. Tubes are made from PVC, polyurethane or silicone. PVC tubes are suitable for short-term feeding (less than 10 days), whereas durable polyurethane or silicone should be used for longer term feeding (up to 6 months). Radio opaque tubes that have markings to ensure accurate identification and documentation of position should be used (NPSA, 2005).

! HOTSPOT

Placement of a Nasogastric Tube

To confirm the length of tube required:

1. Place the tip of the tube at the highest point of the central ribcage and add 5 cm (Fig. 23.5).
2. Pass the tube behind the ear, over the top of the ear and to the tip of the nostril and mark this position (see Fig. 23.5)
3. Placement of the enteral tube to the position of the nostril mark will ensure the tube is in the stomach.

Confirmation of tube placement: before feeding commences, it is vital to confirm that the tube is in the stomach and not the lungs. There have been 11 reported deaths over a 2-year period following the misplacement of nasogastric tubes (NPSA 2005).

The NPSA made the following recommendations:

1. Aspirate contents from the tube and check the contents are acidic with pH strips/indicator. The pH should be <5.5 to confirm position. If a patient is on continuous feeding, there is milk in the stomach, or the person is taking antacids, the pH may be >5.5.
2. X-ray confirmation. This should be carried out if there is any doubt over the position of the tube or difficulty in obtaining aspirate (NPSA, 2005).

Gastrostomy feeding is the creation of an artificial tract between the stomach and abdominal surface and is commonly used for long-term artificial feeding. They can be inserted endoscopically (percutaneous endoscopic astrostomy; PEG), surgically, or radiologically (radiologically inserted percutaneous gastrostomy (RIG) or per-oral image-guided gastrostomy (PIG)). Prior to placement, the suitability should be assessed by a

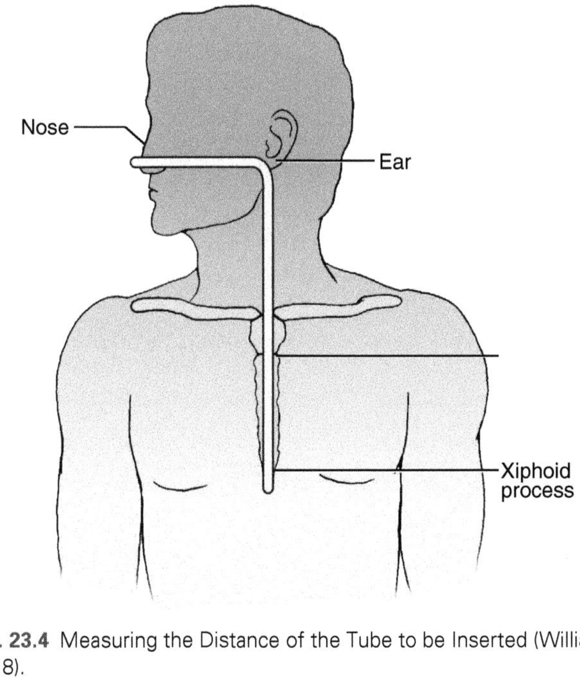

Fig. 23.4 Measuring the Distance of the Tube to be Inserted (Williams, 2018).

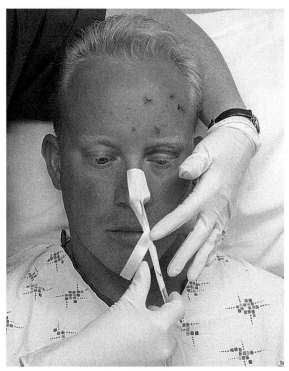

Fig. 23.5 Taping the Tube Securely (Williams, 2018).

BOX 23.1   Types of Feeding

Total parenteral nutrition
Peripheral parenteral nutrition
Intravenous alimentation feeding
Gastrostomy tube
Jejunostomy tube
Nasoduodenal tube
Nasojejunal tube

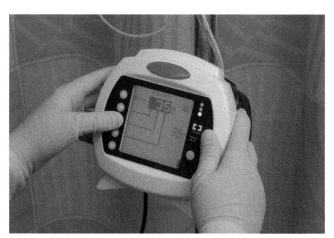

Fig. 23.6 Feeding Infusion Pump (Williams, 2018).

! HOTSPOT

Unblocking of Tubes

The most common causes of feeding tube blocking are coagulation of feed by drug syrups or suspensions, inadequate flushing, or obstruction by particles of crushed oral medications.

This can be minimized by flushing tubes regularly, before and after medication using drugs in syrups or linctus form rather than crushed tablets.

Normal tap water can be used for gastric tubes and should always be tried first. Gastrostomy tubes tend to have a bigger lumen and therefore there is less chance of them blocking.

Methods Used to Unblock Feeding Tubes

Warm water should always be tried first, 5–10 mL at a time – this should be warm to touch.

Pancreatic enzymes are effective and can unblock a feed-blocked feeding tube in 10–20 minutes (Marcuad & Stegall, 1990).

Carbonated drinks, pineapple juice and sodium bicarbonate solution are effective at unblocking tubes but are more anecdotal methods and these substances can damage the tubes (Stroud, 2003).

! HOTSPOT

Nutrient–Drug Interactions

Enteral feeds can interfere with the dosage, presentation and action of many drugs. Oral phenytoin, for example, if given with enteral feeds, forms complexes with calcium and protein reducing its absorption by almost 80%. With oral phenytoin, an enteral feed should be stopped 2 hours pre and post dose. If it is not possible to give that break, then intravenous phenytoin should be given.

*Drugs should not be added to enteral feeds

Liaise with ward pharmacist to ensure optimal administration of medications.

multidisciplinary team: PEG specialist nurse, gastroenterologist and dietician.

Considerations to take into account with gastrostomy placement are that it is a consented procedure with its own risks, that has an increased risk of mortality, peritonitis and bacterial contamination. It is routine to administer prophylactic antibiotics. Tract formation occurs within a few hours and it can be safe to commence feeding four hours after tube insertion (NICE, 2006).

Post-pyloric feeding routes bypass the stomach, feeding into the small bowel. This is commonly used if the patient is unable to tolerate nasogastric feeding, perhaps due to high gastric aspirates. They are more difficult to place (usually performed under radiological conditions) and this should be a multidisciplinary team decision. Box 23.1 shows the different types of feeding routes that would be agreed by the team.

Enteral feed delivery can be administered as a continuous feed using a pump (Fig 23.6), usually for 16–20 hours. Patients may be fed over 24 hours in intensive care to keep blood sugars stable. Bolus feeding is an alternative method, which is a delivery of a volume of feed at several times in the day, for example, 200 mL of feed given every 3 hours. It takes half an hour for the pump to administer it. Gravity feeds can also be given using syringes, but this can be more challenging on a ward environment due to time constraints. Flushes of water should be given 4-hourly to keep feeding tubes patent, and before and after feed and medications are given to prevent them from blocking. Ensure the positioning of the patient is at a 30-degree angle to reduce risk of aspiration.

Parenteral nutrition

NICE indications for parenteral nutrition (PN) (NICE, 2006) are for those people who are malnourished or at risk of malnutrition *and* either inadequate or unsafe for oral and/or enteral intake or have a non-functioning/inaccessible or perforated gastrointestinal (GI) tract. For example, an elderly man who has had bowel surgery for cancer and now has a high output from his stoma post operatively and his weight is reducing drastically due to malabsorption of any food/fluid or enteral feeds given, would be a candidate for PN short-term. Indications for PN include:

Short-term PN
- Critically ill, unable to establish any tolerance with enteral tube feeding/oral intake
- Paralytic ileus
- Gastrointestinal perforation
- High output stoma/fistula
- Obstruction of the gastrointestinal tract mainly from cancer or inflammation
- Severe malabsorption
- Severe acute pancreatitis

Long-term PN (may need PN at home)
- Chronic malabsorption
- Short bowel syndrome
- Inflammatory bowel disease.

Contraindications
- Palliative care
- If the gut is functional

- Low albumin
- PN is not suitable for patients just refusing to eat/have enteral feeding
- If oral diet, supplements and enteral feeding have not been tried first.

Parenteral nutrition is a formulation of carbohydrate, protein, fats, vitamins, minerals, trace elements, electrolytes and fluid made up aseptically by pharmacy. This is time-consuming and costly compared to other types of artificial feeding and carries many more risks than enteral feeding as it requires a central venous access device (CVAD). Central lines are where the tip of the CVAD lies in a central vein (usually the superior vena cava), allowing access to the venous system for blood sampling, intravenous medications and parenteral nutrition.

PN can be used in combination with enteral and oral nutrition to meet nutritional requirements and does not have to be a sole source of nutrition.

There are two main types of central line:
- Skin tunnelled cuffed catheters (Hickman lines)
- Peripherally inserted central catheters (PICC lines).

Other types are:
- Implantable catheters
- Jugular lines (CVP)
- Femoral lines.

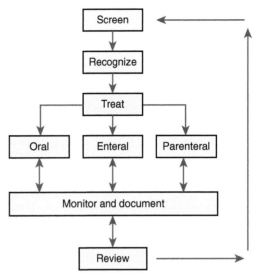

Fig. 23.7 Organization of Nutrition Support (NICE, 2006).

Fig. 23.7 gives an overview of the pathway for nutrition support patients.

CARE IN THE HOME SETTING

Mrs Wright was discharged home from hospital with support from her daughter, when she could get to visit, and community nurses/GP for monitoring of her weight, eating and drinking and general health.

Four weeks after discharge, the community nurse on a review observed that Mrs Wright looked very thin. On asking Mrs Wright if she could weigh her, she noticed that she was quite unsteady on her feet when asked to stand.

Mrs Wright had lost 3 kg since discharge from the ward and it appeared that her mobility and strength was reducing. She had not been able to get to the shops as regularly or cook the kind of meals she enjoyed. She was mainly having biscuits and cups of tea.

Mrs Wright was commenced on milkshake-style oral nutritional supplements that came in pre-mixed bottles. She was advised to sip these between meals to help increase her strength and weight, while advice was given on high-protein and high-calorie snacks and meals that were easy for her to access. The community team also looked into meal deliveries and additional support for Mrs Wright.

She was more closely monitored with weekly weighings and reviews of her dietary intake, and checks that she was taking the nutritional drinks, to prevent the situation worsening and avoiding the need for another hospital admission.

DIABETES MELLITUS

Diabetes mellitus is one of the most common chronic conditions in the UK and the incidence particularly of type 2 diabetes is rising. Diabetes has major complications and, if not managed, can increase mortality and morbidity. Diabetes-associated problems include cardiovascular disease (diabetes being a major contributor to heart disease), stroke, renal failure, blindness, gangrene and amputation if not well controlled.

There has been much emphasis on prevention of diabetes rather than cure. But health promotion on healthy eating, maintaining a healthy weight and reducing risk factors has had little impact, given the emergence of children with type 2 diabetes due to the increase in obesity in this younger age group.

Changes to diet and nutritional intake are the biggest factor in predicting outcome in patients with diabetes mellitus. Many have other chronic conditions, for example heart disease and obesity.

Signs and symptoms

Diabetes results from a lack of the hormone insulin. Insulin is essential in transferring glucose from the blood to the tissues where it is used for energy. Therefore if insulin is lacking or not working effectively, glucose levels in the blood become unusually high (hyperglycaemia). The body tries to get rid of it by passing it into the urine and increasing the amount of urine produced (polyuria). As the glucose in the blood is not being used as an energy source, the body starts to use its fat stores for energy. All these combined lead to signs and symptoms of:

- excessive thirst (polydipsia)
- excessive urine production (polyuria)
- unexplained weight loss
- diabetic ketoacidosis (in severe cases).

Type 1 diabetes

This is known as insulin-dependent diabetes, and is linked to a partial or total failure of insulin production. This is due to the destruction of pancreatic beta cells and usually presents in children or young adults. It is an autoimmune condition and the triggers are still unclear, but there is a genetic susceptibility (NICE, 2002).

Type 2 diabetes

The most common type of diabetes, accounting for up to 75% of cases, is mainly due to insulin insensitivity as a result of obesity, and is predominantly detected later on in life, although because it has less severe symptoms, it can remain undetected for some time. Diet and lifestyle changes have the biggest impact on improving outcomes with this diagnosis, but many people will require oral hypoglycaemic drugs, which increase insulin production, or medication that enhances insulin's effectiveness (NICE, 2002).

Diagnosis

Diagnosis of diabetes was defined by the World Health Organization (WHO) in 2006 and in 2011, WHO made the decision to allow the use of HbA1c testing in diagnosing diabetes: 'use of glycated haemoglobin in the diagnosis of diabetes mellitus'. (WHO, 2011).

If a patient has symptoms of diabetes (e.g., for type 1: polyuria, polydipsia and unexplained weight loss) plus one of the below criteria, diabetes would be confirmed:

- a random venous plasma glucose concentration equal to or greater than 11.1 mmol/L or
- a fasting plasma glucose concentration equal to or greater than 7.0 mmol/L (whole blood equal to or greater than 6.1 mmol/L) or
- two hour plasma glucose concentration equal to or greater than 11.1 mmol/L two hours after 75 g anhydrous glucose in an oral glucose tolerance test (OGTT).

If the patient does not have any symptoms, a diagnosis should not be based on a single glucose test such as this. At least one additional glucose test result on another day with a value in the diabetic range is essential, either fasting, from a random sample, or from the 2-hour post glucose load. If the fasting random values are not adequate, then the 2-hour result should be used.

Care and treatment

Diet is an essential component of diabetes management; weight loss is the key element as 5%–10% weight loss has been shown to improve blood glucose levels, reduce insulin resistance, blood lipids and blood pressure. Healthy eating advice is key, as well as increasing activity levels to optimize weight loss, regular meal patterns and a good balance of protein, carbohydrates and fruits and vegetables. The amount, type and timing of carbohydrate consumption can be important to maintain hunger as well as blood glucose levels.

Key dietary treatment changes:

- regular meal times
- reduce the fat, sugar or salt content of food
- include more fruit and vegetables
- reduce sugary drinks and alcohol
- increase activity levels.

COELIAC DISEASE

Coeliac disease is an autoimmune condition of the small intestine where the body reacts to gluten, a protein found in wheat, barley and rye. A person can be genetically predisposed and diagnosis can be from early childhood to old age, often going undetected for some time in the older age group.

Coeliac disease can be triggered by viruses, and the body produces antibodies to the gluten ingested, which in turn damages the mucosal lining of the gut, mainly in the small intestine where the villi that aid absorption of nutrients become flattened and damaged. Once diagnosed, a permanent change to the diet is required and non-adherence can lead to further complications, including osteoporosis, malignancy, poor growth in children and nutrient deficiencies (NICE, 2015).

Signs and symptoms

- Poor growth in childhood/delayed puberty
- Malabsorption
- Tiredness
- Anaemia

- Irritability
- Depression
- Breathlessness
- Peripheral oedema
- Abdominal discomfort/pain/increased frequency of bowel opening/diarrhoea
- Unexplained weight loss
- Mouth ulcers
- Infertility.

Diagnosis

Initial serological tests should be undertaken to measure blood antibodies; these are IgA endomysial antibodies (EMA) or IgA tissue transglutaminase (tTGA). If these blood levels are elevated, there is high suspicion of coeliac disease and being exposed to gluten on a regular basis, but this would not confirm diagnosis. The gold standard would be an intestinal biopsy following a referral to a specialist gastroenterologist. A biopsy would usually be of the duodenum and would normally reveal the typical flattening of the villi. Although recent guidelines have confirmed that if the tTG levels are ten times the upper limit and the patient has the positive genetic predisposition, then biopsy would not be required to confirm diagnosis (Ludvigsson et al., 2014).

Care and treatment

A strict gluten-free diet is the only treatment for coeliac disease. Some foods are naturally gluten free, for example fruits, vegetables, meat, fish, potatoes and rice, but many packaged and processed foods contain gluten as a hidden ingredient. It is essential people with coeliac disease are referred to a dietician for regular support and advice regarding their diet, symptom improvement, increased growth and the correction of vitamin deficiencies that can occur with adherence to a gluten-free diet. It is routine to recheck antibody levels 6–12 months following diagnosis to ensure these are returning to normal (NICE, 2015).

IRON DEFICIENCY ANAEMIA

The major role of iron is an as oxygen carrier in haemoglobin in blood and myoglobin in muscles. Iron is also required for many metabolic processes within the body.

Dietary iron exists in two forms: haem and non-haem, which are absorbed by different mechanisms. Haem iron is contained within the haemoglobin of animal foods and is very well absorbed (10% of intake) e.g., red meat, liver, offal, poultry and fish, whereas non-haem iron is mainly found in cereal products and green leafy vegetables (accounting for 90% of intake), but how it is absorbed is much more variable.

Non-haem iron interacts with tannins and phytates (for example, tea and wholegrains) in the gut making it unavailable for absorption, but vitamin C can aid the absorption of non-haem iron.

Signs and symptoms

Deficiency can be due to an underlying condition affecting the absorption of nutrients. At-risk groups are children over the age of 6 months and toddlers who are not having a varied weaning diet or drinking large volumes of milk; menstruating women, particularly younger women who require more iron, but intakes may be low; pregnant women; vegetarians and vegans; and people with malabsorption.

Deficiency can affect and delay a child's development if it is not picked up. Typical signs and symptoms may include:

- Pallor
- Lethargy
- Breathlessness
- A change in ability to do normal activities.

Diagnosis

A number of haematological parameters are used to assess iron levels. Low serum ferritin levels can indicate early signs of deficiency as this reflects iron stores within the body and falls prior to the haemoglobin blood levels dropping. It is important to note that ferritin levels can increase with infection and vary during pregnancy, so do not always indicate deficiency.

Other parameters to check for iron depletion are a low serum transferrin, low transferrin saturation and increased total iron-binding capacity (TIBC). As deficiency becomes more prolonged, a drop in blood haemoglobin to less than 130 g/dL in men and 120 g/dL in women would be indicative of iron deficiency anaemia.

Care and treatment

It is essential to look for a cause of the deficiency as it may indicate a chronic condition that has not yet been diagnosed, for example, coeliac disease. If it is found that the diet is lacking in iron, then changes should be suggested to optimize iron intake within the diet, and if necessary, a supplement for the short-term until levels have improved to normal. It is important to note that most iron supplements prescribed can cause abdominal discomfort.

COMMUNITIES OF CARE
Child Development

A 7-year-old boy is brought to the GP surgery for review as his mother is concerned the child is not growing.

On further examination, you notice the child does look thin and you assess their growth on the appropriate growth chart (WHO, 2006) for boys. You notice that at 5 years of age the child's weight and height were perfectly proportional on the 75th centiles for both, but today his height has dropped to the 25th centile and his weight has not increased for 2 years, meaning that this has also dropped down the centile charts.

It is important at this point to gather information regarding his dietary intake; what is a normal day of eating for him? Has this changed recently? Has he had any time off school? Does he manage normal activities for a 7-year-old boy?

It appears he has been very tired and withdrawn, complaining of tummy pains often and going to the toilet much more frequently, mainly after eating; therefore, he has not been eating well.

His bloods are checked and it is noted he is iron deficient. Further investigation into this confirms he has raised antibodies for coeliac disease and a referral to a specialist gastroenterologist and dietician is required to confirm diagnosis as quickly as possible to ensure growth is corrected, as well as development.

COMMUNITIES OF CARE

Maternity: Nutritional Considerations for Breastfeeding Mother

Fetal growth depends on the nutritional status of the mother before conception, during pregnancy and also after birth if mother breastfeeds. Breastfeeding should always be encouraged and supported, where possible, as there are many advantages with regard to the nutritional element of breast milk, as well as the immunological elements and protection against the development of atopic allergies. There are increasing instances of infants with symptoms of cow's milk protein allergy and mothers are making changes to their own diets and restricting certain food groups to help with the symptoms. This can be detrimental to mother and baby if it is not done under guidance from health professionals, as exposure to high-risk foods via breast milk has a positive effect to prevent allergies in later life. It can also affect the nutrition the baby receives, as well as the mother's health.

It is vital that breastfeeding mothers take adequate calcium and vitamin D while breast feeding (1200 mg calcium and 10 micrograms of vitamin D daily) especially if the mother is making changes to her own diet. If there are any concerns regarding allergies from the infant or the mother's diet being restricted, refer to an appropriate health professional for guidance and further support (Venter et al., 2017).

LOOKING BACK, FEEDING FORWARD

The purpose of this chapter was to give you an insight into how important nutrition is in your day-to-day practice, outlining the key role of the Nursing Associate. Everybody eats, and the types of foods that we eat can affect our health and well-being, with a good diet improving health outcomes.

Nutrition and diet play an important role in almost all chronic health conditions. Simple dietary changes can make a significant impact on the recovery of an unwell patient, and either prevent admission to hospital or reduce the length of stay.

There is, however, lots of incorrect and inappropriate nutritional guidance available in the public domain, and therefore it is important that any advice given is evidence-based.

REFERENCES

Dennis, M.S., Lewis, S.C., Warlow, C., 2005. FOOD Trial Collaboration. Effect of timing and method of enteral tube feeding for dysphagic stroke patients (FOOD): a multicentre randomised controlled trial. Lancet 365, 764–772.

Department of Health, 2015. Essence of Care 2010. Benchmarks for Respect and Dignity.

Diabetes UK, 2005. Diabetes in the UK 2004. Diabetes UK, London.

Elia, M. (Ed.), 2000. Guidelines for the Detection and Management of Malnutrition. BAPEN, Maidenhead. Malnutrition Advisory Group (MAG). Standing Committee of BAPEN.

Elia, M. (Ed.), 2003. Screening for Malnutrition; a Multidisciplinary Responsibility. Development and Use of the Malnutrition Universal Screening Tool ('MUST') for Adults. BAPEN, Redditch.

Food Standards Agency (FSA), 2005. Eat Well. Your Guide to Healthy Eating. Eight Tips for Healthier Choices. FSA, London.

Health Education Authority (HEA), 2014. The Balance of Good Health. Introducing the National Food Guide. HEA, London.

Heyland, D.K., Dhawali, R., Drover, J.W., et al., 2003. Canadian Critical Care Clinical Practice Guidelines Committee. Canadian clinical practice guidelines for nutrition support in mechanically ventilated, critically ill adult patients. JPEN J. Parenter. Enteral Nutr. 27, 355–373.

Ludvigsson, J.F., Bai, J.C., Biagi, F., et al., 2014. Diagnosis and management of adult coeliac disease: guidelines from the British Society of Gastroenterology. Gut 63, 1210–1228.

Marcuad, S.P., Stegall, K.S., 1990. Unclogging feeding tubes with pancreatic enzyme. JPEN J. Parenter. Enteral Nutr. 14, 198–200.

National Institute for Clinical Excellence, 2002. Management of Type 2 Diabetes: Management of Blood Glucose. NICE, London.

National Institute for Health and Clinical Excellence, 2006. Nutrition Support in Adults: Oral Nutrition Support, Enteral Tube Feeding and Parenteral Nutrition. Clinical Guideline 32. NICE, London.

National Institute for Health and Clinical Excellence, 2012a. Nutrition Support in Adults. Quality Standard 24. NICE, London.

National Institute for Health and Clinical Excellence, 2012b. Nutrition Support in Adults: Oral Nutrition Support, Enteral Tube Feeding and Parenteral Nutrition. Quality Standard 23. NICE, London.

National Institute for Health and Care Excellence, 2015. NG20 Coeliac Disease; Recognition, Assessment and Management of Coeliac Disease. NICE, London.

National Patient Safety Agency, 2005. Reducing the Harm Caused by Misplaced Nasogastric Feeding Tubes. Patient Safety Alert 05. NPSA, London.

National Patient Safety Agency, 2011. Reducing the Harm Caused by Misplaced Nasogastric Feeding Tubes in Adults, Children and Infants. Patient Safety Alert 002. NPSA, London.

Public Health England, 2016. Government Dietary Recommendations; Government recommendations for energy and nutrients for males and females aged 1–18 years and 19+ years. https://www.gov.uk/government/publications/the-eatwell-guide.

Rassool, G.H., 2015. Cultural competence in nursing muslim patients. Nurs. Times 111 (14), 12–15.

Stratton, R.J., Green, C.J., Elia, M., 2003. Disease Related Malnutrition: An Evidence Based Approach to Treatment. CABI Publishing, Oxford.

Stroud, M., Duncan, H., Nightingale, J., 2003. Guidelines for enteral feeding in adult hospital patient. Gut 52 (Suppl.VII), 1–12.

Venter, C., Brown, T., Rosan, M., et al., 2017. Better recognition, diagnosis and management of non-IgE-mediated cow's milk allergy in infancy: iMAP – an international interpretation of the MAP (Milk Allergy in Primary Care) guideline. Clinical and Translational Allergy.

Whitten, C., Nicholson, S.K., Roberts, C., et al., 2011. National Diet and Nutrition Survey: UK food consumption and nutrient intakes from the first year of the rolling programme and comparisons with previous surveys. Br. J. Nutr. 106, 2.

World Health Organization, 1998. Obesity: Preventing and managing the Global Epidemic. Report of a WHO Consultation on Obesity, Geneva, 3–5 June 1997. WHO.

World Health Organization, 2006. The WHO Child Growth Standards. WHO, Geneva. www.who.int/child-growth.

World Health Organization, 2011. Use of glycated haemoglobin (HbA1c) in the diagnosis of diabetes mellitus. WHO. http://www.who.int/diabetes/publications/diagnosis_diabetes2011/en/.

24

Cancer

Kathy Whayman, Karen Sumpter

OBJECTIVES

By the end of the chapter the reader will be able to:

1. Understand the processes and pathophysiological changes involved in the development of cancerous tumours
2. Understand the signs and symptoms of cancer leading to a diagnosis and explain them for some of the more common cancers
3. Outline the physical, psychological and social care required by individuals who are diagnosed with cancer
4. List and explain the different tests and investigations involved in the staging of cancer
5. Understand the different methods used in the treatment of cancer
6. Review the role of the Nursing Associate (NA) in promoting health and well-being for individuals and families affected by and living with cancer

KEY WORDS

Carcinogenesis	Screening	Support groups
Genes	Cancer staging	Tailored information
Risk factors	Chemotherapy	
Carcinogen	Radiotherapy	

CHAPTER AIM

The aim of this chapter is to provide the reader with an understanding of the skills, knowledge and attitude required to provide safe, effective and compassionate care to people with a diagnosis of cancer.

SELF TEST

1. What does carcinogenesis mean?
2. What is the difference between a malignant tumour and a benign tumour?
3. Name three environmental factors that can cause cancer development.
4. Name three known carcinogens.
5. What types of imaging investigations are used to diagnose cancer?
6. What is a core biopsy?
7. What is the most common cancer in men in the UK?
8. List three common side effects of chemotherapy.
9. Describe two treatments used as complementary therapies in cancer care.
10. Which groups find it difficult to access palliative care services?

INTRODUCTION

In this chapter, the nature and biological basis of cancer is considered. The first part discusses cancer development and the factors that influence it. It is important for the Nursing Associate (NA) to have a comprehensive understanding of cancer development if the treatment and care provided is to be appropriate, person-centred and effective.

The second part of the chapter addresses three common cancers and their impact on the health and well-being of the individual affected and those close to them. The Nursing Associate should be aware that there are many types of cancer and further reading on specific cancers is encouraged. The care and comfort of the patient who is diagnosed with and treated for cancer is described. When offering care and support to individuals and families, the NA is required to be kind and compassionate. Care provision can be complex – the physical and psychological impact of this potentially life-threatening disease can instil fear, anxiety and, in some people, a loss of hope. Effective and compassionate care can make a critical difference to someone affected in this way. When harm or damage occurs to the body as a result of treatment for cancer (for example surgery, or radiotherapy), there can be a lasting impact on a person's body image, identity, self-awareness, self-esteem and confidence.

! HOTSPOT
Fear of Cancer - Compassion in Care

Despite improvements in cancer survival rates in the last two decades, which will be discussed later in this chapter, there remain many negative perceptions about cancer. Experiencing cancer can affect the individual in all aspects of their lives, including their social, cultural and spiritual well-being. Fatalistic associations with cancer (associating cancer with death) can adversely affect help-seeking behaviour for cancer symptoms and engagement in cancer prevention – and has been shown to be most common in the middle aged and older adult groups (Agustina et al., 2017). Information and psychological support is critical at each stage of diagnosis and treatment and the role of the NA is to offer non-judgemental, kind and compassionate support for people affected by cancer as part of the healthcare team. (Please refer to Table 34.2 on p. 428 for important factors in the essence of care that must be embodied by the NA involved in cancer care.)

THE BIOLOGICAL BASIS OF CANCER

Cancer starts when cells start to divide and grow in an abnormal way. It is a disease traditionally characterized by cellular origin. Cancer involving changes and mutations within the body's cells brought about by many factors. These changes can then result in the disruption of normal cell regulation, abnormal cell growth and erratic cell division. Cancer is a very common disease – recent statistics show that 1 in 2 people in the UK will develop cancer in their lifetime (Cancer Research UK, 2014a). Much more is known about cancer now, and with advances in research, prevention, treatments and support services, survival rates are improving.

In the UK – 2014 (Cancer Research UK, 2014a):

- 356,860 new cases of cancer were diagnosed
- 50% people diagnosed with cancer will survive for 10 years or more
- 1.8 million people are living with cancer
- 163,000 deaths from cancer in 2014
- 42% of cancers are preventable.

Types of cancer

There are over 200 types of cancer (Waugh & Grant, 2018), with some being more common than others. They all share similar characteristics of cell changes. Four cancers are the most common, making up 54% of all cancer incidence in the UK (Wyatt & Hubert-Williams, 2015). These are breast, lung, bowel and prostate cancer.

CRITICAL AWARENESS
Will There Be a Cure for Cancer?

Although there are types of cancers that share the same characteristics, each type of cancer, and each person's individual cancer, is unique, and they each come with their own set of challenges. According to Alford (2017), this is why researchers are unlikely to find a single cure that can wipe out all cancers. She reports in a Cancer Research UK science blog that this does not mean individual cases of cancer cannot be cured, and many cancers, in fact, already can be. Testicular cancer, for instance, is sensitive to treatment with drugs (chemotherapy) and most cases can be cured – survival today is as high as 98%, and that is just one example among many.

There are many factors that affect survival rate: for example, advances in treatment, early detection of the cancer, the stage of development of a cancer when it is diagnosed and the success of treatment.

How do cancers start?

To understand how cancers begin and grow, we first need to consider how normal cells work and function.

All living creatures are made up of cells, and most are multi-cellular organisms. Life begins as a single cell, which divides thousands of times to form the embryonic body of the fetus (Marieb, 2015). Within the body, tissues and organs are composed of cells with a specialized structure and function for that particular part of the body. Each cell has a complex physical and chemical structure; it requires food to live and carry out its specific functions, and all have the ability to repair (Wheeldon, 2013). Within most cells (red blood cells are an exception), there are structures called organelles – small 'organs' that enable the cell to function and carry out its job for growth and maintenance of bodily function (Marieb, 2015). A diagram of a simple cell can be seen in Fig. 24.1.

Cells can also reproduce and are designed to grow and divide. Sometimes called the 'brain' of the cell, the organelle called the nucleus houses the genetic material (composed of deoxyribonucleic acid: DNA) located in the chromosomes.

The nucleus assumes responsibility for cell division (Wheeldon, 2013). Each cell has a cycle for cellular growth repair and reproduction, which is governed by control and regulatory processes. A second nucleic acid – ribonucleic Acid (RNA) is located outside the nucleus in the cytoplasm within the ribosomes. This RNA (mRNA) ensures protein synthesis as per instructions in the copying and expression of proteins from the DNA (Marieb, 2015). See Fig. 24.2 for a diagram of the cell cycle. The processes of cell division are known as meiosis and mitosis.

Mitosis

In this part of the cell cycle, cells reproduce, and in doing so, replicate their genetic material to make exact copies of themselves. For cell growth and development, this must be done accurately to avoid abnormalities. There are four phases involved in mitosis:

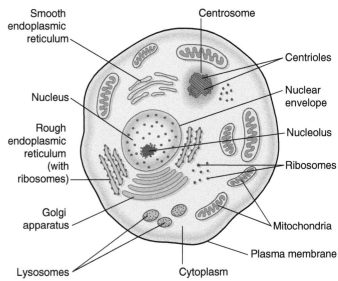

Fig. 24.1 A simple cell (Waugh & Grant, 2018).

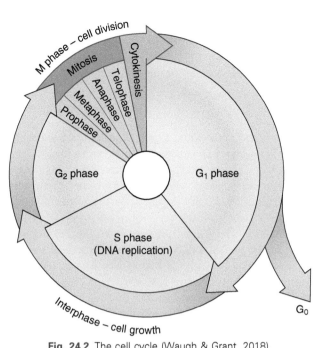

Fig. 24.2 The cell cycle (Waugh & Grant, 2018).

prophase, metaphase, anaphase and telophase, as described below (Waugh & Grant, 2018). These can be seen in Fig. 24.3.

The genetic material within the cell is located in the chromosomes. When the cell is not reproducing, the molecules of DNA make up a threadlike mass called chromatin.

- Prophase: When cells prepare to divide in the prophase stage, the chromatin shortens and forms 23 chromosomes. Each chromosome is now made of two chromatids and these are joined by a centromere. During the cell cycle leading up to this stage, the DNA has been replicated and each chromatid is an exact copy of the other. The membrane around the nucleus breaks down and the cell prepares to split into two.
- Metaphase: Here the 46 chromatids are separated by becoming attached to spindle fibres.
- Anaphase: There is a spindle (pole) at each end of the cell, and one chromatid from each chromosome is drawn to the pole at each end of the cell.
- Telophase: Finally, the cell cytoplasm begins to split, and a new cell membrane is formed around the two daughter cells. A new nuclear membrane then forms around the 23 chromosomes in each new cell, and the division is complete, and each cell has its own nucleus with an exact copy of the DNA.

DNA synthesis and repair

To prepare for this process of cell division, the cell will first enter interphase – as can be seen in Fig. 24.2 in the cell cycle. This is the phase when a cell will grow and prepare for DNA replication (Wheeldon, 2013). Here the DNA is examined for errors, and repaired. If errors are too numerous, or they cannot be repaired, the proteins within the cell will set off instructions to bring about the process of cell death – also known as apoptosis. If a cell has reached a certain age (as errors can be more prevalent in DNA within an older cell) and has reached its set number of reproductions, then regulations within the cell cycle will also

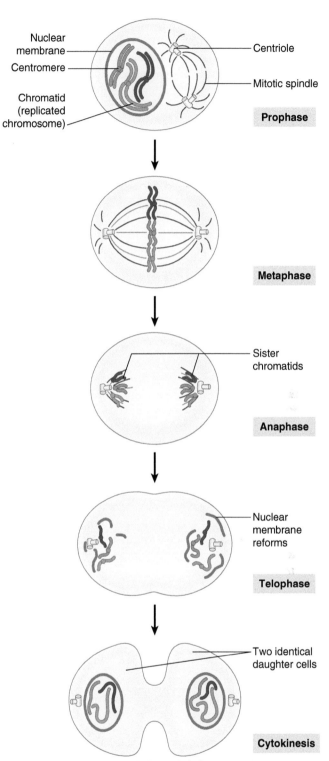

Fig. 24.3 Mitosis (Waugh & Grant, 2018).

trigger apoptosis. Once apoptosis is started, no further replication of that cell's DNA can occur and the cell will not be able to reproduce. Chemicals, such as enzymes and proteins within the cell, will be triggered to break down the cell structures into components. Other types of cells, such as macrophages (a type of white blood cell) will then recognize those components and remove them from the body by excretion.

Understanding the normal cellular activity and control for growth, repair and cell reproduction is necessary for the NA to appreciate what happens when cancers develop. Understanding this biological basis for cancer development has enabled scientists to discover more about when things go wrong within the cell, and about the genetic mutations of different cancers. Over the last few decades, huge advances in molecular biology have helped develop treatments that are now so specific they can be tailored to different types of cancer, and even to the individual tumour itself. This has had an impact on global cancer survival rates and increased the number of people who are successfully treated for cancer. The research has also improved the side-effect profile of many treatments (these will be outlined later in this chapter). Many more people are now living with cancer, and in many cases, it is considered to be a long-term condition.

How do cancers develop?

Most cells have the ability to lose regulation and normal control to form a tumour.

Cancer development and progression is a process known as carcinogenesis. This is a multistep process involving an accumulation of cellular and chemical errors (Corner and Bailey, 2008). This occurs when repair mechanisms in the cell cycle fail, or during cell division when regulatory processes malfunction. This process of cancer development occurs when a single cell has DNA which is damaged for some reason (Clare, 2013). A series of mutations will need to occur, however, before a cancerous tumour will manifest itself and grow. The body has systems that step in to recognize errors and mutations, such as within the cell cycle phases and apoptosis (as discussed previously) or in the inflammatory and immunity response, as discussed in Chapter 27.

CRITICAL AWARENESS

Benign or Malignant?

A tumour can be benign or malignant. A **benign** tumour is a non-cancerous type of tumour and is usually contained within its own structure. This tumour can grow but does not spread to other parts of the body. Problems generally occur when the tumour grows sufficiently to put pressure on other organs or tissue. One example of this is a pituitary adenoma (a benign brain tumour), which can grow large enough to press on the optic nerve and induce blindness.

A **malignant** tumour, by contrast, has properties that enable it to invade other organs (either directly from one organ to another next to it, or via the circulatory or lymphatic systems). Malignant tumours have the ability to metastasize – i.e., spread to a secondary site.

Many cancers take years to develop and will only result when there are billions of replications of a mutated cell (Clare, 2013). Cancer is considered a disease of older age, but due to other factors such as genetic inheritance and family history, mutations and tumour development can occur in children or even in-utero.

CAUSES OF CANCER

Exactly what mechanisms occur to cause cancer are not yet known. However, the involvement of certain factors that promote mutations of particular genes and also the switching off of normal regulatory processes are thought to promote cancer development and disease progression.

There are three stages of carcinogenesis (Marieb, 2015):
- Initiation
- Promotion
- Progression.

Initiation is the phase when a genetic mutation has occurred and there is possibly an interaction with an environmental factor, such as when a person is exposed to a carcinogen. This would explain why some people who smoke go on to develop lung cancer whilst others do not. A genetic change needs to occur as well as the exposure to the carcinogenic agent – in this case cigarette smoke. There does not need to be exposure to a carcinogen as genetic mutations can occur spontaneously – this would also explain why certain people who have never smoked a cigarette go on to develop lung cancer. However, the most common link for the development and progression of lung cancer is smoking, which is linked to a much higher risk of developing the disease.

Examples of carcinogens include:
- Food preservatives
- Pesticides
- Pollution
- Cigarette smoke
- Alcohol
- Certain foods
- Radiation
- Asbestos
- Some substances found within food or produced as a result of cooking.

HOTSPOT

Radiation

There are types of radiation that are known to cause cancer. Sunlight, for example, is ultraviolet light and is directly linked to types of skin cancer, particularly in people with pale skin. The sunlight reacts with cellular development and causes genetic changes in skin cells. Ionising radiation, such as that emitted through x-rays or in the environment, is known to affect the cell cycle and mitosis. Many cancers are linked with this type of radiation including leukaemia, thyroid cancer, breast cancer, lung cancer, gastrointestinal cancers, myeloma and bladder cancer (Clare, 2013). X-rays and radiation treatment are very helpful in diagnosing and treating disease (see later Hotspot on imaging) but are carefully prescribed and planned to reduce the risk of over exposure and damage to cells.

HOTSPOT

Viruses

Some viruses are linked to cancer development where the virus will cause genetic mutations in the host cell's DNA – the virus enters the cell and transfers its DNA or RNA into the cell causing mutation and potential malignant changes (Waugh & Grant, 2018). Examples include the human papillomavirus (HPV) which is linked to cervical cancer and, in rarer cases, anal cancer.

Promotion is the phase where imbalances in the chemical and biological processes of the cells can be disrupted leading to a switch-off of the normal regulations, such as cell repair and cell death. We now have a mutated cell with the potential to replicate and divide. This potential is either as a result of genetic involvement or as a result of further changes in the cell brought about by the environmental factors, or both. Some genes that regulate cell mechanisms are thought to be altered as well by exposure to carcinogens: these are called proto-oncogenes and can be 'switched' to become oncogenes. Another gene thought to be affected in this way is called the tumour suppressor gene.

By the alteration in their chemical make-up, these genes no longer function as they should, and in some cases are switched off, resulting in cell division of a mutated gene which is rapid and out of control.

> **! HOTSPOT**
>
> **Proto-oncogenes** work by telling the cell to replicate and divide – a bit like the accelerator tells a car to go faster. The **tumour suppressor gene** works by telling the cell to slow down the rate of division and growth – such as when the brake is pressed in a car to slow it down. These genes can also slow down the changes in cell mutations as a result of the effect of carcinogens (Marieb, 2015). These genes maintain cellular health and an effective speed of division, keeping them under control. When one or both these genes are altered or switched off, then cells can divide and replicate out of control and rapidly, with a greater degree of mutation.

Other cellular regulations can be altered as a result of this promotion phase and into progression. For example, changed cancer cells can evade recognition by other cells or chemicals by turning off receptors on the cell's surface and affecting communication methods which make the cells recognizable. This can stop these rogue cells being discovered and being 'rested', repaired or destroyed. Usually, cells are recognizable and their replication and division can be slowed or stopped by a mechanism called 'contact inhibition'. As cells mutate and become less characteristic of their normal form, they can lose this contact inhibition and receptors fail, resulting in the rapidly dividing cells clumping together and becoming invasive to surrounding tissues and vessels.

Progression is the phase where cells continue to change and become less well defined, resulting in a loss of differentiation.

If a cancer cell is slow-growing, it may still maintain some of the original characteristics of the cell function, which means it is well differentiated. As time progresses, however, and the mutated cell continues to proliferate, the original features become less recognizable. Thus, a cancer cell that is fast growing it is likely to lose all original characteristics and is thus poorly differentiated. These cells then lose the capacity to function normally. A cancer whose cells are poorly differentiated is more difficult to treat as the cancer is likely to be more advanced. This stage of cancer development is discussed later on in the chapter.

If a cell cannot differentiate, it may lack certain biochemical properties, or may acquire new properties. For example, a mutated group of cells may not be so dependent on oxygen to survive, or it may secrete hormones that it would not normally do. Cells also have a chromosomal instability and are therefore also less genetically stable. If a cell is 'unstable', increasing mutant versions will grow as the cancer cells multiply, proliferate and behave erratically.

In this **progression** phase, cancers also develop the capacity to advance and increase in size. Some cancers are said to be locally advanced and some will have the ability to metastasize.

- **Locally advanced tumours:** These may increase in size and move outside the organ where the cancer started. They may do this by penetrating the walls or vessels of an adjacent organ. One common example is an abdominal tumour, such as ovarian cancer, which invades the peritoneal cavity. Nerves, blood or lymphatic vessels and muscle may be eroded in the process. Some locally advanced cancers like this are considered incurable.
- **Metastases:** By metastasizing, the cancer can spread to distant secondary sites. This can also either be by direct invasion to adjacent sites or vessels, or by transport through the circulatory and lymphatic system (as seen in Fig. 24.5). By now, these cells may be poorly differentiated and have the ability to detach from the original tumour and move to another distant site, where they will develop another cancer. See Table 24.1 for the most common sites of metastatic spread.

Cancer cells become increasingly malignant with each mutation. Malignant tumours can also develop their own energy storage and nutritional source. These tumours can also create their own circulatory system and become independent from the organ from which they originate. This process is known as angiogenesis. The degree of malignancy relates to its ability to metastasize, continuing to act in an uncontrolled way.

All these processes are important because understanding the biological basis of cancer can help develop our knowledge of all stages of a cancer diagnosis and its treatment (see Table 24.2 on the various stages of diagnosing and treating cancer). The NA should also be able to explain or clarify information to the patient and their family about some of these processes if asked to do so, giving information safely and effectively within their level of knowledge.

Table 24.2 lists the possible stages that a person may experience during their diagnosis and treatment for cancer. Not

TABLE 24.1 Common Sites of Metastatic Spread in Relation to a Primary Cancer

Primary tumour	Common sites for metastatic spread
Bronchogenic (lung)	Spinal cord, brain, liver, bone
Breast	Regional lymph nodes, vertebrae, brain, liver, lung, bone
Colon (bowel)	Liver, lung, brain, ovary, bone
Prostate	Bladder, bone (especially vertebrae), liver
Malignant melanoma (skin)	Lung, liver, spleen, regional lymph nodes, brain

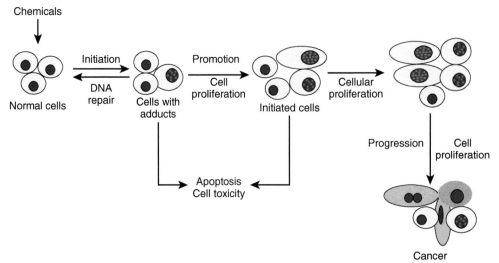

Fig. 24.4 Carcinogenesis. (Oliveira, P.A., Colaço, A., Chaves, R. Guedes-Pinto, H., L. F. De la Cruz, P., Lopes, C., 2007. Chemical carcinogenesis. Am. Acad. Bras. Cienc. 79(4), 593–616).

TABLE 24.2	Stages of Cancer – From Diagnosis to Treatment and Beyond
Stage	**What is involved?**
Prevention	This might involve cancer awareness campaigns, and health promotion activities. Also includes national screening programmes for certain types of cancer – cervical, breast, prostate and bowel cancer
Presentation of symptoms leading to a diagnosis of cancer	Either from a screening programme or reporting signs and symptoms to a healthcare professional, such as GP, practice nurse, or hospital team
Diagnosis and staging	Investigations into signs and symptoms and the extent of disease. Informing the patient and family about the diagnosis
Staging of disease	Using information from patient history and investigations to determine the treatment required
Treatment	May involve surgery, chemotherapy, radiotherapy, immunotherapy or a combination
Survivorship	Involving support and follow-up on the short and long-term consequences of treatment. Often nurse-led, for example by a nurse specialist in a clinic. There are now some patient groups and charities looking at how people cope after treatment (Macmillan Cancer Support, 2014)
Recurrence of the cancer/ advanced disease	Either through presentation of new symptoms or through follow-up – resulting possibly in a new diagnosis of cancer or a diagnosis of advanced disease
Palliative treatment	Designed to stabilize the progression of the cancer, to enhance the person's quality of life and manage their symptoms
End of life care	Focused on controlling symptoms and maximizing the individual's quality of life, for example, when that person's disease cannot be treated or is progressing despite treatment. There is a focus on the needs and wishes of the dying person (DH, 2013)

every person will be screened for cancer and similarly not every person will require palliative treatment or end of life care for cancer. People may get diagnosed and treated successfully in the early stages and some may present with advanced cancer needing palliative treatment from the start. It is vital that every patient is treated as an individual and their holistic needs are assessed and reviewed regularly. The plan of care will involve many different professionals (forming the multidisciplinary team – MDT). MDT working is at the heart of all cancer care and was set out as a standard by the NHS Cancer Plan (DH, 2000), and remains so to this day. Care must be person-centred,

involving the patient and those close to them as much as they wish to improve their experience and the quality of care (NHS England, 2017).

Prevention: According to Cancer Research UK (2014a) nearly half of all cancers are now preventable. Identifying and educating the public about risk factors has been a very important part of national policy in recent years. There are a number of inherited factors and lifestyle choices that are said to heighten a person's risk of developing a cancer. Awareness and modification of these factors is essential, as prevention offers the best long-term strategy in cancer control (WHO, 2017).

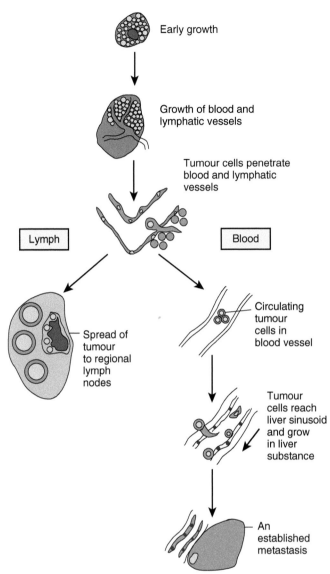

Early growth

Growth of blood and lymphatic vessels

Tumour cells penetrate blood and lymphatic vessels

Lymph

Blood

Spread of tumour to regional lymph nodes

Circulating tumour cells in blood vessel

Tumour cells reach liver sinusoid and grow in liver substance

An established metastasis

Fig. 24.5 Tissue invasion and the development of cancer using liver metastasis as an example (Tobias, J. and Hochhauser, D. (2009) The Biology of Cancer. In Cancer and Its Management, sixth ed. Chichester, John Wiley & Sons, Ltd. Chapter 3, p39, Fig. 3.12).

CRITICAL AWARENESS

Public Health and National Cancer Screening Programmes

In the UK, there are currently three population-based cancer screening programmes: for cervical cancer, breast cancer and bowel cancer. These are identified in the Cancer Strategy (Independent Cancer Taskforce, 2015) and the role of public health and cancer prevention is central to improving early detection, access to treatment and increased survival rates. The screening programmes currently detect around 5% of all cancer cases, including around 30% of breast cancers and 10% of bowel cancers. The Strategy outlines that the cervical screening programme in England, which includes the human papillomavirus (HPV) vaccination programme and cervical smear testing, is the most successful in the world. Over 86% of girls aged 13 have received the vaccination and evidence already suggests a reduction in HPV infection. The Government is currently considering extending this vaccination in the future to homosexual men who are also at high risk of contracting HPV.

MODIFICATION OF LIFESTYLE TO REDUCE CANCER RISK

Diet, alcohol, obesity and tobacco

Excessive alcohol intake has been linked to breast, colon, oesophageal, pharyngeal, liver and oral cancers. Obesity and lack of exercise are also linked to many cancers (and also other diseases that can impact a person's treatment experience and recovery). It is now known that a diet that is high in fat (particularly in animal fat), and low in fish and vegetables, is strongly correlated with a higher risk of bowel cancer. There are protective elements known to exist in vegetables, such as lycopene and flavonoids, which are thought to protect against cancer development.

Smoking is the biggest preventable cause of cancer. According to Cancer Research UK (2014b), reducing the number of people smoking by just 1% could have a large impact on cancer survival rates in the UK. Tobacco use causes cancers of the lung, oesophagus, larynx, mouth, throat, kidney, bladder, pancreas, stomach and cervix and secondary smoke or passive smoking is also linked heavily to the development of many cancers. The World Health Organization (2017) reports that 80% of the world's smokers come from low- or middle-income countries. In the UK, there has been huge investment into smoking cessation clinics, awareness campaigns and reduction in tobacco packaging/advertising.

Radiation

Exposure to manmade or natural radiation increases the risk of many types of cancer. Many countries now promote policies about ultraviolet light radiation, advising the public on taking precautions in strong sunshine, such as the use of sunscreens, and raising awareness of the risk factors for skin cancers (see the Hotspot on radiation as a carcinogen).

Infections

Worldwide, 15% of cancers can be attributed to infections, such as hepatitis B, human papillomavirus (HPV) and gastrointestinal viruses. This varies from country to country, with low incidence reported in Australia, USA and Canada, and a very high incidence in some European and African countries (World Health Organization, 2017). Vaccines are rapidly being developed, such as the hepatitis B vaccine, and there is a comprehensive programme in the UK, which includes a vaccine for the HPV virus as part of the National Screening Programme for cervical cancer. Infections and risk of cancer (particularly cancers involving the HPV virus) can also be linked to sexual health and reproductive behaviour, such as a transmission of a viral infection between sexual partners. Incidence is correlated to number of sexual partners and age of first sexual contact (see Chapter 34 for further information on sexual health).

Occupational hazards

Exposure to carcinogens and raised cancer risk through work has been known for a long time, certainly since Victorian times, for example, boy chimney sweeps (Clare, 2013). Many other carcinogens, however, are also known to expose the worker to risk. Working with asbestos is well-known to cause mesothelioma (cancer of the lining of the lung), but there are over 40 substances or combinations that have been classified as occupational carcinogens. Workplaces have a legal responsibility to employees to have robust policies in place to reduce risk of exposure to hazardous substances.

AT THE GP SURGERY
Routes to Diagnosis

Cancer screening programmes are one of the routes to a diagnosis of cancer. Most people will, however, be diagnosed following presentation and investigations of symptoms to their GP or practice nurse. Some will be seen as part of a clinic setting (such as a well-person service) or having been admitted to hospital as an emergency. The success of treatment and the survival rate can be determined by the stage of the cancer by the time a diagnosis is made. The earlier a cancer is detected, the less likely it is to be advanced which will lead to a better outcome. Therefore, there are national targets for urgent referrals when a person presents to their GP or hospital with symptoms indicative of a possible cancer. Currently, the target is that if a patient presents with 'red flag' symptoms leading to a suspected cancer, they will be seen by a specialist within 2 weeks. (This is sometimes called a '2 Week Wait'.) The target from diagnosis to first treatment is currently set at 62 days. GP and hospital datasets are examined to ensure services are meeting or working to meet these targets. Many people who are referred urgently do not go on to be diagnosed with cancer. This is because symptoms for other conditions can be similar: one example of this is rectal bleeding, accompanied by a change of bowel habit over 6 weeks in length. This can be a symptom of bowel cancer, but may also lead to a diagnosis of ulcerative colitis or haemorrhoids. Investigating this urgently is vital, however, as a missed bowel cancer can have a catastrophic impact on the individual, as it may potentially lead to a diagnosis of advanced cancer in the future.

As the symptoms of cancer can sometimes be vague, there can be a delay in getting a diagnosis, which again can lead to a situation where the cancer has begun to advance and spread. There are many health promotion campaigns now that seek to raise people's awareness of symptoms and to get them investigated by their doctor or practice nurse.

COMMON SYMPTOMS: UNEXPLAINED CHANGES IN THE BODY

There are many different types of cancers and the signs and symptoms can vary depending on the location of the tumour and the organ affected. Some common symptoms of many cancers are as follows:
- Lumps, mass or swelling
- Unexplained pain and/or bruising
- Marked altered bowel habits
- Nausea or vomiting with no known cause
- Bleeding: urine, stool, altered menstrual cycle
- Weight loss
- Loss of appetite, general feeling of being unwell/run down
- Fatigue
- Coughing, chest pain, breathlessness
- Moles: change in shape, size.

Investigating symptoms and staging of cancers

Driven by the national ambition for earlier detection and treatment, the Independent Cancer Taskforce (2015) has identified the need for faster and less restrictive investigative testing, quickly responding to patients who present with symptoms, to rule out cancer or other serious disease. The target is set that by 2020, 95% of patients referred for testing by a GP are definitively diagnosed with cancer, or cancer is excluded, and the result communicated to the patient, within 4 weeks. Many investigations are hospital-based and therefore excellent communication between the hospital services and GP surgeries will be vital.

Investigating cancer further once a diagnosis is made will also enable the MDT to know more about the stage of the cancer and the patient can be told what stage their cancer has reached. This information is very important for the team to decide the best and most appropriate treatment based on the stage of the cancer. Cancers that have started to spread to other parts of the body (metastasize) will have a poorer outcome than a cancer that has not.

Different types of cancers have different staging systems and grading criteria specific to the part of body affected. There are some universal systems, however.

TNM classification: This relates to the **tumour, nodes** and **metastases** criteria. It grades a cancer describing the primary tumour (T) – e.g., how large the tumour is – whether lymph nodes near to the cancer are affected (N), and whether there are any sites the cancer has spread to (M).

Many cancers are graded using **general cancer stages**:
- stage 1: localized to the original organ with no spread
- stage 2: the cancer has spread or is about to spread into neighbouring tissue
- stage 3: the cancer has spread to the local lymph nodes near to the cancer
- stage 4: the cancer has spread to neighbouring tissues and to distant sites in other parts of the body (see Table 24.1 for common sites of metastatic spread).

Some staging criteria use Roman numerals, and some use letters, either for the particular type of cancer or for more specific grading, e.g., stage 2a cervical cancer.

Biopsies

The first step in the management of cancer is usually to establish the diagnosis based on pathological examination under the microscope (World Health Organization, 2017). This tells the histopathologist and the MDT what the cells look like in the tumour, for example, whether they are malignant in appearance, or how well differentiated they are. Obtaining a sample of the tumour is achieved by performing a biopsy or aspiration. This may be done in different ways depending on the site and nature of the suspected cancer. For example, obtaining a tissue sample through biopsy in a breast lump or bowel polyp is achievable, but not for a blood cancer such as leukaemia, where blood cells are examined as no tissue is involved. Biopsies may require an intervention such as an x-ray-guided procedure or endoscopy to locate the tumour (see Hotspot on core biopsy accompanying Case Study 24.1).

There are a number of tests that can be carried to confirm diagnosis or to stage the cancer:

- Biopsies
- Blood tests
- Computer tomography (CT) scans
- X-rays
- Ultrasound scans
- Magnetic resonance imaging (MRI) scans
- Positron emission tomography (PET) scans
- Nuclear imaging techniques
- Urinalysis
- Stool analysis.

⚠ HOTSPOT

Radiology for Diagnosing and Staging Cancer

Huge advances have been made in the use of imaging in the diagnosis, staging, treatment and prediction of cancer development. **Plain film x-rays** are used with or without a substance called a 'contrast' (for example given to the patient to swallow). This x-ray will produce an image through a part of the body, such as the abdomen or chest (Gabriel, 2008). **Ultrasound scans** use radio and sound waves targeted by the operator to examine the density of soft tissues. They are quick and cheap and mostly used to examine the abdomen to create a 2D image – useful in diagnosis of liver metastases. **CT scans** (computer tomography) are a more expensive investigation, using a series of x-rays (with or without contrast) taken as 'slices' to look at the primary tumour, its size, invasion of other tissues and lymph node involvement, as well as distant metastases (Tobias and Hochhauser, 2015). **MRI scans** (magnetic resonance imaging) are a non-invasive investigation which does not use ionising radiation. It uses the properties of nuclei in the body to behave like weak magnets. The nuclei are normally located in a random fashion. The patient lies on a couch in a powerful magnetic field and all the nuclei align themselves within the magnetic field. Pulsing radio waves are used to disturb the alignment and images are taken and interpreted to look at the process (Gabriel, 2008). **PET scans** (positron emission tomography) are an expensive investigation that uses tagged biochemical compounds administered to the patient to investigate the biochemical and metabolic activity of the tissues, which differ in tumours from normal tissue (Tobias and Hochhauser, 2015). **Nuclear imaging** techniques use compounds and material with a radioactive element given to the patient to observe and interpret the uptake of the substance in specific organs and tissues under investigation (Gabriel, 2008).

It is important that the NA has an understanding of what is involved in these imaging investigations to be able to provide advice and information to patients and families safely and effectively. The nursing care, preparation and aftercare for these investigations can be very specific and the NA should follow the advice of the radiology department at all times.

REFLECTION 24.1

If possible, shadow a clinical nurse specialist and attend a cancer multidisciplinary meeting to observe and reflect on the discussions that take place. What types of tests are discussed? What treatment is planned for each person based on the investigation findings and the stage of their cancer?

TREATMENT

The main goal of cancer treatment is to cure the disease or prolong the life of patient and to ensure the best possible quality of life for cancer survivors and those with advanced disease. There are many treatments for the different types of cancers. There are, however, five main treatments that are currently used:

- Surgery
- Chemotherapy
- Radiotherapy
- Immunotherapy
- Hormone therapy.

Surgery

Surgery is very often the first line of treatment for cancer. This would usually be carried out in the secondary care setting of a hospital.

The aim of surgery is to remove the tumour and surrounding tissue where possible. The surgical procedure will usually be localized to the affected area only and may be dependent on the stage of the cancer. The smaller the tumour, the easier/safer the procedure will be. Lymph nodes can also be removed if suspicious looking, and a selection of lymph nodes are removed close to the tumour, again for staging purposes. These are examined by a histopathologist and a report created for the MDT to discuss the stage of the cancer. They then decide on whether further treatment should be offered, such as chemotherapy or radiotherapy.

Depending on the site of the cancer, there may be specialist requirements. One example is breast cancer, where there maybe the option of a cosmetic reconstruction of the breast (depending on site/size) following tumour removal. Another example is a person may require a stoma (colostomy) after removal of part of the bowel for colon cancer.

Surgery may be for prevention purposes if the patient is deemed at high risk of developing cancer. Again, using the example of breast cancer, inherited genes within the family may indicate the person is at high risk of developing breast cancer, and so the person is given the option of a mastectomy to remove the risk. All these requirements require sensitive and holistic nursing care, to support the patient in their decision-making and in managing an altered body image.

As with most cancer treatments, surgery can be used to cure the disease, or to provide palliative therapy for controlling advanced disease and managing symptoms. In palliative surgery, a procedure may be done to remove the bulk of a tumour to alleviate pressure, obstruction or pain, but for whatever reason (usually safety or integrity of another organ), not to remove it.

Chemotherapy

Chemotherapy works by damaging the genes inside the nucleus of cells, either at the point of dividing in mitosis, or in interphase (see Fig. 24.2) while they are making copies of all their genes before they divide. Most often, chemotherapy is given following surgery, depending on the stage of the cancer. It can be given to limit the chance of a cancer returning by targeting any rogue cancer cells that are in the circulation, or to stabilize the cancer and alleviate symptoms when advanced disease cannot be cured (Clare, 2013).

The drugs are usually given in regular cycles, either in hospital or in the community, to allow the body to recover between doses and to minimize the level of side effects. The treatment regimen can last 6 months or more at a time. Chemotherapy drugs can also be given in combination, which allows different drugs to work on different parts of the cell cycle.

Chemotherapy can be given in oral tablet form, intravenously via an infusion, by intramuscular injection or in rare cases, into the spine (intrathecally). A newer method of administration is by installation directly into the organ affected – for example, into the bladder via a catheter in the urinary tract.

The principle of treatment is to damage cancer cells at different stages in the process of cell division. With more than one type of drug, there is more chance of killing more cells. As treatments advance, it is now possible that drugs can even target specific phases of mitosis to induce cell death, or even to stimulate the body's own immune system to kill the cells (this is called immunotherapy) (Gabriel, 2008).

Chemotherapy is a systemic treatment, and so, despite becoming more specific and targeted, side effects do occur, which can be very debilitating for the patient.

Different drugs can have specific side effects, but those that commonly occur are in areas of the body that have rapid cell division: the side effects happen because chemotherapy targets cells that are rapidly dividing and as yet the drugs cannot differentiate between good cells and cancer cells. Therefore, side effects include:

- Hair loss
- Nail and skin changes
- Nausea and vomiting
- Disturbances of the gastrointestinal tract (for example diarrhoea)
- Reduction of the cells in the bone marrow, resulting in lowered resistance to infection (called neutropenia)
- Mouth ulcers (also called mucositis).

Some of the newer cytotoxic chemotherapy drugs bring about a peripheral neuropathy, which can be temporary, but is sometimes permanent. This can result in a person being unable to use their fingers for fine movements, such as unbuttoning a coat, cutting up food, or having difficulty walking because their toes have no feeling.

Communication, support and patient education is vital in the chemotherapy setting – so that a person knows when to report adverse events and seek help. It may be that the dose of treatment needs to be modified to lessen the side effects or that they need medication to help manage the symptoms (see Hotspot).

❗ HOTSPOT

Severe Side Effects

Some side effects can be fatal if not treated – for example, neutropenia if not addressed, can result in severe infection and sepsis very quickly as the person's immune system is suppressed. Usually, if a person receiving chemotherapy reports an infection, rise in temperature (fever), or even just flu-like symptoms, they may well be near to septic shock. They should be brought straight to Accident and Emergency and be given antibiotics within 1 hour of arrival (Williams et al., 2014). Diarrhoea, if acute, can also be fatal, inducing severe dehydration and shock if not treated quickly.

Radiotherapy

The principle of radiotherapy as a treatment for cancer is that it uses ionizing radiation to damage cells' DNA. This is either to kill the cell, induce it into the repair phase of the cell cycle, or expose the cell to be targeted by another treatment, such as chemotherapy. Treatments are meticulously planned to spare good tissue and lessen the side effects.

External radiotherapy

Given externally, radiotherapy destroys cancer cells in the body by damaging the DNA within those cells – similar to a large x-ray. The aim is to give the highest chance of curing or shrinking the cancer while minimizing the side effects of the treatment. Radiotherapy is given over a course of doses (fractions) over a number of days, depending on what is being treated. The effect of the treatment is accumulation of deep x-ray treatment over time. Radiotherapy can either be given before surgery, in combination with chemotherapy, to cure the cancer, or to alleviate symptoms in advanced disease.

Internal radiotherapy

There are two types of treatment: brachytherapy and radioactive liquids. Brachytherapy involves internal radiotherapy implants, which are radioactive metal wires, seeds or tubes put into the body, inside or close to a tumour. The radioactive metal is called a 'source' and is left inside the body for a period of time. This may be a few minutes each time or a few days.

Radioactive liquids to treat cancer can be given either as a drink or by injection. The radioactive part of the liquid is called an isotope. It may be attached to another substance, which is designed to take the isotope into the tumour and destroy the cells that way.

Radiotherapy also puts the individual potentially at risk of experiencing side effects. General side effects may be fatigue, sore skin, ulceration at the site of treatment, and hair loss at the radiation site.

Site specific effects may also be felt – for example, radiotherapy for head and neck cancer may induce loss of taste, mouth ulcers, nausea and voice changes. Skin soreness may be a problem, which can feel like severe sunburn. The NA will be able to advise the patient/carer to take care of the skin site, keep it clean and dry, not to use creams unless prescribed and to avoid soap/perfume. Care must be taken to observe the area for ulceration as this can cause the skin to break down and a wound to form. The NA must communicate any side effects and skin assessment and document it carefully, effectively and safely in the care plan.

Hormone therapy

Many cancers are susceptible to hormone control, and so therapy that changes the cells' receptors to switch this hormone control off can be offered in these cases. One example is breast cancer. Some breast cancers are stimulated to grow by the hormones oestrogen or progesterone. Inducing menopause by ablation or removal of the ovaries can remove the stimulation and thus 'switch off' the hormone and stop the cancer from growing. Drug therapy can also do this, and many women are offered drugs such tamoxifen after treatment to reduce the risk of a cancer returning once it has been removed via surgery.

Hormone therapy is also offered for some prostate cancers to work in the same way.

This type of treatment does come with side effects as well, however, and taking them can seem like a very difficult decision for many people.

Side effects of hormone therapy can include the following:
- Hot flushes
- Weight gain
- Headaches
- Dizziness
- Bone thinning and loss of density
- Permanent infertility.

It is very important for the best possible outcome that any treatment offered for cancer is timely, and equitable in its access – especially for individuals with cancer that is advanced or highly aggressive (for example, where metastatic disease is present or in acute leukaemia – see later).

Cancer and its investigations, treatment and long-term effects, can produce many different symptoms and side effects, which patients may or may not experience. Common drugs used in the management of these are listed in Medicine Trolley 24.1. The Nursing Associate should be aware that medication management of cancer symptoms changes regularly with the introduction of new drugs and technologies. Therefore it is imperative that national and local policies/guidelines are followed.

The Medicine Trolley 24.1

Oral Medications Often Used to Support Side Effects of Cancer Treatments

Drug	Drug classification	Reason for administration	Route of administration	Dose	Contraindications	Common side effects
Lactulose	Laxative	Constipation – stool softener	Oral	15 mL twice daily adjusted according to response	Intestinal obstruction	Abdominal cramps, nausea and vomiting
Senna	Laxative	Constipation – stimulation laxative	Oral	7.5 mg–15 mg daily (usually at night)	Intestinal obstruction, undiagnosed abdominal pain	Abdominal spasm, discoloration of urine, pruritus
Bisacodyl	Laxative	Constipation – stimulation laxative	Oral	5 mg–10 mg daily (usually at night)	Intestinal obstruction, acute inflammatory bowel disease	Intestinal obstruction, severe dehydration
Nystatin	Anti-fungal	Treatment of oral candida (thrush) – a common side effect when undergoing chemotherapy	Oral	100,000 units in 1 mL QDS (liquid preparation)		Nausea
Fluconazole	Anti-fungal	Treatment of oral candida (thrush) – a common side effect when undergoing chemotherapy	Oral	50 mg daily	Acute porphyria	Abdominal discomfort, diarrhoea, flatulence, headaches, rash
Metoclopramide	Antiemetic	Chemotherapy/radiotherapy induced nausea & vomiting. Short term use – up to 5 days only	Oral, intramuscular injection, intravenous	10 mg TDS	3–4 days after gastrointestinal surgery, gastrointestinal haemorrhage, gastrointestinal obstruction, gastrointestinal perforation	Extrapyramidal effects (such as muscle spasms, rigidity, restlessness, jerky movements), Menstrual changes in young adult girls, anxiety, confusion, dizziness
Ondansetron	Antiemetic	Often given pre-chemotherapy to prevent nausea & vomiting, then for 5 days after treatment	Oral, by rectum, intramuscular, intravenous	8 mg BD	Congenital long QT syndrome	Constipation, flushing, headache

Continued

The Medicine Trolley 24.1 (Continued)

Drug	Drug classification	Reason for administration	Route of administration	Dose	Contraindications	Common side effects
Haloperidol	Antiemetic	Nausea & vomiting (NB: also used to treat psychosis in mental health)	Oral, subcuticular injection/ continuous subcutaneous infusion	1.5 mg BD	Bradycardia, central nervous system depression, lesions of the basal ganglia, Parkinson disease	Headache, dizziness, dry mouth, weight gain, diabetes
Paracetamol	Analgesia	Mild pain Reducing of high temperature	Oral	500 mg–1g every 4 hours as needed		Very occasionally patients may experience a skin rash
Codeine	Analgesia	Moderate pain	Oral	30 mg–60 mg every 4 hours as needed	Ulcerative colitis, Acute respiratory depression, raised intracranial pressure, head injury	Bradycardia, constipation, drowsiness, dizziness, nausea & vomiting, dry mouth, dysphoria, euphoria, flushing, hallucinations, headache
Tramadol	Analgesia	Moderate to severe pain	Oral	50 mg–100 mg every 4 hours as needed	Alcohol, Acute respiratory depression, raised intracranial pressure, head injury	Bradycardia, constipation, dizziness, nausea & vomiting, vertigo, sexual dysfunction, oedema, dry mouth, hypotension, sweating
Oral morphine (Oromorph)	Analgesia	Severe pain. Often given in between regular doses of slow release morphine (known as MST)	Oral liquid preparation	5 mg–10 mg every 4 hours. (Higher doses may be given for palliative care patients)	Acute respiratory depression, raised intracranial pressure, head injury	Bradycardia, confusion, constipation, mood changes, sweating, vomiting, hallucinations
Dexamethasone	Steroid	Oral steroid often given during chemotherapy treatments to help prevent side effects of treatment	Oral, subcuticular injection/ continuous subcutaneous infusion	8 mg daily	Live virus vaccines, systemic infection	Increased risk of infection, weight gain as increased appetite, raised sugar levels in the blood, mood changes, swollen hands and feet

PSYCHOLOGICAL SUPPORT FOR CANCER PATIENTS

Receiving a cancer diagnosis can be devastating for a patient and their family. Whilst most people with cancer will receive psychological support from their assigned clinical nurse specialist, the NA may be with the patient and their family when a diagnosis is given in the outpatient setting, or they may be supporting patients during the treatment phase in either the hospital or GP practice. When supporting patients and their families at this time, the use of empathy is important, as well as showing kindness and compassion (Gault et al., 2017). Patients may display feelings of emotion, such as crying or anger, and it is important to know how to support the patient in this situation. When developing communication skills to support patients and families in difficult situations, the use of a model can be of benefit to guide you. The Simple Skills Secret Model has been shown to enhance communication between the nurse and the patient (Jack et al., 2013) and supports the use of open questions, active listening, using silence and supporting the patient to develop their own plan going forward (see Hotspot).

! HOTSPOT

Simple Skills Secret Model

1. Patient gives cue
2. Respond using an open question
3. Listen and use silence
4. Encourage patient to share
5. Summarize
6. Support the patient to make a plan
7. But resist the urge to rush in with a solution.
   (Jack et al., 2013)

Support groups

Some patients find it helpful to talk with other patients in similar situations or receiving similar cancer treatments. Support groups can be of benefit here, either face-to-face or by joining an online chat room. Many cancer charities also have information services where specialist nurses are available to talk to patients and their families. Written information may also be helpful – treatment-specific information can usually be sought from hospital cancer

TABLE 24.3   Various Complementary Therapies and Their Descriptions

Name of therapy	Description of therapy	Indications for use
Massage	A treatment that involves touch – stroking, kneading or pressing soft tissues in the body.	May help to relieve pain. May be used to aid relaxation and sleep.
Aromatherapy	The use of essential oils to enhance well-being. Most commonly used in conjunction with massage.	May be of benefit in reducing side effects of treatment such as nausea or constipation. Also used to aid relaxation or help with breathlessness.
Reiki	Hands on treatment, sometimes called 'healing'. Uses touch to improve well-being.	May be of benefit to reduce anxiety, particularly prior to treatments when patients are nervous.
Acupuncture	The insertion of tiny needles into specific pressure points within the body.	May help with pain; also, to relieve symptoms of nausea.
Reflexology	Pressure is applied to specific areas of the feet (and sometimes the hands) which are believed to be synced to specific areas within the body.	May help with symptoms such as pain, nausea or peripheral neuropathy.

information centres, or from GP practices. It is often helpful to ask patients how much information they would like and in what format – bombarding them with lots of information at once can be overwhelming for some people, so be guided by the individual.

Complementary therapies in cancer care

Complementary therapies can be described as therapies to support patient well-being alongside conventional medical treatments (London Cancer Alliance, 2014). They are sometimes offered in cancer centres or palliative care settings to support patient well-being. Although they are becoming increasingly popular, there remains limited scientific evidence to support the benefits of complementary therapies in alleviating patient symptoms during treatments for cancer. However, anecdotally, patients may report a decrease in symptoms, such as nausea or constipation, together with an increase in general well-being and a reduction in anxiety after receiving complementary treatments (Cancer Research UK, 2017).

The treatments offered can depend on several factors, including the types of practitioners employed by an organization, as well as the types of treatments that may relieve certain symptoms. Table 24.3 outlines a selection of different therapies with a short definition for each, together with how they might be of benefit to patients with cancer.

ACUTE LEUKAEMIA

Leukaemia is a type of cancer of the blood involving white blood cells (WBCs). This cancer can be chronic or acute in nature. Acute leukaemia is classified depending on the blood cells affected – such as acute lymphoblastic leukaemia (ALL) and acute myeloid leukaemia (AML): a disease of the WBCs that are involved in fighting viral or bacterial infections. Bone marrow contains progenitor cells (similar to stem cells), which normally produce infection-fighting WBCs (Tidy, 2016). In acute leukaemia, however, cells in the bone marrow are replaced with ones too immature to fight infections – these are called blast cells. This over-production and the replacement WBCs can limit the amount of other blood cells produced, such as red blood cells or platelets (Meenaghan et al., 2012).

Risk factors for leukaemia include possible genetic family history, exposure to carcinogens, such as cigarette smoke, radiation, previous chemotherapy and a weakened immune system due to viruses (Waugh & Grant, 2018). Symptoms and complications include the patient feeling short of breath, fatigue, pallor, unexplained bruising, excessive bleeding and extreme vulnerability to infection. Chemotherapy is the main first option treatment using cytotoxic drug therapy to kill the leukaemia cells, restore the balance of blood cells in the bone marrow, and control symptoms. Treatment then focuses on killing the remainder of the cells, followed by maintenance to prevent relapse. It is possible that a bone marrow transplant may be required (Clare, 2013). The person with leukaemia may also require blood transfusions and antibiotics during their treatment and remission phases of their illness as supportive therapy. Although quite rare, acute leukaemia can be a particularly aggressive type of cancer, affecting both adults or more commonly children (Tidy, 2016). Its often rapid progression means that treatment is required as soon as possible after diagnosis.

The NA may be involved in providing supportive care at all points during a leukaemia patient's treatment, either in hospital or in the community. Treatment plans for ALL or AML can be long, often requiring prolonged stays in hospital, where the patient is nursed in isolation away from those close to them to protect them from acquiring infections. Care for these patients requires vigilance in anticipating signs of infection and in managing the side effects of the treatment. The main symptoms experienced by patients are infection, anaemia, hair loss, bleeding and bruising, gastric upset and pain, where often profound psychosocial issues are experienced (Meenaghan et al., 2012). The NA will be required to monitor the patient, for example by taking vital sign measurements. Communication of any symptoms or adverse effects to the MDT is essential and should be rapid. Individuals and families will require comfort, good communication and reassurance to help them manage the shock of the diagnosis, and the stress and challenges these treatments can bring on a daily basis (see psychological support section in this chapter).

PROSTATE CANCER

Prostate cancer is the most common cancer in men (Cancer Research UK, 2017). In the UK, 1 in 8 men are at risk of developing prostate cancer; this statistic reduces to 1 in 4 for black men (Prostate Cancer UK, 2017). Prostate cancer mainly affects men over 50 years of age, with the average age of diagnosis between 65 and 69 years old (Prostate Cancer UK, 2017). Black men are more likely to be diagnosed at a younger age (Hussein et al., 2015), and men diagnosed before the age of 50 may have a more aggressive form of the disease (Thorstenson et al., 2017). The risk of prostate cancer is also increased if an individual has either a father or brother who has been diagnosed with the disease or a mother or sister who has had breast cancer (Prostate Cancer UK, 2017).

Prostate cancer symptoms may not appear in early stages of the disease, and the cancer can be very slow growing. A benign enlargement of the prostate (benign prostatic hyperplasia) can produce similar symptoms. Symptoms can include difficulty in passing urine, frequency of urinating at night, urgency and, more rarely, blood or semen in the urine (Macmillan Cancer Support, 2017). Some men experience the first symptoms as pain in the hips or back, that is, the bones – this may be because the cancer has spread to the bones from the prostate and is said then to be advanced.

Treatment options for prostate cancer include surgery, hormonal therapy, brachytherapy and external radiotherapy (see section on radiotherapy) and chemotherapy. Some early tumours are very slow growing and therefore will be placed on a 'watch and wait' surveillance follow-up programme.

> ### CASE STUDY 24.1   Earl – Metastatic Prostate Cancer
>
> Earl is a 59-year-old Caribbean gentleman with advanced metastatic prostate cancer. He lives in a first-floor maisonette with his wife June. They have two grown-up children who do not live at home.
>
> Earl was diagnosed with advanced prostate cancer 18 months ago; the cancer has now spread to his bones. This causes him to have significant pain in his lower spine and reduces his ability to mobilize. He also has some urinary incontinence and wears incontinence pads to help cope with this.
>
> He is aware that no further curative treatment is available. It is important at this stage of his cancer journey that his treatment is tailored to support his needs and manage his symptoms. Part of the nursing role would be to act as a patient advocate and to support his family (Drudge-Coates & Turner, 2012).

> ### REFLECTION 24.3
>
> Using the framework suggested for history taking in Chapter 10 (see Box 10.2, p. 100), how would the Nursing Associate care for Earl at home as his condition deteriorates? Think about the assessments that would be required and how the care would be planned to support his needs. Think about which other health professionals might be involved in supporting Earl and June over the weeks ahead.

> ### CASE STUDY 24.2   Julie – Diagnosing Breast Cancer
>
> Julie is a 33-year-old woman who, having found a lump in her left breast, has been referred to the one-stop breast clinic under the 2-week suspected cancer referral guidance (NICE, 2017). Julie lives with her partner Sangita and they have a 3-year-old daughter, Sky. Julie is the biological mother of Sky.
>
> Julie arrives at the clinic looking very worried. Sangita is with her. Julie will spend the morning in the clinic and will undergo a series of investigations: mammography, ultrasonography, an MRI scan and possibly a biopsy. Dependent on the examination findings, the biopsy may be either a core biopsy or a fine-needle aspiration biopsy. Julie may also have a blood test to check for tumour markers.
>
> Julie will see the consultant first, who will take a medical history and do a physical examination. The NA will accompany Julie and Sangita during this consultation. Following the consultation, the NA is asked to support Julie through the series of tests: mammography, biopsy, and MRI scan, and undertake the blood tests. Julie and Sangita will return to see the consultant at the end of the morning to obtain the results from the tests.

> ### REFLECTION 24.4
>
> As the Nursing Associate, what communication skills might you use to support Julie and Sangita throughout the morning? What questions do you think they might ask you, and how will you respond to these? Would you refer them to any other members of the multidisciplinary team? (Use the communication skills model in the Psychological Care section to guide you.)

LIVING WITH OR BEYOND CANCER

Despite the increases in survival rates and lower death rates from cancer compared with 20 years ago, the incidence is rising. It is very likely that whatever setting the nurse is working in, they will care for someone who has or has had cancer. More people are living longer with the disease and with the consequences of the long-term effects of treatment or psychological difficulty as a result of their experience.

Many organizations have developed packages to support people in managing this difficult transition from being treated for cancer to surviving it or living with it. Macmillan Cancer Support (2014), for example, developed a recovery package to help people rehabilitate and access support when they need it as part of the National Cancer Survivorship Initiative. This has been found to improve outcomes for people living with and after cancer, helping them to recognize signs of concerning symptoms which may lead to recurrence, to access support groups, and get back to work, and their social life. Many of the usual social and work activities for people with cancer can be lost, and they may need help and support from professionals to return to previous activities.

Many more people are now living with cancer and in situations of advanced disease when it is life-limiting. They are potentially vulnerable to many physical, psychological, social and spiritual issues. Mitchell (2011) states that all professional groups have a responsibility to look out for emotional concerns, as many are experiencing unmet needs. The Department of Health reported in 2013 that there is still inequitable access to consistent, high-quality cancer and palliative care for the following vulnerable groups:

- Homeless people: three times more likely to die early from cancer and long-term conditions.
- Black and minority ethnic populations: a lower uptake of palliative services compared to white/majority groups and there is evidence of poorer outcomes.
- Individuals with learning disability: less likely to access services, have poorer pain control, more disorganized and unplanned care.
- People with dementia: one-third of people aged over 60 years have dementia, many with complex physical and psychological needs.

The NA has a responsibility to respond to the needs of patients, particularly those who find it difficult to access care. They can be a key person in providing comfort and care and in informing patients and families about services available to support them. Some groups of people may find accessing these supportive services difficult; some find it difficult to express their wishes – for example, they may not know who to talk to when trying to manage returning to social activities, seeking help with a problematic symptom or coping with an altered body image. Knowledge of these issues and concerns, as well as knowing how to refer to these MDT services, is vital for the NA when becoming part of the workforce helping improve outcomes for patients living with cancer.

LOOKING BACK, FEEDING FORWARD

This chapter has outlined the principles of cancer care in the context of today's healthcare settings. In order to understand the cancer diagnosis, stages of cancers and how treatments work, it is firstly necessary to understand the biological basis for cancer and the processes involved. Developments in cancer care are happening all the time with the advances in treatments, preventative measures and the ambition of successive governments to address inequalities of care.

The NA has a vital role to play in supporting the individual affected by cancer and those close to them. By having an understanding of the biological nature of cancer and the stages of a cancer diagnosis, they can advocate and work in partnership with the patient to help them navigate the information they need to make decisions and participate in their care as much as they wish to.

The NA also must treat each patient as an individual and with dignity and inform those who are responsible for the care of the patient when needs are not met. They also have a central role to play in the multidisciplinary team, as they will often be the person closest to the patient in the clinical setting. Communication with the team and having the knowledge and skill to make appropriate referrals to the wider MDT is crucial, and reporting adverse events and side effects of treatment in a timely manner will assist the patient to receive the best possible care available. More people are living with cancer, and their care can be complex. Having the appropriate knowledge, skills and attitudes to support these people will help the NA provide excellent standard of evidence-based care.

REFERENCES

Agustina, E., Dodd, R.H., Waller, J., Vrinten, C., 2017. Understanding middle-aged and older adults' first associations with the word 'cancer': A mixed methods study in England. Psychooncology 1–7, https://doi.org/10.1002/pon.4569.

Alford, J., 2017. Will There be a Cure for Cancer? http://scienceblog.cancerresearchuk.org/2017/09/21/science-surgery-will-cancer-ever-be-cured/.

BreastCancerCare.org.uk., 2017. Information and Support. https://www.breastcancercare.org.uk/information-support/have-i-got-breast-cancer/referral-breast-clinic/mammograms-breast-scans/fine-needle-aspiration#whatarebiopsies.

Cancer Research UK, 2014a. Cancer Statistics in the UK. http://www.cancerresearchuk.org/health-professional/cancer-statistics-for-the-uk.

Cancer Research UK, 2014b. Beating Cancer Sooner – Our Strategy. http://www.cancerresearchuk.org/sites/default/files/cruk_strategy.pdf.

Cancer Research UK, 2017. Prostate Cancer Incidence. http://www.cancerresearchuk.org/health-professional/cancer-statistics/statistics-by-cancer-type/prostate-cancer#heading-Zero.

Clare, C., 2013. Cancer. In: Muralitharan, N., Peate, I. (Eds.), Fundamentals of Applied Pathophysiology: An Essential Guide for Nursing And Healthcare Students, 2nd ed. Wiley–Blackwell, Sussex.

Corner, J., Bailey, C., 2008. Cancer Nursing: Care in Context. Blackwell Publishing, Oxford.

Department of Health (DH), 2000. The NHS Cancer Plan: A Plan For Investment, a Plan for Reform. Crown Copyright, DH.

Department of Health (DH), 2013. One Chance to Get it Right. https://www.gov.uk/government/uploads/system/uploads/attachment_data/file/323188/One_chance_to_get_it_right.pdf.

Dixon, J.M., 2012. ABC of Breast Diseases, fourth ed. Wiley, Hoboken.

Drudge-Coates, L., Turner, B., 2012. Prostate cancer overview. Part 2: metastatic prostate cancer. Br. J. Nurs. 21 (Suppl. 18), S23–S28.

Gabriel, J.A., 2008. The Biology of Cancer. Wiley & Sons Ltd, Chichester.

Gault, I., Shapcott, J., Luthi, A., Reid, G., 2017. Communication in Nursing and Healthcare: A Guide for Compassionate Practice. Sage, Los Angeles, CA.

Hussein, S., Satturwar, S., Van der Kwast, T., 2015. Young Aged Prostate Cancer. http://jcp.bmj.com/content/68/7/511?utm_source=TrendMD&utm_medium=cpc&utm_campaign=JCP_TrendMD-1.

Independent Cancer Taskforce, 2015. Achieving World Class Outcomes: A Strategy for England 2015–2020. http://www.cancerresearchuk.org/sites/default/files/achieving_world-class_cancer_outcomes_-_a_strategy_for_england_2015-2020.pdf.

Jack, B.A., O'Brien, M.R., Kirton, J.A., et al., 2013. Enhancing communication with distressed patients, families and colleagues: the value of the Simple Skills Secrets model of communication for the nursing and healthcare workforce. Nurse Educ. Today 33 (12), 1550–1556.

London Cancer Alliance, 2014. Guidelines and Criteria for Complementary Therapies. http://www.londoncanceralliance.nhs.uk/media/88226/lca-guidelinesseptember-2014.pdf.

Macmillan Cancer Support, 2014. The Recovery Package. https://www.macmillan.org.uk/aboutus/healthandsocialcare

professionals/newsandupdates/macvoice/summer2014/ sharinggoodpracticesummer2014.aspx.

Macmillan Cancer Support, 2017. Prostate Cancer. https:// www.macmillan.org.uk/information-and-support/ prostate-cancer/early-prostate-cancer/understanding-cancer/sign s-and-symptoms-of-prostate-cancer.html#106006.

Marieb, E.N., 2015. Essentials of Human Anatomy & Physiology, Global Edition. Pearson Education, M.U.A.

Meenaghan, T., Dowling, M., Kelly, M., 2012. Acute leukaemia: making sense of a complex blood cancer. Br. J. Nurs. 21 (2), 76–83.

Mitchell, A.J., Chan, M., Bhatti, H., et al., 2011. Prevalence of depression, anxiety, and adjustment disorder in oncological, haematological, and palliative-care settings: a meta-analysis of 94 interview-based studies. Lancet Oncol. 12 (2), 160–174.

NHS England, 2017. Achieving World-Class Cancer Outcomes: A Strategy for England 2015–2020. Progress Report 2016–17. https://www.england.nhs.uk/wp-content/uploads/2017/10/nationa l-cancer-transformation-programme-2016-17-progress.pdf.

NICE, 2017. Suspected Cancer: Recognition and Referral. NG12. National Institute for Health and Care Excellence. https://www. nice.org.uk/guidance/ng12.

Prostate Cancer UK, 2017. Signs and Symptoms. https:// prostatecanceruk.org/prostate-information/about-prostate-cancer.

Thorstenson, A., Garmo, H., Adolfsson, J., Bratt, O., 2017. Cancer Specific Mortality in Men Diagnosed with Prostate Cancer before Age 50 years: A Nationwide Population Based Study. J. Urol. 197, 61–66.

Tidy, C., 2016. Acute Lymphoblastic Leukaemia. http://patient.info/ doctor/acute-lymphoblastic-leukaemia-pro.

Tobias, J.S., Hochhauser, D., 2015. Cancer and Its Management, seventh ed. Wiley–Blackwell, Chichester.

Waugh, A., Grant, A., 2018. Ross & Wilson Anatomy and Physiology in Health and Illness, thirteenth ed. Elsevier, Oxford.

Wheeldon, A., 2013. Cell and Body tissue physiology. In: Muralitharan, N., Peate, I. (Eds.), Fundamentals of Applied Pathophysiology: An Essential Guide for Nursing and Healthcare Students, second ed. Wiley–Blackwell, Sussex.

Williams, A., Candish, C., Ayrton, C., et al., 2014. Reducing the door to needle time for antibiotics in suspected neutropenic sepsis using a dedicated clinical pathway. Clin. Oncol. 26, S2. DOI. http://dx.doi.org/10.1016/j.clon.2014.04.003.

World Health Organization, 2017. Cancer Prevention. http:// www.who.int/cancer/prevention/en/.

Wyatt, D., Hubert-Williams, N., 2015. Cancer and Cancer Care. Sage, London.

25

Skin Care

Wyn Glencross

OBJECTIVES

By the end of the chapter the reader will be able to:

1. Appreciate the need to understand the anatomy and physiology of the skin
2. Discuss the role the Nursing Associate has to play in ensuring those they offer skin care to are safe
3. Differentiate between a number of common skin conditions
4. Describe some of the causes of skin damage
5. Discuss common internal factors that many result in skin damage
6. Discuss the aims of skin care and appreciate the importance of selecting appropriate skin-care products

KEY WORDS

Comfort	Trauma	Excoriated
Internal	Moisture	Bacteria
External	Protection	
Safety	Macerated	

CHAPTER AIM

The aim of this chapter is to introduce the reader to the structure and functions of the skin and issues surrounding it. It will provide the Nursing Associate (NA) with information on how to care for the skin in order to maintain its integrity, and give insight into the types of skin damage that can occur and how these can be prevented.

SELF TEST

1. How many layers does the skin have?
2. What are the three main functions of the skin?
3. What does the subcutaneous layer consist of?
4. Name six structures that can be found in the dermis.
5. What are the differences between a laceration and a cut and how are each caused?
6. Name the types of burns that can occur to the skin.
7. Name three common internal factors that can cause skin damage.
8. Name three common external factors that can cause skin damage.
9. What is the most effective skin moisturizer?
10. How can certain creams/moisture barriers adversely affect incontinence pad absorbency?

INTRODUCTION

Skin refers to the outer covering of the body. It is the body's first line of defence against external threats, so the main purpose of the skin is a defensive one. It also prevents fluid loss while protecting internal organs from the external world.

The skin is the largest organ of the body, weighing an average of 2.2–3 kg and equates to approximately 5% of total bodyweight. Although it is an essential organ, it is not regarded as a vital organ. It is the most vulnerable organ of all as it is at constant risk of insults from the external world so is often breached by trauma, burning, disease and even by excess moisture. When skin is intact, it is the first-line of defence against bacterial invasion that would otherwise result in infection.

It is therefore essential that we maintain good skin integrity. But first, as the Nursing Associate (NA) will be responsible for maintaining the integrity and health of the skin of their patients, it is important to understand the anatomy and physiology of the skin in order to care for it appropriately.

To aid this understanding, this chapter will focus on the anatomy, physiology and care of the skin, as well as considering the issues that can arise with the skin. It will enable the NA to appreciate the level of care required to maintain skin integrity and how to deal with any issues that arise.

THE FUNCTIONS OF THE SKIN

For the NA to appreciate how to care for their patient's skin, it is first important that the NA understands the main functions of the skin.

1. Protection – it acts as a defence barrier, keeping out external hazards from the environment, for example bacteria and chemicals. It keeps *in* substances the body requires, for example, water and electrolytes. Because of its elasticity and toughness, it protects against mechanical injury. It also keeps the body 'waterproof' thanks to the keratin, fats and oils of the skin.
2. Temperature control – this is achieved through the blood supply travelling over the large surface area of the skin. When hot, the blood vessels dilate increasing the flow of blood to the skin surface, allowing heat loss through radiation and through evaporation of sweat. When cold, the blood vessels constrict, reducing the circulation to the skin. Body hair stands erect by contraction of the erector pili muscles, which then keeps a layer of insulating air around the skin.
3. Sensation – the skin is a sensory organ; it is sensitive to touch, temperature, pressure and pain.
4. Water balance – the skin allows the excretion of waste products and the preservation of water balance.
5. Production of vitamin D – by exchanging solar energy. Vitamin D is essential for the effective absorption of calcium and phosphorus, which maintains healthy bones.

The skin also has a psychosocial impact on how the individual is perceived. It can also reveal how a person is likely to be feeling emotionally if closely observed; for example, a flushed face when embarrassed or nervous, goose bumps when in fear, or a radiant look when happy are everyday occurrences that can reveal much about how we are feeling.

Why is it so important to understand the functions of the skin, and how does this affect how the patient is cared for by the NA? The definition of healthy skin is that it is fulfilling all of its functions so that it is allowing optimum health and quality of life for the patient (Penzer & Finch, 2001) and the NA must appreciate these functions before appropriate observations and care can be provided. Case Study 25.1 shows how knowledge and insight about the functions of the skin can prove to be a positive experience for the patient as well as the NA.

CRITICAL AWARENESS

People with chronic wounds or skin conditions will often face not only physiological challenges, but emotional ones too. For centuries there has been a stigma attached to diseases of the skin. Lepers were considered 'unclean' and cast out from society in biblical and medieval times. Some labelled and persecuted as lepers had other diseases, such as eczema or psoriasis. The stigmatization of lepers was not a public-health measure to control spread of the disease, but a manifestation of fear, ignorance and prejudice.

Skin disease is very often obvious and visible to others. People who have skin diseases not only have to cope with the effects of their disease from a physiological perspective, but also the reaction of others to their condition. There is stigma attached to a number of skin diseases, and many millions of people are affected, from all corners of society and across all ages.

Skin diseases are often incurable and some skin conditions leave scarring, and the aim of treatment is usually to reduce symptoms rather than cure. Whether these conditions are common or rare, the impact on quality of life can be far-reaching and profound. Stigmatization is an expression of prejudice and ignorance, and care providers, including NAs, have a duty to address it with information and education. This should include those with skin diseases and their families, schools, the media, other healthcare providers and the rest of the community.

CASE STUDY 25.1   Josephine

Josephine is a 75-year-old housebound patient, who experienced a stroke (cerebrovascular accident – CVA) two years ago. She lives alone with the support of visiting carers four times a day. She made a reasonable recovery from the stroke, but has been left with left-sided weakness (resulting from a right hemisphere stroke). As the stroke was on the right hemisphere of the brain, the stroke did not affect her speech. However, as a result of the weakness, she had a fall and was admitted to hospital. Unfortunately, as she lay on the floor at home for several hours, she developed an open Grade 2 pressure ulcer on her sacrum with an underlying deep tissue injury, caused by lying on the hard surface of the floor for a prolonged period.

The issues that the NA must deal with in this case are as follows:

Protection: As the skin is no longer intact, Josephine is now at risk of infection via the pressure ulcer. *Patient Safety in the NHS* (NHS England, 2016) states that patients should be treated in clean surroundings with a minimal risk of infection. Indeed, 'Cleanliness is not a luxury in a highly developed country, it is….a basic human right' (Young, 1991).

NHS England's 'Key Improvements' for 2017/2018 and 2018/2019, led by NHS Improvement, aim to prevent healthcare-acquired infections with a view to achieving a fall in such infections by 50% by 2020/2021. This is to be achieved by data collection, national guidance and giving *E. coli* infections the same level of priority as is currently given to MRSA and *Clostridium difficile* infections by displaying numbers of infections on ward information boards.

Therefore, it is vital that the NA appreciates the need for, and ensures, high standards in hand hygiene and strict aseptic, non-touch technique when managing wounds and skin care in general.

Temperature control: Due to her limited mobility and left-sided weakness, Josephine may not be able to control her own body temperature. For example, she may not be able to remove clothes if she feels hot, or put on extra clothing or close a window if she feels cold. She would therefore require assistance to maintain a comfortable body temperature. The skin consists of four nerve receptors: heat, cold, touch and pressure.

Sensation: Unfortunately, as the left side of Josephine's body lacks sensation because of the stroke, this will increase her vulnerability to further skin breaches. For example:

- Pressure damage – she will not be able to respond naturally to the effects of pressure on the skin.
- Burns and scalds – there is an especial risk from hot drinks and spillages.
- Trauma – she will not be aware of sustaining an injury to the left side, for example during moving and handling procedures.

Appreciating and considering the functions of the skin in each individual circumstance, and with adherence to local and national policies and guidelines, will enable the NA to identify and mitigate the risks of skin breaches that would otherwise occur.

STRUCTURE OF THE SKIN

The strength and elasticity of our skin changes over time and in certain circumstances. One individual's skin will not be the same as the next individual's for one reason or another. Understanding the structures of the skin in conjunction with its functions will enable the NA to appreciate the toughness as well as the vulnerability of the skin throughout an individual's lifetime. Having this understanding will ensure that the most appropriate care and advice can be provided at any given time, and for any individual. It will ensure that the NA recognizes and appreciates the need for onward referral to a registered nurse, medical officer or specialized dermatologist in a timely manner.

Epidermis

This outer part of the skin is made up of four or five layers, depending on where it occurs on the body. For example, the 'stratum lucidum' is an extra layer on the palms of the hands and the soles of the feet beneath the 'stratum corneum' that provides a cushioning effect to reduce impact. It consists of dead, flattened cells containing a substance called eleidin. The main layers are detailed below and shown in Fig. 25.1.

Stratum corneum – the outer layer consisting of dead flattened cells filled with keratin. It is waterproof, which provides protection from bacteria. It is constantly replaced due to erosion from normal wear and tear and is generally renewed every fourteen days.

Stratum granulosum – the second layer containing flattened cells in various stages of degeneration.

Stratum spinosum – a layer of several cells thickness that contains live cells tightly packed together by their cell membranes. They move upwards and get flattened; as they do so, new cell production occurs in the layer below (the stratum basale).

Stratum basale – a single layer of cuboidal cells that multiply and move upwards. This is the only living layer of the epidermis as it contains the distant branches of the blood supply (tip of the arterial tree).

Cells of the epidermis

There are four cell types found in this layer.
1. Keratinocytes – these produce keratin (a structural fibrous protein) in 90% of the epidermis.
2. Melanocytes – these are pigment-producing cells that are found in the stratum basale layer. These cells are responsible for giving the skin its colour.
3. Langerhans cells – these arise in the bone marrow and are involved in cell-mediated immune responses in the skin, for example, in dermatitis or allergic reactions.
4. Merkel cells – these are located in the stratum basale, and are closely associated with sensory nerve endings (touch sensation).

The cells of epidermis originate at the cuboidal cells and gradually become flattened and drier as they are forced to the outer surface of the skin by the production of new cuboidal cells, where they eventually shed as dead skin. This entire process takes approximately 28 days, but slows down as we age.

Between the epidermal and the next layer (the dermis) is a cell layer of protein fibres known as the basement membrane. The purpose of this layer is to bond the epidermis and the dermis layers together. When this layer deactivates for any reason (for instance, friction), the two layers of the skin separate, resulting in a blister. The roof of the blister is the entire epidermal layer,

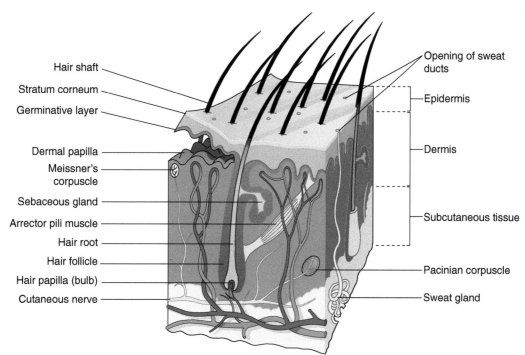

Fig. 25.1 Structure of the Skin (Waugh & Grant, 2018).

which is no longer attached to the blood supply via the cuboidal cells, so becomes a dead layer of skin. Repair of the blister occurs from the migration across the exposed area of dermis by the cuboidal cells until the entire area is once again covered with skin.

The cells in all layers, except the stratum basale, are called keratinocytes. These are dead cells that store the protein keratin. Keratin gives hair, nails and skin their toughness and water-resistant properties. The epidermal layer can regenerate itself and will leave no scarring if damage to the skin is restricted to this layer.

In certain cases, there can be an unwanted buildup of epithelial cells, which can adversely affect the underlying living layers of skin. This is known as hyperkeratosis, and can occur from recent friction, inflammation, recent trauma, corns and in some cases, malignancy.

Such excess layers of skin can place pressure on the blood supply within the cuboidal cells (the only living layer of epithelial cells), which can result in death of the cuboidal cells as the capillaries are compressed, thereby restricting the blood flow. This can result in an open wound, which may be regarded as a pressure ulcer. It is therefore vital that skin is cleaned and hydrated well to prevent this unwanted buildup as far as possible.

The following two case studies demonstrate how the NA can utilize their knowledge and understanding of the epidermal structure and purpose to provide a positive experience for the patient and to mitigate the risks of infection or further damage.

CASE STUDY 25.2   Henry

Henry is a 52-year-old, otherwise healthy, individual who has as yet undiagnosed hyperkeratosis, which he had suffered from for many years. This condition has affected Henry's self-esteem, as it affects large parts of his body and he has been concerned about how others perceive him. This condition had prevented Henry from socializing and working with others and he has become more and more isolated and depressed because of this over the years.

Hyperkeratosis is usually a painless condition that results in an over production of keratin (epidermal cells). In Henry's case, the condition presents as itchy, scaly patches of skin that are often purplish-blue in colour.

He attended the NA at the GP surgery who noted the presenting condition and that the skin was flaking over his clothing and into his hair. Because the NA recognized that this did not present as healthy skin, and she was aware that the skin should not be thickened, itchy, dry and flaky as a result of too many epithelial layers, Henry was referred to the practice nurse. This led to a GP referral to the dermatology department, where Henry received the treatments he required to manage this condition.

Thanks to the NA's recognition of an overproduction of epithelial cells and immediate action, Henry's self-esteem and confidence improved as his skin condition improved.

When Henry attended a review with his GP, the NA saw Henry in the waiting room where she noted his improved skin condition. He informed her that he had been offered a job and was returning to work. She noted that he seemed so much happier, his skin condition had improved immensely, and he was much more confident that the last time she had seen him. It occurred to the NA that Henry had suffered needlessly for many years, and it was her understanding of the structures of the skin that enabled him to obtain the specialist care that he needed.

AT THE GP SURGERY

The core activities of a dermatology service held in a GP surgery will vary, dependent upon local needs and resources available, as well as the skills of the clinician (for example a general practitioner with a special interest in dermatology). The proposed dermatology service will then be accredited in the context of the service to be provided and the competences that are needed to provide it. There are several possible models of care. These include the following:

- dermatology: a general practitioner with a special interest in the diagnosis and management of skin disease
- dermatology and skin surgery: diagnosis and management of skin disease and benign skin surgery
- dermatology, skin surgery and community skin cancer: diagnosis and management of skin disease and skin surgery including skin cancer community services
- skin lesions general practitioner with a special interest in dermatology: skin lesions and skin surgery including skin cancer community services.

CASE STUDY 25.3   Vijay

Vijay is an 83-year-old man with Parkinson disease, a neurodegenerative disorder resulting in bradykinesia, tremors and rigidity. He was admitted to hospital following a bout of pneumonia.

The depletion of dopamine, a critically important neurotransmitter, is the critical pathology of Parkinson disease. Insufficient dopamine can affect the condition of the skin and its appendages (hair, nails), as well as adversely impacting on the wound healing processes. Symptoms include excessive sweating and excessive salivation.

High levels of moisture on the skin from sweat, salivation or other bodily fluids (e.g., faecal matter or urine) for regular or prolonged periods can adversely impact on the quality and integrity of the skin. Maceration (waterlogging of the dead epidermal cells) and/or excoriation (burning of these cells from acidity in the fluids) will occur if control over this moisture is not undertaken.

Susan, an NA, recognized that moisture would potentially harm Vijay's skin if it was not controlled somehow, which could potentially increase the risk of infection via any breaches caused. Because she understood the anatomy of the skin and how Parkinson disease could adversely impact on the skin, she arranged for moisture barrier products to be applied to protect the areas subject to moisture.

Additionally, the tremors caused by Parkinson disease can cause skin to rub on clothing or against furniture resulting in friction burns. Susan became aware that this was happening to Vijay as he sat in his chair – his right elbow was rubbing within the sleeve of his jersey, which was causing the epidermal cells on the outer aspect of his elbow to erode. Susan recognized that this would result in a friction burn, which would make the area vulnerable to pressure damage, and she mitigated the risk of this developing into an open wound by covering the vulnerable area with a film dressing and ensured that Vijay was sitting in a chair where he was supported sufficiently to reduce any pressure on the affected elbow. This reduced the friction on the site and reduced the pressure and tremors. By taking this action, Susan demonstrated a holistic approach to care, and skin care in particular.

❗ HOTSPOT

Changes in the skin are common symptoms of Parkinson disease. A number of people with the disease develop oily or flaky skin, particularly on the face and scalp. Others have issues with dry skin or excessive sweating. They may have an increased risk of skin cancer.

Dermis

This layer is predominantly connective tissue consisting of protein fibres of collagen and elastin. They give this layer a high tensile strength and flexibility. These fibres are surrounded by a gel-like ground substance.

Cells of the dermis:

Fibroblasts – produce collagen, elastic fibres and the ground substance.

Macrophages – fight infection and originate in the bone marrow.

Mast cells – produce histamine and are part of the immune system. They are responsible for signs of allergic reactions.

(Adipocytes – fat cells beneath the dermal layer, often thought of as the third layer of the skin.)

Accessory structures of the dermal layer:

Hair follicles – roots and hair. Used for the thermal regulation within the body.

Sebaceous glands – secrete an oily fluid known as sebum, which 'waterproofs' the skin.

Sweat glands – part of the excretion and temperature control systems.

Erector pili muscles – attached to the hair follicles and the dermis. Their function is to assist thermal regulation. It is these muscles that cause 'goose-pimples' when the hairs stand up from the skin.

Damage to the skin that extends into this dermal layer will usually result in scar formation, as the cells cannot regenerate themselves efficiently.

Subcutaneous layer

This layer consists of loose connective tissue composed of adipose (fat) and connective tissue. It has an important role in controlling body temperature, as well as the storage of energy. It has a minimal blood supply and has pressure sensitive nerve endings. Fibres from the dermis extend into this layer, firmly fixing it to the skin. It is slow to heal due to a minimal blood supply.

THE EFFECTS OF THE AGEING PROCESS ON THE SKIN

All cells of the body (except in the brain) have a natural life-span of around 28 days, after which they are renewed, originating from master (stem) cells, which each have a life-span of around 40 days. Age and poor or insufficient nutrients can restrict the speed of cell regeneration. This in turn will adversely impact on the quality, strength and elasticity of the skin, thereby making it more vulnerable to external insults. It is therefore vital that a good hydration and a nutritionally well-balanced diet and a healthy lifestyle is maintained to improve the rate of cell regeneration and to improve and maintain skin integrity.

As we age, our skin integrity reduces due to the reduced production of collagen and elastin that give the skin its strength and elasticity. Cell regeneration rates slow down and skin takes longer to repair and renew itself. Good nutrition and hydration is therefore very important as we age. However, many elderly people have a reduced appetite and nutritional intake and are often mildly or moderately dehydrated.

COMMUNITIES OF CARE

Elderly Care

Skin health is crucial to the health and well-being of the older person; it is a fundamental feature of nursing care. NAs should regularly assess the skin health of older patients, encourage self-care and promote the use of appropriate products.

As skin ages, it will become less able to perform its barrier functions and when this occurs, skin breakdown becomes more of a risk. Skin breakdown can have a negative impact on the person's quality of life and can have economic implications.

The NA needs to understand that age-related changes decrease the skin's ability to perform its barrier function. The NA is in a unique position as they have frequent opportunities to undertake an assessment of older people's skin. Skin care regimens have to be based on individual needs, ensuring the skin is clean and dry and that suitable and appropriate emollients are used. When possible, the older person should be supported to self-manage their own skin care.

Dehydration can lead to dry, itchy skin that increases the risk of skin breakages from cracking and trauma from scratching. Dry skin is less elastic and is more vulnerable to pressure damage and skin splitting and from external insults. Dehydration can also lead to urinary tract infections that can in turn result in urinary incontinence (and excess sweating due to the infection).

Urinary incontinence can lead to moisture damage around the buttock and groin areas (known as 'continence dermatitis'/'moisture lesions'). Such damage increases the vulnerability to pressure sores if adequate pressure relief is not provided.

As the bacteria that thrive within bodily fluids produce waste products that alter the pH balance in the fluid (urine, faecal matter or sweat), this can cause excoriation when in contact with the skin. This then breaches the surface area of the skin, leaving the patient vulnerable.

Many people with urinary incontinence will restrict their fluid intake, believing this will help control the problem. Unfortunately, this will inevitably lead to dehydrated skin and a vicious cycle of ongoing urinary tract infections and incontinence that would otherwise be avoided if the patient was kept well hydrated.

! HOTSPOT

Beware that fluid intake restriction can lead to urinary tract infection and this can have a negative impact on the person's health and well-being; this will include their skin.

Furthermore, dry skin will absorb moisture from incontinence (and sweating) and will become macerated or excoriated. Maceration presents as white wrinkly skin, whilst excoriation appears as red burning skin. Both mean that the skin has been breached and can potentially lead to the invasion of bacteria.

To maintain good skin integrity throughout our lives, it is crucial that a good nutritional intake is maintained and that we are well hydrated. Indeed, it is widely accepted that good hydration is the skin's most effective moisturizer.

SKIN DAMAGE

The skin can become damaged from many causes, and once the skin has been breached for any reason, the protective barrier from bacterial invasion is lost until such time the skin repairs itself and is once again intact. Skin damage can be caused by external insults or by internal conditions and diseases. Any breach to the skin could deteriorate into an open wound, leaving the area vulnerable to damage from other external insults, such as pressure. It is therefore vital that the NA understands and appreciates the risks to the skin, so the appropriate care can be provided.

> **! HOTSPOT**
>
> Understanding the functions of the skin will assist the NA to care appropriately and safely for patients. Failing to understand the many functions of the skin can lead to injury or disease.

Common external factors that cause skin damage

Cut/Incision – an incised wound caused by sharp edges, such as a knife or glass. The edges of the wound are usually well defined and are often straight with little or no skin loss (Fig. 25.2).

In the example in Fig. 25.2, the farmer cut his arm on dirty machinery, but failed to attend the minor injuries unit for treatment until day 5 of the injury. Upon arrival, the NA recognized that the wound was infected by the surrounding redness, which was hot to touch, and from the patient's report that the pain was worse than it was on the day of the injury. The NA promptly referred the patient to a doctor for antibiotics.

Laceration – usually caused by a blunt force. The edges of the wound are irregular with tearing of the tissue.

Due to the inelastic nature of dehydrated skin, it can burst on impact with any blunt object. If a patient is hydrated, it is highly likely that the injury would be less severe in terms of tearing, or would be restricted to simply bruising (that is, rupture of underlying blood vessels, but with no rupture of the skin).

Penetrating wound – or puncture wound. This is a wound with a fine path made by a pointed object. Cat bites are a common penetrating wound. These can be highly infective due to the 'injection' of saliva during the bite. It is usually the case that the hole in the skin appears uncomplicated; however the NA must be aware of the underlying anatomy that exists below the skin, such as major organs, blood vessels and nerve endings.

Contusion – an area of bruising due to a blunt force where there is no break in the skin but underlying blood vessels rupture, causing leakage of blood and the resulting bruise.

A low platelet count or clotting disorders can lead to an increased risk of bruising. The skin can become thin and papery with the use of steroids. Additionally, the ageing process results in a reduction of collagen, which gives the walls of the blood vessels their strength and elasticity. This reduction can render blood vessels vulnerable to blunt trauma, especially during moving and handling procedures. Any slight knock can result in rupture of blood vessels and leakage of blood that results in bruising.

Pressure – prolonged, unrelieved pressure causes occlusion of the blood vessels resulting in ischaemia of the skin (Fig. 25.3).

Abrasion – caused by a scraping or rubbing (friction) causing damage or a break in the skin. Friction can be superficial, affecting only the epidermis, or it can be deep with full tissue loss, depending on the mechanism of injury (Fig. 25.4). Additionally, friction can occur rapidly (such as when falling off a bike), or slowly (such as the rubbing of the skin during tremors).

Burn – caused by heat, including the sun, frost, chemicals and electricity (Figs 25.5 and 25.6).

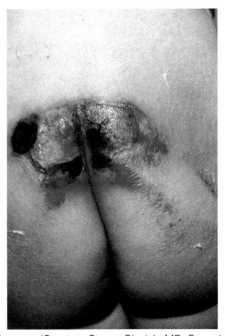

Fig. 25.3 Pressure (Courtesy Steven Binnick, MD. From James et al., 2018).

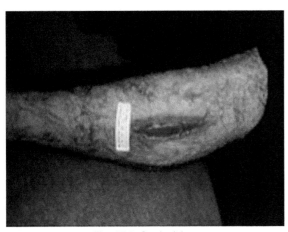

Fig. 25.2 Cut Incision.

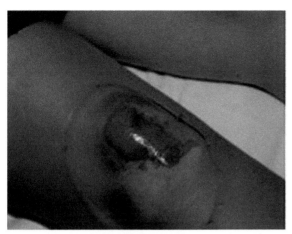

Fig. 25.4 Abrasion.

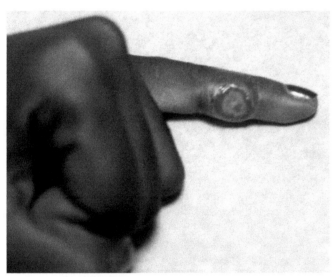

Fig. 25.5 Cigarette Burn (James et al., 2018).

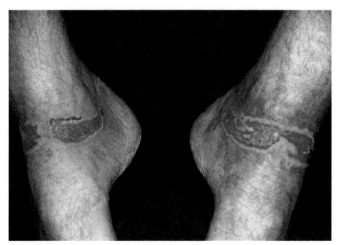

Fig. 25.6 Cement Burn (Courtesy Steven Binnick, MD. From James et al., 2018).

The patient in Fig. 25.6 has sustained a chemical burn. It is recommended that patients with chemical burns attend A&E without any delay so they can be treated immediately, often with many hours of irrigation of the areas under the shower. This will prevent the ongoing burning from the chemical, which would otherwise have eroded down to bone.

Scalds – caused by hot liquids or steam. Often causes blistering.

Moisture – prolonged contact with bodily fluids can cause the skin to become macerated (waterlogged) and/or excoriated (waterlogged and burned/scalded due to high acidity in the bodily fluids, such as urine, faeces or sweat). Once the skin is macerated or excoriated, the immediate line of defence is lost and bacteria can penetrate the dermis. The effects of moisture damage is discussed later.

Scars

A scar is defined as a mark left on the skin after a wound has healed, giving rise to an altered appearance of the skin (Davis et al., 1993). Initially, the scarring is red and raised and after 6 months or so should result in a pale, flat area of skin as the wound progresses through the normal maturative phase of wound healing (Davies, 1985). Scar tissue is said to be between 20%–30% weaker in terms of tensile strength than before the injury took place. Over the course of the following 2 years or so, the collagen and elastin fibres migrate within the healed tissues to optimize the skin's strength and elasticity as far as possible (Singer & Clark, 1999). However, it will always remain vulnerable to external insults, particularly pressure and sunshine.

Hypertrophic and keloid scarring

Occasionally, an abnormal scar develops that becomes raised and itchy. This is defined as a hypertrophic scar. If these symptoms continue, the scar tissue can invade the surrounding tissues, which can develop into a raised scar known as a keloid. Massage and silicone dressings are thought to reduce the effects of scarring. However, a referral to a plastic surgeon may be necessary if a more acceptable cosmetic appearance is required.

Common internal factors that cause skin damage

Arterial insufficiency – caused by the lack of, or reduced blood supply to the skin, which results in tissue death from lack of oxygen (hypoxia). Common causes are peripheral vascular disease, diabetes, tobacco smoking and in those with severe cardiac conditions whereby the circulation is significantly reduced (Fig. 25.7).

Venous insufficiency – caused by a buildup of waste products/fluids (oedema) that seep into the tissues from expanded vein walls (venous hypertension). This seepage results in non-viable tissue that consists of waste products, which can cause a wound to occur spontaneously (due to stretching of the skin) and the waste products will prevent the wound from healing until the waste and oedema has been rectified with compression and/or elevation to drain the fluid from the interstitial spaces.

For similar reasons, if any break to the skin occurs from trauma, the prospect of the wound healing is minimal until such time the underlying venous insufficiency is rectified with compression and/or elevation.

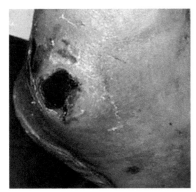

Fig. 25.7 Arterial Insufficiency (James et al., 2018).

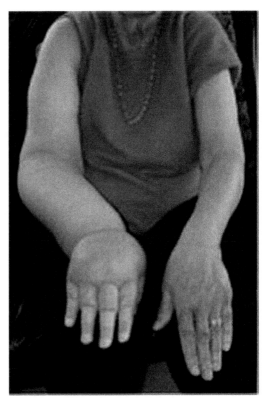

Fig. 25.8 Lymphoedema.

Lymphoedema – caused by the buildup of lymph fluid within the tissues due to ineffective/damaged lymph nodes. Lymphoedema has many causes, one of which is chronic oedema. Chronic oedema applies pressure to lymph nodes rendering them inactive in the affected area (Fig. 25.8).

Dermatological conditions – for example, dermatitis, psoriasis, skin cancers, to name but a few, are discussed in Chapter 26.

GENERAL SKIN CARE

Assessment

Before appropriate skin care can be provided to meet the needs of the individual and their skin, it is vital that the NA undertakes a formal holistic and skin assessment. Once this assessment has been carried out, care plans can be devised that appropriately and effectively meet the needs identified on assessment. It is important that this assessment considers the patient holistically, utilizing appropriate validated assessment tools where necessary, such as a nutrition assessment tool, a pressure ulcer risk assessment tool, a falls risk assessment tool and a skin assessment tool. Any areas of concern on the skin must be recorded in the nursing records and on a body map.

NICE (2014) recommends that the skin assessment should include the following:
- Skin integrity in areas of pressure
- Colour changes or discoloration
- Variations in heat, firmness and moisture (e.g., because of incontinence, oedema, dry or inflamed skin).

It is also important that any unusual scarring, abscesses, lesions or wounds are noted and documented in the nursing records and on the body map.

Regular reassessments need to be carried out, and adjustments made to the care plan(s) as necessary, or alternatively new care plans must be written if significant changes are noted or new problems, needs or risks arise.

Care planning

In 2010, the National Patient Safety Agency (NPSA) NHS England, via NHS Improvement (now NHS England), implemented the 'Stop the Pressure' campaign in the NHS, which continues to date. The purpose of the campaign was to reduce the number of avoidable pressure ulcers developing on patients whilst inpatients in NHS hospitals.

In an effort to achieve this goal, a model of care was introduced across all hospitals known as the 'SSKIN bundle' [of care] (Fig. 25.9). This involves five simple steps for preventing pressure ulcers. SSKIN is an acronym for the following:
- S = Surface – Make sure your patients have the right support
- S = Skin – Inspection: early inspection means early detection. Show patients and carers what to look for.
- K = Keep [your patients] moving.
- I = Incontinence/moisture – your patients need to be clean and dry.
- N = Nutrition/hydration – help patients to have the right diet and plenty of fluids.

The SSKIN bundle is commonly used as a care plan to prevent pressure damage and moisture lesions and/or as a record to evidence that planned care has been provided. However, whilst direction on pressure ulcer prevention may be included on this document, additional care plans are required to direct staff on continence care/moisture management, and nutrition as appropriate, in which case the SSKIN bundle can act as a record to evidence the provision of that care also.

> **REFLECTION 25.1**
>
> Find out more about the SSKIN bundle used in the care area where you have been allocated. Have look at the care plan and identify the key issues associated with SSKIN bundles.

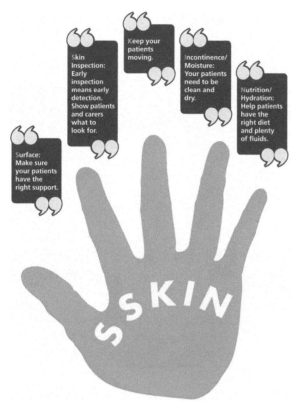

Fig. 25.9 The SSKIN Bundle (© NHS Midlands and East, 2012).

skin is easier to damage than well hydrated skin due to it being less supple. Over-hydration of the skin, such as oedema, can cause the skin to stretch, resulting in it thinning, which will make it more vulnerable to ruptures and even light trauma.

It is therefore extremely important that a good fluid intake is maintained of around 2 litres of fluids per day, and that efforts are made to reduce oedema, such as by elevation, or medical intervention – for instance, in oedema caused by heart failure.

CASE STUDY 25.4   Annie

Annie, an elderly lady with dementia who is resident in a nursing home, was refusing oral fluids over the previous day or two, taking only the occasional sip of water, juice or tea.

Patience, the NA employed at the home, recognized that Annie was not maintaining adequate fluid intake, as all fluids taken were documented on the fluid balance chart and her intake during the previous day was less than 200 mL. Patience also noted that Annie's skin was looking dehydrated, as it was drier and more wrinkly than usual.

Patience recognized that if this situation was not rectified, there was a risk of renal failure, urine infections and skin damage (e.g., moisture lesions, pressure sores and trauma). Patience therefore promptly referred Annie to the nurse in charge, who arranged for a GP to attend. Subcutaneous fluids were prescribed and administered to rehydrate Annie, thus avoiding ill-health and potential hospital admission.

As the SSKIN bundle covers some of the main aspects of care that achieves and maintains healthy, intact skin, it is reasonable to use this document to evidence the provision of skin care. However, where there are specific issues with the skin, such as a wound or medical condition necessitating specific treatments, then a separate care plan needs to be devised that gives clear direction on how this issue should be managed.

The plan should identify the problem, need or risk, set out the aim or goal of the planned care, a step-by-step guide on how that care should be provided, and a date for evaluating/reassessing the care provided for appropriateness and effectiveness.

Types of care that may be provided

The following aspects of care are crucial in maintaining skin integrity and to enable the skin to perform its functions effectively.

Hydration

The human body is made up of approximately 60%–70% water (H_2O), and there is no doubt that water is essential for our survival. Water acts as a carrier of nutrients to various organs; it is a medium for eliminating toxins, a structural support and a thermal regulator. As the largest organ of the body, the skin contains approximately 64% water. Dehydrated skin will become dry, tight, itchy and flaky. It can feel rough and can lack visible radiance.

Any water imbalance in the skin will result in a loss of elasticity and cause thinning of the skin (Potter & Perry, 1995). Dry

---

CARE IN THE HOME SETTING

The NA has a duty to ensure that all patients are adequately hydrated and nourished. This is an important component of care provision and health promotion, regardless of the context of care (and this includes the person's own home). Hydration is crucial for survival. The benefits of good hydration for people to function well are widely known. The recommended amount of fluids suggested for adults varies between 1.2 L to 3.1 L daily per day. Hydration is a fundamental part of care and it must be given the priority it deserves. There is a direct association between poor hydration and patient harm.

Guidelines have acknowledged the problem of poor recognition of dehydration and malnutrition by healthcare staff. This is not only in hospitals, but also in community settings. Predicting problems earlier in the home and care facilities, by identifying those at risk of dehydration at an earlier stage, can help to reduce levels of morbidity and mortality that are associated with this all-too-common problem (NHS England, 2016).

NHS England (2016) *Guidance – Commissioning Excellent Nutrition and Hydration 2015–2018.* https://www.england.nhs.uk/wp-content/uploads/2015/10/nut-hyd-guid.pdf (Last accessed March 2018).

Nutrition

It is vital that any individual receives a well-balanced diet that consists of a variety of nutrients, vitamins and minerals to maintain optimum health and skin integrity so that the functions of the skin can be maintained.

The National Institute of Health and Care Excellence (NICE) states 'Malnutrition has a wide-ranging impact on people's health and wellbeing. Screening for the risk of malnutrition in care settings is important for enabling early and effective interventions. It is important that tools are validated to ensure that screening is as accurate and reliable as possible.'

Screening for malnutrition risk can be undertaken by simply asking about the patient's diet intake (Thomas & Bishop, 2007). A body mass index (BMI) can use used to determine whether or not the patient has a normal weight compared to their height using the following calculation (BAPEN, 2003) as part of the screening process:

$$BMI = \frac{Weight\ (kg)}{Height\ (m)^2}$$

There are also a number of nutrition screening tools available that assist the practitioner to predict those who may be at risk of malnutrition and BAPEN (2003), introduced a screening tool known as the Malnutrition Universal Screening Tool (MUST), which is a validated tool recommended by NICE.

Regular weighing and re-assessment will ensure that a patient's weight is monitored. The frequency of this will be determined by local policy and/or by medical/dietetic direction. Any weight loss or gain must be report to medical staff without delay for a review and ongoing medical management.

Chapter 23 of this text discusses nutritional needs in more detail.

Elimination

When the skin is in contact with moisture for prolonged periods, it loses its protective barrier as it becomes waterlogged (macerated). As the skin is softened with moisture, it becomes penetrable by bacteria and can cause cellulitis to develop. As the skin is no longer resistant to pressure due to the moisture, it will become vulnerable to pressure damage and other traumas.

If the moisture consists of bodily fluids, the waste products can damage the skin by altering the pH levels within the skin. This has the adverse effect of 'burning' or 'excoriating' the skin, making it red, raw and painful.

As maceration and/or excoriation can occur with any type of fluid, especially bodily fluids, such as faecal matter, urine or sweating, NICE (2014) recommend the use of a barrier preparation to prevent skin damage on any area of the body subject to regular contact with moisture.

It is also recommended that incontinent patients are toileted regularly, or that suitable continence pads or, where appropriate, bowel management systems, are utilized to mitigate the risk of any episode of incontinence, as far as possible.

The NA must therefore be vigilant to the causes of moisture on the skin, and must put in place actions to mitigate the moisture damage. The following demonstrates actions that the NA can take to protect the skin from moisture damage.

1. Moisture barriers. In the event there is a risk of moisture damage due to incontinence or sweating, it is important to consider the use of moisture barrier products (creams, sprays). These products protect the skin from contact with, and the impacts of, excess moisture, thereby assisting the waterproofing abilities of the skin while also moisturizing the skin.

2. Care must be taken when selecting appropriate barrier products, as some are thick and sticky to apply and remove, which can result in shearing of the skin (i.e., where the dermis and epidermis can separate, forming a blister).

3. Because of the consistency of such thick and sticky products, they can also block the pores of incontinence pads, which then negates the absorbing abilities of the pad. This results in the urine or faeces sitting against the skin, which in time will result in maceration and/or excoriation, so is counter-productive.

4. In the event that any break appears in the skin for any reason, or if any unusual lesions develop, this will require an assessment by a qualified healthcare professional with experience in wound management, or a doctor, so that the area can be assessed, treated and if necessary referred to the most appropriate specialist for ongoing treatment (e.g., to dermatology).

CASE STUDY 25.5 **Joe**

Joe, a 56-year-old labourer, was admitted to hospital for elective surgery on a back injury sustained during the course of his work. Post-operatively, he was transferred to a rehabilitation unit where he remained for several weeks. During admission, Joe had no problems with eating and drinking.

However, during admission, the NA undertook regular nutrition assessments and weights on a weekly basis (under the direction of the registered nurse), and after 3 weeks, she noted that he was eating and drinking well, but was losing weight. He was not complaining of any pain, nausea or vomiting and neither the NA nor Joe could find any explanation for this weight loss.

The NA also noted that Joe's skin was becoming less radiant, paler in colour and was not as healthy looking as when he was first admitted.

The NA mentioned her observations of Joe's skin and the screening findings to the consultant at the next ward round, and Joe was referred to a gastroenterologist for further investigations.

During the course of these investigations, Joe was unfortunately diagnosed with bowel cancer, but thanks to the regular monitoring of weight and nutrition screening by the NA, the cancer was caught and treated in its early stages. Joe eventually made a full recovery and is now cancer free and back at work.

CASE STUDY 25.6 Jane

Jane is an NA who recognized that one of her patients was pyrexial and sweating because of a urinary tract infection, and was therefore at risk of maceration and excoriation from the moisture that was oozing onto the patient's skin.

Upon washing the patient one morning, Jane noticed that the areas of skin folds were getting red and sore, and realized that this was due to sweating. Jane was concerned that the patient would develop fungal infections in the warm, moist creases of the skin folds, so devised a care plan that would direct others to regularly monitor these areas, and to wash, pat dry the skin folds, and apply a moisture barrier product to protect the skin from any further damage. Jane also made provision in the care plan that instructed staff to observe for signs of a fungal infection (very red, raw, potentially itchy skin that is painful and possibly bleeding and malodorous) and to alert medical staff for treatment should this condition arose.

With regular washing, drying and use of moisture barrier products, and successful treatment of the infection, the patient recovered and suffered no further skin damage, and the redness and soreness originally noted quickly resolved.

Cleansing

Personal hygiene is of paramount importance and consists of the physical act of cleaning the body so that the skin is maintained in an optimum condition and so infection risk is reduced. The Department of Health (2016) states 'Your skin works hard to keep you healthy, and you can return the favour by taking care of it.'

Cleansing the skin must include the following:

- General skin care, including within skin folds
- Hair
- Nails
- Mouth
- Ear lobes/behind the ears
- Genitalia/perianal areas.

REFLECTION 25.2

Hair is an appendage of the skin. There are some conditions when patients may lose their hair, for example, alopecia. How do you think a person might feel if they have alopecia and how might this impact on their health and well-being?

Persistent use of some soaps can cause the skin to dry out and become tight, itchy and flaky. Harsh, alcohol-based products should be avoided as these can irritate and dry the skin. Try to use mild soaps or bath oils instead (DH, 2016). Soap substitutes and emollients can be used to cleanse the skin and maintain suppleness, which reduces the risk of trauma. Hand washing must be carried out by the NA and the patient after assisting the patient with toileting, and especially before eating food.

Fingernails should be kept short and clean, and specialist advice may be required for toenails, particularly with immuno-compromised patients, such as diabetics, who are at increased risk of infection. Special attention should be paid to the feet, especially in between toes where fungal infections commonly occur. Avoid applying moisturizers in between toes to mitigate this risk.

Moisturizing

As stated earlier, the most effective skin moisturizer is good hydration. However, as the outer layers of the skin are dead and compressed epithelial cells, they can become dry due to evaporation of moisture, so require rehydrating with moisturizing products. The use of a non-perfumed moisturizer or emollient will assist in keeping these cells hydrated, which will in turn maintain the suppleness of the skin, thereby reducing the risk of trauma while preventing the buildup of too many epithelial cells, particularly as we age.

Good fluid intake and the use of appropriate moisturizing products will maintain the skin's moisture balance, while maintaining sufficient natural and donated oils to the skin to maintain its waterproofing abilities and suppleness so that it can function as intended.

Sun care

Sunlight includes ultraviolet (UV) rays, which are the main cause of premature skin ageing and can cause skin cancer (DH, 2016). However, the skin requires some time in sunlight so that vitamin D can be produced within the skin.

The Department of Health (2016) advises spending time in the shade between 11:00 and 15:00; covering up with clothes, a hat and sunglasses, and using sunscreen with a sun protection factor (SPF) of at least 15.

Smoking

Smoking is linked to early signs of the skin ageing. Smoking results in fewer nutrients and less oxygen in the blood stream, which is replaced with carbon (carboxyhaemoglobin). It is thought that the carbon in tobacco reduces the skin's natural elasticity by reducing the production of the protein collagen, which is the scaffolding support for the skin, so the skin begins to sag, wrinkle and develop a grey, pale, unhealthy appearance. (DH, 2016).

Alcohol

Alcohol causes dehydration of the skin, leaving it looking old and tired. The Department of Health (2016) recommends no alcohol, or that individuals adhere to the recommended limits.

LOOKING BACK, FEEDING FORWARD

Maintaining a patient's hygiene and caring for skin is an integral part of the role of the NA; it allows the NA to observe the skin and the health of the patient while building trust in the patient/nurse relationship. It must never be regarded as a mundane task, particularly as the skin can tell the NA so very much about the general health and emotional state of the patients under their care. With good observational skills, timely and regular assessment and care planning, close monitoring and timely intervention, many skin issues and health problems can be avoided and the NA can optimize the health and happiness of their patients.

The skin should never be underestimated. It is the largest [non-vital] organ of the body and should be afforded the same respect as any other major organ. The NA is very well-placed to assist their patients and their colleagues to appreciate this fact.

REFERENCES

BAPEN, 2003. Calculating Body Mass Index. Maidenhead, British Association for Parental and Enteral Nutrition. http://www.bapen.org.uk.

BAPEN, 2003. Malnutrition Universal Screening Tool 'MUST' Report. Maidenhead, British Association for Parental and Enteral Nutrition. http://www.bapen.org.uk/screening-and-must/must-calculator.

Davies, D.M., 1985. Plastic and reconstructive surgery. Br. Med. J. 290, 1056–1058.

Davis, M.H., et al., 1993. The Wound Handbook. Centre for Medical Education, Dundee, and Perspective, London.

Department of Health, 2016. Look after your skin. https://www.nhs.uk/live-well/healthy-body/look-after-your-skin/.

James, W.D., Elston, D.M., McMahon, P.J., 2018. Andrews' Diseases of the Skin: Clinical Atlas, first ed. Elsevier, Oxford.

National Patient Safety Agency, 2010. http://www.npsa.nhs.uk/corporate/news/nhs-to-adopt-zero-tolerance-approach-to-pressure-ulcers/?locale=en.

NHS England, 2010. Stop the Pressure: helping to prevent pressure ulcers. http://www.stopthepressure.co.uk.

NHS England, 2016. Patient Safety in the NHS. https://www.nhs.uk/NHSEngland/thenhs/patient-safety/Pages/about-patient-safety.aspx.

NHS England, 2017. Key Improvements: Five Year Plan. https://www.england.nhs.uk/five-year-forward-view/next-steps-on-the-nhs-five-year-forward-view/patient-safety/.

NICE, 2012. Nutrition support in adults. Quality standard [QS24]. https://www.nice.org.uk/guidance/qs24/chapter/quality-statement-1-screening-for-the-risk-of-malnutrition.

NICE, 2014. Pressure ulcers: prevention and management. Clinical guideline [CG 179]. https://www.nice.org.uk/guidance/cg179.

Penzer, R., Finch, M., 2001. Promoting healthy skin in older people. Nurs. Stand. 15 (34), 46–52.

Potter, P.A., Perry, G., 1995. Basic Nursing Theory and Practice. Mosby, London.

Singer, A.J., Clark, R.A.F., 1999. Cutaneous wound healing. N. Engl. J. Med. 341 (10), 738–746.

Thomas, B., Bishop, J., 2007. Manual of Dietetic Practice, fourth ed. Blackwell Publishing, Oxford.

Waugh, A., Grant, A., 2018. Ross & Wilson Anatomy and Physiology in Health and Illness, thirteenth ed. Elsevier, Oxford.

Young, L., 1991. The clean fight. Nurs. Stand. 5 (35), 54–55.

26

Skin Disorders

Linda Castro

OBJECTIVES

By the end of this chapter the reader will be able to:
1. Accurately describe the skin condition using basic dermatology vocabulary
2. Recognize common skin conditions
3. Recognize common benign lesions
4. Recognize the signs of changes that could indicate a skin cancer
5. Provide the reader with an understanding of the psychological impact of skin disorders
6. Review the role of the Nursing Associate in promoting skin care

KEY WORDS

Skin	Psoriatic	Prevention
Dermatoses	Benign	Psychological
Itchy	Malignant	
Excoriated	Inflamed	

CHAPTER AIMS

The aim of this chapter is to provide the knowledge and skills required to recognize a variety of skin conditions and lesions. It will also provide the reader with an understanding of the psychological impact of skin disorders. This will facilitate safe, effective care delivered with sensitivity.

SELF TEST

1. What does keratosis mean?
2. What is eczema?
3. Discuss who is most commonly affected by eczema.
4. What is psoriasis?
5. Where on the body do fungal infections tend to grow and why?
6. Name five common benign lesions.
7. What are the main signs of change that could indicate a skin cancer is developing?
8. What should people do to protect their skin from ultraviolet radiation?
9. How could a skin condition affect someone psychologically?
10. Name and describe the three most common skin cancers.

INTRODUCTION

In this chapter, the largest organ of the body, the skin, is considered. It will commence by looking at appropriate dermatological vocabulary and will discuss common skin conditions and treatments. The second part of the chapter considers benign and cancerous lesions, how to recognize changes and how to protect against ultraviolet (UV) radiation. Throughout the chapter, the role the Nursing Associate has in providing kind and compassionate care is highlighted, as often skin conditions arise in sensitive areas, as well as being very visible to the observer. The final part of the chapter will discuss the psychological impact of skin conditions on an individual and provide opportunities for self-reflection.

CRITICAL AWARENESS

Knowing the Patient as an Individual

Patients appreciate that the Nursing Associate and other healthcare professionals acknowledge individuality and the unique way in which each person experiences a condition and the impact that this has on their life. Patients' values, beliefs and circumstances will all influence their expectations of, their needs for and their use of services and this is no different for the patient with a dermatological condition. The Nursing Associate must recognize that individual patients are living with their condition, which means the ways in which their family and broader life affect their health and care need to be taken into account.

Develop an understanding of the patient as an individual, including how the condition affects the person, and how the person's circumstances and experiences affect their condition and treatment; this is a hallmark of good nursing care.

Ensure that factors such as physical or learning disabilities, sight, speech or hearing problems and difficulties with reading, understanding or speaking English are addressed; this will enable the patient to participate as fully as possible in consultations and care.

The Nursing Associate should ask the patient about and take into account any factors, for example, their domestic, social and work situation and their previous experience of healthcare, that may:
- impact on their health condition and/or
- affect their ability or willingness to engage with healthcare services and/or
- affect their ability to manage their own care and make decisions about self-management and lifestyle choices.

Listening to and addressing any health beliefs, concerns and preferences that the patient has, and being aware that these affect how and whether the patient engages with treatment, can demonstrate care that is truly patient-centred. Respecting the patient's views and offering them support if required to help them engage effectively with healthcare services and participate in self-management as appropriate are hallmarks of a professional nurse–patient relationship.

The Nursing Associate should avoid making assumptions about the patient based on their appearance or other personal characteristics and they must take into account the patient's individuality, making sure services are equally accessible to, and supportive of, all people who use health services.

If it is appropriate, the Nursing Associate should discuss with the patient their need for psychological, social, spiritual and/or financial support. Offer them support and information and/or direct them to sources of support and information; always act within your scope of practice. Review the patient's circumstances and need for support regularly, ensuring the care plan is up to date and appropriate.

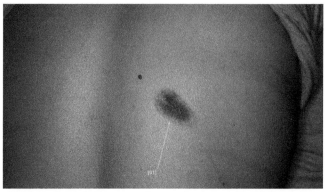

Fig. 26.1 Patch (GHA, 2017; Dermatology photographic database).

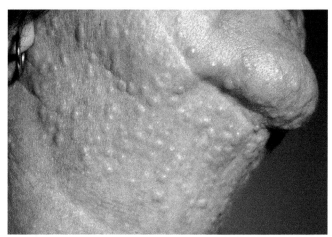

Fig. 26.2 Papules (James et al., 2018).

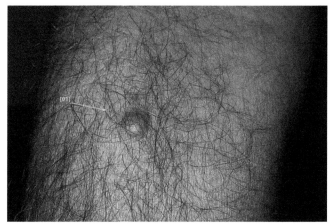

Fig. 26.3 Nodule (GHA, 2017; Dermatology photographic database).

DERMATOLOGICAL VOCABULARY

Macule: A flat area of skin with colour change that is not palpable. It will be less than 1 cm in diameter.

Patch: This is the same as a macule, only larger than 1 cm in diameter (see Fig. 26.1).

Papule: Raised area of skin less than 1 cm which may be smooth or have a crust and can be dome shaped or flat topped (see Fig. 26.2).

Nodule: A solid, elevated lesion, more than 0.5 cm in both width and depth (see Fig. 26.3).

Horn: An outgrowth of keratin, usually longer than its breadth (see Fig. 26.4).

Vesicle: A blister with fluid, less than 1 cm in diameter (see Fig. 26.5).

Pustule: A lesion filled with infected or sterile pus, which is usually larger than 1 cm.

Bulla: A limited elevation of skin, filled with fluid and over 0.5 cm in diameter (see Fig. 26.6).

Plaque: An elevated solid area of skin, more than 2 cm in diameter.

Crust: A scab or accumulation of cellular debris.

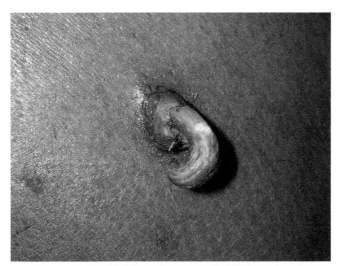

Fig. 26.4 Horn (James et al., 2018).

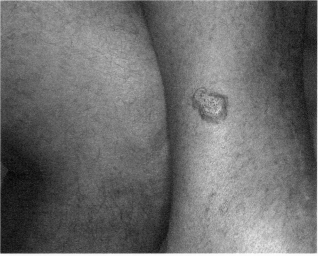

Fig. 26.7 Keratosis (GHA, 2017; Dermatology photographic database).

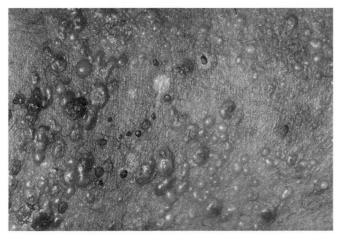

Fig. 26.5 Blister (Courtesy Steven Binnick, MD. From James et al., 2018).

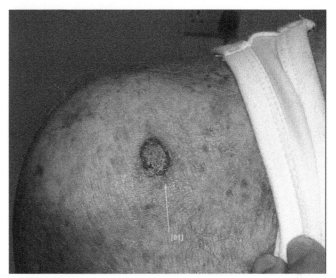

Fig. 26.8 Discoid lesion (GHA, 2017; Dermatology photographic database).

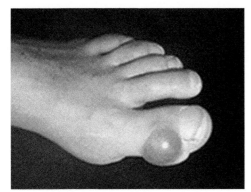

Fig. 26.6 Bulla (James et al., 2018).

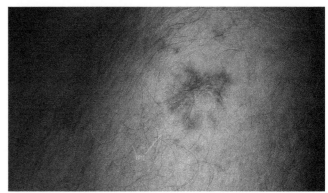

Fig. 26.9 Erosion (GHA, 2017; Dermatology photographic database).

Scale: A flake of skin coming from the horny layer.
Keratosis: A horn-like thickening of the stratum corneum (see Fig. 26.7).
Discoid: Coin shaped (see Fig. 26.8).
Wheal: An itchy, erythematous plaque, firm to touch.
Fissure: A vertical crack in the skin.
Erosion: A partial loss of skin (see Fig. 26.9).

Ulceration: A full-thickness loss of skin (see Fig. 26.10).
Excoriation: An erosion or ulcer caused by scratching.
Erythema: A redness in the skin caused by vassal dilatation.
Erythroderma: A generalized redness of the skin, with or without scaling (see Fig. 26.11).

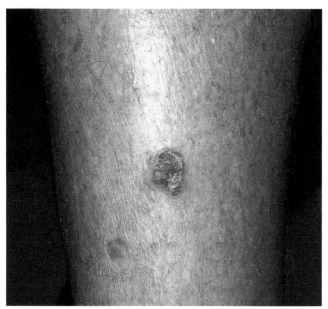

Fig. 26.10 Ulceration (GHA, 2017; Dermatology photographic database).

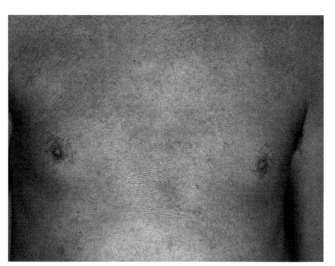

Fig. 26.11 Erythroderma (James et al., 2018).

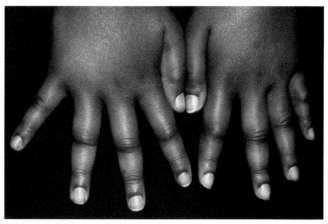

Fig. 26.12 Angiodema (Courtesy Steven Binnick, MD. From James et al, 2018).

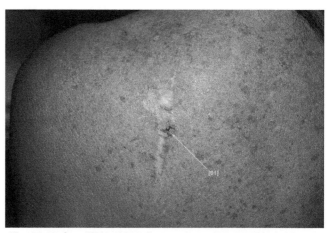

Fig. 26.13 Scar (GHA, 2017; Dermatology photographic database).

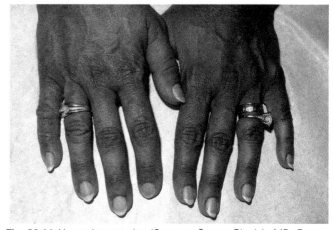

Fig. 26.14 Hyperpigmentation (Courtesy Steven Binnick, MD. From James et al, 2018).

Angioedema: Swelling caused by fluid extending to the subcutaneous tissue (see Fig. 26.12).

Haematoma: Commonly known as a bruise, this is swelling caused by bleeding.

Inflammation: Swelling of the skin tissue caused by multiple reasons.

Scar: The mark left after injury that caused a full-thickness loss of skin (see Fig. 26.13).

Atrophy: A thinning of the skin caused by reduction in the epidermis, dermis or subcutaneous fat.

Lichenification: Marked thickened skin

Stria: Commonly known as stretch marks, they are white, pink or purple and caused by changes in the connective tissue.

Hyperpigmentation: An increase in the pigment of the skin (see Fig. 26.14).

Hypopigmentation: A loss of pigment in the skin (see Fig. 26.15).

Telangiectasia: A visible dilation of small cutaneous blood vessels (see Fig. 26.16).

DOCUMENTATION OF HISTORY

When documenting a history from your examination, it is important to ensure that the patient is provided with privacy in order to discuss their issues and if they need to be examined. Aspects of the history will include:

- Age of patient
- Sex of patient

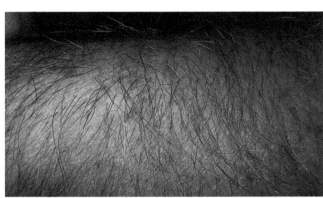

Fig. 26.15 Hypopigmentation (GHA, 2017; Dermatology photographic database).

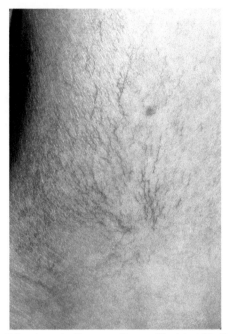

Fig. 26.16 Telangiectasia (Courtesy Steven Binnick, MD. From James et al, 2018).

- Time present
- Size
- Shape
- Colour
- Texture
- Smell
- Temperature
- Site

> **! HOTSPOT**
>
> All patients must be provided with a chaperone of their choice. This must be provided, regardless of pressures that services providers may be experiencing.

COMMON SKIN CONDITIONS

Eczema/dermatitis

Graham-Brown et al. (2017) explain that this is an inflammatory reaction in the skin that can be caused by external or internal factors. Both are names for the same condition.

Signs and symptoms

- Primarily itching
- Redness (erythema)
- Swelling (oedema)
- Weeping lesions (papules, vesicles)
- Scabs (scaling)
- Edges are not clear (ill-defined)

Types of eczema

- Acute (as in new episode)
- Chronic (long-term condition)
- Irritant contact dermatitis (a pre-existing type of dermatitis is irritated by external products, such as shampoo and soaps)
- Allergic contact dermatitis (this is caused by a real allergy to a substance, such as hair dye, rubber, components of cream). This can be confirmed by doing a patch test.
- Atopic dermatitis (there is a genetic predisposition to developing this type)
- Seborrheic dermatitis (this affects the face, scalp, upper back and flexures)
- Discoid eczema (the lesions are round to oval, clearly defined and appear on the trunk or limbs)
- Varicose eczema (occurs on the legs where there is a poor venous supply)
- Eczema of the hands and/or feet
- Eczema craquele (occurs on legs, abdomen and arms. Found in the elderly due to more frequent bathing. It is common to see in elderly hospital patients).

See Fig. 26.17.

Common treatment options

- Use of emollients (moisturizers).
- Application of topical cortisone (ranging from mild to potent depending on severity).
- Antifungal creams (if there is a fungal element, such as in seborrheic dermatitis).
- Administration of oral antifungals, oral steroids in more severe cases.
- Administration of other potent immune suppressive medications (these drugs can cause changes in normal blood values, so require close monitoring of therapeutic levels).
- Biologic therapies (as with immune suppressive medications, these can have major side effects and patients must be closely monitored).

> **! HOTSPOT**
>
> As a Nursing Associate you may be required to apply the topical treatments, so it is important you follow some important rules;
> - Always apply emollients from the top of the limb down.
> - Do not apply emollients to broken skin, as it can cause infections.
> - The rule of cortisone cream is the top third of your finger is enough cream to apply to the equivalent of two palms of hand. Therefore please apply sparingly (Henderson, 2017).
> - Always wash your hands after handling topical cortisone.

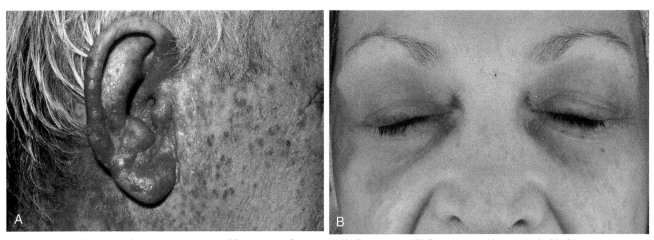

Fig. 26.17 Some Presentations of Eczema and Dermatitis. (A) Ear eczema. (B) Eye eczema. (James et al., 2018.)

NURSING SKILLS

The Fingertip Unit

Unless instructed otherwise by the dermatology nurse specialist or the doctor, the patient should follow the directions on the patient information leaflet that comes with the medication. This gives details of how much to apply and how often.

Sometimes, the amount of medication the patient is advised to use will be given in fingertip units (FTUs). The Nursing Associate is expected to explain what this is to the patient or to advise them to speak with the practice nurse, dermatology nurse specialist, doctor or pharmacist.

An FTU (this is about 500 mg or 0.5 g) is the amount of medication required to squeeze a line from the tip of an adult finger to the first crease of the finger. It should be enough to treat an area of skin double the size of the flat of the hand with the fingers together.

The recommended dosage will depend on what part of the body is being treated. This is because the skin is thinner in some parts of the body and more sensitive to the effects of corticosteroids.

For adults, the recommended FTUs to be applied in one single dose are:
- 0.5 FTU for genitals
- 1 FTU for hands, elbows and knees
- 1.5 FTUs for the feet, including the soles
- 2.5 FTUs for the face and neck
- 3 FTUs for the scalp
- 4 FTUs for a hand and arm together, or the buttocks
- 8 FTUs for the legs and chest, or legs and back .

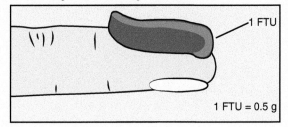

1 FTU

1 FTU = 0.5 g

Fig. 26.18 A Fingertip Unit.

THE MEDICINE TROLLEY 26.1

Drug	Drug classification	Reason for administration	Route of administration	Dose	Side effects	Contraindications	Nursing care
Double base gel	Emollient	Hydration of skin and cleansing	Topical	As required	Itching, burning sensation and allergic reactions	Cuts, infections and known allergies to ingredients	Gain consent prior to administration
E45 Cream		Hydration of skin					Explain the use of the emollient prior to application and answer any questions
Emmolin							
White soft paraffin and liquid paraffin							
Dermol 500	Emollient and bath wash	Hydration of skin and cleansing					
Dermol 200	Emollient shower wash	Hydration of skin and cleansing					Advise on potential side effects
Oilatum	wash	Hydration of skin					

These are just a few choices of emollients and washes available for use.

CARE IN THE HOME SETTING

Safety Advice When Using Emollients

Patients should be advised to follow this general safety advice when using emollients in the home setting:

- Keep away from fire, flames and cigarettes when using paraffin-based emollients. Dressings and clothing soaked with the ointment could be easily ignited.
- Use a clean spoon or spatula to remove emollients from a pot or tub. This reduces the risk of infections from contaminated pots.
- Take care of slipping when using emollients in a bath or shower, or on a tiled floor. Protect the floor with a non-slip mat, towel or sheet. Wearing protective gloves, wash your bath or shower afterwards with hot water and washing up liquid, then dry it with a kitchen towel.
- Never use more than the recommended amount of bath additive. This may cause skin irritation if the concentration is too high, especially when used with antiseptic bath oils.
- Be careful of using aqueous cream. For some people, it can cause burning, stinging, itching and redness, particularly children with atopic eczema.

! HOTSPOT

Apply minimum 30 minutes pre- or postapplication of steroid topical treatments, as it will dilute the potency of steroids if applied at the same time.

These are common topical treatments used for eczema/dermatitis and psoriasis.

! HOTSPOT

Steroid type and strength is determined by the severity of the condition and previous response to milder treatments.

Rule of thumb for choice of treatments is to treat with the mildest dose that works. This means treatment choice may be more potent strengths to achieve clearance faster, ensuring steroids are used for less time, giving fewer side effects.

Psoriasis

This is a chronic, inflammatory, noninfectious skin disorder that rarely affects people under 10 years and affects about 3% of the population. It can appear at any age. It is common for there to be a family history and it causes psoriatic plaques (scaling) to develop. This process is discussed by both Graham-Brown et al. (2017) and Weller et al. (2012).

Signs and symptoms

- Plaques (scales), large or small or both
- Multiple or singular lesions
- Erythematous (redness)
- Silver-like shine on surface
- Itchy
- Bleeding (usually caused by scratching or catching)
- Constant flaking of skin (this often causes embarrassment)

THE MEDICINE TROLLEY 26.2

Drug	Drug classification	Reason for administration	Route of administration	Dose	Side effects	Contraindications	Nursing care
Hydrocortisone	Steroid (mild)	Anti-inflammatory, antipruritic, used for corticosteroid responsive dermatosis	Topical	0.5–2.5 mg once or twice a day	Skin redness, burning, itching, peeling, skin thinness, blistering and steroid induced acne Thinning of skin	Known allergy to ingredients Pregnancy (please inform doctor if pregnant) Broken or infected skin unless also being treated	Gain consent prior to administration Explain the use of the treatment prior to application and answer any questions
Eumovate	Steroid (moderate)			Once or twice a day			
Elocon	Steroid (moderate)						
Betnovate	Steroid (potent)						Advise on potential side effects
Dermovate	Steroid (very potent)						Always wash hands after application
Daktacort	Steroid (mild) and antifungal	Fungal infections in association with dermatosis (i.e., athletes foot and candida)				As above and children under 10 years of age	Do not cover with a dressing unless advised by doctor
Cutivate (fluticasone)	Steroid (potent)					As above	Use fingertip rule to ensure appropriate amount is applied
Protopic (tacrolimus) A calcineurin inhibitor	Non-steroid	Used when topical steroids have not proven effective		Child ≥ 2 years: 0.03%, adult ≥16 years 0.1%		As above	

Types of psoriasis

There are many types of psoriasis and they include:

- Plaque psoriasis
- Scalp psoriasis
- Guttate psoriasis
- Nail psoriasis
- Chronic palmar plantar
- Flexural psoriasis
- Erythrodermic psoriasis
- Brittle psoriasis
- Pustular psoriasis
- Unstable or brittle psoriasis
- Arthropathic psoriasis

See Fig. 26.19.

Common treatment options

Treatment offered will depend on the individual needs of the patient. Treatment options should be discussed with the patient (and if appropriate, family) to ensure the patient makes an informed decision.

- Emollients
- Coal tar preparations
- Topical steroids
- Salicylic acid
- Vitamin D analogues
- Dithranol
- Light therapy
- Cytotoxic drugs
- Biologic drugs

Light therapy (phototherapy/chemotherapy). This is the administration of controlled UVA or UVB light using a light therapy cabinet or hand and foot control panels. This must be supervised with strict control from a dermatologist and fully trained light therapy nurses.

Conditions commonly treated with light therapy are:

- Psoriasis
- Eczema/dermatitis
- Vitiligo
- T-cell lymphoma.

Light therapy may also be used for polymorphic light eruption.

Oral medication and biologics. These medications are used when other methods have proved unsuccessful. There are strict guidelines for each treatment and close monitoring of blood levels, blood pressure and side effects are imperative.

These medications are generally monitored by the dermatology team; some patients, once stable, may be monitored by the practice nurse/general practitioner, but will continue having input from the dermatology department at least yearly. Medications that require very close monitoring of side effects, blood changes (which can be detected through regular blood testing) and changes in blood pressure levels include:

- Methotrexate (Rheumatrex)
- Ciclosporin (Neoral)
- Azathioprine (Imuran)
- Alitretinoin (Toctino)
- Enbrel (Etanercept)
- Adalimumab (Humira)
- Ustekinumab (Stelara).

Vitiligo

This is a pigment disorder where there is a loss (hypopigmentation) of the skin which usually starts in small patches but often spreads to wider areas. It is generally thought to be an autoimmune response and treatments are often unsuccessful.

Signs and symptoms

Loss of pigment in patches, gradually widening to other areas (see Fig. 26.20).

Treatment

Assessment of individual needs is essential prior to commencing treatment. Some treatment regimens include:

- Topical steroids
- Calcineurin inhibitors
- Light therapy: UVB + psoralen UVA

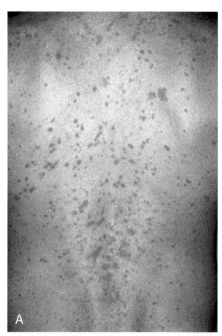

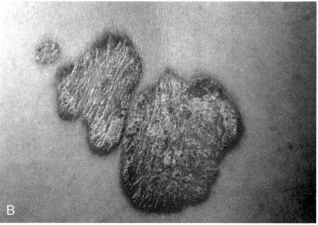

Fig. 26.19 Some Presentations of Psoriasis (Courtesy Steven Binnick, MD. From James et al, 2018).

THE MEDICINE TROLLEY 26.3

Drug	Drug classification	Reason for administration	Route of administration	Dose	Side effects	Contraindications	Nursing care
Capasal shampoo	Shampoo	To treat dry, scaly scalp conditions	Topical	As prescribed (maximum dose is daily)	Irritation, burning sensation, redness, blistering and peeling of skin	Broken or infected skin, unless also being treated	Gain consent prior to administration
Diprosalic (a mix of betamethasone and salicylic acid)	Steroid (potent) and salicylic acid	To treat and soften dry, scaly scalp conditions	Topical	As prescribed (usually applied thinly and left for a determined period of time before washing out	Skin redness, burning, itching, peeling, skin thinness, blistering acne Thinning of skin		Explain the use of the treatment prior to application and answer any questions Advise on potential side effects Always wash hands after application
Dovobet (betamethasone and calcipotriol)	Steroid (potent) vitamin D analogue	Treatment for stable plaque psoriasis	Topical	Daily, initially for 4 weeks		Fungal, viral or bacterial skin infections Erythrodermic, exfoliative or pustular psoriasis	
Dovonex (calcipotriene)	Vitamin D analogue	Treatment for stable plaque psoriasis	Topical	Daily		As above and known allergies to properties High levels of vitamin D High levels of calcium Patient should inform doctor or practice nurse if pregnant	

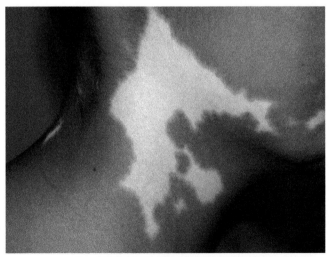

Fig. 26.20 Vitiligo (James et al., 2018).

> ⚠ **HOTSPOT**
>
> Treatment is rarely successful; therefore a compassionate approach is essential.

In difficult cases cosmetic camouflage may be offered. This is offered as a makeup palette that is ordered, and provides a selection of coloured creams that can be mixed to achieve as near to the patient's natural pigment as possible.

Alopecia areata

In this condition, there is a loss of hair, which usually commences with bald patches appearing on the scalp, eyebrows and beard and usually starts in childhood or early adulthood. As with vitiligo, it is thought to be an autoimmune response. This condition sometimes spontaneously resolves but in some cases can cause total hair loss of the scalp and, in extreme cases, of the full body.

Signs and symptoms

There are several signs and symptoms the Nursing Associate should beware of. These include:
- Round or oval patches of hair loss
- Complete loss of hair of scalp (alopecia totalis)
- Complete loss of all body hair (alopecia universalis).

See Fig. 26.21.

Treatment

Treatment options are decided upon in consultation with the patient after a full assessment of needs has been undertaken. Treatment can include:
- Topical steroids
- Intralesional steroids (injected under the skin)
- Calcineurin inhibitors
- Diphencyprone (to desensitize).

THE MEDICINE TROLLEY 26.4

Drug	Drug classification	Reason for administration	Route of administration	Dose	Side effects	Contraindications	Nursing care
Diphencyprone (DCP)	Local irritant	To trigger an immune response	Topical	Small dose, increasing as sensitization is achieved. It is applied weekly; if no response after 6 months, it is stopped; otherwise, applied until full hair growth achieved.	Erythema, burning sensation, blisters, eczema	Pregnancy	This treatment is given by trained professionals and, due to chances of allergy to the person that applies it, the patient or family are trained to do this.

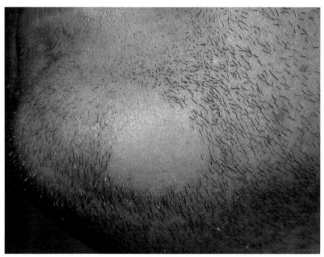

Fig. 26.21 Alopecia Areata (James et al., 2018)

Pityriasis versicolor

This condition is caused by a yeast infection called Malassezia, which is found harmlessly on the skin of 90% of the population. It usually develops when the person lives or has been in a moist, warm environment. It is common in teenagers and young adults, although anyone can develop it.

Signs and symptoms

These may include:
- Itchy skin patches
- Scaly skin patches
- Pigment changes to the skin patches
- Usually develops on trunk, neck, upper arms and back.

Treatment

This can include:
- Application of antifungal cream
- Use of antifungal shampoo
- Administration of antifungal tablets.

Pemphigus vulgaris

Pemphigus vulgaris is a condition that causes flaccid blisters and erosions on the skin and mucous membranes. Graham-Brown et al. (2017) explain that it usually starts in the mouth but affects other mucous membranes, such as the nose, throat and genitals. If untreated, it spreads to other areas of the body and is very debilitating. The lesions can look like someone has been scalded badly. Therefore, it can be extremely painful. It is extremely serious, as it can be fatal. It is most common in middle age but can affect children and the elderly, and it affects both sexes.

Signs and symptoms

These can include:
- Mouth ulcers
- Sore throat
- Blisters
- Erosions on the skin and mucous membranes
- Pain where any lesions develop
- Burning sensation at the site of any lesions
- Dehydration
- Malnutrition
- Infection.

See Fig. 26.22 for examples of pemphigus vulgaris.

Treatment

It is essential if the treatment is to be effective that a detailed physical assessment is undertaken, as well as patient history, prior to deciding upon and commencing treatment.
- Oral prednisolone in high doses
- Immunosuppressant agents
- Intravenous fluids
- Antibiotics if infection present.

> **! HOTSPOT**
>
> Due to the severity of this illness, the patient will initially be nursed in a critical care unit.

THE MEDICINE TROLLEY 26.5

Drug	Drug classification	Reason for administration	Route of administration	Dose	Side effects	Contraindications	Nursing care
Imidazole (clotrimoxazole)	Antifungal	To relieve itch and kill skin fungi	Topical	2–3 times a day	Mild irritation, redness and itch	Discuss with doctor patient if is breast feeding or pregnant	Gain consent prior to administration
Terbinafine (Lamisil)				Once or twice a day for 2–4 weeks		Any allergies to this or similar treatments	Explain the use of the treatment prior to application and answer any questions
Selenium sulphide (Selsun shampoo)				Once a day for 5–7 days		Children under 5 should not use this treatment Do not apply to broken or irritated skin	Advise on potential side effects
Ketoconazole shampoo (Nizoral)				2%, once a day for maximum of 5 days		Do not apply to broken or irritated skin	Always wash hands after application
Itraconazole (Sporanox)			Oral	Usually 200 mg daily for 7 days	Heart failure Liver and kidney problems Allergic reactions	Heart failure Liver and kidney problems Allergy to this or similar medications Pregnancy and breast feeding	Gain consent prior to administration Explain the use of the treatment prior to application and answer any questions Advise on potential side effects and need to report if any occur Advise on importance of review and blood testing whilst on and after taking this medication

CRITICAL AWARENESS

Topical Corticosteroids

Topical corticosteroids (steroids) are medications that are applied directly to the skin and are used to reduce inflammation and irritation. Topical corticosteroids are available in several different forms, including:

- Creams
- Lotions
- Gels
- Mousses
- Ointments

They are also available in four different potencies (strengths):

- Mild
- Moderate
- Potent
- Very potent

Mild corticosteroids, such as hydrocortisone, can often be bought over the counter from pharmacies; however, the stronger types are only available on prescription.

There are other medications that can be used and all require very careful monitoring.

! HOTSPOT

The Nursing Associate should ensure that the patient is aware of the risks of long-term use and that this may raise the chance of developing a cancer.

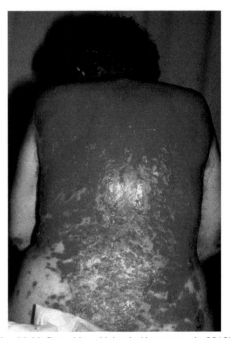

Fig. 26.22 Pemphigus Vulgaris (James et al., 2018).

THE MEDICINE TROLLEY 26.6

Drug	Drug classification	Reason for administration	Route of administration	Dose	Side effect	Contraindications	Nursing care
Prednisolone	Corticosteroid	Reduce and prevent inflammation	Oral	1–2 mg/kg, reduced slowly over 4–6 weeks when blisters have stopped developing	Reduces immune system Raises glucose levels in diabetic patients Weight gain Mood swings	Active fungal infections Inform doctor if diabetic or suffering from any pre-existing condition such as diabetes, ulcers, liver disease. Hypertension and pregnancy	Gain consent prior to administration Explain the use of the treatment prior to application and answer any questions Advise on potential side effects and need to report if any occur Advise on importance of review whilst taking this medication
Azathioprine (Imuran)	Immunosuppressant		Oral or intravenous	1–3 mg/kg of body weight taken daily	Allergic reaction Infections Bleeding Liver damage, pancreatitis, chest pain, upset stomach, cancer	Allergy to ingredients Allergy to other substances Pregnancy and breastfeeding	Gain consent prior to administration Explain the use of the treatment prior to application and answer any questions Advise on potential side effects and need to report if any occur Advise on importance of blood testing whilst taking this medication Advise on importance of contraception as medications harms the unborn child

Bullous pemphigoid

This condition is more common than pemphigus vulgaris and the majority of patients are over 60 years of age. It often initially presents as an eczematous area with itch and the bullae present later. They may occur, rarely, in the mouth but predominately appear on the arms, legs, hands and feet.

Signs and symptoms

These will include:
- Itchy skin prior to the appearance of bullae
- Rash on the skin prior to the appearance of bullae
- Bullae on the skin
- The bullae may be filled with blood
- Varied size.

See Fig. 26.23.

Treatment

Treatment is generally the administration of oral (systemic) medications. Treatment options include:
- Oral steroids
- Doxycycline
- Immunosuppressants.

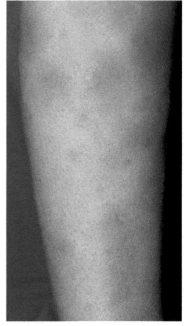

Fig. 26.23 Bullous Pemphigoid (James et al., 2018).

THE MEDICINE TROLLEY 26.7

Drug	Drug classification	Reason for administration	Route of administration	Dose	Side effects	Contraindications	Nursing care
Doxycycline	Antibiotic	To fight infection	Oral	200–300 mg daily	Nausea, vomiting Diarrhoea Allergic reaction Chest pain Vaginal itching or discharge	Allergy to tetracycline Pregnancy Breast feeding	Gain consent prior to administration Explain the use of the treatment prior to administration and answer any questions Advise on potential side effects and need to report if any occur Advise not to get pregnant and that it can affect oral contraceptives

> **! HOTSPOT**
>
> This condition is usually treated with oral steroids, as it is usually less severe than pemphigus vulgaris. It usually responds well to treatment.

Urticaria

There are several forms of urticaria, which is the development of weals (commonly known as hives). These are raised swellings in the skin that disappear, leaving no physical sign.

Signs and symptoms

- Itchy weals
- Stinging
- Presentation of singular weal
- Multiple weals
- Different sizes and shapes of weals

Angioedema may also develop; signs and symptoms of angioedema can include:

- Swelling of the lips
- Swelling of the eyes
- Swelling of the tongue.

> **! HOTSPOT**
>
> Urticaria and angioedema may indicate an anaphylactic reaction to a known or unknown allergy.

Types of urticaria

- Acute (less than 6 weeks)
- Chronic (more than 6 weeks)
- Hereditary
- Physical

Physical urticaria can be triggered by:

- Scratching
- Pressure
- Sweating
- Cold
- Water

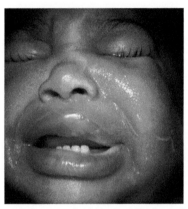

Fig. 26.24 Urticaria (Courtesy Paul Honig, MD. From James et al., 2018).

- Sunlight
- Heat

See Fig. 26.24 for an example of urticaria.

Treatment

Treatment will vary according to the type and length of time present, as well as the severity. In general, acute and chronic urticaria responds to antihistamines, although these may have to be administered in ever increasing doses and taken for a long period of time. If resistant to the antihistamines, other medication can be added, and if an anaphylactic reaction is suspected, adrenaline will be required. Many people also get some relief from using emollient therapies.

SKIN LESIONS

Benign skin lesions

Lentigo

These lesions may be singular or multiple and may occur on any part of the body, at any age; in the elderly, they are more common on sun-exposed areas and are known as solar lentigines. These lesions are small (1–3 mm) and are caused by an increase in melanocytes in the basal layer of the skin. (Schofield and Kneebone, 2006) (see Fig. 26.25).

THE MEDICINE TROLLEY 26.8

Drug	Drug classification	Reason for administration	Route of administration	Dose	Side effects	Contraindications	Nursing care
Fexofenadine	Antihistamine	To treat and prevent formation of hives Relieve signs of allergies	Oral	Varies from 120 mg daily up to 360 mg 3 times a day in severe cases (This is higher than the recommend British National Formulary and at this dose can only be prescribed by a dermatologist)	Allergic reactor Headache Vomiting Palpitations Dry mouth In some people initially may cause drowsiness	Allergies to properties Pregnancy and breast feeding (discuss with doctor) Over 65 Regular consumption of grapefruit or its juices	Gain consent prior to administration Explain the use of the treatment prior to administration and answer any questions Advise on potential side effects and need to report if any occur Inform not to take at same time as antacids

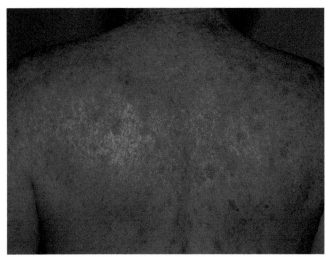

Fig. 26.25 Lentigo (GHA, 2017; Dermatology photographic database).

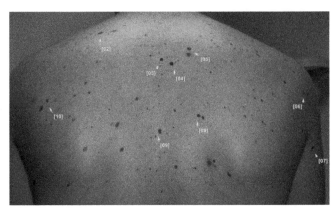

Fig. 26.26 Melanoma (GHA, 2017; Dermatology photographic database).

Atypical mole syndrome (multiple atypical melanocytic naevi)

These pigmented lesions are commonly referred to as moles but the correct term is naevus (singular) or naevi (multiple). When there are multiple naevi of varied shape and size, this is known as atypical mole syndrome or multiple atypical melanocytic naevi. Patients who have this should be seen by a dermatologist or by one of the dermatology team because there is a higher chance of developing a melanoma (see Fig. 26.26).

Blue naevus

A blue naevus is usually singular and usually develops in childhood or early adulthood. They are small (less than 1 cm in diameter) and are slightly raised. They have a blue/grey pigment.

Basal cell papilloma (seborrhoeic keratosis)

These lesions are common to both sexes and tend to develop at around 50 years of age. They are ovoid in shape, raised, crusty and thicken with time. They have a varied colour, ranging from a silver-grey to black. At times parts of them flake off and the

area sometimes bleeds if they catch on clothing or bedding. They can be itchy and most people complain that they are unsightly. They vary in size from millimetres to 3 cm.

Viral warts

Viral warts are caused by becoming infected with the human papilloma virus (HPV). The only exception to this is molluscum contagiosum, which is caused by the pox virus. They can occur anywhere on the body and for most people they are unsightly; if on the feet, they can be painful.

They do tend to resolve spontaneously, between 3 and 6 months, but in some people it can be years before they develop an appropriate immunological response. This is usually the reason why people seek treatment.

Treatment
- Leave alone, as most resolve within a few months
- Salicylic acid topically, in conjunction with regular paring and occlusion
- Salicylic acid in combination with cryotherapy

> **❗ HOTSPOT**
>
> It is important to remember that salicylic acid should not be used on the face and genital warts should be treated only under medical supervision.

See Fig. 26.27, a viral wart.

Molluscum contagiosum

Molluscum are caused by infection from the pox virus. The lesions are small, shiny, white or pink, round, slightly raised and grow slowly. They can be itchy and can develop eczematous patches around them. The incubation period is 2 to 6 weeks and they clear in 6 to 9 months. Some may leave small depressed scars (see Fig. 26.28).

Treatment
- Leave alone, as they will resolve.
- If multiple and large they can be treated with salicylic acid or cryotherapy.
- Due to pain caused by treatments it is not recommended to treat children.

Skin tag (acrochordon)

These are outgrowths of skin that occur in the flexures, around the neck, under arms, under breasts and groin area. They are more common in obese people and the incidence is higher in women than men. There also appears to be a familial factor. They are pigmented pedunculated papules and are soft to touch. They catch on clothing and jewellery and are unsightly. Fig. 26.29 provides an example of a skin tag.

Treatment
- Cryotherapy
- Hyfrecation
- Snip off with small scissors

The choice of treatment will depend on the size.

Dermatofibroma (histiocytoma)

This is a fibrous nodule, commonly thought to be caused by an abnormal reaction to an insect bite. On touch, it feels as if there is a pea-like growth under the skin. Most people complain that it is itchy. Some are flesh coloured and others are pigmented.

Treatment
- Leave alone
- If bothersome remove via ellipse excision

Many of these lesions occur on the lower leg, so caution should be taken before choosing to remove as healing is poor in this area.

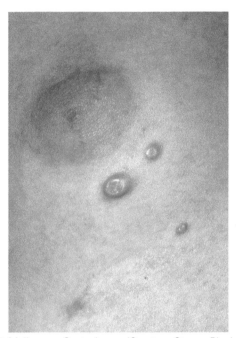

Fig. 26.28 Molluscum Contagiosum (Courtesy Steven Binnick, MD. From James et al., 2018).

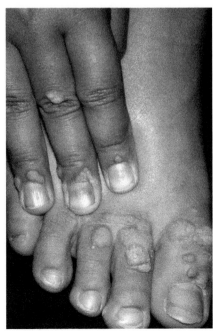

Fig. 26.27 A Viral Wart (Courtesy Scott Norton, MD. From James et al., 2018).

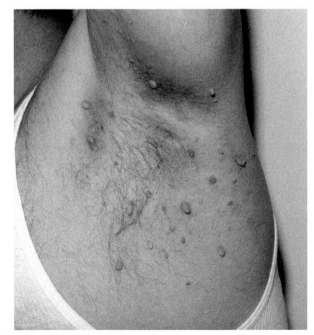

Fig. 26.29 Skin Tag (Courtesy Steven Binnick, MD. From James et al., 2018).

Campbell de Morgan spots

These are very common in middle-aged and elderly people and are caused by an increase of blood vessels in the upper part of the dermis. They are small red spots that grow up to 5 mm. People that develop these usually have multiple lesions and will often develop further lesions in time (see Fig. 26.30).

Treatment

* Leave untreated

Pyogenic granuloma

This is also caused by an increase of blood vessels in the dermis. They usually grow rapidly and many patients can relate it to an injury that occurred within a few weeks of the lesion developing. They are bright red, very vascular, can grow up to 10 cm and bleed easily (see Fig. 26.31).

Treatment

* Curettage and cautery

The histology report will always be checked by the appropriate professionals, as the differential diagnosis is an amelanotic malignant melanoma (Weller et al., 2012). This will not be the responsibility of the Nursing Associate but knowing the diagnosis will be helpful in recognizing the importance of reporting any similar lesions in the future.

Chondrodermatitis nodularis helices

This is an inflammation of the cartilage of the pinna. It is more common in men, but does affect some women. It is a painful nodule that develops on the upper part of the helix, usually on the side the patient sleeps most on. Size is usually between 0.5 mm and 1 cm (see Fig. 26.32).

Treatment

* Cover with a soft dressing or corn plaster
* Surgically excise

Premalignant lesions
Solar keratosis

These lesions are also known as actinic keratosis and develop in sun-exposed areas of the skin (for example, face, head, neck, hands and arms). They are most common in the elderly and in fair-skinned people. Although these are benign, there is the possibility that they may become malignant and as a result, treating them is important (see Fig. 26.33).

Signs and symptoms

* Small scaly patches of skin
* Pink patches of skin before development of, or around the scale
* Usually multiple areas of skin affected

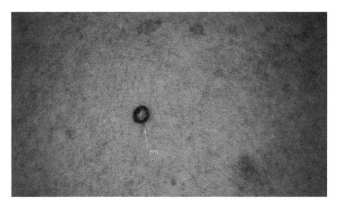

Fig. 26.30 Campbell De Morgan Spots (GHA, 2017; Dermatology photographic database).

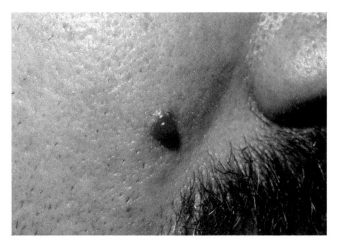

Fig. 26.31 Pyogenic Granuloma (Courtesy Steven Binnick, MD. From James et al., 2018).

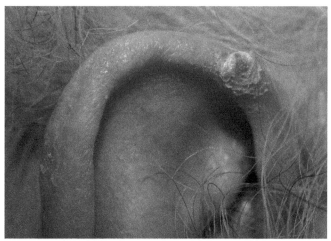

Fig. 26.32 Chondrodermatitis Nodularis Helicis (James et al., 2018).

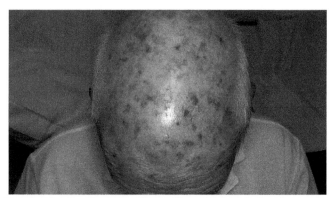

Fig. 26.33 Solar Keratosis (GHA, 2017; Dermatology photographic database).

- Usually small in size, less than 1.5 cm in diameter
- Sometimes itchy at the site of the lesion

Treatment. As these lesions can become malignant, it is essential that a detailed patient history and physical examination are undertaken. If there is uncertainty about diagnosis, a referral must be made and the local referral pathways must be adhered to.

- Can be left alone and observed
- Offer the person sun protection advice, such as using UV-light protection sunscreen creams, wearing a hat, covering skin with light-weight clothing and avoiding the sun between 11 a.m. and 4 p.m.
- Topical therapy of a non-steroidal anti-inflammatory
- Cryotherapy
- Curettage and cautery

Bowen's disease/squamous cell carcinoma (SCC) in situ

Bowen's disease is an SCC in situ, which can become invasive, although this is rare. It is most commonly found on the legs of older women but can also develop in men. It is usually found on sun-exposed sites, such as legs, arms and upper back but can be found in non-sun-exposed areas, such as the lower back (see Fig. 26.34).

Signs and symptoms. These include:

- Red patches of skin
- Scaly patches of skin
- Usually solitary lesions
- Can have multiple lesions
- Can be mistaken for eczema.

Treatment. A referral should be made if a patient presents with Bowen's disease. Treatment options include:

- Biopsy of the lesion
- Excision
- Curettage
- Cryotherapy
- Topical treatments, such as cytotoxic agents.

- Photo dynamic therapy. This is where a light-sensitive cream is applied to the lesion and left for 3 to 6 hours, then a special light is applied at a special wavelength to activate the cream and destroy damaged skin cells
- Radiotherapy

> **! HOTSPOT**
>
> Treatment will be determined by site, size and age of patient.

> **! HOTSPOT**
>
> The Nursing Associate should inform senior staff if the patient becomes too excoriated or is in too much pain during treatment.

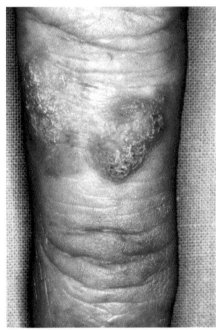

Fig. 26.34 Bowen's Disease (James et al., 2018).

THE MEDICINE TROLLEY 26.9

Drug	Drug classification	Reason for application	Route of administration	Dose	Side effects	Contraindications	Nursing care
Solaraze (Diclofenac)	Non-steroidal anti-inflammatory	To reduce inflammation	Topical	Twice a day for 2–3 months	Burning sensation Redness Itching Allergic reactions	Pregnant or breastfeeding Asthma or allergies Other skin disorders Allergy to similar products	Gain consent prior to administration Explain the use of the treatment prior to application and answer any questions Advise on potential side effects Always wash hands after application Do not cover with a dressing unless advised by doctor Use fingertip rule to ensure appropriate amount is applied

THE MEDICINE TROLLEY 26.10

Drug	Drug classification	Reason for administration	Route of administration	Dose	Side effects	Contraindications	Nursing care
Efudix (5-Fluorouracil)	Cytotoxic agent	To destroy sun damaged skin cells	Topical	Once to twice a day for 3–4 weeks	Inflammation Redness Pain Oozing Crusts Scabs	Pregnancy and breastfeeding Allergy to ingredients	Gain consent prior to administration Explain the use of the treatment prior to application and answer any questions Advise on potential side effects Clean area prior to application Always wash hands after application Do not cover with a dressing unless advised by doctor Use fingertip rule to ensure appropriate amount is applied
Aldara (Imiquimod)	Immune response modifier	To destroy sun damaged skin cells		Five times weekly for 6 weeks			

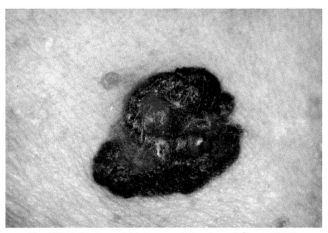

Fig. 26.35 Malignant Melanoma (Waugh and Grant, 2018).

Malignant lesions

Melanoma

This is a type of skin cancer that can spread to other organs and cause secondary cancers, such as breast cancer or cancer of the lung. For the general population, it is the most frightening of all skin cancers. There are several signs and symptoms that are associated with melanoma. If the Nursing Associate understands what these are, they can assist people in a more meaningful and effective manner. Please see Fig. 26.35.

Signs and symptoms

- A new naevus (commonly known as a mole)
- A changing existing naevus
- Melanoma usually occurs on sun-exposed areas
- Change in size
- Irregular shape
- Irregular colour
- Largest diameter ≥ 7 mm
- Inflammation
- Oozing
- Change in sensation

Treatment. The patent must be referred using the appropriate suspected cancer care pathway, which was originally introduced by the National Institute for Health and Care Excellence (NICE, 2005) and was updated in 2017 (NICE, 2017). The pathway establishes that a referral must be made within 1 working day if cancer is suspected and the patient must be seen within 2 weeks of the referral being sent. It also establishes that support must be offered whilst waiting for the appointment. This will consist of explaining to the patient that they are being referred to cancer services and alternative diagnostics, as well as what tests may be done and what to expect from the service.

> **! HOTSPOT**
>
> Ellipse excision will be the treatment of choice if there is any suspicion of melanoma.

Types of excision

- Ellipse excision (this is where an eye-shaped cut around the lesion is made with a predetermined margin, usually 2 mm for melanoma, and the length is three times the width).
- Linear (this is where a straight singular cut is made in line with the skin).
- Shave excision (this is where a lesion is sliced off using a flat blade).
- Snip excision (very small lesions can be cut off with a small pair of scissors).

Superficial spreading melanoma

This is usually a slow-growing lesion that mostly develops on the skin of older people. They are usually very thin and spread outwards. Melanoma pathology (2014) tells us that this type, if caught early, is a low-risk melanoma. However, if this is allowed to grow into a thicker lesion, the prognosis is poor.

Signs and symptoms
- Usually occurs on sun-exposed areas
- Slowly changing in size
- Irregular shape
- Irregular colour
- Largest diameter ≥ 7 mm
- May itch

   Treatment. Referral is made using the appropriate cancer care pathway. These are detailed by NICE (2017).

> **⚠ HOTSPOT**
>
> Ellipse excision will be the treatment of choice if there is a suspicion of melanoma. Sometimes, due to the size or site, plastic surgery may also be required.

Ulcerated basal cell carcinoma

This skin cancer is related to sun exposure and develops on areas of skin most exposed, such as the face, scalp, upper chest and arms (see Fig. 26.36).

   Signs and symptoms. The signs and symptoms include:
- Nodular
- Ulcerated
- May appear cystic
- Telangiectasia
- Crust
- Bleeding
- Itchy.

   Treatment. Referral is made using the appropriate cancer care pathway (NICE, 2017).

> **⚠ HOTSPOT**
>
> An ellipse excision is the usual treatment of choice but, depending on size, site and age of patient, the treatment choice could also be Mohs micrographic surgery (here the lesion is taken away after primary removal in slices, which are frozen and examined under a microscope until the lesion is completely excised). This is usually done on the face, where there is limited tissue to cut through.

Invasive SCC

These lesions are also connected to sun exposure. However, smoking is a contributing factor for lip and mouth cancers (see Fig. 26.37), as is contact with the HPV virus. This virus can also cause SCCs in the genital area. People who have had organ transplants and who take immunosuppressant medications have a higher chance of developing invasive SCCs. As these lesions may metastasize (spread) to the lymph nodes and then to the internal organs such as the liver, they must be treated as urgent when suspected. The Nursing Associate must be familiar with potential signs and symptoms and report any concerns.

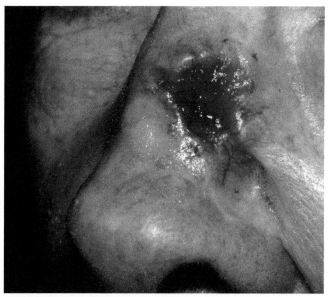

Fig. 26.36 Ulcerated Basal Cell Carcinoma (Courtesy Steven Binnick, MD. From James et al., 2018).

TABLE 26.1 The Weighted Seven-Point Checklist (NICE, 2017)

Feature	Characteristic	Score
Major features of the lesions (scoring 2 points each)	• Change in size • Irregular shape • Irregular colour	
Minor features of the lesion (scoring 2 points each)	• Largest diameter ≥ 7 mm • Inflammation • Oozing • Change in sensation	
Total		

Signs and symptoms
- Keratotic (scaly or flaky patch of skin)
- Pain (at site of lesion)
- Bleeding (on or around lesion)
- Ulceration (on or around lesion)

   Treatment. Refer through the appropriate cancer care pathway (NICE, 2017).

Weighted seven-point checklist

The purpose of this checklist is for a score to be assigned for each of the following features. If the score for the lesion is 4 or more, the lesion must be referred using the 2-week cancer referral guidelines recommended by NICE (2017). See Table 26.1 for an overview of the weighted seven-point checklist.

   NICE (2017) recommends that this checklist is used to assist in diagnosing lesions that are required to be referred urgently through the suspected cancer care pathway.

> **⚠ HOTSPOT**
>
> As a Nursing Associate you will not be expected to make a diagnosis but becoming familiar with the different types of lesions and how to describe them will assist the staff in recognizing when to refer on to the appropriate professional. The weighted seven-point checklist (see Table 26.1) is a particularly helpful tool used for guidance on the important factors to look out for.

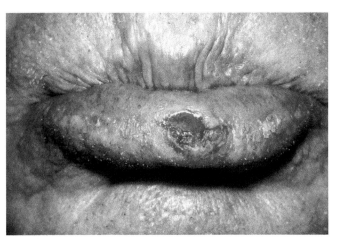

Fig. 26.37 Invasive Squamous Cell Carcinoma (James et al., 2018).

PSYCHOLOGICAL IMPACT OF A SKIN CONDITION ON AN INDIVIDUAL

Few dermatology books look at how a skin condition can affect an individual psychologically but having an understanding of it can help the Nursing Associate approach the service user with care and compassion. The appropriate approach would include attention to the 6Cs:

1. Courage
2. Compassion
3. Competence
4. Communication
5. Care
6. Commitment

The way people react to things in life varies; the same occurs in regards to skin conditions. For some, a small acne spot could mean they are now ugly and for others, a large patch of psoriasis is no bother. Taking this into account, the Nursing Associate must provide holistic care that is patient-centred, ensuring that the patient is at the centre of all that is done.

Skin is the largest organ of the body and it is a 'living biological barrier' (Buxton, 2003) that protects us. It is also the part of us that the world sees. When caring for a person with a skin condition, take into account the individual's perspective of how this is going to affect them and listen to their concerns with compassion and empathy.

REFLECTION 26.1

As part of reflective practice it is valuable to think back at how some things have affected you emotionally in your life. Think how you felt and whether it was proportionate to what was happening. Now think if it had been handled in a different manner, would you have reacted differently? Now, using this, think how you would feel if you had a skin condition or the fear of a skin cancer. How would you like someone to treat you?

It is important to remember that people who use healthcare services need to trust you; they look at the Nursing Associate to be their advocate, as often other professionals are too busy to spend time conversing. The client develops fears of how they look, fears about the possibility of scarring and fears of having a life-threatening disease or cancer. They are also frightened of cross-contamination and this often affects their physical relationships and social relationships. They often isolate themselves from others and can develop depression and anxiety.

The Nursing Associate is in a unique position where they can spend time getting to know these fears, as patients often confide in the front-line workers, who are more easily accessible. They, in turn, can inform their line managers, who can make time available to discuss these fears further and reassure the client in a realistic manner.

CRITICAL AWARENESS
Patient-Centred Care

Any aspect of treatment and care should take into account individual needs and preferences. Patients should be provided with the opportunity to make informed decisions about their care and treatment and they can do this in partnership with those who provide health care. Chapter 5 of this text addresses important issues, such as consent and capacity.

Healthcare teams (Nursing Associates, specialist dermatology nurses and doctors) must work jointly to provide assessment and services to people with suspected or diagnosed skin conditions. Diagnosis, care and management should be reviewed on an ongoing basis.

CASE STUDY 26.1   Alison

Alison Jenks is a 23-year-old woman training to become a Nursing Associate. Ali has been suffering from severe acne on her face and back for the past 7 years. A referral to a dermatology nurse specialist has been made. Past medical history: Ali has acne; she tells the GP she has been low in mood for 2 years, despite being overjoyed to be accepted as a trainee Nursing Associate. It is clear that she is upset with the acne and the way she looks and feels. She tells the nurse that the acne has really been getting her down.

There is no family history to note. Ali is taking the oral contraceptive pill and she has used topical benzoyl peroxide but she has stopped using this.

Ali lives with friends in a flat share; she does not smoke and informs the nurse that she is a moderate drinker. She denies the use of any recreational drugs. The acne is negatively impacting on her social life; she was seeing a man for around 1 year, but the relationship did not last and Ali has put this down to the acne.

Alison reports feeling depressed; she believes that this is linked to the appearance and discomfort of her acne. Recently, the severity of her symptoms has worsened and the acne is more difficult to cover with makeup. Because of this, she is going out less and this is having a negative impact on her social life and studies; she blames this for the relationship breakup with her boyfriend. She tells the nurse that sometimes she does not even want to go to work. She has become tearful as she thinks there no way out of this.

She says a previous face cream had caused redness and itching of her skin (this was the benzoyl peroxide), and that this redness was almost as unsightly as the acne. She would like the acne gone, or to be reduced as much as possible, without scarring.

LOOKING BACK, FEEDING FORWARD

In order to provide people who experience skin conditions (dermatological conditions) with care that is compassionate and, above all, effective, the Nursing Associate must ensure that they have a good understanding of the anatomy and physiology of the skin. They also need to have fundamental understanding of dermatological vocabulary, some of the more common skin conditions and the common treatment options that are available. All of this has to be underpinned by a sound evidence base, ensuring care is safe and truly patient-centred.

This chapter has provided a brief overview of some common skin conditions. It is not possible in a chapter of this size to address all skin conditions. The Nursing Associate is encouraged to delve deep into this fascinating subject area and to develop their knowledge base. The skin is the largest organ of the body; therefore any negative impact on this organ has the potential to impact negatively on a patient's health and well-being. The Nursing Associate is ideally placed to assist people who are experiencing issues with their skin, as they provide care that is empathic and compassionate.

REFERENCES

Buxton, P., 2003. ABC of Dermatology, fourth ed. British Medical Journal Publishing Group, London, Tavistock Square.

GHA, 2017. Gibraltar Health Authority dermatology database.

Graham-Brown, R., Harman, K., Johnston, G., 2017. Dermatology; Lecture Notes, eleventh ed. Wiley and Sons, Sussex, U.K.

Henderson, R., 2017. Fingertip units for topical steroids. Available at https://patient.info/health/fingertip-units-for-topical-steroids.

James, W.D., Elston, D., McMahon, P.J., 2018. Andrews' Diseases of the Skin: Clinical Atlas, first ed. Elsevier, Oxford.

NICE, 2005. National Institute for Health and Clinical Excellence. Guidance on cancer services. Referral guidelines for suspected cancer. Available at https://www.nice.org.uk/guidance.

NICE, 2017. National Institute for Health and Care Excellence. Guidance on cancer services. Melanoma and pigmented lesions. Available at https://www.nice.org.uk/guidance/ng12.

Schofield, J., Kneebone, R., 2006. Skin Lesions: A Practical Guide to Diagnosis, Management and Minor Surgery, second ed. Metro Commercial Printing, U.K.

Waugh, A., Grant, A., 2018. Ross and Wilson Anatomy and Physiology in Health and Illness, thirteenth ed. Elsevier, Edinburgh.

Weller, R., Hunter, J., Savin, J., Dahl, M., 2012. Clinical Dermatology, fourth ed. Blackwell Publishing, Australia.

27

Immunity

Janet G. Migliozzi

OBJECTIVES

By the end of the chapter the reader will:
1. Have an understanding of the anatomy and physiology of the human immune system
2. Describe some common conditions associated with the immune system
3. Review the role of the Nursing Associate in promoting health and well-being
4. Have an understanding of the care of a patient with an immune disorder

KEY WORDS

Pathogen

Innate immunity

Antigen

Memory cells

Antibody

Lymph node

Inflammation

Autoimmune

Defence

Adaptive immunity

CHAPTER AIMS

The primary function of the human immune system is to defend the body from foreign invasion by disease-producing pathogens, such as bacteria and viruses. The aim of this chapter is to provide the reader with an understanding of the skills, knowledge and attitude required to provide safe, effective and compassionate care to people with an immune disorder.

SELF TEST

1. What are the two divisions of the human immune system?
2. How do vaccines work?
3. What are the cardinal signs of inflammation?
4. What is an antibody?
5. What is histamine?
6. What is an autoimmune disorder?
7. What is an allergy?
8. What is urticaria?
9. What is the function of a T lymphocyte?
10. What is lymph?

INTRODUCTION

In this chapter, the immune system is considered, and it is important for the Nursing Associate (NA) to have a comprehensive understanding of the immune system if the care provided to patients with an immune disorder is to be appropriate and effective.

The first part of the chapter discusses the anatomy and physiology of the immune system. The second part of the chapter addresses a selection of common conditions that impact on the health and well-being of the individual, and the care and comfort of the patient who experiences an immune disorder are described.

Many different organs and systems work to keep us alive and healthy, in an external environment that contains a variety of hazards to health. These include not only physical hazards (e.g., poisonous chemicals and sharp objects) but also disease-producing microorganisms, also known as pathogens (e.g., bacteria, viruses and fungi) that can cause inflammation and infection. The immune system, in collaboration with the lymphatic system, provides defence against threats to health and plays a major role in the prevention of disease in man.

THE IMMUNE SYSTEM

The primary function of the immune system is to provide the human body with a defence system that is able to recognize and respond to injury or a wide variety of pathogens. The immune system consists of all the cells, tissues and organs required for an immune response and is divided into the innate/non-specific system and adaptive/specific system, which can be further divided into first-line, second-line and third-line defences. The first- and second-line defences are provided by the innate/non-specific

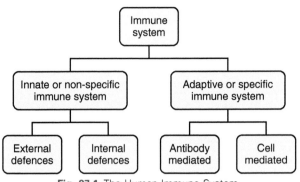

Fig. 27.1 The Human Immune System.

TABLE 27.1	Type of Leucocyte and Mode of Action
Type of leucocyte	Mode of action
Monocytes	Become macrophages and engulf foreign cells/materials
Neutrophils	Attack and kill bacteria and fungi
Eosinophils	Kill parasites
Basophils	Release histamines during allergic reactions

system and the body's third line of defence is provided by the adaptive/specific system (Fig. 27.1).

The innate or non-specific immune system

The innate or non-specific immune system is present from birth and provides general protection against any foreign agent that enters the body.

External defences

The body's first line of defence against foreign invasion is provided through its own physical barriers, which include:
1. The skin: intact skin is the body's primary defence, as it not only provides a physical barrier but also produces chemical barriers to infection. Secretions such as saliva, sweat, tears, stomach acid and oil (sebum) contain chemicals that either destroy or inhibit foreign invaders.
2. The mucous membranes: these are structures that line the passages that open to the outside of the body. The mucous membranes form a barrier against invasion by foreign invaders, by producing mucus which can trap foreign material.
3. Cilia, hairs: these structures are commonly found in the respiratory tract where they help to remove debris and impurities trapped in mucous.

Internal defences

If the external defences are not able to prevent invasion into the body and a pathogen is able to breach the body's physical barriers, then additional internal responses are provided, which include:
- Lysosome, which is contained in tears and saliva
- Gastric acid in the stomach.

White blood cells/leucocytes

The body's innate or non-specific immune system provides a fast, general response to an invading pathogen. It cannot memorize this response, hence repeated exposure to the same pathogen will produce exactly the same response as the first time the pathogen was encountered. Therefore, if an invader is able to bypass the body's physical barrier and enter the body, the white blood cells (leucocytes) are released into the circulation and are responsible for defending the body from invasion. They achieve this by travelling to the invader and undertaking a process known as phagocytosis, to engulf and ingest pathogens or other foreign material. Table 27.1 lists the different types of leucocytes and the role they play in the body's defence.

Natural killer cells

Natural killer (NK) cells: these are found throughout the body and are non-specific in action. They are capable of destroying a variety of foreign cells and also abnormal/altered self-cells (e.g., cancer cells). NK cells 'patrol' the body looking for abnormal cells and directly attack foreign cells.

Mediator cells

A second group of cells of the innate immune system (the basophils and mast cells) are more accurately described as the helper cells of the immune system. They do not actually destroy the invading microorganisms by phagocytosis, but they help the phagocytes to do so. These mediator cells work by releasing various chemicals that have several actions. For example, some of these chemicals improve the inflammatory response to infection and injury, whilst others help the phagocytic cells to reach the microorganisms.

Inflammation

Inflammation is the body's protective tissue response to injury or invasion by foreign invaders and the signs and symptoms include redness, heat, swelling and pain. The purpose of the inflammatory response is:
- Neutralize and destroy harmful agents
- Limit/slow down the spread of foreign invaders to other tissues in the body
- Prepare damaged tissue for repair and regeneration (Williams, 2018).

The process of inflammation (Fig. 27.2) commences with dilatation of the capillaries surrounding the affected area. This allows white and red blood cells to move out from the blood vessels into the tissue. The capillaries also release fibrin, which forms a protective mesh to prevent foreign invaders from spreading further into the tissues. During inflammation, mast cells release histamine and serotonin and this results in localized swelling and pain to the affected area. The release of histamine also paves the way for the repair of the injured tissue. As inflammation continues, dead cells and debris accumulate at the injury site, causing a collection of pus.

Fever

A raised temperature (above 37.2°C), or fever, is a natural protective mechanism and can be a sign that the body is trying to defend itself as it assists the immune system, by inhibiting the growth of pathogens and also stimulating phagocytosis. Within

Local inflammation

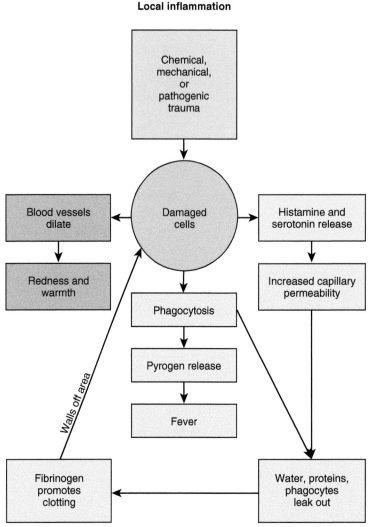

Fig. 27.2 The Inflammatory Response (Williams, 2018).

limits, this raise in body temperature may be beneficial, as it also increases the rate of metabolism and allows for cells and enzymes to act more quickly. In addition, when the phagocytes find and destroy foreign invaders, they release substances known as pyrogens that can reset the body's thermostat (hypothalamus) and raise the body temperature to allow the increase metabolic activity to continue (Zelman et al., 2011).

> ### ❗ HOTSPOT
>
> #### *Sepsis*
> The prevention and recognition of sepsis is now key to the reduction of avoidable deaths in hospitals (Singer et al., 2016) and the early recognition of the signs and symptoms of sepsis is vital to patient survival. Sepsis is usually caused by bacterial, viral or fungal infections that lead to complex inflammatory responses, resulting in tissue injury and poor perfusion of vital organs (Singer et al., 2016).
>
> A systematic assessment of the patient is crucial in identifying the sepsis and ensuring appropriate interventions are commenced. The UK Sepsis Screening Tool (UK Sepsis Trust, 2016) (Fig. 27.3) should be used in conjunction with an early warning system to identify any suspicion of sepsis. Refer to Chapter 20 for information on early warning systems.

Interferons

Interferons are naturally occurring proteins that are produced by cells in response to viral infections. Interferons are released by the virus-infected cell and work by 'interfering' with cells near to the virus-infected cell. This leads to cellular changes occurring within the nearby healthy cells, which help to make them more resistant to the virus.

The complement system

The complement system is a collection of plasma proteins and enzymes in the body that become activated in the presence of a pathogen and assist in the immune response by:
- Attracting phagocytes to the site of invasion
- Enhancing phagocytosis through a process known as opsonization
- Damaging the cell walls of pathogens.

The adaptive or specific immune system

Specific immunity is connected to the body via the lymphatic system and provides the body's third line of defence to foreign invaders/pathogens. Whilst it does not respond to foreign

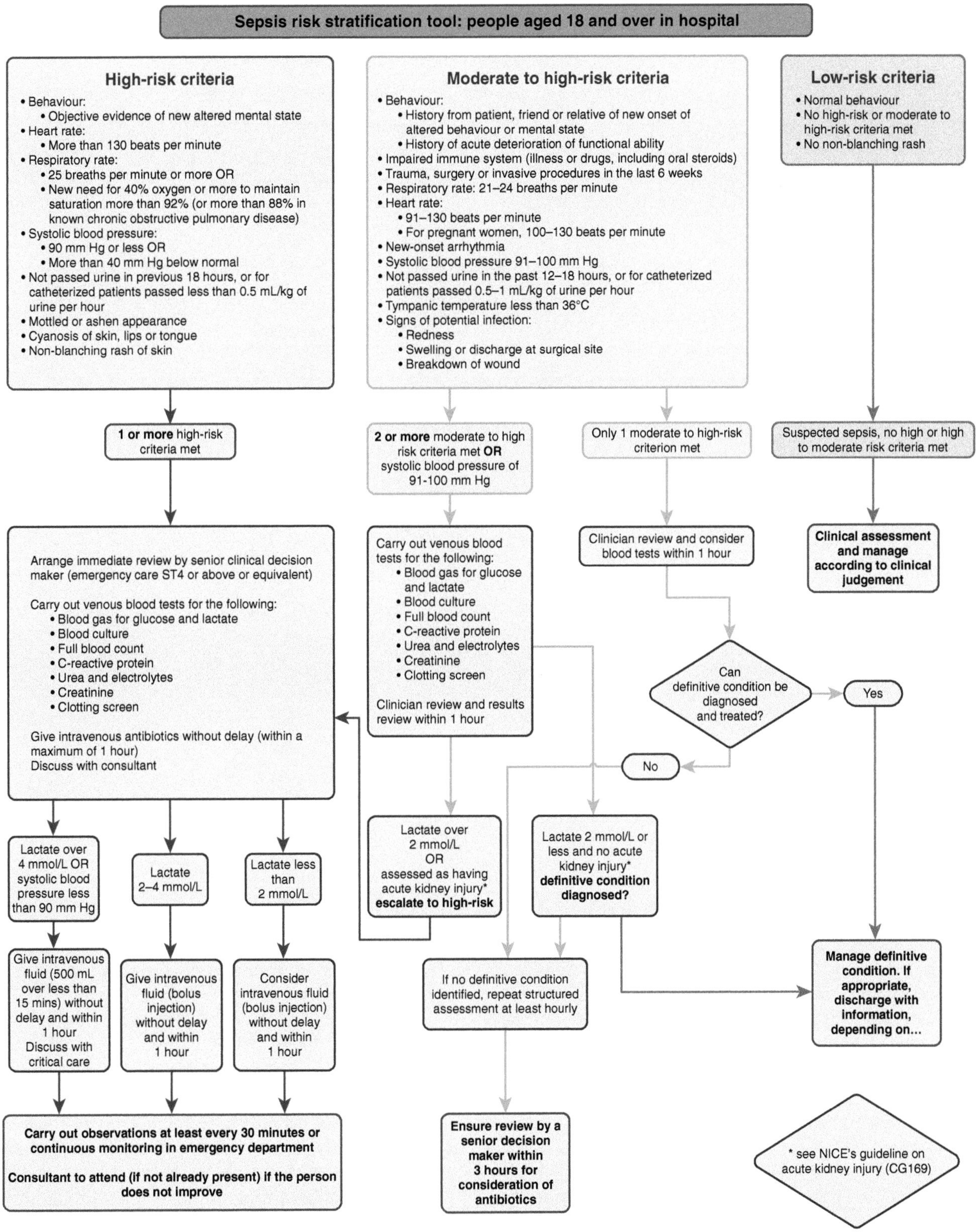

Sepsis risk stratification tool: people aged 18 and over in hospital

High-risk criteria

- Behaviour:
  - Objective evidence of new altered mental state
- Heart rate:
  - More than 130 beats per minute
- Respiratory rate:
  - 25 breaths per minute or more OR
  - New need for 40% oxygen or more to maintain saturation more than 92% (or more than 88% in known chronic obstructive pulmonary disease)
- Systolic blood pressure:
  - 90 mm Hg or less OR
  - More than 40 mm Hg below normal
- Not passed urine in previous 18 hours, or for catheterized patients passed less than 0.5 mL/kg of urine per hour
- Mottled or ashen appearance
- Cyanosis of skin, lips or tongue
- Non-blanching rash of skin

Moderate to high-risk criteria

- Behaviour:
  - History from patient, friend or relative of new onset of altered behaviour or mental state
  - History of acute deterioration of functional ability
- Impaired immune system (illness or drugs, including oral steroids)
- Trauma, surgery or invasive procedures in the last 6 weeks
- Respiratory rate: 21–24 breaths per minute
- Heart rate:
  - 91–130 beats per minute
  - For pregnant women, 100–130 beats per minute
- New-onset arrhythmia
- Systolic blood pressure 91–100 mm Hg
- Not passed urine in the past 12–18 hours, or for catheterized patients passed 0.5–1 mL/kg of urine per hour
- Tympanic temperature less than 36°C
- Signs of potential infection:
  - Redness
  - Swelling or discharge at surgical site
  - Breakdown of wound

Low-risk criteria

- Normal behaviour
- No high-risk or moderate to high-risk criteria met
- No non-blanching rash

---

1 or more high-risk criteria met

2 or more moderate to high risk criteria met **OR** systolic blood pressure of 91-100 mm Hg

Only 1 moderate to high-risk criterion met

Suspected sepsis, no high or high to moderate risk criteria met

---

Arrange immediate review by senior clinical decision maker (emergency care ST4 or above or equivalent)

Carry out venous blood tests for the following:
- Blood gas for glucose and lactate
- Blood culture
- Full blood count
- C-reactive protein
- Urea and electrolytes
- Creatinine
- Clotting screen

Give intravenous antibiotics without delay (within a maximum of 1 hour)
Discuss with consultant

Carry out venous blood tests for the following:
- Blood gas for glucose and lactate
- Blood culture
- Full blood count
- C-reactive protein
- Urea and electrolytes
- Creatinine
- Clotting screen

Clinician review and results review within 1 hour

Clinician review and consider blood tests within 1 hour

Clinical assessment and manage according to clinical judgement

Can definitive condition be diagnosed and treated?

Yes

No

Lactate over 4 mmol/L OR systolic blood pressure less than 90 mm Hg

Lactate 2–4 mmol/L

Lactate less than 2 mmol/L

Lactate over 2 mmol/L OR assessed as having acute kidney injury* **escalate to high-risk**

Lactate 2 mmol/L or less and no acute kidney injury* **definitive condition diagnosed?**

Give intravenous fluid (500 mL over less than 15 mins) without delay and within 1 hour
Discuss with critical care

Give intravenous fluid (bolus injection) without delay and within 1 hour

Consider intravenous fluid (bolus injection) without delay and within 1 hour

If no definitive condition identified, repeat structured assessment at least hourly

Manage definitive condition. If appropriate, discharge with information, depending on...

Carry out observations at least every 30 minutes or continuous monitoring in emergency department

Consultant to attend (if not already present) if the person does not improve

Ensure review by a senior decision maker within 3 hours for consideration of antibiotics

* see NICE's guideline on acute kidney injury (CG169)

Fig. 27.3 An Example of a Risk Stratification Tool for Adults Aged 18 and Over in Hospital (NICE, 2017).

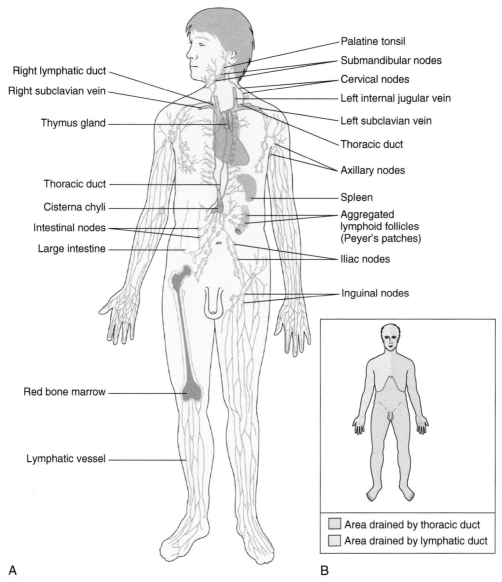

Fig. 27.4 The Lymphatic System (Waugh & Grant, 2018).

invasion as quickly as the innate system, it is able to provide a more targeted response to the invading pathogen through a specific response to an antigen. An antigen is a protein on the cell membrane of microbes, foreign cells or cancer cells that the body does not recognize as 'self'.

Lymphatic system

The lymphatic system plays a central role in maintaining health and includes all the cells, tissues and organs that are responsible for defending the body against pathogens (Fig. 27.4). The immune system consists of lymphoid organs and tissues, lymphocytes and other white blood cells and a significant number of chemicals that help the body to activate a response to destroy foreign material.

Functions of the lymphatic system

The lymphatic system has three interrelated functions:
1. Removal of fluid from tissues
2. Absorption and transportation of fats from the digestive tract to the circulation

3. Transportation of immune cells (lymphocytes) to and from the lymph nodes.

Structure of the lymphatic system

Organs and tissues of the lymphatic system include:
1. Tonsils: the tonsils and adenoids produce antibodies and lymphocytes to help protect the body from pathogens.
2. Lymph nodes: there are approximately 500–600 lymph nodes scattered throughout the body. These are small, oval-shaped structures located in clusters throughout the body, where they act as 'filters' to remove foreign substances from lymph fluid. These substances are then destroyed either by phagocytosis or by the T-lymphocytes (T-cells) of the immune system.
3. Thymus gland: the primary role of the thymus gland is to produce T-cells in the first few months/years of life. Following this, the gland begins to waste away and plays no further role in the immune system during adulthood.
4. Spleen: this is the largest mass of lymphoid tissue in the body and plays a similar filtering role to that of the lymph nodes.

However, instead of filtering lymph, the spleen filters the blood instead. The spleen is also involved in the removal and destruction of abnormal blood cells and components and initiates the responses of B- and T-cells to antigens in the circulating blood.

5. Peyer's patches: these are a cluster of lymph nodes found in the small bowel that provide protection against pathogens and prevent the absorption of toxins from the gastro-intestinal tract.
6. Appendix: the appendix is considered an accessory organ of the lymphatic system.

Bone marrow

The cells of the immune system start life as stem cells made in the bone marrow, from where they then migrate to the lymphoid tissue. Cells destined to become immune system cells can become lymphocytes and are further differentiated into B-cells or T-cells.

Lymphocytes

Specific immunity is dependent on two types of lymphocytes that can target antigen-bearing cells:

1. T-lymphocytes: although these originate in the bone marrow, they migrate to the thymus gland to mature. These kill pathogens and infected cells by direct attack on the foreign cell.
2. B-lymphocytes: these originate in the bone marrow and the main function of these cells is to produce antibodies against specific antigens.

Antibodies

Antibodies (also known as immunoglobulins), are proteins produced by plasma cells in response to foreign antigens and each antibody is specific for only one antigen. Whilst antibodies do not directly kill foreign cells, they mark them for destruction.

There are five types of antibodies (immunoglobulins), each of which has a specific purpose. Table 27.2 provides an outline of these.

TYPES OF IMMUNITY

As previously discussed, natural immunity occurs with prior exposure to foreign invaders and occurs via the adaptive immune system, which creates a 'memory' every time a foreign invader or pathogen is met. This means that when exposed to the same pathogen again, illness does not occur as the body is able to rapidly fight off the invader. However, immunity can also be gained through two other processes:

1. Passive immunity: in this process the individual does not produce their own antibodies; they are obtained from another source. Examples of this include naturally acquired passive immunity, which involves the transmission of antibodies via the placenta from mother to foetus or during breastfeeding. Or preformed antibodies can be injected into the body to stimulate an immune response and prevent disease caused by exposure to a pathogen (e.g., giving a hepatitis B booster vaccination following a needlestick injury etc.). Passive immunity is always temporary, in that antibodies from another source only act for a short while.

2. Active immunity: in this process the individual produces their own antibodies in response to an infection, which leads to the creation of memory cells for a specific pathogen. This means that active immunity to a specific pathogen or disease is much more long-term (in some cases, lifelong). The production of antibodies and memory cells can also be artificially acquired through vaccination against a specific infection/disease.

Vaccination

Effective immunization programmes can prevent and control the spread of infectious disease. Vaccination involves giving a weakened or inactive form of the disease against which protection is required. Once a vaccine is given, it should stimulate antibody production, which can provide protection for years. The overall aim of the UK's routine immunization schedule (DH, 2013) is to provide protection against the following vaccine-preventable infections (Box 27.1).

TABLE 27.2 Classes of Antibodies

Antibody/ immunoglobulin	Location	Function
Ig G	Blood, lymph, extracellular fluid	Provide long-term immunity after illness or vaccination. Cross the placenta and provide passive immunity to the newborn. Account for about 75% of the body's antibodies
Ig A	External secretions – saliva, tears, etc.	Found in secretions of all mucous membranes, including breast milk
Ig M	Blood, lymph	Produced before Ig G during an infection
Ig D	B-cells	Antigen-specific receptors found on B-cells
Ig E	Mast cell or basophils	Mast cells release histamine. Play a part in allergic reactions

BOX 27.1 UK Immunization Schedule (Department of Health, 2013)

Diphtheria
Tetanus
Pertussis (whooping cough)
Haemophilus influenzae type b (Hib)
Polio
Meningococcal disease (certain serogroups)
Measles
Mumps
Rubella
Pneumococcal disease (certain serotypes)
Human papillomavirus types (certain serotypes)
Rotavirus
Influenza
Shingles

NURSING SKILLS

A Skin-Prick Test

This is often the first test to be undertaken when looking for an allergen. It is quick, painless and safe and the results are available within about 20 minutes. The skin is pricked with a tiny amount of the suspected allergen to see if there is a reaction. If there is, the skin around the prick will very quickly become itchy and a red, swollen mark called a wheal appears.

A registered competent nurse performs the skin testing. Local policy and procedure is adhered to throughout. The patient's needs will determine the exact method, procedure and process that is used. There are a number of devices used for prinking the skin (a sharp pointed lancet), as well a range of commercially produced allergens.

Skin-prick testing must always be performed in a medical setting, with the ready availability of medical practitioners competent to treat systemic allergic reactions, and appropriate equipment.

Suggested minimum standards for available emergency equipment and medications:

- Availability of oxygen
- Facility for intravenous cannulation and intravenous fluids for rapid infusion in case of hypotension
- Ready availability of adrenaline for intramuscular injection
- Salbutamol via nebuliser or spacer

The patient's identity is checked, the medical history is reviewed and a physical examination performed. The appropriateness for an allergy skin test is determined to ensure the patient is not put at risk for a bad outcome, for example, severe anaphylaxis or an asthma attack in a poorly controlled asthma patient.

Requirements for skin prick:

- Allergen extracts
- Positive and negative control solutions
- Sterile lancets for skin pricking
- Sharps container for disposal of lancets
- Marker pen for the skin
- Ruler for measuring reactions
- Tissues for wiping solutions
- Recording sheets

- Gloves (as per policy)

The patient needs to be in a comfortable position, with forearms or back at a convenient height to do the test. The procedure explained, patients must have avoided antihistamines and other interfering drugs, as well as skin moisturizers, before the procedure is undertaken.

The area to be tested is exposed (dignity ensured) with no risk of clothing brushing across the test area. The room should be private and at a comfortable temperature. The NA may be required to assist.

The skin site is cleaned, as per policy. Positions for skin pricks are marked by numbers on the skin to identify the allergen, and pricks are made immediately next to the numbers to avoid confusion between allergens. Skin-prick tests should be at least 2 cm apart to avoid overlapping reactions and false-positive results.

In the 'drop then prick approach', a drop of allergen is applied from the dropper bottle onto the skin prior to pricking the skin. It is important not to allow the extract to run onto the next prick site.

It takes around 20 minutes for the reactions to occur. If the test is left for longer than 20 minutes, the histamine and allergen response may diminish or be lost, and if not measured on time, the test may need to be repeated.

A chart should be kept and the wheal (and flare) size in millimetres recorded next to each allergen name. Record wheal diameter in numerical form as the primary reported result. The results are documented in the patient's notes.

Patient care post-test:

Some patients may experience discomfort as a result of itching from the skin test. Numbers should be removed from the skin by cleaning with an alcohol solution (unless contraindicated). Itching from skin-prick testing usually subsides within 15 minutes.

Patients should be told the significance of the test results from the nurse specialist or medical practitioner who ordered the test and receive information on any implications of the test, for example allergen avoidance. The NA may be required to reinforce any information given.

Modified from the Australasian Society of Clinical Immunology and Allergy (2016).

CARE IN THE HOME SETTING

Immunization

The key aims of immunization are threefold. They are to:
1. Protect the individual from infectious diseases, with associated mortality, morbidity and long-term sequelae.
2. Prevent outbreaks of disease.
3. Ultimately eradicate infectious diseases globally, as in the case of smallpox.

Immunization is a safe and highly effective method of preventing infectious disease. Successful immunization, however, depends upon the production of a safe and effective vaccine, the maintenance of the cold chain during vaccine transportation and storage, injection into the correct anatomical site of an appropriate patient and the correct injection technique.

Nurses are the major force in administering vaccinations, not only within the childhood immunization programme, but also increasingly in administering travel vaccines, the annual influenza vaccination campaign and other campaigns.

Annual flu immunization remains the best way to protect against flu; front-line staff, such as Nursing Associates, are advised to have an annual flu vaccine to protect themselves and their patients.

The vaccine changes each year, ensuring it is as suitable as possible for the type of flu viruses that are most likely to be circulating. It is therefore essential to get vaccinated annually.

Seasonal flu vaccines are designed to protect against infection and illness caused by the three or four influenza viruses (depending on vaccine) that research indicates will be most common during the flu season. Flu vaccination is normally able to provide protection in 50%–70% of cases and this could be the difference between life and death.

The vaccine offered to adults in the UK cannot give the person flu as it does not contain any live viruses; however, it can make the person's arm feel a bit sore and sometimes it can cause a slight temperature. Other reactions are very rare.

DISORDERS OF THE IMMUNE SYSTEM

Autoimmune disease

Autoimmune disease occurs when the immune system no longer recognizes the body's normal cells as its own and sees them as foreign invaders. Therefore, it overreacts against the body's own cells and tissues and launches an immune response to destroy them. Several factors are thought to cause or impact on the body's breakdown in self-recognition, including viral infections, hormones and certain types of drugs (Nowak, 2015). There are several hundred different types of autoimmune disease and a few common diseases (e.g., multiple sclerosis [MS], coeliac disease, systemic lupus erythematosus [SLE] and rheumatoid arthritis [RA]).

Multiple sclerosis

MS is a disease of the central nervous system that causes an immune reaction to occur in the protective covering (myelin) of the nerve fibres of the brain, spinal cord and eyes. This causes areas of demyelinated plaques to form in the spinal cord and brain. The reaction leads to weakening of the nerve signals to affected tissue, which may result in permanent loss of function (Amor & van Noort, 2014). The causes of MS are unknown; however, genetic and immune factors are implicated. The incidence of MS is increasing and symptoms are likely to present between the ages of 25 and 35 years (Amor & van Noort, 2014).

Signs and symptoms

The signs and symptoms that the individual experiences varies according to the sites and sizes of demyelinated plaques and the individual is likely to experience periods of relapses and remission of varying time periods. However, each relapse will cause further loss of nervous tissue and progressive loss of function.

Common signs and symptoms include:
- Visual disturbance/loss of vision
- Burning sensation to the hands and feet
- Tingling and numbness
- Weakness or tightness in muscles
- Problems with urinary and bowel function
- Loss of coordination.

Diagnosis

Diagnosis is made based on a combination of clinical presentation of common signs and symptoms, neurological examination and diagnostic tests. These include:
- Magnetic resonance imaging (MRI), which is likely to reveal areas of demyelination and plaque formation in the brain and spinal cord.
- Examination of cerebrospinal fluid, which will contain higher than normal levels of white blood cells and antibodies.

Coeliac disease

Coeliac disease is a common condition that causes inflammation of the small bowel and is associated with intolerance to gluten, a protein found in flour. This leads to poor absorption of nutrients. Coeliac disease may involve an inherited immune dysfunction, as it commonly runs in families, occurs in males and females equally and is more likely to affect the European population/those of a Caucasian background.

Signs and symptoms

Signs and symptoms vary from mild to severe and can be intermittent or constant. Abdominal pain, bloating, diarrhoea, constipation, excessive wind, nausea and vomiting are common symptoms. In addition, the sufferer may experience mouth ulcers, tiredness and fatigue due to iron, B12 and folic acid deficiency. An itchy rash with blisters that burst when scratched may also develop in 20% of sufferers (Pearce, 2016).

Diagnosis

Diagnosis can be made based on the signs and symptoms experienced by the sufferer, blood tests to look for immunological markers and biopsy of the small intestine.

Care and treatment

Lifelong avoidance of foodstuff containing gluten is the most effective measure that can be taken by the sufferer to reduce symptoms of the disease.

Systemic lupus erythematosus

SLE is a chronic autoimmune disease that can affect several of the body's organs, including the central nervous system, skin, joints, kidneys, lungs and the blood. SLE occurs in both sexes but women between the ages of 15 and 45 years are the most likely group to be affected. In addition, being of black ethnicity increases not only the likelihood of contracting the disease but also the severity of symptoms experienced (Childs, 2006).

REFLECTION 27.3

Take some time to think about how having SLE can impact on a person's self-identity.

Signs and symptoms

Common signs and symptoms of SLE are related to wide-spread, chronic inflammation that can affect most of the body's systems and are outlined in Table 27.3.

Diagnosis

A diagnosis of SLE is made on symptoms expressed by the patient, physical examination and blood tests. Two specific tests that look for antibodies in the blood are;

1. Anti-nuclear antibody (ANA) test. About 95% of people with lupus are ANA positive, but the test cannot confirm a diagnosis of SLE as the antibody can also be present in individuals who do not have SLE.
2. Anti-double-stranded DNA (anti-dsDNA) antibody test. About 70% of people with SLE have these antibodies and a positive test means that SLE is highly likely as the test is hardly ever positive in people who do not have lupus. The anti-dsDNA level usually goes up when the disease is more active, so repeat tests may be helpful as a means of monitoring the condition and deciding on treatment.

CASE STUDY 27.1   Amanda

Amanda, a 51-year-old woman who works as a legal secretary, presents to her GP with an 8-week history of joint pain to both wrists. This was initially diagnosed 4 weeks ago as repetitive strain injury and Amanda was advised to rest and take painkillers. Amanda has returned to see her doctor today as the pain in her hands and wrists is worsening; she is also experiencing stiffness in her hands that takes a considerable time to lessen. Amanda also reports feeling constantly tired, and on examination, her hands and wrists are visibly swollen, particularly around the joints. Her GP refers her to a consultant rheumatologist who diagnoses rheumatoid arthritis and initiates treatment.

Rheumatoid arthritis

RA is an autoimmune disorder characterized by progressive destruction and deformity of the peripheral joints. The disease can present at any age but commonly occurs between the ages of 50 and 55 years and is more likely to affect women.

Signs and symptoms

Common signs and symptoms of RA include swelling, stiffness (lasting more than 30 minutes) and joint pain, commonly affecting the hands and feet. Sufferers may also experience weight loss, fatigue and general malaise.

Diagnosis

If RA is suspected, a referral to a specialist Rheumatology Consultant is necessary. Diagnosis is usually made using a variety of diagnostic tests, including blood tests (Table 27.4), physical examination and x-ray of the hands and feet.

REFLECTION 27.4

When might erythrocyte sedimentation rate be used as opposed to C-reactive protein, and vice versa?

TABLE 27.3   Systemic Effects of Systemic Lupus Erythematosus

Body system	Signs and symptoms
Cardiovascular	Heart murmurs, conduction problems, risk of arrhythmias, heart failure, breathlessness
Skin/connective tissue	Loss of hair (alopecia), scarring, skin plaque formation, 'inflammatory lesions to skin (particularly to sun-exposed areas), 'butterfly' rash to face
Musculoskeletal	Painful joints, muscle weakness
Nervous	Memory loss, changes in mental state, mood disorders, seizures, balance, visual and hearing problems
Renal	Acute renal failure
Pulmonary	Pulmonary embolism and hypertension, pleural effusion, generalized inflammation of the lungs
Blood	Low levels of red and white blood cells and platelets, and blood clotting abnormalities

THE MEDICINE TROLLEY 27.1

Drug	Drug classification	Reason for administration	Route of administration	Dose	Side effects	Contraindications	Nursing care
Prednisolone	Corticosteroid	Suppress the immune response and reduce inflammation	Oral	10–20 mg daily – can increase to 60 mg if required for severe disease	Weight gain, elevated blood sugar, oedema	Should be prescribed with care in those with a history of psychiatric disorder. Should be used with caution in those with renal or hepatic impairment	Patient should be educated to not stop steroids suddenly and to take them with food or milk

TABLE 27.4 Blood Tests for the Diagnosis of Rheumatoid Arthritis

Test	Indication
Rheumatoid factor	Rheumatoid factor is present in up to 85% of all cases of RA
Erythrocyte sedimentation rate	A non-specific test for generalized inflammation. A false-negative result may occur if the patient is taking steroids or other anti-inflammatory drugs
C-reactive protein	An abnormal protein found in blood during acute inflammation – this is increased in cases of RA

Care and treatment of the individual with an immune disorder

Due to the long-term nature of most immune disorders, individuals should have ongoing assessment and access to the multidisciplinary team, and measures taken need to address the following:

Improvement in comfort level.
- Incorporation of pain management techniques into daily life.
- Incorporation of strategies necessary to modify fatigue as part of daily living.
- The attainment and maintenance of optimal functional independence.
- Adaption to physical and psychological changes imposed by the immune disorder.
- Use of effective coping behaviours for dealing with actual or perceived limitations and role changes.

Immunodeficiency

Immunodeficiency occurs when the body fails to produce enough of a certain type of immune cell or the cells do not function properly. This results in the individual being more vulnerable to infection and recurrent infections. Immunodeficiency can be primary (genetic) or secondary due to conditions such as diabetes, kidney or liver disease, infection (e.g., human immunodeficiency virus [HIV]), other conditions (e.g., trauma, malnutrition, surgery), extremes of age (newborn and elderly) or due to certain types of medication (e.g., steroids, chemotherapy drugs and other drugs that suppress the immune system) (Thompson, 2015).

Human immunodeficiency virus

HIV is a viral infection that attacks the T-lymphocytes and weakens the immune system, leaving the individual vulnerable to infection. HIV can be acquired through sexual contact or exposure to blood and body fluids. Left untreated, HIV causes acquired immune deficiency syndrome (AIDS). AIDS is the late phase of HIV infection that can develop after a long period of HIV infection and can eventually be fatal, if left untreated. However, the developments in antiretroviral therapy means that HIV is no longer considered a life-ending disease (Williams & Hopper, 2015).

HIV is transmitted from person to person through infected blood, body fluids containing blood, breast milk, vaginal secretions and semen. The virus is surprisingly fragile and requires a direct route into the body or blood stream as it cannot survive for long outside of the body.

In 2015, an estimated 101,200 people (69,500 men and 31,600 women) were living with HIV in the UK, of which 47,000 were gay/bisexual men (Public Health England, 2016).

Signs and symptoms

The initial infection with HIV may not cause symptoms for years (known as the 'clinical latency stage') whilst the virus remains in the lymph nodes, liver and spleen, where it reproduces. However, if the infection is untreated, the cells of the immune system gradually start to become dysfunctional and no longer work together to maintain a healthy immune system. The sufferer will then begin to manifest signs of disease, which initially resemble symptoms of a weakened immune system; however, as the immune system becomes more impaired, opportunistic infections and cancers can occur (Williams & Hopper, 2015). The patient may present with symptoms of weight loss, fatigue, fever, breathlessness, night sweats, skin lesions, oral or vaginal thrush and shingles.

Diagnosis

HIV infection can be diagnosed from blood, urine or saliva. A HIV test works by detecting antibodies and antigens to the HIV virus and results are usually available the same day.

REFLECTION 27.5

Reflect on how you might offer non-judgemental care to a person living with HIV.

Acquired immune deficiency syndrome

AIDS is diagnosed when the cell count of a specific type of T-lymphocyte (CD4+) falls below 200, or opportunistic infections occur (Table 27.5).

THE MEDICINE TROLLEY 27.2

Drug	Drug classification	Reason for administration	Route of administration	Dose	Side effects	Contra-indications	Nursing care
Methotrexate	Disease modifying anti-rheumatic drug (DMARD)	To reduce inflammation and slow the progress of the disease	By mouth for moderate disease or intramuscular or subcutaneous injection in severe disease	7.5–20 mg weekly	Sensitivity to light, diarrhoea, gastric ulceration, risk of fluid accumulation in the lungs or abdomen	Not to be given during active infection, immunodeficiency, ascites or pleural effusion	Patients should be advised to report all signs and symptoms suggestive of infection and attend for blood tests as required

TABLE 27.5 Common AIDS-Defining Conditions in the UK

Pneumocystis carinii pneumonia	Encephalopathy
Tuberculosis	Cytomegalovirus
Kaposi's sarcoma	Cryptosporidiosis
Candidiasis (thrush)	Cryptococcal meningitis
Lymphoma	

Adapted from Public Health England, 2016.

AGEING AND THE IMMUNE SYSTEM

Immune function beings to decline once sexual maturity has been reached and continues to do so as the body ages. As a result, the following occur:

1. The immune system's ability to recognize 'self' as itself declines; therefore the individual is more prone to autoimmune disorders with age.
2. The immune system becomes less able to identify and kill mutant cells, hence the risk of cancer increases with age.

ALLERGY – HYPERSENSITIVITY

Allergic or hypersensitive diseases may occur locally or systemically as a result of the individual's immune response being destructive rather than defensive, and causing tissue damage or disordered function rather than immunity. This results in disease in the individual who is 'allergic' or hypersensitive to an antigen. Abnormal sensitivity to common allergens, such as pollens, dust, animal hair and certain foodstuffs, is a result of over-production of immunoglobulin E and its interaction with the allergens (Zelman et al., 2011). This leads to the breakdown of mast cells

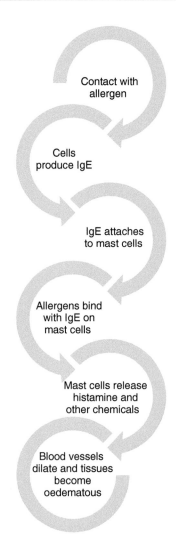

Fig. 27.5 Sequence of Events in an Allergic Reaction. IgE, Immuno-globulin E.

and the release of chemicals, including histamine, which cause localised swelling (oedema) and irritation, itching and hives (see Fig. 27.5).

Anaphylaxis

This is a severe, systemic allergic reaction that presents with sudden, life-threatening signs and symptoms. It is characterized by rapidly developing, potentially fatal airway and/or breathing and/or circulation problems, usually associated with skin and mucosal changes (Working Group of the Resuscitation Council UK, 2008). Therefore, prompt recognition and appropriate treatment by all health professionals is essential (Fig. 27.6).

CRITICAL AWARENESS
Common Causes of Anaphylaxis

Anaphylaxis can be triggered by any of a very broad range of triggers, but those most commonly identified include food, drugs and venom. The relative importance of these varies very considerably with age, with food being particularly important in children and medicinal products being much more common triggers in older people. Virtually any food or class of drug can be implicated, although the classes of foods and drugs responsible for the majority of reactions are well described. Of foods, nuts are the most common cause; muscle relaxants, antibiotics, non-steroidal anti-inflammatory drugs and aspirin are the most commonly implicated drugs. However, it is important to note that, in many cases, no cause can be identified (Working Group of the Resuscitation Council UK, 2008).

CASE STUDY 27.2   Jenny

Jenny Lomax, a 22-year-old art student, has presented to the accident and emergency department with swelling to her face and lips, numerous itchy, red welts over her body and is very anxious. Jenny has no known allergies and she cannot think of anything that may have caused such a reaction. However, on further questioning, it transpires that a few days earlier, Jenny had changed her hair colour using a new hair dye product that she had not used before.

COMMUNITIES OF CARE
Children

From 1 October, 2017, schools in England are allowed to purchase adrenaline auto-injector (AAI) devices without a prescription, for emergency use on children who are at risk of anaphylaxis but whose own device is not available or not working. The Department of Health have issued guidance on this issue (Department of Health, 2017).

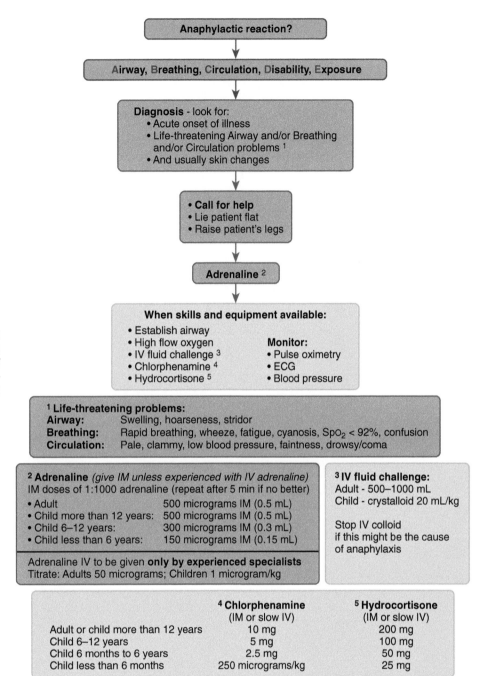

Fig. 27.6 Anaphylaxis Algorithm. (Reproduced with the kind permission of the Resuscitation Council (UK) 2008. https://www.resus.org.uk/anaphylaxis/emergency-treatment-ofanaphylactic-reactions/). IM, Intramuscular; IV, intravenous; SpO₂, oxygen saturation.

Schools may administer their 'spare' AAI, obtained (without prescription) for use in emergencies, but only if a pupil is at risk of anaphylaxis; also, both medical authorization and written parental consent for use of the spare AAI must be provided.

The spare AAI held by the school can be administered to a pupil whose own prescribed AAI cannot be administered correctly without delay.

AAIs can be used through clothes and should be injected into the upper outer thigh, in accordance with the instructions provided by the manufacturer.

If a pupil appears to be having a severe allergic reaction (anaphylaxis), the school MUST call 999 without delay, even if they have already used their own AAI device, or a spare AAI.

In the event of a possible severe allergic reaction in a pupil who does not meet these criteria, emergency services (999) should be contacted and advice sought as to whether administration of the spare emergency AAI is appropriate.

Immunotherapy

Subcutaneous immunotherapy is becoming increasingly popular as a means of desensitizing patients who have long-term allergic symptoms or who have experienced anaphylactic reactions (Williams & Hopper, 2015). Immunotherapy involves injecting small amounts of a very diluted, prepared extract of the offending allergen, initially once or twice weekly. Over a period of 3–6 months, the concentration of the allergen is gradually increased to a point where the individual is no longer hypersensitive to the allergen. The individual will require maintenance injections every few weeks for between 3 and 5 years to ensure hyposensitivity to the allergen is maintained (Williams & Hopper, 2015).

OSCE 27.1

Administration of Subcutaneous Injection

As subcutaneous immunotherapy is becoming increasingly popular, the Nursing Associate will be required to administer these when appropriate. When administering medication the Nursing and Midwifery Council, University and local policy and procedure must be adopted.

Action	Criteria	Achieved/ not achieved
Check the prescription	Check medicine has not already been given	
	Check for any known allergies	
	Gain patient consent to proceed	
Gathering equipment	Equipment tray	
	The medication to be administered	
	The patient's prescription	
7 Rights	1. Right person – check the patient's name band against the name on the prescription. Ask for confirmation of name and date of birth.	
	2. Right drug – select the correct medicine (it may need to have been stored in refrigerator)	
	3. Right dose – calculate the correct dose	
	4. Right time – confirm when the last dose was administered	
	5. Right route – check the route for administration is correct as per medicine prescription (subcutaneous)	
	6. Right to refuse – gain the patient's consent	
	7. Right documentation of prescription	
Drug calculation	Demonstrate how you will calculate the correct amount of drug that you will need to administer to the patient.	
The procedure	Prepares the medication	
	Washes hands	
	Dons gloves	
	Demonstrates the correct size of needle is being used	
	Chooses an appropriate site	
	Positions the patient to provide optimal access to chosen site	
	Uses local policy for cleansing of skin	
	Pierces the skin at the appropriate angle for subcutaneous injection	
	Injects medication	
	Removes needle, disposes into sharps box	
	Disposes of gloves	
	Washes hands	
	Thanks patient	
Completing procedure	Once the medicine has been administered, ensure the drug chart has been signed	
	Explain the effects and side effects that you should assess the patient for	

Pass
Fail

The Nursing Associate must understand the potential side effects associated with the type of medicine being administered.

LOOKING BACK, FEEDING FORWARD

The immune system is a complex system and does not function in isolation; its main system is to help the body fight infection, seeking out and killing invaders. This chapter has provided an overview of this system. It is not possible to address all aspects of the immune system in a chapter of this size. The reader is encouraged to seek out further information to supplement the discussion in this chapter.

A key part of the immune system's role is to differentiate between invaders and the body's own cells. When it fails to make this distinction, a reaction against 'self' cells and molecules causes autoimmune disease. When providing care to those who have immunological conditions, the NA has to understand the risks posed to the patient as a result of a deficient or abnormally functioning immunological system. The person with a condition that impacts on their immune system must be at the centre of what is done and the NA has to provide care that is kind, caring, considerate and responsive to the patient's needs in an appropriate and timely manner.

REFERENCES

Amor, S., van Noort, H., 2014. Multiple Sclerosis. Oxford University Press, England.

Australasian Society of Clinical Immunology and Allergy, 2016. Skin prick testing for the diagnosis of allergic disease. Available at https://www.allergy.org.au/images/stories/pospapers/ASCIA_SPT_Manual_March_2016.pdf.

Childs, S.G., 2006. The pathogenesis of systemic lupus erythematosus. Orthop. Nurs. 25 (2), 140–145.

Department of Health, 2013. UK Immunisation Schedule, the green book. Available at https://www.gov.uk/government/uploads/

system/uploads/attachment_data/file/554298/Green_Book_Chapter_11.pdf.

Department of Health, 2017. Guidance on the use of adrenaline auto-injectors in schools. Available at https://www.gov.uk/government/uploads/system/uploads/attachment_data/file/645476/Adrenaline_auto_injectors_in_schools.pdf.

NICE (National Institute for Health and Care Excellence), 2017. Sepsis: recognition, diagnosis and early management. NICE guideline NG51. https://www.nice.org.uk/guidance/ng51.

Nowak, S.M., 2015. Nursing care of patients with immune disorders. In: Williams, L., Hopper, P. (Eds.), Understanding Medical Surgical Nursing. FA Davis Company.

Pearce, L., 2016. Coeliac disease. Nurs. Stand. 31 (16–18), 17.

Public Health England, 2016. HIV in the UK: 2016 report. Available at https://www.gov.uk/government/uploads/system/uploads/attachment_data/file/602942/HIV_in_the_UK_report.pdf.

Singer, M., Deutschmann, C.S., Seymour, C., 2016. The third international consensus definitions for sepsis and septic shock (sepsis -3). JAMA 315 (8), 801–810.

Thompson, A.E., 2015. The immune system. JAMA 314 (16), 1686.

UK Sepsis Trust, 2016. Inpatient sepsis screening & action tool (non-pregnant adults and children over 12 years). Available at https://sepsistrust.org/.

Waugh, A., Grant, A., 2018. Ross & Wilson Anatomy and Physiology in Health and Illness, thirteenth ed. Elsevier, Edinburgh.

Williams, P., 2018. deWit's Fundamental Concepts and Skills for Nursing, fifth ed. Elsevier, Missouri.

Williams, L.S., Hopper, P.D., 2015. Understanding Medical Surgical Nursing, fifth ed. F.A. Davis, Philadelphia.

Working Group of the Resuscitation Council UK, 2008. Annotated with links to NICE guidance July 2012. Emergency treatment of anaphylactic reactions–guidelines for healthcare providers. UK Resuscitation Council.

Zelman, M., Tompary, E., Raymond, J., et al., 2011. Introductory Pathophysiology for Nursing and Healthcare Professionals. Pearson, England.

Pain Management

Anthony Wheeldon

By the end of the chapter the reader will:

1. Have an understanding of the physiology of pain transmission and sensation
2. Explain the difference between acute and chronic pain
3. Appreciate the impact of personal circumstances and individuals' perspective on the pain experience
4. Outline the care required by people in acute pain and people living with chronic pain
5. List a range of pharmacological and non-pharmacological pain management options
6. Review the role of the Nursing Associate in promoting health and well-being

Acute pain	Somatic pain	Non-steroidal anti-inflammatory
Chronic pain	Visceral pain	Neuropathy
Pain pathways	Analgesia	
Nociceptors	Opioid	

CHAPTER AIMS

This aim of this chapter is to provide the reader with an understanding of the skills, knowledge and attitude required to provide safe, effective and compassionate care to individuals in acute pain and individuals living with chronic pain.

SELF TEST

1. What is pain?
2. What is the difference between acute and chronic pain?
3. How do health professionals assess pain and its impact on well-being?
4. Describe the pain pathway.
5. Explain the difference between deep and superficial pain.
6. Explain the difference between visceral and somatic pain.
7. How might acute pain impact on a patient's recovery from surgery?
8. How might healthcare professionals help an individual living with cancer pain to cope at home?
9. What is an opioid?
10. List five non-pharmacological methods of pain control.

INTRODUCTION

This chapter explores the nature of pain and the pain experience. It also explores the impact of pain on the individual and their physiology. The initial section explores the physiology of pain and reinforces the important concept of holistic pain management, which respects the idea that pain is a personal experience and is whatever the individual in pain says it is. This is important for Nursing Associates who, like all healthcare professionals, must treat people in pain with dignity and compassion if they are to provide care that is appropriate and effective.

The second section explores comprehensive pain assessment and pain management. It is essential that Nursing Associates appreciate the complexities of pain assessment, and also understand the range of treatment options available and how they work. This section will conclude with an overview of common types of pain Nursing Associates may encounter, namely postoperative pain, neuropathy, cancer pain, referred pain and phantom limb pain. Pain can be debilitating and people living with long-term pain often experience difficulties with activities of living, such as eating, socializing and sleeping. Many experience depression and isolation as a result. Nursing Associates, therefore, are required to be kind and considerate when providing care for people living with pain.

PAIN PHYSIOLOGY

Pain is a universal experience. Everyone has pain periodically throughout their life and it is the most likely reason for an individual to seek medical attention. Although pain is ubiquitous, it remains difficult to define. Pain is often described as an unpleasant and uncomfortable sensation, which occurs as a result of injury, inflammation or disease. However, pain can also be a constant presence in individuals living with a long-term health condition, where there is little evidence of tissue damage and healing is complete. Pain is not always associated with injury or tissue damage; it can be associated with emotion, with individuals describing feelings of loss, grief and unrequited love as being painful. Pain physiology explains that pain is an individual and personal experience and the way in which someone expresses and interprets their pain will depend on their culture, life experiences, personality and the meaning they ascribe to their pain. It is no surprise therefore that a popular definition of pain, often cited by healthcare professionals is:

'Pain is whatever the experiencing person says it is, existing when he says it does' (McCaffery, 1979, p. 11).

The physiology of pain is intricate and complex. In some instances, pain transmission and interpretation is not fully understood and pain physiology relies on pain theories to help us understand why individuals in pain may behave as they do. In simple terms, the generation and sensation of pain follows three basic steps:

1. Pain sensation: the peripheral nervous system detects an injury, irritation or inflammation.
2. Pain transmission: messages of pain are transmitted from the site of injury, irritation and inflammation to the central nervous system.
3. Pain interpretation: the brain receives the pain message and assesses the extent and significance of the injury, irritation or inflammation. At this point, the individual feels pain. (Fig. 28.1)

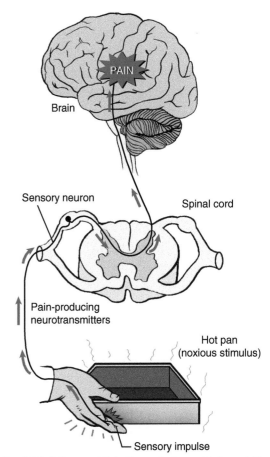

Fig. 28.1 Pathway of Pain Transmission and Interpretation.

PAIN SENSATION

Pain is generated when the peripheral nervous system is stimulated by noxious substances generated by the following:
- Trauma or injury that leads to tissue damage
- Lack of oxygen (i.e., ischaemia and hypoxia)
- Ulceration
- Infection
- Inflammation
- Extreme heat and cold.

Noxious substances are detected by free nerve endings called nociceptors. Nociceptors are found in every tissue in the human body, except the brain. Tissue towards the surface of the body has many nociceptors, whereas tissue deeper within the organs of the body has fewer and more widespread nociceptors.

CLASSIFICATION OF PAIN

There are three classifications of pain, each of which is determined by its duration:
- Transient pain: a short episode of pain, as a consequence of a minor injury.
- Acute pain: debilitating pain, which has a sudden onset and continues until healing begins.
- Chronic pain: pain that continues even though healing is complete.

Transient pain can be intense and can cause upset. However it is short lived and temporary, and the individual will consider the pain to be unimportant and will not seek medical attention.

Acute pain, however, is prolonged and does not ease until healing begins. Acute pain has a sudden onset and can be intense and intolerable. Acute pain is associated with an autonomic nervous system response, such as high pulse rate, high blood pressure, nausea and excessive sweating. Individuals with acute pain often demonstrate specific pain behaviours, such as facial grimace, guarding, irritability, anger and upset.

Chronic pain, however, doesn't always stimulate an autonomous nervous system response, and individuals living with chronic pain may not present with the symptoms of pain. However, their pain may be as intense as acute pain, despite the lack of visible and physical symptoms. For this reason, chronic pain is often considered to be a syndrome – a medical condition in its own right (Melzack & Wall, 1988).

PAIN TRANSMISSION

Messages of pain are transferred from nociceptors to the brain via the ascending pain pathway. The ascending pain pathway carries messages of pain from the site of injury to the thalamus and somatosensory cortex within the brain. The ascending pain pathway consists of three linked neurons, called first, second and third order neurons (Fig. 28.2).

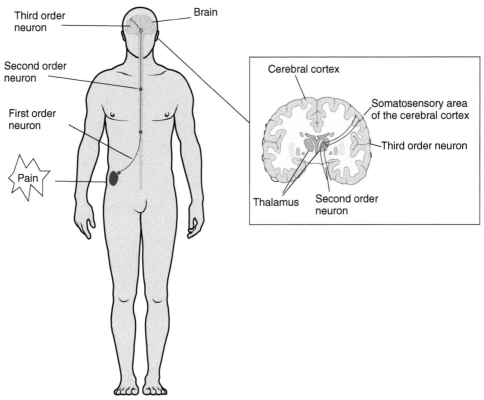

Fig. 28.2 The Ascending Pain Pathway.

- First order neurons carry pain messages from the site of injury to the spine.
- Second order neurons carry pain messages up the spine towards the brain.
- Third order neurons carry pain messages through the brain. The neurotransmitters that transmit pain messages are thought to be substance P and serotonin (MacLellan, 2006). For more information on neurons and neurotransmitters see Chapter 36.

Two first order neurons are responsible for the transmission of the pain messages towards the spine: A-delta (Aδ) fibres and C fibres. The speed of nerve impulses depends upon the diameter of the nerve fibre and presence of a myelin sheath. Neurons with a myelin sheath are capable of transmitting nerve impulses faster because the sheath of myelin that surrounds the axon electrically insulates it (Fig. 28.3). Aδ fibres are thicker and are myelinated, whereas C fibres are thin and non-myelinated (see Fig. 28.3). Aδ fibres can transmit pain signals far quicker than C fibres. The ascending pain pathway follows the same route as transmissions of sensations of heat and cold. The first order neurons that transmit sensations of heat and cold are called A-beta (Aβ) fibres. Aβ fibres are myelinated and thicker than Aδ fibres and can therefore transmit messages of heat and cold quicker than pain impulses. It is for this reason that stimulation of Aβ fibres with heat or cold (e.g., rubbing a mild injury, using a hot water bottle or a cold compress) can alleviate mild pain. The first order neurons that are responsible for transmission of pain, heat and cold are summarized in Table 28.1

There are two phases of pain, often referred to as first and second pain. At the onset of pain, individuals feel a first pain

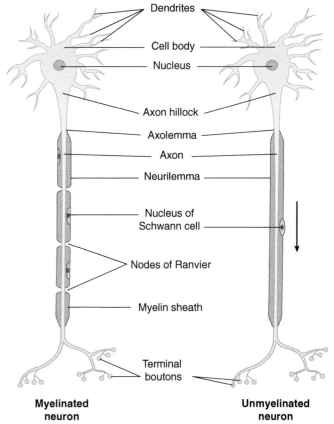

Fig. 28.3 Myelinated and Unmyelinated Nerve Fibres (Waugh & Grant, 2018).

TABLE 28.1 **Speed and Velocity of Transmission of First Order Neurons**

Sensory fibre	Diameter (µm)	Myelinated	Speed of conduction (m/s)
A-beta (Aβ) fibres	6–12	Yes	35–75
A-delta (Aδ) fibres	1–5	Yes	5–35
C fibres	0.2–1.5	No	0.5–2

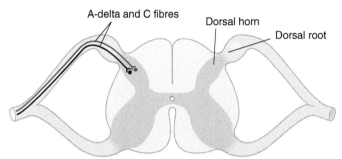

Fig. 28.4 Cross Section of the Spinal Cord.

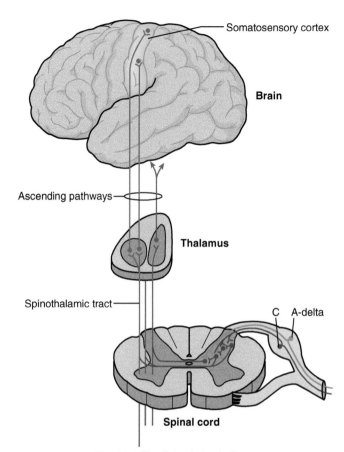

Fig. 28.5 The Spinothalamic Tract.

sensation, which is followed by a more lengthy second pain sensation as follows:

- First pain: sharp or pricking pain
- Second pain: dull, burning, aching pain

First pain is thought to be generated by the action of Aδ fibres, whereas second pain is thought to be generated by C fibres.

The first order neurons carry the pain signal towards the spinal cord, where they connect (synapse) with a second order neuron at a point inside the spinal cord called the dorsal horn (Fig. 28.4). There are two types of second order neurons:

- Nociceptive-specific (NS)
- Wide dynamic range (WDR)

Both NS and WDR second order neurons respond to pain stimulation but WDR second order neurons also transmit signals from Aβ fibres, such as sensations of touch, heat and cold. NS and WDR second order neurons cross over into white matter and travel up the spinal cord towards the brain (Fig. 28.5).

PAIN INTERPRETATION

Pain interpretation occurs in the brain. Pain sensation does not occur until pain signals from second order neurons meet third order neurons in an area of the brain called the thalamus. As third order neurons transport the pain signals from the thalamus towards the outer regions of the brain (called the cortex), pain is interpreted. Pain interpretation involves discerning the location of the pain, a description of the pain, its severity and meaning and producing an emotional response. The location and description of pain is determined by the somatosensory cortex, whereas an area of the brain called the limbic system produces an emotional response, which could range between mild irritation, anger, pleasure or distress. The limbic system is often referred to as the 'emotional brain', as it governs our emotional responses to life events. The limbic system is influenced by our life experiences, personality and culture. The limbic system is also responsible

for determining the seriousness of the pain and its cause. Over time, the limbic system remembers the cause of pain and helps us to learn to avoid painful stimuli in the future (Godfrey, 2005a). The limbic system is a collection of structures found within the cerebrum and diencephalon. Fig. 28.6 shows the main structures within the brain.

Pain is often described as being deep or superficial. Superficial pain occurs in the structures close to or within skin, whereas deep pain occurs within organs and structures deep within the body. The location of the source of pain determines the ease with which the brain can locate it. The skin and nearby structures are well served by nociceptors and therefore the brain can easily locate the source and location of injury. Structures and organs deep within the body, however, are served by fewer nociceptors and therefore the brain often has difficulties locating the source of pain. Deep pain can be divided into two categories: visceral and somatic (MacLellan, 2006):

- Somatic pain: originates in bones, tendons, joints and muscles
- Visceral pain: originates in organs (i.e., kidneys, intestines and gall bladder)

Pain is an individual experience and it is often reported that different people have different thresholds to pain. In reality, the term 'pain threshold' is unhelpful as it is generally accepted that humans have a similar pain threshold. In other words, we will all sense pain and report pain at a similar time. Where humans differ is in the way they express their pain. Individuals express

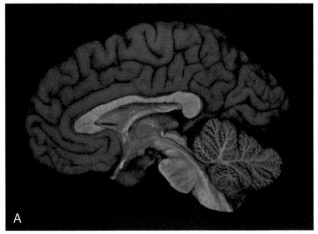

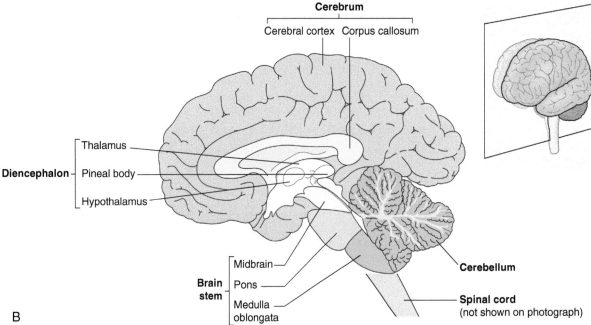

Fig. 28.6 Regions of the Brain (Waugh & Grant, 2018).

pain in various ways because it is influenced by many different factors, such as emotional state, personality, past experience, culture and social status. For that reason, individuals in acute pain may behave irrationally, whereas others may be able to control their emotions if pain occurs when it is socially unacceptable to cry out or complain (Marieb & Hoehn, 2007). States of anxiety or depression can enhance the pain experience and interventions that reduce anxiety can alleviate pain (Carr et al., 2005; Lin & Wang, 2005).

Pain intensity is also closely linked to the meaning the individual ascribes to it. A patient, having undergone surgery to remove a cancer, may be able to tolerate pain because for them pain signifies healing and getting better, whereas an individual with abdominal pain may experience intense pain, exacerbated by the anxiety of not knowing what the cause is and that it could potentially be something serious (Melzack & Wall, 1988). Previous pain experiences could also determine pain intensity. For example, previous exposure to severe pain as a result of a medical procedure could lead to anxiety and greater pain levels as a

result. People also learn how to express pain from others. They way in which an individual expresses pain may be influenced by their culture, upbringing and experiences of family members (Briggs, 2010; Bell & Duffy, 2009).

There are many misconceptions about the pain experience and it is essential that Nursing Associates are able to recognize these misconceptions and ensure that care decisions are based on reality. Some common misconceptions include:

- 'You can teach people to tolerate pain; the longer they have pain the more used to it they become'. This is not true. Tolerance to pain is an individual experience. In reality, people with prolonged pain tend to develop pain hypersensitivity.
- 'Nurses and allied health professionals are the authority on pain and the nature of pain'. This is not true. Only the patient experiencing the pain fully understands how it feels and its impact on their life.
- 'Lying about the existence of pain or malingering is commonplace'. In reality, very few people lie about the existence of pain and fabrication of pain is very rare.

- 'Visible symptoms of pain can be used to verify its severity'. Not always – a lack of pain expression does not equal lack of pain. People living with chronic pain may have the ability to carry on as normal.
- 'Patients should not be given analgesia until a reason for their pain has been diagnosed'. This would not ensure holistic or person-centred care. Pain should be treated even when there is no discernible cause. People seeking assistance for pain have the right to have their pain assessed, accepted and acted upon.

(McGann, 2007)

Pain interpretation leads to an attempt to inhibit the sensation of pain via the descending pain pathway. The descending pain pathway is the release of endogenous opiates, such as endorphins, encephalins and dynorphins, which have pain-reducing properties. Throughout the central nervous system, a range of opiate receptors can be found, including mu (μ), kappa (κ), sigma (σ) and delta (δ). When stimulated by endogenous opiates, opiate receptors can block the actions of substance P, a neurotransmitter responsible for the transmission of pain. Levels of endogenous opiates (endorphins) increase during periods of stress and pain. Stimulation of opiate receptors can also promote feelings of euphoria and pleasure and endogenous opiates are released in response to excitement, such as occurs during thrilling experiences, sexual activity and even exercise.

THE GATE CONTROL THEORY OF PAIN

The gate control theory of pain proposes that pain impulses must pass through a theoretical 'gate' at the dorsal horn of the spinal cord before ascending towards the brain. Pain messages from Aδ and C fibres will push open the gate. However, the descending pain pathway forces the gate to close. The intensity of an individual's pain, therefore, is determined by how wide the gate is opened (McCaffery et al., 2003). Whilst increased Aδ and C fibre activity forces the gate to open, endogenous opiates released via the descending pain pathway push the gate closed. The gate control theory also proposes that pain intensity is governed by the actions of specialist cells in the dorsal horn of the spinal cord. These specialist cells are called transmission cells and substantia gelatinosa (SG) cells. Transmission cells promote the passage of pain signals upwards, towards the brain, and push the gate open, whereas SG cells inhibit transmission cells and push the gate closed. In depressive or anxious states, transmission cell activity is enhanced, whereas in relaxed and contented states, SG cell activity is enhanced. Therefore, nursing and care interventions that seek to promote comfort and reassurance can have a beneficial and therapeutic impact on the well-being of the individual in pain (Melzack & Wall, 1988).

PAIN ASSESSMENT AND MANAGEMENT

Pain assessment

Pain is a complex phenomenon; therefore, effective assessment is a challenge for all healthcare professionals. Pain is a multifaceted, individual experience and close attention must be paid to the physiological, psychological, emotional and social aspects of pain (Manias et al., 2002). Pain is a subjective experience; therefore healthcare professionals are also reliant on the individual's description of their pain. Some people may be unable to verbalize their pain, and in such instances, the Nursing Associate must look for non-verbal indication of pain, such as facial expressions, irritability or guarding.

A comprehensive pain assessment must include the following if the medical team are to select the most appropriate treatments:

- The location of the pain
  - Where is the pain?
  - Can it be easily located?
  - Does it radiate anywhere?
- The duration of the pain
  - How long has the patient had the pain?
- Onset
  - When did the pain start?
  - What was the patient doing at the time?
- Frequency
  - How often does the pain occur?
- Intensity
  - How painful is it?
  - Does the level of pain change?
- Aggravating and relieving factors
  - What makes the pain worse?
  - What makes the pain feel better?
  - How does the individual cope with their pain?
- Other symptoms
  - Does the patient feel dizzy, nauseous or sweaty?
  - Do they feel short of breath?
  - Have they suffered a loss of appetite?
- Sleep
  - Is the patient's sleep disturbed by their pain?
- Expectations
  - What are the patient's expectations of any potential treatments?
  - What are the patient's treatment preferences?
- Concerns
  - What are the patient's concerns regarding the cause of their pain?
  - What are their fears and anxieties?
- Spirituality
  - Does the individual have any personal or spiritual beliefs, which help them to cope with their pain?
- Acceptability
  - What does the individual consider to be an acceptable level of pain?
  - What level of pain would allow the individual to return to work or enjoy personal interests?

(Godfrey, 2005b; MacLellan, 2006).

The most common structured pain assessment tools at the healthcare professional's disposal are rating scales, where the patient is asked to rate their pain. This can take the form of a numerical scale, for example from 1 to 10, where 1 is no pain and 10 is the worst pain imaginable, to visual scales that include pictures of facial expressions.

COMMUNITIES OF CARE

Pain Assessment in Someone with a Learning Disability

Care and attention must be paid when assessing pain in people with learning disabilities. Pain often results in irritability and altered mood. Such changes in behaviour have been misinterpreted as challenging in people with a learning disability, especially in individuals who find it difficult to communicate with others. Often, some behaviours are mistaken for a symptom of their disability rather than as a result of pain. This has, in the past, resulted in pain being ignored and untreated.

Adjustments should be made to pain assessment in people with learning disabilities to ensure holistic care is provided. Nursing Associates must take note of behavioural changes and visible signifiers of pain, such as grimace, irritability and loss of appetite. Patients should be encouraged to tell their pain story, and healthcare staff should avoid the word 'assessment' and use simplified terms. Pain diaries and body maps, which can be completed by service users or carers, can also help establish well-being.

(Adapted from Kingston & Bailey, 2009.)

Pain management

Pain management involves the use of pharmacological or non-pharmacological interventions. Pharmacological pain management involves the use of drugs and is called 'analgesia', whereas non-pharmacological interventions do not utilize any medications. Effective and holistic pain management involves the use of both pharmacological and non-pharmacological interventions (Hader & Guy, 2004).

Pharmacological pain management

Analgesia is classified by its pharmacological action. The two main categories of analgesia are:
- Opioids (or opiates)
  - Strong opioids
  - Weak opioids
- Non-opioid drugs
  - Non-steroidal anti-inflammatories
  - Paracetamol

Opioid drugs. Opioids (opiates) work by mimicking the actions of endogenous opiates. Like endorphins, encephalins and dynorphins, they bind to opiate receptors in the central nervous system and block the transmission of pain. Unlike endogenous opiates, the body does not break down opioid drugs quickly; therefore their pain-killing effects are powerful and long lasting. For that reason, they are often used for intense and severe pain.

Opioids are classified on their strength and are said to be either strong or weak. As their name suggests, weak opioids are not as potent as strong opioids, but they remain, nevertheless, very effective analgesics. Common strong opioids used in the United Kingdom include morphine, diamorphine, oxycodone, fentanyl and pethidine. Popular weak opioids include codeine, dihydrocodeine and tramadol.

❗ HOTSPOT

Side Effects of Opioids

Opioid analgesia has many unwanted side effects. After administration, Nursing Associates should continually assess for the presence of the following side effects:
- Respiratory depression
- Nausea and vomiting
- Constipation
- Bradycardia and hypotension

Opioid analgesia can be self-administered postsurgery via a system known as patient-controlled analgesia (PCA). The opioid is placed into a syringe driver, which is attached to patient via a subcutaneous or intravenous infusion. The syringe is operated by a button, which the patient presses when they are in pain. To protect against overdose, the syringe locks for a short time. PCA has been routinely and safely used for many years (Layzell, 2008).

THE MEDICINE TROLLEY 28.1

Drug	Drug classification	Reason for administration	Route of administration	Dose	Side effects	Contraindications	Nursing care
Dihydrocodeine	Weak opioid	Relief of moderate to severe acute pain	Intramuscular	50 mg every 4–6 hours	Bradycardia Confusion Constipation Drowsiness Hallucinations Hypotension Miosis Mood changes Nausea Pruritus Respiratory depression	Respiratory disease Comatose patients Raised intracranial pressure	Dihydrocodeine is a controlled drug and therefore administration must follow local policy Seek consent prior to administration Explain the use of the drug to the patient, respond to any questions Monitor for side effects and consider use of laxatives for constipation Monitor effectiveness of analgesia, always reassess pain levels

Non-opioid drugs. Non-opioid drugs are used for mild to moderate pain. The most common non-opioid drug is paracetamol (acetaminophen). Other non-opioid drugs include non-steroidal anti-inflammatory drugs. Paracetamol and non-steroidal anti-inflammatory drugs disrupt the action of prostaglandins, which enhance inflammation, stimulate nociceptors and increase pain sensation. Non-opioid drugs can enhance the effectiveness of weak opioids and many common analgesia medications are a combination of weak opioid and non-opioid drugs. Non-opioid drugs also have an antipyretic effect and can be used to effectively reduce high temperatures or fever. Common non-steroidal anti-inflammatory drugs include aspirin, ibuprofen, diclofenac and naproxen. Popular combinations of non-opioid and weak opioid drugs include co-codamol, which is a combination of codeine phosphate and paracetamol, and co-dydramol, which is dihydrocodeine combined with paracetamol.

Non-pharmacological pain management

As the name suggests, non-pharmacological methods of pain control do not involve the use of drugs. There are various non-pharmacological methods of pain management that are utilized by patients and healthcare professionals in the UK. Non-pharmacological interventions are said to be either physical or psychological. Physical non-pharmacological interventions physically manipulate the individual, whereas psychological interventions concentrate on the individual's coping strategies.

Examples of physical non-pharmacological pain management interventions include:

- application of hot and cold substances
- massage
- osteopathy
- transcutaneous electric nerve stimulation (TENS)
- acupuncture

(Wigens, 2006).

Many physical non-pharmacological pain management interventions have a physiological basis. The therapeutic effects of mild heat and ice packs on injuries, saw joints and muscle strains are well known. It is thought that they can stimulate Aβ fibres and disrupt pain messages. The stimulation of large-diameter Aβ fibres also helps explain the therapeutic effects of pressure- and touch-based interventions, such as osteopathy and massage, which has been shown to be potentially effective in patients with low-back pain (Furlan, et al., 2002). TENS (transcutaneous electrical nerve stimulation) machines, for example, are thought to work in a similar way. They could also increase levels of endogenous opiates, such as endorphins (Sluka & Walsh, 2003). Acupuncture is also thought to stimulate the release of endogenous opiates (Lundeberg & Stener-Victorin, 2002); however, there is very little evidence to suggest that it is effective (Lee & Ernst, 2005).

Examples of psychological non-pharmacological pain management interventions include:

- cognitive behavioural therapy (CBT)
- meditation
- relaxation
- distraction
- hypnosis

(Wigens, 2006).

Any non-pharmacological method that can alleviate anxiety, stress or help an individual to cope with their pain could be beneficial. It is not surprising therefore that psychological-based non-pharmacological pain control methods are being increasingly utilized by chronic pain sufferers (Dopson, 2010). Psychological-based pain control interventions range from basic practices, such as relaxation and distraction, to more alternative therapies, such as hypnosis.

A more intense psychological approach is CBT. CBT involves a series of structured, patient-focused sessions that aim to address the individual's psychological and emotional experience of their pain, and enable them to self-manage and control their anxiety (and therefore their pain). CBT should complement rather than replace traditional pharmacology-based therapies. As a pain control method for those in chronic pain, CBT has proved effective (Eccleston et al., 2009).

THE MEDICINE TROLLEY 28.2

Drug	Drug classification	Reason for administration	Route of administration	Dose	Side effects	Contraindications	Nursing care
Paracetamol	Analgesia	Mild to moderate pain	Oral	500 mg to 1 g, up to 4 times a day	Leucopenia Neutropenia Thrombocytopenia	Chronic alcohol consumption Liver disease Severe dehydration Malnutrition	Seek consent prior to administration Explain the use of the drug to the patient, respond to any questions Small overdoses can cause liver failure. Always ensure that doses are at least 4–6 hours apart and do not administer more than 4 g in one 24-hour period Monitor effectiveness of analgesia, always reassess pain levels

ACUTE PAIN

Acute pain is associated with a sudden onset and is an indicator of tissue damage. Acute pain is often excruciating, intolerable and debilitating. However, its presence is often temporary and it reduces as healing progresses. Acute pain is not a diagnosis, it is a symptom of an acute problem, such as burns, injury/trauma or abdominal pain. Patients can also experience acute pain after surgery.

Signs and symptoms of acute pain

Acute pain is stressful and many of the signs and symptoms are as a result of an autonomic nervous system response. Individuals in acute pain may also verbalize their pain and may visually project their suffering.

The major signs and symptoms of acute pain are:
- Tachycardia
- Hypertension
- Excessive sweating
- Altered respiratory rate
- Increased muscle tension
- Cool and clammy skin and peripheries
- Nausea and vomiting
- Anxiety, fear
- Altered facial expressions (i.e., grimace)
- Verbalization of pain
- Agitation, restlessness, anger, irritability
- Guarding.

Care and treatment

The main nursing aims for the patient in acute pain are to reduce discomfort and promote healing and recovery. Unresolved acute pain has a detrimental impact on many body systems and could also lead to the development of chronic pain.

The main care objectives for an individual in acute pain are:
- Perform an accurate pain assessment
- Administer prescribed analgesia safely
- Monitor for evidence of the main side effects of opioid therapy
- Use of psychological interventions, such as relaxation, distraction and imagery to complement pharmacological interventions
- Monitor patient for signs and symptoms of stress
- Regularly reassess pain intensity and evaluate success of pharmacological and psychological interventions.

Postoperative pain

Between 20% and 80% of patients report moderate to severe pain after surgery (Lorentzen et al., 2012). One significant factor in enhanced pain after surgery is anxiety. Anxiety and depression prior to surgery leads to increased levels of pain after surgery (Carr et al., 2005). In order to reduce postoperative pain, Nursing Associates should select appropriate preoperative care interventions that counteract the impact of anxiety, such as patient education (Johansson et al., 2005). The nursing team are ideally placed to minimize postoperative pain, as they are responsible for the safe administration and evaluation of prescribed analgesics.

The main care objective for individuals that have acute post-surgery pain is the minimization of its impact. Not only can unresolved pain lead to the development of chronic pain, it can also lead to a complicated and protracted postsurgical recovery. Unresolved acute pain has an impact on many body systems, but the nursing team must pay close attention to the following:

- The respiratory system: pain in the thorax can lead to reduced muscle contraction in the chest and abdominal area, a phenomenon called 'muscle splinting', which results in muscle contraction on either side of the injury to splint the area and prevent movement. Splinting also reduces the patient's ability to cough and clear secretions. Such changes in respiration, if left untreated, could lead to the development of atelectasis and chest infections.
- The cardiovascular system: stress increases heart rate and blood pressure, which in turn increases the workload of the heart, enhancing the risk of ischaemia and chest pain.
- The musculoskeletal system: acute muscular pain promotes muscle spasm and increased pain on movement. As a result, the patient becomes locked into a vicious circle of increased anxiety, increased pain and lack of mobility. A reduction of mobility is associated with reduced muscle metabolism, atrophy and a delayed return to normal muscle function.
- The digestive system: stress from acute pain can increase intestinal secretions and smooth muscle sphincter tone but simultaneously slow down intestinal motility. This reduced intestinal motility may be detrimental to the patient's nutritional status.

(Macintyre & Schug, 2015).

Acute abdominal pain

Abdominal pain is very common and one of the main reasons why someone would seek emergency attention. Often the cause of abdominal pain is not ascertained and the symptoms subside spontaneously. However, there are a large number of potential causes of abdominal pain and the site and location of the pain can help healthcare professionals diagnose the cause of pain. Table 28.2 lists the common causes of pain based in the abdominopelvic quadrants and Fig. 28.7 shows the location of the abdominopelvic quadrants.

Chest pain

Acute chest pain is a very common cause of admission to emergency departments. Acute central crushing chest pain is synonymous with myocardial conditions (see Chapter 29) but there are many other causes of chest pain that the Nursing Associates must be aware of. Causes of chest pain include:
- Cardiac disorders
  - Acute coronary syndromes (see Chapter 29)
  - Angina
- Respiratory disorders
  - Pleurisy
  - Pulmonary embolism
  - Pneumothorax
  - Pneumonia (see Chapter 31)
- Musculoskeletal disorders
  - Costochondritis
- Gastrointestinal disorders (see Chapter 32)
  - Pancreatitis
  - Gastric ulcers

TABLE 28.2 Potential Causes of Abdominal Pain Based on Location

Location of pain	Potential diagnosis
Right upper quadrant	Acute cholecystitis
	Biliary colic
	Acute hepatic distension or inflammation
	Perforated duodenal ulcer
Left upper quadrant	Perisplenitis
	Splenic infarct
Right lower quadrant	Acute appendicitis
	Mesenteric lymphadenitis
	Infective distal ileitis
	Crohn's disease
	Acute pyelonephritis
	Acute cholecystitis
	Acute rheumatic fever
	Ectopic pregnancy
	Ruptured ovarian cyst
Left lower quadrant	Acute diverticulitis
	Pyogenic sacroiliitis
Central abdominal pain	Gastroenteritis
	Small intestinal colic
	Acute pancreatitis

(Adapted from Blendis, 2003.)

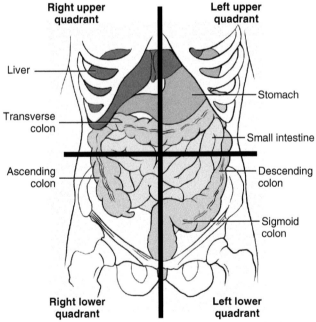

Fig. 28.7 Abdominopelvic Quadrants (Williams, 2018).

- Gallstones
- Reflux
- Psychological
- Anxiety

Adapted from MacLellan (2006).

Burns

Pain control for burn victims presents a significant nursing challenge because there are multiple causes of pain, which constantly change. It is vital that Nursing Associates caring for burn victims fully appreciate and recognize the multiple factors that contribute to the burn victim's pain experience. Pain from burns can be categorized as follows:

- Background pain: the pain generated by the burns and the surrounding areas. This pain is constant and at times excruciating and unbearable.
- Breakthrough pain: pain generated by movement, changing position or breathing. Breakthrough pain exacerbates background pain.
- Procedural pain: pain generated by necessary care interventions and therapies, such as wound cleansing, dressing changes and physiotherapy.
- Pain associated with tissue regeneration: wound healing and nerve regeneration can cause pain, which is often described as an itching or intense tingling sensation.

(Choiniere, 2003)

CHRONIC PAIN

Chronic pain is pain sensation that occurs in the absence of any discernible biological or physical cause. Chronic pain may be insidious, in that it develops over time and is often classified as a psychological phenomenon or syndrome. Such a description suggests that chronic pain occurs as a result of a maladaptive psychological response to prolonged and unresolved pain. Nevertheless, there are a number of chronic health conditions for which chronic pain is a feature. Examples include arthritis, neuropathy, chronic back pain and cancer.

Signs and symptoms of chronic pain

Autonomic stress responses in response to pain are difficult to maintain over sustained periods of time. Therefore, individuals living with chronic pain may not present with the signs and symptoms associated with acute pain. Rather, because chronic pain has debilitating psychological effects, sufferers may measure their pain by reporting its impact on their day to day life. Factors the Nursing Associate must consider are:

- Sleep: does the pain keep the patient awake during the night?
- Diet: does the pain have an impact on appetite?
- Sexuality: does the patient's pain have a negative impact on their libido or relationships?
- Socialization: is the patient able to maintain social activities or do they feel isolated?
- Mood and well-being: does the patient express any feelings of anxiety, depression or despair?

CRITICAL AWARENESS
Lack of Signs and Symptoms of Pain

People living with chronic pain may not present with the classic symptoms of pain seen in people in acute pain. However, while they may not appear to be in pain, their suffering could be as intense as someone in acute care; therefore, a lack of attention and compassion could lead to someone not receiving the care they need.

Remember – 'Pain is what the patient says it is'.

Care and treatment

The care priorities for the individual living with chronic pain are to reduce the impact of pain on the quality of life. The care aims are:

- Perform an accurate pain assessment
- Aadminister prescribed analgesia safely
- Monitor for evidence of the main side effects of opioid therapy
- Use psychological interventions such as cognitive behavioural therapy, relaxation, distraction and imagery
- Consider complimentary therapies
- Establish a pain management plan
- Monitor the individual's quality of care
- Refer to chronic pain services.

Arthritis

Around 100 conditions encompass arthritis (see also Chapter 39 of this text). The two most common are osteoarthritis and rheumatoid arthritis. The chronic pain associated with arthritis is caused by inflammation in the synovial membrane, tendons, ligaments and muscle strain. Arthritis pain can range from mild to severe and can last for weeks, months or even years. The inflammation that causes arthritis is unpredictable, which makes pain management challenging. The care of people living with arthritis should include:

- A comprehensive assessment of pain and function
- Analgesia that is appropriate for the level of pain
  - Paracetamol for mild to moderate pain
  - Non-steroidal anti-inflammatory drugs for moderate to severe pain
  - Opioid drugs for severe pain not alleviated by paracetamol or non-steroidal anti-inflammatory drugs
- Consideration of surgery when analgesic therapy is ineffective
- Promotion of ideal body weight
- Referral to physiotherapy and occupational therapy

MacLellan (2006).

Chronic back pain

Back pain affects most people at some point in their life. Sufferers describe an ache, tension or stiffness in their back, which is at times debilitating. Causes of back pain include poor posture, bending awkwardly or lifting incorrectly. In most cases, back pain is not caused by a serious condition and normally improves within 12 weeks. It can usually be successfully treated by taking painkillers and keeping mobile. In some cases, osteopathy and physiotherapy may be required. Chapter 39 of this text also considers back pain.

Back pain can be classified as follows:

- Transient back pain: back pain of a short lifespan, which does not normally require medical attention. Often the cause is unknown and does not have any long-term issues or any lasting significance to the patient.
- Acute back pain: back pain that is long term (i.e., several days to a few months in duration). Treatments include analgesia and bed rest, and surgery if associated with spinal injury/ inflammation.

- Persistent back pain: back pain that persists for more than 6 months. Sufferers may become preoccupied with the pain and depression and anxiety may occur.

CASE STUDY 28.1   Martin

Martin McGregor is a 40-year-old painter and decorator. He has recently separated from his partner, who has moved 100 miles away with their children. Martin tries to see his children when he can but, due to financial difficulties, he has to work 6 to 7 days a week to make ends meet.

Martin injured his back when he fell off a ladder 6 months ago. Since then, he has suffered intermittently with back pain, which is exacerbated by standing for long periods of time. Lately his pain seems worse than ever. It is an almost constant presence and it has spread to his neck and shoulder. He finds it difficult to sleep and during the day, he finds that he often loses his temper with people. He has tried using anti-inflammatory analgesics and gels and ointments, but they appear to have little effect. Martin visits his GP and confesses that the only thing that seems to work at present is alcohol. Martin is currently drinking every evening to help him sleep. Martin's GP prescribes diclofenac 50 mg three times a day, advises him to reduce his alcohol intake and take a week off work to rest his back. Martin is reluctant to take time off as he is self-employed and if he does not work, he does not earn any money.

REFLECTION 28.1

Depression commonly accompanies and exacerbates chronic pain. How can healthcare professionals help people like Martin? Are analgesics the only pain control option available to healthcare professionals?

Take some time to consider Martin McGregor's situation. What is the impact of Martin's relationship breakdown and financial concerns on his back pain?

Neuropathy

Neuropathic pain occurs when nociceptors and neurons are damaged. This can occur as a result of trauma or numerous conditions. Table 28.3 lists some of the common causes of neuropathic pain. Patients with neuropathy describe their pain as being a burning, electric or a tingling sensation that can be continuous or spasmodic. The nervous tissue is often described as being plastic as it can change in response to different psychological and physical stimuli. Such changes can include altered

TABLE 28.3   Causes of Neuropathy

Cause	Examples
Trauma	Painful scars
	Thoracotomy
	Amputation
	Damage through heat, cold, electricity, radiation
Ischaemia	
Toxins	Thallium
	Arsenic
	Clioquinol
Metabolic effects	Diabetes
Nutritional	Vitamin B_{12} deficiency
Inflammation	Multiple sclerosis
Infection	Human immunodeficiency virus
Cancer	Myeloma
Hereditary	Fabry disease

(Scadding, 2003; Hanna et al., 2011.)

sensitivity of nociceptors, which leads to pain impulses in response to ordinary feelings of touch. The patient may also report pain in response to minimal pressure on injuries, a phenomenon called 'allodynia'. Individuals living with neuropathy may describe pain that appears out of proportion to the level of tissue damage, a phenomenon known as hyperalgesia (Scadding, 2003).

Cancer pain

Up to 96% of patients with cancer experience pain, more than AIDS (80%), heart disease (77%), renal disease (77%) and chronic obstructive pulmonary disease (50%) (Solano et al., 2006). The causes of cancer pain are multiple but the most likely contributing factor is bone metastases. Cancer pain can be classified as being somatic or visceral nociceptor pain or neuropathic pain. Table 28.4 lists the different types of cancer pain and their possible causes.

CASE STUDY 28.2 Luke

Luke Podmore is a 76-year-old retired plumber, who lives alone. For the past 12 months, he has been living with lung cancer. Pain is a constant in his life at present, especially in his left shoulder and his back. Luke has tried over-the-counter analgesics but none of them seem to work. The pain is often debilitating and he has not been able to get out of his flat for several days. He spends the majority of the day on his sofa, watching television. Luke has always enjoyed being outdoors; he visits friends and likes to go walking in the park. Being unable to leave his flat has led to him feeling depressed. The pain also keeps him awake at night and he feels constantly tired during the day. Luke also has little appetite and only eats light snacks.

CARE IN THE HOME SETTING

The Community Palliative Care Nurse

Luke is visited by a community palliative care nurse. Her main care priority is to assess and treat his pain. She refers Luke to his GP, who in turn prescribes an opioid analgesia for his shoulder and back pain. The nurse also advises Luke on the potential side effects, such as nausea and constipation.

In subsequent visits, Luke reports that his shoulder and back pain has eased and that he is able to sleep much better. He does report that he has become constipated, for which the community palliative care nurse prescribes a laxative. She also encourages him to try and go walking in the park again and explores ways in which he can increase his dietary intake.

TABLE 28.4 Types of Cancer Pain, Their Source, Causes and Descriptions

Type of pain	Structures affected	Causes	Patient description
Somatic nociceptor	Muscle and bone	Bone metastases Surgical incisions	Aching, sharp, gnawing or dull Easily located
Neuropathic	Nerves	Chemotherapy Tumours	Burning, itching, numbness, tingling, shooting
Visceral nociceptor	Organs of the abdomen, pelvis and thorax	Tumour	Crampy, colicky, aching, deep, squeezing, dull Less easily located

(Adapted from Kochhar, 2002.)

The aim of palliative care is to minimize pain and its associated distressing symptoms (World Health Organization, 2008). Cancer pain is therefore classified according to when it occurs, or if it becomes more intense and unmanageable. The three main classifications of cancer pain are:
- Breakthrough pain: this occurs in addition to the underlying cancer pain. It is more intense than the patient's normal pain levels.
- Incident pain: is caused by incidental activities (i.e., walking, lifting, climbing stairs, washing and dressing).
- End-of-dose failure pain: this occurs if the therapeutic effects of the patient's prescribed analgesia subside before the next dose is due. Breakthrough and incident pain are common, even in patients whose pain is well controlled. End-of-dose pain, however, is an indicator that the patient's current pain control may need reviewing (Hayden, 2006).

The World Health Organization produced the analgesic ladder in 1986 to help combat cancer pain. The ladder has three steps, each containing a recommended level of pharmacological treatment (Fig. 28.8). If pain persists, the patient's treatment should be moved up to the next step. The goal is for the patient to be pain free at the lowest point on the ladder. Step one involves the use of non-opioid drugs, step two recommends adding a weak opioid and the final step advocates the use of strong opioids. Each step also suggests the use of an adjuvant. Adjuvants are a range of drugs that have analgesic effects, despite being normally prescribed for other conditions. Antidepressants, anticonvulsants, muscle relaxants, corticosteroids and local anaesthetics have all been shown to reduce pain when used in conjunction with opioid and non-opioid drugs.

LOOKING BACK, FEEDING FORWARD

Pain is a personal experience. The way in which the individual in pain will express themselves will be dependent on their state

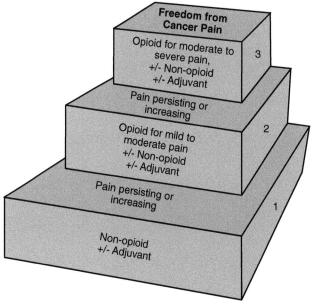

Fig. 28.8 The Analgesic Ladder (World Health Organization (1986) Cancer Pain Relief, WHO, Geneva).

of mind, their personality, their upbringing, culture, life experiences and the meaning they ascribe to the pain. Acute pain can be debilitating but is often short-term; however, it has a significant impact on the human body and, if left unresolved, can become problematic and could potentially lead to the development of chronic pain. Therefore, the management of pain is crucial if homeostasis is to be maintained. There are many forms of analgesia that are at the healthcare teams disposal; however, as pain is an emotional as well as physiological experience, non-pharmacological methods must also be explored. Healthcare professionals, including Nursing Associates, are ideally placed to provide effective care for the patient with pain, as long as they remember that pain is what the patient says it is.

REFERENCES

Bell, L., Duffy, A., 2009. Pain assessment and management in surgical nursing: a literature review. Br. J. Nurs. 18 (3), 153–156.

Blendis, L.M., 2003. Abdominal pain. In: Melzack, R., Wall, P.D. (Eds.), Handbook of Pain Management: A Clinical Companion to Wall and Melzack's Textbook of Pain. Churchill Livingstone, Edinburgh.

Briggs, E., 2010. Understanding the experience and physiology of pain. Nurs. Stand. 25 (3), 35–39.

Carr, E.C.J., Thomas, V.N., Wilson-Barnet, J., 2005. Patient experiences of anxiety, depression and acute pain after surgery: a longitudinal perspective. Int. J. Nurs. Stud. 42, 521–530.

Choiniere, M., 2003. Pain of burns. In: Melzack, R., Wall, P.D. (Eds.), Handbook of Pain Management: A Clinical Companion to Wall and Melzack's Textbook of Pain. Churchill Livingstone, Edinburgh.

Dopson, L., 2010. Role of pain management programmes in chronic pain. Nurs. Stand. 25 (13), 35–40.

Eccleston, C., Williams, A., Morley, S., 2009. Psychological therapies for the management of chronic pain (excluding headache) in adults (review). Cochrane Database Syst. Rev. (2), CD007047.

Furlan, A.D., Brosseau, L., Imamura, M., Irvin, E., 2002. Massage for low back pain. Cochrane Database Syst. Rev. (2), CD001929.

Godfrey, H., 2005a. Understanding pain, part 1: physiology of pain. Br. J. Nurs. 14 (16), 846–852.

Godfrey, H., 2005b. Understanding pain, part 2: pain management. Br. J. Nurs. 14 (17), 904–909.

Hader, C.F., Guy, J., 2004. Your hand in pain management. Nurs. Manage. 35 (11), 21–28.

Hanna, M., Holdcroft, A., Jaggar, S.I., 2011. Neuropathic pain. In: Holdcroft, A., Jaggar, S. (Eds.), Core Topics in Pain. Cambridge University Press.

Hayden, D., 2006. Pain management in palliative care. In: MacLellan, K. (Ed.), Expanding Nursing and Health Care Practice: Management of Pain. Nelson Thornes, Cheltenham.

Johansson, K., Nuutila, L., Virtanen, H., et al., 2005. Preoperative education for orthopaedic patients: systematic review. J. Adv. Nurs. 50 (2), 212–223.

Kingston, K., Bailey, C., 2009. Assessing the pain of people living with a learning disability. Br. J. Nurs. 18 (7), 420–423.

Kochhar, S.C., 2002. Cancer pain. In: Warfield, C.A., Fausett, H.J. (Eds.), Manual of Pain Management, second ed. Lippincott Williams & Wilkins, Philadelphia.

Layzell, M., 2008. Current interventions and approaches to post-operative pain management. Br. J. Nurs. 17 (7), 414–419.

Lee, H., Ernst, E., 2005. Acupuncture analgesia during surgery: a systematic review. Pain 114 (3), 511–517.

Lin, L., Wang, R., 2005. Abdominal surgery, pain and anxiety: preoperative nursing intervention. J. Adv. Nurs. 51 (3), 252–260.

Lorentzen, V., Hermansen, I.L., Botti, M., 2012. A prospective analysis of pain experience, beliefs and attitudes, and pain management in a cohort of Danish surgical patients. Eur. J. Pain 16 (2), 278–288.

Lundeberg, T., Stener-Victorin, E., 2002. Is there a physiological basis for the use of acupuncture in pain? Int. Congr. Ser. 1238, 3–10.

MacIntyre, P.E., Schug, S.A., 2015. Acute Pain Management: A Practical Guide, fourth ed. CRC Press, Boca Raton.

MacLellan, K., 2006. Expanding Nursing and Health Care Practice: Management of Pain. Nelson Thornes, Cheltenham.

Manias, E., Botti, M., Bucknall, T., 2002. Observation of pain assessment and management – the complexities of clinical practice. J. Clin. Nurs. 11, 724–733.

Marieb, E., Hoehn, K., 2007. Human Anatomy and Physiology, seventh ed. Pearson Benjamin Cummings, San Francisco.

McCaffery, M., 1979. Nursing Management of the Patient with Pain, second ed. J.B. Lippincott Company, New York.

McCaffery, R., Frock, T.L., Garguilo, H., 2003. Understanding chronic pain and the mind–body connection. Holist. Nurs. Pract. 17 (6), 281–287.

McGann, K., 2007. Fundamental Aspects of Pain Assessment and Management. Quay Books, Gateshead.

Melzack, R., Wall, P., 1988. The Challenge of Pain, second ed. Penguin, London.

Scadding, J.W., 2003. Peripheral neuropathies. In: Melzack, R., Wall, P.D. (Eds.), Handbook of Pain Management: A Clinical Companion to Wall and Melzack's Textbook of Pain. Churchill Livingstone, Edinburgh.

Sluka, K.A., Walsh, D., 2003. Transcutaneous electrical nerve stimulation: basic science mechanisms and clinical effectiveness. J. Pain 4 (3), 109–121.

Solano, J.P., Games, B., Higginson, I.J., 2006. A comparison of symptom prevalence in far advanced cancer, AIDS, heart disease, chronic obstructive pulmonary disease (COPD) and renal disease. J. Pain Symptom Manage. 31 (1), 58–69.

Waugh, A., Grant, A., 2018. Ross & Wilson Anatomy and Physiology in Health and Illness, thirteenth ed. Elsevier, Edinburgh.

Wigens, L., 2006. The role of complementary and alternative therapies in pain management. In: MacLellan, K. (Ed.), Expanding Nursing and Health Care Practice: Management of Pain. Nelson Thornes, Cheltenham.

Williams, P., 2018. deWit's Fundamental Concepts and Skills for Nursing, fifth ed. Elsevier, Missouri.

World Health Organization, 2008. National Cancer Control Programmes: Policies and Management Guidelines, second ed. WHO, Geneva.

29

Cardiovascular Disorders

Carl Clare

OBJECTIVES

By the end of the chapter the reader will:
1. Have an understanding of the anatomy and physiology of the cardiovascular system
2. Discuss the pathophysiological changes associated with a selection of cardiovascular disorders
3. Understand the relationship between the cardiovascular system and other body systems
4. Outline the care required by people with cardiovascular disorders
5. Describe some common conditions associated with the cardiovascular system
6. Review the role of the Nursing Associate in promoting health and well-being

KEY WORDS

Valve	SA Node	Deoxygenated
Artery	Myocardium	Atria
Vein	Myocyte	
Ventricle	Oxygenated	

CHAPTER AIMS

This aim of this chapter is to provide the reader with an understanding of the skills, knowledge and attitude required to provide safe, effective and compassionate care to people with a cardiovascular disorder.

SELF TEST

1. What are the four chambers of the heart?
2. Blood travelling from the heart to the organs is transported in what type of blood vessels?
3. What is a myocyte?
4. What does stroke volume mean?
5. Discuss the blood supply to the heart muscles.
6. What is the most common heart rhythm disorder in the UK?
7. What is a myocardial infarction?
8. What do you understand by the term 'cardiac rehabilitation'?
9. What is meant by secondary prevention?
10. How can coronary artery disease be prevented?

INTRODUCTION

In this chapter, the cardiovascular system is considered. The first part discusses the anatomy and physiology of the cardiovascular system. It is important for the Nursing Associate to have a comprehensive understanding of the cardiovascular system, to provide appropriate and effective care.

The second part of the chapter addresses a selection of common conditions that impact on the cardiovascular health and well-being of people. The care and comfort of the patient who experiences a cardiovascular disorder are described. The heart is often seen as the source of life and any disorder of the heart will create fear and anxiety. When offering care, the Nursing Associate is required to be kind and compassionate. Care provision must recognize the fear that a cardiovascular condition can instil within a patient and must be sensitive to the anxiety that is often present.

SENSITIVE CARE

When caring for a patient with a cardiovascular disorder, it is essential that the Nursing Associate is sensitive to the physical and psychological effects such a condition can create. Many patients, especially those first diagnosed with a cardiovascular condition, will show evidence of anxiety and, potentially, fear. There can often be a fear of dying and the patient will commonly be concerned about their future life in terms of ability to work, being a family member (for instance mother or father) and such like. This can sometimes make patients, and their relatives, seem demanding, aggressive or distant in their interactions with staff.

It is important to understand in these situations that their response is not personal and requires sensitive and calm handling.

Patients (and relatives of patients) who are suffering from an acute cardiovascular condition will often have a lot of questions, many of which cannot be answered at the time of diagnosis as the information will not be available. For instance, common questions from relatives (and patients) include: will the patient be 'alright'? How bad is it? How long will they be in hospital? When can they go back to work? Unfortunately, the answer to many of these questions is 'we don't know'. Especially in the first hours of an acute cardiovascular emergency, medical staff are unable to give detailed responses as the full effect of the condition is unknown and will only become clear as time passes. In these situations, it is essential that care staff are sensitive, open and honest in their communication. It is not a failure of your ability as a carer to say that you 'don't know' and to offer to either find out or to explain why this information is not yet available. The Nursing and Midwifery Council Code (Nursing and Midwifery Council, 2018) is clear that you must ensure that, if you are unsure, you should always strive to refer the patient to a person who does know; you should only act within the sphere of your competence.

Part of the role of the Nursing Associate is to deliver person-centred holistic care (Health Education England, 2017) and one of the most overlooked aspects of caring for the acutely ill at the time of admission/diagnosis is just to 'be there' for the patient and their relatives. Being an open and empathic presence is just as important to many patients and their relatives as the physical care that we provide.

THE CARDIOVASCULAR SYSTEM

The cardiovascular system can be viewed as a closed transport system (like a road system). The purpose of the system is to deliver oxygen and nutrients to the various parts of the body and to transport waste products for excretion. Any disorder of this system will lead to some disruption of this transportation mechanism and, in some cases, its complete failure.

The components of the cardiovascular system (Fig. 29.1) are the heart, arteries, veins and capillaries (the latter three are known collectively as the blood vessels). Each component is vital to the continuing health of the system as a whole and, whilst the system is considered as one unit, it is useful when learning about the cardiovascular system to separate the anatomy and physiology into two sections: the heart and the blood vessels.

The heart

The heart is a relatively small but very muscular organ, located in the chest, behind and slightly to the left of the breast bone (Fig. 29.2). It sits in a space (the mediastinum) between the

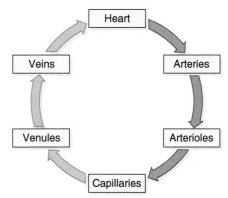

Fig. 29.1 The Heart and the Blood Vessels Make One System (Waugh & Grant, 2014).

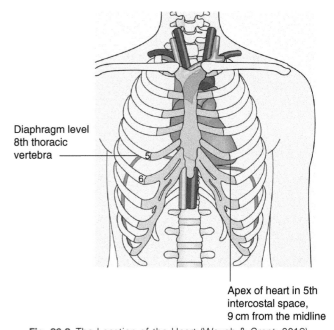

Diaphragm level 8th thoracic vertebra

Apex of heart in 5th intercostal space, 9 cm from the midline

Fig. 29.2 The Location of the Heart (Waugh & Grant, 2018).

lungs and is inverted (it is upside down), with the apex located at the 'bottom', nearest the diaphragm, and the base up towards the head.

The heart contains four chambers made of specialized muscle and is surrounded by a series of layers (known as the pericardium). The pericardium is commonly referred to as though it is a single sac that surrounds the heart but it is actually made up of two membranes, the fibrous pericardium and the serous pericardium.

- The fibrous pericardium is a tough, semi-rigid, membrane that protects the heart, anchors it in place in the chest cavity and prevents the heart from becoming overstretched.
- The serous pericardium is a thinner membrane that folds back on itself to create a double layer around the heart; these two layers are known as the parietal and visceral pericardium. Between the parietal and visceral pericardium is a 'potential space' (i.e., a space so small it is virtually not there), which contains a very thin film of pericardial fluid. The role of the pericardial fluid is to reduce the friction between the

membranes as the heart moves during its normal cycle of contraction and relaxation. Without the fluid, the two layers of the serous pericardium would rub together as the heart expands and contracts, leading to inflammation, pain and eventual damage.

The largest proportion of the heart is made up of myocardium (specialized heart muscle). Myocardium is a not found in any other part of the body and is unlike any other muscle found in the body. Furthermore, the myocardium is split into two types. The majority of the myocardial cells carry out the mechanical work of making the heart contract; the remaining cells are specialized conduction cells that transmit the nerve impulses that coordinate the heartbeat.

The cardiac muscle cells (known as myocytes) are held in bundles that are connected together and look like sheets of cells. Each myocyte is connected end to end to its surrounding myocytes and this allows the rapid passage of electrical impulses, ensuring that all the cells in a 'sheet' contract at the same time. Unlike skeletal muscle, the myocardial cells are not under our conscious control. As the muscles of the heart are never at rest, they are adapted in ways to make sure that they do not tire, like skeletal muscle. For instance, myocytes contain many more mitochondria than skeletal muscle cells and the mitochondria are also much larger. As mitochondria are the energy generators of the cell, the presence of more mitochondria (and the fact they are larger than normal) means that the cardiac muscle has a constant energy supply but it also means that the cardiac muscle requires a significantly greater oxygen supply and is less tolerant of shortages in oxygen than other muscle.

Coating the inside of the myocardium is a smooth, continuous layer known as endocardium. The endocardium also coats the surfaces of the heart valves and the blood vessels.

Even though the heart is referred to as a pump, it is better to think of it as two pumps (Fig. 29.3):

- The right heart pump: deoxygenated blood is returned to the right heart and is then pumped out into the pulmonary circulation (the lungs).
- The left heart pump: oxygenated blood is returned to the left heart from the pulmonary circulation and is then pumped out into the systemic circulation (the rest of the body).

Structurally, the heart is made up of four chambers: two atria and two ventricles. The atria are the smaller chambers of the heart and are above the ventricles (Fig. 29.4).

- The right atrium receives blood from the systemic circulation (blood returning from the majority of the body).
- The left atrium receives blood from the lungs (pulmonary circulation).

Between these two atria, there is a thin dividing wall known as the interatrial septum. Because they have lower pressures to overcome in ejecting the blood they contain, the atria have much thinner walls than the ventricles.

Both atria pump blood out into their respective ventricles (right and left) through atrioventricular valves. The presence of the valves ensures that blood does not flow backwards, from the ventricles into the atria, when the ventricles contract.

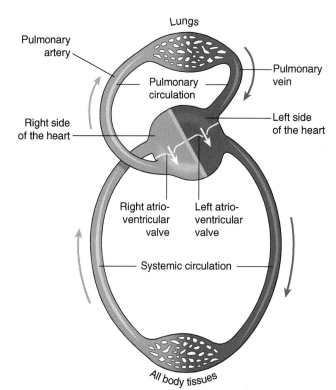

Fig. 29.3 A Simplified Diagram of Blood Flow in the Cardiovascular System Showing the Right and Left Heart Pumps (Waugh & Grant, 2018).

The tricuspid valve lies between the right atrium and the right ventricle.

The bicuspid (mitral) valve lies between the left atrium and the left ventricle.

As noted, each atrium ejects blood into its associated ventricle:

- The right ventricle receives blood from the right atrium and pumps this blood out into the pulmonary circulation (the lungs). As the right ventricle has a lower pressure to overcome, it has a thinner wall than the left ventricle.
- The left ventricle receives blood from the left atrium and pumps this blood out into the systemic circulation (the rest of the body) via the aorta. As the left ventricle has to overcome a higher pressure and pump blood over a greater distance, it has a much thicker (more muscular) wall than the right ventricle.

Between the ventricles is the interventricular septum. Thus, with the septum between the atria and the septum between the ventricles, there is no mixing of blood between the two sides.

At the outlet of each ventricle is a valve. These ensure that blood does not enter the ventricles from the blood vessels whilst the ventricles are filling with blood from the atria.

- The pulmonary valve is located between the right ventricle and the arteries supplying the lungs (the pulmonary arteries) and prevents the backwards flow of blood into the right ventricle from the pulmonary arteries.
- The aortic valve is located between the left ventricle and the main artery supplying the rest of the body (the aorta) and

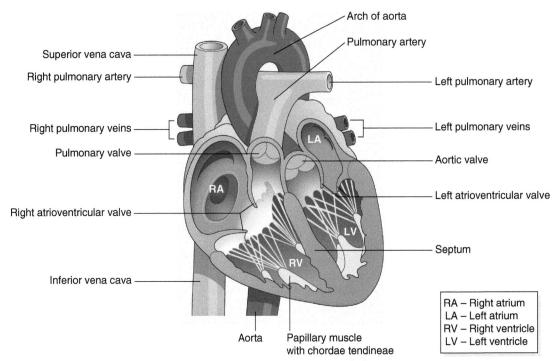

Fig. 29.4 The Structure of the Heart (Waugh & Grant, 2018).

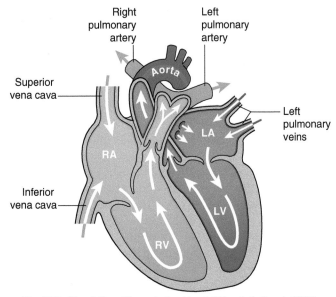

Fig. 29.5 Blood Flow Through the Heart (Waugh & Grant, 2018).

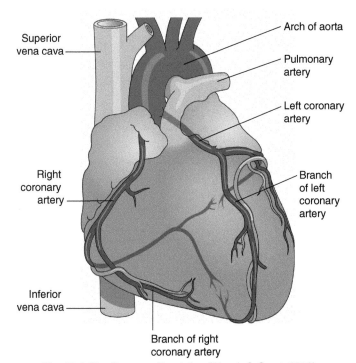

Fig. 29.6 The Coronary Circulation (Waugh & Grant, 2018).

prevents the backwards flow of blood into the left ventricle from the systemic circulation.

The blood flow through the heart can be seen in Fig. 29.5.

Blood supply to the heart

The heart requires a large and uninterrupted blood supply to ensure that it receives the significant amounts of oxygen and nutrients it requires and for the removal of associated waste products. Thus, the heart receives approximately 5% of the total amount of blood it pumps out at every beat. To ensure that the myocardium is well perfused with blood, the heart is interlaced with its own dedicated blood vessel system, known as the coronary circulation.

Just after the point that the main blood vessel to the body (the aorta) meets the heart, there are two openings (ostia) from which the main coronary arteries arise (Fig. 29.6). These main arteries then divide and subdivide into smaller and smaller arteries that dive deep into the heart muscle to ensure that the full thickness of the heart wall is supplied with blood.

To ensure the coordinated contraction of the heart muscle, there is a dedicated network of electrical conduction fibres to transmit electrical impulses rapidly throughout the myocardium. The network is made of specialized myocardial cells whose sole purpose is the generation and transmission of electrical signals. As such, they do not contract like other myocardial cells. A simplified diagram detailing the electrical system of the heart can be seen in Fig. 29.7. One aspect to note (that is not present in the diagram for the sake of simplicity) is that between the atria and the ventricles, there is a layer of nonconducting fibrous tissue. This nonconducting layer splits the heart (electrically) into two halves. Thus, the atria are electrically isolated from the ventricles. This means that both the atria beat as one unit and both the ventricles beat as one unit (but at a different time to the atria). This is often referred to as the atria and the ventricles acting as two syncytia (that is the atria act in a synchronized manner and the ventricles also act as a synchronized whole). The importance of this fact should become clear in the discussion of the cardiac cycle later in the chapter.

In Fig. 29.7, it can be noted that there are two areas of collected cells (known as nodes). These nodes are the basis for the control of the electrical stimulation of the heart. The sino-atrial (SA) node is located in the upper right part of the right atrium and is the 'pacemaker' of the heart. All electrical conduction cells in the heart have the ability to generate an electrical impulse (this is known as 'automaticity' or 'autorhythmicity'); the difference is in how fast these impulses are generated. In the SA node, the cells would create impulses at a rate of approximately 100 per minute if they were not affected by other factors (see the later section on the control of the heart rate for more details). This rate being the fastest 'normal' impulse generation rate in the heart means that the SA node overrides the impulse generation in all other parts of the conduction system. Should the SA node fail for any reason, the atrioventricular (AV) node is the next fastest impulse generator (at 40–60 impulses a minute) and would take over the control of the heart rate.

Electrical impulses generated in the SA node are rapidly spread throughout both atria via tracts of nerve fibres, thus ensuring that the two atria are electrically excited (and thus contract) at same time. Once the electrical impulse arrives at the AV node, it is held there for approximately 100 ms before being passed to the ventricles via the atrioventricular bundle (otherwise known as the bundle of His). This atrioventricular bundle is normally the only tract that communicates, electrically, between the atria and the ventricles. There are certain conditions where a second electrical tract can be present but these are rare and considered to be an abnormality of cardiac anatomy that requires treatment. Because the impulse is delayed by the AV node, this ensures that the atria have completed their contraction before the ventricles begin to contract.

Once the electrical impulse is transmitted through the atrioventricular bundle, it enters into the two bundle branches (one for the left ventricle and one for the right ventricle). From these two bundle branches, smaller and smaller fibres spread out (like tree roots) to ensure that every part of the heart is connected to the electrical system. This branching system of nerve fibres that supply the ventricles is known as the Purkinje system (or Purkinje fibres) and a simplified idea of what the system looks like can be seen in Fig. 29.7.

The cardiac cycle

The cardiac cycle is best understood if the heart is thought about as the two syncytia (the atria and the ventricles) acting separately to each other but in a coordinated manner (controlled by the conduction system). To understand the cardiac cycle, you also need to understand that it relies on two processes or movements: contraction and relaxation.

The contraction of a heart chamber is normally known as systole. Thus, you can refer to ventricular systole (the ventricles contracting) or atrial systole (the atria contracting). This is an active process requiring muscle contraction.

The relaxation of a heart chamber is known as diastole. Therefore, you can refer to ventricular diastole (the ventricles relaxing) or atrial diastole (the atria relaxing). Diastole (relaxation) is a passive process that requires the muscles to relax so that the pressure inside the heart chamber can push the heart walls out to their starting position.

One thing to note is that the cardiac cycle of contraction and relaxation of both the atria and the ventricles is very short and the time taken is related to the heart rate. For instance, at a heart rate of 74 beats per minute, the cardiac cycle will be 0.8 seconds long.

The cardiac cycle can be seen in Fig. 29.8. At section A, the atria are full of blood, the right atrium with blood that has returned from the body's circulation via the inferior vena cava and superior vena cava. This blood is relatively deoxygenated (it still contains oxygen but less than oxygenated blood) as it has supplied the bodily tissues with oxygen and transported away carbon dioxide. The left atrium is filled with blood from the pulmonary circulation (the lungs), which is oxygenated. It is important to note that the colours in the diagram are to help the reader, they do not reflect the colour of real oxygenated and deoxygenated blood (in fact deoxygenated blood is actually a darker shade of red than oxygenated blood). Because the ventricles are relaxed, the AV valves are open, allowing blood to flow through into the ventricles. The aortic and pulmonary valves remain closed at this point and so the blood is contained within the expanding ventricles.

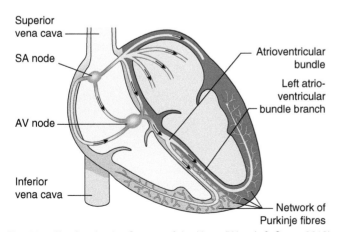

Fig. 29.7 The Conduction System of the Heart (Waugh & Grant, 2018).

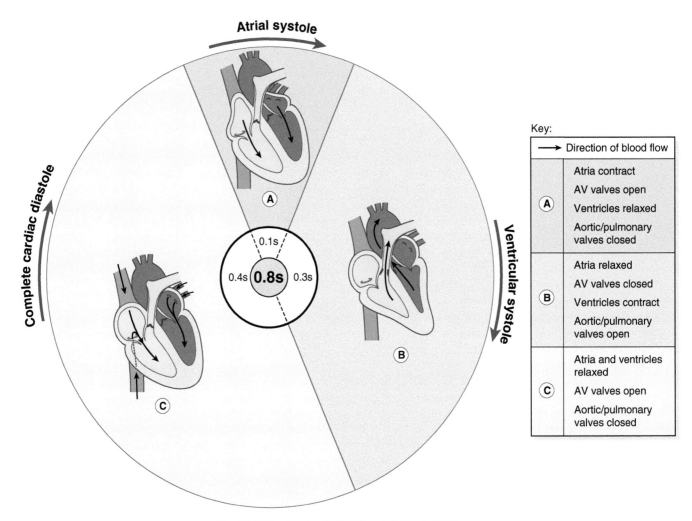

Fig. 29.8 The Cardiac Cycle (Waugh & Grant, 2018).

In section B, the atria relax and the ventricles begin to contract until they generate enough pressure to push the AV valves closed and eventually, as the pressure rises, to open the aortic and pulmonary valves. Thus, blood is pumped out into the pulmonary (lung) and systemic (bodily) circulation.

Finally, in section C, all the heart chambers relax. The aortic and pulmonary valves are pushed closed by the pressure in the aorta and pulmonary arteries and the AV valves open to allow the free flow of blood into the ventricles. When the SA node transmits an impulse, this starts the whole cycle again with section A.

In the simplest terms, the sections of Fig. 29.8 can be summarized as:

A: Atrial contraction (atrial systole)

B: Ventricular contraction (ventricular systole).

C: Whole heart relaxation (atrial and ventricular diastole).

Putting the cardiac cycle and the activity of the conduction system of the heart together, it can be seen that section A is related to the production of an electrical impulse in the SA node being transmitted to the atria. Section B relates to the transmission of the impulse from the AV bundle to the ventricles and section C relates to the time when no electrical activity is being generated.

In everyday practice, the mechanical activity of the heart can be visualized using an echocardiogram (many videos of echocardiograms can be found on the internet) but this is a specialized test that is not seen often in the ward or community environment. The electrical activity of the heart is regularly monitored both in hospital and in the community (for instance in a General Practitioner [GP] surgery) by the use of an electrocardiogram (ECG). The relationship between the ECG and the cardiac cycle can be seen in Fig. 29.9.

In Fig. 29.9, the P wave is the electrical activity of the atrial contraction (section A in Fig. 29.8). The QRS complex is the electrical activity related to the ventricular contraction (section B of Fig. 29.8) and the T wave shows the electrical relaxation (repolarization) of the ventricles (section C of Fig. 29.8); atrial relaxation is electrically small and is hidden by the QRS complex.

> ### ! HOTSPOT
>
> Recording an ECG is a skilled activity and should only be done when you have been appropriately trained and assessed.

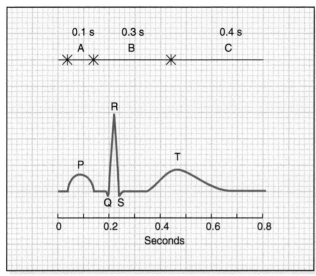

Fig. 29.9 An Electrocardiogram of One Cardiac Cycle (the letters at the top correspond to the sections in Fig. 29.8) (Waugh & Grant, 2018).

Control of heart rate

Heart rate is affected by many factors, such as age, sex, nervous control, circulating hormones, and chemicals, to name a few. Heart rate is controlled by two main mechanisms:

- Autonomic nervous system activity. Sympathetic nervous system activity leads to an increase in heart rate and parasympathetic nervous system activity leads to a decrease in heart rate.
- Hormone activity. The release of adrenaline or large amounts of thyroxine leads to an increase in heart rate.

! HOTSPOT

The normal heart rate for a person is considered to be between 60 and 100 beats per minute (bpm).

A heart rate slower than 60 bpm is known as a 'bradycardia' and a heart rate higher than 100 bpm is known as a 'tachycardia'. Either a bradycardia or a tachycardia may be a cause for concern and should be recorded on the observation/National Early Warning Score (NEWS) chart and reported to senior staff.

OSCE 29.1   Electrocardiograph (ECG)

This test is used to record the electrical activity of the heart from different angles, to identify and locate abnormality. Electrodes are placed on different parts of a patient's limbs and chest to record the electrical activity.

The procedure should be undertaken using local policy and procedure.

Action	Criteria	Achieved/not achieved
Introduction	Washes hands	
	Introduces self	
	Confirms patient details	
	Checks for allergies	
Explain the procedure	Explains rationale for test so patient is able to understand and is able to give informed consent	
	Gains consent to proceed	
Gathers equipment	Hand washing gel	
	• ECG machine and paper	
	• Self-adhesive ECG electrodes (ensure patient is not allergic to the adhesive)	
	• Razor	
Position of patient and electrode placement	Positions patient on examination couch at 45 degrees	
	Exposes the patient appropriately and offers a chaperone	
	• Removes socks from the patient to expose ankles	
	• Exposes patient's chest (preserves dignity)	
	• Correctly places the 6 chest electrodes	
	Ensures good skin contact with the electrodes May need to remove hair at the electrode site	
	• If skin is particularly oily, cleans site with an alcohol wipe, allows to dry prior to electrode application	
	• If skin is visibly soiled, cleans it with soap and water, dries prior to electrode application	
	Once all electrodes have been applied, attaches associated leads	
	• Correctly places the 4 limb electrodes	
Records the trace	Adheres to manufactures instructions and local policy	
	Turns ECG machine on, ensures paper loaded	
	Double checks all electrodes are attached in appropriate positions	
	Asks patient to remain still and not talk during recording	
	Presses appropriate button to record trace	
	If tracing is poor, double checks connections to ensure good skin contact	
Completes procedure	Once trace has been obtained, switches off ECG machine	
	Detaches leads from electrodes	
	Gently removes electrodes	
	Thanks patient and allows them to get dressed or assists if needed	
	Washes hands	
	Labels ECG with patient's details, documents findings according to local policy and procedure	
	Responds to any questions patient may have	
Pass Fail		

The anatomy and physiology of blood vessels

When thinking of the circulatory system, it is first useful to consider the system as a whole before discussing the individual blood vessel types. In Fig. 29.10, the overall structure of a circulatory system can be seen; this shows the relationship between the heart and the blood vessels. It should be noted that this figure shows the overall structure of both circulatory systems (pulmonary and systemic) as they are both the same in structure, even though they differ in size and the pressures within them. It can be seen from the diagram that the heart pumps blood into the arteries, which then branch into smaller vessels, known as arterioles, until eventually the blood reaches the capillaries before being returned to venules and then to larger and larger veins. Thus, the basic principle is the 'closer' to the heart a vessel is the larger it will be and the vessels 'furthest' from the heart (the capillaries) are the smallest blood vessels of all.

Looking at the micrograph (Fig. 29.11), the comparative structures of veins and arteries can be compared.

The anatomy of an artery

• Outer layer (tunica externa or tunica adventitia)

This is a protective layer of fibres that protect the artery and prevent overstretching.

• Thick middle layer (tunica media)

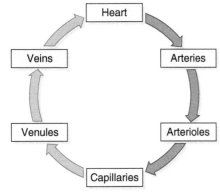

Fig. 29.10 The Structure of a Circulatory System (Waugh & Grant, 2014).

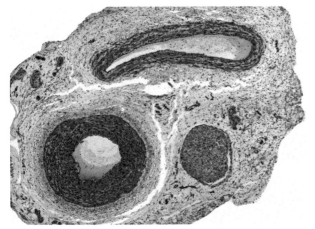

Fig. 29.11 A Light Micrograph of an Artery, a Vein and a Nerve (Waugh & Grant, 2018).

This is a layer of smooth muscle responsible for the control of the diameter of an artery.

• Inner layer (tunica intima)

The tunica intima is a covering of endothelium on the inside of the artery that creates a smooth surface for blood flow.

As the arterioles enter bodily tissues, the blood vessels change and the arteriole divides into multiple tiny vessels, known as capillaries. These collections of capillaries are known as capillary beds. The function of capillaries is to allow the exchange of substances (such as oxygen, carbon dioxide and nutrients) between the tissues and the blood. As the wall of the capillary is only made up of a single layer of cells, substances can easily pass from the blood into the tissues and vice versa. At the end of the capillary beds the capillaries begin to converge into venules.

Whilst the anatomy of a vein is similar to that of an artery there are some notable differences:

• Tunica media.

This is thinner in veins, as they do not have to overcome the higher pressures there are in arteries.

• Valves.

Veins and venules contain one-way valves that arise from the tunica intima, preventing backwards blood flow away from the heart.

Control of blood pressure

The factors associated with the short-term control of blood pressure can be presented as a simple equation:

$$\text{Blood pressure} = \text{Cardiac output} \times \text{Total peripheral resistance}$$

Note: total peripheral resistance is also known as systemic vascular resistance.

Cardiac output is a factor of the heart rate times the stroke volume, where stroke volume is the amount of blood the heart ejects in one beat. The control of the heart rate has been discussed earlier in the chapter. The control of stroke volume is a multifactorial process but one of the main factors is sympathetic nervous system activity. The greater the sympathetic nervous system input to the heart, the harder the heart beats and the greater the amount of the blood pumped by the heart (the greater the stroke volume).

The most important factor in the control of blood pressure is the total peripheral resistance. This refers to the resistance to blood flow created by the arterial system (specifically the arterioles). The resistance a blood vessel creates is derived from the diameter of the inner lumen. The relaxation or contraction of the muscle wall of the arteriole (and thus the lumen) is affected by many mechanisms but one of the most important is the output from the sympathetic nervous system (Fig. 29.12).

Longer-term control of blood pressure is a process of the renin–angiotensin–aldosterone system and the secretion of antidiuretic hormone. Both of these affect total blood volume and thus blood pressure.

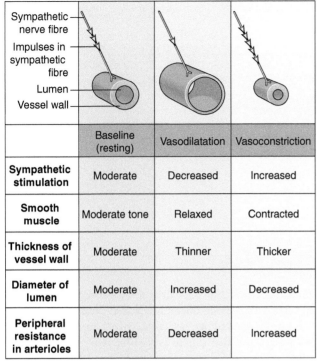

	Baseline (resting)	Vasodilatation	Vasoconstriction
Sympathetic stimulation	Moderate	Decreased	Increased
Smooth muscle	Moderate tone	Relaxed	Contracted
Thickness of vessel wall	Moderate	Thinner	Thicker
Diameter of lumen	Moderate	Increased	Decreased
Peripheral resistance in arterioles	Moderate	Decreased	Increased

Fig. 29.12 The Effects of Sympathetic Nervous System Outflow on the Arteriolar Wall (Waugh & Grant, 2018).

CARDIOVASCULAR DISORDERS

Stable angina

Signs and symptoms

Stable angina is characterized by chest pain/discomfort, jaw pain or pain in the arm (usually the left arm) that usually presents when the patient is exercising or emotionally distressed.

The heart muscle has a high oxygen requirement and the blood supply to the heart muscle is via the coronary arteries. In patients with coronary heart disease (angina or a myocardial infarction), the underlying changes are based on the same processes. Cholesterol and other fatty substances are deposited into the artery wall, creating a structure known as a plaque. As the plaque is in the wall of the artery, the lumen of the artery becomes narrowed, thus reducing blood flow to the heart muscles. In the case of stable angina, the blood flow is sufficient to supply enough oxygen to the heart when it is at rest but when the workload of the heart is increased (for instance by exercise), the oxygen demand of the heart muscle increases. The narrowing within one, or more, coronary arteries means the blood supply to the muscle is insufficient to deliver enough oxygen to meet the demand of the heart muscle and thus pain develops. Resting reduces the work of the heart and thus reduces the oxygen demand, removing the cause of the pain.

Diagnosis

The diagnosis of stable angina can often be made by taking a patient history. If the patient reports chest pain occurring on exertion (which may or may not radiate into the arm), lasting for a short period and relieved by rest, then the diagnosis is almost certainly stable angina. However, investigations and physical examination are still required to make a firm diagnosis and to assess the underlying heart disease:

- 12-Lead ECG: this will often be normal but occasionally changes will be seen that suggest previous damage to the heart muscle.
- Exercise tolerance test: this involves exercising the patient on a treadmill while they are attached to continuous ECG monitoring. Thus, the conditions whereby angina is often experienced (exercise) can be mimicked to see if chest pain occurs.
- Plasma glucose and cholesterol tests are also recommended to assess for two of the risk factors of coronary heart disease (Department of Health, 2000).

Care and treatment

Patients with stable angina will normally be prescribed a nitrate spray for use when they have episodes of pain. The spray is administered under the tongue as required by the patient. However, it is best to warn patients who are new to the use of the nitrate spray that it is best to sit down before using the spray, as it can cause a reduction in blood pressure and then the patient may faint. The patient should be taught that if the pain does not go after the first dose, to use the spray again 5 minutes later. If the pain has not gone 5 minutes after this second dose, then the patient should call an ambulance (NICE, 2016a).

If the patient has been diagnosed with angina, then it is necessary to give them information about their condition and give them time to ask questions. Advice will include resting when pain develops and the use of nitrate sprays.

As well as the nitrate spray, patients will often be prescribed regular medication for long-term control of their angina (SIGN, 2007). These medications include:
- Beta blockers
- Calcium channel blockers
- ACE inhibitors.

CRITICAL AWARENESS

The combination of nitrates with sildenafil is contraindicated. This combination must be avoided as it can produce significant hypotension and is potentially fatal. The guidance from the Committee on Safety of Medicines regarding nitrates and sildenafil states:
- sildenafil and nitrates - it is stated that these should not be used concurrently as there is a risk of severe hypotension. Nitrates are stated as those used for cardiovascular disease, such as glyceryl trinitrate spray, and also recreational compounds (e.g., amyl nitrate).
- sildenafil should not be used in men for whom sexual activity is inadvisable (e.g., patients with severe cardiovascular disorders, such as severe heart failure or unstable angina).

Unstable angina

Signs and symptoms

Unstable angina is characterized by cardiac chest pain (often radiating into the left arm or other areas) that is frequent, more severe and lasting longer than the pain associated with stable angina. Unstable angina pain may begin whilst the patient is resting or sleeping and is not relieved by rest or nitrate spray. Underlying unstable angina is the same narrowing of the

THE MEDICINE TROLLEY 29.1

Drug	Drug classification	Reason for administration	Route of administration	Dose	Side effects	Contra-indications	Nursing care
Atenolol	Beta blocker	Stable angina	Oral	100 mg daily (usually in two doses)	These include: slow heart rate, low blood pressure, dizziness, headache, sexual dysfunction, sleep disturbance, fatigue	Should be avoided in patient with asthma or low blood pressure, very slow heart rate	Seek consent prior to administration Explain the use of the drug to the patient, respond to any questions Monitor for low blood pressure or heart rate (especially with symptoms of dizziness) Maintain patient safety, observe for confusion/drowsiness

coronary arteries but often blood clots have developed in the narrowing, further reducing the blood flow. Often the clots develop and then partially dissolve, leading to the pain increasing and reducing over a short period of time.

Diagnosis

The diagnosis of unstable angina involves taking a medical history (to assess for risk factors) and a history of the present condition. An ECG will be required and blood tests will be taken, including tests for the cardiac enzyme troponin (see later for a discussion of troponin testing).

Care and treatment

Patients experiencing unstable angina should be nursed in bed and encouraged to rest. Pain relief may require the use of opiate analgesia but an intravenous infusion of a nitrate (such as isosorbide dinitrate) is often enough. As the underlying pathophysiology of unstable angina is normally based on the development of blood clots inside the lumen of the coronary artery, some form of anticoagulant drug is normally administered. Definitive treatment of unstable angina will normally include percutaneous coronary intervention (PCI) or coronary artery bypass grafts.

Myocardial infarction

A myocardial infarction is what is commonly referred to as a 'heart attack'. This is what most people immediately think of when they are asked to name a heart problem.

❗ HOTSPOT

Being precise in your use of language and clarifying what a patient or relative means by a particular term is essential. Where possible (and appropriate), use the correct terminology to avoid confusion and explain what it means as necessary.

To the lay person, the term 'heart attack' can be used to refer to a myocardial infarction or a cardiac arrest. As you can see, these are very different things and telling a relative their loved one has had a 'heart attack' may lead to unnecessary distress.

A myocardial infarction happens when the blood supply through a coronary artery is significantly reduced (by narrowing of the artery) or stopped altogether (usually by a thrombus) and the myocardial tissue dies due to lack of oxygen.

REFLECTION 29.2

What advice (evidence-based) might you give to a 68-year-old lady who asks you when it might be safe for her to resume sexual activity after a diagnosis of a myocardial infarction?

Signs and symptoms

The signs and symptoms of a myocardial infarction are related to the lack of blood flow to a part of the heart.

- Pain: most (but not all) patients experiencing a myocardial infarction will have pain. The pain is normally in the central chest and is often described as a crushing pain. It may be described as a tight band across the chest. Pain may radiate into the arms (the left arm is the classic side), the jaw, the neck and the epigastrium (upper abdomen).
- Nausea and vomiting: for reasons that are not clearly understood, many patients experiencing a myocardial infarction will experience significant nausea and may vomit.
- Shortness of breath: after pain, this is the most common symptom of a myocardial infarction.
- Sweatiness (diaphoresis): due to sympathetic nervous system activity.

Diagnosis

The primary test for a myocardial infarction is an ECG. Changes in the shape of the waves in the ECG can give information about the part of the heart affected and the size of the infarction. However, some changes can be subtle and thus the doctor will also take into account the patient's history and symptoms to aid diagnosis (Anderson & Morrow, 2017).

Secondary to the ECG, blood tests are taken for troponin I or troponin T levels. Troponin I and T are chemicals that are exclusively found in heart muscle and, when heart muscle

THE MEDICINE TROLLEY 29.2

Drug	Drug classification	Reason for administration	Route of administration	Dose	Side effects	Contra-indications	Nursing care
Aspirin	Antiplatelet drug	Unstable angina/myocardial infarction	Oral	150–300 mg daily	Bronchospasm, gastro-intestinal bleeding, skin reactions, tinnitus	Known sensitivity to aspirin	Seek consent prior to administration Explain the use of the drug to the patient, respond to any questions Explain to the patient aspirin is best taken with food
Clexane	Anticoagulant (low molecular weight heparin)	Unstable angina	Subcutaneous injection	100–325 mg once daily	These include: bleeding, injection site reactions, headache	Should be avoided in patients who are currently bleeding, suffer from gastric ulcers, have a history of renal impairment	Seek consent prior to administration Explain the use of the drug to the patient, respond to any questions Dispose of syringe in accordance with local policy Note the effect of this drug cannot be reversed easily
Unfractionated heparin	Anticoagulant	Unstable angina	Continuous intravenous infusion	Weight based	These include: bleeding, allergic reaction	Active bleeding, epidural analgesia, gastric ulcer, very high blood pressure	Seek consent prior to administration Explain the use of the drug to the patient, respond to any questions As with all patients receiving intravenous infusions, the cannula site must be monitored for signs of infection
Abciximab	GpIIa/IIIb inhibitor (platelet inhibitor)	Unstable angina	Continuous intravenous infusion	Weight based	These include: back pain, fever, headache, nausea, reduced heart rate	Active bleeding, major surgery within 2 months, very high blood pressure	Seek consent prior to administration Explain the use of the drug to the patient, respond to any questions As with all patients receiving intravenous infusions, the cannula site must be monitored for signs of infection

dies and ruptures, they are released into the blood (Reed et al., 2017). Following this release into the blood, the detection of troponin I or T indicates there has been damage to the heart muscle. Unfortunately, it takes at least 3 hours for detectable levels of troponins to develop in the blood, so they are best seen as a confirmation of a diagnosis and as being useful for judging the size of the damage to the heart muscle.

It should be noted that the use of troponin levels is not completely reliable, as the damage to the heart muscle may not necessarily be a myocardial infarction; thus, a rise in blood levels of troponin I or T are not considered absolute proof that a myocardial infarction has occurred.

Other tests are available for diagnosing a myocardial infarction but they are not readily available and are rarely used in the immediate medical emergency of an acute myocardial infarction.

Care and treatment

! HOTSPOT

Time is critical.

The treatment of a myocardial infarction is time critical. The sooner expert help is summoned and the quicker the treatment commenced, the more heart muscle may be saved.

Therefore, when you suspect a myocardial infarction you must escalate your concern immediately to senior staff (or if you are in the community by calling an ambulance).

As a medical emergency, the treatment of an acute myocardial infarction should begin as soon as possible; therefore, do not be afraid to raise concerns about a patient you think may be suffering from one.

When nursing a patient with any pain from a suspected cardiac origin, it is important to reduce the oxygen demand of the heart by reducing heart rate and the work of the heart. Patients with pain from a suspected cardiac origin should be nursed in a semi-recumbent position when possible and mobility should be restricted to use of the commode only. The semi-recumbent position reduces the return of blood to the heart and thus reduces the workload on the heart; however, if the patient has a low blood pressure, they may need to be nursed flat to prevent loss of consciousness. The patient should be kept calm to reduce heart rate and sympathetic nervous system activity. To help with this, it is important that staff looking after the patient remain calm and give reassurance to the patient.

Pain relief is an essential first-line treatment in any patient experiencing cardiac pain (Parodi, 2016). In the case of myocardial infarction, doctors will normally prescribe morphine or diamorphine. Both are powerful opiate drugs and are very effective at reducing cardiac pain. However, in common with all opiate drugs, both are also known to have the side effect of creating nausea, and potentially vomiting, in patients.

In addition to the potential side effect of opiate medication, many patients suffering from a myocardial infarction will be nauseous and may actively vomit (Anderson & Morrow, 2017). Vomit bowls and tissues should be supplied and, where prescribed, qualified staff should administer antiemetic medication, such as metoclopramide hydrochloride, prochlorperazine or ondansetron.

REFLECTION 29.3

Can you recall a time when you felt nauseous and vomited? How might you help a person who is feeling nauseous or is vomiting? What nursing interventions might you employ to care with compassion for that person?

Psychological care of the patient with myocardial infarction begins before diagnosis and never stops. After the acute event, the patient will require ongoing psychological care throughout their hospital stay and through the rehabilitation period. Depression is common in patients who have suffered a myocardial infarction (Smolderen et al., 2017) and healthcare staff should be ready to signpost services as appropriate.

The definitive treatment for a patient suffering from acute myocardial infarction is PCI, also commonly known as angioplasty (Levine et al., 2016). During the procedure, the patient has a catheter inserted through a hole made in the femoral artery and the catheter is manoeuvred to the artery, where the blockage is situated. A balloon is then passed through and inflated to push the thrombus into the walls of the artery and, if necessary, a metal cage (a stent) is inserted into the artery to keep the artery open.

Health promotion and the rehabilitation of the patient who has suffered from a myocardial infarction begin almost immediately. Patients should be advised to:
- Stop smoking
- Eat a healthy, balanced diet, including reducing fat intake
- Reduce alcohol intake (if appropriate)
- Take regular exercise (with doctor's permission)
- Take medication as prescribed

Once the patient is discharged from hospital they will be referred to a cardiac rehabilitation programme. Uptake and attendance in cardiac rehabilitation should be promoted, especially for patients from an ethnic minority background and women, as both groups show poor levels of uptake for cardiac rehabilitation (Dalal et al., 2015).

COMMUNITIES OF CARE
Black, Asian and Other Minority Ethnic Groups

Some black, Asian and other minority ethnic (BME) groups often face major health inequalities, with a differential risk of disease for various population subgroups:

Some BME groups have a higher incidence of cardiovascular disease when compared with the general population. The incidence of angina is higher amongst Pakistani men of all ages, as well as for Indian women. Pakistani men and women who are aged over 55 years have a higher occurrence of heart attacks. The prevalence of hypertension is highest in black Caribbean groups; Pakistani women, however, have amongst the lowest prevalence.

Type 2 diabetes is significantly higher among Bangladeshi, Pakistani, Indian, black African, black Caribbean and Chinese populations.

There is variation in behavioural risk factors:
- In some black, Asian and other minority ethnic groups, such as black Caribbean and Bangladeshi men and black Caribbean women, smoking rates remain high.
- Pakistani and Bangladeshi groups engage in less physical activity.
- Alcohol consumption is far lower amongst black, Asian and other minority ethnic groups; however, of those people who do drink, a large proportion of men from India, black Caribbean, black African and Chinese populations do drink above the suggested levels.
- Similarly, diet is, on the whole, better amongst black, Asian and other minority ethnic groups, but the use of salt in cooking is high amongst black African and Bangladeshi men, black Caribbean and Indian women.

(Adapted with permission from NICE, 2017.)

AT THE GP SURGERY

The role of the cardiac rehabilitation nurse can occur in the hospital setting or at the GP surgery. They manage a clinical caseload of cardiac patients and take responsibility for direct patient care: assessing, planning, providing and evaluating nursing care needs, including monitoring, diagnostics and investigations.

The cardiac rehabilitation nurse provides information to those with specific cardiac conditions about having a heart-healthy lifestyle, so the person can be as fit as possible for surgery and to help keep them as healthy as possible afterwards. They work as part of a team that often includes dietitians and exercise specialists.

Atrial fibrillation
Signs and symptoms

Atrial fibrillation is a disorder of the normal heart rhythm; its most obvious sign will be an irregular pulse that has no pattern to its irregularity. If the atria of the heart could be seen, they would appear to be wobbling like a bag of jelly as multiple electrical impulses cause the myocardium to contract in a chaotic manner. Some of these impulses will be large enough to pass through the AV node into the ventricles but this is not a regular event. Thus, the irregular passage of electrical impulses through to the ventricles will lead to the irregular heart rate. The heart rate in atrial fibrillation may be fast or slow, either of which may cause the same symptoms in the patient.

In atrial fibrillation, the patient may report feeling drowsy, dizzy (to the extent they may faint), short of breath and having palpitations.

THE MEDICINE TROLLEY 29.3

Drug	Drug classification	Reason for administration	Route of administration	Dose	Side effects	Contra-indications	Nursing care
Diamorphine	Opiate analgesic	Chest pain of a cardiac origin	Intravenous	2.5–5 mg	These include: nausea and vomiting, confusion, constipation, dry mouth, difficulty passing urine, respiratory depression	Should be avoided in patients with acute respiratory depression, head injury and comatose patients	Seek consent prior to administration Explain the use of the drug to the patient, respond to any questions Monitor for signs of respiratory depression (reduced respiration rate) Maintain patient safety, observe for confusion/drowsiness

Diagnosis

The diagnosis of atrial fibrillation will always require an ECG to assess the heart rhythm. In patients with intermittent atrial fibrillation, it may be necessary for the patient to have a 24-hour (Holter) ECG to try and catch an episode of the atrial fibrillation.

CARE IN THE HOME SETTING

ECG Holter Monitor

This test monitors the person's heart rhythm over 1 to 7 days. It is about the size of a mobile phone and the person needs to wear it around the waist, or it can be carried in the pocket. There is no need for the person to stay in hospital; they can continue with their normal daily activities during the test.

The test provides the nurse or doctor with much more information about heart rhythm on which to base any medical decisions about the person's health. The Nursing Associate should explain to the person:

- Throughout the test, the Holter monitor can be stored in a pouch to wear around the neck or clipped to the belt.
- Remember that very strenuous activities may interfere with data recordings.
- Be careful not to get the Holter monitor wet. The person will not be able to shower whilst the monitor is attached.
- At night, place the Holter monitor under the pillow.
- Ensure the leads are still clipped to the electrodes on the chest. If a lead or electrode comes off accidentally, reattach it to the area where it was originally. If necessary, new electrodes may need to be used.

An event diary will be given to the person to help with the analysis and to make a more accurate evaluation of the 24-hour recording. The person should record any symptoms they experience during the test, along with their time, duration and circumstance. Encourage the person to keep the Holter monitor diary and a pen with them at all times.

A follow-up appointment will be made for the monitor to be removed; the person should also bring the completed patient diary to this appointment. The results from the test will be sent to the doctor, who will call the patient in for a further appointment if needed.

The causes of atrial fibrillation are numerous and include: heart valve disease, coronary heart disease, alterations in the blood levels of the electrolytes, thyroid gland disorders and infection. To rule out easily treatable causes, any patient with atrial fibrillation will require blood tests and an echocardiogram.

Because the atria of the heart are not beating effectively, blood is not efficiently ejected and may 'pool' in the atria. This leads to the risk of blood clots developing and being pumped out into the circulation, potentially creating a stroke. Thus, it is common for patients with atrial fibrillation (especially long-standing atrial fibrillation) to undergo a transoesophageal echocardiogram to assess for the presence of blood clots.

Care and treatment

The care and treatment of atrial fibrillation is based on three main components:

1. Rate control.

   Often the effect of atrial fibrillation will be to create a high heart rate and this leads to the feelings of dizziness and palpitations. To control these symptoms, it is necessary to reduce the heart rate with medication. There are several medications used to control the heart rate in atrial fibrillation but the most common is amiodarone, although digoxin may still be used by some doctors.

2. Anticoagulation.

   Due to the risk of a blood clot developing and causing a stroke, patients with atrial fibrillation will often be prescribed warfarin (an anticoagulant). If a patient is prescribed warfarin, they will need to be educated on the reason for the anticoagulation and the importance of regular monitoring of their clotting by blood test. It is also very important that patients are encouraged to always take their warfarin at the same time every day, not to miss doses or change the dose, except when told to by a doctor or anticoagulation nurse. Furthermore, patients must be advised to avoid alcohol, except in moderation, and not to drink cranberry juice as alcohol and cranberry juice can affect the anticoagulant effects of warfarin.

3. Cardioversion.

   Cardioversion is the process of restoring the heart rhythm to normal. It can be attempted by drug therapy (such as amiodarone) or by electrical shock under sedation.

REFLECTION 29.4

How might you feel if you or a member of your family were told that you required cardioversion to restore your heart rhythm to normal? What might be your biggest anxiety? How might a Nursing Associate help to reduce that anxiety?

THE MEDICINE TROLLEY 29.4

Drug	Drug classification	Reason for administration	Route of administration	Dose	Side effects	Contra-indications	Nursing care
Amiodarone	Anti-arrhythmic	Cardiac arrhythmias including atrial fibrillation	Oral unless rapid treatment is required, in which case can be administered by intravenous infusion	Oral: 200 mg three times a day reducing to 200 mg once a day after a few weeks Intravenous: 5 mg/kg	These include: slow heart rate, thyroid disorders, nausea, grey skin discolouration	Should be avoided in patients with thyroid disorders and used with caution in the elderly	Seek consent prior to administration Explain the use of the drug to the patient, respond to any questions In the initial phase of administration monitor blood pressure and heart rate regularly In the initial phase regular blood tests may be required

THE MEDICINE TROLLEY 29.5

Drug	Drug classification	Reason for administration	Route of administration	Dose	Side effects	Contra-indications	Nursing care
Enalapril	ACE inhibitor	Hypertension	Oral	5 mg once a day, up to 40 mg if required	These include: persistent dry cough, low blood pressure, abdominal pain, diarrhoea, joint pain	Should be used with caution in patients with known kidney disease, the elderly, and diabetes	Seek consent prior to administration Explain the use of the drug to the patient, respond to any questions In the initial phase of administration monitor blood pressure regularly In the initial phase regular blood tests may be required

Hypertension

Hypertension is the medical term for what is commonly known as high blood pressure.

Signs and symptoms

Hypertension is known as a 'silent killer', as most patients will not be aware that they are suffering from it. It is common for the patient to have no symptoms of the disease and the diagnosis only to be made when the patient's blood pressure is taken for unrelated reasons.

Diagnosis

The diagnosis of hypertension is always based on a series of blood pressure readings (never a single reading). Current guidance suggests that a blood pressure that is found to be consistently over 140/90 mm Hg should be followed up by a 24-hour automated blood pressure monitor to confirm the hypertension (NICE, 2016b).

Care and treatment

The treatment of hypertension takes place almost exclusively in the community and is managed by the GP. The patient with hypertension should receive guidance on a healthy lifestyle including:
- Losing weight if required
- Exercising regularly
- Eating a healthy diet
- Cutting down on alcohol
- Stopping smoking
- Cutting down on salt and caffeine.

There are three drugs normally used in the treatment of hypertension; these are angiotensin converting enzyme (ACE) inhibitors, calcium channel blockers and thiazide diuretics. The choice of drug will be based on age and ethnic background, as it has been shown that the best treatment for patients under the age of 55 years from a non–Afro-Caribbean ethnic background is different from the treatment of patients over the age of 55 or from an Afro-Caribbean ethnic background (Krause et al., 2011).

Peripheral artery disease

Peripheral artery disease is most common in the legs. For that reason this section will only discuss peripheral artery disease in the legs.

Signs and symptoms

In many cases, peripheral artery disease will not create any symptoms but in others it will lead to a cramp-like pain felt in the calf, thigh or buttock during walking or other exercise. This is known as 'intermittent claudication' and is usually relieved by rest.

Diagnosis

The first element of the diagnosis of peripheral vascular disease is to examine the legs. Often the skin on an affected leg will be shiny and hairless; in the more severe cases, the leg will be cold to touch and there may be ulcers present on the skin. Palpation of the femoral, knee, ankle and foot pulses may find that these pulses are weak or absent.

Definitive diagnosis of peripheral artery disease will involve investigations such as an ultrasound of the peripheral arteries and an angiogram.

Care and treatment

Treatment of peripheral artery disease can be:

Medical: the reduction of risk factors (such as smoking and fatty diet) and the use of medication to relieve symptoms will be used in mild cases of peripheral vascular disease, for instance where the disease has not progressed very far.

Angioplasty: the same treatment as used for coronary heart disease but in the peripheral arteries.

Bypass surgery: the use of veins taken from the patient's leg to use as vessels to bypass the narrowed section of arteries and thus improve blood flow.

Further care of the patient will depend on the treatment option used but after angioplasty or bypass surgery it is essential for the patient's leg to be assessed and for the healthcare practitioner to record and report the limb colour, the temperature of the limb and the peripheral pulses, as blood clots are a risk to the patient's limb.

Varicose veins

Signs and symptoms

Varicose veins are enlarged and swollen veins that are normally found in the legs and ankles. They are often associated with an itching sensation or pain. The symptoms are usually worse when the patient has been standing for a long time and may be reduced by resting and elevating the legs.

Varicose veins can be caused by the failure of the valves inside the veins of the legs, leading to 'backward flow' and pooling of the blood in the veins. Alternatively, they may be caused by small clots in the veins, reducing the flow of blood back to the heart and acting as a 'dam', thus trapping blood in the vein.

There are known risk factors for varicose veins, including: obesity, female sex, family history of varicose veins or having a job that requires long periods of standing.

Diagnosis

The diagnosis of varicose veins involves inspecting the legs. In significant cases, there may be need for an ultrasound scan of the veins.

Care and treatment

The treatment for varicose veins will depend on the severity of the condition. The most common form of treatment is self-care, including losing weight, elevating the legs when resting and avoiding long periods of standing. Compression stockings may be required in more severe cases. Patients should be encouraged to remove the stockings at night and to inspect the legs whilst washing. If dry skin becomes a problem, then emollient creams may help (these can be bought over the counter).

> **! HOTSPOT**
>
> The patient must be encouraged to apply the stockings correctly (i.e., pulled up to the correct level and without creases or rotation) and to be vigilant for the onset of sores and blisters on the leg.

For cases where the symptoms are severe, the patient will be referred to a surgeon who will discuss options with the patient. There are two main treatment options for varicose veins – either the veins can be sealed using various techniques or the veins can be surgically removed.

LOOKING BACK, FEEDING FORWARD

The cardiovascular system is an interconnected system that is responsible for the transport of oxygen and nutrients to the tissue and the removal of waste products for excretion. This chapter has reviewed the anatomy and physiology of the heart and the circulatory system and has gone on to discuss a few cardiovascular disorders that you are likely to come across in your career. The importance of the cardiovascular system to the ongoing physical functioning of the body cannot be underestimated but it should not be the sole focus of the healthcare practitioner, as the psychological impact of cardiovascular disease can have a significant impact on the patient's life.

REFERENCES

Anderson, J.L., Morrow, D.A., 2017. Acute myocardial infarction. N. Engl. J. Med. 376 (21), 2053–2064.

Dalal, H.M., Doherty, P., Taylor, R.S., 2015. Cardiac rehabilitation. BMJ 351, h5000.

Department of Health, 2000. National Service Framework for Coronary Heart Disease. Department of Health, London.

Health Education England, 2017. Nursing Associate Curriculum Framework. NHS, London.

Krause, T., Lovibond, K., Caulfield, M., et al., 2011. Management of hypertension: summary of NICE guidance. BMJ 343 (2), d4891.

Levine, G.N., Bates, E.R., Blankenship, J.C., et al., 2016. 2015 ACC/AHA/SCAI focused update on primary percutaneous coronary intervention for patients with ST-elevation myocardial infarction: an update of the 2011 ACCF/AHA/SCAI Guideline for Percutaneous Coronary Intervention and the 2013 ACCF/AHA Guideline for the Management of ST-Elevation Myocardial Infarction: a report of the American College of Cardiology/American Heart Association Task Force on Clinical Practice Guidelines and the Society for Cardiovascular Angiography and Interventions. Circulation 133 (11), 1135–1147.

NICE, 2016a. National Institute for Health and Care Excellence. Clinical Guideline 126. Management of stable angina https://www.nice.org.uk/guidance/cg126.

NICE, 2016b. National Institute for Health and Care Excellence. Clinical Guideline 127: Hypertension: Clinical management of primary hypertension in adults. https://www.nice.org.uk/guidance/cg127.

NICE, 2017. National Institute for Health and Care Excellence. Black, Asian and other minority ethnic groups: promoting health and preventing premature mortality. Available at https://www.nice.org.uk/guidance/GID-QS10039/documents/briefing-paper.

Nursing and Midwifery Council, 2018. The Code. Professional Standards of Practice and Behaviour for Nurses, Midwives and Nursing Associates. London: NMC. https://www.nmc.org.uk/.

Parodi, G., 2016. Editor's choice-chest pain relief in patients with acute myocardial infarction. Eur. Heart J. Acute Cardiovasc. Care 5 (3), 277–281.

Reed, G.W., Rossi, J.E., Cannon, C.P., 2017. Acute myocardial infarction. Lancet 389 (10065), 197–210.

SIGN, 2007. Scottish Intercollegiate Guidelines Network. SIGN Guideline 96: Management of stable angina. https://www.sign.ac.uk/sign-96-management-of-stable-angina.html.

Smolderen, K.G., Buchanan, D.M., Gosch, K., et al., 2017. Depression treatment and 1-year mortality following acute myocardial infarction: insights from the TRIUMPH registry. Circulation 135 (18), 1681–1689.

Waugh, A., Grant, A., 2018. Ross & Wilson Anatomy and Physiology in Health and Illness, thirteenth ed. Elsevier, Edinburgh.

30

Haematological Disorders

Barry Hill, Joanne Atkinson

OBJECTIVES

By the end of the chapter, the reader will be able to:

1. Understand the anatomy and physiology of the different blood cells and discuss the pathophysiological changes associated with a selection of haematological disorders
2. Understand the relationship between haematology and other body systems
3. Outline the care required for people with haematological disorders
4. Describe some common conditions associated with the haematological system
5. Review the role of the Nursing Associate in promoting health and well-being
6. Review four key haematological conditions in greater detail

KEY WORDS

Blood cell
Haemoglobin
Oxygen transpiration
Clotting

Haemopoiesis
Neutrophils
Anaemia
Blood cancers

Infection
Immune system

CHAPTER AIMS

This aim of this chapter is to provide the reader with an understanding of the skills, knowledge and attitude required to provide safe, effective and compassionate care to people with a haematological disorder.

SELF TEST

1. What are the three primary functions of the blood?
2. What are the three different types of blood cells?
3. What is anaemia?
4. What are the key functions of the red blood cell (RBC)?
5. What is the name of the microorganisms that cause disease?
6. What is the purpose of a neutrophil?
7. Name the different types of blood cancers?
8. What do you understand by DIC?
9. What is the difference between HL and NHL?
10. What is your understanding of Domain 6?

INTRODUCTION

In this chapter, haematological disorders are considered. The first part discusses the anatomy and physiology of a variety of blood cells. It is important for the Nursing Associate to have a comprehensive understanding of haematological conditions to provide appropriate and effective care.

The second part of the chapter addresses a selection of common haematological conditions that affect the health and well-being of people. The care and comfort of the patient who experiences a haematological disorder are described. When offering care, the Nursing Associate must practice with kindness and compassion, and ensure inclusivity and a holistic approach. People with haematological conditions require a dignified approach to their care, as many of these conditions are not generally understood, and stereotyping and stigma still exist around many haematological conditions. Therefore, the Nursing Associate must ensure that they are competent and knowledgeable, to ensure a factual and evidence-based approach to advocate and empower their patient. Additionally, the Nursing Associate must be reflective and utilize appropriate communication skills when treating patients with haematological conditions. Haematological system diseases can have a significant impact on a person's physical and mental health state; this may create both physical and mental symptoms, and therefore must be acknowledged and supported by the Nursing Associate. From a professional viewpoint, this would also be in keeping with the duty of care obligations, which stipulates that: 'Nursing Associates must not act or fail to act in a way that results in harm' (Health Education England (HEE), 2017). Fig. 30.1 provides an overview of some haematological disorders.

DUTY OF CARE, CANDOUR, EQUALITY AND DIVERSITY

The Nursing Associate must employ a nondiscriminatory approach to their clinical practice. The role of the Nursing Associate is to make the patient feel safe and secure and free from judgement. It is imperative that the patient feels as though they can trust the Nursing Associate to build an effective rapport. This is very important when developing a trusting relationship (Bickley et al., 2017). The Nursing and Midwifery Council's (NMC, 2017) equality objectives action plan explains what is being done to promote all equality groups, including age, disability, gender, gender assignment, marriage/civil partnership, pregnancy, race, religion or belief and sexual orientation. Additionally, the Department of Health (DH) are clear in their expectations of what a registrants' duty of care is within the Equality Act 2010 (DH, 2010). The DH (2010) suggests registrants must be mindful in their provision of care, and (1) eliminate discrimination, harassment and victimization; (2) advance equality of opportunity and (3) foster good relations between different parts of the community. This 'duty of care' covers: age, disability, gender reassignment, marital or civil partnership status, pregnancy and motherhood, race (including ethnic or national origin, colour and nationality), religion or belief (including lack of belief), sex and sexual orientation.

THE HAEMATOLOGICAL SYSTEM

The haematological system is made up of blood (blood cells and plasma), bone marrow and lymphoid tissue. The three primary functions of blood are: (1) transportation, (2) regulation of fluid and (3) protection (Box 30.1).

See Fig. 30.2.

BOX 30.1 The Haematological System

(1) Transportation:
The blood transports substances, including oxygen absorbed from the lungs, carbon dioxide, essential nutrients absorbed from the alimentary canal, enzymes and chemical substances (i.e., hormones), around the body through a vast network of blood vessels. In addition, it is the blood cells' job to transport waste material from all cells to the excretory organs for elimination.

(2) Regulation:
Regulation of water, electrolyte and acid–base balance and body temperature.

(3) Protection:
Protection against infection. As blood contains coagulation factors, it also protects the body from excessive blood loss.

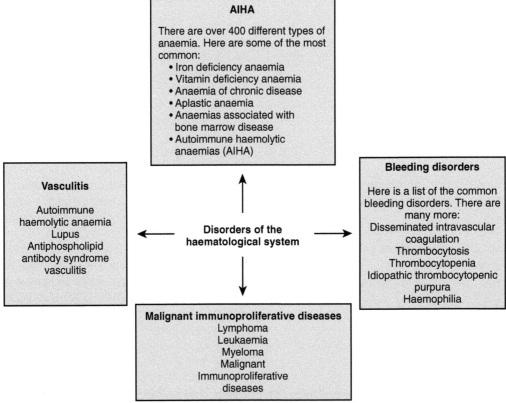

Fig. 30.1 Some Key Haematological Disorders.

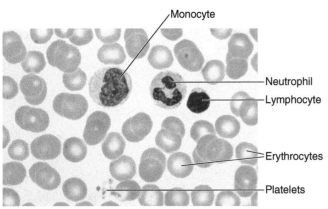

Fig. 30.2 Blood Cells (Waugh & Grant, 2014).

TYPES OF BLOOD CELL

There are three different types of blood cell:
1. The erythrocyte's (red blood cell (RBC)) main function is to transport oxygen and carbon dioxide from the lungs to the body's cells
2. The leukocyte's (white blood cell (WBC)) main function is to protect the body from infection
3. The platelet's (thrombocyte) main function is to support the blood clotting process

The haematological system interacts with all other body systems for the purpose of oxygen and carbon dioxide transportation, protection against infection and blood clotting. The components of the haematological system are:

- Plasma
- Plasma proteins
- Cellular components.

CONTENT OF THE BLOOD

Red blood cells (erythrocytes)

Mature RBCs are the most numerous blood cells in the human body, estimated at approximately 99% of all blood cells (Waugh & Grant, 2014). This accounts for nearly 30 trillion RBCs in the human body; approximately 25% of the body's cell count (Waugh & Grant, 2014). They constitute approximately 45% haematocrit and survive for approximately 4 months prior to being absorbed by the spleen and broken down by phagocytic cells. The RBC has a unique biconcave discoid shape, which allows it to be flexible and fit into tiny blood capillaries, allowing for gas exchange to take place (the attachment of oxygen to haemoglobin [Hb], known as oxyhaemoglobin). These cells contain no organelles, leaving more room in the cell for oxygen to attach to available Hb (Hoffbrand & Moss, 2016). The RBC aims to take oxygen from the lungs to the body's cells, and also to collect carbon dioxide from the body's cells to take back to the lungs for elimination via the respiratory expiration. Hb is characteristic in its bright red colour because it is the oxygen-carrying pigmentation (Hoffbrand & Moss, 2016). Hb is a combination of iron (haem) and protein (globin). Each Hb molecule contains four globin chains and four haem units, each with 1 atom of iron. Each single Hb molecule can carry up to four molecules of oxygen.

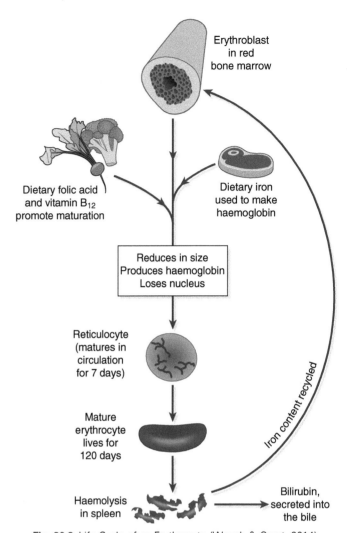

Fig. 30.3 Life Cycle of an Erythrocyte (Waugh & Grant, 2014).

This means that each RBC has a potential capacity of more than 1 billion oxygen molecules (Waugh & Grant, 2014). Hb is the main constituent of the RBC; this is because it lacks a nucleus, ribosomes or mitochondria. Because of this, it is important to understand that protein synthesis is not possible, and the RBC is limited to only an anaerobic glycolytic pathway for its requirement of energy (Pallister & Watson, 2011). It takes approximately 1 week for a stem cell to develop fully into an RBC, a process known as erythropoiesis (Fig. 30.3). After this process, RBCs are unable to divide as they no longer have an available nucleus. (See Table 30.1 for the role of RBCs.)

White blood cells (leukocytes)

A WBC's main function is to defend the body from invasion. They are less numerous than RBCs and are nucleated. Leukocytes are separated into two categories, either granulocytes (multinucleated; these are neutrophils, eosinophils and basophils) or agranulocytes (monocytes and lymphocytes).

Granulocytes

These WBCs are situated in the bone marrow, blood and tissues (Brown & Cutler, 2012). Microorganisms that cause disease are called pathogens. When pathogens enter the body, WBCs called

TABLE 30.1	Red Blood Cells
Oxygen transportation	Oxygen is transported by haemoglobin (Hb) in the red blood cell (RBC). Each molecule of Hb carries up to 4 molecules of oxygen. This means that each RBC has a potential oxygen carrying capacity of over 1 billion oxygen molecules. Oxygen transportation is reliant on available Hb, therefore patients who have active bleeding or bleeding disorders, or those who are anaemic, will potentially have altered oxygen delivery.
Haemopoiesis	The process in which blood cells are formed. See Fig. 30.5.
Destruction of erythrocytes	The lifespan of an erythrocyte is approximately 4 months, after which they break down (haemolysis). The body retains the iron that is released from the broken-down cells and bone marrow uses this to create new cells.
Blood groups	There are four blood groups, known as: A, B, AB, O. Blood group O is usually referred to as 'universal'. When nursing patients that need blood transfusions, it is important to understand the ABO system and send a blood sample for cross matching.

phagocytes pass through the walls of the blood vessels and into the surrounding tissues. The phagocyte can submerge micro-organisms (pathogens) and bacteria utilizing a process known as phagocytosis. This allows them to completely change structure and excrete enzymes capable of absorbing and digesting the pathogen and their toxins. After phagocytes have destroyed a pathogen by releasing enzymes and absorbing the pathogens, they can also send out messages calling on the assistance and support of other types of WBCs. Invading pathogens can be identified by the antigen chemicals on their surface.

Lymphocytes

Lymphocytes are WBCs that carry antibodies, some of which will fit antigens, like pieces of a puzzle. These lymphocytes reproduce rapidly, and many copies of the appropriate antibody are reproduced. Antibodies are able to destroy pathogens directly and/or can make it possible for the phagocytes (the other WBCs) to ingest and destroy the pathogens.

Platelets

Platelets (also known as thrombocytes), are the second most numerous blood cell within the human body. They are a discoid shape and are derived from bone marrow cells called megakaryocytes. Platelets survive for approximately 12 days. The platelet membrane has some similarity to the RBC; however, it has more structures and functions. The platelet is essential for blood clotting and has three fundamental functions to minimize blood loss:
1. Support the constriction of damaged blood vessels.
2. Form haemostatic plugs in injured blood vessels by becoming swollen, spiky, sticky and secretary.

3. Provide a substance that accelerates blood clotting, such as factor 3 and 13, and platelet factor 3.

Haemostasis is a complex process. It involves a dynamic interaction between platelets, plasma and coagulation factors to control active bleeding. When injury occurs to tissue, the surrounding blood vessels will narrow (a process also called vasoconstriction), encouraging platelets to thicken, form a plug and protect the areas.

BLOOD DYSCRASIAS

Blood dyscrasia is an abnormal or pathological condition of the blood cells. RBCs, WBCs and platelets are created in bone marrow. Due to the accelerated rate of production of cells and limited ability to store cells in the marrow, these blood cells are particularly vulnerable to pathological changes. Primary blood disorders present when there are any blood cell problems. Secondary disorders occur from bleeding, and are therefore a result of something other than 'the blood cell' itself (see Fig. 30.4, Clotting).

> **⚠ HOTSPOT**
>
> **Bone Marrow Transplants**
>
> Patients who have diseased bone marrow, or damaged bone marrow that has become ineffective due to medications (such as chemotherapy), may require a bone marrow transplant (BMT). BMT is now a very common procedure, particularly in western culture, with very good results, particularly when bone marrow is matched by family members.

HAEMOPOIESIS

Haemopoiesis refers to the production of blood cells. See Fig. 30.5 for an overview of haemopoiesis.

All cells begin as pluripotent stem cells before changing into either proerythroblasts, megakaryoblasts, myeloblasts, monoblasts or lymphoblasts.

HAEMATOLOGICAL DISORDERS

An understanding of the anatomy of the haematological system is essential for the Nursing Associate to offer care for and give support to patients. Using knowledge, immersing oneself into learning and using evidence-based practice allows practitioners to provide safe care that is holistic and inclusive, with the ability to rationalize what they are doing. This is important, as patients may ask questions and they will expect to be provided with information. They will be expecting a competent and knowledgeable professional person to care for them. As well as understanding the structure of blood cells, the Nursing Associate needs to ensure that the care provided is compassionate, caring and competent. This requires the Nursing Associate to use their interpersonal skills when caring for patients and (if appropriate) their families, as well as anyone advocating on behalf of the patient.

People from adolescence to old age require care for haematological conditions, with concerns regarding a wide range of health issues. The Nursing Associate must aim to be as inclusive as possible, whilst offering care and support, as they work collaboratively with the patient and the wider healthcare and

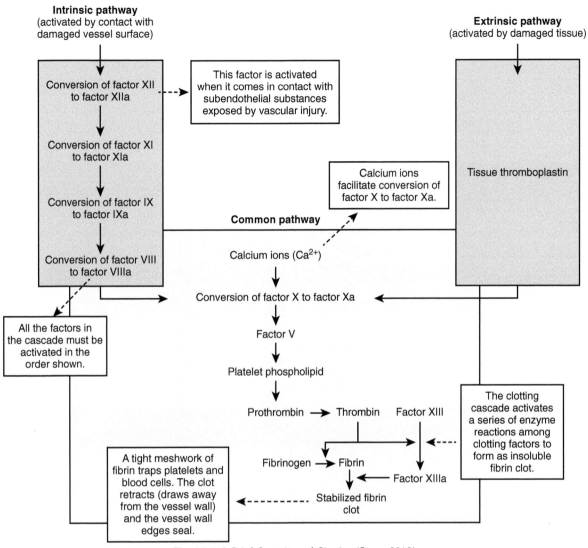

Fig. 30.4 A Brief Overview of Clotting (Scott, 2013).

social care team. Recognizing and respecting the diversity of needs results in care provision that is of a high quality and humanistic. It also empowers people from many perspectives, for example, in being able to access the best available and most appropriate care.

Anaemia

Blood supports all the activities and functions of all of the organs and tissues in the body, providing nutrients, oxygen and hormones, as well as defending the body against infections and getting rid of waste products. The blood cells each have different functions, which sustain life when they work together. Blood cells are produced in the bone marrow. Haematopoiesis ensures that we have the right type of mature functioning blood cells, at the right time and in the right number. When cells are immature and nonfunctioning, we develop diseases and chronic conditions that can seriously impact on quality of life.

Anaemia is a term used to describe a deficiency of the RBCs (erythrocytes) or the Hb that attaches itself to RBCs.

Prevalence

The exact prevalence of anaemia is difficult to estimate, as there are differing causative factors and the pathophysiology will differ.

As anaemia is one of the commonest problems presenting in both primary care and the hospital setting (Howard & Hamilton, 2013), the incidence of anaemia is difficult to quantify. Whilst it is a term used to describe an Hb count below the normal range, Hb is dependent on many factors: ethnicity of the individual, socio-economic factors and gender. It is more common in women than men, and is common in children under 5 years, pregnant women and the elderly (people over the age of 65 years), with 10% of people over 65 years having varying degrees of anaemia (Howard & Hamilton, 2013).

Types and causes of anaemia

There are different causes of anaemia:
- Iron deficiency (ID) anaemia
- Vitamin B$_{12}$ and folate deficiency

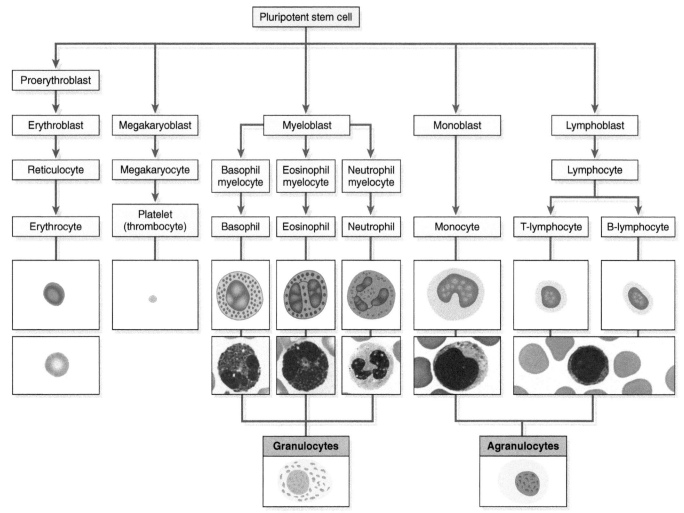

Fig. 30.5 An Overview of Haemopoiesis (Waugh & Grant, 2014).

- Chronic disease, renal disease, liver disease, rheumatoid arthritis
- Autoimmune diseases
- Bone marrow disorders
- Drug side effects
- Infection
- Lead poisoning
- Hereditary causes that reduce Hb production, such as sickle cell disease and thalassaemia
- Acute and chronic blood loss
- Underlying malignancy

Signs and symptoms

The signs and symptoms of anaemia can be of a slow and insidious onset and are often missed. The symptoms are largely dependent on the speed of onset of the anaemia: for example, if the anaemia is due to acute blood loss, the symptoms will be more obvious and of rapid onset. Symptoms are largely due to the lack of oxygen in the tissues due to low Hb and can include the following:

- Shortness of breath
- Palpitations

- Fatigue and lethargy
- Anorexia
- Sensitivity to the cold
- Ankle oedema
- Weakness
- Headaches
- Sore mouth and gums

(Moore et al., 2010; Brown & Cutler, 2012).

REFLECTION 30.1

Anaemia is a chronic condition that, without treatment, can seriously affect the way people live their lives. Consider the impact of living with constant fatigue and tiredness on the following:

1. Role within the family
2. Caring for oneself
3. Activity
4. Motivation
5. Feeling valued
6. Work and leisure activities

THE MEDICINE TROLLEY 30.1

Drug	Drug classification	Reason for administration	Route of administration	Dose	Side effects	Contra-indications	Nursing care
Ferrous sulphate	Supplement	To add iron	Oral Intramuscular Intravenous	200 mg twice per day	Constipation Upset stomach, leading to nausea and vomiting Black stools Teeth staining	Pregnancy consult doctor Alcoholic	Seek consent prior to administration Explain the use of the drug to the patient, respond to any questions Regular medical supervision to monitor full blood counts Do not take with indigestion remedies

Investigation and diagnosis

When examining a patient with suspected anaemia, a careful history is required. The patient who is anaemic may often have a pallor or a yellow tinge, dependent on the type of anaemia they have. The diagnosis is based on a general history, which should include any chronic illness the person may have and medication being taken. A full blood count will reflect the degree of anaemia and further analysis of the blood will uncover the type of anaemia the patient has (Howard & Hamilton, 2013). Further investigations may be undertaken to find the cause of any chronic blood loss if indicated. These would include:

- Urine testing for the presence of blood (haematuria)
- Faecal occult blood
- Endoscopy
- Colonoscopy
- Investigations of the bone marrow.

Making the diagnosis in anaemia is very important and assumptions should not be made about the cause. Signs and symptoms are considered carefully, blood profile is analyzed and treatment is dependent on the type of anaemia. In addition, the patient will be asked detailed questions about:

- Their diet: do they eat iron-rich foods?
- Their medication: do any of the drugs taken cause bleeding into the gastrointestinal tract, for example, non-steroidal anti-inflammatory drugs (e.g., ibuprofen)?
- Pregnancy and menstrual cycle.
- Any pertinent family history, not only for anaemia but also for jaundice, cholelithiasis, splenectomy, bleeding disorders and abnormal Hb.
- Any chronic diseases or history of weight loss, sickness and/or diarrhoea.

Treatment for iron deficiency anaemia

ID anaemia is most often caused by long-term blood loss (Howard & Hamilton, 2013). Patients may describe problems with heavy menstrual periods, indigestion or change in bowel habit. Ferritin is a protein in the body that stores iron. Blood tests may be taken to measure the ferritin in the bloodstream to help confirm ID anaemia. ID anaemia can be the presenting factor for some disorders, such as gastric ulceration, gynaecological problems and underlying cancers. Once all of the investigations have taken place to identify chronic blood loss and treat the underlying cause if there is one, iron supplements are prescribed and the patient is given dietary advice. This will include increasing green leafy vegetables, pulses and beans, eggs, meat and fish to name but a few. Blood monitoring is required and a regular review of the full blood count is recommended, depending on the severity of the anaemia.

Whilst the oral administration of iron supplements is the commonest treatment for ID anaemia, some severe cases may require iron injections. This would be decided in consultation with specialist services.

Vitamin B$_{12}$ (folate) deficiency anaemia

A lack of vitamin B$_{12}$ and folate can cause a malfunction in the RBCs. They become abnormally large and do not function effectively. This lack of vitamins can be caused through a poor diet or vegan diet; certain medications, such as anticonvulsants or proton pump inhibitors can also alter the absorption of these vitamins. Dietary advice should be given and patients advised to eat a good balanced diet, to include meat, salmon, milk and eggs.

Pernicious anaemia

This is a result of vitamin B$_{12}$ and folate deficiency: an autoimmune disorder affects the cells in the stomach and prevents the absorption of vitamin B$_{12}$ and folate, which would normally be absorbed when we eat. It is the commonest cause of vitamin B$_{12}$ deficiency (Howard & Hamilton, 2013). Alongside medication, patients should be advised to eat a balanced diet that includes leafy green vegetables, such as Brussels sprouts and cabbage.

Anaemia in chronic disease

Anaemia is a common disorder, associated with chronic disease such as rheumatoid arthritis, renal failure, heart failure, infections and malignancies. Patients often do not have frank symptoms of anaemia and at times are often over-investigated for the anaemia rather than it being considered a consequence of living with an underlying disease (Howard & Hamilton, 2013). The anaemia is often more pronounced when the disease is more flagrant; for example, if there is a greater degree of infection, or if the cancer is more disseminated, then the degree of anaemia

THE MEDICINE TROLLEY 30.2

Drug	Drug classification	Reason for administration	Route of administration	Dose	Side effects	Contraindications	Nursing care
Hydroxocobalamin	Supplement vitamin B_{12}	To increase vitamin B_{12} Pernicious anaemia	Intramuscular	1 mg three times per week for 2 weeks and then 1 mg every 3 months	Nausea Headache Fever Vomiting Redness Changes in taste	Check if the patient is on any other medication, if so consider if the medicines are compatible and the side effects. Also consider the risks of polypharmacy. Liaise with the multidisciplinary team to provide best practice.	Seek consent prior to administration Explain the use of the drug to the patient, respond to any questions Regular medical supervision to monitor full blood counts Check counts after 2 weeks of treatment
Folic acid	Supplement (folate)	To increase folate (folate deficiency)	Oral	400 µg daily	As above	As above	As above

will be greater. It is important not to treat patients unnecessarily for anaemia in chronic disease. The pathophysiology of this cause of anaemia is complex; however, the aim should be to treat the underlying disease. In particularly difficult cases, when quality of life is affected, then blood transfusion may be indicated.

Haemolytic anaemias

Haemolytic anaemia is a term used to describe many different anaemias that all have a common characteristic: they have an abnormality that destructs red cells. This disorder leads to the reduced lifespan of RBCs, not an underproduction of them. The patient often presents with symptoms of anaemia due to haemolysis and further investigation gives rise to diagnosis of haemolytic anaemia, which requires specialist management.

Thalassaemia

This describes a group of inherited disorders that affects the production of Hb. Depending on the severity of the condition, there is little Hb produced, resulting in a profound symptomatic anaemia. NHS UK (2017) suggests that this affects people primarily of Middle Eastern, Mediterranean and South East Asian origin. It is a genetic disease, often diagnosed soon after birth, with differing degrees of severity dependent on the type. Patients will have severe anaemia and an overload of iron in their haematological system. Patients with thalassaemia should be reviewed by specialist haematology services, take any medications as prescribed, maintain a healthy diet, try to be as healthy as possible, not consume alcohol and be cautious around activities that cause injury, bruising or increase oxygen consumption. Blood transfusions may be required and bone marrow transplant in severe cases.

Sickle cell anaemia

Sickle cell disease and sickle cell anaemia are terms used to describe a group of disorders that are hereditary and largely affect African, Caribbean, Middle Eastern and Asian people. The RBCs are

misshapen, and the lifespan of the RBCs is shorter. Patients may have sickle cell crises, which is very painful and requires hospitalisation, pain relief and hydration. In addition, patients may have anaemia and the associated symptoms and be more predisposed to developing infections. Treatment, like in thalassaemia, is for the lifespan of the patient; blood transfusions, pain relief and antibiotics for infection help manage the disease (NHS UK, 2017).

The complexity of anaemia is clear; when anaemia is discussed in practice it is often considered as a chronic condition. Some types of anaemia are common, particularly iron deficient anaemia; in fact, this is one of the commonest presenting factors in primary and secondary care (Howard & Hamilton, 2013). It is important, however, to recognize that some of the rarer anaemias are, if not life-limiting, very debilitating. In addition, anaemia can herald the start of a chronic disease that itself is very difficult to live with. Offering care to people experiencing anaemia can be a challenge. One of the key challenges is to ensure that care is delivered in such a way that recognizes the impact the symptoms of anaemia can have on quality of life, and to support the patient and their family.

Lymphoma

Another common haematological condition is lymphoma. The term lymphoma covers a variety of malignant blood cancer conditions, usually of B-cell origin. These are characterized as lymphomas because of the production of lymphoid cells, starting in the lymph nodes or lymph tissues within the lymphatic system (Fig. 30.6). Lymphomas belong to two groups, which are Hodgkin's lymphoma (HL) and non-Hodgkin's lymphoma (NHL).

Hodgkin's lymphoma

Data from Cancer Research UK (2018a) for HL reveals that, within the UK, there were 2110 new diagnoses in 2015 (this is approximately six new cases per day based on today's UK population), with 1203 male and 907 female; there were 355 deaths. Survival

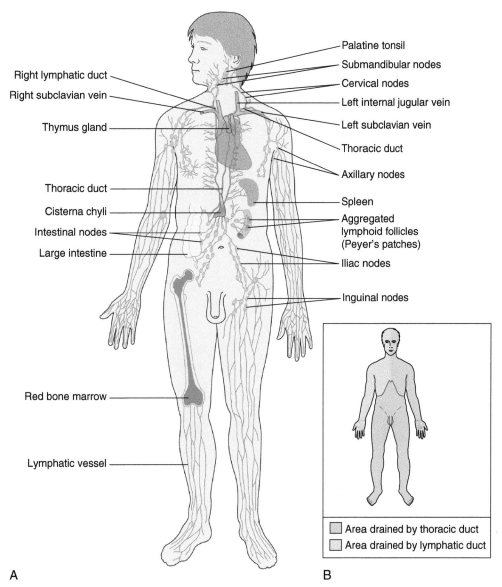

Fig. 30.6 The Lymphatic System (Waugh & Grant, 2018).

Labels (figure A):
- Palatine tonsil
- Submandibular nodes
- Cervical nodes
- Left internal jugular vein
- Left subclavian vein
- Thoracic duct
- Axillary nodes
- Spleen
- Aggregated lymphoid follicles (Peyer's patches)
- Iliac nodes
- Inguinal nodes
- Right lymphatic duct
- Right subclavian vein
- Thymus gland
- Thoracic duct
- Cisterna chyli
- Intestinal nodes
- Large intestine
- Red bone marrow
- Lymphatic vessel

Figure B legend:
- Area drained by thoracic duct
- Area drained by lymphatic duct

A   B

for 10 years or more has risen from 50% in the 1970s to 80% in 2014, with preventable cases being at 45% (Cancer Research UK, 2018a). It is suggested, using current data, that by 2035 there will be a 5% rise in HL, which is an increase of four people per 100,000 population.

Risk factors. The risk factors include age, genetics and lifestyle, with lifestyle accounting for approximate 45% of cases. Epstein–Barr virus (human widespread herpes virus) is the highest-ranking avoidable lifestyle risk factor for HL. As a risk factor, it is weighted at 45% (in the UK population), whilst other conditions such as human immunodeficiency virus (HIV), immunological problems, being overweight and having weight-related conditions, as well as smoking, all increase the risk of developing HL.

Signs and symptoms. 90% of HL patients will identify a palpable nonpainful lump within their lymph nodes (see Fig. 30.6). The clinical term for this is 'painless lymphadenopathy'.

According to Cancer Research UK (2018b), the first symptom of HL is usually a swelling in the neck, axilla or inguinal canal. The swellings are usually painless, but some people may find that they ache. Other symptoms may include any of the following:
- Drenching and/or frequent sweats, especially at night
- Unexplained high temperatures (pyrexia)
- Weight loss
- Tiredness
- A cough or breathlessness
- A persistent itch all over the body.

The most common symptoms are pyrexia, drenching night sweats and weight loss. These are called 'B symptoms'. Other symptoms, such as pain, tenderness and swelling, will depend on where in the body the enlarged lymph nodes are. Some people with HL may have abnormal cells in their bone marrow when they are diagnosed. This can lower the number of healthy blood cells in the blood, which may cause the following symptoms:
- Breathlessness (dyspnoea) and tiredness
- An increased risk of infection

- Excessive bleeding, such as nosebleeds (epistaxis), very heavy menstrual periods in women (menometrorrhagia), or tiny spots of blood under the skin (multiple petechiae).

Very rarely, some people with HL may have pain in the affected lymph node when drinking alcohol. Many of these symptoms are common to many other conditions and most people with these symptoms will not have HL.

❗ HOTSPOT

Pyrexia

Pyrexia is a temperature that is atypically high. A low-grade pyrexia is considered 37.5°C. A true pyrexia is considered 38°C and above. According to NHS Direct (2017) and the 'Sepsis Six' principles, blood cultures must be drawn if a patient presents with a pyrexia above 38°C.

Table 30.2 identifies the staging of lymphomas.

The Cotswolds modification (Table 30.3) maintains the original four-stage clinical and pathological staging framework of the Ann Arbor staging system but also adds information regarding the prognostic significance of bulky disease.

Diagnosis. The diagnosis, staging and risk stratification and pretreatment examinations according to the European Society for Medical Oncology (2014), are shown in Box 30.2.

Nursing care and treatment. The key role and function of the Nursing Associate when offering care to people with HL is to offer the ability to problem solve and make decisions. It is imperative that Nursing Associates demonstrate knowledge and assess the holistic needs of their patients, especially any HL health legislation and care policies (NMC, 2018). To protect the skin receiving radiation, avoid rubbing, powders, deodorants, lotions or ointments (unless prescribed) and application of heat or cold.

- Encourage the patient to keep clean and dry, and to bathe the area affected by radiation gently with tepid water and mild soap.
- Encourage wearing loose-fitting clothes and to protect skin from exposure to sun, chlorine and temperature extremes.

- To protect the oral and gastrointestinal tract mucous membranes, encourage frequent, small meals, using bland and soft diet at mild temperatures.
- Teach the patients to avoid irritants, such as alcohol, tobacco, spices and extremely hot or cold foods.
- Administer or teach self-administration of pain medication or antiemetic before eating or drinking, if needed.
- Encourage mouth care at least twice per day and after meals using a soft toothbrush and mild mouth rinse.
- Assess for ulcers, plaques or discharge that may be indicative of superimposed infection.
- For diarrhoea, consider low-residue diet and administer anti-diarrhoeals as prescribed.
- Teach the patient about risk of infection.
- Advise the patient to monitor temperature and report any fever or other sign of infection promptly.
- Explain to the patient that radiation therapy may cause sterility.

TABLE 30.2 Staging of Lymphomas Using the Cotswolds Modification of Ann Arbor Staging System

Stage	Area of involvement
I	Single lymph node group
II	Multiple lymph node groups on same side of diaphragm
II	Multiple lymph node groups on both sides of diaphragm
IV	Multiple extranodal sites or lymph nodes and extranodal disease
X	Bulk greater than 10 cm
E	Extranodal extension or single, isolated site of extranodal disease
A/B	B symptoms: weight loss greater than 10%, fever, drenching night sweats

(Data from Lister, 1989.)

TABLE 30.3 The Cotswolds Modification

1. Determine stage according to sites involved by lymphoma

Stage	Features
I	Involvement of a single lymph node region* or lymphoid structure
II	Involvement of two or more lymph node regions*, or localized involvement of one extranodal site and one lymph node region, all on the same side of the diaphragm
III	Involvement of lymph node regions* or structures on both sides of the diaphragm
IV	Diffuse or disseminated involvement of one or more extralymphatic organs, OR isolated extralymphatic organ involvement without adjacent regional lymph node involvement, but with disease in distant site(s), OR any involvement of the liver, bone marrow, pleura or cerebrospinal fluid

*Lymph node regions include: right cervical (including cervical, supraclavicular, occipital and preauricular lymph nodes), left cervical, right axillary, left axillary, right infraclavicular, left infraclavicular, mediastinal, hilar, periaortic, mesentery, right pelvic, left pelvic, right inguinal femoral and left inguinal femoral.

2. Add relevant suffixes

Suffix	Meaning
A	Absence of constitutional symptoms
B	Constitutional symptoms: fever (>38°C), drenching sweats, weight loss (10% body weight over 6 months)
E	Involvement of a single, extranodal site contiguous or proximal to a known nodal site (stages I to III only; additional extranodal involvement is stage IV)
S	Splenic involvement
X	Bulky disease, defined as one or more site of disease of >10 cm diameter, or mediastinal widening to >1/3 of the chest width on chest x-ray

Other provisions include designation of involved extranodal site(s): M = marrow, L = lung, H = liver, P = pleura, O = bone, D = skin and subcutaneous tissue; and number of sites of disease (e.g., II_2, II_4).

BOX 30.2 Diagnostic Work-Up in Hodgkin's Lymphoma

Diagnosis
Lymph node biopsy

Staging and risk stratification
Medical history and physical examination
X-ray of the chest
Contrast-enhanced computed tomography (CT) scan of neck, chest and abdomen
Positron emission tomography (PET)
Full blood cell count and blood chemistry
Hepatitis B virus (HBV), hepatitis C virus (HCV) and human immunodeficiency virus (HIV) screening

Pretreatment examinations
Echocardiography (ECG)
Pulmonary function test
Reproductive counselling (in younger patients)
Serum pregnancy test (in younger female patients)
CT scan
PET
HBV
HCV
HIV
ECG

BOX 30.3 Interventions Required to Make a Diagnosis

1. Take a biopsy
2. Utilize laboratory techniques to stratify high-grade B-cell lymphomas
3. Stage the lymphoma using fluorodeoxyglucose–positron emission tomography–computed tomography (FDG–PET–CT)
4. Treatment may consist of 'watch and wait', medications, chemotherapy, surgical intervention, blood and blood product transfusion to treat symptoms, possibly a combination of these
5. Assess responses to treatment
6. Consider end-of-life treatment assessment and survivorship

CARE IN THE HOME SETTING

Patients will continue to have immune defects following their HL treatment, even when cured. When at home, they may be left with complications from both poor immunity and from the side effects of radiation and chemotherapy. It is therefore imperative that they are given information and understand their condition, and receive health promotion around their risk and immunity, risks of anaemia and potential breathlessness from lack of Hb creation. Additionally, following radiation treatment, there is risk of Graves disease, hypothyroidism, thyroid cancer, pulmonary and pericardial fibrosis, coronary artery changes and risk of lung, breast and other solid tumours (Sommers et al., 2007).

Non-Hodgkin's lymphoma

In 2014 there were 13,605 new diagnoses of NHL in the UK (NHS England, 2018). This equates to approximately 37 new cases per day, with 7500 male cases, 6105 female cases and 4801 deaths. Survival is most probable in those aged 15 to 39 years. Only 4 out of 10 aged 80 years and over survive. The survival rate of 10 years or more has risen, showing mortality improvement of 83% when comparing the 1970s with 2014, with preventable cases being at 6% (Cancer Research UK, 2018c). Approximately half of all diagnosis are in people over 70 years, with the highest category being aged 85 to 89 years. It is suggested, using current data, that by 2035 there will be a 2% decrease in HL, which is a decrease of 26 people per 100,000 population.

Risk factors. The risk factors include age, genetics and lifestyle (Cancer Research UK, 2018c). As this blood cancer is so rare, with so many subtypes and variables, most contemporary evidence remains limited. It is suggested that a variety of infections, particularly *Helicobacter pylori* are linked to NHL. Within the UK, lifestyle risk factors include certain occupational exposure, such as constant exposure to diesel fumes, ionizing radiations, and farmer and machinist held occupations (Karunanayake et al., 2008), and medicines (such as chemotherapy) may increase the risk. Additionally, some studies have suggested that certain drugs used to treat rheumatoid arthritis, such as methotrexate and tumour necrosis factor inhibitors, might increase the risk of NHL (American Cancer Society, 2017). Ionizing radiation, HIV, immunological problems, being overweight and having weight-related conditions, as well as smoking, all increase the risk of developing NHL.

Signs and symptoms. According to MacMillian Cancer Support (2017), the most common patient presentation is from painless swelling in the lymph nodes in one area of the body, usually in the neck, axilla or inguinal canal. Some people have other symptoms relating to where the lymphoma is in their body. This could lead to the following symptoms:

- A cough, difficulty swallowing (dysphagia) or breathlessness (dyspnoea) (if the lymphoma is in the chest area)
- Indigestion (dyspepsia), abdominal pain or weight loss (if the lymphoma is in the stomach or bowel).

If NHL spreads to the bone marrow, it can reduce the number of blood cells. This can cause:

- Tiredness (too few RBCs)
- Difficulty fighting infections (too few WBCs)
- Bruising or bleeding (too few platelets).

NHL can also cause general symptoms, including:

- Heavy, drenching sweats at night
- Pyrexia that come and go without any obvious cause
- Unexplained weight loss
- Tiredness
- Itching of the skin (pruritus) that does not go away.

Diagnosis. The most current National Institute for Health and Care Excellence (NICE) guideline for diagnosis and management of NHL is NG52 (NICE, 2017). NG52 covers diagnosis and management of NHL in people aged 16 years and over. It aims to improve care for people with NHL by promoting the best tests for diagnosis and staging and the most effective treatments for six of the subtypes: follicular lymphoma, mucosa-associated lymphoid tissue (MALT) lymphoma, mantle lymphoma, diffuse B-cell lymphoma, Burkitt lymphoma and peripheral T-cell lymphoma. A variety of diagnoses require different management; for specific advice, please refer to NG52 (NICE, 2017).

To make a diagnosis, interventions listed in Box 30.3 are recommended.

Care and treatment of people with NHL. According to Cancer Research UK (2018c), it is typical in all countries to have a '2 weeks wait' standard for a diagnosis of blood cancers, with the highest proportion of cases diagnosed early. Referral is most frequently made by the General Practitioner. Patients in the UK report very good or excellent experiences of their episodes of care, with all patients having a Clinical Nurse Specialist. NICE guideline NG52 (NICE, 2017) recommends tests and treatments, suggesting biopsy, radiotherapy, immunochemotherapy and BMT/stem cell transplantation.

CASE STUDY 30.1 **Ray**

Mr Ray Hill is a 63-year-old driving instructor from London. He has three children and a wife named Tina. Ray was diagnosed with an NHL 6 months ago, after becoming unwell during a routine hospital appointment for a chronic health condition. He was then referred to an oncologist by the hospital medical team. The oncologist obtained a patient history and completed a general physical examination, consequently discovering splenomegaly. Once this was identified, the doctor performed a focused lymphatic system assessment to exclude any notable lumps or bumps, and a range of baseline blood work, including a full blood count. Ray has been taking a range of prescribed pharmaceutical preparations to help manage his condition. His past medical history is complex and includes Ménière's disease, type 1 diabetes mellitus, coronary artery bypass graft (triple heart bypass), hypertension (high blood pressure) and chronic obstructive pulmonary disease.

Ray's presenting complaint was initiated when he mentioned he had been experiencing fatigue, loss of energy and had noticed a paler completion. He believed that this was being caused by a new medication he was taking for his blood pressure, as one of the noted side effects in the patient information leaflet was weight loss. His initial blood results showed his bone marrow neutrophil count to be zero, meaning that he had granulocytopenia (he was neutropenic). Also, it was identified that he had anaemia, as his Hb was only 7.0 g/dL. He was recalled to hospital for further tests and was informed of his NHL diagnosis within 2 weeks. He started treatment for his condition with chemotherapy, and his NHL symptoms (mainly having low Hb) were also treated by receiving a blood transfusion of 3 units of RBCs.

After consultation with the specialist cancer nurse, Ray was given specific information that would enable him to make sense of his situation and become empowered by learning about his NHL condition and its effects on his life. This gave him the ability to make some informed decisions regarding his treatment. Ray visited the oncologists and specialist nurse regularly, who gave various information and explanations as and when required. He also gained support from the multi-disciplinary team on his routine visits for chemotherapy and occasional blood transfusions.

! HOTSPOT

Granulocytopenia

This term is used to indicate an abnormal reduction in the numbers of circulating granulocytes. This is commonly called neutropenia, as up to 75% of granulocytes are neutrophils. In cases that involve splenomegaly (enlarged spleen), a number of these cells get trapped and are unable to circulate through veins and arteries around the body. The consequence of neutropenia is that the body will be susceptible to infections that, if unrecognized or left untreated, may result in sepsis and could lead to death.

! HOTSPOT

Transfusion of Red Blood Cells

The British Society for Haematology suggest that every hospital must have a policy stipulating the procedure regarding blood and blood component transfusions. This must include the essential care and specific monitoring requirements of patients undergoing blood and blood component transfusions. Policy must also govern aspects including correct documentation (i.e., patient identification), sample, any special requirements, storage, collection and transportation of blood. Every step of the blood transfusion process must be traceable for a period of 30 years. Hospitals are also required to be transparent (open and honest) about near misses, transfusion errors, fatalities and never events.

! HOTSPOT

When to Transfuse

An exploration of the cause of anaemia is imperative prior to transfusing RBCs. Currently, there is not an established Hb that warrants blood transfusion. However, within clinical practice, it is accepted that most patients who are in a stable condition can tolerate an anaemia with an Hb level of 70 g/L. Again, remembering the role RBCs have within the human body, if a patient is weak, fatigued, actively bleeding, acutely unstable or breathless with low oxygen saturation, this level of Hb would need to be increased.

OSCE 30.1 **Lymphatic Examination**

Depending on where you are working and your local policy and procedure, you may assist or be performing history taking and physical examination of patients, particularly in a clinic or primary care setting.

Mr Ray hILL had a lymphatic examination. Below is a list specifying the process of lymphatic assessment. You will be marked on the following areas; all areas must be passed in order to achieve an overall pass:

1. Inspect thyroid gland from front of patient – enlarged thyroid – goitre?
2. Inspect patient swallow to inspect isthmus rising?
3. Inspect salivary glands bilaterally – lift tongue.
4. Palpate thyroid gland from behind patient.
5. Palpate salivary glands.
6. Palpate preauricular lymph node bilaterally.
7. Palpate postauricular lymph node bilaterally.
8. Palpate occipital lymph node bilaterally.
9. Palpate superficial cervical lymph node bilaterally.
10. Palpate deep cervical lymph node bilaterally.
11. Palpate tonsillar lymph node.
12. Palpate submandibular lymph node bilaterally.
13. Palpate submental lymph node.
14. Palpate supraclavicular lymph node.
15. Palpate axillary nodes.
16. If breast examination is necessary, use a chaperone. Breast examination may be required to identify lumps or enlarged lymph nodes.
17. Palpate inguinal nodes bilaterally.

When assessing the lymphatic system, if you identify a lump it is important that the points noted in Box 30.4 are considered as part of your data collection. This must be referred to a specialist once completed.

Disseminated intravascular coagulation

Disseminated intravascular coagulation (DIC) is defined as 'a widespread inappropriate intravascular deposition of fibrin with consumption of coagulation factors and platelets that occur as a consequence of disorders which release pro-coagulant material into the circulation or cause widespread endothelial damage or platelet aggregation' (Hoffbrand & Moss, 2016). Therefore, it is suggested that DIC is a thrombo-haemorrhagic disorder characterized by primary thrombotic and secondary haemorrhagic diathesis, causing multiorgan failure.

Signs and symptoms

The main clinical presentation is bleeding, but in approximately 5%–10% of the population it is manifested with microthrombotic lesions, such as gangrenous limbs. In the majority of patients nursed in hospital, excessive bleeding may be seen after venepuncture, or around cannula sites, sutures, wound drains and wounds. Because of the high probability of bleeding, the Nursing Associate must be cautious of nonvisible bleeding. Generalized bleeding in the gastrointestinal tract, mouth, throat, lung and urinary tract and vaginal bleeding may become severe.

Additional signs and symptoms include:
- Infections
- Malignancy
- Vascular abnormalities
- Miscellaneous (see Table 30.4 for the causes of DIC)

BOX 30.4 Points to Note in Lymphatic Assessment

Characteristics of a mass/lump
Does it illuminate?
Size (in cm)
Position/location
Does it have a defined edge?
Depth in tissue
Does it pulsate?
Pain
Shape
Skin colour/condition overlying lump
Consistency
Temperature
Does it indent on pressure?
Mobility
Is it fluctuant (does it move or is it fixed in one place)?
Surface characteristics (e.g., smooth, regular)

- Hypersensitivity reactions
- Obstetric complications.

Less frequently, thrombi may cause acute kidney injury and ischaemia, and can sometimes cause gangrene.

Diagnosis

The diagnosis of DIC is not made from a single laboratory value. It will be made based on the collection of a variety of data, beginning with a characteristic patient history and physical examination, investigations for prolonged clotting times, deranged fibrinogen levels (fibrin degradation and D dimer) and a declining platelet count. The International Society for Thrombosis and Haemostasis DIC scoring system provides objective measurement of DIC. Where DIC is present, the scoring system correlates with key clinical observations and outcomes. It is important to repeat the tests to monitor the dynamically changing scenario, based on laboratory results and clinical observations (British Society of Haematology, 2009).

Pathogenesis is believed to be a key event underlying DIC and comes from the increased activity of tissue factor. Damaged tissue will inevitably be released into the circulating volume from damaged cells or tumours, or because of increased cell release secondary to normal inflammatory processes (such as proinflammatory cytokine release by monocytes and endothelial cells).

It is usual that blood is taken and sent to pathology for clotting-focused testing when:
- Patients present as being pale and complaining of fatigue
- Patients present with abnormal bleeding, such as prolonged bleeding or with an inability to stop bleeding
- When organ function is impaired, in multiorgan failure
- When liver failure is suspected.

In cases such as these, it would be pertinent to explore partial thromboplastin time (PTT) and activated PPT. PTT is a test that measures the overall speed at which blood clots, by means of two consecutive series of biochemical reactions known as the intrinsic and common coagulation pathways.

Care and treatment

The British Society of Haematology (2009), give the following guidelines for the diagnosis and management of DIC:

Transfusion of platelets or plasma (components) in patients with DIC should not primarily be based on laboratory results

---

TABLE 30.4 Causes of Disseminated Intravascular Coagulation

Infections	Malignancy	Obstetric complications	Hypersensitivity reactions	Widespread tissue damage	Vascular abnormalities	Miscellaneous
Gram-negative septicaemia	Widespread mucin-secreting adenocarcinoma Acute promyelocytic leukaemia	Amniotic fluid embolism Premature separation of placenta Eclampsia Retained placenta Septic abortion	Anaphylaxis Incompatible blood transfusion	Postoperative complications Secondary to trauma Following severe burns	Kasabach-Merritt syndrome Leaking prosthetic valves Cardiac bypass surgery Vascular aneurysms	Liver failure Pancreatitis Poisonous invertebrate venoms Hypothermia Pyrexia Excessive blood loss

(Hoffbrand & Moss, 2016.)

and should in general be reserved for patients who present with bleeding.

In patients with DIC and bleeding or at high risk of bleeding (e.g., postoperative patients or patients due to undergo an invasive procedure) and a low platelet count, transfusion of platelets should be considered.

Nurses and Nursing Associates must ensure that patients are monitored appropriately and that they use early warning score (EWS) to recognize deterioration and escalate concerns as they arise.

Patients who are actively bleeding and have an inability to clot are at greater risk of hypoxia and bleeding, as well as anxiety and fear about their condition.

Nurses must observe for any obvious bleeding, including lower gastrointestinal tract (such as melena) and upper gastrointestinal tract (such as hemoptysis) and observe patient for non-obvious bleeding (such as colour changes, temperature, abdominal distention and new bruising) as this might indicate bleeding within the body.

LOOKING BACK, FEEDING FORWARD

The haematological system is made up of the blood and bone marrow. The blood delivers oxygen and nutrients to all of the body's tissues, removes wastes and transports gases, blood cells, immune cells, antibodies and hormones throughout the body. This chapter has provided an insight into this complex system.

Nursing Associates may be required to provide nursing care for patients with blood diseases or disorders. Some of the more commonly known blood diseases and disorders a Nursing Associate may encounter include: anaemia, leukaemia, lymphoma and sickle cell anaemia. In order to provide care that is safe and effective, the Nursing Associate must have insight and understanding of the key issues associated with the haematological system.

The pathological processes underlying common haematological disorders have been examined and contemporary management strategies explored. The Nursing Associate is encouraged to delve deeper to ensure that their practice is up to date and based on the best available evidence and guidelines, and to consider individual patient needs relating to diagnosis of chronic/life-threatening diseases.

REFERENCES

American Cancer Society, 2017. Non-Hodgkin's lymphoma risk factors. Available at https://www.cancer.org/cancer/non-hodgkin-lymphoma/causes-risks-prevention/risk-factors.html.

Bickley, L.S., Szilagyi, P.G., Hoffman, R.M., 2017. Bates' Guide to Physical Examination and History Taking, 12th ed. Wolters Kluwer.

British Society of Haematology, 2009. Diagnosis and management of disseminated intravascular coagulation (1). Available at http://www.b-s-h.org.uk/guidelines/guidelines/diagnosis-and-management-of-disseminated-intravascular-coagulation-1/.

British Society of Haematology. 2017. Guidelines. Available at http://www.b-s-h.org.uk/guidelines/?category=Transfusion&p=1&search=#guideline-filters__select__status.

Brown, M., Cutler, T., 2012. Haematology Nursing. Wiley Blackwell, London.

Cancer Research UK, 2018a. Hodgkin lymphoma: incidence statistics. https://www.cancerresearchuk.org/health-professional/cancer-statistics/statistics-by-cancer-type/hodgkin-lymphoma/.

Cancer Research UK, 2018b. Hodgkin lymphoma symptoms. https://www.cancerresearchuk.org/about-cancer/hodgkin-lymphoma/symptoms.

Cancer Research UK, 2018c. Non-Hodgkin lymphoma statistics. Available at http://www.cancerresearchuk.org/health-professional/cancer-statistics/statistics-by-cancer-type/non-hodgkin-lymphoma.

Department of Health (DH), 2010. Equality and diversity: Equality Act 2010. Available at https://www.gov.uk/government/organisations/department-of-health/about/equality-and-diversity.

European Society for Medical Oncology, 2014. Clinical practice guidelines: Hodgkin's lymphoma: ESMO clinical practice guidelines for diagnosis, treatment and follow-up. Ann. Oncol. 25 (3), 70–75.

Health Education England (HEE), 2017. Nursing Associate Curriculum Framework. https://www.hee.nhs.uk/sites/default/files/documents/Nursing%20Associate%20Curriculum%20Framework%20Feb2017_0.pdf.

Hernadez-Ilizaliturri, J., 2016. Hodgkin lymphoma staging. Classification and staging systems for Hodgkin lymphoma. Available at https://emedicine.medscape.com/article/2007081-overview.

Hoffbrand, V., Moss, P., 2016. Hoffbrand's Essential Haematology, seventh ed. Wiley Blackwell.

Howard, M.R., Hamilton, P.J., 2013. Haematology, fourth ed. Churchill Livingstone, London.

Karunanayake, C., McDuffie, H.H., Dosman, J.A., et al., 2008. Occupational exposure and non-Hodgkin's lymphoma: Canadian case-control study. Environmental Health. Available at: https://ehjournal.biomedcentral.com/articles/10.1186/1476-069X-7-44#Bib1.

Lister, T.A., Crowther, D., et al., 1989. Report of a committee convened to discuss the evaluation and staging of patients with Hodgkin's disease: Cotswolds meeting. J. Clin. Oncol. 7 (11), 1630–1636.

MacMillian Cancer Support, 2017. Signs and symptoms of non-Hodgkin's lymphoma (NHL). Available at https://www.macmillan.org.uk/information-and-support/lymphoma/lymphoma-non-hodgkin/understanding-cancer/signs-and-symptoms.html.

Moore, G.W., Knight, G., Blan, A.D., 2010. Haematology. Oxford University Press, Oxford.

NHS Direct, 2017. Sepsis. Available at http://www.nhsdirect.wales.nhs.uk/encyclopaedia/s/article/sepsis/.

NHS England, 2018. Clinical commissioning policy: Bendamustine with rituximab for first line treatment of advanced indolent non-Hodgkin's lymphoma (all ages). https://www.england.nhs.uk/wp.../1605-bendamustine-with-rituximab-for-nhl.pdf.

NHS UK, 2017. Thalassaemia. Available at https://www.nhs.uk/conditions/thalassaemia/.

NICE, 2017. National Institute for Health and Care Excellence. Non-Hodgkin's lymphoma: diagnosis and management. Available at https://www.nice.org.uk/guidance/ng52/chapter/Recommendations.

Nursing and Midwifery Council (NMC), 2017. Equality, diversity and inclusion framework. Available at https://www.nmc.org.uk/about-us/our-equality-and-diversity-commitments/framework/.

Nursing and Midwifery Council (NMC), 2018. Standards of Proficiency for Nursing Associates. London: NMC. https://www

.nmc.org.uk/globalassets/sitedocuments/education-standards/nursing-associates-proficiency-standards.pdf.

Pallister, C.J., Watson, M.S., 2011. Haematology, second ed. Scion, Banbury.

Scott, W.N., 2013. Pathophysiology Made Incredibly Easy, fifth ed. Lippincott Williams & Wilki, Philadelphia.

Sommers, M., Johnson, S., Beery, T., 2007. Diseases and disorders: A nursing therapeutics manual. In: Dickinson, S. (Ed.), Handbook for Brunner and Suddarth's Textbook of Medical-Surgical Nursing, eleventh ed. Lippincott Williams & Wilkins, Philadelphia.

Waugh, A., Grant, A., 2018. Ross and Wilson Anatomy & Physiology in Health and Illness, thirteenth ed. Elsevier, Edinburgh.

Respiratory Disorders

Anthony Wheeldon

CHAPTER AIMS

The aim of this chapter is to provide the reader with an understanding of the skills, knowledge and attitude required to provide safe, effective and compassionate care to people with a respiratory disorder.

SELF TEST

1. Name five major anatomical structures of the lower respiratory tract.
2. What is the main function of the respiratory system?
3. How are oxygen and carbon dioxide transported around the human body?
4. What are the care priorities for a patient requiring oxygen therapy?
5. What do you understand by the term 'breathlessness'?
6. What physiological observations would you use to assess a patient's respiratory status?
7. Describe the main signs and symptoms of pneumonia.
8. List the main differences between obstructive and restrictive lung disorders.
9. List the main medications and therapies used for patients experiencing an exacerbation of asthma.
10. What is the main cause of chronic obstructive pulmonary disease?

INTRODUCTION

This chapter explores respiratory disorders commonly encountered in clinical practice. The initial section explores respiratory anatomy and physiology, which is important for Nursing Associates, who require an in-depth understanding of breathing if the care they provide is to be appropriate and effective.

The second section addresses a selection of common respiratory conditions that impact on the health and well-being of people living with respiratory disease, with emphasis on the care and comfort that people require. When offering care, the Nursing Associate is required to be kind and compassionate. Symptoms associated with respiratory disorders, such as breathlessness, pain and cough, can be exhausting, debilitating and often cause anxiety. Often, people living with respiratory disease experience difficulties with activities of living, such as shopping, eating, washing, dressing and socializing. Many suffer feelings of depression, isolation and embarrassment as a result. Nursing Associates therefore are required to be kind and considerate when providing care for people living with a respiratory disorder (see Table 31.1).

RESPIRATORY ANATOMY

The respiratory system is divided into the upper and lower respiratory tracts. The upper respiratory tract consists of the oral and nasal cavities, the pharynx and the larynx. The lower respiratory tract includes the trachea, bronchi, bronchioles and alveoli. Many of the structures within the lower respiratory tract are very fragile and easily damaged by infection. For this reason, both the upper and the lower respiratory tracts are equipped to fight off any invading airborne pathogens. Fig. 31.1 shows the main structures of the respiratory tract.

The upper respiratory tract

The upper respiratory tract consists of the oral and nasal cavities, the pharynx and the larynx (Fig. 31.2). The main functions of the upper respiratory tract are:

- Provision of sense of smell
- Speech
- Humidification of inhaled gases
- Protection of lower respiratory tract

The spaces just inside the nostrils are lined with course hairs that filter inhaled air. This ensures that large dust particles do not enter the upper and lower respiratory tract. The walls of the nasal cavity are also lined with a mucous membrane made from pseudostratified ciliated columnar epithelium, which contains mucus-secreting goblet cells and capillaries. Inhaled air is warmed by the blood flowing through the capillaries and moistened by

mucus as it passes through the nasal cavity. Dust particles that pass through the nasal hairs are captured in the mucus and propelled by cilia towards the pharynx, where they can be swallowed or expectorated. Also found on the roof of the nasal cavity is olfactory epithelium, which is a specialist tissue that is involved with the sensation of smell.

The pharynx is the region underneath the nasal cavity, behind the oral cavity and just above the larynx and is more commonly referred to as the throat. The pharynx contains five tonsils, whose primary function is to protect the lower respiratory tract from infection. The two tonsils visible when the mouth is open are the palatine tonsils; behind the tongue are the two lingual tonsils and the pharyngeal tonsil or adenoid sits on the upper back wall of the pharynx. Tonsils are lymph nodules and part of the body's defence system. Their epithelial lining has deep folds, called crypts, which trap and entangle bacteria, which are then engulfed and destroyed.

The larynx is more commonly referred to as the voice box and its main function is the formulation of speech. This is of particular importance for health professionals as the ability to speak relies on a fully functioning respiratory system. Individuals who are experiencing difficulties breathing, for example, will also find speaking in full sentences challenging. The ability to speak in full sentences therefore forms part of a comprehensive respiratory assessment (British Thoracic Society and Scottish Intercollegiate Guidelines Network, 2016).

The oral cavity and pharynx are also major structures of the digestive system and the larynx provides protection against the inhalation of food and drink. The larynx occupies the space between the pharynx and the trachea, the first section of the lower respiratory tract, which is adjacent to the oesophagus (the structure that propels food towards the stomach). Attached to the top of the larynx is a leaf-shaped piece of epithelial-covered

TABLE 31.1	Common Respiratory Disorders
Obstructive lung disorders	Chronic obstructive pulmonary disease
	Asthma
Restrictive lung disorders	Pneumoconioses
Infection	Pneumonia
	Tuberculosis
Cancer	Lung cancer

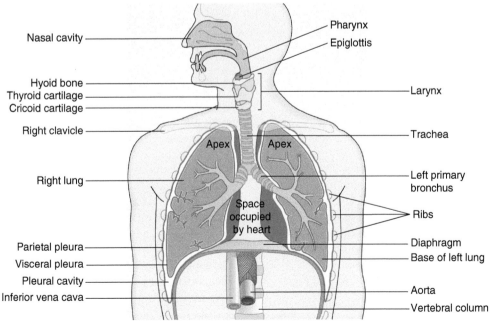

Fig. 31.1 The Respiratory Tract (Waugh & Grant, 2018).

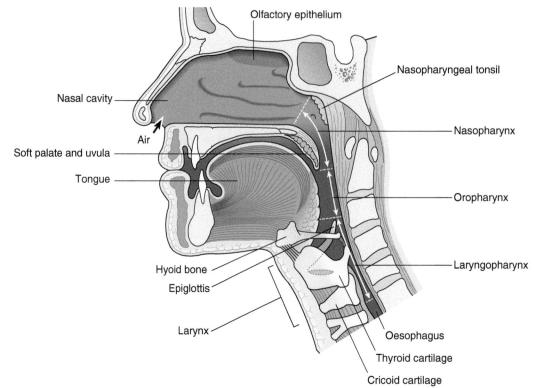

Fig. 31.2 The Upper Respiratory Tract (Waugh & Grant, 2018).

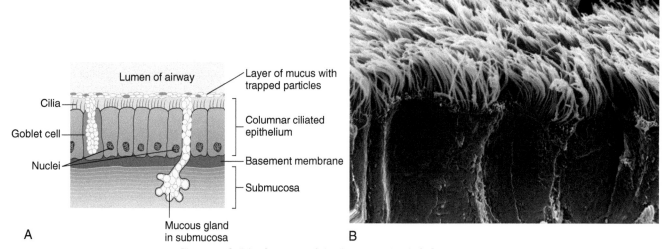

Fig. 31.3 Cellular Structure of the Trachea (Waugh & Grant, 2018).

elastic cartilage, called the epiglottis. On swallowing, the epiglottis blocks entry to the larynx and solid and liquid food matter are pushed towards the oesophagus.

To add further protection, the upper respiratory tract is lined with irritant receptors, which when stimulated by invading particles (e.g., dust or pollen) force a sneeze, ensuring the offending material is ejected through the nose or mouth.

The lower respiratory tract

The lower respiratory tract consists of the trachea, the right and left primary bronchi and the constituents of both lungs. The

trachea is commonly referred to as the windpipe, as it carries air from the larynx down towards the lungs. The trachea is a tubular vessel that is lined with pseudostratified ciliated columnar epithelium that can trap inhaled debris and propel it up towards the oesophagus and pharynx to be swallowed or expectorated (Fig. 31.3). The trachea and the right and left primary bronchi also contain irritant receptors that generate coughs when stimulated, forcing larger invading particles upwards. The outermost layer of the trachea is made of connective tissue, reinforced by a series of 16–20 C-shaped cartilage rings, which prevent the trachea from collapsing.

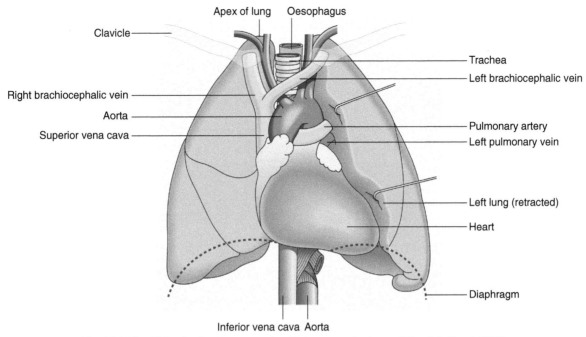

Fig. 31.4 The Major Cardiac Structures that Sit between the Lungs (Waugh & Grant, 2018).

The lungs are two cone-shaped organs. They are protected by the thoracic cage: a skeletal structure made up of the ribs, sternum (breast bone) and vertebrae (spine). The apex (tip) of each lung protrudes just above the clavicle (collar bone), whilst their wide bases sit just above the diaphragm, a concave muscle that plays a vital role in breathing. The lungs are divided into five lobes, three on the right and two on the left. Each lobe is named after its location:

- Superior lobe of right lung
- Middle lobe of right lung
- Inferior lobe of right lung
- Superior lobe of left lung
- Inferior lobe of left lung

Each lung is surrounded by two thin protective membranes called the parietal and visceral pleura. The parietal pleura lines the walls of the thoracic cage and the visceral pleura lines the lungs themselves. The space between the two pleurae (the pleural space) is minute and contains a thin film of lubricating fluid. This reduces friction between the two pleura, allowing both layers to slide over one another during breathing. The fluid also helps the visceral and parietal pleura to adhere to one another, in the same way two pieces of glass stick together when wet.

The heart, along with major blood vessels such as the aorta, vena cava, pulmonary veins and arteries, sit in a space between the two lungs called the cardiac notch (see also Chapter 29). Fig. 31.4 shows the major cardiac structures that sit between the two lungs.

The structures that make up both lungs are a series of airways of decreasing size that eventually terminate with a lobule, which is a microscopic structure whose primary function is to supply the blood with oxygen. The dividing nature and ever decreasing size of the airways is often compared to the branches and twigs of a tree. Indeed, the airways are often collectively referred to as

the 'bronchial tree', and the points at which the airways divide are called 'branches'. The airways begin with the trachea, which divides into the right and left primary bronchi. The right and left primary bronchi then divide into the secondary bronchi, of which there are five branches, one for each lobe. The secondary bronchi divide again into a series of tertiary bronchi, which continue to divide into smaller and smaller fourth and fifth generation airways. Airways which are less than 1 mm in diameter are called bronchioles, which continue to divide into a network of tinier bronchioles approximately 0.5 mm in diameter, called terminal bronchioles. The lobules are found beyond the terminal bronchioles. Lobules consist of a series of respiratory bronchioles, alveolar ducts and alveoli. Alveoli are sphere-like structures, which are clustered together to form alveolar sacs (Fig. 31.5). There are approximately 490 alveoli in a pair of human lungs (Ochs et al., 2004). Fig. 31.6 shows the structure of the bronchial tree and the passage of airflow from the trachea down towards the lobule.

RESPIRATORY PHYSIOLOGY

The respiratory system has several functions:

- Respiration
- Sense of smell
- Speech production
- Acid–base balance
- Aid fluid balance
- Aid temperature control.

The first of these six functions is the primary function of the respiratory system, whilst the remaining five are often referred to as secondary functions. Respiration describes the inhalation of oxygen and the expulsion of carbon dioxide. All human cells require a continuous supply of oxygen. Fortunately, there is a

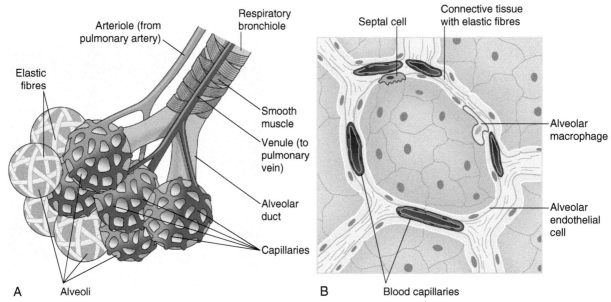

Fig. 31.5 Anatomical Structure of a Lobule (Waugh & Grant, 2018).

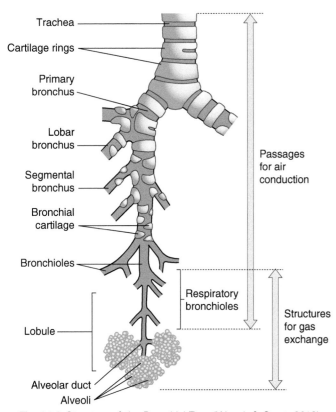

Fig. 31.6 Structure of the Bronchial Tree (Waugh & Grant, 2018).

plentiful supply, as it constitutes around 21% of our atmosphere. As cells use oxygen, a waste gas is produced: carbon dioxide. If allowed to build up within circulation, large levels of carbon dioxide can disrupt cellular homeostasis and lead to respiratory failure. Respiration is extraction of oxygen from the atmosphere and simultaneous disposal of excess carbon dioxide. It encompasses the following four distinct processes:
- Pulmonary ventilation: breathing

- External respiration: gaseous exchange, the transfer of oxygen from the lungs into blood and the transfer of carbon dioxide from blood into the lungs
- Transport of gases: the ways that oxygen is carried from the lungs to the cells and carbon dioxide is carried from cells to the lungs
- Internal respiration: the transfer of oxygen from blood to the cells and carbon dioxide from cells to blood

All four processes of respiration are explored in this chapter; however, only pulmonary ventilation and external respiration are the sole responsibility of the respiratory system. Oxygen and carbon dioxide are transported around the human body in circulation, therefore, effective respiration is reliant upon a fully functioning cardiovascular system (see Chapter 29).

Pulmonary ventilation

Pulmonary ventilation describes the movement of air in and out of the lungs. The way gases behave helps explain how this movement of air occurs. Gases always flow from areas of high pressure to low pressure. The gases that constitute air collectively exert atmospheric pressure. The air within the lungs also exerts a pressure, which is known as alveolar pressure. During inspiration (breathing in), the thorax expands, and alveolar pressure falls below atmospheric pressure. Because alveolar pressure is now less than atmospheric pressure, air will naturally move into the airways until the pressure difference no longer exists. During expiration (breathing out) respiratory muscles relax and the thorax springs back to its normal shape and air is forced out of the lungs. Breathing in and out is produced by the action of a range of respiratory muscles, which are shown in Fig. 31.7.

For normal quiet inhalation (breathing in), the external intercostal muscles pull the rib cage outwards and upwards and the diaphragm pulls the lungs downwards. Normal quiet exhalation (breathing out) is a passive process, where the external intercostal muscles and the diaphragm relax and return to their normal

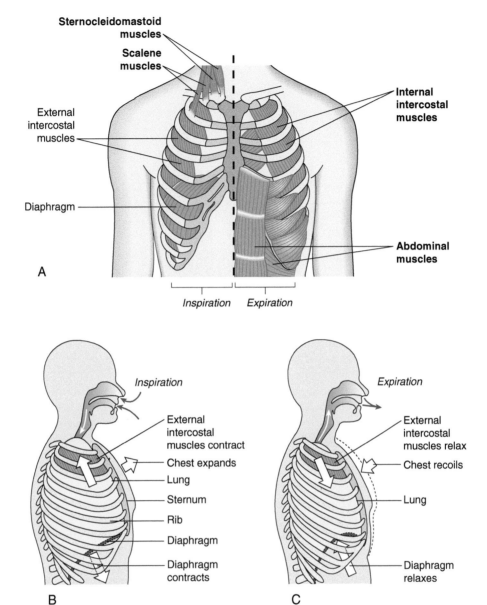

Fig. 31.7 The Respiratory Muscles in Action (Waugh & Grant, 2018).

shape; as a result, the rib cage moves downwards and inwards and the diaphragm pushes the lungs upwards. Fig. 31.7 also shows the muscular processes of normal quiet exhalation and inhalation. Other muscles can also be utilized to enhance breathing. The internal intercostal and abdominal wall muscles can be used to achieve a forceful exhalation beyond a normal breath, for example when blowing candles out on a birthday cake or playing a musical instrument. The sternocleidomastoid and scalenes can also increase the size of the upper lobes and can be used to produce a deeper forceful inspiration. These muscles are also referred to as the accessory muscles of breathing, as they are rarely used in normal quiet breathing (Wheeldon, 2016).

The lungs have a large capacity for air. The volume of air a pair of lungs is capable of housing will vary from individual to individual, depending on the size. However, in physiological terms, the average human male is said to have the capacity to house around 6 L of air. This volume of air is referred to as 'total

vital capacity'. Normal quiet breathing, however, involves much smaller volumes of air. On average, normal resting breathing totals around 500 mL of air inhaled and exhaled each breath. This volume of air is called 'tidal volume'. After a normal inspiration, a space will remain within the lungs for further inhalation of air; this capacity for larger intakes of breath is referred to as the 'inspiratory reserve volume', which in healthy individuals is around 3100 mL. Likewise, after normal resting expiration, a volume of air that could be expelled by force remains in the lungs. This volume of air is called the 'functional residual capacity', which is around 2400 mL in volume. However, not all this volume of air can be exhaled. A small volume of air always remains in the lungs. This volume is referred to as 'residual volume' (RV) and is around 1200 mL. The remaining portion of functional residual volume, around 1200 mL, is called the 'expiratory reserve volume' (ERV), which is the maximum amount of air you could forcefully breathe out if required. Because residual

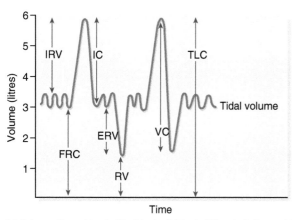

Fig. 31.8 Lung Capacities in Healthy Individuals (Waugh & Grant, 2018). ERV, Expiratory reserve volume; FRC, functional residual capacity; IC, inspiratory capacity; IRV, inspiratory reserve volume; RV, residual volume; TLC, total lung capacity; VC, vital capacity.

volume cannot be exhaled, it is not considered in measurements of lung capacity for purposes of diagnosis. Instead, the total of inspiratory reserve volume, tidal volume and expiratory reserve volume is used. This accumulated capacity is referred to as 'vital capacity', the potential capacity for the volume of air that the lungs can breathe in and out. In the average healthy adult male, this is approximately 4800 mL. Fig. 31.8 shows a diagrammatical representation of how vital capacity is divided.

At rest, a tidal volume of 500 mL is enough to provide oxygen for cells and to expire newly generated carbon dioxide. On exercise, when the body's demand for oxygen rises and more carbon dioxide is generated, breathing becomes deeper, tidal volume increases and inspiratory and expiratory reserve volumes decrease. This increases the volume of air inhaled and exhaled and increases the surface area of the lungs used for the extraction of oxygen and the expulsion of carbon dioxide. In ill health, if airways are obstructed by respiratory disease, this increases residual volume and reduces vital capacity.

External respiration

External respiration is the process by which oxygen diffuses from the alveoli into circulation and carbon dioxide diffuses from circulation and enters the alveoli to be breathed away. External respiration only occurs in the lobules and for this reason this portion of the bronchial tree is referred to as the 'respiratory zone'. The air present in the remainder of the bronchial tree plays no part in external respiration; therefore, these structures are collectively referred to as the 'conducting zone'. The diffusion of oxygen between the alveoli and circulation and carbon dioxide between circulation and the alveoli occurs because gas molecules always move from areas of high pressure to low pressure. Each lobule has its own arterial blood supply; this blood supply originates from the pulmonary artery, which stems from the right ventricle of the heart (Fig. 31.9). Because the blood flowing through the arterioles supplying the lobules of the lungs originates from the pulmonary arteries, it is low in oxygen and relatively high in carbon dioxide. The amount (and therefore partial pressure) of oxygen in the alveoli is far greater, around 12–13 kPa (90–97 mm Hg), than that in the passing arterial blood supply,

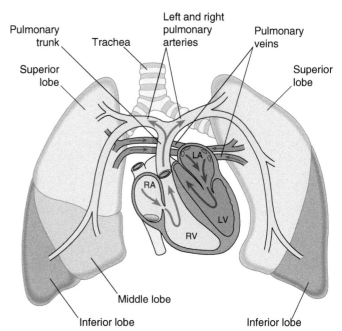

Fig. 31.9 Blood Flow through the Heart and Lungs (Waugh & Grant, 2018).

which is around 5.3 kPa (40 mm Hg). Oxygen therefore diffuses out of the alveoli, into the pulmonary circulation and onwards toward the left side of the heart via the pulmonary veins. Simultaneously, because there is less carbon dioxide (around 5.3 kPa (40 mm Hg)), in the alveoli than in pulmonary circulation, approximately 5.8–6 kPa (44–45 mm Hg) carbon dioxide diffuses into the alveoli, ready to be exhaled (Fig. 31.10A).

Transport of gases

Transport of gases describes the methods by which respiratory gases are transported between the lungs and cells. Most oxygen, around 98.5%, is transported between the lungs and cells attached to haemoglobin (Hb) in erythrocytes. The remaining 1.5% is dissolved in plasma. Healthcare professionals can measure the amount of oxygen attached to Hb in arterial blood by the use of a pulse oximeter, which measures oxygen saturation (SpO_2). In healthy individuals, SpO_2 should be between 97% and 99%. Carbon dioxide is transferred from cells to the lungs in three ways. Around 10% is found dissolved in plasma and 20% is attached to Hb in erythrocytes. The remaining carbon dioxide combines with water to form carbonic acid, which then dissociates into hydrogen ions and bicarbonate ions. The volumes of oxygen and carbon dioxide dissolved in plasma provide another useful measure of respiratory health. Arterial blood gas tests provide an accurate measure of volumes of oxygen and carbon dioxide dissolved in plasma and provide members of the healthcare team with sensitive measures of respiratory function. In healthy individuals, the partial pressure of oxygen dissolved in plasma ranges between 11 and 13.5 kPa and the partial pressure of carbon dioxide should be between 4.5 and 6 kPa. Arterial blood gas readings outside of these ranges indicate respiratory failure, caused by an acute or long-term respiratory disorder. Table 31.2 highlights some of the main measures used by health professionals to determine external respiration and transport of gases.

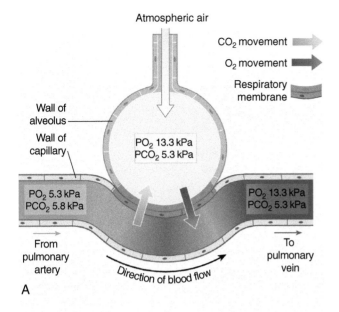

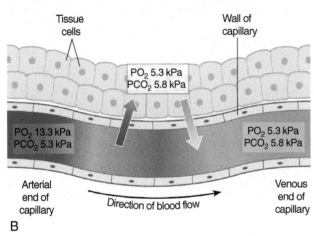

Fig. 31.10 External and Internal Respiration (Waugh & Grant, 2018). PCO_2, partial pressure of carbon dioxide; PO_2, partial pressure of oxygen.

CRITICAL AWARENESS

Pulse-Oximeters and Inaccurate Readings

Nursing Associates need to be mindful that there are factors that can lead to inaccurate pulse-oximeter readings. Tremors, anaemia and polycythaemia (low and high haemoglobin levels), cold fingers and the presence of nail varnish can all lead to inaccurate readings.

Internal respiration

Cells continually use oxygen as part of their manufacture of adenosine tri-phosphate (ATP), which is their prime energy source. In addition to ATP, cells also produce water, heat and carbon dioxide. Internal respiration is the exchange of oxygen and carbon dioxide between blood and cells. This process is governed by the same principles as external respiration. Cells are continually using oxygen and, as a result, its concentration (pressure) within the cells is always lower than within circulation. Simultaneously, the constant production of carbon dioxide ensures increased levels within cells in comparison with circulating blood. As blood flows through the capillaries, oxygen and carbon dioxide follow their concentration/pressure gradients and continually diffuse between blood and cells (see Fig. 31.10B).

CONTROL AND WORK OF BREATHING

In addition to respiration, the physiological principles of control of breathing and work of breathing can help Nursing Associates to understand the nature of respiratory disorders and their impact on well-being.

Control of breathing

The rate and depth of breathing are controlled by the respiratory rhythmicity centre within the medulla oblongata (in the brain stem) and the cerebral cortex in the brain. Fig. 31.11 shows the main neurological structures that control the rate and depth of

TABLE 31.2 Common Measures of External Respiration and Transport of Gases Used by Healthcare Professionals to Determine the Effectiveness of a Patient's Respiratory System			
Measurement	Notation	Normal parameters	Explanation
Oxygen saturation via pulse-oximeter	SpO_2	97%–99%	The percentage of haemoglobin in arterial blood that is carrying oxygen molecules.
Oxygen saturation via arterial blood gas analysis	SaO_2	97%–99%	The percentage of haemoglobin in arterial blood that is carrying oxygen molecules. Considered to be a more accurate reading due to the drawbacks of pulse-oximetry (see Critical Awareness)
Partial pressure of oxygen via blood gas analysis	PaO_2	11–13.5 kPa	The pressure exerted by the small amount of oxygen dissolved in plasma. The greater the pressure exerted, the greater the amount of oxygen will be bound to haemoglobin.
Partial pressure of carbon dioxide via blood gas analysis	$PaCO_2$	4.5–6 kPa	The pressure exerted by the small amount of carbon dioxide dissolved in plasma. The greater the pressure exerted, the greater the amount of carbon dioxide will combine with water to form hydrogen ions.

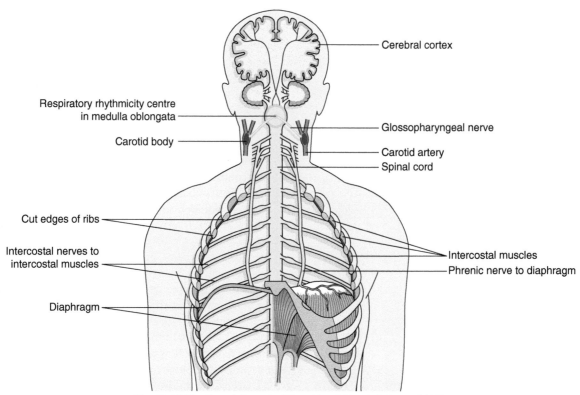

Fig. 31.11 The Neural Control of Breathing (Waugh & Grant, 2018).

breathing. The respiratory rhythmicity centre continually analyses carbon dioxide levels within the cerebrospinal fluid. As levels of carbon dioxide rise, neural messages are sent via the phrenic and intercostal nerves to the diaphragm and intercostal muscles, instructing them to contract. Within the aorta and carotid arteries there are chemoreceptors (the aortic and carotid bodies) that also analyse levels of carbon dioxide, as well as oxygen, in arterial blood. If arterial oxygen levels fall or arterial carbon dioxide levels rise, neural messages are sent to the respiratory rhythmicity centre via the glossopharyngeal nerve and vagus nerve, stimulating further contraction.

Normal quiet breathing is a subconscious activity. However, its rate and depth can be controlled voluntarily or even stopped altogether by the cerebral cortex, when swimming under water for example. This voluntary control is limited as the respiratory rhythmicity centre has a strong urge to ensure breathing is not interrupted. A person's state of mind can also influence the rate and depth breathing. Fear, anxiety or even the anticipation of stressful activities can cause an involuntary increase in the rate and depth of breathing. Further factors that can affect breathing include high temperature/fever (pyrexia) and pain. It is important for Nursing Associates to appreciate that breathing is largely beyond an individual's control and therefore any changes in respiration rate are clinically significant.

Work of breathing

When breathing in, respiratory muscles must overcome the elastic recoil of lung tissue and resistance to airflow through tiny airways. Work of breathing describes the muscle energy required to overcome elastic recoil and resistance to airflow. In healthy individuals,

very little energy is required to overcome work of breathing. This is because the lungs have compliance, which is aided by the production of a detergent-like substance called surfactant. Surfactant is produced by type 2 alveolar cells within the alveoli and reduces the surface tension that occurs where the alveoli meets pulmonary capillary blood flow in lobules. Many lung disorders can affect lung compliance and airway resistance and increase work of breathing as a result. In acute respiratory failure, work of breathing could account for up to 30% of total body energy expenditure (Levitzky et al., 1990).

CASE STUDY 31.1   Emily

Emily is a 67-year-old woman who has been admitted to her local accident and emergency department with shortness of breath and difficulty in breathing. Emily is a retired school cook and lives alone in a high-rise council flat. Emily's husband died 3 years ago from lung cancer and her only daughter lives abroad. Emily has smoked 20 cigarettes a day since she was a teenager and currently drinks alcohol every day. She has had a productive cough for several weeks, which has become progressively worse in the last 48 hours. This morning she couldn't catch her breath after coughing for several minutes and now complains of feeling short of breath and a tight chest. On assessment, she has a bluish tinge to her lips, is using accessory muscles of breathing and is expectorating rust-coloured sputum. Her respiratory rate is 28 respirations per minute and her breaths are shallow. Her temperature is 38.8°C and she is complaining that breathing is painful and that she feels exhausted. A pulse-oximeter shows an oxygen saturation of 88%.

She is commenced on oxygen therapy and sent for an urgent chest x-ray. Emily is diagnosed with pneumonia and is admitted to the respiratory unit for bed rest, intravenous antibiotics, intravenous fluids and analgesia.

NURSING SKILLS

Respiratory Rate

It is paramount that the Nursing Associate can establish the severity of a patient's condition. The respiratory rate provides a quick and significant measure of someone's well-being and cardiorespiratory stability. Respiratory rates differ throughout the lifespan (Table 31.3). Low respiration rates (less than 12 respirations per minute at rest) are associated with opiate overdose, respiratory fatigue, central nervous system depression and hypothermia. Tachypnoea, however, is a key indicator of acute deterioration and associated with high mortality rate.

To take a respiratory rate, count the number of times the patient's chest rises and falls in 1 minute. One rise and fall equals one respiration. It is advisable to measure a patient's respiratory rate after the pulse rate has been recorded, to ensure the patient does not subconsciously change their breathing pattern (Smith & Rushton, 2015). It is vital that the Nursing Associate counts respirations for 1 full minute and that this figure is accurately recorded. In addition to the respiratory rate in respirations per minute, the Nursing Associate must also check the following:

- Inspiration/expiration ratio
- Shape of chest expansion
- Rhythm of breathing
- Use of accessory muscles
- Added sounds
- Signs of respiratory distress or dyspnoea
- Ability to speak in full sentences
- Signs of central cyanosis

In normal quiet breathing, exhalation should be approximately twice as long as inspiration: an inspiration/exhalation ratio of 1:2. Any changes in chest expansion are abnormal. For example, hypoventilation will result in a reduction in inhaled oxygen and asymmetrical breathing could indicate that a lung is not inflating, as occurs as a result of a pneumothorax or flail chest. Hyperventilation could lead to a rapid reduction in carbon dioxide and can cause feelings of dizziness, headache and fainting. The use of accessory muscles of breathing is regarded as a cardinal sign of respiratory distress (Cox, 2001), as are added sounds, such as a wheeze or stridor, which occurs in the presence of an obstructed airway.

TABLE 31.3 Respiration Rates by Age

Age	Respiratory rates in respirations per minute at rest
Less than 12 months	30–40
1–2 years	25–35
2–5 years	25–30
5–12 years	20–25
12 years and over	15–20

(Advanced Life Support Group, 2011.)

DISORDERS OF THE RESPIRATORY SYSTEM

The atmosphere we breathe is contaminated by many pollutants, from exhaust fumes and industrial gases to cigarette smoke. As a result, respiratory diseases account for 5 of the top 30 causes of death worldwide (Forum of International Respiratory Societies, 2017). The most common respiratory disorders include lung cancer, asthma, chronic obstructive pulmonary disease (COPD), pneumonia and tuberculosis (TB). In the United Kingdom, 12 million people have been diagnosed with a respiratory disorder and around 700,000 hospital admissions each year are the result of respiratory disease. Respiratory disease places a heavy burden on the National Health Service, costing an estimated £11 billion per annum, with asthma alone estimated to cost around £965 million a year (British Thoracic Society and British Lung Foundation, 2017).

Respiratory failure

Respiratory failure has been defined as the inability of the respiratory system to meet the metabolic needs of the body (Schwartzstein & Parker, 2006). A simpler way of expressing this is to state that, due to lung disease, the alveoli are unable to extract sufficient amounts of oxygen during breathing. As the respiratory system also expels excess carbon dioxide, respiratory failure can also lead to a build-up of this waste gas, which can cause an acid–base imbalance and severely disrupt homeostasis.

There are two types of respiratory failure. When respiratory disease leads to a reduction in oxygen levels within arterial blood, the patient is said to be in respiratory failure type 1. A reduced amount of oxygen in arterial blood is referred to as hypoxaemia. In severe cases, respiratory failure can also lead to an increase in arterial carbon dioxide, at which point the patient is said to be in respiratory failure type 2. An increased amount of carbon dioxide in arterial blood is called hypercapnia. Table 31.4 describes the main differences between respiratory failure type 1 and 2.

Respiratory failure type 1

All major respiratory disorders can lead to respiratory failure type 1 and it is important that the Nursing Associate is able to identify the main signs and symptoms, as highlighted in Table 31.4. The Nursing Associate may also encounter terminology such as hypoxaemia and hypoxia and it is important to determine the major differences between the two. As explained earlier, hypoxaemia is a low level of oxygen in arterial blood. Hypoxia is low amounts of oxygen in tissues. Naturally, hypoxaemia will lead to the development of hypoxia. However, hypoxia can occur even if there is a plentiful supply of oxygen in arterial blood. Effective transport of gases also relies upon a fully functioning cardiovascular system (see Chapter 29). Any cardiovascular disorder, therefore, could cause a lack of oxygen delivery, even if the lungs are working normally. Haemorrhage or heart failure, for example, could lead to hypoxia, as both could result in a poor distribution of blood to cells.

Respiratory failure type 2

Respiratory disease often leads to respiratory muscle fatigue. This, in turn, could lead to a weak respiratory effort and shallow breathing (hypoventilation). Hypoventilation will lead to a reduced expulsion of carbon dioxide. Because most carbon dioxide is transported as hydrogen ions and bicarbonate ions, excess carbon dioxide can disturb arterial acid–base balance. Whereas in respiratory failure type 1, entrained oxygen could be used to decrease hypoxaemia, the only way to reduce carbon dioxide levels is to enhance weak respiratory effort via ventilation. You may therefore witness patients with respiratory failure type 2 being placed on a mechanical ventilator to increase their depth of breathing. One common example of mechanical ventilation

TABLE 31.4   Summary of Respiratory Failure Type 1 and 2, Observations and Interventions

Type of respiratory failure	Physiological changes	Physical symptoms that should be noted	Treatments and nursing interventions
Type 1	SpO$_2$ <92% PaO$_2$ <8 kPa (Hypoxaemia)	Central cyanosis Tachypnoea Dyspnoea Use of accessory muscles of breathing	Oxygen to maintain SpO$_2$ above 92% Nurse in upright position Comfort and reassure
Type 2	SpO$_2$ <92% PaO$_2$ <8 kPa (Hypoxaemia) PaCO$_2$ >6 kPa (Hypercapnia) Decreased arterial blood pH (acidosis)	Central cyanosis Dyspnoea Use of accessory muscles of breathing Weak respiratory effort Hypoventilation	Oxygen to maintain SpO$_2$ above 92% Nurse in upright position Comfort and reassure Medical team may consider non-invasive ventilation

used in both hospital and community settings is non-invasive positive pressure ventilation (British Thoracic Society, 2016).

! HOTSPOT

Non-Invasive Ventilation

Non-invasive ventilation involves patients wearing a tight-fitting mask over their nose and/or mouth. The mask is attached to a ventilator via a flexible hose. As they breathe, each inhalation is increased and lengthened, allowing greater time for gaseous exchange.

Commencing non-invasive ventilation is a frightening and uncomfortable experience, especially in the early stages. Nursing Associates must appreciate their patient's fears and anxieties and care for the individual with sensitivity and patience. Patients requiring non-invasive ventilation will require a lot of comfort, reassurance, explanations and constant monitoring.

Because effective non-invasive ventilation requires the mask to be tight-fitting the Nursing Associate must be vigilant for the formation of pressure ulcers, especially on the bridge of the nose.

Respiratory infections
Influenza

Influenza is a common viral respiratory infection that is highly infectious. Influenza can be contracted throughout the year but is most active in the winter months in the UK. Although common, new strains of the influenza virus can lead to epidemics and pandemics due to low immunity in populations.

The influenza virus is expelled in aerosol particles and droplets in the infected individual's coughs and sneezes. Other people can inadvertently become contaminated by inhaling the virus or by touching infected areas, such as door handles and surfaces. The viruses that cause influenza are called orthomyxoviruses, of which there are three types: type A, type B and type C. Type A influenza viruses are most likely to cause a severe infection, whereas type B and C are less severe; type C viruses may only produce mild or even no symptoms. The outer lipoprotein layer of the type A influenza virus normally displays three proteins: haemagglutinin, neuraminidase and M2. There are 16 identified subtypes of haemagglutinin and 9 subtypes of neuraminidase, and type A influenza viruses are classified according to which subtypes are present. The most common variation of type A influenza has haemagglutinin subtype 1 and neuraminidase

BOX 31.1   Individuals Most at Risk of Contracting Influenza and Secondary Infections

- Children under 5 years old
- The older person
- Immunocompromised individuals
- Women in the later stages of pregnancy
- People with chronic health conditions, such as diabetes; respiratory, heart and renal disease; cancer
- Young adults (in flu pandemics)

subtype 1 on its outer lipoprotein layer and is commonly referred to as H1N1. Type A influenza viruses are found in both animals and humans and infections can potentially transfer between species. Recent examples include a variation of H1N1 called 'swine flu' and H5N5 or 'bird/avian flu' (Driver, 2012). In most cases, influenza is a debilitating but short-lived illness, which has no long-lasting effects. However, in certain circumstances, influenza can lead to the development of more severe lower respiratory tract infections, such as bronchitis and pneumonia. Death as a result of influenza is almost exclusively as a result of secondary lower respiratory tract infection.

Everyone is at risk of contracting flu. However, some individuals are more susceptible than others, and some are at greater risk of developing more severe secondary respiratory infections. Box 31.1 lists the individuals most at risk of contracting influenza and secondary infections.

Signs and symptoms. The signs of symptoms of influenza are:

- Fever (sudden onset)
- Headache
- Sore throat
- Muscle aches
- Dry cough
- Weakness and malaise
- Fatigue
- Loss of appetite

Care and treatment. Mild and uncomplicated cases of influenza can be treated with rest, drugs that can reduce fever (such as paracetamol and ibuprofen) and plenty of fluids. When caring for individuals with influenza, effective hand washing and appropriate use of tissues should be promoted. Antiviral drugs such as oseltamivir or zanamivir are available but they are only usually prescribed to vulnerable or 'at risk' individuals as per Box 31.1. The most effective management strategy for the minimization of the impact of influenza is vaccination and a major role of healthcare professionals is to encourage the uptake of influenza vaccines in the most vulnerable and 'at risk' groups in society.

Pulmonary tuberculosis

Pulmonary TB is a lower respiratory tract infection, which is most commonly caused by an airborne, slow-growing bacillus called *Mycobacterium tuberculosis*. Pulmonary TB normally occurs in two phases, referred to as primary and secondary infections. During the primary infection, lymphocytes and neutrophils congregate at the infection site within the lungs. The bacilli are enveloped and walled off by fibrous tissue and as a result the individual is no longer contagious. During the primary infection phase of TB, the infected person may display no symptoms and be unaware they have contracted TB. As the bacilli are very hardy, they can survive trapped in fibrous tissue for long periods. Sometimes individuals can remain unaware that they have TB for many years. The secondary infection occurs at some point after primary infection and is caused by the re-exposure to TB or another form of bacteria. On re-infection, the bacilli are reactivated and quickly multiply and spread within the lung. As a result, the infected individual rapidly becomes symptomatic and infectious. In recent times, some strains of TB have become resistant to the antibiotics commonly used to treat it. TB that is resistant to one or more first choice treatments is referred to as 'multi-drug resistant TB' or MDR-TB. It has become clear in recent years that a small number of TB strains have become resistant to almost all available pharmacological treatments, a condition referred to as 'extensively drug-resistant TB' or XDR-TB.

Signs and symptoms. The signs and symptoms of pulmonary TB are:

- Chronic cough
- Haemoptysis
- Weight loss
- Pyrexia
- Fatigue
- Night sweats.

Diagnosis. Pulmonary TB is diagnosed by chest x-ray and an investigation called an 'acid-fast staining test', which determines the presence of the bacteria that cause TB in a patient's sputum. Further culture tests will determine whether the species of TB infection is *M. tuberculosis*, *Mycobacterium bovis*, or *Mycobacterium africanum*. If the patient has a positive result for an acid-fast bacillus and culture, they will need to be nursed in isolation as they will be contagious, whereas patients with a negative acid-fast bacillus and a positive culture test may not be contagious and do not need to be placed in isolation (Gough & Kaufman, 2011).

Care and treatment. In the main, pulmonary TB is treatable and individuals can soon recover, be symptom free and return to work. However, the treatment process takes 6 months; therefore, one of the main care considerations is compliance with treatment. Nonadherence to the pharmacological treatment regimen is associated with the development of drug resistant strains of TB. The first-line treatment for pulmonary TB is a 6-month medication regimen that consists of 2 months of rifampicin, isoniazid, pyrazinamide and ethambutol, followed by a further 4 months of rifampicin and isoniazid. Infective patients will remain infective for the first 2 weeks of treatment and, if admitted to hospital, would be nursed in a negative pressure isolation room. The vast majority of individuals diagnosed with pulmonary TB are cared for in the community. Only when there are medical or socio-economic reasons are people with pulmonary TB admitted to hospital.

COMMUNITIES OF CARE

Under-Served and High-Risk Groups

The National Institute for Health and Care Excellence points out that there are under-served and high-risk groups of people that are more likely to contract tuberculosis.

High-risk groups could be any age and may come from any ethnic background; they include the following:

- Those living in close contact or caring for people infected with TB.
- People who have moved to the UK recently from countries with a high prevalence of TB.
- People with suppressed immune systems, for example, those who are living with human immunodeficiency virus.

There are individuals in our society who are considered to be at risk of contracting TB as they are 'under-served' by healthcare providers. Examples include:

- Homeless people and their children.
- People misusing substances and their children.
- Those who are detained in the prison system and their children.
- Vulnerable migrants and their children.
- Those children who are from gypsy or travelling communities.
- Looked-after children.

Adapted with permission from NICE (2016).

CASE STUDY 31.2   Bashiir

Bashiir Bakoo is a 28-year-old asylum seeker from Somalia, who is currently waiting for indefinite leave to remain in the UK. Bashiir would like to go to university to study medicine and would like to get a job as a doctor. He currently lives alone in a small bedsit in East London. He has not been able to secure employment at present but he volunteers at the local community centre during weekdays, helping fellow asylum seekers adjust to life in the UK. Four weeks ago, he contracted a cough, which became progressively worse. He has been waking up in the night soaking wet with sweat and has been feeling very tired during the day, to the extent that he has not been able to help at the community centre. Today he presented at his local accident and emergency after coughing up blood. Bashiir does not drink alcohol or smoke tobacco.

After a chest x-ray, Bashiir receives a provisional diagnosis of pulmonary tuberculosis. A sputum sample is requested and he is commenced on a 6-month course of rifampicin and isoniazid and a 2-month course of pyrazinamide and ethambutol.

CARE IN THE HOME SETTING

As most patients with tuberculosis (TB) are cared for in the community, the main focus of the primary care team looking after Bashiir would be:

- Supporting Bashiir with adherence to the 6-month course of tablets. Bashiir will hopefully feel much better after a short space of time; however, despite feeling well, it is essential he continues to take his medication to ensure the TB is eradicated and that he does not develop drug resistant TB.
- Advising Bashiir on reducing the risk of transmission by restricting visitors to his bedsit, especially young children, in the first 2 weeks of treatment.
- Remaining away from the community centre for the first 2 weeks of treatment and avoiding using public transport.
- Discuss cough etiquette with Bashiir, ensuring he always covers his mouth when coughing or sneezing and that he disposes of tissues safely.
- Discussing handwashing and maintaining good hand hygiene with Bashiir.
- Encouraging Bashiir to maintain good ventilation at home by opening his windows.

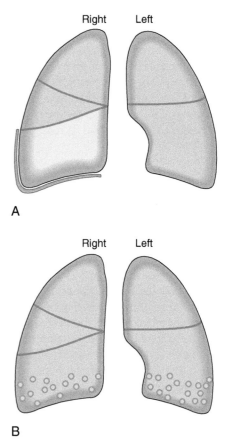

Fig. 31.12 Lobular and Diffuse Pneumonia (Waugh & Grant, 2018).

Pneumonia

Pneumonia is a lower respiratory tract infection caused by inhalation of bacterial, viral or fungal pathogens. Pneumonia can also be the result of aspiration of fluid, such as drink or vomit, or by the transfer via blood of pathogens from an infection elsewhere in the body. Some pneumonia infections are present in one or more of the lobes and are described as being lobular (Fig. 31.12A). Other pneumonias are spread throughout the lungs and are described as being diffuse (see Fig. 31.12B). Most pneumonia infections are caught in the community and, as a result, are called 'community-acquired pneumonia'. This is to differentiate them from pneumonia contracted whilst in hospital. Hospital-acquired (nosocomial) infections affect patients with low immune resistance, such as the older person or immunosuppressed individuals. Such cases are normally caused by bacterial infections, such as *Klebsiella pneumonia* or *Pseudomonas aeruginosa* (Gould, 2006).

Lobular pneumonia is normally caused by bacterial infections, such as *Streptococcus pneumoniae* (pneumococcus) and characteristically has a sudden and acute onset. Once the invading pathogens reach the lower respiratory tract beyond the trachea, they multiply quickly in the warm and moist surroundings of lung tissue. The ensuing inflammatory response causes vasodilation of capillaries, causing the alveoli to fill with debris and exudate. The exudate quickly fills with white blood cells, red blood cells and fibrin, and a solid mass called 'consolidation' is formed. This consolidation in the alveoli disturbs external respiration and less oxygen is able to diffuse into pulmonary circulation.

Pneumonia that is diffuse through both lungs is often referred to as bronchopneumonia (see Fig. 31.12B). It is characterized by a gradual onset with symptoms developing over time. There are many pathogens that can cause bronchopneumonia, but the infection normally starts in the bronchi before spreading to the alveoli. As with lobular pneumonia, inflammation causes a build-up of exudate within the alveoli, reducing gaseous exchange.

Other less common pneumonia infections include Legionnaire's disease, primary atypical pneumonia (PAP) and *Pneumocystis jiroveci* pneumonia (PJP) (formally known as *Pneumocystis carinii* pneumonia). Legionnaire's disease is caused by bacteria called *Legionella pneumophila*, which are found in natural water sources. Contraction of Legionnaire's disease usually occurs in people who have come into contact with infected in-built water sources (i.e., cooling systems). Legionnaire's disease can cause severe lung necrosis and has a high risk of mortality. PAP is commonly caused by bacterial infections such as *Chlamydia pneumoniae* and *Mycoplasma pneumoniae*, a minuscule bacterium found within the upper respiratory tract. PAP can also be the result of viral infection, as a result of influenza for example. PJP is considered to be a fungal infection. It is an opportunistic and often deadly infection, which preys on individuals with weakened immune systems (Gould, 2006).

All humans are susceptible to pneumonia but some individuals are more vulnerable to infection than others. Factors that healthcare professionals must be aware of include:

- Age: the very young and the older person are at greater risk
- Individuals living with chronic cardiorespiratory disease
- Individuals with weakened immune systems
- Individuals who smoke tobacco
- Alcoholics
- Individuals who abuse drugs and substances

- Intubation: unconscious patients have increased risk of developing pneumonia
- Patients at risk of aspiration (i.e., patients with dysphagia, individuals who have suffered a stroke and people living with gastric reflux).

Signs and symptoms. The signs of symptoms of pneumonia are:

- Low SpO_2 readings (hypoxaemia)
- Fast and/or laboured breathing (tachypnoea and dyspnoea)
- Elevated heart rate
- Pyrexia
- Dehydration: pyrexia causes fluid loss, also the body loses humidified air on breathing out
- Weak respiratory effort: consolidation makes it difficult to breathe in
- Pain: inflammation could spread to the pleura, causing pleuritic pain while breathing
- Productive cough: patients with pneumonia may cough up rusty-coloured sputum
- Lethargy and tiredness.

Diagnosis. A diagnosis of pneumonia is normally confirmed by sputum cultures, which identify the pathological agent (i.e., *S. pneumoniae*). An x-ray can also establish the extent of lung tissue damage and blood tests can also be used to indicate infection. For example, an increased white blood cell count of above 11×10^9/L can indicate inflammation, infection or an immune system response. Raised urea levels of greater than 7 mmol/L are another indicator of severe infection (Hoare & Lim, 2006).

Care and treatment. Pneumonia is treated with antibiotics. Most people with pneumonia are cared for in the community. When people are admitted to hospital with pneumonia, the main care goal for the nursing team is the early detection of acute deterioration. The care of an individual with pneumonia must include:

- The safe administration of prescribed antibiotics.
- The safe administration of prescribed oxygen, to correct hypoxaemia and maintain SpO_2 above 90%.
- Nursing the patient in an upright position to promote diaphragm and intercostal muscle activity and enhance ventilation.
- Assessing pain levels.
- Administering prescribed analgesia, to make the patient more comfortable and enhance respiratory effort.
- Managing body temperature, for example, safe administration of antipyretic agents, such as aspirin, paracetamol or ibuprofen, using electric fans and reducing bed clothing.
- Close monitoring of vital signs. Respiratory rate, blood pressure, temperature and pulse should be recorded hourly until the patient's condition stabilizes.
- Close attention to the patient's fluid balance because they may become dehydrated. A minimum of 2.5 L every 24 hours is required, intravenously if necessary (Dunn, 2005).
- Sensitive communication at all times, to reduce anxiety and promote comfort.

CRITICAL AWARENESS

Acute Deterioration in Patients with Pneumonia

Patients with pneumonia are at risk of mortality. This risk increases with age and Nursing Associates therefore need to be aware of the signs and symptoms that would indicate that an individual over the age of 65 is developing a life-threatening pneumonia. The following signs and symptoms in patients over the age of 65 are indicative of acute deterioration and should be reported to the medical team as soon as possible:

- Respiratory rate greater than 30 respirations per minute.
- New hypotension: systolic less than 90 mm Hg or a diastolic less than 60 mm Hg.
- New mental confusion or disorientation.
- Adapted from the National Institute for Health and Care Excellence (2014).

Obstructive lung disorders

Obstructive lung disorders are diseases which lead to a degree of airway obstruction. The hallmark of obstructive lung disorders, such as COPD and asthma, is obstructed airflow due to narrowed airways or increased airflow resistance. If the lumen of an airway is halved in size, the resistance to airflow increases 16 times. In narrow airways, gas molecules begin to collide with one another, generating a characteristic wheeze that is often heard in people with an exacerbation of a respiratory disease (Meredith & Massey, 2011). Increases in airway resistance are overcome by an increase in work of breathing. This increase in respiratory muscle activity requires greater energy expenditure. In obstructive lung disorders, normal passive expiration may not adequately empty the alveoli. Patients with an obstructive lung disorder may need forced expiration, which can increase pressures within the airway and force smaller airways to close, trapping air in the chest.

REFLECTION 31.1

People living with long-term obstructive lung disorders use more calories breathing than those with healthy lungs and airways. Replacing these calories can be difficult when someone is experiencing breathlessness. Imagine jogging for a short while and then sitting down to eat a meal immediately afterwards. This may be how it feels to eat when you are finding it difficult to breathe. Think about how healthcare professionals such as nurses, Nursing Associates and dieticians can increase the calorie intake of people living with long-term obstructive lung disorders.

Diagnosis

Airway obstruction and air trapping can be measured by spirometry and peak flow. Spirometry measures the force and volume of the individual's maximum expiration after a full inspiration. Spirometry involves the patient taking as deep a breath as they can and then blowing into a spirometry device via a flexible hose as fast as they can for as long as they can. The spirometry device provides doctors and nurses with two important measures of lung capability. Firstly, the spirometry device measures the individual's forced vital capacity (FVC), which is the volume of air the patient is able to exhale (see Fig. 31.8). People with obstructive lung disorders are unable to fully exhale their vital capacity, and the proportion of the vital capacity they can exhale provides doctors and nurses with an indication of the extent of airway obstruction. A further measure is the proportion of FVC that can be exhaled in the first second of the test. This volume of exhaled air is referred to as the 'forced expiratory volume in the first second' (FEV_1). By comparing FEV_1 with FVC (the FEV_1:FVC ratio), the severity of airway obstruction can be ascertained. Healthy individuals should be able to exhale 80% or more of their vital capacity in the first second of the test. An individual with an FEV_1:FVC ratio of less than 80%, therefore, has obstructed airways (Sheldon, 2005).

Peak expiratory flow rate (PEFR) provides another quick method of measuring airway obstruction and resistance. PEFR or 'peak flow' measures the force of expiration in litres per minute. Rather than volume of air expelled, 'peak flow' measures the speed or velocity of expelled air. The velocity at which an individual can force air out of the lungs and through their mouths can be predicted based on age, sex and height. A peak flow reading less than predicted can indicate airway obstruction.

NURSING SKILLS

Recording Peak Expiratory Flow Rate (PEFR)

To record an individual's peak expiratory flow rate (PEFR), you will need a peak flow meter and a disposable mouthpiece. Always wash your hands before taking someone's peak flow. Introduce yourself to the patient and explain what you need them to do and gain consent before proceeding. Before asking the patient to use the peak flow meter, always ensure that it is set to zero. Insert a clean disposable mouthpiece. Ask the individual to stand or sit upright. Ask them to take as deep a breath in as they can manage, then place the disposable mouthpiece into their mouth and form a tight seal with their lips. Ask them to then blow into the peak flow meter as hard and as fast as they can. Remove the meter from the patient's mouth and note the peak flow reading in litres per minute. This process needs to be repeated three times and the highest of the three readings should be recorded as the patient's peak flow. Ensure your patient is comfortable and answer any questions they may have. The disposable mouthpiece should be disposed of appropriately and you must wash your hands. Report your reading to the nurse or doctor responsible for the patient.

! HOTSPOT

Accuracy in Peak Flow Readings

Peak flow readings are effort dependent, and poor technique can produce inaccurate readings. Nursing Associates need to fully understand peak flow technique and monitor the patient's effort to ensure accuracy.

Furthermore, regular measurements are more revealing than single readings, so constant monitoring of a patient's peak flow is essential.

Asthma

Asthma is a chronic inflammatory disorder of the lungs that causes periodic inflammation in the bronchi and bronchioles. Airflow becomes obstructed as a result, often producing a characteristic wheeze. Asthmatics normally react to substances or situations that would not normally cause airway inflammation in an asthma-free person's airways. Such substances or situations

are referred to as 'triggers'. Asthma can be either extrinsic or intrinsic, depending upon the triggers. In extrinsic asthma, for example, airway inflammation is triggered by allergy (i.e., pollen, dust mites or foodstuffs). Intrinsic asthma, however, is triggered by other stimuli (e.g., infection, sudden exposure to cold, exercise, stress or cigarette smoke). Many asthma sufferers, however, have a combination of both types and it can be difficult to discern the trigger for an individual's asthma attack. Nevertheless, irrespective of the trigger, the physiological changes, symptoms and treatments are the same.

The pathophysiological changes that occur in the airway during an asthma attack are complex. The bronchi and bronchioles contain smooth muscle and are lined with mucous-secreting glands and ciliated cells. There are also large quantities of mast cells close by, which, once stimulated, release cytokines that cause physiological changes to the lining of the airways. Three such cytokines are histamine, kinins and prostaglandins, which cause smooth muscle contraction, increased mucus production and increased capillary permeability. As a result, the bronchioles and bronchi begin to narrow and become clogged with mucus and fluid leaking from capillaries (Fig. 31.13). In response the patient finds it increasingly difficult to breathe out and to expectorate mucus (Sims, 2006).

Signs and symptoms. The main symptoms of an exacerbation of asthma are:

- Cough, which may become productive with thick sticky mucus
- Dyspnoea and chest tightness
- Wheeze
- A peak flow that is less than predicted or best

Exacerbations of asthma are reversible if treated correctly. If unresolved, fatigue soon leads to a weak respiratory effort, causing hypoxaemia and, in severe cases, hypercapnia. In the UK, around 14% of people admitted to hospital with an exacerbation of asthma are reviewed by the critical care team and just less than 1% of asthma admissions die (British Thoracic Society, 2017). Therefore, it is essential that the Nursing Associate is fully aware of the signs and symptoms of acute and life-threating asthma. Table 31.5 details the distinctions between moderate acute asthma and life-threatening asthma.

Care and treatment. Asthma is reversible and care should focus on close monitoring and health promotion. The main treatment aims are:

- Close and continuous monitoring of respiratory rate, pulse, blood pressure, SpO_2 and peak flow until the patient is stabilized.
- Safe administration of prescribed oxygen to maintain SpO_2 above 92%.
- Safe administration of prescribed medications (Medicine Trolley 31.1 and 31.2)
- Assessment of speech: speaking requires a constant flow of air; patients experiencing acute breathlessness are able to talk only for very short periods before the need to breathe interrupts them. The patient's inability to complete a sentence, therefore, provides a sensitive measure of the extent of a patient's respiratory distress (Higginson & Jones, 2009).
- Comfort and reassurance: dyspnoea can be a traumatic experience and fear and anxiety also promote hyperventilation.

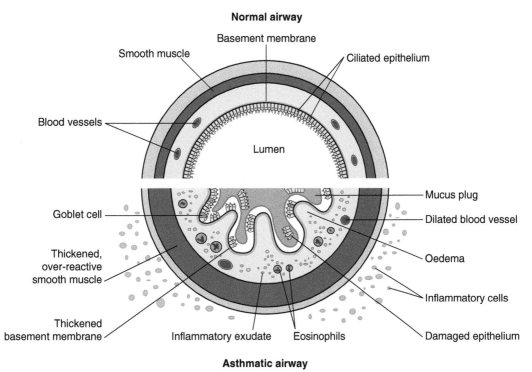

Normal airway

Smooth muscle
Basement membrane
Ciliated epithelium
Blood vessels
Lumen
Goblet cell
Mucus plug
Dilated blood vessel
Thickened, over-reactive smooth muscle
Oedema
Inflammatory cells
Thickened basement membrane
Inflammatory exudate
Eosinophils
Damaged epithelium

Asthmatic airway

Fig. 31.13 Cellular Structure of the Airways in Health and during Status Asthmaticus (Waugh & Grant, 2018).

TABLE 31.5 Distinctions between Moderate, Acute and Life-Threatening Asthma

Moderate acute asthma	Increasing symptoms PEF >50%–75% best or predicted
Acute severe asthma	Any one of: • PEF 33%–50% best of predicted • respiratory rate ≥25/min • heart rate ≥110/min • Inability to complete sentences in one breath
Life-threatening asthma	Any one of the following in a patient with severe asthma:

Clinical signs	Measurements
Altered conscious level	PEF <33% best or predicted
Exhaustion	SpO$_2$ <92%
Arrhythmia	PaO$_2$ <8 kPa
Hypotension	'normal' PaCO$_2$ (4.6–6.0 kPa)
Cyanosis	
Silent chest	
Poor respiratory effort	

Near-fatal asthma	Raised PaCO$_2$ and/or requiring mechanical ventilation with raised inflation pressures

(Reproduced from British Thoracic Society [BTS] and Scottish Intercollegiate Guidelines Network [SIGN], 2016. British Guideline on the Management of Asthma, by kind permission of the British Thoracic Society.)
kPa, kilopascals; PaCO$_2$, partial arterial pressure of carbon dioxide; PaO$_2$, partial arterial pressure of oxygen; SpO$_2$, oxygen saturation measured by a pulse oximeter

- The patient's anxieties should be listened to and continuous explanations provided for the multidisciplinary team's actions.
- Collection of sputum samples for analysis.
- Health promotion, discuss the following with the patient:
  - How to avoid triggers
  - Adherence with prescribed pharmacological therapies
  - Inhaler technique
  - Smoking cessation if applicable
  - Weight reduction in obese patients to reduce the frequency of asthma attacks.

CASE STUDY 31.3 Emma

Emma Granger is an 18-year-old woman who lives at home with her parents. Emma is currently studying for her 'A' levels and hopes to go to university to study architecture. She enjoys horse riding and playing tennis. Recently, Emma contracted a cold, which has left her with a dry cough that is worse during the night. She often feels short of breath when she is walking to school and has not been able to enjoy her tennis lessons as she has to keep stopping to catch her breath.

Emma visits her GP with her Mum. He asks her to do a peak expiratory flow rate test, which shows her peak flow is less than predicted for someone of her age and height. The GP explains that he thinks Emma may have asthma and that he would like her to monitor her peak flow at home, particularly in the morning, take a steroid inhaler twice daily, take a salbutamol inhaler when she feels short of breath and to make an appointment to see the respiratory nurse. Emma is asked to return for a review appointment in 4 weeks.

THE MEDICINE TROLLEY 31.1

Drug	Drug classification	Reason for administration	Route of administration	Dose	Side effects	Contra-indications	Nursing care
Salbutamol	Bronchodilator	To open the airway and reduce airway inflammation	Inhaler or nebulizer	Inhaler: 100–200 μg up to 4 times a day Nebulizer: 2.5–5 mg 4 times a day	Tremor Tachycardia Lowered potassium	Salbutamol is contraindicated in pregnancy if given intravenously Caution is also needed for patients with heart failure or pulmonary hypertension	Seek consent prior to administration Explain the use of the drug to the patient, respond to any questions Ensure patient follows correct inhaler technique Advise that drug may cause a tremor in their hands

OSCE 31.1

Administration of an Inhaler for a Newly Diagnosed Patient

Ben Baines has been recently diagnosed with asthma and has been prescribed a salbutamol inhaler. He is to take two puffs via a spacer when he is feeling short of breath.

You will be marked on the following areas; all areas must be passed in order to achieve an overall pass:

Action	Criteria	Achieved/not achieved
Making an introduction	Introduce yourself Wash hands Confirm the patient's details Explain how to use the inhaler Check the patient's understanding of the inhaler, and that they can explain when they need to use it Check for allergies Gain consent to proceed	
Gathering equipment	Equipment tray A salbutamol inhaler A spacer Nonsterile gloves	
7 Rights	1. Right person: check the patient's arm band against the name on the prescription. Where possible, aim to use two identifiers (e.g., from the patient and the arm band) 2. Right drug: check the labelled drug against the prescription, ensure expiry date is appropriate 3. Right dose: check the dose against the prescription 4. Right time: confirm when the last dose was given 5. Right route 6. Right to refuse: has the patient consented? 7. Right documentation of prescription and allergies: does the patient have any allergies?	
Inhaler technique	1. Wash hands 2. Don gloves and apron 3. Ask patient to sit upright with chin lifted 4. Remove cap from the mouthpiece and shake the inhaler 5. Test the inhaler by pressing the canister and checking for a spray 6. Attach the inhaler to the spacer correctly 7. Explain to the patient to place the mouthpiece of the spacer in their mouth and form a solid seal around it with their lips 8. Ask the patient to keep breathing normally and to press the canister in the inhaler down when ready 9. Ask the patient to press the inhaler and inhale as deeply as they can and hold for 10 seconds 10. Ask the patient to repeat step 9 11. Ensure the patient waits 30 seconds before their second puff 12. Detach the inhaler from the spacer and replace the cap	
Completing procedure	Thank the patient Discuss post inhaler care: • Warn them that a hand tremor and fast heart rate are normal side effects Wash hands Document that the medication has been given on the medication chart and in the patient's notes Have the patient observed for 15–30 minutes for adverse effects	
Pass Fail		

Chronic obstructive pulmonary disease

COPD is defined as airflow obstruction that is progressive, not fully reversible and does not change markedly over several months. It is an umbrella term used to describe traditional diagnosis of chronic bronchitis and emphysema. Chronic asthma sufferers are also at risk of developing COPD as their airways become remodelled over time. Furthermore, their symptoms are often indistinguishable from COPD and many COPD patients may also have asthma, making accurate diagnosis difficult. Whatever the underlying condition, the major cause of COPD is smoking (Devereux, 2006).

Signs and symptoms. The signs and symptoms of COPD are:

- A FEV_1/FVC ratio which is less than the predicted value
- Dyspnoea, due to airway obstruction and air trapping
- Productive cough
- Reduced exercise tolerance
- Respiratory failure
- Cor pulmonale: chronic hypoxia causes hypertension within pulmonary circulation, which leads to right ventricular failure and ultimately oedema.

Emphysema. Emphysema is the permanent enlargement of airspaces beyond the terminal bronchiole and the destruction of the alveolar wall. The cause of this destruction of lung tissue is thought to be related to the actions of destructive enzymes called proteases, which are present during respiratory infections. In healthy airways, lung tissue produces a substance called alpha-1 antitrypsin, which can counteract the destructive action of protease. Cigarette smoke reduces the effect of alpha-1 antitrypsin and the destructive actions of protease are allowed to continue (Hogg & Senior, 2002). The destructive actions of proteases include the breaking down of the elastic fibres within respiratory bronchioles and alveoli. Elastic fibres are essential for the elastic recoil required on passive exhalation. This loss of elasticity causes the alveoli to become overinflated as air becomes trapped within the lung. The resulting increased volume of air within the lungs forces the diaphragm downwards, making breathing difficult. Frequent infections can also develop as the individual finds it increasingly difficult to cough up retained secretions (Gould, 2006). There are two types of emphysema: centrilobar and panacinar. In panacinar emphysema, the alveoli are most affected, whereas in centrilobar emphysema the respiratory bronchioles are the most affected area. Fig. 31.14 compares healthy lobules with lobules of individuals with panacinar and centrilobar emphysema.

Chronic bronchitis. Chronic bronchitis is defined as the presence of a productive cough, lasting for 3 months in each of 2 consecutive years, when other pulmonary and cardiac causes of cough have been ruled out (Braman, 2006). Chronic bronchitis results in increased mucus production and damaged cilia in the bronchi; as a result, the bronchi become blocked by mucus that continuously irritates the airways, producing a chronic cough. The continuous irritation leads to inflammation and the thickened bronchial wall which causes airway obstruction. Because the cilia are ineffective, mucus clearance becomes difficult and mucus collects and clogs the smaller airways. Blocked and clogged

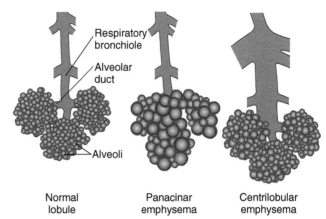

Fig. 31.14 Lobules Destroyed by Emphysema Compared with Healthy Lobules (Waugh & Grant, 2018).

smaller airways lead to secondary infections, which cause yet more irritation and inflammation. Over time, more and more airways become blocked, external respiration becomes impaired and less oxygen is transferred into the bloodstream. The major cause of increased mucus production and cilia dysfunction is an inflammatory response to cigarette smoke (MacNee, 2006).

Care and treatment of chronic obstructive pulmonary disease. Wherever possible, people living with COPD should be managed by the multidisciplinary team in their own home. However, they remain susceptible to acute exacerbation and factors that may necessitate an admission to hospital include:

- An inability to cope at home
- Poor social circumstances (i.e., damp or crowded living conditions)
- Cyanosis
- A rapid onset of symptoms
- Impaired level of consciousness
- Individuals requiring long-term oxygen therapy
- Individuals who are confused or disorientated
- SpO_2 less than 90%
- Respiratory failure type 2
- Chest x-ray changes
- Co-morbidities, such as diabetes and heart disease (National Institute for Health and Care Excellence, 2010).

COPD is a long-term condition. Its impact on the person will differ from individual to individual and symptoms can be diverse and varied. The Nursing Associate must appreciate that the care of people living with COPD requires a person-centred, holistic care plan that focusses on the promotion of coping, self-management and symptom control. The main care goals are:

- Advice on smoking cessation.
- Education on the appropriate use of prescribed oxygen and bronchodilator therapies, to maximize relief of breathlessness.
- Encouraging the uptake of immunisation (i.e., pneumonia and influenza).
- Advice on diet: severe weight loss is a feature of both emphysema and chronic bronchitis.
- Referral to pulmonary rehabilitation.
- Promotion of self-management techniques: COPD is associated with high levels of anxiety and depression.

THE MEDICINE TROLLEY 31.2

Drug	Drug classification	Reason for administration	Route of administration	Dose	Side effects	Contra-indications	Nursing care
Prednisolone	Steroid	To reduce airway inflammation in COPD	Oral	30 mg for 7–14 days	Bruising Candidiasis Cushing's syndrome Dyspepsia Hirsutism Hyperglycaemia Insomnia Impaired healing Increased appetite Irritability Sodium retention Water retention Weight gain	Congestive heart failure Diabetes Glaucoma Tuberculosis Hypertension Ulcers	Seek consent prior to administration Explain the use of the drug to the patient, respond to any questions Advise that drug may cause a variety of side effects Monitor blood glucose levels Advise not to stop medication suddenly

AT THE GP SURGERY

The Respiratory Nurse

The role of the respiratory nurse is vital for the promotion of health and the prevention of exacerbations. People living with long-term respiratory conditions can benefit from the advice and guidance that the respiratory nurse can provide. Such guidance will include:

- Advice on smoking cessation
- Education on the patient's respiratory disease
- Self-management and coping techniques
- The importance of correct use of mediations
- The importance of correct use of inhalers
- The importance of a healthy diet and exercise

Restrictive respiratory disorders

Restrictive respiratory disorders restrict the expansion of the lungs. The main reasons why an individual may experience difficulties expanding their chest are disorders that restrict the thorax, such as kyphosis or scoliosis, and diseases that reduce lung compliance. Conditions that reduce lung compliance include poliomyelitis and botulism, which cause respiratory muscle paralysis, and muscular dystrophy, which causes muscle weakness. Chronic inhalation of industrial and commercial pollutants can also cause a loss of lung compliance. Pneumoconiosis is a collection of respiratory disorders that lead to a loss of lung compliance and therefore restricted breathing. Pneumoconioses are often named after the job or pastime that generated them. Examples include coal worker's lung, bird fancier's lung, asbestosis or silicosis, which is caused by exposure to silica through stone cutting or sand blasting (Gould, 2006). The constant exposure of lung tissue to pollutants leads to repeated inflammation within the airways and, as a consequence, fibrous tissue develops. As the development of fibrous tissue spreads through the lungs, lung expansion becomes difficult and lung tissue loses much of its compliance.

Signs and symptoms of pneumoconiosis

- Progressive and worsening dyspnoea
- Increased respiratory effort at rest
- Chronic cough
- Recurrent chest infections

Care and treatment

Pneumoconioses are long-term conditions and, like other chronic respiratory diseases, their management requires a person-centred, holistic approach, centred upon self-management and symptom control. The main management goals are:

- Referral to pulmonary rehabilitation
- Antibiotic therapy for recurrent chest infections
- Oxygen
- Promotion of self-management techniques.

Lung cancer

Lung cancer has the highest mortality rate of all known cancers in the Western world (British Thoracic Society, 2006). The most significant causative agent is cigarette smoke. Ex-smokers' risk of developing lung cancer subsides over time and non-smokers are at risk of developing lung cancer as a result of passive smoking. Certain chemicals present within cigarette smoke are carcinogenic and they promote the development of tumours within the lung tissue. Most lung cancers are bronchial carcinomas of which there are two major types: non-small cell and small cell. Non-small cell carcinomas can be divided into squamous cell carcinomas, which tend to develop within the larger bronchi, and adenocarcinomas and large cell carcinomas, which are found in the smaller airways. As they develop in the smaller airways, their detection is much harder. Small cell carcinomas tend to grow near bronchi and are the most aggressive lung carcinomas.

Diagnosis

There are no specific signs of lung cancer, but a diagnosis is usually made in smokers who present with the following symptoms:

- Chronic cough
- Haemoptysis
- Dyspnoea
- Chest pain
- Wheeze
- Finger clubbing (National Institute for Health and Care Excellence, 2011).

LOOKING BACK, FEEDING FORWARD

The respiratory system ensures that the body receives enough oxygen whilst disposing of excess carbon dioxide. In doing so, respiration plays a vital role in the maintenance of homeostasis. The respiratory system has a complex anatomical structure and therefore there are a multitude of respiratory diseases. TB and pneumonia, for example, are infections which disrupt the actions of alveoli, whereas COPD and asthma obstruct the airways.

Whatever the cause of the respiratory disorder, individuals living with respiratory disease present with a multitude of debilitating symptoms, such as dyspnoea, tachypnoea, pleuritic pain, reduced PEFR, low SpO_2, cyanosis and an inability to speak in complete sentences being just a few examples. Therefore, care and attention need to be paid to the implementation of a person-centred and holistic care management plan, which can help people living with respiratory disease to live the best life they can.

REFERENCES

Advanced Life Support Group, 2011. Advanced Paediatric Life Support The Practical Approach, fifth ed. BMJ, Chichester.

Braman, S.S., 2006. Chronic cough due to bronchitis: ACCP evidence-based clinical practice. Chest 129, 104S–115S.

British Thoracic Society, 2006. The Burden of Lung Disease. BTS, London.

British Thoracic Society, 2016. BTS/ICS guideline for the ventilator management of acute hypercapnic respiratory failure in adults. Thorax 71, ii1–ii35.

British Thoracic Society, 2017. Adult asthma audit report national audit period 1st Sept – 31st October 2016. Available at https://www.brit-thoracic.org.uk/publication-library/bts-reports/.

British Thoracic Society and British Lung Foundation, 2017. Literature review: the economic costs of lung disease. Available at blf.org.uk/policy.

British Thoracic Society (BTS)/Scottish Intercollegiate Guidelines Network (SIGN), 2016. British Guideline on the Management of Asthma. QRG 153. SIGN, Edinburgh. http://www.sign.ac.uk.

Cox, C.L., 2001. Respiratory assessment. In: Esmond, G. (Ed.), Respiratory Nursing. Bailliere Tindall, Edinburgh.

Devereux, G., 2006. ABC of chronic obstructive disease definition, epidemiology and risk factors. Br. Med. J. 332, 1142–1144.

Driver, C., 2012. Pneumonia part 3: management and prevention of influenza virus. Br. J. Nurs. 21 (6), 362–366.

Dunn, L., 2005. Pneumonia: classification, diagnosis and nursing management. Nurs. Stand. 19, 50–54.

Forum of International Respiratory Societies, 2017. The Global Impact of Respiratory Disease, second ed. European Respiratory Society, Sheffield.

Gough, A., Kaufman, G., 2011. Pulmonary tuberculosis: clinical features and patient management. Nurs. Stand. 25 (47), 48–56.

Gould, B.E., 2006. Pathophysiology for the Health Professions, third ed. Elsevier, Philadelphia.

Higginson, R., Jones, B., 2009. Respiratory assessment in critically ill patients: airway and breathing. Br. J. Nurs. 18 (8), 456–461.

Hoare, Z., Lim, W.S., 2006. Pneumonia: update on diagnosis and management. Br. Med. J. 332, 1077–1079.

Hogg, J.C., Senior, R.M., 2002. Chronic obstructive pulmonary disease 2: pathology and biochemistry of emphysema. Thorax 57, 830–834.

Levitzky, M.G., Cairo, J.M., Hall, S.M., 1990. Introduction to Respiratory Care. WB Saunders, London.

MacNee, W., 2006. ABC of chronic obstructive pulmonary disease pathology, pathogenesis and pathophysiology. Br. Med. J. 332, 1202–1204.

Meredith, T., Massey, D., 2011. Respiratory assessment 2: more key skills to improve care. Br. J. Cardiac Nurs. 6 (2), 63–68.

NICE (National Institute for Health and Clinical Excellence), 2010. Clinical Guideline 101. Chronic obstructive pulmonary disease. Management of chronic obstructive pulmonary disease in primary and secondary care. Available at https://www.nice.org.uk/guidance/cg101/.

NICE (National Institute for Health and Clinical Excellene), 2011. Clinical Guideline 121. Lung cancer: Diagnosis and treatment of lung cancer. Available at https://www.nice.org.uk/guidance/cg121/.

NICE (National Institute for Health and Care Excellence, 2014. Pneumonia in adults: Diagnosis and management CG191. Available at https://www.nice.org.uk/guidance/cg191/.

NICE (National Institute for Health and Care Excellence, 2016. Tuberculosis – NICE Guidance NG33. Available at https://www.nice.org.uk/guidance/ng33.

Ochs, M., Nyengaard, A.J., Knudsen, L., et al., 2004. The number of alveoli in the human lung. Am. J. Respir. Crit. Care Med. 169, 120–124.

Schwartzstein, R.M., Parker, M.J., 2006. Respiratory Physiology: A Clinical Approach. Lippincott Williams & Wilkins, Philadelphia.

Sheldon, R.L., 2005. Pulmonary function testing. In: Wilkins, R.L., Sheldon, R.L., Krider, S.J. (Eds.), Clinical Assessment in Respiratory Care, fifth ed. Elsevier Mosby, St. Louis.

Sims, J.M., 2006. An overview of asthma. Dimens. Crit. Care Nurs. 25 (6), 264–268.

Smith, J., Rushton, M., 2015. How to perform a respiratory assessment. Nurs. Stand. 30 (7), 34–36.

Waugh, A., Grant, A., 2018. Ross & Wilson Anatomy and Physiology in Health and Illness, thirteenth ed. Elsevier, Edinburgh.

Wheeldon, A., 2016. The respiratory system. In: Peate, I., Nair, M. (Eds.), Fundamental Anatomy and Physiology for Student Nurses, second ed. Wiley-Blackwell, Chichester.

32

Gastrointestinal Disorders

Louise McErlean

OBJECTIVES

By the end of the chapter the reader will:

1. Have an understanding of the anatomy and physiology of the gastrointestinal system
2. Discuss the pathophysiological changes associated with a selection of gastrointestinal system disorders
3. Understand the relationship between the gastrointestinal system and other body systems
4. Outline the care required by people with gastrointestinal disorders
5. Describe some common conditions associated with the gastrointestinal system
6. Review the role of the Nursing Associate in promoting health and well-being

KEY WORDS

Chemical digestion	Melena	Accessory organs
Mechanical digestion	Haematemesis	Peristalsis
Emesis	Anorexia	
Diarrhoea	Enzymes	

CHAPTER AIMS

This aim of this chapter is to provide the reader with an understanding of the skills, knowledge and attitude required to provide safe, effective and compassionate care to people with a gastrointestinal disorder.

SELF TEST

1. What is the name of the enzyme involved in the digestion of carbohydrates?
2. What are proteins broken down into?
3. Name the inflammatory bowel diseases.
4. What does oesophagitis mean?
5. Describe peristalsis.
6. What is the difference between a stoma occurring in the small intestine and a stoma occurring in the large intestine?
7. Where does the majority of absorption of the products of digestion occur in the digestive system?
8. List the functions of the liver.
9. Describe the signs and symptoms of irritable bowel disease.
10. Discuss the nursing assessments associated with eating and drinking.

INTRODUCTION

In this chapter, the gastrointestinal system is considered. The first part discusses the anatomy and physiology of the gastrointestinal system. It is important for the Nursing Associate to have a comprehensive understanding of the gastrointestinal system if the care provided is to be appropriate and effective.

The second part of the chapter addresses a selection of common conditions associated with the gastrointestinal system. Nursing Associates will be guided with regard to the care required by those with gastrointestinal system conditions. It is important to remember that eating and drinking are not only physical body requirements for health but are a big part of the psychosocial activities of individuals. Many social activities are centred on eating out. Eating out is not limited to restaurant visits but includes going to the cinema, bowling and visits to stately homes, which invariably include some form of eating and/or drinking. Disorders of the gastrointestinal system will not only lead to physical signs and symptoms for those affected but can also affect their psychosocial well-being.

THE GASTROINTESTINAL SYSTEM

The gastrointestinal system is also known as the digestive system, or the alimentary canal. It is a long, continuous system,

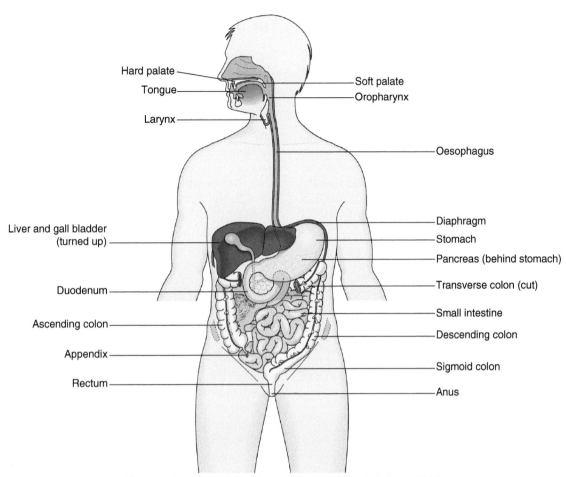

Fig. 32.1 Overview of the Digestive System (Waugh & Grant, 2018).

TABLE 32.1	Digestive System Processes	
	Process	**Description**
1	Ingestion	Taking food and drink into the body.
2	Propulsion	The movement of food through the length of the digestive tract.
3	Mechanical digestion	The physical breakdown of food in preparation for the chemical breakdown of food.
4	Chemical digestion	The action of enzymes breaks complex food molecules down into smaller molecules in preparation for absorption.
5	Absorption	The end products of digestion are transported into the blood or lymph. Most absorption occurs in the small intestine.
6	Defaecation	Any unused products or indigestible substances are eliminated from the body as faeces.

(Data from Marieb, 2015.)

beginning at the mouth and ending in the anus. The digestive system is supported by accessory organs (Fig. 32.1). Food and fluid passes through the digestive system and is processed by the actions and activities that occur. Once broken down, the products of digestion are used for cell metabolism, tissue repair and the creation of new molecules required by the body. Any remaining wastes are excreted via the digestive system.

There are six digestive processes, summarized in Table 32.1.

THE DIGESTIVE SYSTEM STRUCTURE

There are four layers, or tunicae, that form the structure of the digestive tract from the oesophagus to the anus. This allows each structure of the digestive tract to have similarity of function.

The mucosa

The inner layer that comes into contact with the products of digestion is called the mucosa. This layer is divided into three further sublayers: the lining epithelium, the lamina propria and the muscularis mucosa. The lining epithelium is composed of epithelial tissue. It is a mucous membrane, containing goblet cells that secrete mucus. The function of the mucus is twofold: it eases the passage of food and it protects the structures of the digestive system from the action of digestive enzymes. Within the stomach and small intestine, the mucosa also secretes enzymes and hormones required for digestion. The lamina propria is composed of loose areolar connective tissue. This layer has a good capillary network and is therefore involved in the absorption of the products of digestion. The lamina propria contains lymph nodules which help defend the digestive tract from invading pathogens. This lymph tissue forms part of the mucosa associated lymph tissue (MALT), to which the appendix and tonsils also belong. The final layer is the muscularis mucosae which is a thin layer of smooth muscle.

The submucosa

The submucosa layer is connective tissue layer with a blood, lymph and nerve supply.

The muscularis externa

The muscularis externa is smooth muscle layers under involuntary control and is responsible for the movements required for the mechanical digestion of food (peristalsis) and the activity of the large intestine (segmentation). As this is involuntary, it is impossible to control the rumblings and gurglings associated with the digestive system. To prevent backflow of the products of digestion within the digestive tract, the muscularis externa has sphincters located along its length.

The serosa

The serosa is the outermost layer of the digestive tract. Its role is to protect the structures below. Within the abdominal and pelvic cavities, this layer is known as the visceral peritoneum, which is a single layer of squamous epithelia. In the oesophagus, the serosa is fibrous connective tissue and helps anchor the oesophagus to its surrounding structures.

The peritoneum is the serous membrane that lines the abdominal cavity and covers the abdominal organs.

BLOOD SUPPLY

The digestive tract receives its blood supply from the splanchnic circulation. This includes the hepatic portal system and arteries that serve the abdominal organs branching form the descending aorta. The hepatic portal system delivers the nutrients absorbed via the digestive system for processing at the liver.

NERVE SUPPLY

The nerve supply to the digestive system is both sympathetic and parasympathetic. During resting and digesting, the parasympathetic nervous system is active. When the sympathetic nervous system is more active, there is a decrease in smooth muscle activity, such as peristalsis.

⚠ HOTSPOT

Bowel Sounds

The parasympathetic and sympathetic nervous system work together to balance the amount and timing of activity occurring within the digestive system. However, when listening with a stethoscope pressed against the abdominal wall, it is clear that the bowel is always gurgling. This noise is called 'bowel sounds'. Although abdominal auscultation is a useful assessment tool, there is a lack of guidance as to normal expectations (Jacob, 2017). However, an absence of bowel sounds is abnormal and often associated with conditions of the digestive system, including paralytic ileus, which is a commonly occurring postsurgery phenomenon. The treatment for paralytic ileus is to rest the gut for a day or two before introducing diet again.

THE ORAL CAVITY

Digestion begins in the mouth (also known as the oral cavity). The lips form the entrance to the mouth. The lips contain many sensory receptors of the nervous system, making them good gate keepers to the oral cavity. Very small hairs can be detected by the lips and prevented from entering the oral cavity. The cheeks form the sides of the oral cavity, the hard and soft palate form the roof and the tongue forms the floor of the oral cavity. The oral cavity (Fig. 32.2) is lined with stratified squamous epithelial tissue. The many layers of this tissue offer protection to the oral cavity from the wear and tear associated with eating and drinking.

The tongue is a voluntary muscle. It contains many sensory receptors, which are responsible for taste. The tongue's functions include taste, speech, swallowing (also known as deglutition) and chewing (also known as mastication).

Teeth begin to appear in children from around 6 months of age. There are 20 temporary (deciduous) teeth and by adulthood there should be 32 permanent teeth (Fig. 32.3). There are four different types of teeth: incisors and canine teeth used for biting and cutting, and molars and premolars used for chewing and grinding. The actions of the tongue and teeth on the food begins the mechanical digestion of food.

There are three pairs of salivary glands: the parotid glands, the submandibular glands and the sublingual glands (Fig. 32.4). They secrete approximately 1 litre of saliva per day. Saliva has many functions:

- Protection. Saliva contains immunoglobulin A antibodies, lysozyme and defensins, which protect the digestive tract from invading pathogens. Saliva is usually (but not always) slightly acidic, which is not a microorganism-friendly environment. The epithelial lining of the oral cavity is kept cleansed by the saliva; the saliva offers additional protection to the epithelial layer, which is often subject to abrasion by food.
- Lubrication of food and taste. Saliva mainly consists of water and has a role in lubrication of the food that enters the oral cavity. This eases the movement of food around the oral cavity,

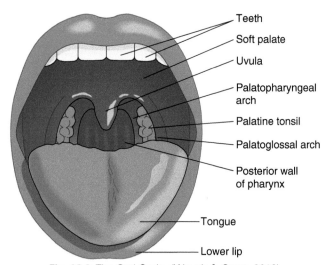

Fig. 32.2 The Oral Cavity (Waugh & Grant, 2018).

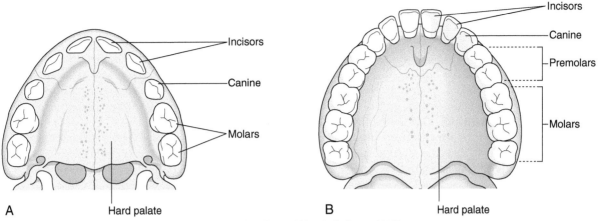

Fig. 32.3 The Teeth (Waugh & Grant, 2018).

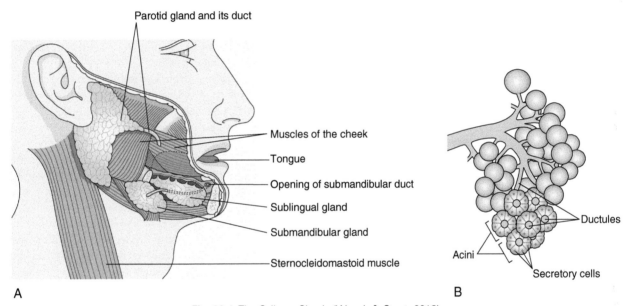

Fig. 32.4 The Salivary Glands (Waugh & Grant, 2018).

preparing the food for swallowing. Dry food needs to be lubricated by saliva for the taste buds to be able to sense specific tastes.

- Chemical digestion of carbohydrates. Saliva contains the enzyme salivary amylase. Salivary amylase begins the process of the chemical digestion of carbohydrates.

The oral cavity also contains the uvula, which is a small muscular tissue tag hanging from the soft palate. The uvula has a role in protecting the respiratory system during swallowing. The palatopharyngeal arches and the palatoglossal arches are folds of mucous membrane. The palatine tonsils are located bilaterally between these arches. The palatine tonsils are lymphoid tissue and part of the immune system. They are thought to have a role in protecting the body from respiratory infections.

THE OESOPHAGUS

The oesophagus is a muscular tube that carries food from the laryngopharynx to the stomach. When there is no food in the oesophagus, it collapses. Entry to the upper oesophagus is controlled by the upper oesophageal sphincter. This sphincter prevents air entering the oesophagus and digestive tract during breathing. Mucus is secreted from the oesophageal glands and this lubricates the passage of the food bolus through the oesophagus. The oesophagus has a mixture of skeletal muscle superiorly and smooth muscle inferiorly.

Swallowing (deglutition)

It is important that swallowing is controlled, as the trachea lies in front of the oesophagus and any food entering the trachea could have devastating consequences for the individual. Food is prepared into a bolus by the digestive processes that occur in the oral cavity. The food is moved toward the back of the mouth and the tongue contracts against the hard palate, pushing the food into the oropharynx. At the same time the pharynx contracts, occluding the nasopharynx, and the epiglottis moves down, preventing the food bolus from entering the larynx or trachea. This is called the oropharyngeal phase and it is under voluntary control. This phase usually lasts 1 second.

The oesophageal phase occurs next. The food bolus then enters the oesophagus and waves of contraction called peristalsis propel the bolus down the oesophagus toward the lower oesophageal or cardiac sphincter. This phase is not under voluntary control and usually lasts for 5–10 seconds. Peristalsis continues the process of mechanical digestion that began in the oral cavity. The cardiac sphincter has a role in preventing the acidic contents of the stomach from backflowing and damaging the lower oesophagus.

THE STOMACH

The stomach lies just below the diaphragm in the abdominal cavity. It is a hollow, muscular organ. The stomach is divided into three regions: the fundus, the body and the antrum (Fig. 32.5).

The food bolus enters the stomach via the cardiac sphincter from the oesophagus and leaves as chyme via the pyloric sphincter. Here it enters the duodenum, which is the first section of the small intestine. The action of contraction and relaxation of the muscles of the stomach churns the stomach contents and continues the process of mechanical digestion, as well as mixing the food bolus with the stomach secretions to continue the chemical digestion of the food. The smooth muscles of the stomach are involuntarily controlled by the nerves of the parasympathetic nervous system. Activation of the sympathetic nervous system opposes this. The stomach has an arterial blood supply originating from the coeliac artery, forming the right and left gastric arteries. Venous drainage leads to the hepatic portal vein.

The stomach contains many gastric glands. The secretions from these glands form gastric juice. Approximately 2–3 L of gastric juice are secreted per day. Gastric juice is composed of water and mineral salts.

Hydrochloric acid is secreted by the parietal cells located in the gastric glands. The secretion of hydrochloric acid makes the stomach an acid environment, with a pH of 1.5–3.5. The acidic nature of the stomach ensures that pathogens that enter the digestive tract are likely to be destroyed. Proteins are denatured by the acid environment, making them easier to break down. The acidic environment assists in the actions of pepsin, which is a protein-digesting enzyme. The action of salivary amylase is halted by hydrochloric acid.

Parietal cells also secrete intrinsic factor, which is necessary for the absorption of vitamin B_{12}. Absorption of vitamin B_{12} occurs in the small intestine.

Inactive enzyme precursors are produced by the chief cells. Pepsinogen is the inactive form of pepsin. In the presence of hydrochloric acid, the pepsinogen is converted to pepsin and begins the breakdown of proteins. Enteroendocrine cells secrete many hormones involved in digestion, including gastrin and cholecystokinin. The mucous neck cells produce a thin mucus, which is different from the mucus produced by goblet cells.

The harsh acidic environment of the stomach means that it requires some protection from autodigestion by the action of pepsins and hydrochloric acid. The simple columnar epithelium lining the stomach contains goblet cells, which secrete a thick layer of mucus. This is a double layer of mucus; the layer closet to the stomach is alkaline, which would help neutralize any acid that should breach this barrier. This helps to protect the stomach.

The functions of the stomach can be summarized as follows:
- The stomach acts as a store for food. When empty it has a volume of 50 mL but can hold 1.5 L (adult stomach).
- The acidic environment in the stomach kills many of the pathogens ingested with food.
- Mechanical digestion of food continues as waves of muscular activity mix the food with digestive enzymes in gastric juice. This liquefies the food bolus and breaks it down into chyme.
- Chemical digestion of proteins begins with denaturing by hydrochloric acid and the activity of the enzyme pepsin.
- The action of salivary amylase is halted.
- Some absorption occurs in the stomach, specifically some drugs, water and fat-soluble substances.
- Secretion of intrinsic factor, which is required for the absorption of vitamin B_{12} in the duodenum.
- Secretion of hormones involved in digestion.

The stomach produces approximately 2–3 L of gastric juice per day. It is secreted in three phases:
1. The cephalic phase. The thought, smell, sight or taste of food triggers the secretion of gastric juice and this occurs before food enters the stomach. The sensory input from the special senses, the taste buds and the olfactory receptors are relayed to the central nervous system. The motor response is via the

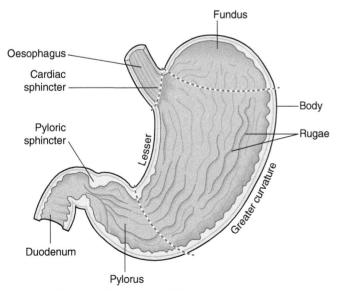

Fig. 32.5 The Stomach (Waugh & Grant, 2018).

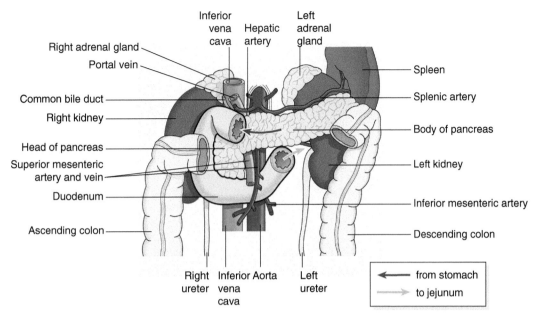

Fig. 32.6 The Duodenum in Relation to Associated Digestive System Organs (Waugh & Grant, 2018).

parasympathetic vagus nerve, which stimulates the stomach glands to secret gastric juice. This phase lasts for a few minutes.

2. The gastric phase. This phase can last for 3–4 hours and occurs when food reaches the stomach. This stimulates the enteroendocrine cells to secrete the hormone gastrin, which is secreted directly into the blood. The action of gastrin is to stimulate the gastric glands to produce more gastric juice. A reduction in the pH stops the secretion of gastrin.

3. The intestinal phase. When chyme is delivered to the small intestine, two hormones are secreted: cholecystokinin and secretin. The action of these hormones is to slow down the secretion of gastric juice. They also have a role in slowing down the rate of gastric emptying, therefore controlling the amount of chyme entering the small intestine. Given the acidic nature of the chyme entering the small intestine, controlling the amounts of emptying allows the small intestine to safely deal with the acidic chyme.

Food can be in the stomach for 2 to 4 hours, depending on the nature of the meal.

THE SMALL INTESTINE

The small intestine extends from the pyloric sphincter in the stomach to the ileocecal valve, where the small intestine meets the large intestine. The small intestine is divided into three segments: the duodenum (Fig. 32.6), the jejunum and the ileum (Fig. 32.7).

Digestion in the small intestine

Chyme leaves the stomach and enters the duodenum. The pancreas produces pancreatic juice, which is delivered to the duodenum via the pancreatic duct. The liver produces bile, which is stored and concentrated in the gall bladder. Bile is delivered to the duodenum via the bile duct. Bile and pancreatic juice enter the duodenum via the hepatopancreatic ampulla. The

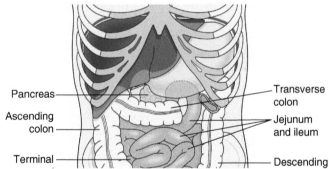

Fig. 32.7 The Jejunum and Ileum and Their Position in the Abdominal Cavity (Waugh & Grant, 2018).

control of entry of bile and pancreatic juice is controlled by the muscular sphincter of Oddi.

Fig. 32.8 demonstrates the position in the abdominal cavity of the pancreas and gall bladder.

The walls of the small intestine contain glands which secrete intestinal juice, 1–2 L of which is secreted daily. Intestinal juice is mainly water and mucus, with some electrolytes. It is alkaline, with a pH ranging from 7.4 to 8. The hormone secretin and the presence of chyme in the duodenum stimulate the secretion of intestinal juice.

The pancreas produces 1.5 L of pancreatic juice per day. Pancreatic juice contains water, enzymes and electrolytes and it is alkaline, with a pH of 8 due to the presence of bicarbonate ions. Pancreatic juice contains the enzymes amylase and lipase and

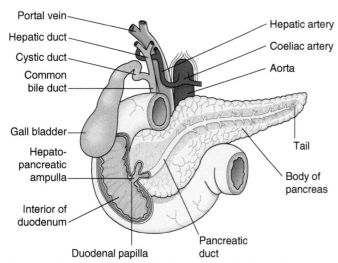

Fig. 32.8 The Pancreas and Gall Bladder and Their Position in the Abdominal Cavity (Waugh & Grant, 2018).

the inactive enzyme precursors trypsinogen, chymotrypsinogen and procarboxypeptidase. The secretion of pancreatic juice is stimulated by the presence of chyme in the duodenum and the hormones secretin and cholecystokinin, which is produced by the enteroendocrine cells within the duodenum.

Bile is produced by the liver. It is composed of bile salts, bile pigments (mainly bilirubin), cholesterol, electrolytes and water. It is yellow-green in colour. The pH of bile is also alkaline, pH 8. The liver produces 0.5–1 L of bile per day. It is carried from the liver via the hepatic duct, then enters the gall bladder via the cystic duct.

The bilirubin in bile salts is a product of erythrocyte recycling. When it eventually enters the large intestine it is acted upon by microbes and converted to urobilinogen. Urobilinogen that is not reabsorbed or excreted in the urine is converted to stercobilin, which is responsible for giving faeces its distinctive colour.

In the gall bladder, bile is stored and concentrated. The function of bile is to emulsify fats. It is also responsible for making cholesterol and fatty acids soluble. This allows them to be absorbed. Secretion of bile is stimulated by the hormones secretin and cholecystokinin, as well as the presence of chyme with a high fat content entering the duodenum.

The mixing of the acidic chyme with the alkaline pancreatic and intestinal juices and bile neutralizes the chyme and increases the pH to 6–8, thus protecting the duodenum from the digestive action of the acid.

> **! HOTSPOT**
>
> The duodenum is a common site for the formation of ulcers. The most common cause for this is a bacterium called *Helicobacter pylori* or *H. pylori*. The bacteria destroy the protective mucous layer of the duodenum and allows the action of the acidic chyme to cause an ulcer. *H. pylori*, when identified, can be easily treated by a course of antibiotics.

Mechanical digestion in the small intestine

The smooth muscle layer within the small intestines mixes the chyme with bile, intestinal juice and pancreatic juice. It also moves the products of digestion along the length of the small intestine by peristalsis. This allows for the greatest opportunity for absorption to occur.

Chemical digestion in the small intestine

Carbohydrates. The chemical digestion of carbohydrates continues in the small intestine by the action of pancreatic amylase. Disaccharides are eventually converted to glucose.

Proteins. The microvilli of the small intestine produce an enzyme called enterokinase. This enzyme converts the inactive enzyme precursors trypsinogen to trypsin, chymotrypsinogen to chymotrypsin and procarboxypeptidase to carboxypeptidase. These act on proteins, breaking them down into amino acids. The pancreas produces the inactive enzyme precursors because if it were to produce the enzymes themselves, they would digest the pancreas.

Fats. Once fats have been emulsified by the action of bile, they are acted upon by lipase. Fats are converted to fatty acids and glycerol.

Absorption in the small intestine

The inner mucosa layer of the small intestine contains many folds, known as villi. This greatly increases the surface area of the small intestine. This is a useful feature within the small intestine as it increases the surface area for the absorption of the products of digestion. The largest amount of absorption occurs in the small intestine. Blood supply is required for the transport of the products of digestion. The small intestine receives its arterial blood supply from the superior mesenteric arteries. Blood leaves the small intestine via the mesenteric veins and goes on to the hepatic portal vein. Then, the nutrient-rich blood reaches the liver, where some processing occurs. The small intestine is served with a capillary network, known as lacteals. Towards the end of the small intestine, where there are larger numbers of bacteria, there are more areas of lymph tissue, known as Peyer's patches. Peyer's patches help prevent the bacteria from entering the bloodstream. As well as the absorption of monosaccharides, amino acids, fatty acids and glycerides, water, some mineral salts and vitamins are also absorbed via the length of the small intestine.

THE LARGE INTESTINE

The food residue leaves the ileum of the small intestine via the ileocaecal valve and enters the caecum of the large intestine. The large intestine is wider in diameter and shorter than the small intestine (Fig. 32.9). The caecum extends superiorly to the ascending colon. It also has a small opening into the vermiform appendix. This structure contains lymphoid tissue and is not thought to have a digestive system physiological function.

The ascending colon curves at the hepatic flexure to form the transverse colon. The transverse colon curves at the splenic flexure to form the descending colon. The descending colon curves toward the centre of the body at the sigmoid colon and the remaining waste products of digestion exit the body as faeces via the rectum and down the anal canal.

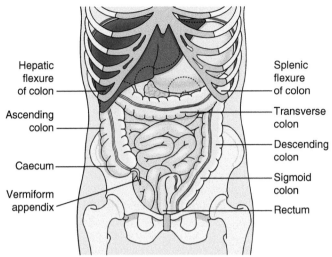

Fig. 32.9 The Large Intestine (Waugh & Grant, 2018).

The longitudinal muscle layer in the large intestine is not continuous with the colon but instead forms bands called taeniae coli. This arrangement gives the large intestine its distinctive puckered appearance. Smooth muscle also forms the internal anal sphincter, whereas the external anal sphincter is made of skeletal muscle. The external anal sphincter is under voluntary control. These sphincters control the exit of faeces from the body.

Absorption in the large intestine

The large intestine is colonized by many bacteria. When located in the colon, these bacteria form the commensals expected in the large intestine but if transferred to another area of the body, they can become pathogenic. The submucosal layer of the large intestine contains lymphoid tissue, more than is located elsewhere in the digestive system. The lymphoid tissue has a role in protecting the large intestine from invading pathogens.

The role of bacteria in the large intestine is to synthesize folic acid and vitamin K.

Water absorption has already occurred within the small intestine, but the food residue that enters the large intestine still contains fluid. As the food residue passes along the length of the large intestine, more water is absorbed by osmosis until eventually faeces are formed (the faeces are semi-solid). As well as water, some drugs, electrolyte and minerals are absorbed in the large intestine.

A unique type of peristalsis occurs within the large intestine. Stimulated by food entering the stomach, a wave of contraction spreads along the large intestine, moving the contents along toward its end. These waves of contraction are called 'mass movements'. Mucus secreted from the mucous layer lubricates the faeces as it moves through the large intestine.

Defaecation

Defaecation is an involuntary action from birth until 2–3 years old. The individual can learn to inhibit the reflex to defaecate. The external anal sphincter is under voluntary control and so can remain closed until a convenience is found or until the next mass movement occurs. Faeces consists of water, indigestible food parts such as fibre, bacteria, mucus, dead cells and fatty acids.

> **! HOTSPOT**
> *Infection Prevention*
>
> An important role undertaken by Nursing Associates is to assist patients with personal cleansing and dressing. When patients have been incontinent of faeces, it is important to ensure that the faeces do not contaminate the urethra, as large intestine commensals, such as *Escherichia coli*, can become pathogenic and could lead to urinary tract infection.

THE LIVER, GALL BLADDER AND PANCREAS

The liver is the largest organ in the body. It receives its blood supply from the hepatic artery. Additionally, blood from the hepatic portal vein is also delivered to the liver. Venous return is via hepatic veins that drain into the vena cava. The liver has many functions which include:
- Metabolism of nutrients
  - Protein metabolism
  - Carbohydrate metabolism
  - Fat metabolism
- Breakdown of erythrocytes
- Production and secretion of bile
- Detoxification of drugs
- Heat production
- Storage
  - Fat soluble vitamins (A, D, E and K)
  - Vitamin B_{12}
  - Glycogen
  - Iron and copper.

The gall bladder

The gall bladder lies on the surface of the liver. Bile is stored in the gall bladder. The mucosa of the gall bladder absorbs water and electrolytes, concentrating the bile.

The pancreas

The pancreas has both endocrine and exocrine functions. The endocrine pancreas secretes insulin, glucagon and somatostatin. Chapter 35 of this text discusses the endocrine system further. The exocrine function of the pancreas is to produce pancreatic juice. Small clusters of secretory cells, called acini, are responsible for the production of pancreatic juice.

An understanding of the anatomy and physiology of the digestive system is essential to care for patients who have conditions associated with the digestive system.

The remainder of this chapter will focus on commonly occurring digestive system conditions.

Disorders of the digestive system often have many signs and symptoms in common that warrant some explanation. As a Nursing Associate you will be assessing your client group for these signs and symptoms, which may be due to a digestive system disorder or a symptom of another condition or medication.

NAUSEA AND VOMITING

Nausea is the unpleasant sensation associated with the feeling of needing to vomit. Nausea can be associated with many conditions, including gastric infections, motion sickness, migraines, ear infections and pregnancy (morning sickness). It is also a side effect of many medications that patients are prescribed.

Nausea is often, but not always, followed by vomiting. Vomiting often, but not always, occurs after the sensation of nausea. Vomiting is the forceful emptying of the stomach and sometimes intestinal contents via the oral cavity. Vomiting is a reflex initiated from the vomiting centre, which is located in the medulla oblongata in the central nervous system. The sympathetic nervous system is stimulated and the heart rate increases (tachycardia), breathing increases (tachypnoea) and sweating occurs (diaphoresis). The parasympathetic nervous system stimulates the salivary glands to produce copious amounts of secretions prior to vomiting. It also increases gastric motility and relaxes the upper and lower oesophageal sphincters. The act of vomiting is usually preceded by a deep inspiration. The glottis closes to protect the respiratory system and intrathoracic pressure drops as the diaphragm contracts. The abdominal muscles also contract. This change in pressure and wave of contraction squeezes the stomach. The stomach contents are pushed up the oesophagus and out of the mouth.

Retching is the same as vomiting but without the vomit, which may be because the stomach is empty or as a precursor to vomiting. Projectile vomiting is not usually associated with nausea. It is vomiting that occurs very suddenly and with great force. Projectile vomiting can occur as a result of bowel obstruction, paralytic ileus or disorders of the nervous system, for example, a brain tumour or raised intracranial pressure.

Care and treatment

The Nursing Associate should stay with the patient who is vomiting and offer them a sick bowl. Consider the position of the patient and reposition if there is a risk to the patient's airway through aspiration of vomitus. Ensure that suction is available; a Yankauer sucker can be used to assist with removing vomitus from the patient's mouth. Vomit is documented as a loss on the patient's fluid balance chart. Not only is the patient losing fluid, they are unlikely to want to drink to replace this fluid, which can lead to dehydration in the long term. Vomitus contains electrolytes, such as sodium and potassium. Checking the patient's blood results for the level of electrolytes will allow the Nursing Associate to assess the effect of the vomiting. Lost fluid and electrolytes can be replaced either orally or intravenously. Other signs of dehydration should be observed for and these include:
- Hypotension
- Tachycardia
- Decreased urine output (less than 0.5 mL/kg per min)
- Increased capillary refill time (more than 2 seconds)
- Cool peripherals.

Treatment for nausea and vomiting is to treat the cause. However, anti-emetic medication can be given to reduce the symptoms.

> **REFLECTION 32.1**
>
> Think about a patient who has had symptoms of nausea and vomiting for 2 days. What essential assessments should the Nursing Associate consider implementing?
>
> Should the patient be allowed to eat or drink?
>
> If the nurse administers the anti-emetic medication and the patient is still experiencing nausea and vomiting 30 minutes later, what action do you take?

THE MEDICINE TROLLEY 32.1

Drug	Drug classification/ action	Reason for administration	Route of administration	Dose	Side effects	Contraindications	Nursing care
Cyclizine	Histamine H₁-receptor agonist	To treat nausea and vomiting	Oral/IV/IM IV should be given slowly as the patient may experience tachycardia	50 mg 8 hourly	Dry throat and mouth Drowsiness	Avoid in hepatic encephalopathy and prostatic hypertrophy	Explain the use of the drug to the patient, respond to any questions. A qualified nurse may have to administer IV medication if vomiting prevents oral administration.
Ondansetron	Serotonin 5-HT₃-receptor antagonist	To treat nausea and vomiting	Oral or IV	4–8 mg 8 hourly	Constipation Diarrhoea Headache	Prolonged Q-T interval ECG	
Metoclopramide	Dopamine D₂-receptor antagonist	To treat nausea and vomiting	IM/IV	10 mg 3 times daily	Diarrhoea	Should not be used in patients with gastrointestinal obstruction or young adults due to movement abnormalities Avoid in children	Monitor to ensure nausea and vomiting reduces. If it does not, request that an alternate anti-emetic be prescribed.

ECG, Electrocardiograph; IM, intramuscular; IV, intravenous.

CASE STUDY 32.1 Robert

Robert Mphoko is 67 years old and has described symptoms of vomiting lasting for 2 days. He has a history of type 2 diabetes mellitus, which is controlled by diet and medication. His wife is concerned because he appears to be confused. They were both unwell after having a meal out and Mrs Mphoko has recovered.

At the GP Surgery

Mr Mphoko has his observations recorded by the practice nurse:

Respiratory rate 18 breaths per minute, oxygen saturation 97% on room air.

Temperature 38°C, heart rate 110 beats per minute, blood pressure 100/65 mm Hg.

No urine output for 4 hours.

Neurologically alert but disorientated, blood sugar 12 mmol/L.

Skin turgor poor, oral cavity dry, lips are cracked.

Mr Mphoko is no longer vomiting but is retching.

The practice nurse and GP advise that Mr Mphoko attends the emergency room as they are concerned that he is dehydrated.

Care in the acute setting

The doctor suspects a gastric infection and commences Mr Mphoko on intravenous fluid, ondansetron and intravenous antibiotics.

The Nursing Associate is asked to plan the care that Mr Mphoko will require.

National Early Warning Score (NEWS) observations and a fluid balance chart are commenced. Initially observations are hourly and Mr Mphoko is nil by mouth. Oral hygiene is commenced. Initially Mr Mphoko refuses oral hygiene because he feels that it is making him feel sick. Four hours after commencement of intravenous fluids, anti-emetics and antibiotics, Mr Mphoko's observations show:

Respiratory rate 14 breaths per minute; oxygen saturation 97%.

Temperature 37°C, heart rate 98 beats per minute, blood pressure 105/67 mm Hg. He has passed urine.

Mr Mphoko is alert and less confused. His blood sugar is 9 mmol/L. His nausea is settling and he is able to tolerate oral hygiene.

The doctor reviews Mr Mphoko and advises the Nursing Associate to introduce fluid, which Mr Mphoko tolerates. Mr Mphoko spends 2 days on the ward and is discharged home.

Knowledge and skills – oral assessment and care
Purpose

To maintain the health of the oral cavity and lips

To prevent oral infections

Always ask the patient for consent before carrying out oral assessment and care

Assessment

Inspect the lips and oral cavity, identify any issues such as halitosis, tooth or gum problems, presence of dentures, gingivitis, dry mucous membranes, cracked lips, oral ulcers, cracked tongue

Gather Equipment and Implement

Gloves, apron, kidney dish, towel, wipes, denture bowl, cup of warm water, toothbrush, toothpaste, foam swabs, suction catheter if needed

Procedure
- Explain what you are going to do.
- Wash hands, wear gloves and apron.
- Consider patient privacy (close doors or curtain).
- Position patient in a comfortable position, upright if able.
- Consider the patient's ability, he may be able to carry out his own oral hygiene.
- If dentures are present, remove and wash them.
- Place the towel under the chin and place the curved kidney dish under the patients chin.
- If the patient has teeth, then gently clean the teeth using the toothbrush and tooth paste or assist the patient to do so.
- Rinse the mouth by asking the patient to sip some of the warm water and rinse, spitting into the kidney dish, or assist by syringing about 10 mL of water into the mouth and gently suctioning it out. This step should be repeated until the mouth is rinsed.
- Use the foam swabs soaked in warm water to clean the tongue, lips and mucous membranes. Be aware that this could make the nauseous patient feel worse.
- If the patient has dentures, these should be returned to the patient.

Evaluation
- Inspect the oral cavity and document your findings

CONSTIPATION

Constipation is when stools are being passed less frequently than normal for that individual (Grossman & Porth, 2014). There is usually an associated dry stool, which may be very large or very small. Constipation can affect all age groups but it is common in the elderly and it affects more women than men. Chronic constipation is constipation that has lasted for more than 3 months. In developed countries, 10%–15% of adults are thought to have experienced constipation (COMPASS, 2016).

Constipation can be associated with lifestyle:

- Sedentary lifestyle
- Poor diet: refined foods
- Poor hydration habit

Or associated with the colon itself:
- Slow transit time
- Evacuation disorders

Or secondary to another condition or medication. For example:
- Spinal cord injury
- Multiple sclerosis
- As a side effect of medications, for example, codeine.

THE MEDICINE TROLLEY 32.2

Drug	Drug classification/ action	Reason for administration	Route of administration	Dose	Side effects	Contra-indications	Nursing care
Lactulose	Osmotic laxative Holds water in the stool and stimulates peristalsis	Constipation Hepatic encephalopathy	Oral	Depends on response but 15 mL twice daily	Flatulence Abdominal cramps Diarrhoea	Intestinal obstruction	Explain the use of the drug to the patient, respond to any questions.
Senna	Stimulant laxative Increases water and electrolyte secretion into the bowel and stimulates peristalsis	Constipation	Oral	1–2 tablets twice daily	Abdominal cramps Diarrhoea	Intestinal obstruction	

Signs and symptoms

The signs and symptoms of constipation are linked to the function of the large intestine. The function of the large intestine is to absorb water. During dehydration, there is an increase in the amount of water reabsorption through the colon. This leads to the faecal material becoming more solid and less fluid. The transit of the faecal material is less easy when it is solid and the eventual evacuation can lead to tearing of the anal canal (anal fissure). Anal fissure can lead to defaecation becoming painful, which further exacerbates constipation as the patient associates defaecation with pain.

Regular exercise not only improves the functioning of skeletal muscles but improves the action of smooth muscles in the gut wall. This can slow down the transit of the faecal material through the large intestine, which in turn means that more water can be absorbed, leading to the issues discussed earlier. Lack of fibre in the diet also slows down transit times in the large intestine. The patient with constipation may complain of the following signs and symptoms:

- Infrequent bowel movements (two or less per week)
- Straining
- A feeling of incomplete emptying of the bowel
- Lumpy or hard stools
- Change in bowel habit
- A feeling of fullness
- Discomfort
- Rectal bleeding
- Anal fissures.

The Nursing Associate should assess the patient's bowel habit to include:

- Normal bowel habit
- Hydration status
- Lifestyle
- Pain
- Bloating
- The use of a Bristol stool chart
- Presence of blood in or on the stool.

Treatment of constipation is to treat the underlying cause. To prevent further dehydration, recommend bowel retraining, increase fibre intake and advise moderate exercise. In the short term, laxatives may be useful.

REFLECTION 32.2

Geeta Sharma is 68 years old and has a history of back pain following a car accident. Her doctor has recommended she take co-codamol for back pain that she has currently. Geeta is visiting the practice nurse for her flu vaccination, when she mentions to the nurse that since taking the co-codamol, she is very constipated. This is causing her some discomfort and she does not feel like eating or drinking or going out.

What advice should the practice nurse provide Mrs Sharma to help resolve the constipation?

DIARRHOEA

Diarrhoea is an increase in the frequency of stools, which are watery in consistency. Acute diarrhoea usually lasts for less than 14 days and is self-limiting. Persistent diarrhoea can last for between 14 days and 4 weeks (Huether et al., 2017). Chronic diarrhoea lasts for more than 4 weeks and is likely to need further investigations (Royal College of Nursing, 2013). Diarrhoea can be osmotic, inflammatory and secretory or associated with abnormal gut motility.

Osmotic diarrhoea can occur in malabsorption disorders, such as pancreatic insufficiency. It can also be associated with the ingestion of a nonabsorbable substance, for example, sweeteners that contain sorbitol and magnesium-containing laxatives or indigestion remedies.

Inflammatory diarrhoea is due to damage to the mucosa of the intestines, caused by inflammatory bowel conditions. This leads to poor absorption of water and diarrhoea.

Secretory diarrhoea is when there is a decrease in absorption, accompanied by an increase in mucosal secretions. Secretory diarrhoea often occurs as a result of infections, such as antibiotic-associated colitis or E. coli infection.

Abnormal gut motility diarrhoea occurs due to the faecal material passing through the intestine at a faster than normal rate, reducing the opportunity for the absorption of water. It can be associated with diabetic neuropathy, hyperthyroidism, small intestine resection or laxative abuse. Signs and symptoms associated with diarrhoea include dehydration due to a decreased absorption of water and electrolyte loss, particularly sodium (hyponatraemia) and potassium (hypokalaemia). If secretory diarrhoea is due to infection, then the patient may have the clinical manifestations of this, such as pyrexia and elevated white cell count. The patient with diarrhoea may complain of abdominal pain, which may be 'crampy' in nature.

The Nursing Associate should assess the patient for signs and symptoms. Treatment may include fluid and electrolyte replacement, treatment of infection and treatment for inflammatory bowel disease if appropriate (Dinesen & Harbord, 2013).

DYSPHAGIA

A person with dysphagia has difficulty swallowing. Dysphagia can occur due to a mechanical obstruction, for example, caused by an oesophageal tumour or stricture, or it could be functional, caused by a cerebrovascular accident (stroke), Parkinson disease or multiple sclerosis.

Patients who have difficulty swallowing are at risk of dehydration, weight loss and aspiration of food and fluid into the lungs. Speech and language therapists will assess the patient's ability to swallow and can help patients with swallowing therapy. They will also offer postural advice with regard to swallowing and may suggest nutritional support (NICE, 2013a; 2017).

CRITICAL AWARENESS

Activities of Living

Eating and drinking
  Nursing Associates have a role in assisting patients with eating and drinking.
  As dehydration and malnutrition are associated with poor outcomes for patients, the importance of assisting patients with eating and drinking cannot be underestimated.
  The Malnutrition Universal Scoring Tool (MUST) (BAPEN, 2011) is an assessment tool used to determine a patient's risk of malnutrition.
  Accurate monitoring of food intake should be documented on a food chart, and fluid intake and output on a fluid balance chart.
  Elderly patients are at greater risk of malnutrition. Age Concern (2006) have seven recommendations to improve nutrition for the elderly patients. These include:
1. Listen to patients and carers.
  The Nursing Associate should therefore consider finding out the patient's nutritional likes and dislikes; consider using pictures of food instead of menus.
2. Staff caring for patients should be food aware.
  As a Nursing Associate, ensure that you attend nutritional training and research strategies to improve nourishment for your patients.
3. Assess for the signs of malnourishment.
  Ensure that you can use the MUST assessment tool to accurately assess your patient's nutritional status. Assess weights and accurately complete food intake charts. Nutritional advice from dieticians should be followed.
4. Protected meal times.
  Protected meal times are an initiative that have been in place for some time and should continue to be properly observed to allow time for patients to eat their food at the correct temperature and free from interruptions.
5. Red tray initiative.
  Following assessment, those patients who require assistance with food and fluid intake should be identified by having their food arrive on a red tray. All staff are then aware that this patient will require assistance and may take a bit longer over their meal.
6. Use of trained volunteers to help with nutrition. This strategy has been shown to be very useful in assisting patients with their nutritional needs.

As a Nursing Associate you will be communicating and assisting the volunteers in addressing the nutritional needs of the patient.
7. Follow guidance from professional codes and other professional bodies. As registered practitioners there is an expectation that Nursing Associates will include good evidence to guide their practice and keep up to date with nutritional advice for patient care.
  Consider also: how can we prepare patients for discharge from hospital and ensure their nutritional needs continue to be met?

CHOLELITHIASIS AND CHOLECYSTITIS

In the UK, it is thought that 10%–15% of the population have cholelithiasis or gall stones (AUGIS & RCS, 2016). Although many of these people may have very general and nonspecific symptoms that they do not have investigated, some will have symptoms that do require further investigation and treatment.

Aetiology

People who are more at risk of developing gall stones are:
• Women: usually those who have had children
• Overweight or obese
• Over 40 years old with the risk increasing with age
• A genetic predisposition to gall stones
• High blood cholesterol
• Diabetes mellitus.

Pathophysiology

The formation of gall stones occurs as a result of the impaired metabolism of some of the constituents of bile, for example bilirubin, calcium salts or cholesterol. The salts crystalize to form stones. The stones usually form in the gall bladder and may lie dormant there (Fig. 32.10). The person with gall stones located

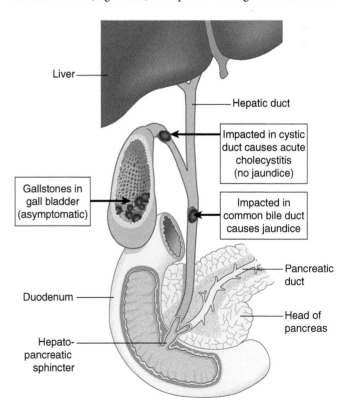

Fig. 32.10 Gall Stones (Waugh & Grant, 2018).

in the gall bladder may be asymptomatic. However, if the stone/s move out of the gall bladder, they can become lodged in the cystic or bile duct. This can lead to inflammation of the gall bladder or cystic duct, which is known as cholecystitis, and can be acute or chronic.

Signs and symptoms

Signs and symptoms are not always present but when patients do have them, the main symptom is pain. The pain may occur following a fatty meal. It is usually located in the right upper quadrant of the abdomen, radiating into the back. Some patients report other gastric symptoms, including heartburn, flatulence and general abdominal pain.

The pain is known as biliary colic. If the patient has jaundice, this would suggest that the stone is occluding the bile duct.

Diagnosis

The diagnosis is usually based on the presenting symptoms and an abdominal ultrasound scan. Liver function test should be ordered to look for complications associated with gall stones, such as pancreatitis. Intravenous cholangiography can determine if other causes of obstruction, such as tumour, can be ruled out. A magnetic resonance imaging (MRI) scan will more accurately determine the position of the gall stones.

Treatment

The presence of gall stones does not always lead to treatment. Some patients may benefit from a low-fat diet. However, if the patient has symptoms, then surgery to remove the stones and gall bladder may be required; this is called cholecystectomy. Cholecystectomy is more usually a laparoscopic procedure; if there is a risk of complications occurring, an open cholecystectomy may be required.

Gall stones that move into the common bile duct have the potential to cause serious complications for the patient, such as infection and ulceration of the tissues. The complications include cholangitis, pancreatitis and jaundice. These patients require urgent assessment and intervention.

REFLECTION 32.3

A female patient aged 58 years visits her GP and complains of right-sided abdominal pain radiating into her back; she has a history of indigestion and previous myocardial infarction.

Although the doctor suspects gall stones, what are the other potential illnesses the patient may have that need to be ruled out? Which investigations would have to be ordered?

INFLAMMATORY BOWEL DISEASES

Inflammatory bowel diseases include ulcerative colitis and Crohn's disease. These are the main inflammatory bowel disorders. In the UK, there are thought to be 300,000 people living with inflammatory bowel disease (Crohn's and Colitis UK, 2017a)

Inflammatory bowel diseases are characterized by periods of relapsing disease and periods of remission. They can occur in any age range but often it is the 10–35 year age range. There can

be a family link with inflammatory bowel disease. Both diseases carry an increased risk of developing cancer in the future.

Ulcerative colitis

Chronic inflammation in ulcerative colitis affects the large intestine. The rectum and sigmoid colon are most often affected (McCance et al., 2014).

Pathophysiology

Ulcerative colitis is thought to be linked to the immune system and it could be triggered by environmental factors, such as infection (bacterial or viral) and diet.

The ulcers or lesions begin in the mucosa layer, often in the rectum, and can spread back from the rectum into the sigmoid colon and beyond. If the entire colon is involved, this is known as pancolitis. The ulcers can begin as small erosions that join to form large continuous areas of ulcer. The ulceration can give the mucosa a red and velvety appearance (erythema) and abscesses can form. As part of the inflammatory process, oedema occurs and the muscularis mucosa layer of the large intestine becomes thicker but the lumen of the large intestine gets narrower.

Crohn's disease
Pathophysiology

Crohn's disease can affect any part of the digestive tract from the mouth to the anus. It frequently occurs in the ileum of the small intestine (McCance et al., 2014). The inflammation begins in the submucosa. It does not spread continuously across the length of submucosa but instead the inflammation appears in patches known as 'skip lesions'. Small areas of inflammation, or granulomas, give the mucosa a cobblestone appearance. The ulcers formed are often deep and can lead to the formation of fistulas. Fistulas can form between one loop of bowel and another; between a loop of bowel and rectum, vagina or bladder. Stricture formation increases the risk of obstruction.

REFLECTION 32.4

John Appleton is 19 years old and has been ill for about 6 months. He is about to commence a degree in medicine at university. Many of his symptoms are associated with stress due to studying. His GP referred him to the gastroenterology department, where a diagnosis of Crohn's disease has been confirmed.

Consider the implications of this diagnosis on the following:
John's psychological health.
John's social health.
John's physical health.

The signs and symptoms for ulcerative colitis and Crohn's disease are similar and are listed here.

Signs and symptoms

- Pain. The pain can be mild to severe, depending on the severity of the relapse. It is described as cramping abdominal pain.
- Bleeding. Some bleeding from the ulcers can be evident in the stool.

- Anaemia. Loss of blood from the ulcers. May be more pronounced in Crohn's disease if vitamin B_{12} (essential for the production of haemoglobin) is not absorbed.
- Fatigue. Low haemoglobin and exhaustion
- Presence of purulent mucus in the stool.
- Pyrexia.

- Elevated pulse rate (due to low haemoglobin and/or pyrexia and dehydration).
- Frequent diarrhoea. This can be 10–20 times per day. Loss of bowel function leads to increased transit times.
- Urgency.
- Dehydration. Loss of absorptive surface reduces the amount of water reabsorbed in the large intestine. The increased transit time reduces the opportunity for water reabsorption. The amount of diarrhoea increases the risk of dehydration. Additionally, the patient may be feeling too unwell to eat or drink.
- Weight loss. May be more pronounced in Crohn's disease as the absorptive surface of the small intestine may be lost if affected.
- Mouth ulcers in Crohn's disease.

Complications

There are complications associated with both ulcerative colitis and Crohn's disease. These include obstruction of the colon if the disease process leads to strictures and fibrosis and the oedema is severe. Perforation can occur but is unusual. People with ulcerative colitis can develop anal fissures and rectal abscesses can occur.

Diagnosis

Ulcerative colitis and Crohn's disease are often suspected based upon the patient's symptoms. Blood tests would show raised inflammatory markers, such as C-reactive protein, low haemoglobin and elevated white cell count. Stool samples can be tested for signs of bleeding, inflammation or infection.

Upper gastrointestinal investigations, such as gastroscopy, are useful in diagnosing or eliminating Crohn's disease if a person has ulcerative colitis. Capsule endoscopy is useful in Crohn's disease. The patient swallows a small camera in the form of a capsule and the camera takes a series of images from the digestive tract. The camera is eventually passed out of the body with the stool. This allows a more detailed view of the length of the digestive tract.

Assessing the lower gastrointestinal tract via colonoscopy or sigmoidoscopy is more useful in ulcerative colitis or if the patient with Crohn's disease has lower gastrointestinal symptoms Biopsies can be sent to the laboratory for further analysis to help confirm diagnosis.

MRI and computed tomography scans can more accurately pinpoint areas of inflammation.

Treatment

The aim of treatment for ulcerative colitis and Crohn's disease is to manage the symptoms of the conditions using medicines to induce remission and to try and avoid surgery. Table 32.2 summarizes the medications used. Symptom management may include rehydration, replacement of electrolytes, pain management, anti-inflammatory medications in acute flare-ups and nutritional assessment. Parenteral nutrition may be required if there is evidence of extreme malnutrition (McCance et al., 2014).

Surgery is considered if the patient's quality of life is affected by repeated flare-ups. The types of surgery required for ulcerative colitis include:

TABLE 32.2 Medications Used in Inflammatory Bowel Disease

Drug classification	Example of the medication	Mode of action	Ulcerative colitis or Crohn's disease
Aminosalicylates	Mesalazine Sulfasalazine	Reduce inflammation	Both
Corticosteroids	Prednisolone Budesonide	Modify the immune response, suppressing the action of inflammatory cells	Both
Immunosuppressants	Azathioprine Methotrexate	Reduce the effects of the immune system, and therefore reduce levels of inflammation	Both
Biological drugs	Infliximab	Blocks the action of tumour necrosis factor, preventing inflammation	Both
Antibiotics	Metronidazole Ciprofloxacin	Antibiotics are used to treat abscesses or fistulas	Crohn's disease
Analgesia	Paracetamol	Inhibits prostaglandin metabolism which increases the pain threshold	Both if required and with discussion with the treating IBD team
Antispasmodics	Hyoscine Butylbromide	Reduces smooth muscle tone and therefore reduces abdominal cramping and spasms	Both if required and with discussion with the treating IBD team

(Crohn's and Colitis UK 2017b; Page et al., 2009.)
IBD, Inflammatory bowel disease.

- Subtotal colectomy with ileostomy. Subtotal colectomy is the removal of the colon but not the rectum. The end of the ileum is formed into a stoma: an ileostomy. The ileostomy may be permanent or there could be an option to form an ileo-anal pouch.
- Restorative proctocolectomy with ileal pouch–anal anastomosis (IPAA). This procedure begins with a subtotal colectomy and ileostomy, removing the rectum and leaving the anus. A pouch is created from the ileum and joined to the anus. A further ileostomy is formed. When the pouch has healed, the ileostomy is closed. Patients should be warned that there is a risk of pouch failure (Perry-Woodford, 2013).
- Proctocolectomy with ileostomy. This surgery is often required in severe disease. Proctocolectomy is the removal of the large intestine, including the rectum and the anus. The ileostomy formed is permanent.
- Colectomy with ileorectal anastomosis. This procedure involves removal of the colon and joining the end of the ileum to the rectum.

Although these types of surgery are seen in ulcerative colitis, they are sometimes applicable to Crohn's disease if the colon is affected. Bowel resection is more common in Crohn's disease, where the very ulcerated or diseased part of the intestine is removed and the two ends are joined together. As stricture is common in Crohn's disease, balloon dilation (NICE, 2016) or strictureplasty can be carried out to widen the area of intestine where the stricture is.

Nursing assessment and care

REFLECTION 32.5

Claire Davis is 27 years old. She has had ulcerative colitis for several years. She has not been able to hold down a job because of her persistent symptoms. When she was 20, she began her midwifery degree but could not complete it because of her condition.

After a bad year of persistent flare-ups, Claire and her consultant have decided that surgery is the best course of action for Claire. Claire is anxious as she is worried about the stoma and the implications of this. She asks the Nursing Associate to help her consider the positive benefits of the surgery that she is about to have. Make a list of the positive benefits of the surgery and consider where you could find support for Claire.

CASE STUDY 32.2 Claire

Claire has her surgery and she has had a subtotal colectomy with ileostomy formation. Claire's surgeon has advised that there is a possibility that Claire can progress to have the restorative proctocolectomy with ileal pouch–anal anastomosis (IPAA) surgery. Following surgery, Claire is seen by the stoma nurse, who is concerned that the stoma looks a little 'dusky'. The surgeon is called and Claire returns to theatre.

Wound care

In the case study above, discuss the importance of wound and stoma care for the postoperative patient. What are the complications and how would assessments help us recognize them?

Claire's stoma is now functioning well and you are asked to help Claire with stoma care.

Knowledge and skills – stoma care
Purpose
Assess and care for the stoma and the skin surrounding the stoma
Assess the amount and type of effluent from the stoma
Change the stoma bag
Prevent leakage from an overfull stoma bag

Assessment
Type of stoma bag currently being used
Barrier products that are being used
Leaks
Surrounding skin where the stoma bag is stuck and beyond
The stoma: colour, size, shape, position, bleeding

Amount and type of faeces

Presence of blood or pus in the faeces

Pain

Patient's ability to manage stoma

Gather Equipment and Implements

Gloves, apron

Container to hold and measure faeces

Yellow bag

Cleaning materials: warm water, mild soap, wipes, skin barrier

Stoma measuring guide and new stoma bag

Procedure

- Ensure the patient is pain free.
- Explain the procedure to the patient and gain consent.
- Encourage the patient to participate if possible.
- Ensure the patient's privacy by closing doors/curtain.
- Assess the current stoma bag for any evidence of leakage and assess the skin surrounding the bag before removing it.
- Assess the patient by asking if there are any concerns, for example, pain or discomfort from the stoma.
- If the stoma bag is intact and there are no obvious reasons to remove the bag, then the bag should be emptied and left in place, and documentation completed.
- If the stoma bag is to be replaced: wash hands, wear gloves and apron.
- Empty the stoma bag into a bedpan to prevent risk of spilling contents when removing bag.
- Assess the amount, consistency, presence of blood and pus in the effluent.
- Gently remove the stoma bag and place in yellow bag.

- Use warm water and soap (optional). If soap is used, a mild soap is preferred. Clean the skin around the stoma and gently clean the stoma.
- Dry the area by gently patting with a dry tissue.
- Inspect the skin surrounding the stoma for any signs of irritation, such as redness or swelling.
- Inspect the stoma for colour, shape, size or bleeding and check the position of the stoma. It should not have retracted but should be sitting proud of the surface of the skin.
- If required, apply the barrier cream.
- Measure the stoma: the stoma plate needs to be cut to size, allowing room for the smooth muscle of the stoma to move when active.
- Remove the backing and apply to the stoma.
- Ensure the bag is closed at the bottom.
- Remove all of the materials and dispose of according to the policy.

Evaluation

Discuss the procedure with the patient.

Document your findings in the patient's notes, the stool chart or fluid balance chart as appropriate. Compare with previous care episode.

The outcome and healing

The stoma is pink and healthy. Claire has been allowed to commence on oral fluids and diet. As Claire has lost a considerable amount of weight prior to her surgery, she has been referred to the dietician, who has prescribed nutritional supplements. This will help with wound healing and weight gain. Claire is allowed to go home with follow-up appointments made. She expresses to the Nursing Associate that she is now nervous about the surgery to come, as she had a complication with the original surgery.

How can the Nursing Associate help Claire with this?

CARE IN THE HOME SETTING

The ward team have arranged for Claire to be visited by the community stoma nurse to ensure she is supported with her stoma at home. Claire reports that she has pain in the peristomal skin. The stoma nurse examines this and on assessment there is an area of excoriated skin. Claire tells the stoma nurse that the bag has leaked on a couple of occasions. The stoma nurse selects some alternative stoma products for Claire, to try and avoid the excoriated skin and to achieve a better fit. She arranges to see Claire again in a week. A week later, the skin has improved, and Claire is managing the stoma well. The stoma nurse has many roles and can also help Claire with concerns about how the stoma and ulcerative colitis can affect lifestyle

(Adapted from NICE, 2013b.)

LOOKING BACK, FEEDING FORWARD

The digestive system is a large system and there are many opportunities for disease to occur along its length. The Nursing Associate has an important role to play in ensuring the patient's fluid and nutritional needs are met. Digestive health has an impact, not just in preventing malnutrition, but it is also essential for tissue repair and healing. Eating and drinking is a social activity that impacts on the mental health of the patient also. Most people have experienced being too ill to eat and nausea or diarrhoea. Caring for a patient with these symptoms is easy to relate to and it is important that the person's needs are met. From ensuring oral hygiene needs are met, to spending time helping a

person with their meal, this will ensure not only that nutritional needs are met but that psychological and social needs are also addressed.

REFERENCES

Age Concern, 2006. Hungry to be Heard: The Scandal of Malnourished Older People in Hospital. Age Concern, England.

AUGIS (Association of Upper Gastrointestinal Surgeons of Great Britain and Ireland) & RCS (Royal College of Surgeons), 2013. Commissioning Guide. Gallstone disease. Available at: https://www.rcseng.ac.uk/library-and-publications/rcs-publications/docs/gallstones-commissioning-guide/.

BAPEN (British Association for Parenteral and Enteral Nutrition), 2011. The 'MUST' Explanatory Booklet. A Guide to the Malnutrition Universal Screening Tool (MUST) for adults. Available at: https://www.bapen.org.uk/screening-and-must/must/must-toolkit/the-must-explanatory-booklet.

COMPASS, 2016. Therapeutic notes on the management of chronic constipation in primary care. Available at: https://www.medicinesni.com/assets/COMPASS/constipation.pdf.

Crohn's and Colitis UK, 2017a. Understanding IBD. Available at: http://s3-eu-west-1.amazonaws.com/files.crohnsandcolitis.org.uk/Publications/understanding-IBD.pdf.

Crohn's and Colitis UK, 2017b. Drugs to treat IBD. Available at: https://www.crohnsandcolitis.org.uk/about-inflammatory-bowel-disease/treatments.

Cronin, E., 2010. Prednisolone in the management of patients with Crohn's disease. Br. J. Nurs. 19 (21), 1333–1336.

Dinesen, L., Harbord, M., 2013. Acute diarrhoea. Medicine (Baltimore) 41 (2), 104–107.

Grossman, S.C., Porth, C.M., 2014. Porth's Pathophysiology. Concepts of Altered Health States. Lippincott, Williams & Wilkins, London.

Huether, S.E., McCance, K.L., Brashers, V.L., Rote, N.S., 2017. Understanding Pathophysiology, sixth ed. Elsevier, St Louis.

Jacob, L., 2017. Auscultation of bowel sounds in critical care: the role of the nurse. Br. J. Nurs. 26 (17), 962–963.

Marieb, E.N., 2015. Essentials of Human Anatomy and Physiology, eleventh ed. Harlow, Pearson.

McCance, K.E., Huether, S.E., Rote, N.S., 2014. Pathophysiology: The Biologic Basis for Disease in Adults and Children, seventh ed. Elsevier, St Louis.

NICE, 2013a. National Institute Health and Care Excellence. Clinical Guideline CG162. Stroke rehabilitation in adults. Available at: https://www.nice.org.uk/guidance/cg162/chapter/1-recommendations#swallowing-2.

NICE, 2013b. National Institute for Health and Care Excellence. Clinical Guideline CG166. Ulcerative colitis management. Available at: https://www.nice.org.uk/guidance/CG166/chapter/1-Recommendations#information-about-treatment-options-for-people-who-are-considering-surgery-2.

NICE, 2016. National Institute for Health and Care Excellence. Clinical Guideline CG51. Crohn's disease management. Available at: https://www.nice.org.uk/guidance/cg152/chapter/Recommendations#maintaining-remission-in-crohns-disease-after-surgery.

NICE, 2017. National Institute for Health and Care Excellence. Clinical Guideline CG 32. Nutrition support for adults: Oral nutrition support, enteral tube feeding and parenteral nutrition. Available at: https://www.nice.org.uk/guidance/cg32.

Page, C.P., Greenstein, B., Gould, D., 2009. Trounce' s Clinical Pharmacology for Nurses, eighteenth ed. Churchill Livingstone, Elsevier, Edinburgh.

Perry-Woodford, Z.L., 2013. Quality of life following ileo-anal pouch failure. Br. J. Nurs. 22 (16), S23–S28.

Royal College of Nursing, 2013. The management of diarrhoea in adults. RCN guidance for nursing staff. Available at: https://my.rcn.org.uk/__data/assets/pdf_file/0016/510721/004371.pdf.

Waugh, A., Grant, A., 2018. Ross & Wilson Anatomy and Physiology in Health and Illness, thirteenth ed. Elsevier, Edinburgh.

33

Urinary Disorders

Karen Nagalingam

OBJECTIVES

By the end of the chapter the reader will:

1. Have an understanding of the anatomy and physiology of the urinary system
2. Discuss the pathophysiological changes associated with a selection of urinary disorders
3. Understand the impact on other body systems of certain urinary disorders
4. Outline the care required by patients with urinary disorders
5. Review the role of the Nursing Associate in promoting health and well-being

KEY WORDS

Nephron	Hormones	Kidneys
Acute kidney injury (AKI)	Fluid	Urethra
Chronic kidney disease (CKD)	Blood pressure	
Glomerulus	Bladder	

CHAPTER AIMS

The aim of this chapter is to provide the reader with an understanding of the function of the renal system and the manifestation and management of patients with a range of disorders affecting the urinary system.

SELF TEST

1. The urinary system consists of four main structures; name these structures.
2. What is the function of the glomerulus?
3. What is nitrogenous waste?
4. Erythropoietin is a hormone that stimulates what?
5. Name some causes that are pre-renal and cause the development of acute kidney injury (AKI).
6. What are the signs of fluid overload in a patient?
7. What is pyelonephritis?
8. Renal calculi (stones) can cause urinary tract infection. Why is this a risk factor?
9. Nephrotoxic drugs can damage the nephron. Name a nephrotoxic drug.
10. How much urine should an adult excrete in 1 hour?

INTRODUCTION

In this chapter the structure and function of the urinary system will be discussed. This comprises of the kidneys, ureter, bladder and urethra. It is important to understand the anatomy and physiology of the urinary system in order to understand normal physiological processes.

The second part of the chapter will look at a range of diseases of the urinary system (Box 33.1). This section will include identification of disease and the causes. The impact of the disease on the patient, including signs and symptoms and consideration with regard to managing or avoiding problems, will be highlighted. Patients with urinary problems may need a variety of supportive care, including monitoring physical signs and consideration of managing a patient in discomfort. If a patient is unwell, the Nursing Associate will need excellent communication skills. This is important when reassuring the patient and calming a patient who may be in discomfort.

> **! HOTSPOT**
>
> Good communication skills are also essential for informing other members of the team about the patient and your findings.

THE URINARY SYSTEM

The urinary system consists of the following structures:
- Kidneys
- Ureters
- Urinary bladder
- Urethra.

BOX 33.1   **Some of the Disorders of the Renal System**

Urinary disorders

Infections and inflammation: cystitis, urethritis, pyelonephritis

Reduced blood flow to kidneys (hypovolaemia/reduced cardiac output/sepsis): acute kidney injury

Blockages: renal calculi, tumour (kidney, bladder, prostate) prostate enlargement (benign prostatic hyperplasia)

Progressive loss of nephrons (hypertension/diabetes/autoimmune disease/nephrotoxins): chronic kidney disease

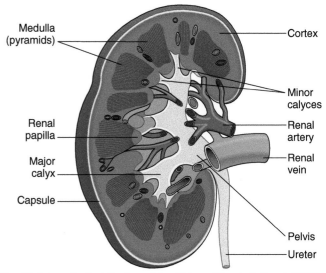

Fig. 33.2 Longitudinal Section of the Kidney (Waugh & Grant, 2018).

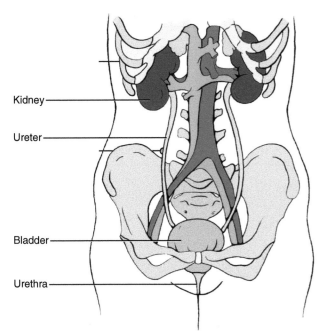

Fig. 33.1 The Structures Associated with the Urinary System (Williams, 2018).

See Fig. 33.1 for the structures associated with the urinary system.

The kidneys are paired organs that are on either side of the vertebral column, with the right kidney slightly lower than the left. This is due to the liver being present on this side. The kidneys are roughly 11 cm long and weigh around 150 g (Chalmers, 2013). Each kidney is bean-shaped and is protected via its location on the back behind the ribs. The outer convex surface is covered in a fibrous capsule and the surface of the kidney is covered in fat to try and protect the kidney from damage.

The inner border of the kidney is the hilus, which is where the renal blood vessels and nerves access the kidney. Approximately 1200 mL of blood flows through the kidney every minute (Nair, 2017), which is roughly 20% of the total cardiac output (Gerhard et al., 2016). This means that the kidney requires a good blood supply and sufficient pressure (Fig. 33.2).

Internal structures of the kidney

The cross section of the kidney shows the differing regions of the kidney. These can be divided into three regions:

- The renal cortex
- The renal medulla
- The renal pelvis.

The renal cortex contains the capillaries and parts of the nephron that are primarily involved in filtering and reabsorption. The renal medulla consists of several renal pyramids and it is within this section that filtrate is concentrated and diluted. The urine is then funnelled through the renal pelvis to the ureters on its way to the bladder.

The nephron

Each kidney contains approximately 1 million nephrons and it is these nephrons that are responsible for producing urine (Fig. 33.3). The main structures of the nephron are the Bowman's capsule, convoluted tubules (proximal and distal), loop of Henle and collecting ducts. Each has a critical function in the management of waste products and regulation of electrolytes and fluid.

The Bowman's capsule is where filtration takes place. A dense network of capillaries called the glomerulus is contained within the capsule. The filtrate then drains into the proximal convoluted tubule, where the bulk of reabsorption occurs. Active reabsorption of ions, nutrients and fluid occurs here. The concentration and dilution of urine mainly occurs in the loop of Henle and this leads to the distal convoluted tubule. It is within this portion that concentration of solutes and other substances is fine-tuned, with active secretion of ions and acids, as well as selective reabsorption of sodium, calcium and water. Once the filtrate leaves the distal convoluted tubule, it enters the collecting ducts, which drain into the renal pelvis. The filtrate is termed urine and will drain from the renal pelvis to the ureters and then to the bladder.

Figs 33.4 and 33.5 outline the glomerulus.

The functions of the kidney

The functions of the kidney are numerous, and it is important to understand this when looking after a person who may have problems with their kidneys (Box 33.2).

Excretion of nitrogenous wastes

Nitrogenous waste refers to metabolic waste products that contain nitrogen. Urea is a by-product of protein metabolism and

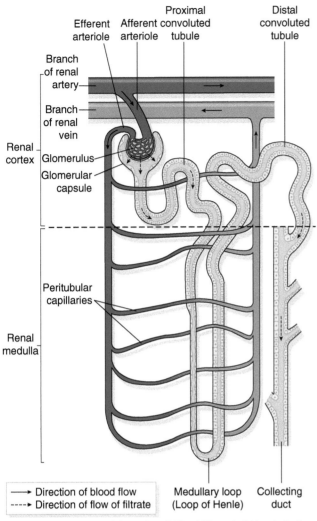

Fig. 33.3 A Nephron and Associated Blood Vessels (Waugh & Grant, 2018).

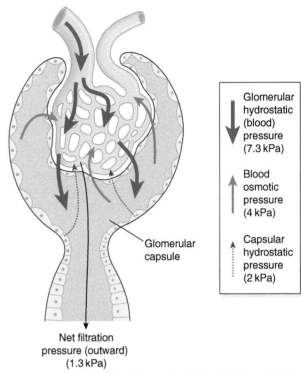

Fig. 33.5 Filtration in the Glomerulus (Waugh & Grant, 2018).

BOX 33.2 Functions of the Kidney

1. Excretion of nitrogenous wastes: urea and creatinine
2. Fluid homeostasis
3. Electrolyte homeostasis
4. Control of blood pressure
5. Acid–base balance
6. Erythropoiesis
7. Vitamin D conversion
8. Calcium and phosphate homeostasis
9. Excretion of drugs and toxins

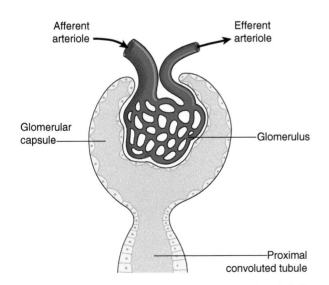

Fig. 33.4 The Glomerulus and Glomerular Capsule (Waugh & Grant, 2018).

creatinine is produced by the skeletal muscle cells. The kidneys excrete creatinine and urea, the levels of which are therefore a useful measure to identify how well the kidneys are working.

! HOTSPOT

Changes in levels of creatinine can indicate if the patient has acute kidney injury or chronic kidney disease.

Fluid homeostasis

The kidneys regulate fluid management within the body. The use of negative feedback loops and hormones aids this process and this is linked with levels of sodium. The three hormones that have an effect on sodium and therefore fluid are:

- Aldosterone
- Antidiuretic hormone
- Atrial natriuretic peptide.

Electrolyte homeostasis

Sodium levels are controlled by the hormones mentioned previously. Potassium is also regulated by the kidney but only the hormone aldosterone controls potassium content. Increased levels of potassium stimulate the adrenal cortex to excrete aldosterone, which increases the excretion of potassium in the urine. Aldosterone reabsorbs sodium in exchange for potassium or hydrogen.

Control of blood pressure

There is a small group of cells, called the macula densa, that detect pressure changes in the arterioles leading to the glomerulus. Any fall in pressure results in the hormone renin being released. It is responsible for ensuring that there is sufficient flow of blood received by the glomerulus. The renin–angiotensin system is triggered to produce vasoconstriction of the efferent arteriole, peripheral vasoconstriction and aldosterone excretion to increase sodium and water. This results in an increase in blood pressure.

Acid–base balance

Acids are constantly being produced (release of hydrogen ions (H^+)) as a result of normal cell metabolism. The body needs to maintain a balance between acids and bases and this is tightly controlled between pH 7.35 and pH 7.45. In healthy individuals, there are a number of ways the body can maintain the acid–base balance. These are:

1. Buffers: these help control the number of hydrogen ions in a solution. Plasma proteins and bicarbonate are examples of these.
2. Respiratory control mechanism: chemoreceptors detect changes in CO_2, H^+ and O_2 and will increase or decrease the respiratory rate to control pH.
3. Renal control mechanism: this takes longer to react to changes in pH but it works by reabsorbing bicarbonate ions and excreting H^+.

The renal control mechanism secretes hydrogen ions into the filtrate via the proximal convoluted tubule, where they combine with bicarbonate to form carbonic acid.

$$H^+ + HCO_3^- \rightarrow H_2CO \rightarrow H_2O + CO_2$$

Carbonic acid is converted to carbon dioxide and water. The carbon dioxide is retained and converted back to bicarbonate and transferred into the plasma. Hydrogen is excreted in the urine. The pH of urine can range from 4.5 to 8, depending on factors such as diet and time of day (Waugh & Grant, 2018).

Erythropoiesis

The hormone erythropoietin is primarily produced by the kidney. Its function is to increase the production of red blood cells.

Hypoxia stimulates its release and when oxygen levels return to normal, levels of erythropoietin decrease. It is essential in the prevention of anaemia and is an example of a negative feedback loop.

Vitamin D conversion

Vitamin D can be attained directly from sunlight, but it can also be ingested from various food items. Increasingly, it is added to items such as cereals, breads and butter (Black et al., 2012). This needs to be converted via the liver and kidneys to the active form. Vitamin D increases calcium and phosphate absorption from the gut.

Calcium and phosphate homeostasis

Reduced calcium absorption from the gut can lead to hypocalcaemia. This is detected by receptors in the parathyroid gland, which releases parathyroid hormone (PTH). PTH causes bone breakdown to help increase calcium levels in the blood.

Excretion of drugs and toxins

Drugs and metabolites may be fully or partially excreted by the kidney. This is important to understand when looking after a patient who may have problems with their kidneys, or if you are aware that the drug may be nephrotoxic (toxic to the nephrons).

The ureters

Urine from the renal pelvis is funnelled along to the ureters. The ureters are approximately 30 cm long and 5 mm in diameter and lead directly to the bladder. They are surrounded by muscle cells, which enables peristaltic movement of the urine into the bladder.

The bladder

The bladder is made up of smooth muscle fibres with the function of storing urine. As the bladder fills up with fluid, the fibres stretch and thin, and information is transmitted to the surrounding nerves and muscle cells (Huether, 2012). The detrusor muscle is the muscle of the bladder, whereas the trigone is a triangular-shaped muscle situated between the ureter openings and the urethra.

The urethra

At the junction of the bladder and the urethra, there is a sphincter that is under involuntary control. When the bladder has approximately 250–300 mL of urine, this muscle will relax, and the patient will feel the urge to pass urine. In older children and adults, this urge can be overridden and is under control of the external urethral sphincter. The urethra is a muscular tube that is approximately 3–4 cm in women and 18–20 cm in men.

URINARY DISORDERS

In this next section, the anatomy and physiology of the urinary system will aid the Nursing Associate in identifying how to care and manage a patient with urinary problems. The patient that presents with urinary problems will require understanding and good communication to enable them to understand the assessments and the interventions that may be required. The disorders that will be covered in this next section are: acute kidney injury (AKI), chronic kidney disease (CKD), urinary tract infection (UTI) and renal calculi.

TABLE 33.1 Causes of Pre-Renal Acute Kidney Injury

Causes of pre-renal AKI	
Volume	Blood loss from trauma or surgery, vomiting, diarrhoea, burns, sweating, diuresis from medication/hyperglycaemia. Reduced intake.
Cardiac	Heart failure, arrhythmias, myocardial infarction, shock
Vascular	NSAIDs, shock, antihypertensive treatment, thrombosis, stenosis

COMMUNITIES OF CARE

Learning Disabilities

When caring for or offering support to people with learning disabilities, you should always ensure that the language you use is understood by the person you are offering care to. The most important thing you should do is assess the person's needs and tailor care provision to those needs, particularly with the language that is used. For example:

A urinary tract infection is sometimes referred to as a 'water infection' or 'UTI'. It is a common condition that occurs when germs get into the person's bladder or urethra.

If you have a UTI, you might experience any of the following symptoms:

- pain or burning when you pass water
- an urgent need to go to the toilet often
- being unable to pass water
- pain in the lower back or lower tummy
- running a temperature

Turning Point is an organization that had produced a healthcare tool kit: https://www.turning-point.co.uk/_cache_96dc/content/TP-Health-Toolkit-2016%20(web)-5090910000025942.pdf.

Acute kidney injury

AKI is a rapid decline in kidney function, with increased urea and creatinine levels and with or without reduction in urine. It can range from mild impairment to advanced and can be life-threatening. AKI occurs in 10%–20% of patients in hospital and can often be the result of hypovolaemia, hypotension, sepsis and nephrotoxins (Ostermann & Sprigings, 2018). Mortality in the UK is estimated at between 25% and 30%, depending upon the severity and other factors (NICE, 2013a). A study undertaken in 2009 identified that only 50% of patients who acquired AKI and subsequently died received good care (NCEPOD, 2009). This means that improvements in identification and management of AKI are needed.

AKI can also be found in the community and therefore knowledge and understanding of the risk factors, signs and symptoms, as well as the management of AKI, are essential.

Causes of acute kidney injury

When identifying what may have caused the AKI, it is often differentiated into pre-renal, intrarenal and post-renal. This refers to where the cause of the problem affecting the kidney is.

Pre-renal. This refers to factors that occur before the kidney (Table 33.1). AKI is a secondary event and is caused as a result of a primary insult somewhere else in the body. Falling blood flow to the kidney (either relative or actual) can cause pre-renal AKI. The kidney receives approximately 1000 mL of blood per minute; this equates to approximately 20%–25% of the cardiac output (Huether, 2012). To maintain perfusion to the kidneys, there needs to be:

1. Effective circulating volume (including blood oxygenation and volume)
2. Effective pump (how effective the heart is at pumping the blood)
3. Sufficient blood pressure
4. Patent vessels

(Bevan, 2016).

The major cause of AKI in individuals is reduced volume; therefore, improving fluid deficit has the potential to halt deterioration of renal function. AKI is reversible, but this depends upon the extent and cause of the damage and timely management.

! HOTSPOT

About 25% of patients with sepsis and roughly 50% with severe sepsis will have AKI (Yaqoob & Ashman, 2017).

Intrarenal (intrinsic/renal). Intrinsic means that the problem has occurred within the kidney itself. This is where damage to various parts of the nephron occurs. This can be caused by acute tubular necrosis, which can occur from continued reduction in renal blood flow and perfusion to the tubules. Other causes include inflammation of the nephron from drugs, infection and systemic disease. Certain antibiotics can be a cause of intrarenal AKI in patients.

REFLECTION 33.2

Make a list of six commonly used antibiotics; then, next to each antibiotic, make a note to identify if the antibiotic can cause intrarenal AKI.

Post-renal. This is where the flow of urine is disrupted from the renal pyramids to the urethra. Common causes include renal calculi (stones) and prostatic hypertrophy.

CASE STUDY 33.1   Jasmin

Yasmin Shaan is a 56-year-old woman who is usually fit and active. She runs her own business and manages the household, whilst running around after her elderly father who lives nearby. She has been admitted for an elective radical hysterectomy, as she was recently diagnosed with early stage cervical cancer.

There were no complications during surgery; however, later that evening after transfer to the postsurgical unit (PSU) there was a lot of blood found in the drain and around her dressing. She was taken back to theatre to halt the bleeding. She lost approximately 2 L of blood. She was given 3 units of blood in theatre and has an intravenous catheter running with normal saline 500 mL, at present for over 4 hours.

She returns to PSU several hours later. The next day the nurse who is looking after Yasmin undertakes a thorough assessment. She is scoring high on the National Early Warning Score chart: her blood pressure is 100/56 mm Hg, pulse is 100 beats per minute and respiratory rate is 19 breaths per minute. She has not passed urine for at least 10 hours. Yasmin is very lethargic and she is complaining of feeling nauseous and cold.

The specialist registrar comes to review Yasmin and diagnoses her with acute kidney injury secondary to hypovolaemia.

Weight 85 kg
Height 1.75 metres
Can you calculate the minimum amount of urine that Yasmin should pass?

	Results	Normal range
Haemoglobin	70 g/L	110–180 (female) g/L
		130–170 (male)
Urea	19 mmol/L	3.0–9.2 mmol/L
Creatinine	186 μmol/L	75–125 μmol/L
Potassium	5.9 mmol/L	3.5–5.1 mmol/L
Sodium	136 mmol/L	136–145 mmol/L

What can be determined from the blood results?

REFLECTION 33.3

In the place where you work, what is the policy and procedure for taking blood results by telephone? How do you document the blood results received?

Signs and symptoms and establishing a diagnosis

AKI is usually secondary to something else that is occurring, such as sepsis, myocardial infarction or hypovolaemia. The focus is on managing the deteriorating patient; therefore measures to assess or avoid AKI may be minimal.

Airway. Depending on the cause of the AKI, the airway should be monitored in case of reduced consciousness caused by hypovolaemia, dehydration, sepsis and uraemia.

Breathing. The breathing may be elevated. This may be due to acidosis caused by the reduced ability of the kidneys to reabsorb bicarbonate, termed Kussmaul's respirations. The lungs will try and manage the AKI by increasing the breathing rate and thereby exhaling carbon dioxide in an attempt to correct the acidosis.

Circulation. The blood pressure may be low due to volume loss or reduced pressure from the heart. Or it may be elevated if the patient is fluid overloaded. This will need to be documented to assess for trends and escalated as appropriate. Identifying the pulse rate, rhythm and strength will aid evaluation of potential cause and management of the patient. A weak and thready pulse

may suggest volume depletion and peripheral vasoconstriction. Changes in potassium levels can lead to life-threatening arrhythmias; therefore the patient will need to be monitored continually. High urea levels are toxic to the body and can cause palpitations, nausea, vomiting and diarrhoea, among other symptoms.

Urine output may reduce and may be the only indication that the kidneys are not working effectively. 0.5 mL/kg per hour is identified as the minimum amount of urine that should be excreted by the kidneys (Yaqoob & Ashman, 2017).

REFLECTION 33.4

What should you do if you feel the person you are caring for has had a reduction in their urinary output or is not passing urine?

Disability. The patient may have reduced consciousness due to deterioration as well as specific renal causes. Urea levels can cause problems with neurological function and continued high levels can lead to coma and death (Bevan, 2016).

⚠ HOTSPOT

When assessing a deteriorating patient, ABCDE refers to airway, breathing, circulation, disability (measurement of conscious level) and exposure (everything else). This is a systematic approach to assessment and aids the healthcare worker in undertaking a rigorous assessment in an attempt to establish potential causes of deterioration.

Exposure (everything else). Rashes on the skin, dry skin and oedema can all help identify potential causes of AKI.

CRITICAL AWARENESS

Consider urgent referral for review for patients with the following:
- Inability to pass urine
- Severe renal colic with inability to pass urine or reduced urine output
- Hyperkalaemia (over 6.0 mmol/L)
- The patient is scoring on the National Early Warning Score chart or the trend indicates that the patient is deteriorating.
- There is an indication that the patient may be volume depleted (e.g., from nausea and vomiting, blood loss, diarrhoea or excess urine output).
- The patient has suspected sepsis.

Diagnosis

Estimating the level of kidney function requires blood tests to identify levels of creatinine in the blood. Creatinine is a by-product of muscle metabolism and is a useful measure of glomerular filtration, as it is only excreted by the kidney. Kidney function can be determined through identifying a rise in creatinine from the baseline or within a given time frame (Table 33.2).

Urine output can also be the first indicator that AKI is present. Robust fluid management may help identify AKI early.

It is useful to identify the stage of AKI, as this determines the management and care of the patient. A stage 1 AKI may require minimal intervention and may be managed on the ward. A stage 3 AKI may require management in an higher acuity bed and possible renal replacement (Connell & Laing, 2015).

TABLE 33.2 Staging for Acute Kidney Injury Can Determine the Severity of the Damage

	Creatinine	Urine output
AKI stage 1	A rise of creatinine of >1.5× baseline level, or of >26 µmol/L within 48 hours	Or a urine output <0.5 mL/kg per hour for more than 6 hours
AKI stage 2	A rise in creatinine which is >2× baseline	Or a urine output ≥0.5 mL/kg per hour for ≥12 h
AKI stage 3	A rise in creatinine of >3× baseline or a rise of >1.5 baseline to >354 µmol/L	A urine output of <0.3 mL/kg per hour for ≥24 h or anuria for ≥12 h

(KDIGO, 2012.)

TABLE 33.3 Treatment and Causes of Acute Kidney Injury

STOP AKI	
Sepsis	Sepsis Six care bundle, including oxygen, fluid, bloods (cultures, lactate and haemoglobin), urine output, antibiotics
Toxins	Drugs which could affect the kidney and lead to further damage. Non-steroidal anti-inflammatory (NSAID), gentamicin
Optimize blood pressure	Consider promoting fluid intake and intravenous fluid. Omit taking blood pressure lowering medication
Prevent harm	Identify the cause of the AKI and treat.

(Reproduced from: Royal College of Physicians. Acute kidney injury and intravenous fluid therapy. London: RCP, 2015.)

TABLE 33.4 Factors Influencing Dehydration

Factor	Example
Reduced intake	Nausea and vomiting
	Nil by mouth
	Poor appetite
Increased output	Vomiting
	Diarrhoea
	Sweating
	Fever
	Drains
Functional	Ability to grasp/reach drink
	Age: thirst response diminishes
	Ability to swallow (stroke)
Medications	Diuretics
Disease	Diabetes insipidus
	Sepsis

Care and treatment

The care and treatment of a patient with AKI will need to take into consideration the cause of AKI. The Royal College of Physicians (2015) uses the acronym 'STOP' to help manage an individual with AKI: Sepsis, Toxins, Optimize blood pressure, Prevent harm. STOP AKI is an acronym which aids the healthcare professional in identifying causes and treating AKI (Table 33.3). A patient with sepsis will need management of the infection as well as supportive measures for their AKI.

Fluid balance

Patients who are at risk of dehydration need interventions in place to identify and prevent it. There are several factors that influence fluid status and therefore dehydration (Table 33.4). Identifying factors that may lead to dehydration are important from a patient safety perspective. In the Francis report (2013) it was found that patients were not receiving adequate support with hydration. This could have an impact on patient recovery, as well as cognitive and physical impairment (Francis, 2013). The Health Foundation report on nutrition and hydration in the elderly concluded that these factors contributed to avoidable harm in patients and management of these is frequently overlooked by healthcare professionals (Lecko, 2013).

To tackle the problem of dehydration, identification of hydration status, a simple but effective tool, can be used to highlight fluid input and output of a patient.

Some factors influencing dehydration are highlighted in Table 33.4 and Table 33.5 provides information on undertaking a fluid balance.

It is important that fluid imbalances are identified promptly; adding up total input and total output should provide relatively

TABLE 33.5 Undertaking a Fluid Input and Output Measurement

Skills: Fluid input and output measurement

Actions

Inform patient of need to undertake a fluid balance. Explain the rationale and what will be undertaken.

Attain the fluid balance chart and clearly label with name and date of birth.

Consider what inputs may need to be documented on the chart:

Drinking and certain foods (e.g., soup)

Intravenous fluids

Nasogastric feed/peg feed/parental feed

Consider what outputs need to be documented on the chart:

Urine (catheterized or not)

Bowels (diarrhoea)/stoma

Vomiting

Drains (postsurgery)

equal figures. However, if input is less than output, then this is a negative fluid balance and could signify dehydration. In severe cases this can put the patient at risk of shock and circulatory collapse (Porth, 2015). If input is greater than output, then this could signify overhydration and this could put the patient at risk of pulmonary oedema (Porth, 2015).

CRITICAL AWARENESS

Signs of Moderate Dehydration

Reduced urine output, increasingly darker colour and stronger odour

Increasingly dry mouth, cracked lips

Dry eyes as a result of a reduction in tears

Lethargy and increased sleepiness

Mild or increased confusion

Irritability and agitation

Worsening constipation

Postural hypotension (drop of systolic blood pressure by 20 mm Hg), resulting in dizziness, often causing falls

Sunken eyes

Unexpected reduction in wound exudate

Reduced skin elasticity/turgor

Signs of Acute Dehydration

Low systolic blood pressure (100 mm Hg or less)

Rapid, thready pulse

Increase in respiratory rate

Extremities are cold

Reduced capillary refill time as a result of peripheral shutdown

Hyper- or hypo-delirium (agitation and severe confusion, or the opposite: increased sleepiness and reduced responsiveness)

Level of consciousness reduced

Greatly reduced urine output (oliguria)

CASE STUDY 33.1 Yasmin (Continued)

Yasmin Shaan was given further intravenous fluids. Her input and output was closely monitored using a fluid balance chart. After 24 hours, Yasmin was passing moderate amounts of urine, her blood pressure was returning to her presurgical values and her pulse was within normal limits.

Yasmin's blood results were in normal ranges and she was discharged 4 days later.

OSCE 33.1

Undertake a Handover of a Patient Using the Situation, Background, Assessment and Recommendation Framework (SBAR)

When handing information over to other colleagues and healthcare professionals, it is useful to have a structured approach to communication. SBAR is a structured approach to managing communication and ensuring the right information is handed over. Poor communication could result in delays and errors occurring in care.

Using the case study, practise handing over the information that you know.

Action	Criteria	Achieved/ not achieved
Situation	Nursing Associate identifies the following:	
	1. Name and ward/location	
	2. Patient's name	
	3. Area of concern/headline	
Background	Nursing Associate identifies the following:	
	1. Admission date/length of stay	
	2. Diagnosis	
	3. Previous medical history	
	4. ABCDE assessment (airway, breathing, circulation, disability, exposure)	
	5. Observations that are abnormal as part of ABCDE	
	6. Early Warning Score (EWS)	
Assessment	Nursing Associate identifies the following:	
	1. The problem	
	2. What they have done so far	
	3. Their level of concern	
Recommendation	The Nursing Associate identifies the following:	
	1. What is required to be done	
	2. What they should be doing	

Pass
Fail

Chronic kidney disease

CKD is the gradual progressive destruction of renal function over a period. This is associated with systemic disorders, such as diabetes and hypertension, or it can be as a result of kidney disease, such as glomerulonephritis or chronic pyelonephritis. The gradual destruction of nephrons may not produce any symptoms until CKD is well advanced. This is because the kidneys have a significant reserve to be able to cope with this. Symptoms may only be evident when the patients renal function declines to 25% of normal (Huether, 2012). In advanced renal failure, the progression can be slowed but it cannot be stopped.

Signs and symptoms

When considering the signs and symptoms, it is useful to consider the nine functions of the kidney (Table 33.6). Uraemic toxins build up in the blood and it is these toxins that are known to cause uraemic symptoms. Symptoms occur when urea is frequently over 40 mmol/L (Yaqoob & Ashman, 2017).

TABLE 33.6 Signs and Symptoms of Chronic Renal Failure

Functions of the kidney	Effects of chronic kidney disease: signs and symptoms
Excretion of nitrogenous wastes: uraemia	Deposits in skin can cause itching and tinting
	Deposits in salivary glands causing metallic taste
	Nausea and vomiting
	Loss of appetite and weight
	Suppression of bone marrow function causing:
	• Reduced red blood cell production and lifespan (anaemia)
	• Reduced white blood cell production (prone to infection)
	• Reduced platelet production (prone to bleeding)
	Neurological effects:
	• Nerve irritation
	• Short-term memory loss and poor concentration
	• Personality changes
	• Confusion, fitting, coma and death
	Malaise and loss of energy
Fluid homeostasis	• Hypertension
	• Oedema: peripherally and pulmonary (shortness of breath)
	• Cardiac failure
	• Increased urine output (early sign)
	• Oliguria (late sign)
Electrolyte homeostasis: potassium	• Muscle irritability, motor muscle spasms/weakness
	• Cardiac arrhythmias
	• Chest pain
	• Cardiac arrest
Control of blood pressure	• Hypertension
	• Headache
	• Nose bleeds
	Long-term effects of hypertension:
	• Cardiac hypertrophy
	• Cardiac failure causing oedema
	• Blood vessel damage (visual changes)
Acid–base balance	**May be acidotic but will be asymptomatic**
Erythropoiesis	Anaemia
	• Shortness of breath
	• Tired and lethargic
	• Reduced appetite
	• Cold pallor
	• Hypoxic
Vitamin D conversion	• Vessel damage
Calcium and phosphate homeostasis	• Itching
	• Calcium deposits in skin, joints and eyes
	• Increased risk of fractures

TABLE 33.7 Classification of Stages of Chronic Kidney Disease

Stage	Description	GFR (mL/min per 1.73 m^2)
1	Kidney damage with normal or increased GFR	≥90
2	Kidney damage with mild decrease in GFR	60–89
3	Moderate decrease in GFR	30–59
4	Severe decrease in GFR	15–29
5	Kidney failure	<15 (or dialysis)

(KDIGO, 2013a.)
GFR, Glomerular filtration rate.

Diagnosis

A blood test to identify levels of urea and creatinine, as well as glomerular filtration rate (GFR), is considered the best measure of the function of the kidneys. A normal GFR is approximately 130 mL/min per 1.73 m^2, but various factors affect the GFR, including age, sex and weight (Porth, 2015). The Kidney Disease Outcome Quality Initiative (KDIGO, 2013) staging system is commonly used to classify CKD (Table 33.7).

CKD is classified as stage 3–4 with sustained reduction in GFR for 3 months or more.

Care and treatment

The level of kidney impairment will influence the care required for a patient with CKD. Initial management may be to slow the rate of progression down and reduce symptoms associated with CKD. Avoiding drugs that may be nephrotoxic or may reduce the blood flow to the kidney is essential.

A patient with CKD has an increased risk of cardiovascular disease (Thomas, 2013); therefore, a variety of interventions can reduce the risk and help the patient manage the disease. The role of the Nursing Associate may be to educate the patient on the importance of taking their medication and offering support to the patient. A patient with CKD may require renal replacement therapy in the future and therefore they may need advice and support. Where possible, the patient should be empowered to manage their CKD, so understanding the management of CKD is required. It is well known that vascular disease and diabetes are causes of CKD (SIGN, 2008) but other factors known to influence CKD include age, race, smoking and chronic use of non-steroidal anti-inflammatory drugs (NSAIDs) (NICE, 2014).

Educating a patient and supporting them to manage their CKD may reduce the progression to end-stage renal failure. Important influences include:

- The target blood pressure for a patient with CKD is below 140/90 mm Hg (NICE, 2014). If the blood pressure is consistently high, a review of blood pressure medication may be needed.
- Blood sugar levels should be maintained within normal ranges for patients with diabetes to avoid further destruction of the nephrons.
- Reduction in salt may help with fluid and blood pressure management.

- Weight reduction and regular exercise is recommended (Thomas, 2013).
- Education on taking over the counter medications, such as NSAIDs.
- Advice on stopping smoking.
- Educating the patient on possible need for dialysis and the lifestyle changes that may occur with this.

Renal replacement therapy

As the renal function deteriorates, a patient may need renal replacement therapy. This is when the kidney can no longer sustain life and therefore treatment is required. The gold standard for renal replacement is having a kidney transplant before dialysis is required (Thomas, 2013). However, this is not always possible due to availability of a donor kidney (cadaveric or live-related), late referral to the renal team and patient factors that may mean that the patient is not suitable for transplantation.

Haemodialysis is the cleaning of the blood using an artificial kidney which is a filter with a semi-permanent membrane. Peritoneal dialysis is the indirect method of cleaning the blood by infusing dialysate into the abdomen, which removes waste molecules from the bloodstream through osmosis and diffusion.

CARE IN THE HOME SETTING

Home Dialysis

Home dialysis means the patient doing either haemodialysis or peritoneal dialysis in their home. Some patients find it helpful to have a partner or friend to help then with their dialysis; however, this is not essential.

Those who are interested in doing haemodialysis at home will need to be willing and able to learn how to do their own treatment. Support may be needed, and this can come from family, friends or carers, although some patients can manage independently. The home dialysis team can help in finding the best solution for you.

A home dialysis machine is smaller than those used in dialysis units. Practically, there is a need to have enough space at home to carry out the dialysis and store the supplies that come with it. A home visit will be needed to ensure that the accommodation is suitable; some adaptations will need to be made to ensure the home is able to accommodate the equipment. The hospital provides the dialysis machine and most of the equipment supplies will be delivered to the person's home.

The advantages and disadvantages of haemodialysis and peritoneal dialysis are highlighted in Table 33.8.

Urinary tract infection

UTIs include infection relating to all aspects of the urinary system. Lower UTIs affecting the bladder and the urethra are less serious than upper UTIs, due to the potential for renal damage. Most UTIs are caused by the bacteria *Escherichia coli* (Porth, 2015), which is found in faeces. Bacteria enters through the urethra and travels upwards, where it attaches to the mucosa of the bladder. *E. coli* has projections termed pili and fimbriae, which allow it to adhere to the bladder and prevent it from washing away. Other organisms that can cause UTIs include

TABLE 33.8 The Advantages and Disadvantages of Haemodialysis and Peritoneal Dialysis for Renal Replacement Therapy

	Haemodialysis	Peritoneal dialysis
Access	Patient will need a fistula forming, which is when an artery and a vein are joined together. Needles are then inserted into the vein. A tunnelled line can also be used	A small tube is inserted into the abdomen and into the peritoneal cavity
Length of time	Usually 3 times a week for 4 hours	Can be 4 times a day for half an hour. Sometimes it can be undertaken at night whilst the patient sleeps
Location	Usually in a dialysis unit but can be undertaken at home eventually	Anywhere. but space needed to store the equipment
Suitability	All patients that are suitable for dialysis	Patients will need to have the dexterity to undertake this, as well as the physical ability. This may limit people with certain co-morbidities

Klebsiella, *Proteus* and *Staphylococcus saprophyticus* (Yaqoob & Ashman, 2017).

However, certain patients have an increased risk of UTI. These risk factors include:

- Diabetes mellitus
- Sexually active woman
- Postmenopausal women
- Men with prostate enlargement
- Age
- Renal calculi/bladder calculi
- Neurogenic disorders that stop the bladder from emptying
- Reflux
- Catheterization

Women are at an increased risk of UTIs due to a short urethra (men have a much longer urethra) and the proximity to the anus. Irritation caused to the area by hygiene products, soaps and sexual activity also increase the risk of UTI. Any disruption in the flow of urine can contribute to the increased risk of UTI. In older males, prostatic hypertrophy can lead to the retention of urine due to constriction of the urethra. Urine that remains in the bladder is a prime host for bacteria to grow as the urine is not flushed out.

Foreign objects, such as the presence of a catheter or calculi, can increase the risk of UTI due to possible trauma to the bladder wall.

Fig. 33.6 shows the pelvic organs associated with the bladder and urethra in females and males.

Signs and symptoms

The signs and symptoms of a UTI vary, depending upon the location of the infection. If the location of the

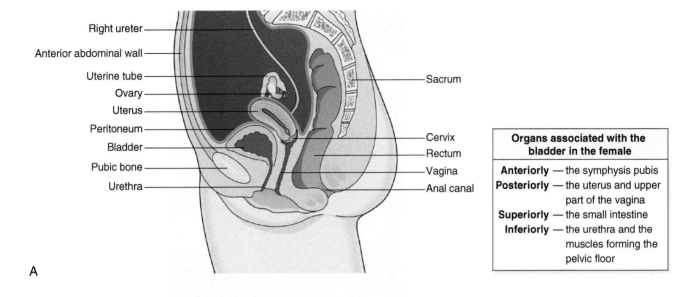

Organs associated with the bladder in the female	
Anteriorly	— the symphysis pubis
Posteriorly	— the uterus and upper part of the vagina
Superiorly	— the small intestine
Inferiorly	— the urethra and the muscles forming the pelvic floor

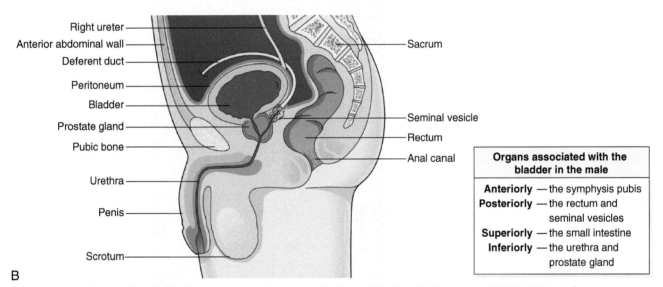

Organs associated with the bladder in the male	
Anteriorly	— the symphysis pubis
Posteriorly	— the rectum and seminal vesicles
Superiorly	— the small intestine
Inferiorly	— the urethra and prostate gland

Fig. 33.6 The Pelvic Organs Associated with the Bladder and Urethra (A) Female and (B) Male (Waugh & Grant, 2018).

infection is within the bladder, it is termed cystitis; if the infection has ascended to the kidneys, then it is known as pyelonephritis.

Diagnosis

Diagnosis of a lower UTI is based upon signs and symptoms. If a patient presents with two out of three signs of: dysuria, frequency and urgency with no vaginal discharge then treatment should commence (Yaqoob & Ashman, 2017). If the patient is pregnant, is a man, has recurrent infections, has suspected pyelonephritis or has failed antibiotic treatment, a urine sample is recommended for culture and sensitivity (Public Health England, 2017). This should be a clean-catch sample, midstream and preferably taken in the morning. Cloudy urine or the presence of pus can indicate infection. If the patient presents with mild symptoms, a urinary dipstick can provide further evidence of infection.

CASE STUDY 33.2 Anne

There is a planned visit to Anne, an 82-year-old lady who requires a dressing change for amputation of one of her left toes. This is the second visit from the team. When you go to the house, her daughter lets you in. Anne is complaining of back pain and appears generally unwell.

The patient has recurrent urinary tract infections (UTIs); this is her third in the last 9 months. She is finding it difficult to mobilize and is concerned that she will not recover from this operation. She feels her mobility has reduced greatly over the last year and does not venture out of the house unless assisted.

Anne's daughter lives nearby but she is busy with her own family and grandchildren. She isn't always around.

1. Consider some of the social and physical factors that may increase Anne's risk of UTI.
2. What interventions could potentially help reduce the reoccurrence of another UTI?

THE MEDICINE TROLLEY 33.1

Drug	Drug classification	Reason for administration	Route of administration	Dose	Side effects	Contra-indications	Nursing care
Trimethoprim	Antibiotic	Treatment of urinary tract infection	Oral	200 mg twice daily	Allergic reaction can occur Nausea, vomiting, hyperkalaemia, rashes	Can affect red blood cells and white cells	Seek consent prior to administration Explain the use of the drug to the patient, respond to any questions If the patient is taking the contraceptive 'pill' at the same time as this medicine, effectiveness of the 'pill' can be reduced if the patient is vomiting or has diarrhoea lasting for more than 24 hours. If this happens, seek advice from a doctor or pharmacist about what additional contraceptive precautions to use over the following few days. No need to use additional precautions for bouts of sickness or diarrhoea lasting for less than 24 hours.

TABLE 33.9 Signs and Symptoms of Urinary Tract Infection

Location Terminology	Bladder Cystitis	Kidneys Pyelonephritis
Specific signs and symptoms that may be present	• Pain in the lower abdomen • Painful urination • Dysuria • Urgency • Frequency • Nocturia • Cloudy urine • Unusual smell to the urine • Haematuria	• Dull aching pain in the lower back • Painful urination • Dysuria • Urgency • Frequency • Nocturia • Cloudy urine • Unusual smell to the urine • Haematuria
General symptoms	May have signs of systemic infection	Symptoms of systemic infection: • Fever • Malaise • Nausea
Signs of urosepsis		• Elevated respiratory rate ≥22 breaths per minute • Low systolic blood pressure ≤100 mm Hg • Altered conscious level

Care and treatment

Some patients will require antibiotics. For patients with uncomplicated (no other risk factors) UTI, then a short 3-day course of antibiotics may be sufficient, such as trimethoprim or nitrofurantoin (Haddock & MacDonald, 2013). However, antimicrobial treatment should be based on local prescribing guidelines.

The Nursing Associate has an important role in educating a patient regarding managing their symptoms and trying to reduce further incidences of UTI. Symptoms such as lower abdominal pain associated with UTI may require pain relief, such as paracetamol or ibuprofen, to ease the pain and discomfort associated with inflammation of the urinary tract. Paracetamol and ibuprofen are both antipyretic drugs, which reduces the body temperature in patients with a fever. In acute pyelonephritis, avoid ibuprofen as it can impair renal function (NICE, 2013b). They should only be given if required by the patient.

If the patient does not require admission, the Nursing Associate can advise on the importance of staying hydrated. Hydration is also important in a patient who has a UTI, as increasing the amount of fluid drunk by a patient will help flush out the bacteria from the urinary tract.

REFLECTION 33.5

A male patient has received his oral trimethoprim 10 minutes ago. He then informed you that he has vomited. What should you do about the dose of trimethoprim he has taken and then may have vomited?

CASE STUDY 33.2   Anne (Continued)

Anne has had mobility issues over the last year and this may influence how much fluid intake she has. She may find it difficult to get herself drinks regularly and this means that she has a reduced urine output. Bacteria in the urinary tract may not be flushed away and this can lead to a urinary tract infection (UTI).

Anne may also be concerned about getting to the toilet in time. Where the toilet is and how easy it is for Anne to mobilize may influence how much she drinks. A commode may be necessary, especially whilst she is convalescing. Involving other health professionals, such as physiotherapists to help with mobility issues and occupational therapists to help with aids around the house, may enable Anne to manage.

The Nursing Associate can educate Anne about using gentle soaps with no perfume and cleaning front to back will help reduce irritation and bacteria. Promoting drinking and ensuring that it is easy to get to the toilet should help reduce the reoccurrence of a UTI. However, further investigations may be needed.

Renal calculi

Urinary stones are a cause of morbidity. They can cause pain and lead to other complications, such as urinary tract obstruction and infections. Urinary stones are also known as 'calculi' and can be found anywhere in the urinary system. Fig. 33.7 shows the ureters and their relationship to the kidneys and bladder.

Stone formation is more common in males than females and it is increasingly more common in the Western world. It is thought that diets high in refined carbohydrates, animal proteins and salt increase the development (McCann et al., 2014). Contributing factors include heredity, infection, metabolic disorders and urine stagnation. Most calculi (75%) are composed of calcium salts and the rest are formed from uric acid, struvite, urates or cystine (VanMeter & Hubert, 2014). The type of stone will influence the treatment and prevention of reoccurrence.

Signs and symptoms

The signs and symptoms include pain, nausea and vomiting, fever and haematuria. The location of the calculi influences the type of pain and the volume of pain. Bladder stones may not cause pain, whereas stones located within the ureters can cause severe intense pain known as renal colic. This can be debilitating and the patient may be unable to lie still. Sweating and rapid pulse linked to the intensity of the pain may be present.

UTI may be an early sign of stone formation and recurrent infections would need investigating.

Diagnosis

If a patient presents with suspected renal stones, investigations undertaken include:
- Urine dipstick: checking for blood, glucose and protein
- Urine sample (midstream): for culture and microscopy
- Bloods: electrolytes, urea, creatinine (estimated GFR) and calcium levels
- Ultrasound
- Computed tomography scan

Care and treatment

The Nursing Associate has a vital role to play in managing a patient who may present with renal stones, especially if renal colic is present. Pain is controlled through medication, such as an NSAID and possibly an opiate analgesic, and the severity of pain is identified through observation, discussion and using a pain score. Medication can also be given to relax the smooth muscles of the ureters, which will help with the pain (McCann et al., 2014).

> **❗ HOTSPOT**
>
> **Pain Assessment**
>
> A pain assessment can include asking the patient to rate their pain on a scale of 1 to 10, where 10 is the most severe and 1 is the least. This enables the Nursing Associate to identify if pain medication is working and whether an alternative or a further dose of medication is required (see also Chapter 28 of this text for further discussion of pain management).

To help with the excretion of small stones, it is important to promote increased fluid intake. Ensuring that the patient is well hydrated and has 2–2.5 L of fluid in a day will help with the passing of the stone. Dietary advice may be needed to prevent stones reoccurring or growing but this depends upon the stone analysis.

If the stone is unable to be passed, then other treatments include:
- Shock wave lithotripsy: this is where the stone is broken up with shock waves. It is then small enough to be excreted in the urine.
- Ureteroscopy: a small scope is inserted into the bladder and up through the ureters to look at the stones. It can also remove stones by capturing them.
- Stents can be inserted in the ureters to help with the excretion of the stone.
- Surgery may be the only option if the stone cannot be broken up or excreted.

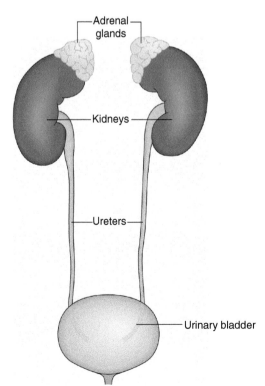

Fig. 33.7 The Ureters, Kidneys and Bladder (Waugh & Grant, 2018).

LOOKING BACK, FEEDING FORWARD

This chapter has outlined the anatomy and physiology of the urinary system, with an overview of the functions of the kidney and the importance of these functions. Some of the conditions that can affect the urinary system have been discussed. This gives the Nursing Associate opportunities to explore the diagnosis, signs and symptoms and the care and management associated with the illness.

REFERENCES

Bevan, M., 2016. Acute kidney injury. In: Clarke, D., Malecki-Ketchell, A. (Eds.), Nursing the Acutely Ill Adult, second ed. Palgrave, London.

Black, L.J., Seamans, K.M., Cashman, K.D., Kiely, M., 2012. An updated systematic review and meta-analysis of the efficacy of vitamin D food fortification. J. Nutr. 142 (6), 1102–1108.

Chalmers, C., 2013. Applied anatomy and physiology and the renal disease process. In: Thomas, N. (Ed.), Renal Nursing. John Wiley & Sons, Hoboken.

Connell, A., Laing, C., 2015. Acute kidney injury. Clin. Med. (Northfield Il) 15 (6), 581–584.

Francis, R. 2013. Report of the Mid Staffordshire NHS Foundation Trust Public Inquiry Volume 3: Present and future annexes. Available at https://assets.publishing.service.gov.uk/government/uploads/system/uploads/attachment_data/file/279121/0898_iii.pdf.

Gerhard, G., Windhager, E., Aronson, P., 2016. Organisation of the urinary system. In: Boron, W.F., Boulpaep, E.L. (Eds.), Medical Physiology E-Book. Elsevier. Available at: https://www.dawsonera.com:443/abstract/9781455733286.

Haddock, G., MacDonald, A., 2013. Managing simple lower UTI in women under 65. Practice Nursing 24 (6), 283–287.

Huether, S., 2012. Structure and function of the renal and urological systems. In: Huether, S., McCance, K. (Eds.), Understanding Pathophysiology, fifth ed. Elsevier Mosby, Missouri.

KDIGO, 2012. Kidney Disease Outcome Quality Initiative. KDIGO clinical practice guideline for acute kidney injury. Kidney Int. Suppl. 2 (1), 1–138.

KDIGO, 2013. Kidney Disease Outcome Quality Initiative. 2012 KDIGO clinical practice guideline for the evaluation and management of chronic kidney disease. Kidney Int. Suppl. 3 (1), 1–150.

Lecko, C. 2013. Patient safety and nutrition and hydration in the elderly. Available at http://patientsafety.health.org.uk/sites/default/files/resources/patient_safety_and_nutrition_and_hydration_in_the_elderly.pdf.

McCann, M., White, C., Fleur, L., 2014. Nursing care of conditions related to the urinary system. In: Brady, A., McCabe, C., McCann, M. (Eds.), Fundamentals of Medical-Surgical Nursing: A Systems Approach. John Wiley & Sons, Oxford.

Nair, M., 2017. The renal system and associated disorders. In: Peate, I. (Ed.), Fundamentals of Applied Pathophysiology: An Essential Guide for Nursing and Healthcare Students. John Wiley & Sons, Chichester.

NCEPOD, 2009. Acute kidney injury: adding insult to injury. In: NCEPOD (Series Ed.) National Confidential Enquiry into Patient Outcome and Death. http://www.ncepod.org.uk/2009report1/Downloads/AKI_report.pdf.

NICE, 2013a. National Institute for Health and Care Excellence. Acute kidney injury: prevention, detection and management (CG169). https://www.nice.org.uk/guidance/cg169/resources/acute-kidney-injury-prevention-detection-and-management-35109700165573.

NICE, 2013b. National Institute for Health and Care Excellence. Pyelonephritis. https://cks.nice.org.uk/pyelonephritis-acute#!scenario.

NICE, 2014. National Institute for Health and Care Excellence. Chronic kidney disease in adults: assessment and management (CG182). Available at https://www.nice.org.uk/guidance/cg182/resources/chronic-kidney-disease-in-adults-assessment-and-management-pdf-35109809343205.

Ostermann, M., Sprigings, D., 2018. Acute kidney injury. In: Sprigings, D., Chambers, J. (Eds.), Acute Medicine: A Practical Guide to the Management of Medical Emergencies, fifth ed. John Wiley & Sons, Chichester.

Porth, C.M., 2015. Essentials of Pathophysiology, fourth ed. Wolters Kluwer, Philadelphia.

Public Health England, 2017. Diagnosis of urinary tract infections (UTIs). Quick reference guide for primary care: For consultation and local adaptation. Available at https://assets.publishing.service.gov.uk/government/uploads/system/uploads/attachment_data/file/619772/Urinary_tract_infection_UTI_guidance.pdf.

Royal College of Physicians, 2015. Acute kidney injury and intravenous fluid therapy. Available at https://www.rcplondon.ac.uk/guidelines-policy/acute-care-toolkit-12-acute-kidney-injury-and-intravenous-fluid-therapy.

SIGN, 2008. Scottish Intercollegiate Guidelines Network. Diagnosis and management of chronic kidney disease. Available at http://www.sign.ac.uk/assets/sign103.pdf.

Thomas, N., 2013. Renal Nursing. John Wiley & Sons, Hoboken.

VanMeter, K., Hubert, R., 2014. Gould's Pathophysiology for the Health Professions, fifth ed. Elsevier, Missouri.

Waugh, A., Grant, A., 2018. Ross & Wilson Anatomy and Physiology in Health and Illness, thirteenth ed. Elsevier, Edinburgh.

Williams, P., 2018. De Wit's Fundamental Concepts and Skills for Nursing, fifth ed. Elsevier, St Louis.

Yaqoob, M., Ashman, N., 2017. Kidney and urinary tract disease. In: Kumar, P., Clark, M. (Eds.), Clinical Medicine, ninth ed. Elsevier, London.

34

Reproductive Disorders

Ian Peate

OBJECTIVES

By the end of the chapter the reader will:
1. Have an understanding of the anatomy and physiology of the male and female reproductive systems.
2. Discuss the pathophysiological changes associated with a selection of male and female reproductive disorders.
3. Understand the relationship between the reproductive systems and other body systems.
4. Outline the care required by men and women with reproductive disorders.
5. Describe some common conditions associated with the reproductive systems.
6. Review the role of the Nursing Associate in promoting health and well-being.

KEY WORDS

Sensitivity	Spermatogenesis	Breasts
Hormones	Oogenesis	STIs
Menopause	Infertility	
Infection	Dysfunction	

CHAPTER AIMS

This aim of this chapter is to provide the reader with an understanding of the skills, knowledge and attitude required to provide safe, effective and compassionate care to people with a reproductive disorder.

SELF TEST

1. What are the steroid hormones that control the expression and maintenance of male sexual characteristics?
2. What are the steroid hormones that control the development and maintenance of female sexual characteristics?
3. What is pelvic inflammatory disease?
4. What does cryptorchidism mean?
5. Discuss the menstrual cycle.
6. What is the most commonly diagnosed sexually transmitted infection in the UK?
7. What is the 'suckling reflex'?
8. What do you understand by 'safer sex'?
9. What is meant by the menarche?
10. How can paraphimosis be prevented?

INTRODUCTION

In this chapter, the male and female reproductive systems are considered. The first part discusses the anatomy and physiology of the male and female reproductive systems. It is important for the Nursing Associate to have a comprehensive understanding of the reproductive systems if the care provided is to be appropriate and effective.

The second part of the chapter addresses a selection of common conditions that impact on the health and well-being of men and women. The care and comfort of the patient who experiences a reproductive disorder are described. When offering care, the Nursing Associate is required to be kind and compassionate. Care provision can be intimate (this, for example, may include examination of the vagina and the testes) and may instil fear, apprehension and embarrassment in some people (for the patient and the Nursing Associate). When harm or damage occurs to the reproductive system, this can impact on a person's body image, identity, self-awareness, confidence and their ability to reproduce. Table 34.1 provides an overview of some reproductive disorders.

COMPASSIONATE CARE

The Nursing Associate must employ an open and nonjudgemental attitude to those they care for, maintaining confidentiality at all times. The role of the Nursing Associate is to offer support and reassurance; there is no place in a contemporary healthcare system for judgemental attitudes. Rassool (2015) points out how important it is to have an understanding of spiritual and cultural values when offering care; this applies to all aspects of care provision,

TABLE 34.1.	Some Reproductive Disorders
Tumours	Testicular cancers
	Prostate cancer
	Benign prostatic hypertrophy
	Breast cancer
	Uterine cancers (endometrial, cervical)
	Fibroids (leiomyomas)
Infection and inflammatory conditions	Orchitis
	Epididymitis
	Prostatitis
	Phimosis
	Oophoritis
	Salpingitis
	Pelvic inflammatory disease
	Vaginitis
	Sexually transmitted infections
Trauma	Inguinal hernia
	Testicular torsion
	Penile injury
Congenital disorders	Cryptorchidism
	Imperforate hymen
Ovarian/uterine-associated disorders	Endometriosis
	Amenorrhoea
	Premenstrual syndrome
	Dysmenorrhoea

TABLE 34.2.	Benchmarks for Respect and Dignity	
Factor	**Best practice**	
Attitudes and behaviours	People and carers feel that they matter all of the time	
Personal world and personal identity	Patients experience care in an environment that actively encompasses individual values, beliefs and personal relationships	
Personal boundaries and space	People's personal space is protected by staff	
Communication	People and carers experience communication with staff, which respects their individuality	
Privacy – confidentiality	People experience care that maintains their confidentiality	
Privacy, dignity and modesty	People's care ensures their privacy and dignity and protects their modesty	
Privacy – private area	People and carers can access an area that safely provides privacy	

(Department of Health, 2010.)

including care related to those who may have a disorder of the reproductive system. The Nursing Associate must be aware of the need to promote modesty and privacy, employ appropriate use of touch and maintain confidentiality. When the Nursing Associate does this, then she/he is going some way to providing culturally competent care. Table 34.2 outlines the Essence of Care Benchmark for Privacy and Dignity (Department of Health, 2010); these factors are particularly important when caring for people with disorders of the reproductive system.

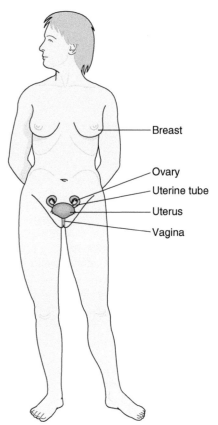

Fig. 34.1 The Female Reproductive Organs (Waugh & Grant, 2018).

THE FEMALE REPRODUCTIVE SYSTEM

The female reproductive system can be divided into internal and external genitalia. See Fig. 34.1 for the female reproductive organs.

The reproductive system interacts with nearly every other body system for the purpose of reproduction. The internal genitalia are:
- Vagina
- Uterus (womb)
- Ovaries
- Fallopian tubes (uterine tubes)
- Cervix

See Fig. 34.2 for the internal female reproductive organs and their associated structures.

The internal genitalia
The vagina
The vagina is an elastic, muscular tube. It is the area between the lower part of the uterus (the cervix) and the outside of the body. The vagina receives the penis during sexual intercourse (coitus). It is also a passageway for childbirth and serves as a channel for menstrual flow from the uterus.

The vagina is approximately 7.5–10 cm long. The walls of the vagina are usually in a relaxed state, they touch each other and contain many folds (these are called rugae). During sexual intercourse, the vagina opens and expands. The vagina will stretch during childbirth to facilitate delivery of the baby.

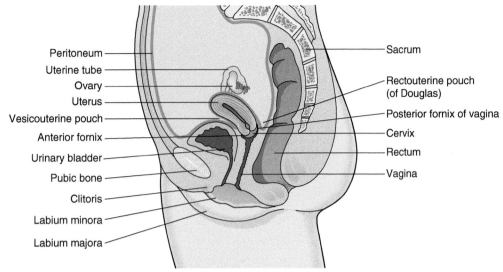

Fig. 34.2 Internal Female Reproductive Organs and Their Associated Structures (Waugh & Grant, 2018).

The vagina is made up of tissue layers. These include the following:
- The epithelial tissue layer: a thin layer of tissue made up of the squamous cells lining the vaginal walls
- The connective tissue layer: a layer underneath the epithelium, made of fibrous tissue with muscle, lymph vessels and nerves.

The surface of the vagina is kept lubricated by small cervical glands secreting mucus. Bacteria is produced between puberty and menopause, keeping the pH of the vagina between 3.5 and 4.9 (this is acidic), helping to inhibit the growth of a number of microorganisms that may enter the vagina.

The hymen is a thin membrane of tissue, partially occluding the vaginal opening. The hymen may be torn or ruptured by sexual activity, the insertion of a tampon, exercise or child birth.

The uterus

The uterus is responsible for a number of reproductive functions, including menses, implantation of the ova, gestation, labour and delivery. It receives a fertilized egg, protects the fetus as it grows and develops, and contracts to push the baby out of the woman's body during birth. It is a hollow, muscular pear-shaped organ, with two parts:
- The cervix, the lower part that opens into the vagina
- The main body of the uterus, known as the corpus

The corpus easily expands to hold a developing baby. A channel through the cervix permits sperm to enter and menstrual blood to exit. It is located above the vagina, between the bladder and rectum, and is about 7 cm long and 5 cm across at the widest point. The uterus is held in place within the pelvis by a number of ligaments; it has three parts:
- The fundus at the top of the uterus
- The body (the main part of the uterus), including the uterine cavity
- The cervix is the lower, narrow part of the uterus.

The walls of the uterus have three layers of tissue:
- Endometrium: the inner layer lining the uterus, made up of glandular cells producing secretions. This is the most active layer, responding to ovarian hormone changes

- Myometrium: the middle and thickest layer, made up mainly of smooth muscle
- Perimetrium: the outer serous layer, which secretes a lubricating fluid helping to reduce friction. This is also part of the peritoneum, covering some of the organs of the pelvis.

Fig. 34.3 shows the three layers of the uterus.

The fallopian tubes

These narrow tubes are attached (bilaterally) to the upper part of the uterus (also known as the uterine tubes); each uterine tube is approximately 10 cm in length and 1 cm in diameter. They serve as channels for the ova to travel from the ovaries to the uterus each month. The fertilization of an ovum by a sperm (conception) usually occurs in the uterine tubes. The fertilized ovum is propelled to the uterus, where it is implanted into the lining of the endometrium.

A uterine tube is made up of three parts:
- The first segment, closest to the uterus, is called the isthmus.
- The second segment is the ampulla, becoming more dilated in diameter. It is the most common site for fertilization.
- The final segment, located farthest from the uterus, is the infundibulum. The infundibulum gives rise to the fimbriae: finger-like projections responsible for picking up the egg released by the ovary.

Fig. 34.4 depicts the various parts of the uterine tubes.

The ovaries

These are small, oval-shaped glands, located on either side of the uterus. Also known as the female gonads, they are 2.5–3.5 cm long and 2 cm wide. The ovaries produce ova (an ovum is one egg and ova means multiple eggs), as well as the sex hormones. It is the ovaries that also produce the main female sex hormones released into the bloodstream. There are two ovaries, one on either side of the body. Each month an ovum is produced in women of childbearing age. In Fig. 34.5, a section of an ovary shows the stages of development of one ovarian follicle.

Women are able to have children between puberty (when the periods start, called the menarche) and the menopause (when

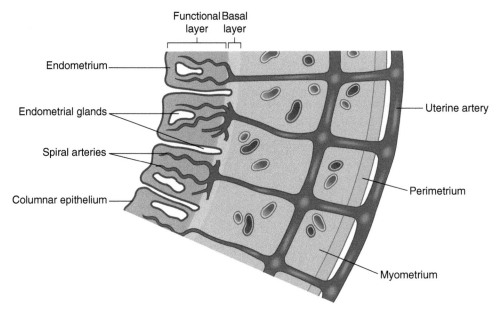

Fig. 34.3 The Three Layers of the Uterus (Waugh & Grant, 2018).

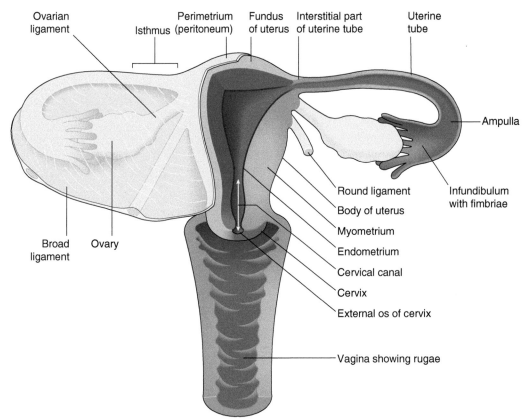

Fig. 34.4 The Female Reproductive Organs, Including Detail of the Uterine Tubes (Waugh & Grant, 2018).

the periods stop, sometimes called 'the change'). The age of the woman when menarche begins and the menopause starts varies a great deal. During the middle of each menstrual cycle (the midway point between periods), an ovum will travel down one of the fallopian tubes into the uterus (womb). The lining of the uterus (the endometrium) becomes thicker and thicker as blood vessels grow throughout the endometrium. At this point, the endometrium is now ready to receive the fertilized ovum. If the ovum does not become fertilized by sperm, the thickened endometrium that lines the uterus is shed as a period. Then the whole cycle begins again.

Ovarian hormones. Activity of the female reproductive system is controlled by hormones released by the brain and the ovaries. The combination of all these hormones gives women their

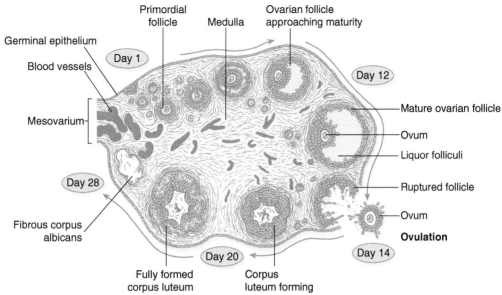

Fig. 34.5 Section of an Ovary Showing Stages of Development of One Ovarian Follicle (Waugh & Grant, 2018).

TABLE 34.3.	Hormones that Control the Reproductive Cycle	
Name of hormone	**Where produced**	**Role**
Gonadotrophin-releasing hormone (GnRH)	Made by a part of the brain called the hypothalamus	GnRH travels to another part of the brain where it controls the release of FSH and LH.
Follicle stimulating hormone (FSH)	Released by a part of the brain called the anterior pituitary	FSH is carried by the bloodstream to the ovaries. Here it stimulates the immature ova to start growing.
Luteinizing hormone (LH)	LH is also released by the anterior pituitary and travels to the ovaries	LH triggers ovulation and encourages the formation of a special group of cells called the corpus luteum.
Oestrogen	Produced in the ovaries by the growing ova and by the corpus luteum	In moderate amounts, oestrogen helps to control the levels of GnRH, FSH and LH. This helps to prevent the development of too many ova. Oestrogen also helps to develop and maintain many of the female reproductive structures.
Progesterone	Mainly released by the corpus luteum in the ovary	Works with oestrogen; progesterone thickens the endometrium ready for the implantation of a fertilized ovum. Progesterone also helps to prepare the breasts for releasing milk. High levels of progesterone will control the levels of GnRH, FSH and LH.

(Data from Waugh and Grant, 2018.)

reproductive cycle. Hormones produced by the ovaries are the female sex hormones:

- Oestrogen
- Progesterone.

These hormones are produced throughout the years when a woman can become pregnant. As a woman ages and gets closer to the menopause, the ovaries produce less and less of these hormones; eventually, the periods will stop.

A small amount of the male sex hormone testosterone is also produced by the ovaries; the role of testosterone in a woman is not fully understood. It is thought it helps with bone and muscle strength; it could have a role to play in a woman's sex drive (libido). Five main hormones control the reproductive cycle: three are produced in the brain, the other two are made in the ovaries (oestrogen and progesterone; Table 34.3).

> **! HOTSPOT**
>
> Many women will notice changes in their vagina and genital area after the menopause. These changes may include dryness and discomfort during sex. These can all usually be improved with treatment. Treatment options include hormone replacement therapy, oestrogen cream, vaginal tablets and lubricating gels.

THE EXTERNAL GENITALIA

The external genitalia are also known collectively as the vulva, and include:

- Labia majora and minora
- Mons pubis

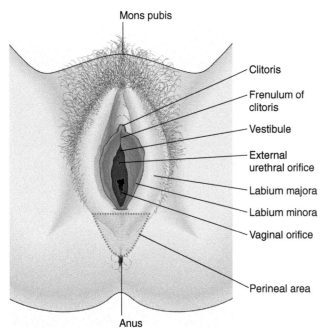

Fig. 34.6 External Female Genitalia (Waugh & Grant, 2018).

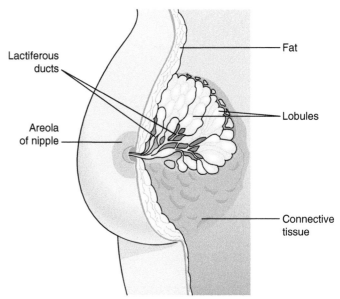

Fig. 34.7 The Breast (Waugh & Grant, 2018).

- Vaginal meatus (opening)
- Urethral meatus
- Clitoris
- Bartholin's glands.

See Fig. 34.6 for the external female genitalia.

Labia majora and minora

These are large, fleshy folds of tissue, enclosing and protecting the other external genital organs. They are analogous to the scrotum in males. The labia majora contain sweat and sebaceous glands, producing lubricating secretions.

The labia minora can be very small or up to 2.5 cm wide and lie just inside the labia majora, surrounding the openings to the vagina and urethra. A rich supply of blood vessels gives the labia minora a pink colour. During sexual stimulation, these blood vessels become engorged with blood, causing the labia minora to swell and become more sensitive to stimulation.

The mons pubis

Sometimes called the mons veneris, it is a rounded fatty bulge above the labia, covered with hair after puberty. It covers the pubic bone, acting as a cushion or pad providing protection to the pubic bone. The mons pubis contains sebaceous (oil-secreting) glands that release substances that are involved in sexual attraction; these are called pheromones.

The clitoris

A small projection of erectile tissue located at the top of the labia, usually 1–2 cm in length, but size can vary. It contains thousands of nerve endings, making it an extremely sensitive organ. During sexual excitement it becomes full of blood (the clitoris is analogous to the penis). The clitoris is very sensitive and is the main source of female sexual pleasure.

Bartholin's glands

These are the vestibular glands, about the size of a pea. The two glands are located on either side of the opening of the vagina. Their primary function is to produce a sticky substance to lubricate the vagina for sexual intercourse.

The female breast

In the female, these are classed as accessory glands. Women's breasts are milk-producing, pear-shaped glands, composed of fat, connective tissue and gland tissue divided into lobes. They contain no muscle. A network of ducts spreads from the lobes towards the nipple (Fig. 34.7).

It is usual for one breast to be smaller than the other. Younger women have more glandular tissue than fat in their breasts, making the breasts dense. After the menopause, the glandular tissue is gradually replaced by fat, which is less dense.

There is a network of lymph nodes located close to the breast, part of the lymphatic system running throughout the body. Lymph nodes and lymph vessels contain lymph that flows through the lymphatic system. Lymph collects waste products and drains into the veins for waste removal. The lymph glands in the axilla are known as the axillary lymph glands. There is also a chain of lymph nodes running up the centre of the chest, close to the sternum (breastbone), called the internal mammary chain.

> ### ❗ HOTSPOT
>
> If a person decides to get part(s) of the body pierced, the Nursing Associate should encourage the person to go to a licensed body-piercing shop or piercer. As with all body art, infection is a risk. To reduce these risks, take advice from the piercer or body artist regarding aftercare.
>
> Piercing is a fairly safe procedure, as long as it is carried out by a licensed practitioner and the person takes care to avoid infection. Healing times for piercing will vary with the type and position of the piercing and vary from person to person. For the first few weeks, it is normal for the area to be red, tender and swollen.

The healing time for a genital piercing can be from 2 to 12 weeks. Remember, these times are approximate and will depend on how healthy the person is and if they look after the piercing properly until healed.

To reduce the risk of a piercing becoming infected, good hygiene is important. Hands should always be washed and dried thoroughly before touching the area around the piercing. The person should avoid fiddling with the area and should not turn the piercing. If a crust develops over the piercing, this should not be removed as it is the body's way of protecting the piercing.

The piercing may bleed when first done, and it may bleed for short periods over a few days afterwards. It may also be tender, itchy and bruised for a few weeks.

THE MALE REPRODUCTIVE SYSTEM

The function of this system is to produce sperm and transfer them to the female reproductive tract; it is a network of external and internal organs, functioning to produce, support, transport and deliver viable sperm for reproduction. Sperm is produced in the testes, transported through the epididymis, ductus deferens, ejaculatory duct and urethra. The seminal vesicles, prostate gland and bulbourethral gland produce seminal fluid, accompanying and nourishing the sperm as it is discharged from the penis during ejaculation and throughout the fertilization process. The male reproductive organs and associated structure are highlighted in Fig. 34.8.

The scrotum

The scrotum is a skin-covered, highly pigmented, muscular sack, extending from the body behind the penis. This location is important with regards to sperm production within the testes; sperm production is more effective when the testes are kept 2°C to 4°C below core body temperature.

Within the subcutaneous muscle layer of the scrotum is the dartos muscle, which continues internally, making up the scrotal septum. Two cremaster muscles descend from the internal oblique muscle of the abdominal wall, covering each teste like a muscular net. The dartos and cremaster muscles contract simultaneously, elevating the testes, for example in cold weather, moving the testes closer to the body and decreasing the surface area of the scrotum in order to retain heat. As the environmental temperature increases, the scrotum relaxes and the testes descend, scrotal surface area increases and heat loss is promoted.

The testes

The testes are necessary components in sperm production, producing sperm and androgens (the male reproductive hormones). The most important male androgen is testosterone. There are several accessory organs and ducts assisting in the process of sperm maturation and transportation of the sperm, as well as other seminal components to the penis. The penis delivers sperm to the female reproductive tract.

The testes (the male gonads) are paired oval structures, approximately 4–5 cm long located in the scrotum, surrounded by two layers of protective connective tissue. The tunica vaginalis is an outer serous membrane with a parietal and a thin visceral layer. The tunica albuginea is beneath the tunica vaginalis, covering the teste. The tunica albuginea also invaginates to form septa, dividing the teste into 300 to 400 structures: the lobules. Within the lobules, sperm develop in the seminiferous tubules (Figs 34.9 and 34.10).

Sperm

Sperm (spermatozoa) are smaller than the majority of cells. The male produces around 100–300 million daily after puberty, continuing throughout life, as opposed to the female who produces no gametes after birth. A mature sperm is composed of a head, midpiece and tail region (Fig. 34.11). The tail of the sperm is used for motility.

Epididymis and duct system

From the seminiferous tubules, immotile sperm are surrounded by testicular fluid moving to the epididymis, which is a tightly coiled tube, approximately 6 m in length, where the newly formed sperm continue to mature (see Fig. 34.10). Sperm is moved along

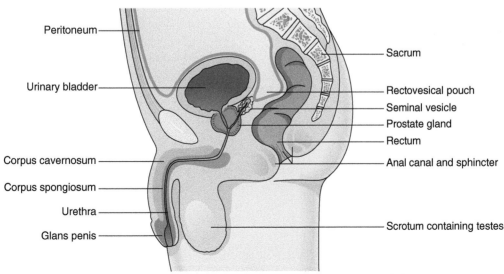

Fig. 34.8 The Male Reproductive Organs and Related Structures (Waugh & Grant, 2018).

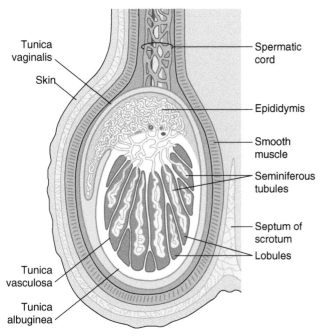

Fig. 34.9 Section of a Testis (Waugh & Grant, 2018).

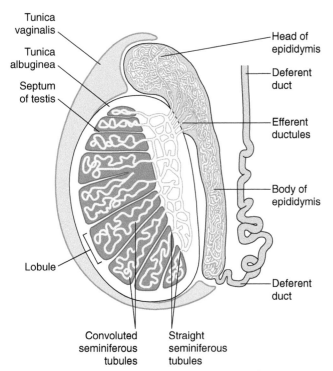

Fig. 34.10 A Longitudinal Section of a Testis (Waugh & Grant, 2018).

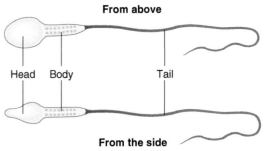

Fig. 34.11 A Spermatozoon (Waugh & Grant, 2018).

> **! HOTSPOT**
>
> Vasectomy (male sterilization) is not the right operation for all men and it is a decision that the man should not make lightly. He should be encouraged to consider all options and discuss things fully with the practice nurse, GP, surgeon and (if appropriate) his family.

From each epididymis, each ductus deferens extends into the abdominal cavity through the inguinal canal in the abdomen. Here, it continues to the pelvic cavity, ending towards the back (posterior) of the urinary bladder.

Only 5% of the final volume of semen is made up by sperm (semen is the thick, milky fluid the man ejaculates). There are three essential accessory glands of the male reproductive system that produce the bulk of semen:
- The seminal vesicles
- The prostate
- The bulbourethral glands.

Fig. 34.12 depicts the route taken by spermatozoa during ejaculation.

Seminal vesicles

As sperm pass through the ductus deferens at ejaculation, they mix with fluid from the seminal vesicle. Seminal vesicles are glands contributing to around 60% of the semen volume. Seminal vesicle fluid is made up of large amounts of fructose, used by the sperm to allow movement through the female reproductive tract.

The fluid, which is now made up of sperm as well as seminal vesicle secretions, moves into the associated ejaculatory duct. The paired ejaculatory ducts move the seminal fluid into the next structure: the prostate gland.

Prostate gland

The prostate gland is centrally located towards the front of the rectum, at the base of the bladder, surrounded by the prostatic urethra. Fig. 34.13 provides an illustration of a section of the prostate gland and the associated reproductive structures.

The prostate gland is around the size of a walnut and is made up of muscular and glandular tissues. It adds an alkaline, milky fluid to the seminal fluid, which has now become semen. During puberty, the prostate gland usually doubles in size, weighing around 8 g. By the age of 60 years, approximately 40% of men have some degree of prostate enlargement (benign prostatic

the length of the epididymis, further maturing and acquiring the ability to move. Once inside the female reproductive tract, sperm use this ability to mobilize independently toward the unfertilized egg.

During ejaculation, sperm exit the tail of the epididymis and are propelled (by the peristaltic action) to the ductus deferens (also known as the vas deferens). This is a thick, muscular tube bundled together inside the spermatic cord.

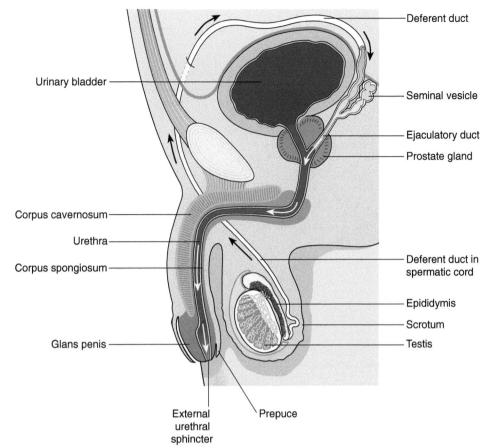

Fig. 34.12 The Route Taken by Spermatozoa During Ejaculation, Indicated by Arrows (Waugh & Grant, 2018).

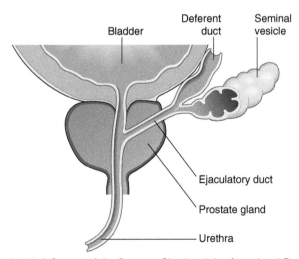

Fig. 34.13 A Section of the Prostate Gland and the Associated Reproductive Structures (Waugh & Grant, 2018).

hypertrophy) and the gland can weigh up to 40 g; by 80 years, most men will have prostatic enlargement.

Bulbourethral glands

The paired bulbourethral glands (Cowper's glands) make the final addition to the semen. These glands release a thick, salty fluid, lubricating the end of the urethra and (during coitus) the vagina. These accessory glands release the fluid when the male becomes sexually aroused, shortly before semen is released; this is pre-ejaculate.

The penis

The penis is the male organ of copulation and is flaccid for non-sexual actions, such as urination via the urethra. When erect, the stiffness of the organ allows it to penetrate into the vagina, depositing semen. The penis has a shaft and root (Fig. 34.14).

The shaft surrounds the urethra and is composed of three chambers of erectile tissue spanning the length of the shaft. The two larger chambers on either side (laterally) are the corpora cavernosa. The corpus spongiosum is a smaller chamber surrounding the spongy, or penile, urethra and can be felt as a raised ridge on the erect penis (Fig. 34.15).

At the end of the penis is the sensitive glans penis. The skin from the shaft extends down over the glans, forming a collar known as the foreskin or prepuce in those men who have not been circumcised.

Vasocongestion, or engorgement of the tissues (often due to sexual arousal), causes arterial blood to flow into the penis, resulting in reduction in the amount of blood leaving the penis via the veins, causing erection. During sexual arousal, nitric oxide is released from nerve endings close to blood vessels within the corpora cavernosa and spongiosum, usually resulting in relaxation of the smooth muscles surrounding the penile arteries, causing them to dilate. The rapid increase in blood volume fills

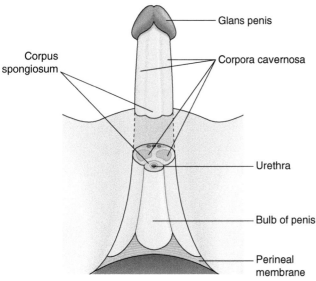

Fig. 34.14 The Penis (Waugh & Grant, 2018).

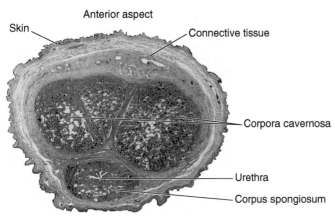

Fig. 34.15 Transverse Section of the Penis (Waugh & Grant, 2018).

the erectile chambers and the increased pressure of the filled chambers compresses the thin-walled penile venules, preventing venous drainage of the penis. This usually leads to erection.

FEMALE REPRODUCTIVE DISORDERS

Women's health

An understanding of the anatomy of the female reproductive system will help you in ensuring that the women you offer care and support to will receive care that is safe and provided in a woman-centred way. As well as having an understanding of the structure of the female reproductive system, the Nursing Associate needs to ensure that the care provided is compassionate, caring and competent. This requires the Nursing Associate to use their interpersonal skills when caring for women and (if appropriate) their families, as well as anyone advocating on behalf of the woman.

Women who require care come from across the lifespan, with concerns regarding a wide range of health issues from adolescence to old age. The Nursing Associate must aim to be as inclusive

as possible, whilst offering care and support as they work collaboratively with the woman, as well as the wider health and social care team. Recognizing and respecting the diversity of needs results in care provision that is of a high quality and humanistic, as well as empowering women from a number of perspectives, for example, in being able to access the best available and most appropriate care.

Endometriosis

Endometriosis is a very common condition, the pathogenesis of which is unknown (Hickey et al., 2014), and currently there is no cure. Endometriosis is defined as the presence of endometrial-like tissue outside the uterus, often in the pelvis and around the uterus, ovaries and fallopian tubes. It usually affects women during their reproductive years and all social ethnic groups can be affected. It is rare to find the condition in girls who have not experienced the menses. The condition is not an infection; it is not transmissible nor is it cancer.

Endometriosis causes a chronic, inflammatory reaction that can be debilitating (Royal College of Nursing, 2015; Dunselman et al., 2014). Some women with endometriosis may experience painful symptoms and/or infertility, whilst others have no symptoms.

The exact prevalence of endometriosis is not known; estimates range from between 2% and 10% of the general female population but up to 50% in infertile women. Endometriosis is the second most common gynaecological condition; approximately 1.5 million women in the UK have endometriosis (Endometriosis UK, 2017).

Box 34.1 provides facts and information related to endometriosis.

Signs and symptoms

The tissue responds to the hormonal cycle (the menses), but instead of being shed, the tissue remains within the body where it may bleed, resulting in lesions, cysts and adhesions (scar tissues) (de Wit et al., 2017). This then leads to:

- Inflammation.
- Chronic severe pain that may be cyclical, usually before or during menstruation. Pain may be lower abdominal or back pain.
- Dysmenorrhoea (including heavy menstrual bleeding).
- Dyspareunia (painful sexual intercourse).
- Infertility.
- Rectal pain (there may be bleeding and/or dyschezia).
- Bladder problems.

Often, the location of symptoms will depend on the location of the disease. The woman may feel lethargic and if there is excessive bleeding, there may be evidence of anaemia.

REFLECTION 34.1

Think about the activities of living (Roper et al., 2000) and how having endometriosis might impact on a woman's ability to perform these activities independently. How might the Nursing Associate and other health and care agencies help the woman (and her family) if she is unable to perform the activities independently?

Also give consideration to the five influencing factors and how these may be implicated:

1. Physical
2. Psychological
3. Environmental
4. Sociocultural
5. Politico-economic

Diagnosis

Making a diagnosis can be difficult. It takes on average 7.5 years to make a diagnosis. Endometriosis UK (2011) undertook an endometriosis diagnosis survey, a summary of which can be found in Box 34.2.

Diagnosis is based on the history the woman offers, symptoms and signs. The diagnosis is confirmed by physical examination and imaging techniques (such as transvaginal sonography, magnetic resonance imaging [MRI]) and finally proven by histology of either a directly biopsied vaginal lesion, from a scar, or of tissue collected during laparoscopy (European Society of Human Reproduction and Embryology, 2013). Laparoscopy and the histological confirmation of endometrial glands is the best way to make a diagnosis of the condition.

BOX 34.2 The Summary Findings for the Endometriosis Diagnosis Survey

- On average, it takes over 7.5 years to diagnose endometriosis.
- Women wait nearly 2 years before visiting their GP about their symptoms.
- GPs then take on average 4 years to refer the patient to a specialist.
- It then takes a further 1 year 9 months to get a formal diagnosis.
- Over 50% of participants waited more than 6 years for a diagnosis.
- Less than 20% of those who responded received a diagnosis within 2 years.
- One-third of respondents waited at least 10 years, and 15% waited for over 15 years, to be diagnosed.

(Endometriosis UK, 2011.)

CRITICAL AWARENESS

On clinical examination, with regards to endometriosis, a vaginal examination should not be performed as it can cause pain and discomfort. Rectal examination may assist in making a diagnosis.

Care and treatment

Treatment will depend on the severity of symptoms, reproductive plans and medical history. It must be remembered that endometriosis is a chronic and incurable condition. Treatment aims to offer relief of pain symptoms and often symptoms recur after therapy is discontinued. Medical treatments reduce pain by suppressing the endometriosis and surgical intervention aims to eliminate endometriotic lesions, divide adhesions and interrupt nerve pathways.

Medical treatment

If endometriosis is suspected, this can be managed in a primary care setting. Referral to a gynaecologist or a specialist endometriosis centre should be considered, particularly in severe cases of pain or if a woman is presenting with issues regarding her fertility.

Analgesia will be required to help relieve pain. This must be based on the woman's need, for example, simple or nonsteroidal anti-inflammatory drugs can be used in combination and, especially around the time of the period, these are first-line treatments.

There are a number of other approaches to pain relief that the Nursing Associate should be aware of (see Table 34.4).

CRITICAL AWARENESS

The Nursing Associate must ensure that the woman is made aware of the potential dangers of using a hot water bottle and the application of heat directly onto skin. An assessment of need must be carried out.

TABLE 34.4. Some Pain-Relieving Modalities

Modality	Comment
Physiotherapy	Exercise and relaxation techniques strengthen pelvic floor muscles, reduce pain and manage stress and anxiety. Physiotherapy may also be required postoperatively as rehabilitation. A physiotherapist can develop a programme based on the woman's individual needs.
Heat and comfort	A hot water bottle or hot bath can help some women in relieving pain.
Pain modifiers	Pain modifiers work by altering perception of the pain.
	An antidepressant (e.g., amitriptyline) has an impact on the nervous system and how the body manages pain.
Transcutaneous electrical nerve stimulators (TENS)	TENS machines are an alternative to pain killers. Electrodes are attached to the skin, sending electrical pulses into the body. They work by blocking the pain messages as they travel through the nerves or by helping the body produce endorphins (natural pain-fighters).

THE MEDICINE TROLLEY 34.1

Drug	Drug classification	Reason for administration	Route of administration	Dose	Side effects	Contra-indications	Nursing care
Naproxen	Non-steroidal anti-inflammatory (NSAID)	Pain relief	Oral	500 mg initially, then 250 mg every 6–8 hours as required; maximum dose after first day: 1.25 g daily	Gastrointestinal disturbances, including discomfort, nausea, diarrhoea and occasionally bleeding and ulceration occur NSAIDs should be used with caution during breastfeeding	Should be avoided in the elderly and those with renal or cardiac impairment Caution with those who have shown hypersensitivity to NSAIDs previously Active or bleeding peptic ulcer	Seek consent prior to administration Explain the use of the drug to the patient, respond to any questions Use lowest effective dose for shortest duration needed to control symptoms Regular medical supervision to monitor for adverse events. Taking with milk or food may reduce gastrointestinal irritation

THE MEDICINE TROLLEY 34.2

Drug	Drug classification	Reason for administration	Route of administration	Dose	Side effects	Contra-indications	Nursing care
Amitriptyline	Tricyclic antidepressant	To treat neuropathic pain	Oral	Initially 10 mg daily at night, gradually increased if necessary to 75 mg daily	Can cause cardiac arrhythmias Abdominal pain, stomatitis, palpitation, oedema, hypertension, restlessness, fatigue, mydriasis and increased intraocular pressure Anxiety, dizziness, agitation, confusion, sleep disturbances, irritability, drowsiness	Contra-indicated in the immediate recovery period after myocardial infarction, in arrhythmias	Seek consent prior to drug administration Explain the use of the drug to the patient, respond to any questions Advise not to drink alcohol with this drug May impair alertness. Instruct not to drive or operate machinery

It should always be remembered that the woman may have her own methods of relieving her pain, and these methods should be respected. The role of the Nursing Associate is to assist the woman in managing her pain.

As endometriosis responds and grows when it is exposed to the hormone oestrogen, hormone treatments that block or reduce the production of oestrogen in the body may assist. The use of oestrogen therapy means the endometriosis will be unable to continue growing and, in so doing, can help to alleviate symptoms.

Any treatment decisions must be made in consultation with the woman. She should be provided with information in a format that is acceptable to her, to help make an informed choice. Time should be provided during a consultation to answer any questions the woman may have regarding the various options. See Table 34.5 for some medical treatment options.

Surgical intervention

Just as there are several medical approaches to the care and treatment of the woman with endometriosis, this is also the case when surgery is indicated (Cotton & Steggle, 2011). Surgical treatment is carried out in the secondary care setting (i.e. the hospital).

Laparoscopy is often used as a diagnostic tool but it can also be used as a surgical procedure to remove the endometriosis; this is referred to as 'minimal access surgery' (Cotton & Steggle, 2011). Surgery can be used as a treatment for endometriosis as it can help in alleviating pain by removing the endometriosis, dividing adhesions or removing any cysts.

Laparoscopy. Laparoscopy is only one type of surgery, aiming to remove or destroy the endometrial deposits. The surgeon can cut out the endometriosis (excision) or destroy it using heat or

TABLE 34.5. Medical Options Available for Women with Endometriosis

Option	Comments
Oral hormone treatments	This is the combined oral contraceptive pill, which contains a mixture of oestrogen and progesterone, suppressing ovulation and affecting the production of female hormones in the ovary. Causes the endometrium to become thinner and menstruation becomes shorter, reducing the symptoms associated with endometriosis.
Intrauterine hormones	The coil: can provide relief from pain and is also a long-term treatment. The Mirena coil is a small plastic T-shaped intrauterine device. It contains progestogen (progesterone-like substance) that is released into the uterus over a period of 5 years.
Progesterones	Thought to relieve the symptoms of endometriosis as they suppress the growth of endometriosis deposits; may also reduce endometriosis-induced inflammation. During treatment, a woman will stop ovulating and menstruating. Drugs containing progesterones that are typically used to treat endometriosis are usually taken orally, for example, medroxyprogesterone (Provera), norethisterone (Primolut). Depo-Provera (medroxyprogesterone) is injected as opposed to taken orally.

(Endometriosis UK, 2011; Royal College of Nursing, 2015.)

TABLE 34.6. Hysterectomy and Oophorectomy

Type of surgery	Description
Hysterectomy	Removal of the uterus, performed under a general anaesthetic. The ovaries can be left in place or may also be removed. If the ovaries are left in situ, then the possibility of endometriosis returning is increased. The ovaries may need to be removed in another operation at another time. If the cervix is removed, it is total hysterectomy; if it remains, then it is a subtotal hysterectomy. Abdominal hysterectomy: when the uterus is removed through an abdominal incision. Vaginal hysterectomy: when the uterus and cervix are removed via the vagina (there is no abdominal incision). Laparoscopic hysterectomy: when a laparoscope (a camera) is inserted into a small cut in or near the umbilicus; it will enable the surgeon to see inside and laparoscopically perform the procedure. The uterus, and sometimes the ovaries, are freed and (along with the cervix) are removed through the vagina.
Oophorectomy	Removal of the ovaries; bilateral oophorectomy refers to the removal of both ovaries, unilateral refers to the removal of one ovary. An instant and irreversible menopause occurs when a bilateral oophorectomy is performed.

(Endometriosis UK, 2011; de Wit et al, 2017.)

laser (ablation). Electrocoagulation/diathermy can destroy the endometriosis through application of heat. Surgery has the potential to provide relief from symptoms, however they can recur. Laparoscopic surgery for endometriosis is often performed as a day case.

Complex surgery. Depending on the severity of the endometriosis, there may be a need for the woman to undergo more complex surgery that can involve other organs, for example, the bowel or the bladder. These types of surgery are often carried out using a laparoscopic approach.

Radical surgery. When a woman has not responded to medical treatment or the conservative surgical approach and she is not planning on starting a family, a more radical approach may be needed, for example, hysterectomy or oophorectomy (Table 34.6). There are many reasons why these procedures are considered; to proceed with either is a big decision as both are irreversible. The advantages and disadvantages of each type of surgery should be discussed in full with the woman.

! HOTSPOT

Hysterectomy is not the right operation for every woman and it is not a decision that the woman should make lightly. It is a huge decision to make. The woman does not have to do it all on her own, but it is her body and the final choice is hers. The Nursing Associate can act as the woman's advocate if required. The woman should be encouraged to consider all options and discuss things fully with the practice nurse, GP, gynaecologist and her family (if appropriate). It should be remembered that a hysterectomy is irreversible.

AT THE GP SURGERY

Practice nurses very often have a great degree of involvement in women's health. Much of this is in the areas of preventive medicine and also general health checks.

Practice nurses are able to highlight the benefit of routine screening programmes. They provide women with verbal and/or written information concerning health awareness (such as breast awareness/breast screening/cervical screening), explain what is normal and emphasize the importance of seeing a nurse or doctor early on if they notice or are concerned about any abnormality or change in their health and well-being. Opportunities can arise when women attend for cervical screening, contraception checks, sexually transmitted infection discussions, well woman checks and for other health and well-being related activities.

Fibroids

Another common gynaecological condition is fibroids (also known as uterine myomas, leiomyomas or leiomyomata) (NICE, 2015). Fibroids are benign tumours originating from smooth muscle of the uterus. They are the most common form of pelvic tumour, occurring in one of every four or five women over 35 years of age (Porth, 2015).

These benign tumours arise from anywhere within the myometrium of the uterus, developing in women of reproductive age; they do not occur in prepubescent girls. Fibroids are promoted and maintained by exposure to oestrogen and

TABLE 34.7.   Classification of Fibroids

Position	Description
Intramural (within the walls of the uterus)	Most are located intramurally, they usually present as an enlargement of the uterus.
Submucosal (under the mucosa)	These grow into the uterine cavity. They may be pedunculated (attached to a stalk or stem) and may protrude through the cervix. They displace endometrial tissue, and are more likely to cause bleeding and infection than the other types.
Subserosal (growing outside of the uterus)	Lying beneath the serous lining of the uterus, projecting into the peritoneal cavity. They may become pedunculated and displace or compress the ureter or bladder.

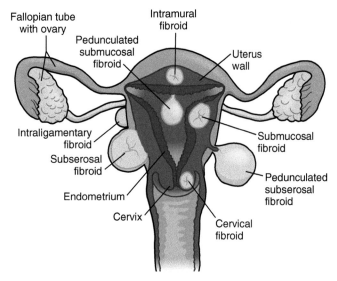

Fig. 34.16 Types of Fibroids.

progestogen; they cannot grow without the presence of these hormones. After puberty, the prevalence of fibroids progressively increases until the woman reaches menopause (Haney, 2008).

It is not known exactly why fibroids develop. The risk of fibroids is increased by early puberty, obesity and increasing age. Black women are more likely to develop fibroids than their white counterparts. In addition, they tend to occur at an earlier age, are larger and they are more likely to be symptomatic. The risk of fibroids is reduced by pregnancy and decreases with an increasing number of pregnancies; therefore women who have never been pregnant are more at risk.

Fibroids, often multiple, are classified according to their position within the uterine wall (Table 34.7 and Fig. 34.16).

CASE STUDY 34.1   Tamanqa

Tamanqa is a 42-year-old bank clerk. She has two children and is a single parent. She was diagnosed with an intramural, small fibroid 3 years ago, after being referred by her GP to a Consultant Nurse (gynaecology) who took a patient history, full blood count and performed an abdominal and transvaginal ultrasound. Tamanqa has been taking a range of prescribed pharmaceutical preparations to help manage her condition.

Tamanqa was experiencing stomach cramps and heavy periods and was originally prescribed tranexamic acid and the combined oral contraceptive pill. This was then changed to a levonorgestrel intrauterine system (a coil). Despite this, Tamanqa continued to have heavy bleeding and she was becoming very tired.

After consultation with the Consultant Nurse and being provided with information that would enable Tamanqa to make an informed decision, she decided to opt for a myomectomy. Tamanqa visited the gynaecologist who explained the various surgical options. Minimally invasive surgery (laparoscopic surgery) was deemed the most appropriate option. Tamanqa was sent an appointment for a preoperative assessment; she made an informed decision, consented to surgery and she was sent a date for surgery in 3 months as a day case.

CARE IN THE HOME SETTING

In Case Study 34.1, during Tamanqa's period of illness, arrangements were made at home for Tamanqa's sister and her mother to look after her children and to stay with Tamanqa for a few weeks after surgery so she could gently recover.

However, on the 4th day postoperatively, Tamanqa was feeling very warm and she appeared flushed. Jamillia, Tamanqa's sister, called the general practice and explained what was happening.

The general practice arranged for a community nurse to visit Tamanqa in her home. The community nurse undertook an assessment of Tamanqa's needs and found her to be pyrexial (37.8°C), tachycardic (98 beats per minute), respiratory rate of 18 breaths per minute and blood pressure 125/70 mm Hg. Tamanqa was flushed and warm to touch and felt pain in the abdomen. A wound swab was taken and sent for microbiological assessment. The multiple incision sites on the abdomen were assessed and they appeared swollen, red and inflamed, with some discharge from two of them. The community nurse made a diagnosis of wound infection and a course of antibiotics was commenced. The community nurse made subsequent visits to assess and evaluate the outcome of care, and was supportive of Tamanqa and her family.

Four weeks after the myomectomy, Tamanqa went to see the Occupational Health Nurse at her place of work and she is now on a phased return to work and is progressing well.

NURSING SKILLS

Taking a Wound Swab

Wound care is an important aspect of care provision; any wound will present risk to the patient. The Nursing Associate has to be knowledgeable about all elements of the wound healing process and be cognisant of the risk of infection and acute onset of deterioration.

The results from a wound swab can direct treatment; therefore, the Nursing Associate must be able to carry out the swabbing of a wound effectively, in a safe, compassionate and evidence-based manner.

The right specimen, taken using the correct method and supported by sound clinical information recorded on a microbiology request form, will mean the patient can receive the most appropriate treatment for the infection. Anything that falls short of this will mean that the person may receive inappropriate antibiotics for an incorrectly diagnosed infection.

The specimen should be obtained prior to dressing or any cleaning process of the wound. A sterile swab is used to gently collect exudate and the specimen is placed in the transport medium.

The Nursing Associate must seek consent from the patient to undertake the procedure, explain the reason for the test, what will happen to the specimen and when the results will be available.

Explain that the test is done when an infection is suspected. A wound swab can also help to decide which antibiotic, if required, will work best.

Explain that the test only lasts a few seconds.

Equipment needed:
- Gloves/apron
- Sampling material (swab attached to plastic stick in transport medium)
- Sterile saline
- Microbiology form (and attached bag)

Procedure

The procedure should be carried out in line with local policy and procedure.

1. Check patient identity, label the pot used for transporting the swab to the laboratory.
2. Ensure a good light source.
3. Ensure all equipment is gathered prior to carrying out the procedure.
4. Wash/decontaminate hands.
5. Don disposable gloves and apron.
6. Expose (and maintain dignity) the area to be swabbed.
7. Open sampling pack. Remove top of the transport medium and place the top upside down on a clean surface.
8. Moisten swab with sterile saline.
9. Do not permit any part of the swab to touch any surface except the wound.
10. Using a zig zag movement, swab the surface of the area of the wound, so that a sufficient amount of exudate is transported to the swab.
11. Place the swab into the special tube with the transport medium.
12. Redress wound as per care plan.
13. Ensure the patient is comfortable.
14. Remove gloves/apron.
15. Wash/decontaminate hands.
16. Dispose of packing and other equipment safely.
17. The specimen should be stored and transported according to local policy and procedure.
18. Document and record the procedure in the patient's notes.

Signs and symptoms of fibroids

The speed at which the fibroid grows varies; they may increase in size during pregnancy or with the use of oral contraceptives or hormone replacement therapy. Smaller fibroids may be asymptomatic; some women may have only one, others can have more. Fibroids usually cause symptoms if they impact on the function of the uterus, and they can disturb the menstrual cycle. With heavy menstrual bleeding, the woman may experience iron deficiency anaemia leading to fatigue, exhaustion and pallor.

The larger fibroid tumours can cause crowding of other organs, resulting in pelvic pressure, pain, dysmenorrhoea, menorrhagia and tiredness. Depending on the location and the size of the fibroid, there may be constipation and urinary urgency and frequency. Typical symptoms include:
- Severe or prolonged menstrual bleeding
- Severe, cramp and period-like pain
- Diffuse pain and tension in the lower abdomen

- Abdominal swelling
- Dyspareunia.

Diagnosis

The woman will be asked to give a history of her symptoms and what it is she is experiencing; a physical examination will be required. Sometimes a diagnosis is made incidentally, for example, if the woman is being investigated for another gynaecological condition. A pregnancy test may be indicated and a full blood count is taken to assess for iron deficiency anaemia, amongst other things.

Pelvic ultrasound may be performed to exclude other causes of a pelvic mass, to confirm the presence and size of a fibroid, as well as excluding possible complications, for example, urinary tract obstruction. A transvaginal ultrasound is a more accurate investigation as it can indicate the number of fibroids, shape, position and size. MRI may occasionally be required if ultrasound is not definitive. A laparoscopy may assist in diagnosis in visualizing subserosal fibroids.

Care and treatment

Fibroids only usually need to be treated if they are symptomatic or if causing symptoms that affect the woman's fertility or if they might cause problems during pregnancy. The choice of treatment must reflect the woman's needs, often dependent on whether the woman still wishes to have children. The severity of the symptoms and the size and position of the fibroids can also establish which treatments are an option.

The woman must be given time to make her decision. The Nursing Associate has a role to play in ensuring the woman has all the information she needs to help her come to a decision. Treatment options usually aim to achieve one or more of the following goals:
- Reduce menstrual bleeding
- Relieve pain, cramps and tension
- Help with difficulties in emptying the bladder and with digestion
- Preserve or improve fertility.

Pharmacological treatment. Moroni et al., (2014) discusses the use of pharmaceutical agents in the treatment of women with fibroids, emphasizing the need to ensure that each woman is assessed and treated as an individual. The larger the fibroid, the less effective a pharmaceutical approach will be.

The main hormone therapies used are hormonal contraceptives and hormones for relieving the symptoms of heavy menstrual bleeding, acting to prevent the production of oestrogens. See Table 34.8 for some pharmaceutical approaches.

> **! HOTSPOT**
>
> Osteoporosis (thinning of the bones) is an occasional side effect of taking gonadotrophin-releasing hormone (GnRH) agonists. The practice nurse can provide the woman with more information about this and it may be possible to prescribe additional medication to minimize the osteoporotic effect of this type of medication.
>
> A GnRH agonist is only prescribed on a short-term basis (a maximum of 6 months at a time).

TABLE 34.8. Some Pharmaceutical Treatments of Fibroids

Drug	Function
Non-steroidal anti-inflammatory agents (such as ibuprofen)	Can reduce menstrual blood loss when the cause is unknown.
Antifibrinolytic agents (i.e., tranexamic acid)	May also reduce menorrhagia.
Combined hormonal contraception (CHC)	CHC can help to shrink the fibroids, helpful if the patient requires contraception.
Levonorgestrel intrauterine system (LNG-IUS)	LNG-IUS reduces the amount of menstrual loss, reduces the uterine size in women with fibroids.
Gonadotrophin-releasing hormone agonists	Reduces the size of fibroids but, once discontinued, fibroids regrow to former size within about 2 months. Associated with side effects, including significant menopausal symptoms and bone loss, can lead to osteoporosis in long-term use. Their use is usually short term/temporary.
Mifepristone	A progesterone receptor inhibitor, effective at reducing fibroid-related bleeding and size of fibroid.

(Adapted from McCance et al, 2014.)

TABLE 34.9. Some Surgical Procedures Used to Treat Fibroids

Procedure	Description
Uterine artery embolization	May be recommended for women with large fibroids and is carried out by a radiologist. It involves blocking the blood vessels that supply the fibroids, causing them to shrink. This is carried out under local anaesthetic. A special solution is injected through a catheter, guided by x-ray through a blood vessel in the femoral artery to the uterus. Tiny particles are injected into the artery supplying the fibroid, cutting off the blood supply. This usually requires an overnight hospital stay, returning to normal activities in 1 week.
Endometrial ablation	The procedure involves removing the lining of the uterus and is mainly used to treat small fibroids. The affected lining can be removed in a number of ways, for example, by laser energy, a heated wire loop or hot fluid in a balloon. The procedure can be carried out under local anaesthetic or general anaesthetic, taking around 20 minutes and is provided as a day case. The woman may experience some vaginal bleeding and abdominal cramps for a few days afterwards; some women can have a bloody discharge for 3 or 4 weeks.

(Adapted from the Royal College of Gynaecologists and Obstetricians, 2015.)

OSCE 34.1

Intramuscular injection

Intramuscular injections administer medication deep into the muscle tissue. Local policy and procedure must be adopted.

Mrs Sally Malone has been prescribed a gonadotrophin-releasing hormone (GnRH) agonist intramuscularly as part of her treatment.

You will be marked on the following areas; all areas must be passed in order to achieve an overall pass:

Action	Criteria	Achieved/not achieved
Making an introduction	Introduce yourself Wash hands Confirm the patient's details Explain the procedure Check the patient's understanding of the medication being given and explain the indication for the medication Check for allergies Check if the patient has a bleeding disorder or takes anticoagulant medication (possible contraindications) Gain consent to proceed	
Gathering equipment	Equipment tray The medication to be administered Patient's prescription Syringe Needle Antiseptic swab Sharps container Apron Nonsterile gloves	
7 Rights	1. Right person: check the patient's arm band against the name on the prescription. Where possible aim to use two identifiers (e.g., from the patient and the arm band). 2. Right drug: check the labelled drug against the prescription, ensure expiry date is appropriate. 3. Right dose: check the dose against the prescription. 4. Right time: confirm when the last dose was given. 5. Right route. 6. Right to refuse: has the patient consented? 7. Right documentation of prescription and allergies: does the patient have any allergies?	

OSCE 34.1 – cont'd

Action	Criteria	Achieved/not achieved
Injection steps	1. Wash hands.	
	2. Don gloves and apron.	
	3. Draw up the appropriate medication into the syringe using a drawing needle.	
	4. Remove the drawing needle and attach the needle to be used for injection.	
	5. Choose an appropriate site.	
	6. Position the patient to provide optimal access to your chosen site.	
	7. Swab the site with an antiseptic swab and wait until it is dry.	
	8. Gently place traction on the skin with your nondominant hand away from the injection site, continuing the traction until the needle has been removed from the skin.	
	9. Warn the patient of a sharp scratch.	
	10. Holding the syringe like a dart in your dominant hand, pierce the skin at a 75- to 90-degree angle. Insert the needle quickly and firmly, with the bevel facing upwards, leaving approximately 1/3 of the shaft exposed (however this varies between sites and patients).	
	11. Aspirate to check the location of the needle. If blood appears, remove the syringe and prepare a new injection (explaining what occurred to the patient).	
	12. If no blood appears on aspiration, inject the contents of the syringe while holding the barrel firmly. Inject the medication slowly at a rate of approximately 1 mL every 10 seconds.	
	13. Remove the needle and immediately dispose of it appropriately (into a sharps container).	
	14. Release the traction on the skin.	
	15. Apply gentle pressure over the injection site with a cotton swab or gauze. Do NOT rub the site.	
Completing procedure	Replace cotton swab with a plaster.	
	Thank the patient	
	Discuss postinjection care:	
	o Warn the patient that the injection site may be sore for 1 or 2 days, but this is normal.	
	o Other potential complications include: haematoma, persistent nodules, local irritation (and rarely anaphylaxis).	
	o Advise the patient to watch for a developing rash, breathing difficulty or other relevant concerning symptoms. They should discuss this with a doctor if concerned.	
	Wash hands	
	Document that the medication has been given on the medication chart and in the patient's notes.	
	Have the patient observed for 15–30 minutes for adverse effects.	
Pass Fail		

Surgical intervention

Referral to a gynaecologist may be required if a pharmaceutical approach is ineffective. Surgery to remove fibroids may be considered if the woman's symptoms are particularly severe and medication has been ineffective. Several procedures may be used to treat fibroids. The woman should be provided with an opportunity to discuss the options she will have, including benefits and any associated risks.

Myomectomy. This type of surgery removes fibroids from the wall of the uterus. This intervention may be considered as an alternative to a hysterectomy if the woman is still contemplating having children.

Myomectomy is not suitable for all types of fibroid; factors such as the size, number and position of fibroids must be considered. Depending on the size and position, a myomectomy may require either minimally invasive surgery (laparoscopic surgery) or a single larger incision (open surgery).

The woman will have to undergo a general anaesthetic and she usually stays in hospital for 2–3 days postprocedure. The woman is advised to rest for several weeks after myomectomy to recover. Myomectomy is usually an effective treatment for fibroids but there is a chance the fibroids may grow back and further surgery may be required.

Hysteroscopic resection of fibroids. A hysteroscope is a thin telescope, equipped with small surgical instruments used to remove fibroids (resected). The procedure can be used to remove submucosal fibroids; this is suitable for women who wish to have children in the future.

There are no incisions made when this method is used; the hysteroscope is inserted through the vagina and into the uterus through the cervix. A number of insertions are required, ensuring that as much fibroid tissue as possible is removed. Usually, this is undertaken with general anaesthetic; however, a local anaesthetic can also be used. Typically, the procedure is carried out as a day case.

BOX 34.3 An Outline of the Pre- and Postoperative Care Required for the Woman Undergoing Hysterectomy

Preoperative care

- Undertake an assessment of the woman's understanding of the procedure. Offer explanation, clarification and emotional support as needed. Explain that the anaesthetic will eliminate any pain during the procedure and medication will be offered postoperatively to reduce pain and discomfort.
- Preoperative skin preparation must be carried out in alignment with an evidence-based local policy and protocol.
- Preoperative bowel preparation must be carried out in alignment with an evidence-based local policy and protocol; ask the woman to empty her bladder.
- Administer preoperative medications.
- Ensure that informed consent has been given and that a consent form has been signed.
- Carry out local procedures with regards to a preoperative check list.

Postoperative care

- Assess for signs of haemorrhage, for presence of bleeding, low blood pressure, tachycardia, pallor.
- Monitor and record vital signs as requested and as the woman's condition dictates and in line with local policy and procedure, monitor, measure and record intake and output.
- If a urinary catheter has been inserted, output must be monitored and documented. When the catheter has been removed, note when urine was passed, measure and record amount.
- Assess for potential complications, for example, infection, paralytic ileus, shock or haemorrhage, thrombophlebitis and pulmonary embolus.
- Assess vaginal discharge; assist the woman with perineal care.
- Assess dressing (incision) and bowel sounds as per local policy and procedure.
- Encourage mobility, turning, coughing and deep breathing.
- Encourage fluid intake as tolerated.
- Teach to splint the abdomen with a pillow and cough deeply.
- Advise the woman to limit physical activity for 4 to 6 weeks after the operation. Heavy lifting, climbing stairs, douching, tampons and sexual intercourse should be avoided. Advise the woman to shower as opposed to taking a bath, until bleeding has ceased.
- Explain she may feel tired for several days after surgery and she should rest periodically.
- Explain that she may not have an appetite and bowel movements may be sluggish.
- Explain to the woman the signs of complications that should be reported to the nurse or doctor which might be:
  o Temperature over 37.7°C
  o Vaginal bleeding greater than a typical menstrual period or bright red
  o Urinary incontinence, urgency, burning or frequency
  o Severe pain
- Encourage the woman to express feelings that may indicate she has a negative self-concept and discuss this with her.
- Provide information concerning the risks and benefits of hormone replacement therapy, if specified.
- Encourage the woman to attend for any out-patient appointments she might have.

(Adapted from Cotton & Steggle 2011; de Wit et al., 2017).

Postoperatively the woman may experience stomach cramps, which usually last for 1–2 hours. There may also be a small amount of vaginal bleeding, which should stop within a few weeks.

Hysteroscopic morcellation of fibroids. Hysteroscopic morcellation of fibroids is a new procedure and evidence about its overall safety and long-term effectiveness is limited (NICE, 2015).

Hysterectomy. Hysterectomy is the most effective way of preventing fibroids returning. It may be recommended if the woman has large fibroids or severe bleeding and does not wish to have any more children.

There are around 55,000 hysterectomies performed in the UK each year. Between 30,000 and 40,000 of these take place in the National Health Service. Globally, 1.2 million women can expect to undergo this form of surgery (Hysterectomy Association UK, 2017). The care required for a woman undergoing a hysterectomy is outlined in Box 34.3.

Nonsurgical procedures

Nonsurgical treatments to treat fibroids are also available, as well as traditional surgical techniques (Table 34.9).

COMMUNITIES OF CARE
Offender Health

Prison nurses are employed in prisons in the UK (including open prisons, high-security prisons, young offenders' institutions, women's prisons). These nurses assume a number of roles.

Those in detention (offenders) receive the same healthcare and treatment as anyone outside of prison. Treatment is free; however, this has to be approved by a prison doctor or a prison nurse. There are no hospitals in prisons, although a number of them have in-patient beds. Most issues are managed by the healthcare team. If they (the team) cannot manage any issues, the prison may:

- get an expert to visit the prison
- arrange for treatment in an outside hospital.

Only if the offender agrees, can prison healthcare staff approach the offender's family doctor for their records.

MALE REPRODUCTIVE DISORDERS

Men's health

Men do not enjoy the best of health. There are a number of male health inequalities that result in poor health outcomes for men, their families and society. The Nursing Associate has a role to play in helping men make a healthier lifestyle choice, assisting them when ill health occurs and providing them with psychological and physical support.

Providing care and support to men who are experiencing problems related to their reproductive system gives the Nursing Associate a chance to offer physical, emotional and practical help. When the Nursing Associate takes the time to explain things to the man (and if appropriate his family) in a language the person understands, as well as actively listening, they can help relieve the embarrassment the man may be feeling when discussing intimate issues, or at least make it more bearable.

Male sexual dysfunction

There are a number of issues that can impact on male sexual function, which can result in dysfunction. Erectile dysfunction (ED) is one of these issues that can have a physical and psychological impact on the man and his partner.

Erectile dysfunction

The British Society for Sexual Medicine (2009) and Wespes et al. (2012) define ED as the man's persistent inability to attain and maintain an erection that is sufficient to permit satisfactory sexual performance. Qaseem et al. (2009) add that any symptoms the man has that last at least 3 months deserve evaluation and consideration of treatment. The degree of severity of this particular condition varies widely. While some men are completely unable to achieve an erection sufficient for sex, others may experience difficulties to sustain physical arousal during moments of intimacy.

Corona et al. (2011) note that ED is a very common disorder, affecting men globally. It is predicted that by 2025, there will be 322 million men with ED (Qaseem, 2009). The prevalence of ED increases greatly in older men and severity increases with aging.

CASE STUDY 34.2   Alec and Maite Cortes

Alec Cortes is a 59-year-old man who has been married to Maite for 32 years. They have two children. He works as an auditor in the local hospital.

Alec is being seen at the general practice by Linda the practice nurse. Alec tells Linda that he has run out of his medications and needs a repeat prescription. Linda says to Alec: 'Just before we look at what you need prescription-wise, are there any other problems?' Alec replies jovially: 'No, not at all. I am fighting fit, but as happens with age, things in the department downstairs (he points to his groin) are not working as well as they used to'. Linda picks up on this cue and respectfully and tactfully asks Alec what does he mean?

Alec explains to Linda that he cannot 'get it up' as he used to and that this is causing him some anxiety and he does not know if not being able to initiate and maintain an erection is a problem or that he can't 'do the job' anymore.

Alec and Maite have enjoyed a happy and what they consider to be a good sex life together. Two years ago, Alec was diagnosed with hypertension (his blood pressure was consistently measuring around 190/90 mm Hg); he was overweight, smoked and he reported being a 'social' drinker. At that time, Alec weighed 88.5 kg, his height was 1.73 m, his waist circumference measured 102 cm, his BMI was 29.5, he smoked 10 cigarettes a day and was drinking in excess of 30 units of alcohol per week.

At this point, his GP prescribed Alec antihypertensive medication (methyldopa) and a diuretic (spironolactone). He was referred to the smoking cessation clinic and he agreed to join a gym. Progressively, he reports a loss of sexual drive and he confides in the practice nurse that it is taking him longer to establish and sustain an erection. This is problematic, as he can't be as sexually intimate with Maite as he once was and this is something they are both missing.

Signs and symptoms

ED is a symptom, not a disease, and as such it is important to identify any underlying disease or condition which may be causing it. Many illnesses affect ED and it is associated with a number of issues (Table 34.10).

The signs and symptoms of ED are varied and each man has to be assessed individually. A detailed holistic assessment is required; assessment is based on the man's physical, psychological and social needs, an integrated approach.

Assessing a man's overall health history may reveal ED. Once a problem is known, information and emotional support can be offered and referral made. Those men who lose erectile function may not be aware of the cause, and not knowing the cause leads to anxiety. The man with ED may believe himself to be 'less than a man'. The Nursing Associate can help alleviate anxiety by using a nonjudgemental approach.

Diagnosis

Often, for many men, all that will be required to make a diagnosis will be a patient history and a physical examination. If, however, the man has any chronic health conditions or it is suspected that an underlying condition might be involved, further tests or referral to a specialist may be required.

History. A detailed account of the man's personal details and his interpretation of the problem are needed. It is important to try to establish if the nature of the dysfunction is physical or psychological. Questions should also be asked in a respectful and tactful manner regarding the man's current and past medical, surgical and mental health history. Assessment of any psychological (or emotional) factors and medications being taken for concurrent health conditions should be determined (Table 34.10). The following may need to be asked but, only if appropriate:

TABLE 34.10. Some Important Issues Associated with Erectile Dysfunction

Physical causes	Vasculogenic: cardiovascular disease, hypertension, hyperlipidaemia, diabetes mellitus, smoking
	Neurogenic: multiple sclerosis, muscle weakness, Parkinson's, stroke, alcoholism, nerve damage as a result of surgery (i.e., pelvic), spinal injury
	Anatomical: Peyronie's disease, penile fracture, micro penis, hypospadias, epispadias, congenital curvature of the penis
	Hormonal: disorders of hormonal makeup, for example, hypogonadism, hyperthyroidism, hypothyroidism
Psychological or emotional causes such as relationship problems or mental health problems	Relationship problems
	Past sexual problems
	Family or social pressures
	Religious or cultural beliefs
	Other sexual health problems in the man or his partner
	Restrictive upbringing
	Unclear sexual or gender preference
	Physical or mental health problems
	Previous sexual abuse
The use of certain drugs	Diuretics (e.g., spironolactone, bendroflumethiazide)
	Antihypertensive (e.g., methyldopa, verapamil)
	Antipsychotics (e.g., chlorpromazine, haloperidol)
	Antidepressants (e.g., amitriptyline, fluoxetine)
	Histamine antagonists (e.g., cimetidine, ranitidine)
	Cytotoxic (e.g., cyclophosphamide, methotrexate)
	Antiarrhythmics (e.g., disopyramide)
	Anticonvulsants (e.g., carbamazepine)
	Hormones (e.g., estradiol, prednisolone, cyproterone acetate)

(Adapted from Wespes et al, 2012; Albersen et al, 2011: Hackett et al., 2018.)

- Current and past relationship status, sexual orientation.
- Present and previous quality of erection (including quality of erections during sexual relations, as well as awakening and masturbatory erections) and if there is any ejaculatory and orgasm dysfunction.
- Issues with sexual aversion or pain, or issues for his partner (including menopause or vaginal pain).
- Lifestyle factors, including use of alcohol, tobacco and illicit drug use and any treatments already tried.
- Energy levels, loss of libido, loss of body hair, or spontaneous hot flushes (may indicate testosterone deficiency hypogonadism).

REFLECTION 34.3

How might you begin to ask a patient about her/his sexual/reproductive health?

What do think might be barriers that would prevent you from assessing this important activity in depth? Remember the barriers may come from both you and the patient.

How might you develop and improve your skills to ensure that when next required to assess a person's sexual/reproductive health, you could do this with more confidence?

Physical examination. A physical examination is required for all men; weight, waist circumference, heart rate and blood pressure form the basis of the physical examination. The genitalia are examined, which can reveal signs of hypogonadism (there may also be evidence of gynaecomastia and reduced body hair) or physical malformation, for example, Peyronie's disease.

Investigations. A series of blood tests are required, which will be determined on individual needs. An assessment of levels of testosterone is required, usually taken in the morning between 9 a.m. and 11 a.m. Other blood tests include checking for signs of heart disease, diabetes and other health conditions. Urinalysis is undertaken for signs of other underlying health conditions.

Ultrasound may be performed. The transducer (a wand-like instrument) is held over the blood vessels supplying the penis. This helps to establish if there are any problems with blood flow. This test may be carried out in combination with an injection of medications into the penis (penile arteriography) to stimulate flow of blood and produce an erection.

Overnight erection test (nocturnal penile tumescence) may be required. Most men have erections during sleep without recollecting them. The test involves wrapping a special device around the penis prior to going to bed; this measures the number and strength of erections achieved overnight, helping to determine if ED is related to psychological or physical causes.

Questions may be asked of the man to screen for depression and other possible psychological causes of ED.

Care and treatment

The aim of care is to ensure the man (and his partner) receive care that is appropriate and effective. Understanding what this care incorporates helps the Nursing Associate help the person being cared for. The care of men with ED is growing in importance; the population as a whole is ageing and so the incidence is increasing. There is also more willingness of men and their partners to discuss sexual worries. Although sexuality may still be seen by some as very sensitive and personal, the increase in knowledge and understanding and help available is encouraging men to seek answers. Importantly, loss of erectile function should not be seen as an inevitable part of ageing.

An interdisciplinary approach to care is needed and this is essential in identifying key steps in the care of the person. The multidisciplinary team can include:

- Practice nurse
- General Practitioners
- Physiotherapist
- Psychosexual counsellors.

A uni-professional approach to care (i.e., care provided by one professional group only) is unacceptable. Prior to treatment, an assessment of current medication is undertaken to determine if the man is taking any drugs for associated condition(s), and if any of these drugs may cause ED (see Table 34.10). If this is the case, consideration should be given to substituting with another drug if a link can be demonstrated (Wespes et al., 2012).

Men experiencing ED should be encouraged to address lifestyle and dietary habits (Esposito & Guigliano, 2011). Being overweight or obese is associated with an increased risk of ED, increased physical activity may have a protective effect on ED and smoking increases the risk for ED.

It has been identified (Hackett et al., 2018) in those men who cycle for more than 3 hours per week that this is a risk factor for ED. This is possibly due to nerve damage caused by contact with the saddle. This damage is usually reversible; a trial period of not cycling, with the aim of enabling nerve repair is recommended.

Pharmaceutical approaches to the treatment of erectile dysfunction

ED can be treated with medications that are taken orally, injected directly into the penis or inserted into the urethra at the tip of the penis. Phosphodiesterase inhibitors (sildenafil, tadalafil, vardenafil and avanafil) are oral pharmaceutical agents that improve the relaxation of smooth muscle.

Sildenafil (Viagra) and vardenafil (Levitra), when taken an hour before sexual activity, facilitate relaxation of the smooth muscle in the penis during sexual stimulation, increasing blood flow. Both drugs should be taken no more than once a day, and should not be taken by those men who are prescribed nitrate-based drugs or alpha-blockers (used to treat hypertension and prostate enlargement). Tadalafil (Cialis) is a selective phosphodiesterase type 5 inhibitor, permitting smooth muscle relaxation and facilitating inflow of blood into the penis, lasting for 36 hours. Erection only occurs with sexual stimulation. Tadalafil should not be taken if the man is also taking nitrates, alpha-blockers, erythromycin or rifampicin (antibiotics), ketoconazole or itraconazole (antifungal medication), or protease inhibitors (for human immunodeficiency virus [HIV]). See Table 34.11 for an overview of some oral pharmaceutical treatments.

There are increasing numbers of products available via the internet, all unlicensed, and they have a number of adverse effects. They include yohimbine, maca, horny goatweed and gingko biloba (Corazza et al., 2014). Men should be advised not to use these internet products.

Non-oral pharmaceutical treatments. Non-oral pharmaceutical treatments include injectable medications. Injectable medications, including papaverine and prostaglandin E injections, are injected directly into the penis. Papaverine relaxes the arterioles

---

TABLE 34.11 Some Oral Pharmaceutical Treatments for Erectile Dysfunction

Drug (generic)	Drug (brand)	Contraindications	Comments/dose
For Viagra see the Medicine Trolley 34.3			
Tadalafil	Cialis	Contraindicated in men receiving nitrates, can cause severe hypotension, which may lead to acute myocardial infarction, stroke and even death.	Has a longer half-life, therefore a longer action and therefore greater spontaneity (effective after 30 minutes, with peak efficacy at 2 hours and lasting up to 36 hours). Start at 10 mg (change according to response).
Vardenafil	Levitra	Contraindicated in men receiving nitrates, can cause severe hypotension, which may lead to acute myocardial infarction, stroke and even death.	Effective after 30 minutes. Its effect is reduced by a fatty meal but it has less interaction with food. A rapidly absorbed preparation is available. For most men, the recommended dose is 10 mg per day taken 60 minutes before intercourse. If no response or side effects, dose may be increased to 20 mg or, if there are side effects, reduced to 5 mg.
Avanafil	Stendra	Contraindicated in men receiving nitrates, can cause severe hypotension, which may lead to acute myocardial infarction, stroke and even death.	Effective after 30 minutes. Effect may be delayed when administered with food but can be taken with or without food. For most men, the recommended starting dose is 100 mg per day taken about 30 minutes before sexual activity. Depending on the adequacy of the response or side effects, the dose may be increased.

THE MEDICINE TROLLEY 34.3

Drug	Drug classification	Reason for administration	Route of administration	Dose	Side effects	Contraindications	Nursing care
Sildenafil (Viagra)	Phosphodiesterase type 5 inhibitors	To treat erectile dysfunction	Oral	50 mg is the recommended starting dose	Stuffy nose Indigestion Nausea Headache Dizziness Changes in vision (blue tint or blurring) Skin flushes on the face	Can exacerbate use of antihypertensive drugs and therefore any patient using antihypertensives should not use Viagra	Explain the use of the drug to the patient, respond to any questions Efficacy is reduced after fatty meals

and smooth muscles of the cavernosum (the columns of erectile tissue in the penis), inducing tumescence. Erection usually lasts 30 minutes to 4 hours. Prostaglandin E performs in a similar way to papaverine, but has fewer side effects. Mode of delivery can be problematic: some men report dissatisfaction with lack of spontaneity, loss of interest in sex, physical limitations and occasionally, pain. Alprostadil (Caverject), another injectable medication, can be used to treat ED.

Intraurethral alprostadil (prostaglandin E1) is inserted as a medicated pellet into the urethral meatus, producing an erection after about 15 minutes. Barrier contraception must be used if the man's partner is pregnant. Intraurethral alprostadil is less effective than intracavernous injections. The most common side effect is mild penile pain.

Topical alprostadil (prostaglandin E1) is a cream licensed for topical use, applied 5–30 minutes before intercourse. The medication is administered using a plunger, delivering the cream to the tip of the penis and the surrounding skin.

! HOTSPOT

Priapism is a persistent penile erection that continues hours beyond, or is unrelated to, sexual stimulation. Typically, only the corpora cavernosa are affected and this can be a side effect of using intraurethral alprostadil (prostaglandin E1). If priapism occurs:

- The man should be referred urgently to hospital.
- Patients are advised to seek medical advice if the erection has lasted longer than 4 hours.
- Treatment should not be delayed for more than 6 hours. Initial treatment is by aspiration of blood from the corpus cavernosum.
- If this is unsuccessful, cautious intracavernosal injection of a sympathomimetic (e.g., phenylephrine or adrenaline (epinephrine)) may be required.
- If sympathomimetics are unsuccessful, urgent surgical referral is required.

Vacuum constriction devices for erectile dysfunction. A vacuum constriction device is an external mechanical device that can be used for the treatment of ED, drawing blood into the penis with a vacuum, resulting in engorgement of the penis. Keeping the blood there is achieved by the use of a constricting band at the base of the penis. When the device is removed, a single small band, (an O-ring), is left at the base of the penis to maintain the erection.

Surgery for erectile dysfunction

Surgical treatment involves revascularization procedures (procedures requiring reconstruction of arteries and/or veins) or implantation of prosthetic devices. Semi-rigid, malleable or inflatable devices are surgically inserted to produce an erect state.

! HOTSPOT

Remember that erectile dysfunction (ED) can be encountered in any healthcare setting. Routine examinations or careful assessment of men can identify their conditions, and treatments that may incidentally cause ED. The Nursing Associate may encounter men in various healthcare settings.

Chlamydia

Nursing Associates working in a number of disciplines and settings have the opportunity to help reduce the incidence of this infection. Genital chlamydia infection is caused by the *Chlamydia trachomatis* bacterium, the most common bacterial sexually transmitted infection (STI) in the UK. The prevalence of infection is highest in young sexually active adults (15–24 years). Often, chlamydia has no symptoms (sometimes referred to as the 'silent epidemic'); it can, however, lead to a wide range of complications, including pelvic inflammatory disease, ectopic pregnancy and tubal factor infertility in women and epididymitis in men. Chlamydia represents a substantial public health problem (Public Health England, 2016).

Improving awareness of chlamydia is key to preventing the infection. If the Nursing Associate is to play a role in prevention and onward transmission, they have to have a deeper understanding of the infection and develop their interpersonal skills to care for people effectively. Those requiring care come from all walks of life; the Nursing Associate is required to provide care that is sensitive and informed. When chlamydia remains untreated or the person has repeated chlamydial infection, it can result in serious complications for the man and his partner's health and well-being; it has a specific impact on the reproductive system.

The bacterium *C. trachomatis* is an intracellular pathogen, which means that the pathogen is unable to reproduce outside of its host cell. Reproduction of the pathogen is totally dependent on resources within the cell. Chlamydia was originally thought to be a virus because of the way it developed.

The ways in which chlamydia develops (its pathogenesis) are not fully understood. This bacterium is found in the semen and vaginal fluid of those who have the infection. The bacterium infects the tissues lining aspects of the urinary and reproductive tract.

Transmission

Chlamydia is transmitted from person to person through vaginal, anal and oral sex without condoms. It can also be transmitted if:

- Sex toys are shared and they are not washed or covered with a condom each time they are used
- A pregnant woman has chlamydia and she passes the infection on to her baby during childbirth (vertical transmission).

It is unclear whether chlamydia can be transmitted through touching another person's genitals if there is infected semen or vaginal fluid on the fingers. Chlamydia cannot be transmitted through kissing or sharing things such as toilets or towels with another person who has the infection.

Signs and symptoms

In most people, this infection is asymptomatic and often it is only detected during screening or during investigations of other genitourinary illnesses. In the male, where there are symptoms, these can include:

- Dysuria
- Urethral discharge

- Epididymo-orchitis (presents as testicular pain and/or swelling)
- Pyrexia.

Other symptoms that may be suggestive of chlamydial infection include:

- Sexually acquired reactive arthritis, particularly in young people (a triad of urethritis, arthritis and conjunctivitis)
- Upper abdominal pain due to perihepatitis (called Fitz-Hugh-Curtis syndrome)
- Proctitis (inflammation of the rectum) with mucopurulent discharge, may be due to rectal chlamydia following anal intercourse
- Pharyngeal (throat) infection
- Chlamydial conjunctivitis in adults is usually sexually acquired.

Signs of the condition in men may include:

- Epididymal tenderness
- Mucoid or mucopurulent discharge.

Diagnosis

It is essential to always obtain a sexual health history, either at the time of testing or when becoming aware of or receiving a positive chlamydia test result. Obtaining a sexual health history requires time. Time must be set aside for this important activity and the man must be put at ease; a nonjudgemental approach is essential. Many of the skills required to undertake a sexual health history are already used by healthcare workers when making assessments of a person's general health, for example, asking open-ended questions and not making any assumptions. As well as a sexual history, a number of laboratory tests are also required to make a definitive diagnosis.

For men, the test of choice is a first catch urine specimen. The man is advised he should not have passed urine for at least the previous hour and then catch the first 20 mL of the sample for testing. If urethral samples are taken, the swab should be inserted 2–4 cm into the urethra and rotated once before removal. Rectal, throat and conjunctival swabs may need to be taken (Nwokolo et al., 2015), see Fig. 34.17. The Nursing Associate may be required to take these swabs or assist in taking them. Samples are taken for nucleic acid amplification tests, currently the most sensitive and specific method of testing for chlamydia (Nwokolo et al., 2015), although no test is 100% accurate.

NURSING SKILLS

Throat Swab

This test is a safe and easy to tolerate test. In some people, the sensation of gagging may lead to an urge to vomit or cough.

A throat (a throat swab culture) is a laboratory test that is done to identify the presence of infection and to identify the causative organisms that may cause infection in the throat. It can be used to diagnose pharyngeal chlamydia.

The patient should not have used antiseptic mouthwash prior to this test. Determine if the patient has taken or is taking any antibiotics and document this.

Seek consent from the patient to undertake the procedure, explain the reason for the test, what will happen to the specimen and when the results will be available.

Explain that the test is done when a throat infection is suspected. A throat culture can also help to decide which antibiotic will work best.

Explain that the throat may be sore when this test is done and the person might feel like gagging when the back of the throat is touched with the swab, but the test only lasts a few seconds.

Equipment needed:

- Gloves/apron
- Tongue depressor
- Sampling material (swab attached to plastic stick in transport medium)
- Microbiology form and attached bag

Procedure

The procedure should be carried out in line with local policy and procedure.

1. Check patient identity, label the pot used for transporting the swab to the laboratory.
2. Ensure a good light source.
3. Ensure all equipment is gathered prior to carrying out the procedure.
4. Wash/decontaminate hands.
5. Don disposable gloves and apron.
6. Open sampling pack. Remove top of the transport medium and place this upside down on clean surface.
7. Do not permit any part of the swab to touch any surface except the throat/tonsil, including the oral mucosa.
8. Ask the patient to tilt the head back and open the mouth wide.
9. Keep the tongue down (if needed with the tongue depressor).
10. Using a rolling movement, swab the surface of the area of the tonsils, so that a sufficient amount of mucosal secretion is transported to the swab.
11. Encourage the patient to resist gagging and closing the mouth while the swab touches this area.
12. Pull the swab out carefully so as to avoid any contamination and place in the special tube with the transport medium.
13. Remove gloves/apron.
14. Wash/decontaminate hands.
15. Dispose of used packing and other equipment safely.
16. The specimen should be stored and transported according to local policy and procedure.
17. Document and record the procedure in the patient's notes.

    After the procedure thank the patient

    Explain that the specimen is to be transported to the laboratory for analysis, when the results will be available (this may take several days) and how these will be communicated.

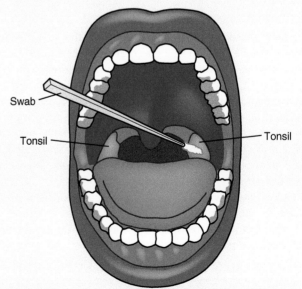

Fig. 34.17 The Throat is Swabbed in the Area of the Tonsils.

> **BOX 34.4 Those Normally Included in a Chlamydia Screening Programme (England)**
>
> - Men or women with symptoms which could indicate infection.
> - Sexual partners of people with proven or suspected chlamydia.
> - All sexually active people younger than 25 years of age, annually, or more frequently if they have changed their partner, as a part of the national screening programme. Testing should be offered opportunistically in England to this group when they visit their GP.
> - People under 25 years of age who have been treated for chlamydia in the past 3 months.
> - Those who have concerns about sexual exposure (if exposure was in the previous 2 weeks)
> - People who have had two or more sexual partners in the past year.
> - All women presenting for termination of pregnancy.
> - All those presenting at a genitourinary medicine clinic.
> - Mothers of infants with chlamydial infection (e.g., neonatal chlamydial conjunctivitis or pneumonia).
> - Women who are about to be fitted with an intrauterine contraceptive device or intrauterine system who are identified as at risk of sexually transmitted infection.

(Adapted from Nwokolo et al., 2015.)

Screening

Those who should be screened for chlamydia is dependent on local guidelines and policy (Nwokolo et al., 2015). See Box 34.4 for an overview of those who should be included in screening in England.

AT THE GP SURGERY

Testing should be offered opportunistically in England to young people when they visit their GP.

Testing kits are available at some pharmacies, GP practices, genitourinary medicine clinics and are also available by post, where the envelope is delivered unmarked and contains full instructions for use. The service is free and confidential when National Health Service packs are used.

Care and treatment

Treatment should be provided in such a way that it is effective, easy to take, has limited side effects and has least impact on a man's lifestyle. The Nursing Associate may be required to provide the man with advice about the impact chlamydia can have on his health and well-being, as well as the implications of having this infection on his partner(s) and also the long-term complications. This information should be provided verbally and supplemented with written information in such a way that it is suited to the needs of the person. Partner notification (notification of sexual partners) will also be required.

Those people with a suspected or confirmed diagnosis of chlamydia should be offered screening for other STIs and an HIV test. Hepatitis screening and, if appropriate, vaccination should also be provided.

Treatment regimens are based on national guidelines (Nwokolo et al., 2015) and should be started prior to the outcome of test results in those who present with signs or symptoms that would strongly suggest they have chlamydia. Antibiotic therapy is the first-line recommended regimen for uncomplicated chlamydial infection. Doxycycline, 100 mg twice daily for 7 days, or a single dose of 1 g of azithromycin is recommended. If these antibiotics are contraindicated, alternative regimens are erythromycin 500 mg twice daily for 10–14 days or ofloxacin 200 mg twice daily or 400 mg once daily for 7 days.

In ensuring that the man is receiving the treatment that has the greatest chance of treating the infection effectively, the Nursing Associate should reinforce safer sex practices (as chlamydia is an STI), for example, correct and regular use of condoms. Provide clear written advice and instructions for taking the prescribed medications. Reinforce the fact that often chlamydia is asymptomatic and it is important that their sexual partner(s) are also tested. The man should be advised to abstain from sexual intercourse (including oral, anal and vaginal sex and mutual masturbation) even with a condom, until they and their partner(s) have completed their therapy. If patients are receiving the one-off dose of azithromycin, it is important that they do not have sexual contact for 7 days after their treatment.

Prevention and control

The principles underpinning the prevention and control of chlamydia focus on primary prevention and secondary prevention. Primary prevention is aimed at keeping those people who are uninfected from being infected. The role of secondary prevention is to prevent onward transmission of the infection of an infected person. Partner notification is also an essential aspect of the management of STIs.

Primary prevention activities are concerned mainly with education to modify knowledge, skills, attitudes and behaviours. This activity takes place at a number of levels: individual, organizational and community levels. The Nursing Associate, as part of the multidisciplinary team, should offer appropriate and timely education that aims to minimize risk associated with sexual intercourse and other sexual activities, drawing on social psychology, risk theory and up to date research.

Secondary prevention is concerned with reducing the risk of transmitting the infection from one person (or community) to another. When using this preventative method, screening (or testing), treating and reinforcing safer sex activity is required. Early diagnosis and effective treatment is the basis of secondary prevention. If, for example, chlamydia was well controlled, then the serious long-term effects associated with the sequelae can be prevented.

Partner notification (an aspect of secondary prevention) is essential to ensure that those sexual partners of a man who is diagnosed with chlamydia can be contacted and made aware of the risks they have undertaken and the possibility of developing complications or infecting others.

Everyone has a right to enjoy good sexual health. There are some instances, however, where people and populations are at risk of developing some infections more than others; chlamydia is an example of this. This infection is increasing and specifically impacts on the young heterosexual population in the UK.

Chlamydial infection is often asymptomatic; therefore, the risk of transmitting the infection unbeknown is high. There are some serious complications associated with chlamydial infection that can have a severe impact on a person's health and well-being. The Nursing Associate can only help others when they understand the modes of transmission, signs and symptoms (where present) and the potential treatment regimens. Offering people sexual health education by encouraging the consistent use of condoms may help in reducing the damaging physical and psychological sequelae of chlamydia on individuals and society. See Box 34.5 for some general points concerning chlamydia.

LOOKING BACK, FEEDING FORWARD

The purpose of the reproductive systems is to produce offspring. When the mature egg with its 23 chromosomes and the sperm with its 23 chromosomes unify, this union provides a fertilized egg with 46 chromosomes. In tandem with other body systems (e.g., the functions of the endocrine system, the musculoskeletal system, the neurological system and the urological system), the reproductive systems are complex and as such are prone to harm and disease and also dysfunction. Female and male reproductive health has an impact on individuals and communities, locally, nationally and internationally and affects individuals across the lifespan.

Many people also derive pleasure from the reproductive system. Reproductive health implies that people are able to have a satisfying and safe sex life and that they have the capability to reproduce and the freedom to decide if, when and how often to do so.

Women and men have the right to be informed and to have access to reproductive health services of their choice. Reproductive health includes sexual health, the purpose of which is the enhancement of life and personal relations, and not just about counselling and care related to reproduction and STIs.

Reproductive health is a central component of general health and a central feature of human development. It is a reflection of health during childhood and is key during youth and maturity. It sets the scene for health beyond the reproductive years for women and men and will impact on the health of the next generation.

The Nursing Associate has a crucial role to play in advocating the availability of information that will help to develop policy and practice and inform those who are responsible for the commissioning of reproductive health services. They also have a central role to play in offering people support in an unbiased nonjudgemental way, as well as having the knowledge and skill to make appropriate referrals. Having the appropriate knowledge, skills and attitudes can help those we have the privilege to care for to make well-informed decisions that are based on a reliable evidence base.

REFERENCES

Albersen, M., Mwamukonda, K.B., Shindel, A.W., Lue, T.F., 2011. Evaluation and treatment of erectile dysfunction. Med. Clin. North Am. 95 (1), 201–212.

British Society for Sexual Medicine, 2009. Guidelines on the management of erectile dysfunction. Available at: www.bssm.org.uk.

> **BOX 34.5 Some General Points Regarding Chlamydia**
>
> Provide a clear explanation of the condition and its long-term implications for the patient and their partner(s). Key points include:
> - Chlamydia is primarily sexually transmitted.
> - Infection is very often asymptomatic and may have persisted for many months or even for years.
> - No diagnostic test is 100% sensitive.
> - The potential complications of not treating chlamydia.
> - The importance of investigating and treating sexual partners. Agree on the method of partner notification.
> - The importance of complying with treatment.
> - Antibiotic side effects and interactions.
> - Avoidance of sexual intercourse (genital, oral and anal sex) even with a condom for 1 week after single-dose therapy or until finishing a longer regimen. The patient should not resume sex with their partner(s) until they too have completed treatment (or for 1 week following a one off dose of azithromycin) or received negative test results; otherwise there is a high risk of reinfection.
> - It is important to test for other sexually transmitted infections, including human immunodeficiency virus (HIV) and hepatitis B.
> - Advice on safer sexual practices, contraception and condom use.
> - Reinforce with clear written information.

Corazza, O., Martinotti, G., Santacroce, R., et al., 2014. Sexual enhancement products for sale online: raising awareness of the psychoactive effects of yohimbine, maca, horny goat weed, and ginkgo biloba. Biomed Res. Int. 2014, 841798.

Corona, G., Mondaini, N., Ungar, A., et al., 2011. Phosphodiesterase type 5 (PDE5) inhibitors in erectile dysfunction: the proper drug for the proper patient. J. Sex. Med. 8, 3418–3432.

Cotton, C., Steggle, M., 2011. Nursing patients with disorders of the breast and reproductive system. In: Brooker, C., McNicol, M. (Eds.), Alexander's Nursing Practice, fourth ed. Elsevier, Edinburgh, pp. 193–272.

Department of Health, 2010. Essence of care 2010. Benchmarks for respect and dignity. Available at: https://www.gov.uk/government/uploads/system/uploads/attachment_data/file/216702/dh_119966.pdf.

de Wit, S.C., Stromberg, H.K., Dallred, C.V., 2017. Medical-Surgical Nursing, Concepts and Practice, third ed. Elsevier, St Louis.

Dunselman, G.A., Vermeulen, N., Becker, C., et al., 2014. ESHRE guideline: management of women with endometriosis. Hum. Reprod. 29 (3), 400–412.

Endometriosis UK, 2011. Endometriosis diagnosis survey 2011: Jan 19th – Feb 4th 2011. Available at: https://www.endometriosis-uk.org/sites/default/files/files/Endometriosis%20Diagnosis%20Survey%20Feb2011%20Report%20final.pdf.

Endometriosis UK, 2017. Endometriosis annual report 2016/17. Available at: https://www.endometriosis-uk.org/sites/default/files/files/AnnualReport2016-2017.pdf.

Esposito, K., Giugliano, D., 2011. Lifestyle/dietary recommendations for erectile dysfunction and female sexual dysfunction. Urol. Clin. North Am. 38 (3), 293–301.

European Society of Human Reproduction and Embryology, 2013. Management of women with endometriosis. Available at: https://

www.eshre.eu/Guidelines-and-Legal/Guidelines/Endometriosis-guideline.aspx.

Hackett, G., Kirby. M., Wylie, K., et al., 2018. British Society for Sexual Medicine Guidelines on the Management of Erectile Dysfunction in Men – 2017. J. Sex. Med. 15 (4), 430–457.

Haney, A.F., 2008. Leiomyomata. In: Gibbs, R.S., Karlan, B.Y., Haney, A.F., Nygaard, I. (Eds.), Danforth's Obstetrics and Gynecology, tenth ed. Lippincott Williams & Wilkins, Philadelphia, pp. 916–931.

Hickey, M., Ballard, K., Farquhar, C., 2014. Endometriosis. Br. Med. J. 348, 1752.

Hysterectomy Association. UK, 2017. Hysterectomy Association UK. Available at: https://www.hysterectomy-association.org.uk.

McCance, K.E., Huether, S.E., Rote, N.S., 2014. Pathophysiology: The Biologic Basis for Disease in Adults and Children, seventh ed. Elsevier, St Louis.

Moroni, R., Viera, C., Ferriani, R., et al., 2014. Pharmacological treatment of uterine fibroids. Ann. Med. Health Sci. Res. 4 (3), S185–S192.

NICE, 2015. National Institute of Health and Care Excellence. Hysteroscopic morcellation of uterine leiomyomas (fibroids). Available at: https://www.nice.org.uk/guidance/ipg522.

Nwokolo, N.C., Dragovic, B., Patel, S., et al., 2015. UK national guideline for the management of infection with Chlamydia trachomatis. Int. J. STD AIDS 27 (4), 251–267.

Porth, C.M., 2015. Essentials of Pathophysiology: Concepts of Altered Health States, fourth ed. Wolters Kluwer, Philadelphia.

Public Health England, 2016. Chlamydia: Surveillance, data, screening and management. Available at: https://www.gov.uk/government/collections/chlamydia-surveillance-data-screening-and-management.

Qaseem, A., Snow, V., Denberg, T.D., et al., 2009. Hormonal testing and pharmacologic treatment of erectile dysfunction: A clinical practice guideline from the American College of Physicians. Ann. Intern. Med. 151 (9), 639–649.

Rassool, G.H., 2015. Cultural competence in nursing Muslim patients. Nurs. Times 111 (14), 12–15.

Roper, N., Logan, W.W., Tierney, A.J., 2000. The Roper-Logan-Tierney Model of Nursing: Based on Activities of Living. Churchill Livingstone, Edinburgh.

Royal College of Gynaecologists and Obstetricians, 2015. Information for you after an endometrial ablation. Available at: https://www.rcog.org.uk/globalassets/documents/patients/patient-information-leaflets/recovering-well/endometrial-ablation.pdf.

Royal College of Nursing, 2015. Endometriosis fact sheet. Available at: https://www.rcn.org.uk/professional-development/publications/pub-004777.

Waugh, A., Grant, A., 2018. Ross and Wilson Anatomy and Physiology in Health and Illness, thirteenth ed. Elsevier, Edinburgh.

Wespes, E., Amar, E., Eardley, I., et al., 2012. Guidelines on Male Sexual Dysfunction: Erectile Dysfunction and Premature Ejaculation. European Association of Urology. Available at: https://uroweb.org/wp-content/uploads/14-Male-Sexual-Dysfunction_LR.pdf.

35

Endocrine Disorders

Carl Clare

OBJECTIVES

By the end of the chapter the reader will:

1. Have an understanding of the anatomy and physiology of the endocrine system.
2. Discuss the pathophysiological changes associated with a selection of endocrine disorders.
3. Understand the relationship between the endocrine system and other body systems.
4. Outline the care required by people with endocrine disorders.
5. Describe some common conditions associated with the endocrine system.
6. Review the role of the Nursing Associate in promoting health and well-being.

KEY WORDS

Secrete	Steroid	Endocrine
Receptor	Feedback	Homeostasis
Hormone	Metabolic	
Regulation	Adherence	

CHAPTER AIMS

This aim of this chapter is to provide the reader with an understanding of the skills, knowledge and attitude required to provide safe, effective and compassionate care to people with an endocrine disorder.

SELF TEST

1. What is an endocrine organ?
2. Name four endocrine organs.
3. Name the hormones produced by the pancreas.
4. What is a 'target cell'?
5. Discuss the transportation of hormones.
6. What is the most common endocrine disorder in the UK?
7. What is type 2 diabetes mellitus?
8. What do you understand by the term 'upregulation'?
9. What is the most common cause of disorders of the thyroid gland?
10. What is meant by the term 'negative feedback loop'?

INTRODUCTION

In this chapter, the endocrine system is considered. The first part discusses the anatomy and physiology of the endocrine system. It is important for the Nursing Associate to have a comprehensive understanding of the endocrine system if the care provided is to be appropriate and effective.

The second part of the chapter addresses a selection of common conditions that impact on the endocrine system and thus the health and well-being of people. The care and comfort of the patient who experiences an endocrine disorder are described. When offering care, the Nursing Associate is required to be kind and compassionate. Care provision must recognize the anxiety that an endocrine condition can instil within a patient and be sensitive to this anxiety. The information needs of the patient with an endocrine condition are high and the Nursing Associate should be aware of the resources available for a patient who is managing an endocrine condition as part of their everyday life.

SENSITIVE CARE

When caring for a patient with an endocrine disorder, it is essential that the Nursing Associate is sensitive to the physical and psychological effects such a condition can create. Many patients, especially those first diagnosed with an endocrine condition, will show evidence of anxiety and will have a high need for information regarding their condition and its everyday management. There can often be a fear of the effect the condition will have on everyday life and the patient will commonly be concerned about their future life in terms of ability to work, sexual activity, self-management of the disorder and the potential complications that can arise. This can sometimes make patients, and their relatives, seem demanding and excessively worried. It is important to understand in these situations that this condition is new to the patient and, whilst many people manage their endocrine condition in daily life with little difficulty, the diagnosis is new to this patient. Thus patients must be dealt with patiently and with sensitive and calm handling.

> ### REFLECTION 35.1
> How might you help a person who has been given a diagnosis of an endocrine disorder? How can you ensure that you have given due consideration to their health, well-being and information needs?

Patients (and relatives of patients) who are suffering from an endocrine disorder will often have a lot of questions. In these situations, it is essential that care staff are sensitive, open and honest in their communication. It is not a failure of your ability as a carer to say that you 'don't know' and to offer to either find out or to signpost the patient to a reliable source of information (such as NHS Choices). The Nursing and Midwifery Council Code (Nursing and Midwifery Council, 2018) makes clear that if you are unsure you should always strive to refer the patient to a person who does know; you should only act within the sphere of your competence.

Part of the role of the Nursing Associate is to deliver person-centred holistic care (Health Education England, 2017) and one of the most overlooked aspects of caring for the newly diagnosed is just to 'be there' for the patient and their relatives. Being an open and empathic presence is just as important to many patients and their relatives as the physical care that we provide.

THE ENDOCRINE SYSTEM

The endocrine system is a system of glands and organs that can be found throughout the body (Fig. 35.1). In contrast to the nervous system, the endocrine system is relatively slow-acting but it has a powerful effect in maintaining homeostasis. In the human body, homeostasis refers to the regulation of the internal systems to maintain the normal balance and functioning of the body's physiology. In attempting to maintain homeostasis, the endocrine and nervous systems act together to manage several mechanisms, such as fluid balance and blood pressure. The nervous system reacts rapidly to changes and is thus involved in the immediate and short-term maintenance of homeostasis. Due to its speed of action, the nervous system controls bodily processes, such as breathing and movement, which require second-by-second input. The endocrine system controls the longer-term regulation of homeostasis; some of the hormones released can exert an effect within several seconds but the effect of most hormones has an onset of hours or days. In contrast to the nervous system, the effect of hormones is often longer lasting;

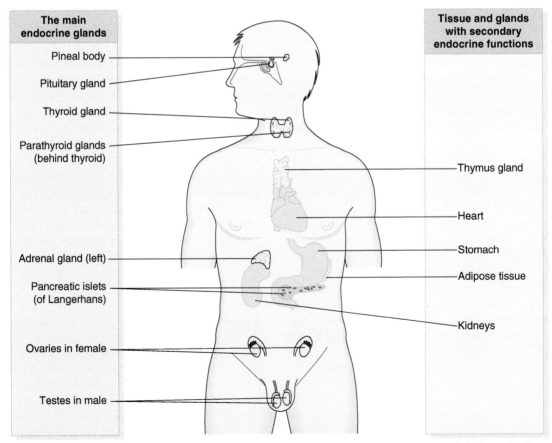

The main endocrine glands	Tissue and glands with secondary endocrine functions
Pineal body	
Pituitary gland	
Thyroid gland	
Parathyroid glands (behind thyroid)	
	Thymus gland
	Heart
	Stomach
Adrenal gland (left)	Adipose tissue
Pancreatic islets (of Langerhans)	
	Kidneys
Ovaries in female	
Testes in male	

Fig. 35.1 The Location of the Endocrine Glands and Organs that Secrete Hormones (Waugh & Grant, 2018).

in fact, some hormones can have an effect that lasts for hours or days.

The structures of the endocrine system can be split into three main types:

- The endocrine glands: these are organs whose only function is the production and release of hormones. These include:
  - The pituitary gland
  - The thyroid gland
  - The parathyroid glands
  - The adrenal glands.
- Organs that are not pure endocrine glands (in that they have other functions as well as the production of hormones) but contain areas of hormone-producing tissue. These include:
  - The hypothalamus
  - The pancreas.
- Organs and other tissues that produce hormones: areas of hormone-producing cells are found in the small intestine, the stomach, the heart, the liver and the skin.

The endocrine system has many effects within the human body. The major functions the endocrine system can have an impact on are:

- Homeostasis: helps to manage the internal body systems to maintain physiological balance
- The storage and metabolism of carbohydrates, proteins and fats
- The regulation of growth and development
- The regulation of reproduction and the sexual functioning of the body (see Chapter 34).
- Control of the body's responses to external stressors.

HORMONES

The nervous system transmits its impulses via nerves and thus the 'message' that is sent is constrained by the pathway the nerves take and the areas of tissue they supply. In this, it is rather like a telephone attached to a landline; the message (impulse) can only travel to receivers (telephones) also attached to the same wires. Hormones, however, are routinely secreted into the blood, or extracellular fluid, and are then dispersed throughout the body. Once secreted into the bodily fluid, the hormone travels wherever that bodily fluid is distributed, and all cells that are in contact with that fluid come into contact with the hormone. However, the cells must contain the receptors for that hormone if the hormone is to have any effect on the cell. Thus, the release of hormones is like the broadcast of a signal from a two-way radio (walkie-talkie). The signal (hormone) is broadcast into the air (body fluid) and travels indiscriminately wherever it can but the signal is only received by radios tuned to that particular channel (cells with receptors for that hormone). If the radio (cell) is not tuned to that channel (has a receptor for the hormone), then the signal is not received (the hormone has no effect).

This concept of receptors is very important in the understanding of the endocrine system, as in many endocrine conditions the receptors on a cell can be upregulated or downregulated. In other words, the number of receptors for a hormone can be increased or decreased, thus making the cell more or less receptive to a hormone.

As well as the number of receptors present, the effect of a hormone is also regulated by the amount of hormone produced, the rate of delivery of the hormone (for instance the rate of blood flow to the target cell) and the half-life of the hormone.

Hormones can have an effect on their target cells even at low levels of concentration; thus it is essential that they are removed from circulation efficiently. Some hormones are broken down within the cells; however, most are inactivated by enzymes in the liver and the kidneys and then excreted.

The effects a hormone can have on a cell are many and varied but include:

- Changing the electrical state of the cell
- Changes in the permeability of the cell wall membrane
- The creation of proteins or enzymes within the cell
- Activating or deactivating enzyme systems
- Stimulating the secretion of other hormones
- Stimulating cell division.

The control of hormone production and secretion

The creation and release of most hormones is in response to an external or internal stimulus; for instance, a reduction in blood glucose levels or exposure to a cold environment. The further synthesis and release of hormones is then usually controlled by a negative feedback system. Negative feedback systems are very common in the endocrine system and rely on the effect of a hormone changing the stimulus for the release of that hormone, thus reducing the stimulus for the release of more hormone. An example of a simple negative feedback system can be seen in Fig. 35.2. In this diagram, the system is the central heating in a home. The drop in room temperature is detected by the thermostat, leading to increased electrical signals to the boiler control to have the boiler produce more hot water. The hot water is pumped out to the radiators, with the effect that the room

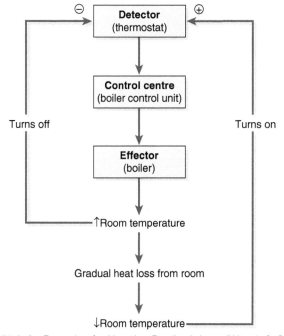

Fig. 35.2 An Example of a Negative Feedback Loop (Waugh & Grant, 2014).

temperature rises. This rise in heat is detected by the thermostat, which reduces its signals to the boiler control system; thus the boiler stops producing hot water. More negative feedback systems will be seen as this chapter reviews the different hormonal systems.

As noted in the preceding paragraph, the production and secretion of a hormone requires an initial stimulus. This stimulus is usually one of three types:

• Humoral

A response to a change in the levels of certain ions and nutrients in the blood. For example, glucagon secretion is stimulated by a drop in blood glucose levels.

• Neural

A response to direct stimulation by the nervous system; however, it should be noted that there are very few endocrine organs that are stimulated in this way. An example would be increased impulses from the sympathetic nervous system to the adrenal medulla, resulting in the release of catecholamines (adrenaline and noradrenaline).

• Hormonal

A response to hormones released by other glands or organs. An example of hormonal control would be the release of thyroxine, which is directly stimulated by the secretion of thyroid stimulating hormone (TSH) from the anterior pituitary gland.

THE ANATOMY AND PHYSIOLOGY OF THE INDIVIDUAL ENDOCRINE GLANDS

The hypothalamus and the pituitary gland

The hypothalamus is a small structure within the brain that is directly connected to the pituitary gland by the pituitary stalk (or infundibulum). By the use of hormonal or electrical mechanisms, the hypothalamus is responsible for almost all the stimuli that lead to the release of hormones from the pituitary gland.

The hypothalamus receives signals from many parts of the nervous system and part of its role is to connect the nervous and hormonal systems via the output from the pituitary gland. The hypothalamus is also under negative feedback control, mediated by the hormones secreted by the pituitary gland.

Though very small (about the size of a pea), the pituitary gland secretes at least nine major hormones. The pituitary gland is divided into two parts:

The posterior lobe

The posterior lobe is mostly made up of nerve fibres, which begin in the hypothalamus and end on the surface of capillaries in the posterior lobe (Fig. 35.3). The posterior lobe receives two hormones directly from cells in the hypothalamus, which are

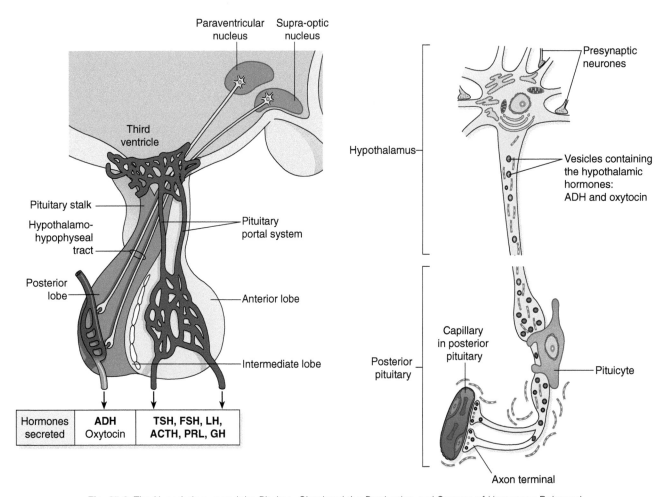

Fig. 35.3 The Hypothalamus and the Pituitary Gland and the Production and Storage of Hormones Released by the Posterior Pituitary Gland (Waugh & Grant, 2014).

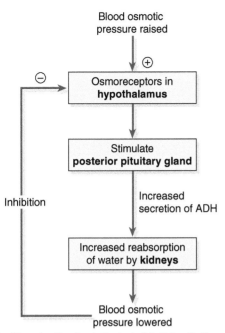

Fig. 35.4 The Negative Feedback Control of Antidiuretic Hormone (ADH) Secretion. (Waugh & Grant, 2014).

TABLE 35.1 **Hormones of the Hypothalamus and Anterior Pituitary and Their Target Tissues**		
Hypothalamus	**Anterior pituitary**	**Target gland or tissue**
GHRH	GH	Most tissues
		Many organs
GHRIH	GH inhibition	Thyroid gland
	TSH inhibition	Pancreatic islets
		Most tissues
TRH	TSH	Thyroid gland
CRH	ACTH	Adrenal cortex
PRH	PRL	Breast
PIH	PRL inhibition	Breast
LHRH or	FSH	Ovaries and testes
GnRH	LH	Ovaries and testes

ACTH, Adrenocorticotrophic hormone; CRH, corticotrophin-releasing hormone; FSH, follicle-stimulating hormone; GH, growth hormone (somatotrophin); GHRH, growth hormone-releasing hormone; GHRIH, growth hormone release-inhibiting hormone (somatostatin); GnRH, gonadotrophin-releasing hormone; LH, luteinizing hormone; LHRH, luteinizing hormone-releasing hormone; PIH, prolactin-inhibiting hormone (dopamine); PRH, prolactin-releasing hormone; PRL, prolactin (lactogenic hormone); TRH, thyrotrophin-releasing hormone; TSH, thyroid-stimulating hormone.

transported down the axons of the nerve bundles connecting the hypothalamus and the pituitary gland (the hypothalamic–hypophyseal tract). These hormones are then stored and released into the bloodstream in response to a stimulus. Thus, the posterior pituitary gland is actually a storage area as opposed to a gland.

The hormones that are secreted by the posterior pituitary are:
- Oxytocin. Oxytocin has an effect on uterine contraction in childbirth and is responsible for the 'let down' response in breast-feeding mothers. It also has a role in sexual arousal and orgasm.
- Antidiuretic hormone (ADH). The effect of ADH is to increase water retention by the kidneys. The control of the release of ADH can be seen in Fig. 35.4.

Osmosis is a complex concept that is best understood through examples. In the case of ADH, the increased osmotic pressure may be caused by dehydration. The lower levels of water in the body increases the levels of electrolytes and other chemicals in the blood (there is less water to dilute them). This increase in osmotic pressure is detected by specialist receptors (osmoreceptors), which leads to the release of ADH. ADH then causes several changes in the body (including a reduction in the production of urine), so that water is retained and the levels of water in the body increase, thus reducing osmotic pressure.

The anterior lobe

The anterior lobe of the pituitary gland (adenohypophysis) is much larger than the posterior lobe. Unlike the posterior pituitary gland, the anterior pituitary gland and the hypothalamus have no direct nerve connections, but they do have a dense vascular (blood vessel) connection known as the hypothalamo-hypophyseal portal system. Thus, the hypothalamus controls the anterior pituitary gland by releasing hormones that promote or inhibit the secretion of other hormones from the anterior pituitary gland.

The hormones secreted by the anterior pituitary gland and the releasing or inhibiting hormones from the hypothalamus that influence their production and release are summarized in Table 35.1.

Growth hormone

The secretion of growth hormone is controlled by the release of growth hormone-releasing hormone and growth hormone release-inhibiting hormone (somatostatin) by the hypothalamus. Growth hormone promotes the growth of bone, cartilage and soft tissue.

Prolactin

Prolactin stimulates the secretion of milk in the breast.

Follicle stimulating hormone and luteinising hormone (gonadotrophins)

The gonadotrophins are involved in the regulation of the reproductive system and control of their release is regulated by the release of gonadotrophin-releasing hormone.

Thyroid stimulating hormone

The release of thyrotrophin-releasing hormone (TRH) from the hypothalamus stimulates the production and release of TSH. TSH then stimulates the activity of the cells of the thyroid gland, leading to an increased production and secretion of the thyroid hormones.

Adrenocorticotropic hormone

Corticotrophin-releasing hormone (CRH) is released by the hypothalamus in response to any form of stress and this leads

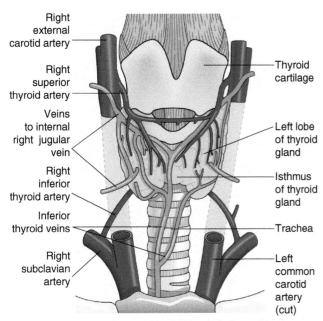

Fig. 35.5 The Thyroid Gland (Waugh & Grant, 2014).

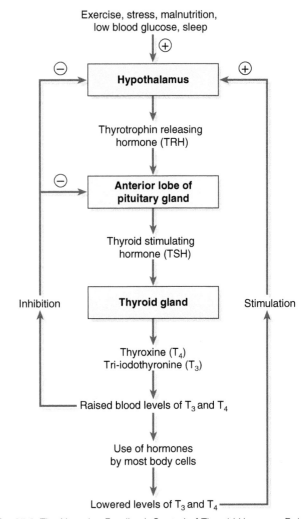

Fig. 35.6 The Negative Feedback Control of Thyroid Hormone Release (Waugh & Grant, 2014).

to the production and release of adrenocorticotropic hormone (ACTH). ACTH stimulates the production of cortisol and androgens from the adrenal gland. It also leads to the production of aldosterone.

The thyroid gland

The thyroid gland is a butterfly-shaped gland located in the front of the neck on the trachea, just below the larynx (Fig. 35.5). It is made up of two lobes that are joined by a narrow strip (this strip is known as an 'isthmus'). Each lobe is made up of hollow, spherical follicles surrounded by capillaries. The rich capillary network surrounding the follicles ensures that, when released, thyroid hormone rapidly enters the bloodstream.

One unusual aspect of the thyroid gland is that it can store up to 100 days' supply of the hormone it releases. The thyroid gland releases two forms of thyroid hormones:

* Thyroxine (T_4): the primary hormone released by the thyroid gland; it is converted into T_3 by the target cells.
* Triiodothyronine (T_3): created in smaller amounts than T_4 but has a more potent effect on cell receptors.

Thyroid hormone affects virtually every cell in the body, except:

* The adult brain
* Spleen
* Testes
* Uterus
* Thyroid gland.

In the target cells, thyroid hormone has the effect of stimulating enzymes that are involved with glucose use. This is known as the 'calorigenic effect' and its general effects are:

* An increase in the basal metabolic rate
* An increase in oxygen consumption by the cell
* An increase in the production of body heat.

Thyroid hormone also has an important role in the maintenance of blood pressure.

Like most of the individual endocrine systems, the control of thyroid hormone release is regulated by a negative feedback system (Fig. 35.6).

Thyroid hormone levels in the blood are monitored by the hypothalamus and by cells in the anterior lobe of the pituitary gland. When thyroid hormone levels in the blood are low, it is detected by the hypothalamus and this leads to the release of TRH. The effect of TRH is to promote the production and release of TSH from the anterior pituitary gland. In response to stimulation by TSH, the follicle cells of the thyroid gland release the thyroid hormones T_3 and T_4 into the bloodstream. As the levels of thyroid hormones in the bloodstream increase, this change is detected by the hypothalamus and anterior pituitary gland, leading to a gradual inhibition of the release of TRH and TSH and thus a reduction in the release of thyroid hormones.

In addition to the thyroid follicles, there are C cells in the thyroid gland, which secrete calcitonin. Calcitonin is involved in the regulation of calcium and phosphorous within the body.

The parathyroid glands

On the posterior (back) of the thyroid gland are a set of small glands, usually found in two pairs. These are the parathyroid

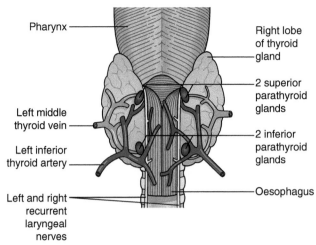

Fig. 35.7 The Parathyroid Glands (Waugh & Grant, 2014).

glands (Fig. 35.7). As with the thyroid gland, the cells that produce parathyroid hormone (known as chief cells) are surrounded by a dense capillary network that ensures a rich blood supply. Parathyroid hormone is the most important hormone for the control of the calcium balance in the body. The effects of parathyroid hormone include increasing absorption of calcium from the intestine, increasing calcium absorption in the kidneys and promoting the release of calcium from the bones.

Calcium is important for the human body as it is involved in the transmission of nerve impulses, muscle contraction and is also a major factor in the creation of clotting elements in the blood. As with most hormones, the control of the production and release of parathyroid hormone is regulated by a negative feedback loop based on the calcium levels in the blood.

Along with a decrease in calcium ions in the blood, the release of parathyroid hormone also stimulates the release of the hormone calcitriol from the kidneys. When calcitriol levels achieve a high enough level, its presence in the blood inhibits the release of parathyroid hormone. This prevents an uncontrollable increase in calcium in the blood.

The adrenal glands

There are two adrenal glands and they are located one on the top of each of the two kidneys. In common with the other glands, adrenal glands have a rich blood supply helping to ensure the rapid transportation of the hormones secreted to the target organs.

Functionally, each of the adrenal glands is comprised of two major regions:
- Adrenal medulla
- Adrenal cortex.

Adrenal medulla

The adrenal medulla is the internal (centre) section of the adrenal gland. The function of the adrenal medulla is the secretion of the catecholamines:
- Adrenaline
- Noradrenaline.

The adrenal medulla receives sympathetic nervous system input, which means that hormone release can occur rapidly if there is a stimulus such as:
- Pain
- Anxiety
- Excitement
- Hypovolaemia
- Hypoglycaemia.

Adrenaline and noradrenaline have several effects:
- Stimulating the nervous system
- Metabolic effects: for instance, the breakdown of glycogen to create glucose in the liver and skeletal muscle
- Increasing metabolic rate
- Increasing heart rate
- Increasing alertness
- Noradrenaline causes significant vasoconstriction
- Adrenaline causes vasoconstriction in the skin and viscera but vasodilation in skeletal muscles.

Adrenaline and noradrenaline have a very short half-life in the blood and they are rapidly degraded by blood-borne enzymes.

Adrenal cortex

The outer section of each adrenal gland is responsible for the production of three hormones types:
- Mineralocorticoids
- Glucocorticoids
- Adrenal sex hormones (androgens).

Mineralocorticoids. The role of the mineralocorticoids is the regulation of electrolyte levels in the blood. Approximately 95% of the synthesized mineralocorticoids are aldosterone, with a small amount of other mineralocorticoids also being produced. Aldosterone increases the reabsorption of sodium in the kidneys, leading to an increase in the blood levels of sodium. Aldosterone is also important in the regulation of water levels in the blood and the levels of several other ions (such as potassium and bicarbonate). The control of aldosterone secretion is primarily related to the blood concentrations of sodium, the mean arterial blood pressure and blood volume. Reduced blood concentrations of sodium and a reduction in blood pressure stimulate the release of aldosterone via the renin–angiotensin–aldosterone system (Fig. 35.8).

Glucocorticoids. There appears to be no cell within the body that does not have receptors for the glucocorticoid hormones and their effect is important in many bodily systems. Glucocorticoid hormones appear to have a significant effect on metabolism and the inflammation and immune systems. Thus the glucocorticoids are a necessary part of the bodily response to a stressor (such as an injury).The glucocorticoid hormones have several effects including:
- Influencing the metabolism of most body cells
  - Promote glycogen storage in the liver
  - During fasting, they stimulate the generation of glucose
  - Increase blood glucose levels
- Helping provide resistance to stressors
- Enhancing the vasoconstrictor effect of adrenaline and noradrenaline

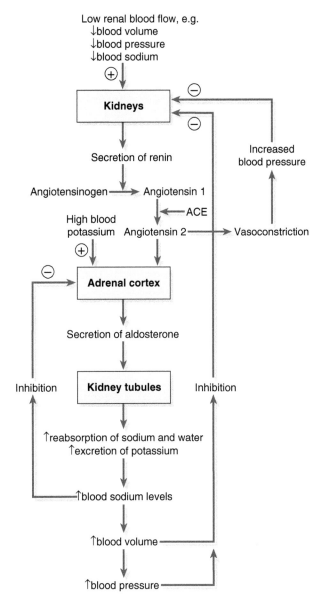

Low renal blood flow, e.g.
↓blood volume
↓blood pressure
↓blood sodium

Fig. 35.8 Control of Aldosterone Release (Waugh & Grant, 2014).

in sympathetic nervous system activity in response to an acute stressor triggers greater CRH release regardless of blood concentrations of cortisol; thus there is a significant increase in subsequent cortisol production (Fig. 35.9).

Pancreas

The pancreas is composed of two different types of tissues; the majority of the pancreas is made up of exocrine tissues (acini). This tissue produces and secretes a fluid rich with digestive enzymes into the small intestine (see Chapter 32). Distributed throughout the exocrine tissue are multiple clusters of cells known as islets of Langerhans. These are the site of the endocrine cells of the pancreas. Each islet has three major cell types, each of which produces a different hormone:
- Alpha cells, which secrete glucagon
- Beta cells, which secrete insulin
- Delta cells, which secrete somatostatin.

Insulin

The main action of insulin is well known: it reduces the blood glucose levels in the blood by:
- Facilitating the passage of glucose into muscle, adipose tissue and several other tissues. The exceptions to this are the brain and the liver, which do not use insulin.
- Insulin stimulates the storage of glucose (as glycogen) in the liver.

Insulin is also known to have an effect on protein, mineral and lipid metabolism. As glycogen storage in the liver rises to approximately 5% of the total liver mass, further glycogen creation is suppressed. Glucose is then diverted into the production of fatty acids and triglycerides for further storage in the tissues.

The main stimulus for insulin creation and secretion is a rise in blood glucose levels, but other stimuli include a rise in the levels of amino acids and fatty acids in the blood. It appears that some nervous system stimuli, for example the sight and smell of food, also increase insulin secretion, possibly as the body prepares for the intake of food.

The control of insulin synthesis and secretion is via a negative feedback loop: as blood glucose levels fall, there is a corresponding fall in the production and secretion of insulin. Enzymes that break down glycogen become active, leading to an increase in the levels of glucose in the blood.

Glucagon

Glucagon has the opposite effect to insulin and thus plays an important role in maintaining normal blood glucose levels. The effect of glucagon is to increase blood glucose levels by:
- Stimulating the breakdown of the glycogen stored in the liver to create glucose
- Activating the creation of glucose in the liver.

The production and secretion of glucagon is stimulated in response to a reduction in blood glucose concentrations. Whilst glucagon production and secretion appears to be controlled by a negative feedback loop, it is unknown whether a decrease in glucagon release is a direct effect of the increasing blood glucose levels or a response to rising levels of insulin. When a person exercises, the resulting increase in sympathetic nervous system

- Promoting the repair of damaged tissues
- Suppressing the immune system and inflammatory responses.

There are three main glucocorticoid hormones: cortisol, cortisone and corticosterone. Of these three, cortisol is the only one produced and secreted in any significant amounts.

Cortisol release is controlled by a negative feedback loop. A reduced level of cortisol in the blood stimulates the release of CRH from the hypothalamus. This promotes the release of ACTH from the anterior pituitary gland, which has the effect of increasing the production and secretion of cortisol from the adrenal glands. As cortisol levels in the blood increase, there is a negative feedback effect on both the hypothalamus and the pituitary gland, which inhibits the release of both CRH and ACTH. In situations of acute physiological stress (for instance in situations of trauma, infection or haemorrhage) or mental stress, this negative feedback system can be overridden. An increase

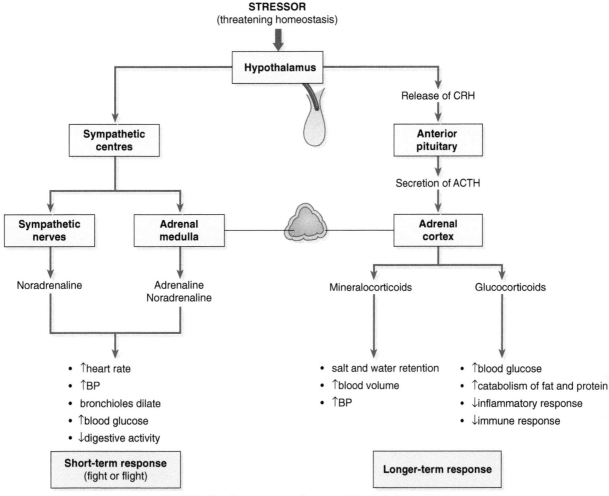

Fig. 35.9 The Response to a Stressor (Waugh & Grant, 2014).

activity stimulates the production and release of glucagon, which releases glucose stores for muscle use.

ENDOCRINE DISORDERS

Hypothyroidism

Hypothyroidism is a disorder characterized by the inadequate production of thyroid hormone.

Signs and symptoms

The causes of hypothyroidism include radiation therapy of the neck, treatment for hyperthyroidism and viral destruction of the thyroid gland. However, the most common cause of hypothyroidism is autoimmune destruction of the tissues of the thyroid gland, known as Hashimoto's thyroiditis (Biondi & Cooper, 2008).

The signs and symptoms of hypothyroidism include:

- Confusion, memory loss, depression
- Lethargy
- Bradycardia
- Constipation
- Weight gain
- Muscle cramps, myalgia (generalized muscle aches), stiffness
- Dry, cool skin
- Brittle nails
- Coarse hair, hair loss
- Oedema of hands and eyelids
- Cold intolerance
- Vacant expression
- Hoarse voice

(Gaitonde et al., 2012).

Diagnosis

The diagnosis of hypothyroidism generally occurs in general practice. The patient will often attend the GP surgery with a vague collection of symptoms that can often be mistaken for symptoms of aging or other, normal processes that may have developed over years. If, following history-taking and examination, there is clinical suspicion of hypothyroidism, current guidelines recommend that a blood sample is taken and sent for thyroid function tests (Garber et al., 2012).

Care and treatment

The treatment of hypothyroidism is thyroid hormone replacement with levothyroxine (Jonklaas et al., 2014). Levothyroxine

THE MEDICINE TROLLEY 35.1

Drug	Drug classification	Reason for administration	Route of administration	Dose	Side effects	Contra-indications	Nursing care
Levothyroxine	Thyroxine replacement	Hypothyroidism	Oral	50–100 µg daily	Angina Diarrhoea Excitability Fever Headache Insomnia Muscle cramps Rash	Should be used with caution in patient with heart disease, diabetes, the elderly	Seek consent prior to administration Explain the use of the drug to the patient, respond to any questions Information on when to take levothyroxine and what to do in the event of severe gastrointestinal illness is essential Close monitoring of thyroxine levels are required during pregnancy (and preferably before conception)

should be taken at the same time each day and, if possible, about an hour before breakfast (Weetman, 2013). Patients should be informed that their symptoms will not be resolved immediately and the amount of levothyroxine they take should only be altered on medical advice. Patients must be advised that it may take months to find the correct dose of levothyroxine for them and frequent blood tests will be required in the first year.

Once the correct dose for a patient has been found, annual blood tests will be taken to ensure that the required levels of replacement therapy have not changed.

Many patients are reluctant to take long-term thyroxine therapy (Crilly, 2004). The monitoring of adherence with hormone replacement therapy and the use of strategies to encourage and maintain adherence are an important part of the role of the healthcare professional. It is important that patients are informed of the possible side effects of thyroid replacement therapy, including temporary hair loss (Roberts & Ladenson, 2004), as this will affect their adherence with treatment. Patients should be given information regarding the need to take their replacement therapy as prescribed and what to do in the event of prolonged gastrointestinal problems that prevents them taking their daily levothyroxine dose.

CRITICAL AWARENESS

Levothyroxine Interactions

Levothyroxine is known to interact with multivitamin preparations; these should be taken 4 hours apart.

Antacids and proton pump inhibitors are known to reduce the absorption of levothyroxine and should be taken several hours apart.

Levothyroxine enhances the anticoagulant effect of warfarin.

COMMUNITIES OF CARE

Hypothyroidism is the most common endocrine disorder in primary care. Unfortunately, it is frequently undiagnosed because the symptoms are vague, and in the elderly, both the patient and the doctor may attribute the signs and symptoms to the ageing process. Primary care staff should be alert for the possibility of hypothyroidism in patients with more than one potential symptom.

Most patients with hypothyroidism are managed in primary care. Elderly patients may require regular community nursing follow up to assess pill counts or to review dosset boxes.

Patients will often be referred to specialist care if they:
- Are younger than 16
- Are pregnant or trying to get pregnant (hypothyroidism in the mother can have significant effects on the foetus)
- Have just given birth
- Have another health condition, such as heart disease
- Are taking amiodarone or lithium medication (both these drugs interfere with blood tests for TSH).

Elderly patients and those with heart disease will require a lower starting dose of levothyroxine.

Hyperthyroidism

Hyperthyroidism is the production and release of excessive levels of thyroxine.

Signs and symptoms

Hyperthyroidism is commonly caused by an autoimmune disorder known as Graves disease (Weetman, 2013). In Graves disease, antibodies mimic the effect of TSH. This leads to the overproduction of thyroid hormone from the thyroid gland. The reason for the onset of production of the antibodies is unknown but it appears to have a genetic cause. The most likely time in life to develop Graves disease is between 20 and 40 years of age (Weeks, 2005). There are other causes of hyperthyroidism, including thyroid cancer, thyroid nodules, viral thyroiditis (inflammation of the thyroid gland), postpartum thyroiditis and patients taking iodine-containing drugs (such as amiodarone) but these are much less common than Graves disease.

The signs and symptoms of hyperthyroidism are directly related to the activity of the excess thyroid hormone and include:

- Nervousness, restlessness
- Tremors
- Fatigue
- Insomnia
- Tachycardia, palpitations (atrial fibrillation is common in the elderly)
- Shortness of breath
- Weight loss despite an increased appetite
- Frequency of passing stools
- Nausea and vomiting
- Muscle weakness, tremors
- Warm, moist flushed skin
- Fine hair
- Staring gaze, exophthalmos (bulging or protrusion of the eyes) – only related to Graves disease
- Goitre (swelling of the neck, usually due to a swollen thyroid gland)
- Heat intolerance.

! HOTSPOT

Exophthalmos is often very slow to develop and it may not be noted by the patient or their relatives. Taking a photograph of the patient at each clinic visit may be a useful method of assessing development and progression.

Diagnosis

As with hypothyroidism, diagnosis relies on taking a detailed history, a physical examination and diagnostic tests.

Blood will be taken to assess TSH and free T_4 levels in the blood. Free T_4 levels may be normal or raised; therefore a reduced TSH level in the blood is the most useful result for diagnosing hyperthyroidism. This is because the high levels of thyroid hormone in the blood will lead to negative feedback to the hypothalamus and pituitary gland, causing a reduction in TSH production.

It is also common to undertake isotope thyroid scans to assess the cause of the hyperthyroidism. In this test, the patient is asked to swallow small amounts of a mildly radioactive substance and a scan is undertaken to assess how much of the isotope is absorbed by the thyroid gland. A high level of absorption indicates Graves disease or thyroid nodules, whereas low uptake may suggest an inflammatory disease process, excess iodine in the diet or thyroid cancer. If cancer of the thyroid is suspected, then fine-needle aspiration cytology (taking cells from the swollen lump) may be undertaken to assess for the presence of cancerous cells.

Care and treatment

There are three main methods for treating hyperthyroidism:

- Anti-thyroid drugs
  Anti-thyroid drugs (such as carbimazole) have a slow onset of action due to the continued release of stored thyroxine in the thyroid gland. All anti-thyroid drugs have a significant side effect profile and this means that many patients will not tolerate taking them for long.
- Radioactive iodine
  As the most active cells within the thyroid gland will take up the most iodine, they will be the cells exposed to the highest doses of radiation and be destroyed. There is often a need to take anti-thyroid drugs in the first few weeks after treatment, as large amounts of the thyroxine stored in the thyroid gland may be released. Following radioactive iodine treatment, the patient may become hypothyroid, as there is little control over the amount of thyroid gland that is destroyed. Radioactive iodine is contraindicated in pregnancy.
- Surgical removal of part, or all, of the thyroid gland
  Thyroidectomy or partial thyroidectomy is the least used of the treatment options as it carries risks of damage to the parathyroid glands and the vocal cords and, as the thyroid gland is very vascular, there is also a risk of a major haemorrhage.

THE MEDICINE TROLLEY 35.2

Drug	Drug classification	Reason for administration	Route of administration	Dose	Side effects	Contra-indications	Nursing care
Carbimazole	Anti-thyroid drug	Hyperthyroidism	Oral	15–40 mg daily	Joint pains Fever Headache Jaundice Malaise Mild gastrointestinal disturbances Nausea Pruritus Rash Taste disturbance	Severe blood disorders	Seek consent prior to administration Explain the use of the drug to the patient, respond to any questions Carbimazole crosses the blood–placenta barrier and the lowest dose possible should be used in pregnancy Patients should be asked to report symptoms and signs suggestive of infection, especially sore throat, as there is a risk of agranulocytosis (suppression of white blood cell production).

REFLECTION 35.2

How might you feel if you or a member of your family were told that you required treatment for hyperthyroidism? What might be your biggest anxiety? How might a Nursing Associate help to reduce that anxiety?

Before treatment is started, or during treatment, there may be a need for symptom relief from the effects of hyperthyroidism.
- Atrial fibrillation, increased heart rate and heart failure should all be treated with appropriate medication.
- Frequent snacks should be encouraged to prevent weight loss. Remember that thyroxine is responsible for the basal metabolic rate; therefore high levels of thyroxine will increase the basal metabolic rate and thus calorie consumption. A high-calorie, high-protein diet should be encouraged until thyroid function is normalized and vitamin supplements (particularly A, thiamine, B_6 and C) should be recommended (Weeks, 2005).
- Anxiety can be managed with the use of beta-blocking drugs, which may also be of use in the treatment of tremors.
- Provision of a quiet, calm environment will also be of value.

If the patient has developed exophthalmos, they will require monitoring by an ophthalmologist and may require treatment. It may also be useful to suggest that patients:
- Raise the head of their bed, for example, by using extra pillows. This may help reduce some of the puffiness around the eyes.
- Stop smoking. Smoking can significantly increase the risk of the thyroid condition affecting the eyes.
- Wear sunglasses if they have photophobia (sensitivity to light).
- If the patient has dry eyes, the use of over the counter eye drops may be beneficial.
- Wear a patch over one eye if they have double vision.
- If the eye disease is recent in onset and mild, then the patient may wish to take selenium supplements as this is thought to help (selenium is a mineral found in Brazil nuts, meat and fish).

COMMUNITIES OF CARE

Patients with hyperthyroidism will normally be under the care of an endocrinologist but primary care staff still have a role in the management of these patients. The regular monitoring of thyroid hormone levels, education and advice regarding the treatment and control of hyperthyroidism are all appropriate roles for the primary care team.

Primary care providers will also need to monitor other bodily changes that can occur with hyperthyroidism, such as high cholesterol levels, high blood glucose levels and electrolyte disturbances.

Cushing's syndrome

Cushing's syndrome is a form of hypercortisolism, a condition where there is excessive levels of cortisol in the blood.

Signs and symptoms

Whilst Cushing's syndrome can be caused by a tumour of the adrenal gland or the pituitary gland, the most common cause is the use of high levels of corticosteroid medication for conditions such as arthritis, asthma and other inflammatory diseases.

The most common signs and symptoms of Cushing's syndrome can be seen in Fig. 35.10 and include:

- Weight gain
- High blood pressure
- Poor short-term memory
- Irritability
- Excess hair growth (women)
- Red, ruddy face
- Extra fat deposition at the neck and shoulders (buffalo hump)
- Round face (otherwise referred to as a 'moon face')
- Fatigue
- Poor concentration
- Menstrual irregularity
- Slow wound healing
- Depression and rapid mood swings
- Insomnia
- Recurrent infections (especially fungal infections, such as thrush)
- Thin skin and stretch marks (often showing as purple striations)
- Easily bruising skin
- Weak bones
- Acne
- Hair loss (women)
- Hip and shoulder weakness
- Swelling of feet/legs due to oedema
- Diabetes mellitus.

Diagnosis

The diagnosis of Cushing's syndrome, like the diagnosis of all endocrine disorders, is based on taking a detailed history, performing a physical examination and a number of diagnostic investigations.

History-taking should focus on the development of the symptoms and must include a full drug history to review the patient for the use of steroid medication. The signs and symptoms of Cushing's syndrome, but an absence of a history of steroid use, will potentially lead on to a number of investigations:
- Late night salivary cortisol. Cortisol levels at midnight should be very low; if they are high, then this suggests Cushing's syndrome.
- 24-hour urine collection that is then tested for cortisol levels.
- Dexamethasone suppression test. The patient is administered a synthetic version of cortisol and the cortisol levels in the blood are measured after a suitable time period. The administration of dexamethasone should suppress the production of cortisol by the body. If cortisol levels do not fall, then it is likely the patient is suffering from Cushing's syndrome.

Further investigations may include scanning the pituitary and adrenal glands for tumours.

Care and treatment

! HOTSPOT

Patients who have been taking steroids for more than a few days must never stop their steroids suddenly, as this may precipitate a hypoadrenal crisis. Patients who take steroids for more than 3 weeks must be issued with, and carry, a steroid treatment card.

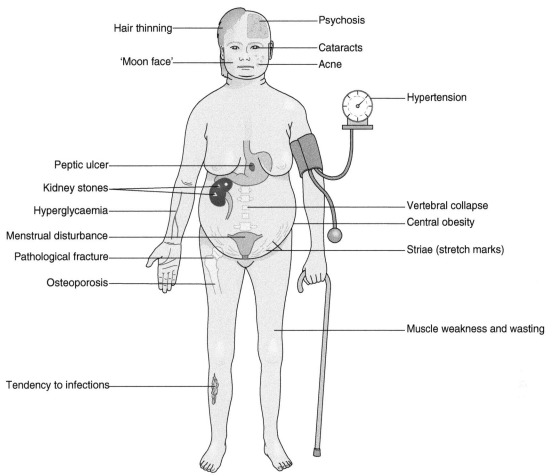

Hair thinning —
'Moon face' —
Psychosis
Cataracts
Acne
Hypertension

Peptic ulcer —
Kidney stones —
Hyperglycaemia —
Menstrual disturbance —
Pathological fracture —
Osteoporosis —

Vertebral collapse
Central obesity
Striae (stretch marks)

Muscle weakness and wasting

Tendency to infections —

Fig. 35.10 The Signs and Symptoms of Cushing's Syndrome (Waugh & Grant, 2014).

For those patients with Cushing's syndrome caused by extended use of high-dose steroid medication, the treatment is to gradually reduce the dose of steroids. However, the dose of steroids will be dictated by the progress of the disease the steroids are being used to treat. In patients with a tumour of the adrenal gland or pituitary gland, treatment will usually be by radiotherapy or surgery.

Other management of the patient with Cushing's syndrome may include:

- Decreasing the risk of injury by removing slip and trip hazards and helping unstable patients to mobilize. In the community, a visit to the patient's home may be advised to assess for slip and trip hazards.
- It may be appropriate to refer the patient to the dietician for advice on diet to promote muscle mass and bone density.
- Minimize the risk of infection. If the patient has not had chicken pox, they are best advised to avoid people suffering from chicken pox or shingles.
- Promote moderate exercise to reduce muscle wasting.
- Maintain good skin care and avoid adhesive tapes, which may tear skin. Monitor vulnerable areas of skin, such as the shins, for damage.
- Explain to the patient and their family the reasons for the patient's mood swings.

- Provide information and support for issues such as changes in body image.
- Ensure patients who are reducing steroid doses understand the need to follow the reduction plan and not stop the steroids suddenly.
- Ensure patients taking steroids have been given, and carry, the steroid treatment card.

COMMUNITIES OF CARE

Primary care practitioners have a vital role to play in the prevention of, and monitoring for, Cushing's syndrome.

Cushing's syndrome is often missed as a diagnosis, as it is slow in onset with a vague set of symptoms that are easily confused with other conditions, such as obesity and high blood pressure. As the commonest cause of Cushing's syndrome is the use of steroid medication, primary care staff should be alert for the syndrome in any patient taking high-dose or long-term steroid medication.

Courses of steroid treatment are often used in the community and primary care health professionals should be aware of the need to use the lowest effective dose.

Prolonged use of steroids can make patient susceptible to developing diabetes mellitus. Therefore, patients should have blood sugar levels taken once a year.

Adrenal insufficiency

CASE STUDY 35.1   John

John is a 33-year-old man who has presented to his GP for an urgent appointment. On questioning, he reports a history of lethargy, tiredness, abdominal pain, alternating diarrhoea and constipation. The doctor notes that John appears to have darkened skin in his skin creases (such as the creases in the palms, on the knuckles, between the top of the leg and the groin) and at the waistband.

Vital Signs

The GP noted the following vital signs:

Vital sign	Observation	Normal
Temperature	37°C	36.1–38.0°C
Pulse	80 beats per minute	51–90 beats per minute
Respiration	14 breaths per minute	12–20 breaths per minute
Blood pressure	112/58 mm Hg	111–219 mm Hg
O_2 saturation:	99%	≥96%

A full blood count and U&Es* were taken and sent to the hospital laboratory.

Test	Result	Guideline normal values
Sodium	137 mmol/L	135–145 mmol/L
Potassium	5.0 mmol/L	3.5–5.5 mmol/L
White blood cells	10×10^9/L	$4–11 \times 10^9$/L
Neutrophils	8.0×10^9/L	$2.0–7.5 \times 10^9$/L
Lymphocytes	3.5×10^9/L	$1.3–4.0 \times 10^9$/L
Red blood cells	4.0×10^{12}/L	$3.8–5 \times 10^{12}$/L
Haemoglobin	16.0 g/dL	13.0–18.0 g/dL
Platelets	350×10^9/L	$150–440 \times 10^9$/L
Blood glucose	100 mg/dL	65–110 mg/dL

*Urea and Electrolytes

Take some time to reflect on this case and then consider the following:
1. What is the likely diagnosis for John?
2. What test could the GP perform to confirm the potential diagnosis?
3. Who should the GP refer John to at the hospital?
4. What medication might be prescribed for John?

CRITICAL AWARENESS

Investigation: Short Synacthen Test

The use of an artificial version of ACTH (synacthen) to stimulate the adrenal gland is used in patients with suspected adrenal insufficiency (Addison disease), who are not critically ill.

Before the injection of the synacthen, a baseline blood cortisol level is taken and labelled accordingly. The patient is then administered the synacthen by intramuscular injection. A second blood test for blood cortisol levels is then taken 30 minutes later and labelled appropriately.

Samples should be sent to the laboratory the same day and kept at room temperature. If the samples cannot be sent the same day, they should be refrigerated overnight. It is not advisable to store the samples for more than 24 hours.

A cortisol level of >420 nmol/L at 30 minutes post-synacthen administration indicates an adequate adrenal response. Responses lower than this indicate probable Addison disease and the patient should be prescribed hydrocortisone and fludrocortisone to replace the corticosteroids no longer being produced by the adrenal glands.

Adrenal insufficiency is a condition characterized by the reduced production of mineralocorticoid and glucocorticoid steroids by the adrenal glands.

Adrenal insufficiency is divided into two types (Arlt & Allolio, 2003):
- Primary adrenal insufficiency (Addison disease) due to a disorder of the adrenal glands. The leading cause of Addison disease in the UK is autoimmune destruction of the glands.
- Secondary adrenal insufficiency. This is most commonly due to the patient suddenly stopping steroid therapy; however, disorders affecting the hypothalamus or the pituitary gland can also be a cause of secondary adrenal insufficiency.

Signs and symptoms

Regardless of the cause of adrenal insufficiency, the signs and symptoms are the same and include:
- Fatigue, lack of stamina, loss of energy
- Reduced muscle strength
- Increased irritability
- Nausea
- Weight loss
- Muscle and joint pain
- Abdominal pain
- Low blood pressure
- Reduction in or loss of libido.

In Addison disease, along with the loss of aldosterone synthesis and high levels of ACTH, the patient may also present with:
- Dehydration
- Hypovolaemia
- Postural hypotension
- Low levels of blood sodium
- High levels of blood potassium
- Hyperpigmentation of the skin: often a darkening in the skin creases (such as the palms, knuckles, inner elbow) or the waist (where clothes rub) but may be an all-over sun tan
- Vitiligo (pale patches of skin).

Diagnosis

The signs and symptoms of Addison disease are vague and may be slow and subtle in onset. The patient may have signs and symptoms for several months. In the event of acute trauma or infection, the added stress to the body may cause an acute adrenal crisis and the patient will present with acute symptoms of severe hypotension, dehydration, hypovolemic shock, acute abdominal pain and vomiting.

The definitive test for Addison disease is a synacthen (artificial ACTH) test. Blood cortisol level is measured before and after the administration of intramuscular synacthen. If the adrenal glands are working, there will be a rise in blood cortisol levels in response to the synacthen. If there is little or no response, then the adrenal glands are no longer functioning properly (or at all).

If secondary adrenal insufficiency is suspected, then blood ACTH and renin levels will be assessed by blood test. Both of these will be high in Addison disease but in secondary insufficiency, ACTH will be low and renin levels will be normal.

THE MEDICINE TROLLEY 35.3

Drug	Drug classification	Reason for administration	Route of administration	Dose	Side effects	Contra-indications	Nursing care
Hydrocortisone	Steroid	Adrenal insufficiency	Oral	15–30 mg daily in divided doses	Cushing's syndrome Indigestion Bruising Headache Impaired healing Increasing appetite Menstrual irregularities Susceptibility to infection (particularly thrush)	None but use with caution in: diabetes mellitus, heart failure, hypertension, hypothyroidism, osteoporosis	Seek consent prior to administration Explain the use of the drug to the patient, respond to any questions Explain the importance of a steroid treatment card Advise patients who have not had chicken pox to avoid people with chicken pox or shingles Advise patients who have not had measles to avoid people with measles Any suggestion the patient has developed chickenpox or measles means they must be referred to urgent specialist care

Care and treatment

Treatment of adrenal insufficiency is often commenced by an endocrinologist but will be continued in primary care with routine follow up in outpatient's clinic.

Treatment for Addison disease is based on the replacement of glucocorticoid and mineralocorticoid hormones. Androgen replacement is not usually prescribed in the UK, as there is limited evidence for its effectiveness. In secondary adrenal insufficiency, only glucocorticoid hormones are required for treatment.

COMMUNITIES OF CARE

The role of the primary care staff in the diagnosis and management of adrenal insufficiency is of great importance. Undiagnosed Addison disease is universally fatal and deterioration can be rapid.

Primary care practitioners should have a suspicion of Addison disease if the patient presents with being constantly fatigued, losing weight without dieting, has postural hypotension, unusual skin pigmentation and low blood sodium levels.

Once diagnosed, patients must be prescribed an extra month's supply of hydrocortisone as a 'backup' and an emergency injection kit for the first-line treatment of potential crisis.

Patients with adrenal insufficiency should be strongly advised to wear a medic alert talisman and carry a steroid card as emergency treatment in the event of a traumatic event must include intravenous steroids or the situation may become rapidly fatal.

Diabetes mellitus

Diabetes mellitus is a disorder of the endocrine system, characterized by high blood glucose levels.

There are two types of diabetes:

- Type 1 diabetes
  Type 1 diabetes is associated with development in childhood or early adulthood and is responsible for about 15% of the total incidence of diabetes in the UK; however, the prevalence of type 1 diabetes is increasing, particularly in children less than 5 years of age (Department of Health, 2001). The cause of type 1 diabetes is normally autoimmune destruction of the beta cells of the pancreas. Therefore, it is associated with a large reduction in, or complete loss of, insulin production (Daneman, 2006).
- Type 2 diabetes
  Type 2 diabetes is the most common form of diabetes and is normally considered to develop in patients over the age of 40. Over the last 20 years, the rates of juvenile onset type 2 diabetes appear to be rising (Haines et al., 2007). Type 2 diabetes is normally associated with the development of resistance to the effects of insulin in the tissues (especially body fat and skeletal muscles) and the continued production and release of glucose by the liver. Due to the insulin resistance, the fatty tissues and muscles are unable to respond effectively to insulin and absorb glucose from the blood, leading to an increasing blood glucose level. Following this, there is an associated reduction in the ability of the pancreatic beta cells to increase the production of insulin to meet the demands created by the increased insulin resistance in the body (Stumvoll et al., 2005). As levels of blood glucose rise, this is associated with toxic damage of the beta cells, leading to a reduction in the production of insulin. Risk factors for type 2 diabetes include being overweight, lack of exercise, genetic inheritance and increasing age. Genetic predisposition to type 2 diabetes appears to be especially strong in patients from south Asian or Afro-Caribbean backgrounds (Oldroyd et al., 2005).

Signs and symptoms

The signs and symptoms of diabetes are common to both forms of diabetes and are associated with increased blood glucose levels:

CASE STUDY 35.2   Sarah

Sarah Pope is a 17-year-old student who was found unconscious in her flat this morning by her flat mate. Sarah was diagnosed with type 1 diabetes 4 months ago and is struggling to accept the diagnosis. She has received education on managing her diabetes, including advice on her diet and the use of alcohol. Last night was her birthday and Sarah went out to celebrate with her friends. After eating at home, Sarah went out and is known to have consumed a large amount of alcohol. No one knows if Sarah adjusted her insulin or measured her blood sugar between eating and the following morning.

When her friend tried to wake Sarah this morning, Sarah was found to be unarousable. The paramedics were called, and on examination they found Sarah to be extremely pale and cold; her bed was wet from excessive sweating. Finding a Medic Alert talisman, the paramedics realized Sarah was diabetic and took a capillary blood sugar by finger prick. They found Sarah's blood sugar to be 1.5 mmol/L and immediately administered glucagon by an intramuscular injection. She was brought to A&E but remains unconscious.

Vital Signs

On admission to the A&E department, the following vital signs were noted and recorded:

Vital sign	Observation	Normal
Temperature	35.5°C	36.1–38.0°C
Pulse	110 beats per minute	51–90 beats per minute
Respiration	20 breaths per minute	12–20 breaths per minute
Blood pressure	100/58 mm Hg	111–219 mm Hg
O_2 saturation	98%	≥96%

A full blood count was performed.

Test	Result	Guideline normal values
White blood cells	6×10^9/L	$4–11 \times 10^9$/L
Neutrophils	3.0×10^9/L	$2.0–7.5 \times 10^9$/L
Lymphocytes	1.5×10^9/L	$1.3–4.0 \times 10^9$/L
Red blood cells	4.0×10^{12}/L	$3.8–5 \times 10^{12}$/L
Haemoglobin	13.0 g/dL	13.0–18.0 g/dL
Platelets	160×10^9/L	$150–440 \times 10^9$/L
Blood glucose	30 mg/dL	65–110 mg/dL

Take some time to reflect on this case and then consider the following.
1. What is the immediate care required by Sarah?
2. Why was Sarah's blood sugar so low?
3. Once Sarah's blood sugar has been stabilized, who would you refer Sarah to?
4. Why do you think Sarah behaved the way she did?

NEWS

Physiological parameter	3	2	1	0	1	2	3
Respiration rate				20			
Oxygen saturation (%)				98			
Supplemental oxygen				No			
Temperature (°C)			35.5				
Systolic BP mm Hg		100					
Heart rate				110			
Level of consciousness				U			
Score	3	2	2				
Total	7						

BP, Blood pressure. NEWS, National Early Warning Score.

- Passing urine more often than usual, especially at night
- Increased thirst
- Extreme tiredness
- Unexplained weight loss (usually only in type 1 diabetes)
- Genital itching or regular episodes of thrush
- Slow healing of cuts and wounds
- Blurred vision
- Abdominal pain
- Increased blood glucose
- Glucose in the urine
- Ketones in the urine.

Diagnosis

Type 1 diabetes is normally quite rapid in its development and this means that patients rarely remain undiagnosed for long, as symptom onset is rapid and noticeable. Many patients will go to their GP due to their symptoms; however, in some cases, the onset is rapid or is precipitated by an acute illness, so that the patient develops diabetic ketoacidosis and is admitted to hospital as an emergency.

Type 2 diabetes is slower and more subtle in its development and many patients will remain unaware of the fact that they have diabetes for years before they are diagnosed (Department of Health, 2001). Unfortunately, by the time some patients are diagnosed, they have been suffering from diabetes for years and complications have already developed.

The diagnosis of type 1 diabetes is based on the presence of high blood glucose on finger prick test, weight loss, thirst and increased urine output. Formal diagnosis is confirmed by one laboratory blood glucose measurement.

Type 2 diabetes is often diagnosed after an opportunistic finger prick or urine dipstick test, or a blood glucose is added to the normal blood tests a patient is undergoing, especially if blood tests are being taken for the management of another condition. Current guidance is focused on identifying people at risk of developing type 2 diabetes and encouraging those patients to have a risk assessment and risk identification (NICE, 2017).

Treatment and care

The treatment of type 1 diabetes is based on the replacement of insulin by subcutaneous injection. There are several forms of insulin but they are all classified by:
- How soon it starts working (onset)
- When it works the hardest (peak time)
- How long it lasts in the body (duration).

The decision regarding the appropriate insulin for an individual patient is made by an endocrinologist and will take into account factors such as lifestyle, blood glucose levels and the doctor's experience. Patients who are recently diagnosed with type 1 diabetes will require education regarding self-injection and insulin doses. This should be reviewed regularly with the patient to ensure they are maintaining best practice. Patients should also be advised regarding the storage of insulin and the rotation of injection sites.

Newly diagnosed type 1 diabetics have a high need for information and often have a lot of questions. The patient should be

OSCE 35.1 Urine Dipstick

This test is used to test for substances in the urine. They are relatively quick to use and the test can be performed on the ward, in the GP surgery or in the home.

The procedure should be undertaken using local policy and procedure

Action	Criteria	Achieved/not achieved
Introduction	Washes hands. Introduces self. Confirms patient details.	
Explain the procedure	Explains rationale for test so patient is able to understand and is able to give informed consent. Gains consent to proceed.	
Gathers equipment	• Gloves • Dipsticks • Watch • Fresh urine sample	
Assess the ability of the patient to produce a urine sample.	The patient may have recently emptied their bladder and may need to drink some water and then wait for the bladder to fill.	
Open the dipstick container, remove one without touching the squares. Place lid back on the container.	Touching the reagent squares may affect the test result. Closing the container promptly reduces the risk of the remaining dipsticks being exposed to moisture.	
Dipstick the urine	The dipstick must be completely immersed in the sample and then quickly removed. Tap the dipstick on the edge of the sample container to remove excess urine.	
Begin timing	Different tests require different lengths of time to ensure an accurate result.	
Compare the reagent strip to the colour charts on the side of the container	Allows for comparison of the colours for each square on the stick with the colour chart on the container.	
Dispose of equipment appropriately	In line with local policy.	
Remove gloves and wash hands	Infection control.	
Record results accurately	Maintain accurate records for patient safety.	

Pass
Fail

offered a structured programme of education and information should be offered on a regular basis (NICE, 2016).

REFLECTION 35.3

Imagine you, or a close relative, is newly diagnosed with type 1 diabetes. How would you feel? What sort of information would you want?

As a Nursing Associate, how can you support the newly diagnosed type 1 diabetic patient? Where could you advise them to find good quality advice and support for their condition?

The dietary advice given to all type 1 diabetic patients should include:
• Discussion of the effects of different foods and ensuring they have adequate insulin
• Type, timing and amount of snacks taken between meals and at bedtime
• Healthy eating to reduce the risk of complications
• If the person wants it, information on:
  • effects of alcohol-containing drinks on blood glucose and calorie intake
  • use of high-calorie and high-sugar 'treats'
  • use of foods with a high glycaemic index

CARE IN THE HOME SETTING

Self-monitoring of blood glucose levels in the home setting is essential in type 1 diabetes. The patient should be provided with a capillary blood glucose monitor. Education about testing (with specific guidance on the particular monitor supplied) should be offered at diagnosis and skills reassessed regularly. The patient should be advised to:

1. Wash their hands with warm, soapy water, and dry them well with a clean towel.
2. Put a clean needle (lancet) in the lancet device.
3. Check the expiry date of the test strips.
4. Get a test strip from the bottle of testing strips. Put the lid back on the bottle immediately to prevent moisture from affecting the other strips.
5. Get the blood sugar meter ready. Follow the manufacturer's instructions for the specific meter.
6. Use the lancet device to stick the side of the fingertip with the lancet. Some devices and blood sugar meters allow blood testing on other parts of the body, such as the forearm, leg, or hand, but this must be confirmed before the patient is advised to do this.
7. Put a drop of blood on the correct spot of the test strip.
8. Using a clean cotton ball or piece of gauze, stop the bleeding by applying pressure.
9. Wait for the results.
10. Record the results as directed by the doctor or diabetes specialist nurse.

THE MEDICINE TROLLEY 35.4

Drug	Drug classification	Reason for administration	Route of administration	Dose	Side effects	Contra-indications	Nursing care
Glucagon	Anti-hypoglycaemic	Hypoglycaemia	Subcutaneous or intramuscular injection	500 µg	Hypersensitivity reaction	Pheochromocytoma	As an emergency medicine, it may not be possible to gain consent for the administration of glucagon Once it is safe for the patient to eat, the patient should be encouraged to eat some carbohydrates to prevent further hypoglycaemia

! HOTSPOT

Hypoglycaemia is a potentially life-threatening condition characterized by a low blood sugar. The patient will present with:
- Hunger
- Nervousness and shakiness
- Perspiration
- Dizziness or light-headedness
- Sleepiness
- Confusion
- Difficulty speaking
- Feelings of anxiety or weakness

If safe to do so, the patient should be encouraged to eat glucose (in the form of jam, chocolate, etc.) or glucose paste can be rubbed into the gums. The glucose will be short acting and must be followed up with a longer acting carbohydrate (such as brown bread) if the patient is able to eat safely.

Semi-conscious and unconscious patients will require the administration of glucagon or intravenous glucose.

Patients with type 1 diabetes will also require education on the recognition and management of hypoglycaemia (often called 'hypos').

! HOTSPOT

Women of child-bearing age who are pregnant (or wish to become pregnant) will require close management of their diabetic control, as there is an increased risk of miscarriage and still birth.

The treatment of type 2 diabetes will depend on the severity of the condition. Treatment will always include advising the patient on making dietary adjustments (healthy diet with reduced fat and sugar) and lifestyle changes (such as exercising and losing weight if required). Dietary advice for patients with type 2 diabetes includes:
- Include high-fibre, low-glycaemic index sources of carbohydrate (such as porridge, beans, pulses and brown bread).
- Using low-fat dairy products and eating oily fish.
- Reduce the intake of foods containing saturated fats and trans-fatty acids.
- Moderate the use of foods marketed specifically for people with diabetes. These foods often contain fructose as a substitute for sucrose; fructose still affects blood glucose levels.

However, the treatment of type 2 diabetes may require the use of oral medication. Medication for type 2 diabetes generally has one of three potential actions:
- Reduces the amount of glucose released by the liver
- Increases the cells' ability to utilize insulin (decreasing insulin resistance)
- Promotes the production of insulin by the pancreas.

Self-monitoring of type 2 diabetes may be advised. If this is the case, the patient will need to be educated in the use of capillary blood measurement of glucose. However, it is more common for the primary care provider to monitor the HbA1C (long-term blood glucose measurement) every 2–6 months.

Patients with both types of diabetes will require advice on:
- Undertaking regular physical activity but be aware that strenuous exercise can reduce blood glucose levels and patients with type 1 diabetes will need to monitor blood glucose levels and adjust insulin doses accordingly.
- Stopping smoking. Smoking is a risk for all patients, but diabetic patients have an increased risk of cardiovascular disease, which is compounded by smoking.
- Managing cholesterol intake.
- Reducing salt intake.
- Weight loss, if required, as weight loss improves diabetic control in both types of diabetes.

COMMUNITIES OF CARE

Black, Minority Ethnic Groups

The incidence of type 1 diabetes is not known to be substantially different between groups with different ethnic backgrounds; however, the incidence of type 2 diabetes is three to five times higher in people with an Afro-Caribbean or south Asian ethnic background (Oldroyd et al., 2005).

There are many reasons for these differences, and cultural differences in dietary patterns and exercise are suggested as two possible mechanisms. Yet, when populations are matched for the same risk factors, Afro-Caribbean and south Asian populations have a greater incidence of type 2 diabetes than the white population, suggesting a genetic or gestational predisposition to the development of diabetes (Oldroyd et al., 2005).

Once the onset of diabetes is confirmed, it is clear that some patients from a minority ethnic background face difficulties in accessing healthcare and maintaining self-care activities due to socio-economic barriers, cultural and language barriers and low health literacy (Creamer et al., 2016). Culturally appropriate and accessible health education is essential for patients from an ethnic minority background, as research has clearly shown that improvements in the long-term control of blood glucose in these groups of patients is possible and is almost certainly just as beneficial for longer-term morbidity and mortality as for patients from a white background.

Recommendations for creating health education for patients from a minority ethnic background include:

- Using both group and individual support mechanisms
- Using lay workers in a supportive role
- Ensuring advice is tailored to take into account the patient's socio-economic status and cultural background
- Asking the target population to help in designing the health promotion

LOOKING BACK, FEEDING FORWARD

The endocrine system is essential for the maintenance of homeostasis. It is also involved in metabolism and energy management, the maintenance of electrolyte and water levels in the blood and responses to stress. This chapter has reviewed the anatomy and physiology of the various endocrine systems and their control and has gone on to discuss a few endocrine disorders that you are likely to come across in your career. The importance of the endocrine system to the ongoing physical functioning of the body cannot be underestimated, but it should not be the sole focus of the healthcare practitioner as the psychological impact of any endocrine disorder can have a significant impact on the patient's life.

REFERENCES

Arlt, W., Allolio, B., 2003. Adrenal insufficiency. Lancet 361 (9372), 1881–1893.

Biondi, B., Cooper, D.S., 2008. The clinical significance of subclinical thyroid dysfunction. Endocr. Rev. 29 (1), 76–131.

Creamer, J., Attridge, M., Ramsden, M., et al., 2016. Culturally appropriate health education for type 2 diabetes in ethnic minority groups: An updated Cochrane Review of randomized controlled trials. Diabet. Med. 33 (2), 169–183.

Crilly, M., 2004. Correspondence: Thyroxine adherence in primary hypothyroidism. Lancet 363 (9420), 1558.

Daneman, D., 2006. Type 1 diabetes. Lancet 367 (9513), 847–858.

Department of Health, 2001. National service framework for diabetes: Standards. Department of Health, London. Available at: https://assets.publishing.service.gov.uk/government/uploads/system/uploads/attachment_data/file/198836/National_Service_Framework_for_Diabetes.pdf.

Gaitonde, D.Y., Rowley, K.D., Sweeney, L.B., 2012. Hypothyroidism: an update. S. Afr. Fam. Pract. 54 (5), 384–390.

Garber, J.R., Cobin, R.H., Gharib, H., et al., 2012. Clinical practice guidelines for hypothyroidism in adults: cosponsored by the American Association of Clinical Endocrinologists and the American Thyroid Association. Thyroid 22 (12), 1200–1235.

Haines, L., Wan, K.C., Lynn, R., et al., 2007. Rising incidence of type 2 diabetes in children in the UK. Diabetes Care 30 (5), 1097–1101.

Health Education England, 2017. Nursing associate curriculum framework. NHS, London. Available at: https://hee.nhs.uk/sites/default/files/documents/Nursing%20Associate%20Curriculum%20Framework%20Feb2017_0.pdf.

Jonklaas, J., Bianco, A.C., Bauer, A.J., et al., 2014. Guidelines for the treatment of hypothyroidism: prepared by the American thyroid association task force on thyroid hormone replacement. Thyroid 24 (12), 1670–1751.

NICE, 2016. National Institute for Health and Care Excellence. NG17 Type 1 diabetes in adults: Diagnosis and management. Available at: https://www.nice.org.uk/guidance/ng17.

NICE, 2017. National Institute for Health and Care Excellence. PH38 Preventing type 2 diabetes: Risk identification and interventions for individuals at high risk. Available at: https://www.nice.org.uk/Guidance/PH38.

Nursing and Midwifery Council, 2018. The Code. Professional Standards of Practice and Behaviour for Nurses, Midwives and Nursing Associates. London: NMC. https://www.nmc.org.uk/standards/code/.Oldroyd, J., Banerjee, M., Heald, A., Cruickshank, K., 2005. Diabetes and ethnic minorities. Postgrad. Med. J. 81 (958), 486–490.

Roberts, C.G.P., Ladenson, P.W., 2004. Hypothyroidism. Lancet 363 (9411), 793–803.

Stumvoll, M., Goldstein, B.J., van Haeften, T.W., 2005. Type 2 diabetes: Principles of pathogenesis and therapy. Lancet 365 (9467), 1333–1346.

Waugh, A., Grant, A., 2018. Ross & Wilson Anatomy and Physiology in Health and Illness, thirteenth ed. Elsevier, Edinburgh.

Weeks, B.H., 2005. Graves' disease: The importance of early diagnosis. Nurse Pract. 30 (11), 34–45.

Weetman, A., 2013. Current choice of treatment for hypo- and hyperthyroidism. Prescriber 24 (13–16), 23–33.

36

Neurological Disorders

Julie Derbyshire and Barry Hill

OBJECTIVES

By the end of the chapter the reader will:

1. Develop an understanding of the anatomy and physiology of the central nervous system
2. Discuss the concept of raised intracranial pressure
3. Outline the components of a neurological assessment
4. Discuss the pathophysiological changes associated with a selection of neurological disorders
5. Describe the treatment and nursing management of common neurological disorders
6. Demonstrate an awareness of the role of the Nursing Associate and their contribution as a member of the multi-disciplinary team, caring for people with neurological disorders

KEY WORDS

Brain	Competence	Reflex
Spinal cord	Confidence	Nerves
Assessment	Central and peripheral nervous	Rehabilitation
Multi-disciplinary	systems	

CHAPTER AIMS

The aim of this chapter is to provide the reader with an understanding of the skills, knowledge and attitude required to provide safe, effective and compassionate care to people with a neurological disorder.

SELF TEST

1. What are the four lobes of the cerebral cortex and can you name a function of each lobe?
2. What is the function of the hypothalamus?
3. Where is the pituitary gland situated and can you name two hormones released from the gland?
4. What is the function of the cerebellum?
5. What are the three parts of the brainstem?
6. What is the main protection for the brain?
7. What are the three layers of the meninges?
8. What is contained in the ventricles of the brain?
9. What colour is CSF and how would a sample be obtained?
10. What are the two main arteries that supply the brain?

INTRODUCTION

In this chapter, neurological disorders are considered. The first part of this chapter will discuss the anatomy and physiology of the central nervous system (CNS), which consists of the brain and spinal cord. It is important for the Nursing Associate to have a comprehensive understanding of neurological disorders if the care provided is to be appropriate and effective. The second part of the chapter addresses a selection of common neurological disorders that affect the health and well-being of people and will begin by addressing the concept of intracranial pressure (ICP) and the importance of neurological observations. A selection of acute and chronic neurological disorders will be discussed, including the epidemiology and aetiology, signs and symptoms and the management of the condition. It is hoped that the information in this chapter will raise awareness of this specialist field of nursing and help Nursing Associates to deliver safe and effective care to patients with a neurological disorder. The care and comfort of the patient who experiences a neurological disorder are described. When offering care, the Nursing Associate must practice with kindness and compassion, and ensure inclusivity and a holistic approach. People with neurological disorders require a dignified approach to their care, as many neurological disorders result in personality, cognitive and behavioural changes. As neurology is so complex, the Nursing Associate must ensure that they are competent and knowledgeable to ensure a factual and evidence-based approach to advocate and empower their patient. Additionally, the Nursing Associate must be reflective and utilize appropriate communication skills when treating patients with neurological disorders. Neurological system diseases can have a significant impact on a person's physical and mental health state; this may create both physical and disordered conditions, and therefore must be acknowledged and supported by the Nursing Associate. From a professional viewpoint, this would also be in keeping with the duty of care obligations, which stipulates that 'Nursing Associates must not act or fail to act in a way that results in harm' (Health Education England, 2017).

NEUROLOGICAL DISORDERS

An understanding of the anatomy of the neurological system is essential to ensure that the Nursing Associate can offer care for and give support to people. Using knowledge, immersing oneself into learning and using evidence-based practice allows practitioners to provide safe care that is holistic and inclusive, with the ability to rationalize what they are doing. This is important, as patients may ask questions and they will expect to be provided with information. They will be expecting a competent and knowledgeable professional person to care for them. As well as understanding the structure of the neurological system, the Nursing Associate needs to ensure that the care provided is compassionate, caring and competent. This requires the Nursing Associate to use their interpersonal skills when caring for patients and (if appropriate) their families, as well as anyone advocating on behalf of the patient.

People who require care for neurological disorders come from across the lifespan, with concerns regarding a wide range of health issues, from childhood to old age. The Nursing Associate must aim to be as inclusive as possible, whilst offering care and support, as they work collaboratively with the patient as well as the wider health and social care team. Recognizing and respecting the diversity of needs results in care provision that is of a high quality and is humanistic, as well as empowering people from many perspectives, for example, in being able to access the best available and most appropriate care.

THE NEUROLOGICAL SYSTEM

It is important to understand neurological anatomy, organization, how the neurological system communicates and what happens when the neurological system is damaged. The three fundamental principle functions of the neurological system are:

- Sensory input
- Integration
- Motor output.

For example, sensory receptors would detect stimuli such as touch. The nervous system would then process the sensory input and make decisions as to what to do with the information (this is called 'integration'). The motor output is the response that occurs when the nervous system activates certain parts of the body. Therefore, it is recognized that the neurological system is highly complex, as it must continuously detect, process and act on data. When learning about the nervous system, it is pertinent to know that there are several levels of organization, starting with two main parts: the central (CNS) and peripheral nervous systems (PNS).

The CNS is the brain (cerebrum and cerebellum; see Fig. 36.1) and spinal cord, which is the main control centre (Fig. 36.2).

The cerebrum

The cerebrum (see Fig. 36.1) is supported on the brainstem and forms the bulk of the brain. The surface of the cerebrum is composed of grey matter and is referred to as the cerebral cortex. The convoluted cerebral cortex is made up of billions of nerve cell bodies. Beneath the cerebral cortex lies the cerebral white matter, which consists of myelinated nerve axons plus the basal ganglia. The cerebrum determines intelligence and personality and other functions include interpretation of sensory impulses, motor function (Fig. 36.3), planning and organization and touch sensation.

Functions of the brain
Key functions of the lobes

The frontal lobe is responsible for motor functions, higher order functions, planning, reasoning, judgement, impulse control, memory and speech. The parietal lobe is responsible for cognition, information processing, pain and touch sensation, spatial awareness, speech and visual perception. The occipital lobe controls vision and colour recognition. The temporal lobe is responsible for emotional responses, hearing, memory and speech (Fig. 36.4).

The cerebellum

The cerebellum (little brain) and associated structures (Fig. 36.5) play an important role in the integration of sensory perception and motor control. It receives input from muscles, tendons and joints. There is constant interaction with the motor cortex, which facilitates smooth coordination and fine tuning of muscle activity. The cerebellum also functions in maintaining balance and posture.

Medulla oblongata

The medulla oblongata is a continuation of the upper part of the spinal cord and forms the inferior part of the brainstem. The medulla contains all ascending and descending 'tracts' (white matter) that communicate between the spinal cord and various parts of the brain. Just above the junction of the medulla with the spinal cord, most of these 'tracts' cross over (decussation). Therefore, motor areas of one side of the cerebral cortex control muscular movements on the opposite side of the body. Within the medulla there are three vital centres:

1. Cardiac centre: regulates the heartbeat and force of contraction
2. Rhythmicity centre: adjusts the basic rhythm of breathing
3. Vasomotor centre: regulates the diameter of blood vessels.

There are also five non-vital centres:

1. Swallow
2. Cough
3. Vomit
4. Sneezing
5. Hiccupping

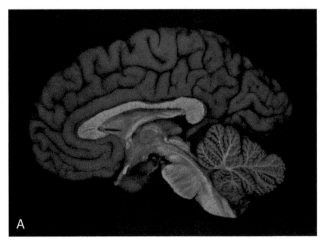

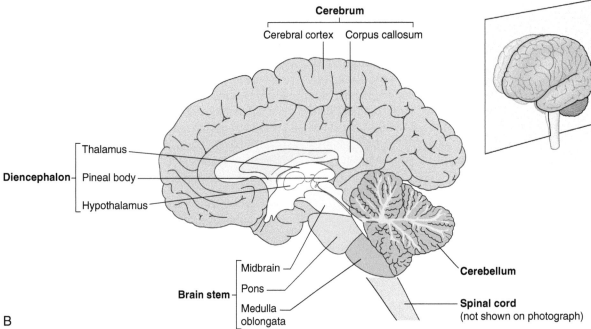

Fig. 36.1 A Midsagittal Section of the Brain Showing the Main Parts (Waugh & Grant, 2018).

Part of the reticular formation is within the medulla, which helps control consciousness and arousal. Several pairs of cranial nerves originate in the medulla.

Pons

The pons is a bridge connecting the spinal cord with the brain and parts of the brain with each other. The transverse fibres in the pons connect with the cerebellum, whilst the longitudinal fibres belong to the sensory and motor tracts that connect the spinal cord with the upper parts of the brainstem. Part of the reticular formation is within the pons and the pneumotaxic and apneustic areas help to control respiration. Several pairs of cranial nerves originate in the pons.

Midbrain (middle brain)

Within the midbrain there are reflex centres which cause eye, head and neck responses to visual and other stimuli (blink) and movements of the head and trunk in response to auditory

stimuli. The third and fourth cranial nerves originate in the midbrain. The substantia nigra (basal ganglia) are situated in the midbrain. The cerebral aqueduct passes through the midbrain, connecting the third and fourth ventricles.

The cranial nerves

There are 12 pairs of cranial nerves. These are sensory, motor or both (Fig. 36.6). The 12 cranial nerves, general functions and key functions are listed in Table 36.1.

Cranial nerve mnemonics can sometimes support the ability to remember the order of the cranial nerves and whether the cranial nerve is sensory, motor or both (Box 36.1).

The spinal cord

'The spinal cord transmits and manages the flow of information continuously between the brain and the rest of the body therefore it facilitates homeostasis in response to changes within and without the body' (Woodward & Mestecky, 2011). The spinal

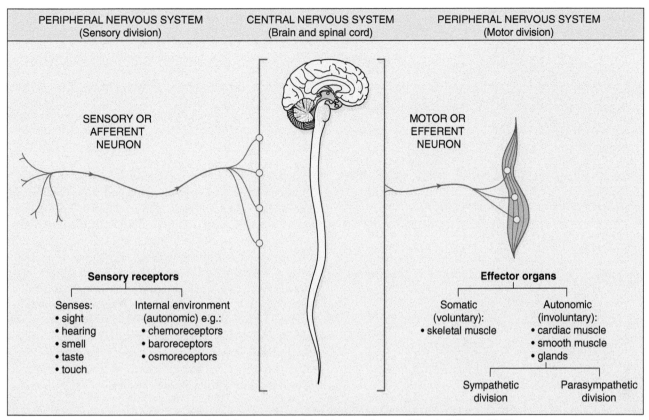

Fig. 36.2 Functional Components of the Nervous System (Waugh & Grant, 2018).

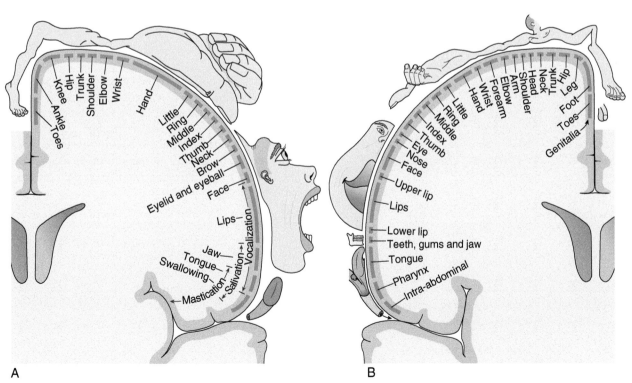

A

B

Fig. 36.3 Functional Areas of the Cerebral Cortex. (A) The motor homunculus, showing how the body is represented in the motor area of the cerebrum. (B) The sensory homunculus, showing how the body is represented in the sensory area of the cerebrum (Waugh & Grant, 2018).

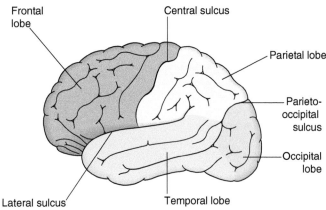

Fig. 36.4 The Lobes and Principal Sulci of the Cerebrum. Viewed from the left side (Waugh & Grant, 2018).

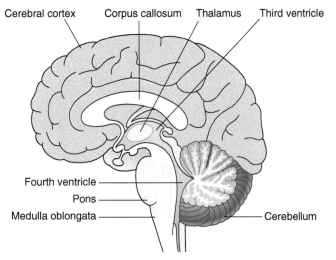

Fig. 36.5 The Cerebellum (Little Brain) and Associated Structures (Waugh & Grant, 2018).

cord originates at the lower (inferior) end of the medulla oblongata. It leaves the skull via a large opening called the foramen magnum and extends about two-thirds of the way down the spine, as far as the first lumber vertebra. Connecting with the cord are 31 pairs of spinal nerves (Cervical 1–8, Thoracic 1–12, Lumbar 1–5, Sacral 1–5, Coccyx 1), which feed sensory impulses (afferent) into the spinal cord, which in turn relays them to the brain (Fig. 36.7). Motor impulses (efferent) generated in the brain are relayed by the spinal cord to the spinal nerves, which pass the impulses to muscles and glands. The spinal cord mediates the reflex responses to some sensory impulses directly (i.e., without recourse to the brain, such as when a person's leg is tapped, producing the knee jerk reflex).

REFLECTION 36.1

You may have been privileged to witness and assist during a neurological examination as part of your work, or you may have experienced one as a patient.

You may also have seen on television or other such media where the examiner uses a patella hammer to test knee or ankle reflexes. Why do you think the examiner carries out this test?

The skin over the body is supplied segmentally by spinal nerves. The skin segment supplied by the dorsal root of the spinal nerve is called a 'dermatome'. Most of the face and scalp is supplied by the fifth cranial nerve (the trigeminal). In the neck and trunk, the dermatomes form consecutive layers. In the trunk, there is overlap of adjacent dermatome nerve supply; therefore, there is little loss of sensation if only a single nerve supply is interrupted.

Grey matter

Grey matter in the spinal cord consists of nerve cells which are divided into regions called 'horns':
- Anterior or ventral column
- Posterior or dorsal column
- Lateral column

White matter

White matter in the spinal cord consists of myelinated and non-myelinated nerve fibres, which are organized in columns:
- Ventral column
- Dorsal column
- Lateral column

TABLE 36.1 Cranial Nerves

No.	Nerve	General function	M, S, B
1	Olfactory	Sense of smell	Sensory
2	Optic	Sense of vision	Sensory
3	Oculomotor	Eye movements	Motor
4	Trochlear	Eye movements	Motor
5	Trigeminal	Sensation of face, scalp, teeth, chewing	Both
6	Abducens	Eye movement	Motor
7	Facial	Sense of taste, facial muscle movements (expression)	Both
8	Vestibulocochlear	Hearing; sense of balance	Sensory
9	Glossopharyngeal	Sensations of throat, taste, swallowing movement, saliva	Both
10	Vagus	Sensations of throat, larynx, thoracic and abdominal organs, swallowing, voice productions, slows heart rate, peristalsis	Both
11	Accessory	Accessory shoulder and head movements	Motor
12	Hypoglossal	Tongue movements	Motor

M, Motor; S, sensory; B, both.

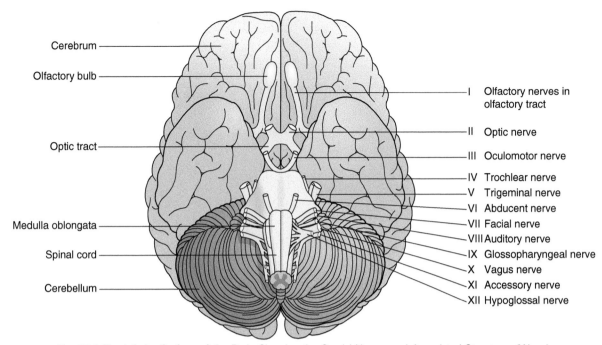

Fig. 36.6 The Inferior Surface of the Brain Showing the Cranial Nerves and Associated Structures (Waugh & Grant, 2018).

Labels: Cerebrum, Olfactory bulb, Optic tract, Medulla oblongata, Spinal cord, Cerebellum

I Olfactory nerves in olfactory tract
II Optic nerve
III Oculomotor nerve
IV Trochlear nerve
V Trigeminal nerve
VI Abducent nerve
VII Facial nerve
VIII Auditory nerve
IX Glossopharyngeal nerve
X Vagus nerve
XI Accessory nerve
XII Hypoglossal nerve

Organization of the nervous system

The PNS is composed of all the nerves that branch off from the brain and spine that allow the CNS to communicate with the rest of the body; this includes 31 pairs of spinal nerves that originate from the spinal cord. There are 8 cervical, 12 thoracic, 5 lumbar, 5 sacral and 1 coccygeal (Waugh & Grant, 2018). Since the main function of the PNS is communication, the PNS can work in both directions; the sensory (or afferent) division detects sensory stimuli. The motor (or efferent) division is the part of the brain that sends directions from the brain to the muscles and glands (Figs 36.8 and 36.9). The motor division also includes the somatic (or voluntary) nervous system, which manages skeletal muscle movement, and the autonomic (or involuntary) nervous system, which keeps the vital organs such as the heart, lungs and stomach functioning constantly (Table 36.2). Finally, the autonomic system has its own complementary forces. Its sympathetic division mobilizes the body into action (sometimes referred to as 'fight or flight'), whilst the parasympathetic division relaxes the body. That is the organization of the nervous system (Fig. 36.10).

Cell types

The nervous system is made up of nervous tissues, which are densely packed with cells. The different cells include neurons (nerve cells), which respond to stimuli and transmit signals (Fig. 36.11).

These cells only make up a small proportion of cells, as they are surrounded by and protected by neuroglia (or glial cells). Different glial cell types serve many important functions, such as providing support, nutrition, insulation and help with signal transmission in the nervous system. They also make up half of

TABLE 36.2 Somatic Versus Autonomic Systems	
Somatic	**Autonomic**
• Consists of efferent neurons that conduct impulses from the central nervous system (CNS) to skeletal muscle tissue	• Consists of efferent neurons that conduct impulses from the CNS to smooth muscle tissue, cardiac muscle tissue and glands
• Produces movement only in skeletal muscle tissue	• It produces responses only in involuntary muscles and glands and is therefore considered to be an involuntary system
• Under conscious control and is therefore voluntary movement	• There are two divisions to the autonomic nervous system: • Sympathetic • Parasympathetic

the brain mass, outnumbering neurons by 10 to 1. Astrocytes for example, are the most versatile glial cells; they connect neurons to the blood supply and support the exchange of materials between neurons and capillaries. Also in the CNS are the protective microglial cells. They are much smaller and act as the main source of immune defence against invading microorganisms in the brain and spinal cord. The ependymal cells line cavities in the brain and spinal cord and create, secrete and circulate cerebrospinal fluid (CSF), which fills cavities and cushions organs. Finally, the CNS oligodendrocyte cells wrap around neurons, producing an insulating barrier called the myelin sheath.

In the PNS there are only two kinds of glial cells. Satellite cells do the same in the peripheral system as astrocytes in the CNS, meaning they surround and support neuron cell bodies,

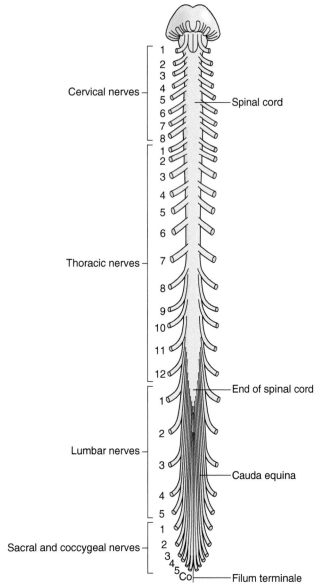

Fig. 36.7 The Spinal Cord and Spinal Nerves (Waugh & Grant, 2018).

TABLE 36.3	Glial Cells
Central nervous system	**Peripheral nervous system**
Astrocytes	**Satellite cells**
• Support and regulate ions	• Surround neuron
	• Cell bodies
Microglial cells	**Schwann cells**
• Defend	• Insulate, help for myelin sheath
Ependymal cells	
• Line cavities	
Oligodendrocytes	
• Wrap and insult	
• Form myelin sheath	

whilst Schwann cells are like oligodendrocytes; they wrap around axons and make the insulating myelin sheath (Table 36.3).

Neuron cells share distinctive features. They are the longest living cells in the body. Neurons are irreplaceable (they are amitotic), reaching full maturity approximately 21 days after birth. As they are irreplaceable, damage to neurons will lead to necrosis and organ failure. Waugh and Grant (2018) suggest that changes are associated with infections, hypoxia, nutritional deficiencies, trauma, ageing and hypoglycaemia. Neurons have a high metabolic rate and 25% of the daily food intake provides energy for the neuron. Additionally, neurons share the same basic structure (Fig. 36.12). The cell body (or soma), is the cell's life support. It has a nucleus, mitochondria, ribosomes, cytoplasm and dendrites. Dendrites act as listeners; they transport messages from other cells and convey information to the cell body. The neuron's axon acts as a talker and is the fibre that transmits electrical impulses away from the cell body to other cells.

Cell functions

Sensory neurons (afferent neurons) transmit impulses from sensory receptors towards the CNS. Most sensory neurons are unipolar. Motor neurons (efferent neurons), do the opposite, and are mostly multipolar, transmitting impulses away from the CNS and out to the body's muscles and glands. Finally, there are interneurons (or association neurons), which live in the CNS. These transmit impulses between sensory and motor neurons. Interneurons are the most abundant of the body's neurons and are mostly multipolar.

Intracranial pressure

ICP is the total force exerted by the contents of the skull. Normally ICP measures between 0 and 10 mm Hg but above 15 mm Hg is considered abnormally elevated. The skull is a closed, rigid box and is filled by brain tissue (80%), CSF (10%) and blood (10%). These components remain constant and are essentially incompressible, which means that if one of the components increases in volume the others must decrease in volume to keep the pressure inside the skull steady (Hickey, 2009; Brooker & Nichol, 2011). For example, if a patient has a brain tumour, there is extra tissue volume. Blood and CSF must decrease in volume to keep the pressure from rising. If a patient has excess CSF (hydrocephalus), then blood and tissue must decrease in volume to prevent the ICP from rising. This is known as the 'Monroe-Kellie hypothesis', which enables the mechanism of compensation to manage changes in volume without a rise in ICP. However, there comes a point when ICP exceeds the limits of this compensatory mechanism and will rise, which is recognized as a critical point (Fig. 36.13).

Accurate monitoring and measurement of ICP enables timely interventions for those patients with raised ICP (Box 36.2). A typical invasive monitor consists of a fibreoptic transducer-tipped catheter, placed in the lateral ventricle, subdural space or extradural space (Fig. 36.14). The ICP measurement is displayed as a waveform on a digital monitor (Brooker & Nichol, 2011). This requires invasive monitoring on a critical care unit, but not all patients can be monitored in this way, which is why Nursing Associates have an integral role to play in detecting rises in ICP

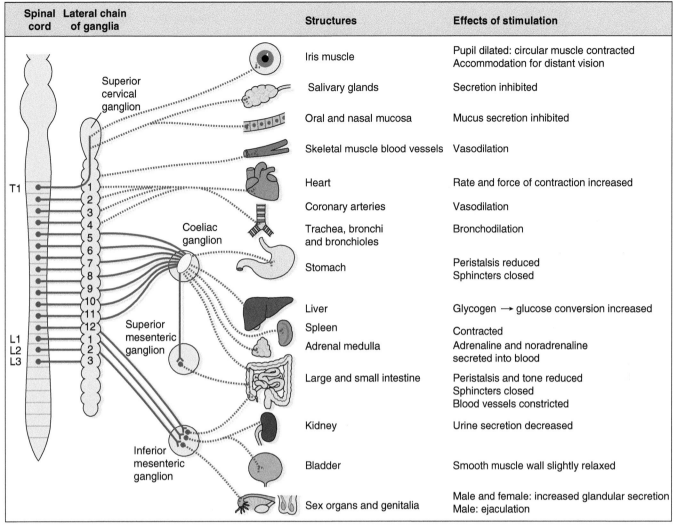

Spinal cord	Lateral chain of ganglia		Structures	Effects of stimulation
	Superior cervical ganglion		Iris muscle	Pupil dilated: circular muscle contracted Accommodation for distant vision
			Salivary glands	Secretion inhibited
			Oral and nasal mucosa	Mucus secretion inhibited
			Skeletal muscle blood vessels	Vasodilation
T1	1		Heart	Rate and force of contraction increased
	2		Coronary arteries	Vasodilation
	3		Trachea, bronchi and bronchioles	Bronchodilation
	4 Coeliac 5 ganglion			
	6		Stomach	Peristalsis reduced Sphincters closed
	7			
	8			
	9		Liver	Glycogen → glucose conversion increased
	10		Spleen	Contracted
	11		Adrenal medulla	Adrenaline and noradrenaline secreted into blood
	12 Superior mesenteric			
L1	1 ganglion		Large and small intestine	Peristalsis and tone reduced Sphincters closed Blood vessels constricted
L2	2			
L3	3		Kidney	Urine secretion decreased
	Inferior mesenteric ganglion		Bladder	Smooth muscle wall slightly relaxed
			Sex organs and genitalia	Male and female: increased glandular secretion Male: ejaculation

Fig. 36.8 The Sympathetic Outflow, the Main Structures Supplied and the Effects of Stimulation. *Solid red lines* denote preganglionic fibres; *broken lines* denote postganglionic fibres. There are right and left lateral chains of ganglia (Waugh & Grant, 2018).

BOX 36.2 Signs of Raised Intracranial Pressure

Early signs	Later signs
• Decreased conscious level • Motor weakness, often one sided • Headache • Papilloedema (swelling of the optic disc seen on ophthalmoscope)	• Continued deterioration in conscious level • Pupillary changes • Vomiting • Progressive motor weakness • Alteration in vital signs • Respiratory distress • Impaired brainstem reflexes

BOX 36.3 Factors that Increase Intracranial Pressure

Low oxygen levels (hypoxia) and high carbon dioxide levels (hypercapnia)
Anatomical body positioning (i.e., being prone, flexion at the neck or hip)
Experiencing loud sounds and undergoing painful procedures (noxious stimuli)
The effects of constipation (including straining at stool)
Rapid eye movement sleep
Exposure to emotional upset
Waking from sleep

(Data from Hickey, 2009.)

---

through effective nursing assessment and neurological observations. In addition, Nursing Associates need to be aware of the contributing factors that can cause rises in ICP and must deliver care to patients to avoid these factors (see Boxes 36.3 and 36.4 for factors and causes).

NEUROLOGICAL OBSERVATIONS

Neurological observations involve collection of the information that indicates the function and integrity of the patient's CNS. Neurological observations should only be performed by appropriately trained staff and recorded accurately (NICE, 2014).

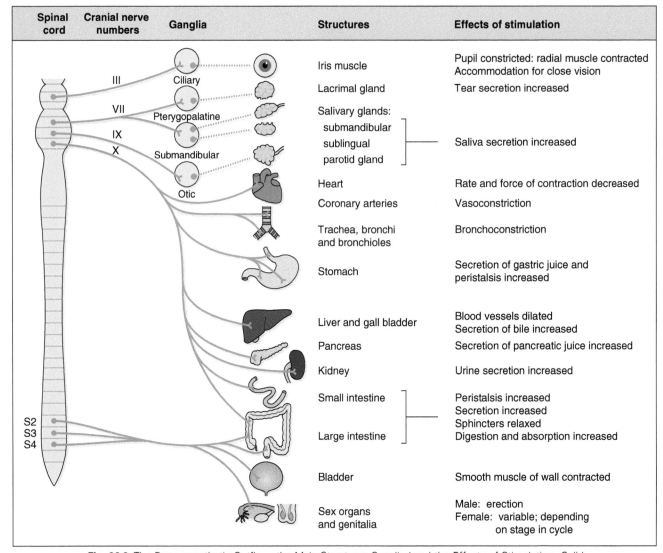

Spinal cord	Cranial nerve numbers	Ganglia	Structures	Effects of stimulation
	III	Ciliary	Iris muscle	Pupil constricted: radial muscle contracted Accommodation for close vision
	VII		Lacrimal gland	Tear secretion increased
		Pterygopalatine	Salivary glands: submandibular sublingual parotid gland	Saliva secretion increased
	IX			
	X	Submandibular		
		Otic	Heart	Rate and force of contraction decreased
			Coronary arteries	Vasoconstriction
			Trachea, bronchi and bronchioles	Bronchoconstriction
			Stomach	Secretion of gastric juice and peristalsis increased
			Liver and gall bladder	Blood vessels dilated Secretion of bile increased
			Pancreas	Secretion of pancreatic juice increased
			Kidney	Urine secretion increased
			Small intestine	Peristalsis increased Secretion increased Sphincters relaxed
S2 S3 S4			Large intestine	Digestion and absorption increased
			Bladder	Smooth muscle of wall contracted
			Sex organs and genitalia	Male: erection Female: variable; depending on stage in cycle

Fig. 36.9 The Parasympathetic Outflow, the Main Structures Supplied and the Effects of Stimulation. *Solid blue lines* denote preganglionic fibres; *broken lines* denote postganglionic fibres. Where there are no broken lines, the postganglionic neuron is in the wall of the structure (Waugh & Grant, 2018).

BOX 36.4 **Causes of Raised Intracranial Pressure**

- Brain tumours
- Subdural, extradural and intracerebral haematoma
- Skull fracture
- Cerebral oedema
- Cerebral abscess
- Hydrocephalus
- Benign/idiopathic intracranial hypertension
- Meningitis
- Subarachnoid haemorrhage
- Contusion
- Diffuse axonal injury

BOX 36.5 **AVPU**

AVPU scale
A – Alert
V – Responds to voice
P – Responds to pain
U – Unresponsive

AVPU can be used quickly and is an objective tool that can be readily used to communicate information. It is incorporated into the standardized patients' observation chart and the National Early Warning Scoring tool (NEWS2, see Chapter 20). However, if patients are recorded as anything other than alert, or there is a deterioration in their conscious level, then it is essential that the Glasgow Coma Scale (GCS) is used. The GCS was developed in 1974 by neurosurgeons Dr Brian Jennett and Dr Graham Teasdale in Glasgow and is now adopted internationally in more than 80 countries as a standardized tool for assessment of conscious level (Teasdale, 2014). The GCS reflects diffuse brain

Neurological observations should be performed on patients with an altered level of consciousness or those at risk of neurological deterioration. AVPU (Box 36.5) is a simplified assessment tool to assess the conscious level in an emergency, used by first aiders, ambulance crews and accident and emergency staff.

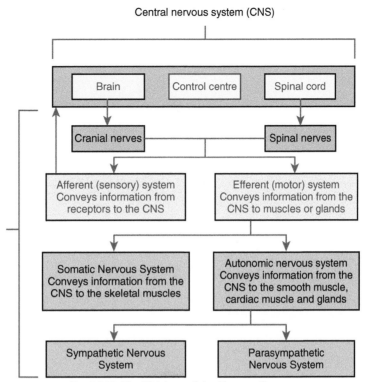

Fig. 36.10 The Divisions of the Nervous System.

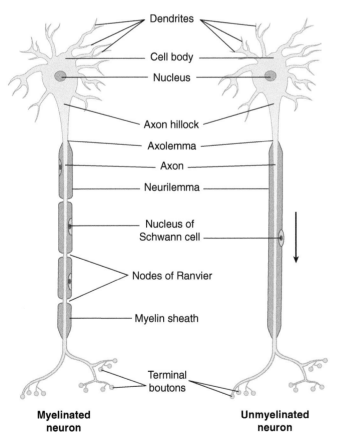

Fig. 36.11 The Structure of Neurons (Waugh & Grant, 2018).

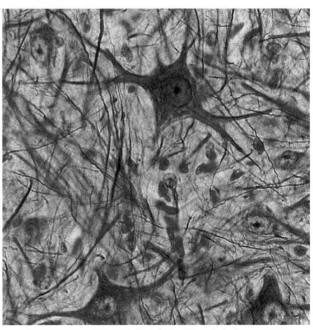

Fig. 36.12 Neurons and Glial Cells (Waugh & Grant, 2018).

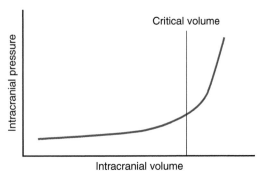

Fig. 36.13 Intracranial Pressure.

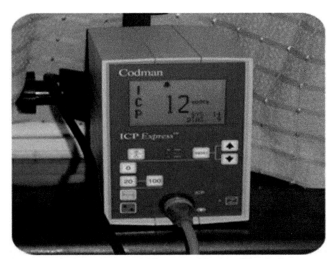

Fig. 36.14 Codman Intracranial Pressure Monitor. (Permission granted by Integra LifeSciences Corporation, Plainsboro, NJ).

TABLE 36.5 **Verbal Response**

Verbal response

5 Orientated: to time, place and person; questions might include who they are, their job, where they are, where they live, the month and year.

4 Confusion: the patient gives incorrect answers to any of the above questions but can speak in sentences.

3 Inappropriate words: the patient can speak words but not in a coherent way or in response to questions asked.

2 Incomprehensible sounds: the patient moans or groans with no clear words, more in response to stimulus.

1 None: no verbal response.

CRITICAL AWARENESS

The Glasgow Coma Scale provides a baseline against which changes can be evaluated.

The Glasgow Coma Scale is used to score the neurological examination and to quantify the patient's neurological condition.

The Nursing Associate must be competent and confident with its use and how to interpret and report findings.

Verbal response is used to assess higher cerebral function, including awareness of time, place and person and is assessed in the following way (Table 36.5):

Factors influencing the score but not necessarily indicating lack of awareness or cognitive function would be dysphasia (difficulty in speech), recorded as 'D', or the presence of a tracheostomy, which can be documented as 'T'.

REFLECTION 36.2

Take some to time to think about what it might mean for person who has a tracheostomy. How might this impact on their activities of living?

Assessment of the motor response is recognized as the most significant component of the GCS in predicting patient outcome and is shown to be the most difficult to assess accurately (Woodward & Mestecky, 2011). Motor response assesses the ability to understand language and simple commands and indicates integrity of the motor cortex. Motor response is assessed in the following way (Table 36.6):

When recording the motor response, if the patient is doing anything other than obeying commands, it is the best arm response that is recorded, so only one limb needs to respond for the score of 5 or less. Factors influencing motor response include sedatives and muscle relaxants.

Once the GCS is assessed, the information is plotted on a recording chart using dots to represent a visual perspective of the deterioration, improvement or stability. Based on the score, healthcare professionals can determine the severity of the condition or the level of consciousness. For example, a patient with a score of 15 would be fully alert and orientated, whereas a score of 3 is indicative of deep coma (Hickey, 2009). The frequency

TABLE 36.4 **Eye Opening**

Eye opening

4 Spontaneously: eyes are open when approaching the patient

3 Speech: the eyes open in response to verbal stimuli/speech

2 Pain: the eyes open in response to painful stimuli (e.g., trapezius pinch/squeeze or side of fingernail [not the nail bed])

1 None: no eye opening

function and impairment of the conscious level in a patient with raised ICP; how much it is impaired is dependent on how much pressure is present. The GCS is divided into three subscales, with each subscale given a score that is added together to give an overall score of between 3 and 15. The three key areas of the GCS are: eye opening (1–4), verbal response (1–5) and motor response (1–6). Eye opening is a measure of arousal rather than awareness and is assessed in the following way (Table 36.4):

Factors influencing the score but not necessarily indicating lack of arousal may be a patient who is deaf or if their eyes are closed by swelling and in this instance a 'C' will be documented.

TABLE 36.6 Motor Response

6	Obeys commands: the patient can obey commands and instructions (e.g., lifts arms, puts thumbs up or sticks out tongue).
5	Localize to pain: the patient can localize to the point of where the central painful stimuli is being applied by trying to push away the source, moving their arm across the midline. The use of the trapezius pinch/squeeze is the recommended method. It is performed by using the thumb and two fingers to pinch the muscle between the neck and shoulders.
4	Flexion to pain: using the trapezius pinch, the patient will flex their arm to towards the source of the pain but no rotation of the wrist.
3	Abnormal flexion: using the trapezium pinch, the patient bends their arm and rotates wrist, often described as a decorticate movement.
2	Extension: using the trapezius pinch, the patient straightens their elbows and rotates their arms toward their body, often described as decerebrate movement.
1	None: no motor response to central stimulus.

TABLE 36.7 Limb Assessment

Arms	Normal power: the patient has normal power and strength in both arms.
	Mild weakness: the patient can lift arm but not fully and not normally; they find it difficult to move against resistance.
	Severe weakness: the patient can move arms but not lift them and cannot move against gravity or resistance.
	Spastic flexion: if the patient cannot obey commands, trapezium pinch is used to assess the response. In this category, the arm is drawn away from the body, elbow is flexed but more often the forearms and hands are held against the body in a spastic flex, with muscles stiff.
	Extension: using the trapezium pinch, the patient will straighten and extend, external rotation of the shoulders and forearms.
	No response: no evidence of arm movements.
Legs	Normal power: the patient has normal power and strength in both legs.
	Mild weakness: the patient can lift leg but not fully and not normally; they find it difficult to move against resistance.
	Severe weakness: the patient can move legs but not lift them and cannot move against gravity or resistance.
	Extension: using the trapezium pinch, the patient will straighten and extend their leg and foot.
	No response: no evidence of limb movements.

of neurological observations will be dictated by the condition of the patient and reviewed regularly by a registered practitioner. Any deterioration must be reported promptly, which is essential to reduce the risk of complications and damage to the brain (NICE, 2014).

⚠ HOTSPOT

Remember that the non-alert or comatose patient also needs emotional support. The 6Cs are just as important for the person who is unconscious, as well as the person's family, if appropriate.

Focal signs include the pupillary response and limb power, which are also important in assessing the function and integrity of the CNS and are assessed once the GCS has been completed. Careful examination of the pupil size and reactivity to light is an important part of the neurological assessment and assesses the third cranial nerve function. Normal function of the third cranial nerve would be for the pupils to constrict briskly, with an equal size of 2–5 mm. The pupils are assessed using a bright pen torch and pupillary size is compared with the scale printed on the torch or the neurological observation chart, before and after the light source is shone into the eye. It is important when recording the pupil size that each pupil is assessed separately, with the light applied from the side of the eye being assessed, as this overcomes the accommodation response in which pupils constrict to a nearing object (Iggulden, 2006).

The pupil size should be recorded using the number in millimetres and the reaction recorded using a positive sign for a brisk response, sluggish for a slow reaction and a negative sign for no reaction or fixed pupil. If one pupil is fixed, dilated and unreactive to light, this could indicate raised ICP on one side of the brain; however, it is more serious if both pupils are fixed and dilated, indicative of brain herniation. Factors influencing abnormal pupillary size, shape and reactions, in the absence of raised ICP, include previous eye surgery, medication and hormonal disorders, which is why it is important to observe the pupils first before applying a light source.

Assessment of limb power and movement is an important indicator of motor response and may give clues to the location and extent of the neurological dysfunction. Starting from the upper limbs to lower limbs, each limb is assessed individually for its strength, as each side of the brain controls the limbs on the opposite side, so they are recorded using left (L) and right (R) if they are different (Table 36.7).

Vital signs are also an important aspect of the neurological assessment, with Dougherty and Lister (2011) recommending that respirations are recorded first, as they give the clearest indication of how the brain is functioning, followed by temperature, blood pressure and pulse. Recording of rate, depth and rhythm of breathing are important, as any deterioration or abnormal patterns can indicate poor functioning of the vital centres of the brain. A raised temperature may indicate infection, but it can also indicate hypothalamic damage because of the role of the hypothalamus in temperature regulation (Hickey, 2009). A slow pulse and rising blood pressure are indicative of raised ICP in patients with conditions that may cause the pressure inside the skull to rise. Whilst routine observation of vital signs is important for all patients, abnormal changes in respirations, blood pressure and pulse are late signs in the neurological patient, often after the patient's consciousness level has deteriorated.

STROKE

Epidemiology and aetiology

Stroke is defined as 'a clinical syndrome consisting of rapidly developing clinical signs of focal (at times global) disturbance of cerebral function, lasting more than 24 hours or leading to death with no apparent cause other than that of vascular origin'

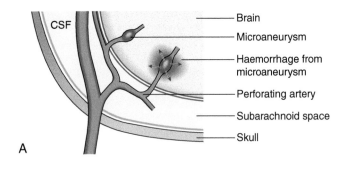

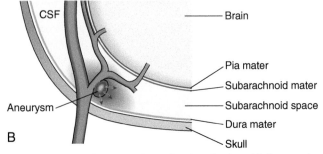

Fig. 36.15 Types of Haemorrhage Causing Strokes. (A) Intracerebral haemorrhage. (B) Subarachnoid haemorrhage (Waugh & Grant, 2018).

TABLE 36.8	FAST
F	Face: Is the person able to smile? Do they have any signs of facial drooping?
A	Arms: Can the person raise both arms, or is one side obviously weaker?
S	Speech: Ask the person to repeat a simple phrase. Do they have slurred speech, or is their speech unusually strange?
T	Time: If any of these signs are observed, it's time to call for help. Dial 999 and save a life.

(Data from the National Stroke Association, 2017.)

(World Health Organization, 2017a). It is generally caused by cerebrovascular disease, causing cerebral infarction or spontaneous intracranial haemorrhage (intracerebral and/or subarachnoid haemorrhage) (Fig. 36.15).

NICE (2016c) states that stroke is a major health problem in the UK. The Stroke Association's report, State of the Nation (2017a), highlighted that stroke accounted for around 40,000 deaths in the UK in 2015, which represents 7% of all deaths. Each year there are approximately 152,000 cases of stroke in the UK, of which about 25%–33% are recurrent strokes. Most people survive a first stroke, but often have significant morbidity. About 1.2 million people in the UK live with the effects of stroke, and over a third of these are dependent on other people.

The State of the Nation (2017a) report highlights that stroke is estimated to cost the UK economy around £9 billion a year. This comprises direct costs to health and social care of £4.38 billion, costs of informal care of £2.4 billion, costs because of lost productivity of £1.33 billion and benefits payments totalling £841 million.

Development of stroke services, and particularly access to acute stroke care on a stroke unit, has resulted in improvements in mortality and disability outcomes post-stroke. However, many people who have a stroke need long–term support to help them manage any difficulties they have, participate in society, and regain their independence. Stroke rehabilitation aims to help people to restore or improve their physical and mental functioning, adapt to any loss of function and work towards regaining a meaningful role for the individual. It involves many different specialists for different areas of care, depending on the person's needs.

In April 2016, NICE updated their 'Stroke in adults' (quality standard 2 QS2), which recommends evidence-based practice for diagnosing and managing stroke for those aged over 16 years.

It includes the initial management and long-term rehabilitation and support required by people who have suffered from a stroke (NICE, 2016c).

Classification

Types of strokes

The three types of stroke are:

Ischaemic (clots). Resulting from occlusion of the blood vessel supplying blood to the brain. This accounts for approximately 87% of all stroke cases (Stroke Association, 2017b).

Haemorrhagic (bleeds). This results from a rupture of an already weakened blood vessel. There are two types of blood vessel that result in this type of stroke: aneurisms and arteriovenous malformations. The Stroke Association (2017b) states that the most common type of stroke is the result of uncontrolled hypertension.

Transient ischemic attacks. This is usually identified as a mini-stroke and is a result of a small temporary clot in the blood vessels of the brain.

The acronym FAST

The word 'FAST' is used as an acronym to remind people to look out for the most common symptoms of stroke. By recognizing these signs (Table 36.8), the patient will receive prompt help and treatment.

Nursing considerations

Diagnosis of stroke is based on clinical symptoms that would help to identify if a stroke has occurred. Patients are assessed using a validated stroke assessment tool in an admission unit, for example 'Recognition of stroke in the emergency room' (NICE, 2017). For all suspected strokes, the patient will require a computed tomography (CT) scan to identify the type of stroke, as treatment is different depending on whether it is a haemorrhagic stroke or ischaemic stroke. For ischaemic strokes, which account for 87% of all strokes, pharmacological treatment using thrombolysis can significantly improve outcome, using a drug called alteplase, which is an anticoagulant administered to dissolve the clot. NICE (2017) recommend that thrombolysis is given within 4.5 hours of stroke onset by healthcare professionals trained in its administration. For other patients with acute ischaemic stroke, aspirin 300 mg is recommended. On occasions, the clot can be removed using x-ray techniques or neurosurgery.

Nursing Associate skills in this emergency phase will include assessment of conscious level and recognition of neurological deterioration, fluid management (nil by mouth if suspected absence of swallowing), oxygen therapy, blood pressure monitoring and maintenance of blood glucose between 4 and 11 mmols (NICE, 2017). Care on the specialist stroke unit should be provided by a 'core multi-disciplinary team (MDT) who have the knowledge, skills and behaviours to work in partnership with people with stroke and their families and carers to manage the changes experienced as a result of a stroke' (NICE, 2013). A Nursing Associate is an important part of this MDT and will provide care to ensure that patients with strokes are encouraged to be as independent as possible and that rehabilitation is aimed at maximizing the potential for each patient. Some of the long-term complications of stroke can include physical and psychological problems and this will depend on the area of the brain involved. The Stroke Association is a dedicated website which has useful resources and guidance on all aspects of stroke for patients, families and healthcare professionals to provide safe and effective care for all.

TRAUMATIC BRAIN INJURY

Epidemiology and aetiology

Traumatic brain injury (TBI) is defined as injury caused by trauma to the head, including the effects upon the brain or other possible complications of injury (Headway, 2013). Each year, 1.4 million people attend hospital accident and emergency departments in the UK following a head injury. Around 200,000 people will be admitted to hospital in the UK because of the severity of the injury and it is the commonest cause of death and disability in the 1–40-year-old age group worldwide (NICE, 2014). The main causes of TBI are falls, road traffic collisions, assaults, injuries at work and sporting activities, with drugs and alcohol often contributing factors to the actual incidents. The incidence of TBI is three times greater in males than female and it is estimated that across the UK there are over 500,000 people living with long-term disabilities as the result of TBI (NICE, 2014; Headway 2013). For this reason, TBI can be considered as a long-term neurological disorder (Department of Health, 2005). It is now widely accepted that not all neurological damage and long-term disability is attributed to the primary injury that occurs at the time of impact. It occurs over the hours and days following the injury because of delayed complications, such as uncontrollable rises in ICP, cerebral oedema, ischaemia and infection (Woodward & Mestecky, 2011).

CRITICAL AWARENESS

Brain Death

All human death will involve the permanent loss of the capacity for consciousness, along with the irreversible loss of the ability to breathe.

A definition of brain death includes the absence of any brain activity as depicted by the absence of waves on an electroencephalograph. There are three key findings that determine brain death, these are:

1. Coma
2. Absence of brainstem reflexes
3. Apnoea (cessation of breathing)

Data from Williams (2018)

BOX 36.6 Classification of Traumatic Brain Injury

Focal damage
Scalp: laceration, contusion
Skull injuries: fracture (e.g., basal skull, depressed)
Between skull and brain: extradural, subdural haematomas
Brain: contusions, intracerebral haemorrhage, penetrating brain injury

Diffuse damage
Brain: concussion, contusion, cerebral oedema and diffuse axonal injury

---

Classification of traumatic brain injury

Clinical severity of TBI may be classified based on the GCS at time of injury and following initial treatment, with a GCS of 13–15 indicating mild injury, a GCS of 9–12 moderate injury and a GCS of 3–8 severe injury. Mechanism of injury and CT scan results can also be an indicator of injury severity, as well as length of post-traumatic amnesia (Woodward & Mestecky, 2011). It can also be categorized as closed or open TBI. Closed head injury is where there is no break of the skin and no open wound is visible. This is a frequent occurrence with rapid acceleration or deceleration injuries. An open head injury is where the skull is penetrated and the brain is exposed and damaged (e.g., bullet wound or collision with a sharp object) (Swann, 2013). The impact of the injury can be described as a coup and contrecoup injury. A TBI that causes damage directly below the site of the impact is a coup injury and one that causes damage at the opposite side of the impact is a contrecoup injury, often caused by rapid movement of the brain within the rigid cranium vault (Hickey, 2009).

Classification of TBI (Box 36.6) is most often based on whether the damage to the brain is localized or diffuse.

Main types of traumatic brain injury
Skull fractures

Skull fractures indicate that the skull and brain have received significant impact, often occurring as a result of direct blunt trauma. A linear fracture is the most minor and resembles a line or single crack in the skull and is often treated conservatively. A depressed skull fracture is characterized by inward depression of the bone, which can result in bony fragments lacerating into the dura and tearing blood vessels, with the increased risk of underlying damage to the brain (Woodward & Waterhouse, 2006; Woodward and Mestecky 2011). Basal skull fractures occur at the base of the skull, usually affecting the frontal and temporal bones. They are more common and more serious because of the location and the fragility of the bones and the dura in this area. A dural tear in this area can cause CSF leakage from the nose (rhinorrhoea) or the ear (otorrhoea), with the potential for meningitis because organisms have direct access to the cranium. The treatment for skull fractures depends on the type of fractures, but most fractures are treated conservatively, with close nursing observations of changes in patient condition and symptom control (Hickey, 2009). Depressed skull fractures often require surgical elevation and debridement of bony fragments. It is important to note that skull fractures are often accompanied by more significant brain injuries, which take priority in the management of the TBI.

Extradural haematoma

An extradural haematoma refers to bleeding in the potential space between the skull and the dura mater, most often in the temporal region as a result of a skull fracture and laceration of the middle meningeal artery. Extradural haematomas strip the dura away from the inner skull and accumulate very quickly, and, whilst the patient can present neurologically intact immediately after the injury, they can deteriorate quickly as the clot enlarges (Woodward & Mestecky, 2011). The haematoma compresses the brain, causing midline shift and raised ICP and requires immediate surgical removal.

REFLECTION 36.3

Reflect on the care that a family might need when they have learned that their relative has sustained a traumatic brain injury. Their relative requires surgical intervention at a hospital 50 miles from the patient's home. How might you provide care that is sensitive and compassionate?

Subdural haematoma

Subdural haematomas can be categorized as acute, subacute and chronic, which are all an accumulation of blood in the space between the dura and the arachnoid mater due to the tearing of cortical veins. Acute subdural haematomas occur within 48 hours of the initial injury and are often accompanied by other injuries (Hickey, 2009). They are associated with road traffic collisions, falls and assaults. A subacute subdural haematoma most often develops after 48 hours and up to 2 weeks as a result of another injury, such as a contusion. A chronic subdural haematoma can present many weeks after the initial injury (minor and not often remembered), presenting more frequently in the elderly, where the cortical veins are more fragile.

For small haematomas, the treatment can be conservative but for larger haematomas the treatment involves surgical evacuation (Fig. 36.16).

Diffuse axonal injury

Diffuse axonal injury (DAI) refers to a TBI that causes widespread neurological dysfunction due to the impact of the injury and rotational forces and acceleration–deceleration that cause axonal damage, commonly in the corpus callosum and brainstem. It is most often caused by high-speed road traffic collisions or falls. DAI is characterized by an immediate and prolonged loss of consciousness at initial impact (more than 6 hours) and is accompanied by diffuse brain swelling, often without any focal lesion. If the patient survives, they often remain in a coma for approximately 3 months, with severe neurological disabilities (Hickey, 2009). There is evidence to suggest that axonal damage from DAI is not always associated with neuronal death; therefore some functional recovery is possible as undamaged nerves recover (Woodward & Mestecky, 2011).

Assessment and management of people with traumatic brain injury

The assessment and management of TBI are influenced by a range of guidelines, which all have the aim of improving patient outcomes following TBI. The National Institute for Health and Care Excellence (NICE, 2014) produced guidelines on the triage, assessment, investigation and early management of head injury in infants, children and adults. Local policies, protocols and use of clinical judgement must also be taken into consideration in the assessment and management of TBI.

The aim of initial management is for effective resuscitation, early detection and timely intervention, which have been enhanced since the establishment of major trauma centres in the UK. Patients with major trauma can be taken by ambulance or airlifted directly to specialist centres rather than local hospitals, which enables timely assessment and interventions (NICE, 2016a). Patients who have sustained a head injury should receive immediate care based on the principles of airway, breathing, circulation,

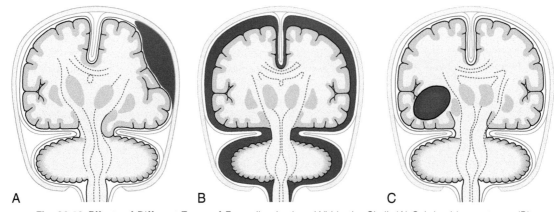

Fig. 36.16 Effects of Different Types of Expanding Lesions Within the Skull. (A) Subdural haematoma. (B) Subarachnoid haemorrhage. (C) Tumour or intracerebral haemorrhage (Waugh & Grant, 2018).

BOX 36.7   Criteria for Computed Tomography Scan

- Glasgow Coma Scale (GCS) less than 13 on initial assessment in the emergency department.
- GCS less than 15 at 2 hours after the injury on assessment in the emergency department.
- Suspected open or depressed skull fracture.
- Any sign of basal skull fracture
- Post-traumatic seizure.
- Focal neurological deficit.
- More than one episode of vomiting.

(NICE, 2014.)

BOX 36.8   Types of Neurosurgical Approaches

Burr hole is a surgical operation where a small hole is made into the skull to access the contents of the skull. It can be used to place a drain in the brain, remove a small subdural haematoma or for a biopsy of a tumour.

Craniotomy is a surgical operation where an opening is made into the skull using several burr holes to access the contents (e.g., to remove a large extradural haematoma).

Craniectomy is the removal of part of the bone (temporarily) to relieve raised intracranial pressure.

disability and exposure (ABCDE), with identification of any cervical injury excluded in this initial assessment. Prompt assessment in accident and emergency is essential, where these patients will be triaged and assessed within 15 minutes. History of injury is important in the assessment of TBI and should include mechanism of injury, period of loss of consciousness, seizure activity, GCS at time of injury, presence of other signs and symptoms and pupillary response. CT scanning is the main diagnostic tool for identifying TBI; however, there are set criteria for its use (Box 36.7).

Criteria for admission to hospital for close monitoring include:
- Patients with a CT scan that confirms presence of abnormalities
- Patients with a GCS of less than 15
- Those with contributing factors that delay the assessment process (e.g., substance misuse).

Indications for referral to a neurosurgical unit and discussion with a neurosurgeon are identified in the guidelines (NICE, 2014).

Current management of TBI will depend on the age of the patient, extent of head injury, incidence of other injuries, pre-existing conditions and physiological state, including conscious level. However, early diagnosis, immediate transfer to a specialist neurosurgical centre and surgical intervention will significantly improve outcome for patients with head injuries (NICE, 2014). There is a range of different types of neurosurgical approaches (Box 36.8).

Those patients with TBI are often admitted to a critical care unit for intensive management, which will involve close monitoring of the patient's airway, breathing and circulation and their neurological function to prevent secondary complications. Those with GCS of 8 or less, or those with progressive neurological deterioration, should be intubated and ventilated. ICP monitoring is also recommended for patients with GCS of 8 or less, midline shift, cerebral oedema and intracranial haematomas (NICE, 2014).

Nursing considerations

Nursing management of severe TBI in all healthcare settings revolve around the activities of living (Mattar, 2011). Respiratory assessment and support relates to appropriate airway management and adequate oxygenation, which is crucial in preventing secondary brain damage. This might include caring for the intubated patient via an endotracheal tube or a tracheostomy. In addition, the patient may need suctioning. As their respiratory status improves, it is important to encourage the patient to cough and expectorate.

Neurological observations are an important part of the Nursing Associate's role in all healthcare settings, as detecting deterioration early will ensure prompt treatment for patients.

REFLECTION 36.4

What communication strategies might you employ when caring for a person with a tracheostomy, who is unable to speak?

TBI patients require the commencement of nutritional support early due to the increased metabolism and stress response triggered by major trauma. A person who has experienced a TBI on average will require 3000–4000 calories per day, calculated by a dietician and based on the body weight of the patient (Woodward & Waterhouse, 2006). Depending on the patient's physiological status, this may be via enteral feeding (i.e., nasogastric feeding or a percutaneous endoscopic gastrostomy tube). Nursing Associates work closely with the dieticians to ensure the nutritional needs of patients are met. Adequate cerebral perfusion is also important through strict monitoring of fluid input and electrolyte status (Hickey, 2009). As the patient stabilizes, they may need assistance with diet and fluids.

Elimination is recorded in relation to urine output, often via a urinary catheter initially until the patient is stable. Avoidance of constipation is an important care consideration as this can increase ICP (Brooker & Nichol, 2011).

Early mobilization is important in promoting normal postural tone, alignment of joints and prevention of complications of immobility, such as pressures sores. Mobility might initially include frequent positional changes and head tilt of 30 degrees to reduce ICP (Brooker & Nichol, 2011). Passive exercises on limbs should be performed by the Nursing Associate and involvement of the physiotherapist is important (Woodward & Mestecky, 2011). Splinting of the limbs is often required to prevent muscle wasting, foot drop and spasticity. To prevent deep vein thrombosis, anti-embolic stockings should be applied. As the patient's condition improves further, movement should be encouraged, such as sitting in the chair and walking to the toilet. This will be assessed by the physiotherapist initially, with support of the Nursing Associate and other care staff.

Attending to the needs of the patient's personal hygiene is an important part of the Nursing Associate's role, as TBI patients are often dependent on assistance for personal care to skin, eyes, mouth and hair (Mattar, 2011). As soon as the patient is able, they should be encouraged to attend to their own personal hygiene needs.

> **! HOTSPOT**
>
> A person who is unconscious requires complete oral care; they will require assistance with all of their activities of living.

NURSING SKILLS

Administering Oral Care to the Unconscious Patient

Unconscious patients require frequent mouth care. Cleansing is especially important for these patients because they often breathe through their mouths, which leads to dryness and crusting of the area.

Supplies
- Toothbrush and toothpaste
- Mouthwash
- Mouth suction device
- Gloves
- Water-soluble lubricant
- Water
- Paper towels
- Tongue blade and 4 × 4 gauze pads
- Towel or toothettes
- Emesis basin
- Irrigation syringe

Action (rationale)
Assessment (Data Collection)
1. Assess for gag reflex. (Identifies risk of aspiration.)
Planning
2. Gather supplies and place on paper towels on the over-the-bed table. (Provides easy access to equipment. Paper towels keep table clean.)
3. Explain the procedure to the patient. (Provides stimulation because unconscious patients may be able to hear.)
4. Close door or pull curtain. (Provides privacy.)
Implementation
5. Raise bed level to a comfortable working height. Turn patient laterally on side of bed nearest you. Lower side rail. (Promotes good body mechanics; work is at your centre of gravity.)
6. Turn on the suction and place the suction device under the corner of the pillow near you. Put a towel under the patient's head and the emesis basin beneath patient's mouth and chin. (Readying suction device provides for immediate use of suction in case patient gags. Towel and basin keep gown and linens clean.)
7. Wear gloves. Use toothettes or toothbrush and toothpaste to cleanse the teeth and mouth. Use mouthwash or water to clean the interior of the cheeks, roof of the mouth, teeth and tongue. A 4 × 4 gauze pad may be wrapped around an index finger or tongue blade to remove crusts. Repeat as necessary. (Observes standard precautions. Mouthwash and water are good cleansing agents. Removing crusting and debris maintains a healthy mouth.)
8. Floss by holding a 24 to 30 cm piece of floss, with the ends wrapped around the middle finger of each hand. Using index fingers and thumbs, gently work floss between each tooth, moving down to gum line and back up to tooth edge. (Removes tartar and plaque.)

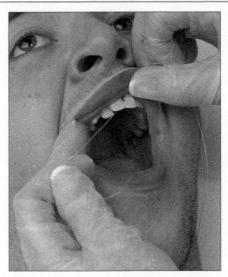

Fig. 36.17 Step 8.

9. With patient's head turned to the side, intermittently rinse the mouth by gently squirting water in with the syringe; use the suction device to remove water and debris. (Using small amounts of water and turning the head to the side promote drainage and reduce risk of aspiration.)
10. Wipe patient's mouth and lubricate the lips and corners of the mouth with water-soluble lubricant. (Prevents drying and cracking of lips.)

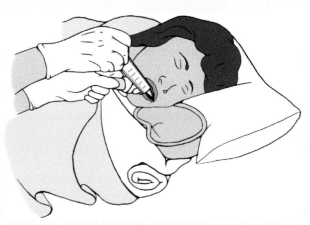

Fig. 36.18 Step 9.

11. Explain to the patient that you have finished the procedure. (Provides stimulation because the unconscious patient may be able to hear.)
12. Remove gloves and dispose of them properly. Reposition patient, raise side rail and lower bed. (Proper removal and disposal of gloves prevents spread of microorganisms. Repositioning patient and restoring unit promote safety and comfort.)
13. Clean supplies and tidy unit. (Readies equipment for next use and straightens patient's environment.)

Evaluation
14. Put on gloves and inspect mouth to check effectiveness of procedure. (Determines if other actions are needed.)
Documentation
15. Note procedure done and assessment of mouth before and after care. (Notes any abnormalities.)

(Reproduced with permission from Williams, 2018.)

Agitation is a common complication during the first 6 months following severe head injury and is the most challenging for healthcare professionals and families. Environmental and behavioural modifications are recommended, with avoidance of restraint and antipsychotic medication wherever possible (Pangilinan et al., 2008). Good pain assessment and management is important, particularly management of headache, with codeine phosphate being the drug of choice rather than opioid medication (Brooker & Nichol, 2011).

A calm and reassuring approach by the Nursing Associate is essential when caring for people with TBI, with avoidance of unpleasant stimuli (such as noise, bright lights) and avoidance of excessive and unwarranted interventions (such as touching, rolling and excessive position changes or suction); such activities will increase ICP (Hickey, 2009). The Nursing Associate should work in collaboration with family members and support them in communicating with the patients as often they are anxious about this, particularly if the patient is unconscious. Non-verbal communication (such as the use of touch), should also be encouraged by the patient and the family. The future is often unknown with TBI, so information and support to patients and their families throughout the patient's journey is crucial.

Rehabilitation is defined as 'appropriate measures, including through peer support, to enable persons with disabilities to attain and maintain their maximum independence, full physical, mental, social and vocational ability and full inclusion and participation in all aspects of life' (World Health Organization, 2011). Rehabilitation plays a crucial role in the recovery process for patients with TBI, maximizing quality of life and reducing long-term disability and should begin as soon as the patient is clinically stable (Hickey, 2009). The role of the MDT in the care of TBI patients is essential and will include Nursing Associates, doctors, physiotherapists, occupational therapists, dieticians, speech and language therapists and clinical psychologists (Department of Health, 2005; NICE, 2014). Rehabilitation is often delivered in specialist units, day hospitals, outpatient departments and in the community. The aim is that people with long-term conditions are provided with appropriate rehabilitation and ongoing support to work and are provided with alternative occupational/educational opportunities (Department of Health, 2005; Woodward & Mestecky, 2011). Ongoing support for patients, families

TABLE 36.9 Long-Term Consequences of Traumatic Brain Injury	
Physical	• Poor mobility • Loss of sensation • Communication deficits • Loss of smell • Poor vision
Cognitive and executive functions	• Poor memory • Lack of concentration • Inability to solve problems • Lack of understanding
Emotional and behavioural	• Agitation • Irritability • Frustration • Lack of self-awareness • Mood changes • Disinhibited • Depression

and carers is also crucial in the rehabilitation process as the long-term consequences of a TBI can be life changing, and there are many long-term consequences of TBI (Table 36.9) This should include access to relevant support agencies, such as Headway and the Brain and Spine Foundation (Department of Health, 2005; Headway, 2013).

CRITICAL AWARENESS

Go to www.headway.org.uk
Headway is a charity that promotes understanding of all aspects of brain injury and provides information, support and services to survivors, their families and carers. Headway also campaigns to reduce the incidence of brain injury.

The Headway Brain Injury Identity Card is designed to help police officers and staff more easily identify brain injury survivors, ensuring that they receive an appropriate response and support. The card can also provide brain injury survivors with added confidence during every day social scenarios. The card is personalized, helping the card holder to explain the effects of their brain injury and ask for any support they may require.

CASE STUDY 36.1 John – Traumatic Brain Injury

John Smith is a 38-year-old man who was found by his brother following a fall at home. The initial assessment in the accident and emergency department involved a quick history of events, assessment of the airway, breathing and circulation, followed by a neurological examination. John was able to maintain his own airway but was found to be drowsy, agitated, with confused speech, obeying commands and all limbs appeared to have normal power (GCS 13). Pupillary size and reactions were tested and found to be size 3, equal and reacting to light. His vital observations were recorded and were all within normal parameters. A comprehensive physical examination was also undertaken at this time and John was found to have no other injuries.

Within 1 hour a computed tomography scan was performed, which diagnosed a left frontal subdural haematoma and a frontal contusion. The patient was referred to a neurosurgeon and immediately transferred to the Regional Neurosciences Centre. On admission to the ward, the patient was assessed by a Nursing Associate, who recorded his neurological observations as: eyes opening to pain, incomprehensible sounds and localizing to pain (GCS 9). It was also noted that he had a left dilated pupil, which was sluggish to light and a right-sided limb weakness. The patient was hypertensive, with a blood pressure of 180/100 mm Hg, pulse 60 beats per minute, respirations 22 breaths per minute, a temperature of 38.6°C and oxygen saturations of 96% (on 28% oxygen via a face mask). The patient was transferred to the intensive care unit for intubation and ventilation and had his intracranial pressure (ICP) monitored. Within 1 hour he was taken to theatre and underwent a craniotomy and removal of the subdural haematoma in an attempt to decrease ICP.

The principles of care during this phase revolved around preventing and minimizing secondary neurological complications to optimize recovery. Maintenance of John's airway was important through ventilation and periodic suctioning. The Nursing Associate also maintained an accurate fluid balance with the monitoring of input through adherence to the 2500 mL fluid intake as ordered by the medical staff, with intravenous therapy only at this stage. A urinary catheter was also inserted to monitor urine output. John's positioning was also very important, with his head elevated to 30 degrees, the head, neck and chest maintained in alignment and positions of extreme flexion avoided. The promotion of sleep, care to personal hygiene, administration of prescribed medication and wound care to the craniotomy were also considered. John was fed at this stage through a nasogastric tube and he was given high calorie enteral feeds over a 24-hour period. The family were encouraged to visit and spoke regularly to the medical and nursing staff whilst John was being cared for in the intensive therapy unit (ITU). After spending 4 days on ITU, John was extubated and transferred to a ward.

On transfer to the ward, John was able to maintain his own airway and was able to cough and expectorate independently. Neurologically, John was able to open his eyes to speech, he was able to respond with conversation, although confused, and he obeyed commands (GCS 13). John's pupils were equal and reacting to light and he had a right-sided limb weakness. John was assessed for swallowing and within 24 hours was allowed soft diet and fluids. John found it difficult to come to terms with his right limb weakness initially; however, within a week he was able to walk with one Nursing Associate following input by the physiotherapist. John's speech continued to improve but it was clear that he had some cognitive impairment and a poor short-term memory.

John was accepted by the rehabilitation unit but was able to walk short distances with a walking stick and managed his hygiene needs with assistance. He was taking a normal diet. He continued anticonvulsants as he had experienced two seizures prior to transfer, but no other medication was prescribed at this stage. In terms of the outcome, John made a moderate recovery, meaning that he hadn't quite managed to be back to his baseline functions with motor and sensory function. He managed to be discharged from the local hospital 12 weeks after initial injury, attending as a day patient only. He is unable to work in his previous capacity and is on disability benefit. He was referred to a social worker for support and advice; he is also restricted in social and leisure activities. He has family support and his practice nurse and GP take much interest in health needs.

EPILEPSY

Epidemiology and aetiology

Epilepsy is one of the most common chronic neurological disorders (World Health Organization, 2017b) and is characterized by recurrent and unprovoked seizures originating in the brain, with the dysfunction caused by excessive and abnormal neuronal discharge (Hickey, 2009). Accurate estimates of incidence and prevalence are difficult to achieve because identifying people who may have epilepsy is difficult. It is estimated that approximately 600,000 people in the UK have epilepsy (Epilepsy Research UK, 2017). One in 20 people will have a seizure at some point in their life, but this does not mean that they have epilepsy and not everyone with epilepsy will have it for life (Epilepsy Society, 2017). Epilepsy varies in its clinical presentation and presents very differently in each patient; this can be dependent on the age at which epilepsy develops. The causes of epilepsy can be complex and therefore difficult to identify but can include one of the following:

- Genetic tendency
- A structural change in the brain, such as the brain not developing properly
- Previous cerebral trauma or a neurological condition

In many of the cases, a cause of the epilepsy is not identified and is referred to as 'unknown' (ILAE, 2017), previously described as idiopathic or cryptogenic. It is recommended that patients suspected as having epilepsy must be seen by a specialist within 2 weeks to ensure early diagnosis and initiation of therapy as appropriate to their individual needs (NICE, 2016b).

Classification of seizures and diagnosis

Seizures are classified by the International League Against Epilepsy, which is a worldwide organization of epilepsy professionals (Epilepsy Action, 2017). They are most often categorized into focal and generalized seizures (Box 36.9).

Focal seizures present with signs and symptoms representative of the location where the seizure occurs, with some patients experiencing one symptom and others experiencing several symptoms. The symptoms of focal seizures can be split into two groups (Table 36.10).

Most focal aware seizures are brief, usually lasting between 2 and 3 minutes, with full recovery 10 minutes after the seizure but occasionally people are tired and confused following the seizure (Woodward & Mestecky, 2011).

Generalized seizures are characterized by diffuse and widespread abnormal electrical activity throughout the brain. A

BOX 36.9 Classification of Seizures

Focal
- Focal aware seizures, without impaired conscious level
- Focal impaired awareness, seizures with impaired conscious level

Generalized seizures
- Absence seizures
- Myoclonic seizures
- Clonic seizures
- Tonic seizures
- Tonic–clonic seizures
- Atonic seizures

TABLE 36.10 Motor and Nonmotor Symptoms

Motor symptoms	Nonmotor symptoms
• Brief irregular jerking movements of parts of the body • Lip smacking • Chewing • Running	• Feelings of anxiety • Fear • Changes to smell, vision or hearing

(Epilepsy Action, 2017.)

BOX 36.10 Nursing Care and Management of a Seizure

- Stay calm
- Protect patient from injury without restraint
- Use bedrails if in bed and at risk of injury from a fall
- Maintain privacy and dignity
- Loosen tight clothing around the neck
- Administer oxygen if necessary
- Record the seizure activity, including time of event, warning signs, evidence of limb movements, duration of seizure, level of consciousness
- Administer medication as prescribed, with the aim of stopping the seizure if necessary or to reduce the risk of further seizures
- Monitor the airway, have oxygen and suction nearby and monitor vital signs
- At the end of seizure, place patient in recovery position and allow them to sleep
- Stay with the patient
- If this is the first seizure or it lasts more than 5 minutes, call for help

(Data from Hickey, 2009.)

BOX 36.11 Potential Seizure Triggers

- Not taking epilepsy medicine as prescribed
- Feeling tired
- Not sleeping well
- Stress and anxiety
- Alcohol and recreational drugs
- Flashing or flickering lights (in only 5% of people)
- Monthly periods
- Missing meals
- Having an illness which causes a high temperature

(Epilepsy Action, 2017.)

tonic–clonic seizure is a generalized seizure and is the one that most people observe. It often begins with a period of irritability and tension, or what is described as an 'aura' preceding the seizure, with a sudden loss of consciousness. Tonic stiff movements of the limbs are followed by a clonic phase, which is characterized by rhythmic jerking movements of the limbs. Grunting, foaming at the mouth, tongue-biting and incontinence are also signs seen during this type of generalized seizure, referred to as a tonic–clonic seizure (Epilepsy Action, 2017). These seizures can last from seconds to 3 minutes and after the seizure the limbs become limp, breathing is quiet and when the patient awakes they may be disorientated, complain of headache and are fatigued. Because the seizure frequently occurs without warning, it is possible for injury to occur, and if the tonic–clonic seizure lasts more than 5 minutes or the patient experiences another seizure without recovery it is considered a medical emergency (Hickey, 2009). Nursing care and management of a seizure can be seen in Box 36.10.

Absence seizures are the other main type of generalized seizure, characterized by an abrupt stop to normal activity and short loss of consciousness from 10 to 30 seconds. The person does not move, their eyes become vacant and they often stare straight ahead. Absence seizures often go unnoticed because of their short duration but can occur several times a day, with a full recovery after the seizure (Epilepsy Action, 2017). Many potential seizure triggers exist, which can be seen in Box 36.11.

Diagnosis

Diagnosis of epilepsy can be complex, as there are many underlying causes of seizure activity; therefore assessment involves an accurate patient history and a reliable account of what occurs before, during and after a seizure, from both the patient and a witness (Woodward & Mestecky, 2011). A physical and neurological examination will also be performed and an electroencephalogram will identify patterns of electrical activity that can be linked to the type of seizure (Hickey 2009). Additional investigations may be performed to identify differential diagnoses. These can involve electrocardiograph, magnetic resonance imaging and blood tests, including levels of electrolytes (substances in the body such as sodium and potassium), kidney and liver function and blood cell counts (such as white blood cells, red blood cells and platelet counts). NICE (2016b) recommends that all adults having a first seizure should be seen as soon as possible by a specialist in epilepsies, so that prompt diagnosis and appropriate treatment can be initiated.

Management and care of a person with epilepsy

The underlying cause of the seizure will determine treatment interventions but if there is no underlying condition causing the epilepsy, the mainstay of treatment is directed at management of seizures through medication. The anti-epileptic drug (AED) treatment strategy should be individualized according to the seizure and epilepsy type, comorbidity, the person's lifestyle and the preferences of the person, their family and/or carers, as appropriate (NICE 2016b). Hickey (2009) states that 75% of patients with epilepsy can have their seizures reduced or controlled effectively by medication.

AEDs work by controlling the electrical activity in the brain that causes seizures, and work best if they are taken regularly, around the same time each day. The aim of AED treatment is to take the lowest dose of the fewest number of AEDs and with the least side effects. When they are introduced, they are given at a low dose, with gradual increase until seizures are controlled. If seizures are not controlled with a single drug, another drug might be added until optimum management is achieved (Epilepsy Society, 2017). NICE (2016b) provide information to clinicians about which AEDs should be used for different types of epilepsy and this changes as more AEDs become licensed for use in the management of seizures. For example, findings of recent studies show that lamotrigine should be the first-line treatment for focal seizures. When AEDs are not effective, surgery may be considered for focal seizures where specific lesions causing the seizure can be removed in an attempt to prevent further seizures and improve quality of life (Woodward & Mestecky, 2011).

The role of the Nursing Associate in epilepsy is not limited to management of seizures but one of the key roles is the provision of effective education for the patient and their family.

Information needs are dependent on the patient's age, lifestyle, job and how long they have had epilepsy (Woodward & Mestecky, 2011). Whilst epilepsy can be a hidden disability, it is a chronic long-term condition that can have a significant impact on the patients' daily life and well-being, including their mood, relationships, driving and employment. It is important to signpost the patient and their families to agencies such as the Epilepsy Society and Epilepsy Action for ongoing support and up to date information and research on the condition. However, it is the epilepsy nurse specialist who is often the coordinator of the care and the key point of access on an ongoing basis and who is the identified expert who conducts the yearly reviews (NICE 2016b).

CRITICAL AWARENESS

When assessing the patient's neurological status, the nursing and medical notes should be reviewed first, and the medical diagnosis and any other previous symptoms or diseases noted. The patient may have a known neurological disease, for example, multiple sclerosis, or they could have had a previous cerebrovascular accident; these could impact on the outcome of the assessment. It is important to also note what medications/drugs may have been taken or administered. Some drugs, for example, benzodiazepines and opioids, could alter a person's level of consciousness.

CASE STUDY 36.2   Annie – Epilepsy

Annie is a 24-year-old woman who was admitted to accident and emergency following what was believed to have been her first seizure. She was unable to give much of a history; she was at her boyfriend's house, sitting and chatting on the sofa, and the next thing she remembers is collapsing to the ground. The seizure lasted about 3 minutes. She regained consciousness after about a minute but had bitten her tongue. She was confused for a further hour or so and she could not recall the event.

A full screening was undertaken in the accident and emergency, which included a physical examination to assess neurological and cardiac status and rule out any underlying conditions and/or injuries. It was important at this stage to speak to Annie's boyfriend, who witnessed the event, and from this history the seizure was suggestive of a generalized tonic–clonic seizure. A variety of baseline blood tests were obtained, including levels of electrolytes (substances in the body such as sodium and potassium), kidney and liver function and blood cell counts (such as white blood cells, red blood cells, platelet counts). An electroencephalogram and an electrocardiograph were also performed. A computed tomography scan was also performed, which was normal, but referral to a neurologist specializing in epilepsies was made.

Annie had a further generalized tonic–clonic seizure in accident and emergency that was witnessed by the Nursing Associate. Details of the seizure were recorded by the Nursing Associate and she maintained Annie's safety throughout the seizure. The seizure lasted 2 minutes and she was incontinent of urine. Vital signs were recorded at the end of the seizure and Annie was placed in the recovery position. Other than oxygen, no other medication was administered during or after the seizure. Annie's boyfriend was upset after witnessing Annie having a further seizure, so the Nursing Associate rang Annie's parents on request for additional support.

Once stabilized, Annie was commenced on lamotrigine as the first-line treatment and information was provided to Annie and her boyfriend about the medication. In addition, information was provided on epilepsy, potential triggers, first aid and safety during a seizure, lifestyle issues, driving and employment, and they were provided with contact details for support services. Annie was discharged home that day and an appointment was made to visit the epilepsy clinic in 1 month.

(Adapted from tools and resources accessed from NICE, 2016b.)

CARE IN THE HOME SETTING

Epileptic Seizure Risk

The home is the most common place for seizure-related accidents. Activities such as bathing and cooking place the person with seizures at risk for injury. Making simple changes in household activities or the environment may create a safer home. The individual's seizure type and frequency will dictate the type of changes that may help them stay safe.

Bathroom safety
Bathrooms, which have mirrors, sinks, shower doors, baths and hard floors, can be a risk for those with uncontrolled seizures. Bathroom activities are generally

private matters and assessing the need for privacy and safety is important for people with seizures.

A Few Safety Tips:
- To give some privacy, place an occupied sign on the bathroom door as opposed to locking it.
- Hang the bathroom door so that it swings outward (into the hall or bedroom). This prevents the door from being blocked if a person falls during a seizure.
- Encourage showers instead of baths.

- Ensure shower and bath drains work properly so water does not build up.
- Keep water temperature low to avoid burns.
- Use nonskid strips in the bath or shower.
- Use a shower curtain instead of a shower door, it is easier to get in and help someone if they have a fall in the shower.
- Use bath rails or grab bars.
- For those who fall during a seizure or have frequent seizures:
  - Use a shower chair or sit on bottom of the bath and use a hand-held shower nozzle.
  - Encourage the person to take a shower when someone else is in the house.

General Home Safety Tips:
- Use an electric razor to avoid cuts.
- Use shatterproof glass for mirrors.

- Avoid glass tables.
- Avoid scatter rugs. Wall-to-wall carpeting or soft flooring may reduce injuries for individuals who fall.
- Use protective or padded covers on tap handles, nozzles or the edges of countertops to help cushion falls and reduce injuries.
- Use covers on enclosed heating units or radiators.
- Electrical equipment, such as hair dryers or razors, should be used away from any water source.
- Secure televisions, computers or other things that could fall off tables.
- At all times use fireplace screens.
- Avoid clutter in rooms. Also look around and make sure there is room to fall safely.
- Devise a way to call for help if the person is alone. Consider alarm systems, medic alerts and other safety devices.

AT THE GP SURGERY

Key to the care and management of people with epilepsy is a structured system in which primary and secondary care can share responsibility and communicate effectively, ensuring the patient is at the centre of all that is done. Each of the individuals within the primary care team, the practice nurse, the Nursing Associate and the healthcare assistant has an essential role to play in coordinating the system of managed care for those with epilepsy.

Many patients are seen and cared for within primary care and this is the same for people with neurological disorders. Those people who have epilepsy, for example, are often (not exclusively) cared for and managed solely within the primary care setting by the practice nurse and GP. Patients with epilepsy who require medication are often reviewed by the primary care team. Their role is to ensure that the patient's epilepsy is well controlled, unnecessary side effects

are noted (and when possible prevented and not experienced) and they give the support and information needed to the patient concerning issues such as employment and driving.

When a new diagnosis of epilepsy is suspected in primary care, then an urgent referral should be made to an epilepsy specialist. The primary care team can provide essential information to aid the diagnosis, as the practice nurse and GP are often the first to suspect epilepsy and are in an ideal position to obtain a first-hand witness account and record the diagnostic features.

An important aspect of ensuring a system of structured management in primary care is to develop a register of those patients in the practice who have epilepsy and require treatment with anti-epileptic medications.

COMMUNITIES OF CARE

Maternal Health

Pre-eclampsia
Pre-eclampsia is a chief cause of maternal mortality and morbidity, preterm birth, perinatal death and intrauterine growth restriction. The pathophysiology of this multisystem disorder, which is characterized by abnormal vascular response to placentation, remains unclear. Pre-eclampsia may be life-threatening for mother and child; this increases fetal and maternal morbidity and mortality.

Pre-eclampsia is defined as pregnancy-induced hypertension in association with proteinuria (greater than 0.3 g in 24 hours), with or without oedema. Essentially any organ system may be affected. It is characterized by maternal hypertension, proteinuria, oedema, foetal intrauterine growth restriction, as well as

premature birth. Eclampsia is defined as the occurrence of one or more convulsions that are superimposed on pre-eclampsia.

All pregnant women should be made aware of the need to seek immediate advice from a healthcare professional if they experience symptoms of pre-eclampsia. Symptoms include:
- Severe headache
- Problems with vision, such as blurring or flashing before the eyes
- Severe pain just below the ribs
- Vomiting
- Sudden swelling of the face, hands or feet

(NICE, 2008.)

LOOKING BACK, FEEDING FORWARD

To offer care to those people with neurological disorders it is essential that the Nursing Associate has an understanding of the very complex neurological system. This chapter has provided the Nursing Associate with some insight of the neurological system.

The brain informs almost every other part of the body what to do. It does this continually, regardless of whether the person is aware of it or not. The brain controls what a person thinks

and feels, how an individual learns and remembers, as well as the way in which a person moves. It also controls many bodily functions that the person might not be consciously thinking about. The beating of the heart and whether the person is sleeping or awake is under the influence of the brain. Any injury or damage caused to the neurological system can have devastating effects on the individual and their family. The spinal cord is a long bundle of nerve tissue, extending from the lower part of the brain down through the spine, with various nerves branching out to the entire body.

Various conditions can affect the nervous system, and the role and function of the Nursing Associate is to assist the person in those activities that they are unable to do for themselves. There is also a need to promote independence, engaging the person in the rehabilitative process if appropriate, whilst at the same time ensuring safety. A change in a person's neurological status can be subtle and may occur very quickly; the Nursing Associate must be aware of the importance of neurological assessment, what the results of assessment may mean and how to manage the findings. The reporting and documentation of findings are essential if the action to be taken is to be effective.

It is impossible in a chapter of this size to address all neurological conditions. The Nursing Associate is advised to delve deeper into this fascinating subject and develop their knowledge and skills in their growing repertoire of expertise.

REFERENCES

Brooker, C., Nichol, M., 2011. Alexanders Nursing Practice, fourth ed. Churchill Livingstone, London.

Department of Health, 2005. National Service Framework for long term conditions. London, Department of Health. https://assets.publishing.service.gov.uk/government/uploads/system/uploads/attachment_data/file/198114/National_Service_Framework_for_Long_Term_Conditions.pdf.

Dougherty, D., Lister, S., 2011. The Royal Marsden Hospital Manual of Clinical Nursing Procedures. Wiley-Blackwell, London.

Epilepsy Action, 2017. Seizure classification. https://www.epilepsy.org.uk/info/seizure-classification.

Epilepsy Research UK, 2017. What is epilepsy? https://www.epilepsyresearch.org.uk.

Epilepsy Society, 2017. About epilepsy. https://www.epilepsysociety.org.uk/what-epilepsy#.WgOQ-7p2vIU.

Headway, 2013. Brain injury statistics. www.headway.org.uk.

Health Education England (HEE), 2017. Nursing Associate Curriculum Framework. The NHS Constitution. Heath Education England.

Hickey, J.V., 2009. The Clinical Practice of Neurological and Neurosurgical Nursing, sixth ed. Lippincott, Philadelphia.

Iggulden, H., 2006. Care of the Neurological Patient. Blackwell, London.

ILEA (International League Against Epilepsy), 2017. Definitions and guidelines on epilepsy from ILAE. http://www.ilae.org/Visitors/Centre/Definition_Class.cfm.

Mattar, I., 2011. Using the Roper, Logan and Tierney model in the management of traumatic brain injury in a critical care setting. Singapore Nurs. J. 11 (38), 14–19.

National Stroke Association, 2017. Act Fast. http://www.stroke.org/understand-stroke/recognizing-stroke/act-fast.

NICE, 2008. Antenatal care for uncomplicated pregnancies. National Institute for Health and Clinical Excellence clinical guideline CG62. https://www.nice.org.uk/guidance/cg62.

NICE, 2013. Stroke rehabilitation in adults. National Institute for Health and Care Excellence clinical guideline CG162. https://www.nice.org.uk/guidance/cg162.

NICE, 2014. Head injury: assessment and early management. National Institute for Health and Care Excellence clinical guideline CG176. https://www.nice.org.uk/guidance/cg176.

NICE, 2016a. Major trauma: assessment and initial management. National Institute for Health and Care Excellence guideline NG39. https://www.nice.org.uk/guidance/ng39.

NICE, 2016b. Epilepsies: diagnosis and management. National Institute for Health and Care Excellence clinical guideline CG137. https://www.nice.org.uk/guidance/cg137.

NICE, 2016c. Stroke in adults. National Institute for Health and Care Excellence quality standard QS2. https://www.nice.org.uk/guidance/qs2/chapter/Introduction.

NICE, 2017. Stroke and transient ischaemic attack in over 16s: diagnosis and initial management. National Institute for Health and Care Excellence clinical guideline CG68. https://www.nice.org.uk/guidance/cg68.

Pangilinan, P.H., Kishner, S., Kelly, B.M., et al., 2008. Classification and complications of traumatic brain injury https://emedicine.medscape.com/article/326643-overview.

Stroke Association, 2017a. State of the nation: Stroke statistics in January 2017. https://www.stroke.org.uk/sites/default/files/state_of_the_nation_2017_final_1.pdf.

Stroke Association, 2017b. Types of stroke. http://www.strokeassociation.org/STROKEORG/AboutStroke/TypesofStroke/Types-of-Stroke_UCM_308531_SubHomePage.jsp#.

Swann, J.I., 2013. Understanding head injuries. Br. J. Healthcare Assistants 7(4), 174–179.

Teasdale, G., 2014. Forty years on - updating the Glasgow Coma Scale. Nurs. Times 110(42), 12–16.

Waugh, A., Grant, A., 2018. Ross & Wilson Anatomy and Physiology in Health and Illness, thirteenth ed. Elsevier, Edinburgh.

Williams, P., 2018. deWits Fundamental Concepts and Skills for Nursing, fifth ed. Elsevier, St Louis.

Woodward, S., Waterhouse, C., 2006. Oxford Handbook of Neurosciences Nursing. Oxford University Press, London.

Woodward, S., Mestecky, A.M., 2011. Neurosciences Nursing: Evidence Based Practice. Wiley, London.

World Health Organization, 2011. Rehabilitation. http://www.who.int/rehabilitation/en/.

World Health Organization, 2017a. The global burden of cerebrovascular disease. http://www.who.int/healthinfo/statistics/bod_cerebrovasculardiseasestroke.pdf.

World Health Organization, 2017b. Epilepsy. http://www.who.int/mental_health/neurology/epilepsy/en/.

37

Ear, Nose and Throat Disorders

Carl Clare

OBJECTIVES

By the end of the chapter the reader will:
1. Have an understanding of the anatomy and physiology of the ear, nose and throat
2. Discuss the pathophysiological changes associated with a selection of ear, nose and throat disorders
3. Outline the care required by people with an ear, nose and throat disorder
4. Describe some common conditions associated with the ear, nose and throat
5. Review the role of the Nursing Associate in promoting health and well-being

KEY WORDS

Membrane	Tympanic	Epiglottis
Eustachian	Nasopharynx	Cricoid
Semicircular	Ciliary	
Sebaceous	Turbinates	

CHAPTER AIMS

This aim of this chapter is to provide the reader with an understanding of the skills, knowledge and attitude required to provide safe, effective and compassionate care to people with an ear, nose and throat disorder.

SELF TEST

1. What is the purpose of ear wax?
2. Name the bones of the ossicular chain.
3. What are the two labyrinths in the inner ear?
4. What are the functions of the nose?
5. What are the turbinates?
6. What is the other name for the Adam's apple?
7. What is the purpose of the false vocal cords?
8. Name one method for removing ear wax from the middle ear.
9. What is an epistaxis?
10. Explain the difference between a tracheostomy and a laryngectomy.

INTRODUCTION

In this chapter, the ear, nose and throat are considered. The first part discusses the anatomy and physiology of the ear, nose and throat. It is important for the Nursing Associate to have a comprehensive understanding of the ear, nose and throat if the care provided is to be appropriate and effective.

The second part of the chapter addresses a selection of common conditions that impact on the ear, nose and throat and thus the health and well-being of people. The care and comfort of the patient who experiences a disorder of the ear, nose or throat are described. When offering care, the Nursing Associate is required to be kind and compassionate. Care provision must recognize the concern that a condition of the ear, nose or throat can instil within a patient and be sensitive to this. The health promotion needs of the patient with an ear, nose and throat condition are high and the Nursing Associate should be aware of the resources available for a patient who is managing their everyday life whilst experiencing an ear, nose or throat condition.

SENSITIVE CARE

When caring for a patient with an ear, nose or throat disorder, it is essential that the Nursing Associate is sensitive to the physical and psychological effects such a condition can create. Many patients living with a condition affecting the ear, nose or throat will require support and will have needs for information regarding their condition and its everyday management or recovery.

There can often be effects the condition will have on everyday life and the patient will commonly be concerned about returning to a normal life as soon as possible. It is important to understand in these situations that this condition is new to the patient and, whilst it may seem like a minor condition to you, it can have a significant impact on the patient. Thus, patients must be dealt with patiently and requests for information dealt with sensitively.

Patients suffering from an ear, nose or throat condition, and their relatives, may have a lot of questions and a significant need for information. Care staff must be sensitive, open and honest in their communication. It is not a failure of your ability as a carer to say that you 'don't know' and either to offer to find out or to signpost the patient to a reliable source of information (such as NHS Choices). The Nursing and Midwifery Council Code (Nursing and Midwifery Council, 2018) makes clear that in any circumstance in which you are unsure, you should always strive to refer the patient to a person who does know; you should only act within the sphere of your competence.

Part of the role of the Nursing Associate is to deliver person-centred holistic care (Health Education England, 2017) and you must make yourself aware of the impact an ear, nose or throat condition can have on an individual's everyday life. Being an open and empathic listener is just as important to many patients as the physical care that we provide.

ANATOMY AND PHYSIOLOGY OF THE EAR

The ear is divided into three sections (Fig. 37.1):
- External
- Middle
- Inner

Each of these three sections is essential to the process of hearing and the inner ear is also essential to the maintenance of the sense of balance.

External ear

The external ear is made up of the pinna, the external ear canal and the tympanic membrane.
- Pinna: a flap of elastic cartilage covered in skin. It is shaped like the end of a horn and it surrounds the end of the external auditory canal.
- External ear canal: this is a slightly 's'-shaped tube lined with skin, fine hairs, oil-producing glands (known as sebaceous glands) and ceruminous glands (glands that produce wax). The oils and the wax created by the two types of gland help to lubricate the ear canal, kill bacteria and, along with the hairs, keep the canal free of debris.
- Tympanic membrane: this membrane is made up of epithelial cells, connective tissue and mucous membrane. It acts as a barrier between the external and middle ears and is responsible for the transfer of sound from the external to the middle ear.

Middle ear

The middle ear is lined with mucous membrane; it is connected to the upper airways by a duct known as the eustachian (or auditory) tube. This connection between the ear and the airways means that air pressure between the middle ear and the throat (and therefore atmospheric air) is equal, allowing for free movement of the tympanic membrane. If one side of the tympanic membrane was under higher pressure than the other side, this

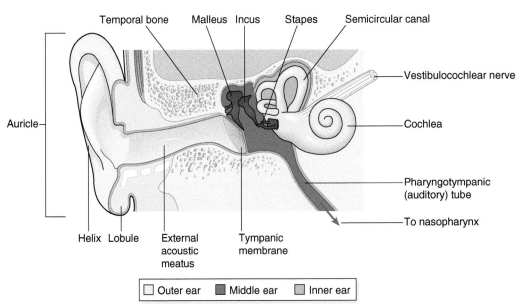

Fig. 37.1 The Structures of the Ear (Waugh & Grant, 2018).

would lead to a reduction in the movement of the membrane and thus a loss of hearing.

Within the middle ear are three bones (the ossicles or ossicular chain):

- Hammer (malleus)
- Anvil (incus)
- Stirrup (stapes)

These three bones interlink (Fig. 37.2) and are connected to the tympanic membrane and the oval window. Thus, when the

tympanic membrane vibrates, the bones transmit the vibrations to the oval window and through to the fluid of the inner ear.

Inner ear

The inner ear is also known as the labyrinth due to the complicated series of canals it contains. The inner ear is made up of two fluid-filled parts (Fig. 37.3):

- Bony labyrinth: within the temporal bone are a series of cavities that contain the main organs responsible for our sense of balance (the semicircular canals and the vestibule) and the main organ responsible for hearing (the cochlea).
- Membranous labyrinth: inside the bony labyrinth are a series of fluid-filled sacs and tubes known as the membranous labyrinth. Movement of the fluid within the membranous labyrinth that is contained within the cochlea leads to stimulation of the hearing receptors. This leads to the generation of nerve impulses that are transmitted to the hearing centres of the brain via the cochlear nerve.

The sense of balance is partially controlled by the ear. The receptors in the semicircular ducts of the membranous labyrinth and the vestibule (the utricle and the saccule) have an important role to play in maintaining balance when we are moving. The receptors are active during movement but inactive when the body is motionless. The sensory receptors in the ducts respond to rotational movements of the head. There are three of these ducts and each has a different orientation:

- Lateral
- Posterior
- Anterior

Each semicircular duct contains an expanded section known as the ampulla and this is where the majority of the receptors for balance can be found. The impulses from the balance receptors are transmitted to the brain via the vestibular nerve.

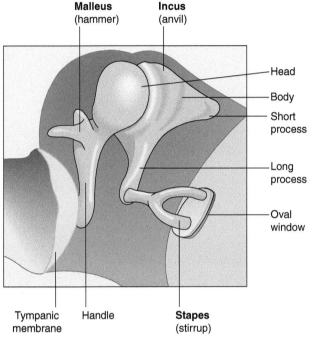

Fig. 37.2 The Three Bones of the Ossicular Chain (Waugh & Grant, 2018).

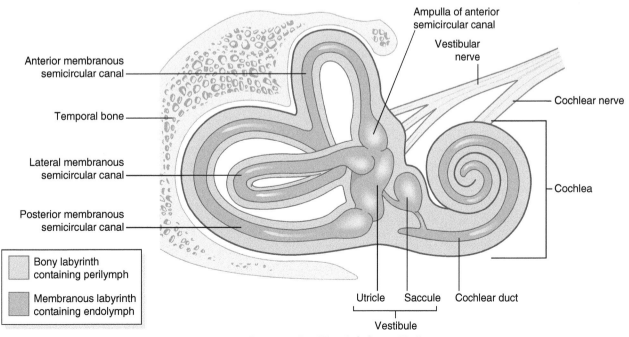

Fig. 37.3 The Inner Ear (Waugh & Grant, 2018).

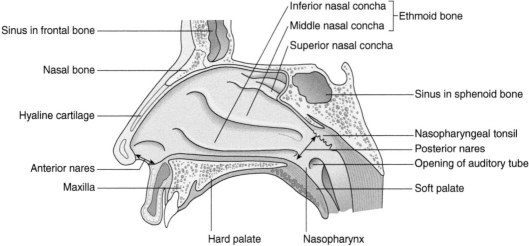

Fig. 37.4 The Nose (Waugh & Grant, 2018).

ANATOMY AND PHYSIOLOGY OF THE NOSE

As well as being the first part of the respiratory tract, the nose also contains the receptors for the sense of smell. The functions of the nose are:

- Warming, moistening and filtering inhaled air
- Detecting smells
- Resonance chamber that modifies the quality of speech.

The nose can be divided into an external and an internal section (Fig. 37.4):

- External nose: a bone and cartilage structure covered by muscle and skin and lined with a mucous membrane. This structure is attached to the bones of the skull. The external nose is divided into two airways (known as nares or nostrils) by the septum.
- Internal nose: a chamber lined with ciliated mucous membrane and containing coarse hairs that filter out large particles from inhaled air. The sticky mucus created by the membrane traps finer particles that enter the nose. These particles are then transported to the nasopharynx by the ciliary system. The internal nose is also divided into two by a continuation of the septum. Each side of the internal nose contains three 'shelves' (concha) made of bone, known as the turbinates; these increase the surface area that inhaled air must pass over. The internal nose has an extremely rich blood supply, which, in combination with the turbinates, increases the humidification and warming of the air passing through. Within the internal nose there are also openings (ostia) from cavities contained within the bones of the skull (known as the sinus cavities).

ANATOMY AND PHYSIOLOGY OF THE THROAT

The throat consists of the oropharynx and the hypopharynx (Fig. 37.5).

Oropharynx
Tonsils

The tonsils are collections of lymphatic nodules, mostly located around the junction of the oral cavity and the oropharynx. The role of the tonsils is to participate in the fight against inhaled or ingested foreign antigens.

Hypopharynx
Larynx

The larynx is a short tube that connects the lower hypopharynx with the trachea. It is composed of a mucous membrane covering several pieces of cartilage, including:

- Thyroid cartilage (Adam's apple)
- Epiglottis: a large piece of cartilage that covers the opening of the glottis during swallowing, thus protecting the airway
- Cricoid cartilage: a ring of cartilage that forms the inferior wall of the larynx and connects to the first cartilage ring of the trachea.

> **⚠ HOTSPOT**
>
> Everyone has an Adam's apple; it is just less prominent in women.

The mucous membrane of the larynx is formed to create two pairs of folds:

- Ventricular folds (false vocal cords): when brought together, these enable the holding of the breath against the pressure in the thoracic cavity. You may do this when lifting a heavy object or women may do this when pushing in childbirth.
- Vocal cords (or vocal folds; the true vocal cords): situated below the false vocal cords, the vocal cords are essential for the production of speech. Sound is generated by the vibration of these cords, but recognizable speech requires the sound to be modified by the mouth, nasal cavity and nasal sinuses.

DISORDERS OF THE EARS, NOSE OR THROAT

Ear
Ear wax

Signs and symptoms. Ear wax can become impacted in the external ear canal. This is often associated with a patient's attempts to remove ear wax with fingers or cotton buds and is more common in the elderly who tend to produce more ear wax. The

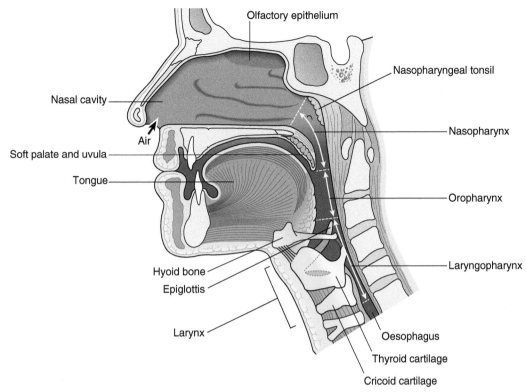

Fig. 37.5 The Throat (Waugh & Grant, 2018).

effect of impacted ear wax is to reduce the ability of sound to travel the length of the external ear canal and it also reduces the responsiveness of the tympanic membrane to sound waves. Thus, patients will report a reduction in the ability to hear, a feeling of 'stuffiness' in the ear and potentially tinnitus.

Diagnosis. The diagnosis of ear wax is based on taking a patient history and the inspection of the ear canal by a trained practitioner using an otoscope.

Care and treatment. There are two main methods for the removal of ear wax. Both methods are normally preceded by the use of a substance that actively helps to break down wax or a wax softener (such as olive oil). One method for the removal of ear wax is the syringing of the external ear canal using water; the other method is the use of micro-suction (Loveman et al., 2011). Both of these methods require specialist training and should not be attempted by the patient themselves.

AT THE GP SURGERY

Impacted ear wax is often treated in the GP surgery, often by ear syringing. Ear syringing is a procedure that should only be undertaken by suitably qualified staff but the Nursing Associate has a role to play in assisting the doctor or nurse.

Ear syringing should not be carried out if the patient:

- Has a perforation of the ear drum or there is a history of mucous discharge in the last year
- Has had a history of middle ear infection in the last 6 weeks
- Has had previous ear surgery (except grommets)

- Has grommets in place
- Has evidence of otitis externa
- The patient has a cleft palate (repaired or not).

The Nursing Associate may be asked to prepare the equipment prior to the procedure:

- Waterproof cape and disposable towel
- Otoscope with a number of different sized disposable specula and spare batteries
- Head mirror and light or mobile light
- Irrigation machine and disposable tips
- Water heated to 37°C
- Receiving bowl for the waste water

During the procedure, you may be asked to stay with the patient or to assist by passing equipment.

Otitis externa

Signs and symptoms. The condition is associated with pain, itching and a discharge from the ear canal caused by inflammation of the external ear. The discharge is usually watery at the beginning but becomes pus-filled as the condition progresses. Otitis externa is often associated with people who swim a lot and is therefore also known as 'swimmer's ear' (Kaushik et al., 2010).

The spread of infection can lead to pyrexia and general symptoms such as a generalized feeling of being tired and unwell.

Diagnosis. Diagnosis of otitis externa is based on taking a patient history and physical inspection of the ear. The infection is usually caused by a mixture of bacteria and swabs should be sent for laboratory culture and sensitivity testing.

Care and treatment. The care of this condition includes:
- Careful removal of any debris from the external ear canal.
- The administration of antibiotics and a steroid preparation into the ear canal.

- If the infection has entered the bloodstream or is extensive, the patient may require oral antibiotics, pain relief and bed rest.
- The patient should be discouraged from scratching the affected ear and advised to prevent water from entering the ear canal (Pankhania et al., 2011).

OSCE 37.1   Instillation of Ear Drops

The procedure should be undertaken using local policy and procedure

Action	Criteria	Achieved/not achieved
Introduction	Washes hands. Introduces self. Confirms patient details.	
Explain the procedure	Explains rationale for the ear drops so patient is able to understand and is able to give informed consent. Gains consent to proceed.	
Gathers equipment	Gloves. Ear drops. Cotton wool.	
Ask the patient to lie on their side with the affected ear uppermost	The ear drops will flow into the ear through gravity.	
Draw the medication into the dropper	Squeezing the bulb of the dropper and letting go draws the fluid into the dropper by suction.	
Straighten the ear canal	In an adult, pull the pinna up and backwards; for children under three, pull the earlobe down and backwards.	
Insert the tip of the dropper into the beginning of the ear canal. Instil the drops.	Ensures the ear drops go to the correct place. Inserting the dropper too far may cause damage.	
Ask the patient to lie on their side for 5–10 minutes	Allows the ear drops to travel the length of the ear canal.	
Place cotton wool at the opening of the ear canal	Stops the ear drops coming out of the ear and getting on to the patient's clothing.	
Ensure dropper/bottle are labelled with the patient's name	To avoid cross contamination to another patient.	
Dispose of equipment appropriately	In line with local policy.	
Remove gloves and wash hands	Infection control.	
Record actions accurately	Maintain accurate records for patient safety.	

Pass
Fail

THE MEDICINE TROLLEY 37.1

Drug	Drug classification	Reason for administration	Route of administration	Dose	Side effects	Contra-indications	Nursing care
Chloramphenicol	Broad spectrum antibiotic	Otitis externa	Topical (ear drops)	2–3 drops 2–3 times a day	There is a high incidence of local reactions to the carrier fluid the chloramphenicol is dissolved in.	None	Use separate bottles/droppers for each ear to avoid cross contamination. Avoid prolonged use. Patients will often be expected to administer these drops at home. Educate the patient as to the correct technique for administration.

Tympanic membrane rupture

Signs and symptoms. Rupture of the tympanic membrane can be due to improper ear syringing technique, blows to the side of the head or blast injuries. Symptoms include:

- Ear pain that may subside quickly
- Clear, pus-filled or bloody drainage from the ear
- Hearing loss
- Ringing in the ear (tinnitus)
- Spinning sensations (vertigo)
- Nausea or vomiting that can result from vertigo.

Diagnosis. Diagnosis is based on taking a patient history and physical examination of the tympanic membrane by a trained practitioner.

Care and treatment. Tympanic membrane rupture often heals without intervention as long as there is no infection present. Whilst natural healing occurs, patients should be advised to avoid:

- The entry of water into the ear
- Introducing foreign objects, such as cotton buds, into the ear.

If there is persistent deafness, this may be due to damage or displacement of the ossicular chain and may require surgery to repair.

Otitis media

Signs and symptoms. Acute otitis media is a condition that is often a complication of upper respiratory tract infections or sinusitis. The infection travels up into the middle ear via the eustachian tube, leading to infection and the collection of pus. The infection and the pressure resulting from the collection of pus may lead to a range of potential symptoms, including (Gopen, 2010):

- Pain
- High temperature
- A generalized feeling of being unwell
- Headache
- Nausea and vomiting
- Tinnitus
- Reduction in hearing

Diagnosis. Diagnosis is based on taking a patient history and physical examination of the ear.

Care and treatment. The treatment for otitis media includes:

- Antibiotics
- Pain relief
- Antipyretics
- Application of warmth to the affected ear in order to reduce pain
- Avoiding water entering the ear canal.

Untreated or repeated episodes of acute otitis media may lead to chronic infection of the middle ear. In chronic infection, tympanic membrane rupture is common and destruction of the bones of the ossicular chain is also possible. Symptoms include:

- Pus-filled discharge
- Pain: may be associated with redness and swelling of the bone behind the pinna

- High temperature
- Hearing loss
- Nausea and vomiting
- Vertigo.

The chronic complications of otitis media are usually treated by surgery:

- Myringoplasty: repair of the tympanic membrane
- Ossiculoplasty: reconstruction of the ossicular chain
- Tympanoplasty: myringoplasty and ossiculoplasty performed at the same time
- Mastoidectomy: removal of infected tissue from the middle ear and mastoid bone; often performed with a tympanoplasty.

Following surgery on the ear, there are certain types of care that are common, regardless of the actual operation:

- In the immediate recovery period the patient should be nursed with no pillows, lying on the side opposite to the ear the surgery was performed on.
- Advise the patient to avoid sudden movements of the head.
- Pain relief should be administered as prescribed.
- Pillows can be used for comfort when the patient feels able to tolerate them; most patients are able to tolerate sitting up after 24 hours.
- Following operations on the inner ear, neurological observations must be carried out at least 4 hourly for the first 24 hours.
- Facial nerve damage may occur at the time of the operation or may occur afterwards due to inflammation. The patient should be asked to show their teeth or smile to assess for facial weakness.
- Patient should be advised to avoid coughing, sneezing and blowing their nose, or straining during bowel movements for 7–10 days after the operation, as this will lead to an increased pressure in the ear. If coughing or sneezing cannot be avoided, then the patient should be advised to keep the mouth open to reduce the pressure on the middle ear.
- Most patients are discharged after 2–3 days. All patients should be advised to avoid water entry into the ear, crowded places (where respiratory infections may be contracted) and changes in air pressure (such as flying or high altitudes) until advised by the surgeon.

Otosclerosis

Signs and symptoms. Otosclerosis is the formation of new bone around the footplate of the stapes. It is often hereditary and is associated with a gradual deterioration in hearing.

Diagnosis. Diagnosis will begin with the taking of a patient history, including family history. Tests may include audiometry, measuring the pressure in the inner ear and a computed tomography scan.

Care and treatment. As the condition is progressive, the use of hearing aids is possible but eventually surgery will be required. The surgery involves the removal of part of the stapes and insertion of a prosthesis.

THE MEDICINE TROLLEY 37.2

Drug	Drug classification	Reason for administration	Route of administration	Dose	Side effects	Contra-indications	Nursing care
Betahistine dihydrochloride	Anti-vertigo medication	Vertigo associated with Ménière's disease	Oral	16 mg three times a day increasing to 24–48 mg daily	Gastrointestinal disturbances, headache, rash	Pheochromocytoma	Should be taken with food. Explain the reason for the medication. Gain consent before administering.

Ménière's disease

Symptoms. Ménière's disease is a disorder of the inner ear. Symptoms include:

- Vertigo
- Nausea and vomiting
- Tinnitus
- Varying hearing loss
- 'Drop attacks': a feeling of being pulled to the ground; alternatively some patients feel as though they are whirling through space.

Diagnosis. The diagnosis of Ménière's disease is based on taking a patient history and the presence of symptoms suggestive of the disease in the absence of any other cause.

Care and treatment. The duration of an episode can last for hours or days. Patients having an acute episode of Ménière's disease need:

- Reassurance
- A quiet, darkened environment
- A comfortable position (often semi-recumbent)
- To avoid sudden head movements
- To avoid fluorescent and flickering lights, and watching television
- Vomit bowls should be provided
- The bedside call bell should be put in the patient's reach and the patient advised not to get out of bed without assistance

Treatment of the disease requires lifestyle changes and long-term medication.

Patients who do not respond to medical treatment may require surgery.

REFLECTION 37.2

- How would you feel when the world feels like it is spinning and you cannot stand upright?
- What reassurance would you want to be given?
- Imagine being dependent on others in order to be able to get out of bed safely. How would it feel to be dependent on others who cannot see or know what you are experiencing?
- How can the Nursing Associate ensure that the patient feels safe and well cared for?

COMMUNITIES OF CARE
Learning Disabilities

Many conditions of the ear are nonspecific and do not have external signs that are easy to see. Therefore it is likely that carers would not notice many ear conditions in their everyday interactions with the people they care for. Pain from an ear infection or loss of hearing may lead to changes in behaviour or the worsening of behaviours that are already present. Often these changes are put down to the learning disability and healthcare professionals will fail to look for physical causes that may be treatable. This is known as 'diagnostic overshadowing'.

Diagnostic overshadowing is a common problem for patients with learning disabilities and can be made worse when the patient is not compliant with diagnostic examinations and has difficulty communicating symptoms.

Avoiding diagnostic overshadowing takes time and requires the healthcare practitioner to create a bond of trust and a rapport with the patient. Often this is not possible for medical staff; therefore, it becomes the role of the Nursing Associate to develop this relationship and become an advocate for the patient in the care setting (Nursing and Midwifery Council, 2018).

Furthermore, if the Nursing Associate has developed a rapport with the patient then they can chaperone the patient for any examinations or diagnostic procedures and help to keep the patient calm and compliant.

Nose
Epistaxis (nose bleed)

Signs and symptoms. A nose bleed is often associated with a blow to the nose or, in some cases, with upper respiratory tract infections. The signs are bleeding from the nose.

Diagnosis. The diagnosis of a nose bleed is based on the physical signs. A doctor may inspect the inside of the nose with a nasal endoscope.

Care and treatment. Controlling the bleeding requires the pinching of the upper part of the nose between the finger and the thumb whilst the patient sits with their head tilted forward. Tilting the patient's head forward stops blood draining into the throat and being swallowed, making the patient nauseous. Nasal packing may be required in severe nose bleeds. In some cases, the use of a Foley catheter or postnasal pack, to provide a firm base against which to pack the nose, may be required (Tikka, 2016). Further care for nose bleeds may include:

- Cold compresses applied to the nose and back of the neck to reduce blood flow to the nose.

- Cauterization of the bleeding point with silver nitrate stick or electrocautery.
- The surgical ligation of blood vessels may be used in cases that are resistant to other treatment (Tikka, 2016).

> **! HOTSPOT**
>
> Silver nitrate sticks degrade over time. They must be kept in an airtight and light-proof container. If the silver nitrate stick has no effect on the bleeding, it may be worth trying a new stick in case the previous one has degraded.

Deviated nasal septum

Signs and symptoms. This is a condition that a patient may be born with (congenital) or acquire due to trauma. The septum dividing the nose into the two nostrils is significantly off centre or crooked. Patients may report repeated infections, snoring, nasal obstruction or difficulty breathing. Pain is common, especially after traumatic deviation.

Diagnosis. Diagnosis is based on a physical examination of the nose. A patient history will be taken to explore the effects of the deviation on the patient's life and help to decide if treatment is necessary.

Care and treatment. Treatment is normally surgical:
- Submucous resection: removal and resection of the parts of the septum causing the deviation
- Septoplasty: septum is completely freed from the surrounding structures and repositioned.

The care of patients following surgery of the nose is detailed here.
- In the period immediately after surgery, patients will normally have a nasal pack in situ (in place).
- Monitoring of the patients' airway due to the risk of blood or nasal packing entering the respiratory tract must be carried out until the patient is alert enough to report complications themselves.
- When the patient is fully conscious, their head should be raised above the level of the heart and they should be encouraged to sleep semi-upright. This reduces bleeding and swelling.
- The patient should be advised to avoid sneezing, blowing their nose and straining during bowel movements for 10–14 days, as this may lead to bleeding. If sneezing is unavoidable,

then the patient should keep the mouth open to reduce the pressure on the nose.
- After the removal of nasal packs, steam inhalations or a saline spray will help to keep the nasal mucosa moist and loosen any crusts.

Sinusitis

Signs and symptoms. Following a viral infection of the nose, the natural resistance of the mucosa is reduced and a secondary bacterial infection can develop. This can rapidly spread into the sinuses, causing swelling of the mucosa. If the mucosa swells enough, then the ostia (openings) of the sinuses can become blocked and infected mucus is unable to escape. The trapping of infected mucus and the swelling leads to symptoms such as:
- Pain
- Nasal obstruction
- A generalized feeling of being unwell and tired
- High temperature
- Tenderness.

If sinusitis remains untreated, there is the possibility of complications such as:
- The spread of infection to the eyes
- The development of an intracranial infection or abscess
- Infection of the bone.

Diagnosis

The diagnosis of sinusitis is based on patient history and physical examination of the patient.

Care and treatment. The treatment of sinusitis includes:
- Nasal decongestants to reduce the swelling of the mucosa and allow drainage
- Antibiotics, such as amoxicillin (Rosenfeld et al., 2015)
- Pain relief
- Saline washouts to relieve symptoms
- Any abscess would require surgical intervention.

The care of patients with sinusitis includes:
- Looking after the patient in a warm, well-ventilated environment
- Encouraging a fluid intake of at least 3 L a day
- Encouraging good oral hygiene
- The use of a humidifier/steam inhalations
- Bed rest may be required
- During recovery the patient should avoid extremes of temperature, crowded environments and smoking.

THE MEDICINE TROLLEY 37.3

Drug	Drug classification	Reason for administration	Route of administration	Dose	Side effects	Contra-indications	Nursing care
Amoxicillin	Antibiotic	Sinusitis	Oral	500 mg three times a day	Allergic reaction, diarrhoea, nausea, vomiting, joint pains, rashes, itchy skin.	Penicillin allergy	Amoxicillin is a member of the penicillin family of antibiotics. Ensure the patient has no history of allergies to penicillin. Explain the purpose of the medication and gain consent before administering. Patients must always complete the course of antibiotics.

Throat

Tonsillitis and quinsy

Signs and symptoms. Tonsillitis is a condition caused by inflammation of the tonsils. The patient may present with:

- Sore throat (often both sides of the throat)
- Difficulty in swallowing
- High temperature
- A general feeling of being unwell.

Diagnosis. The diagnosis of tonsillitis is based on patient history and physical examination by a qualified practitioner.

Care and treatment. Treatment is usually:

- Antibiotics
- Encouraging a fluid intake of 1–3 L per day
- Pain relief
- Good oral hygiene
- Repeated episodes of tonsillitis may require surgical removal of the tonsils (tonsillectomy).

In severe cases, a peritonsillar abscess (quinsy) may develop and patients may present with:

- An inflamed tonsil that is swollen due to the collection of pus
- A worsening inability to swallow (often the patient will be unable to swallow saliva)
- A history of worsening pain on one side of the throat
- Trismus: an inability to open the mouth due to spasm of the jaw muscles.

This is considered a much more serious condition and is treated by removing the pus with a needle attached to a syringe (this is known as needle aspiration). Needle aspiration will always require antibiotic cover. Severe cases may require surgical incision and drainage, or complete removal of the tonsil. Needle aspiration is often preferred, as it does not normally require a general anaesthetic and thus the patient can be discharged home after a few hours.

Tracheostomy

Tracheostomies are created for several reasons:

- The creation of a new airway to relieve upper-airway obstruction
- Protection of the lungs from the aspiration of food or regurgitation of the stomach contents where the normal anatomical protection has failed or been removed
- Long-term artificial ventilation
- After a laryngectomy.

Most tracheostomies are temporary and a tube (often plastic but can be made of metal) is inserted into the stoma to maintain the patency of the airway. Following a laryngectomy, the trachea is brought to the surface of the neck and a permanent stoma is formed.

Potential complications following tracheostomy creation include:

- The tracheostomy tube becomes dislodged. This can be avoided by correctly securing the tube with tapes or a specialized tracheostomy-securing device.
- The tracheostomy tube becomes blocked. This is normally due to the build-up of dried secretions or the formation of a mucous plug, which is then coughed into the tube. This can be avoided by regular cleaning of the tube, the use of humidified oxygen and encouraging a good fluid intake to keep mucus fluid.
- Surgical emphysema: the escape of air into the soft tissue of the neck. This can be detected when the neck is palpated, as there is a crackling noise when pressure is applied to the skin.
- Pneumonia: the protective mechanisms of the upper airway are bypassed by a tracheostomy.
- Tracheo-oesophageal fistula: these are created by inflating a cuffed tracheostomy tube too high or leaving a cuffed tracheostomy tube inflated for too long. Either of these situations can lead to damage to the tracheal wall and the development of a hole (fistula) between the trachea and the oesophagus. The fistula allows the entry of food and fluids into the lungs. This can be avoided by using a pressure gauge to avoid over inflation of the cuff and good care and record-keeping to prevent the cuff being left inflated for too long.

The care of a patient following the creation of a tracheostomy includes:

- Care for the patient in an upright position to reduce swelling.
- Frequent observations must be carried out: blood pressure, pulse, respirations and oxygen saturations should be recorded every 15 minutes for the first 2 hours, then half hourly for 2 hours and then hourly for 24 hours.
- A low-pressure cuffed tracheostomy tube will be placed by the surgeon in the operating theatre. This should be left inflated for the first 24 hours to reduce the chance of bleeding. To reduce the chance of pressure damage, the cuff pressure should be checked every 8 hours using a pressure gauge.

> **! HOTSPOT**
>
> Patients who have a long-term tracheostomy will often have an uncuffed tracheostomy tube in place but it is recommended in the acute setting that a cuffed tracheostomy tube of the correct size is kept by the patient's bedside for use in the event of an emergency (such as cardiac arrest).

- Suctioning: this is dependent on patient requirements (patients will produce secretions at different rates).
- Humidification: as the upper airway has been bypassed, the air entering the patient's lungs is no longer warmed and humidified. It is important that the patient is given humidified oxygen to prevent the formation of crusts, which may block the tracheostomy tube.
- Dressings should be kept clean and dry (and replaced as necessary), as wet dressings encourage the growth of bacteria and may lead to wound infections or, if inhaled, respiratory infections.

> **! HOTSPOT**
>
> All tracheostomy changes (or dressing changes) must involve two people, one of whom is experienced in tracheostomy care. Never try to change a tracheostomy tube alone.

- The tracheostomy tube is first changed after 48 hours.

Longer-term care of the patient with a tracheostomy is aimed towards enabling the patient to perform their own care (including tube care, tube changes, suctioning and dressing changes). It is important that family and other potential care givers are also trained in the care of the tracheostomy.

Laryngectomy

CASE STUDY 37.1   Mohammad

Mohammad is a 37-year-old man who has undergone a laryngectomy for cancer of the throat. He still has a tracheostomy tube in place at present. He is frequently visited by his wife and 11-year-old daughter. Whenever they visit, the daughter does not stay at the bedside for long and is often to be found alone in the day room. Mohammad was a paramedic and will not be returning to work, as he has been advised to retire on health grounds. He is obviously worried and anxious about the future but he finds it hard to communicate and thus he can become quite frustrated.

Though Mohammad has been encouraged to use the humidified oxygen, he is reluctant to do so as he feels that it upsets his daughter. He has also been reluctant to get involved with the care of his tracheostomy and at times refuses to let normal care be carried out.

You make time to see Mohammad as he is sitting at the side of the bed and appears to be finding it hard to breathe.

VITAL SIGNS

Vital sign	Observation	Normal
Temperature	37°C	36.1–38.0°C
Pulse	100 beats per minute	51–90
Respiration	24 breaths per minute	12–20 breaths per minute
Blood pressure	120/58 mm Hg	111–219 mm Hg
O$_2$ saturation:	92%	≥96%

NEWS

Physiological parameter	3	2	1	0	1	2	3
Respiration rate		24					
Oxygen saturation %		92					
Supplemental oxygen				No			
Temperature °C				37			
Systolic BP mm Hg				120			
Heart rate				100			
Level of consciousness				A			
Score			4	1			
Total		5					

BP, Blood pressure.

REFLECTION 37.3

Take some time to reflect on this case and then consider the following.
1. Why do you think Mohammad may be having difficulty breathing?
2. What is the immediate care required by Mohammad?
3. Should you care for Mohammad alone? If not, who would you call to help you?
4. What can be done about Mohammad's reluctance to take responsibility for his care?
5. Who could you refer Mohammad to that could help him with his current dislike of his tracheostomy?
6. Who could you refer Mohammad to that could help him with his financial situation in the future?

Laryngectomy is the removal of the entire structure of the larynx and is the treatment for advanced laryngeal cancer where partial laryngectomy is not possible (NICE, 2016).

Following a laryngectomy, the patient breathes through a stoma created when the trachea is brought to the surface of the neck. As the trachea is brought to the neck, all connections between the trachea and the upper airway (mouth and nose) are severed and air entry to the lungs is directly through the neck. Therefore, air that passes into the lungs will be colder and drier than if it had passed through the upper airways; without artificial aid this leaves the lungs at higher risk of infection. Immediately after the surgery, the stoma will be protected by a tracheostomy tube and the care of the patient is similar to that of a patient with a temporary tracheostomy. There is, however, greater trauma to the trachea in laryngectomy surgery and this raises the risk of bleeding and oedema formation, potentially leading to compromise of the airway. Due to this increased risk, it is common practice for oxygen saturations to be monitored with pulse oximetry continuously for 24 hours post laryngectomy surgery. After 24 hours, pulse oximetry is only used continuously at night and this is done for a further 3 nights (note: oxygen saturations are still taken with every set of observations during the day as well). Once the risk of bleeding and oedema formation has reduced, which is usually about 5–10 days postoperatively, the tracheostomy tube is removed and replaced with a silicone stoma button or stud to prevent the closure of the stoma as scar tissue forms. Patients are normally discharged 14 days after surgery.

As noted, the loss of the normal humidification and warming mechanisms of the mouth and nose will lead to the drying of the mucous lining of the lower respiratory tract and a significant increase in water loss via exhaled air. This leads to changes in the normal respiratory mechanisms and there is a significantly increased risk of respiratory infection. The loss of moisture in inspired air will also lead to the creation of thick secretions and crust formation, which may completely block the stoma and thus threaten life. Humidification is essential for a laryngectomy patient and once the patient is discharged, they must use a passive heat and moisture exchanger (HME) worn over the stoma; these are usually made of foam that traps the heat and moisture in expired air, which are then transferred into the inspired air.

The loss of the patient's voice following laryngectomy can have significant emotional and psychological effects. At first, patients will often use pen and paper to communicate but all patients are encouraged to work towards regaining speech. There are several communication methods available and the choice will depend on the type of surgery undertaken and patient choice:
- Voice prostheses (speaking valve): a valve placed between the trachea and the oesophagus, which diverts expired air into the oesophagus when the tracheostomy is manually blocked; thus air passes into the mouth.
- Electrolarynx: a battery-powered device held against the mouth that creates speech with the use of sound waves.
- Artificial larynx: similar to an electrolarynx, except the device is held to the neck rather than the mouth.
- Oesophageal speech: this involves the patient swallowing air, trapping it in the oesophagus and releasing it to create sound.

It is important that laryngectomy patients wear a medical alert bracelet identifying them as a 'neck breather' in the event of an emergency situation.

REFLECTION 37.4

Imagine being without the ability to speak and trying to communicate your needs to a carer who does not know you.

How do you think this would make you feel?

What methods of communicating could you introduce for a patient in the early stages after a laryngectomy?

How could you as a Nursing Associate ensure that you prevent your patient from becoming socially isolated and feeling abandoned?

! HOTSPOT

In the event of an emergency in a patient who has undergone a laryngectomy, it is important that any airway management/ventilation is performed via the stoma (not the mouth). As normal airway patency no longer exists, any attempt to deliver oxygen or ventilate the patient via the mouth will not be effective. Thus, it is essential that oxygen is delivered via the neck stoma. In an emergency, normal oxygen masks or bag-valve-masks may be used by holding them over the stoma (usually sideways) but specialist equipment will be more effective.

In patients who have undergone a tracheostomy, the upper airway may be patent and therefore it may be possible to ventilate the patient via the mouth. It is vital that information on how to deliver oxygen in an emergency is handed over to all staff looking after the patient and that an emergency guide/care plan is kept by the patient's bedside.

Note: If you are unsure if the upper airway is patent, then it is advised that you apply oxygen to both the mouth and the stoma until expert staff arrive.

LOOKING BACK, FEEDING FORWARD

Disorders of the ear, nose or throat range from the minor (ear wax) to the life-threatening (laryngectomy) but all have the potential to have a huge impact on a person's life. Disorders of the ear or throat can leave a patient virtually disabled or socially isolated. It is important that the nursing assistant is aware of the impact a disorder of the ear, nose or throat can have on an individual patient and understand how they can help to care for a patient with one of these conditions. This chapter has reviewed the anatomy and physiology of the ear, nose and throat and has gone on to discuss a few endocrine disorders that you are likely to come across in your career.

REFERENCES

Gopen, Q., 2010. Pathology & clinical course: Inflammatory diseases of the middle ear. In: Gulya, A.J., Minar, L.B., Poe, D.S. (Eds.), Glassock-Shambaugh Surgery of the Ear, sixth ed. Peoples Medical Publishing House, Beijing, pp. 425–436.

Health Education England, 2017. Nursing Associate Curriculum Framework. Available at https://hee.nhs.uk/sites/default/files/documents/Nursing%20Associate%20Curriculum%20Framework%20Feb2017_0.pdf.

Kaushik, V., Malik, T., Saeed, S.R., 2010. Interventions for acute otitis externa. Cochrane Database Syst. Rev. (1), CD004740.

Loveman, E., Gospodarevskaya, E., Clegg, A., et al., 2011. Ear wax removal interventions: A systematic review and economic evaluation. Br. J. Gen. Pract. 61 (591), e680–e683.

NICE, 2016. National Institute for Health and Care Excellence. NG:36 Cancer of the upper aerodigestive tract: assessment and management in people aged 16 and over. Available at https://www.nice.org.uk/guidance/ng36.

Nursing and Midwifery Council, 2018. The Code. Professional Standards of Practice and Behaviour for Nurses, Midwives and Nursing Associates. London: NMC. https://www.nmc.org.uk/standards/code/

Pankhania, M., Judd, O., Ward, A., 2011. Otorrhea. Br. Med. J. 342, d2299.

Rosenfeld, R.M., Piccirillo, J.F., Chandrasekhar, S.S., et al., 2015. Clinical practice guideline (update): Adult sinusitis. Otolaryngology. Head Neck Surg. 152 (2), S1–S39.

Tikka, T., 2016. The aetiology and management of epistaxis. Otolaryngology Online Journal. Available at http://www.alliedacademies.org/articles/the-aetiology-and-management-of-epistaxis.html.

Waugh, A., Grant, A., 2018. Ross & Wilson Anatomy and Physiology in Health and Illness, thirteenth ed. Elsevier, Edinburgh.

38

Ophthalmological Disorders

Yvonne Needham

OBJECTIVES

By the end of the chapter the reader will:

1. Have an understanding of the anatomy and physiology of the eye and visual pathway
2. Discuss the pathophysiological changes associated with a selection of ophthalmic disorders
3. Understand the effect on the eye of other systemic disorders
4. Outline the care required by people with ophthalmic disorders
5. Describe some common conditions associated with the eye and vision loss
6. Review the role of the Nursing Associate in promoting health and well-being

KEY WORDS

Eye	Cataract	Age-related macular degeneration
Visual pathway	Diabetic retinopathy	Systemic conditions affecting the eye
Visually impaired	Glaucoma	

CHAPTER AIMS

This aim of this chapter is to provide the reader with an understanding of the skills, knowledge and attitude required to provide safe, effective and compassionate care to people with ophthalmic disorders.

SELF TEST

1. What are the key points to consider when guiding a visually impaired person?
2. What are the common refractive errors and how are refractive errors corrected?
3. What are tears made of and how do they support keeping the eye healthy?
4. What systemic disorders may affect the eye?
5. What is glaucoma and how may loss of sight be prevented?
6. What is a cataract and how may sight be restored?
7. How does diabetes affect the eyes?
8. What is macular degeneration and how can this be treated?
9. What conditions may lead to a red eye?
10. What actions can an individual take to maintain visual health?

INTRODUCTION

In this chapter, the first part considers how the loss of vision impacts on a person's life. The second part identifies the anatomy and physiology of the eye and visual pathway and the third part identifies common ophthalmic conditions. When harm or damage occurs to vision, this can impact on a person's body image, identity, self-awareness, confidence and their ability to live independently. It is important for the Nursing Associate to have a comprehensive understanding of the eye and vision to care for all, as there are over 2 million people in the UK living with sight loss (Access Economics, 2009).

For the purpose of this chapter the term 'visual impairment' refers to a person whose vision cannot be corrected to normal levels (i.e., 6/6) (Field et al., 2014). This list provides an overview of some ophthalmic disorders that will be discussed:

- Glaucoma
- Cataract
- Macular degeneration
- Diabetic retinopathy.

REGISTRATION FOR THE SIGHT IMPAIRED OR SEVERELY SIGHT IMPAIRED

The Certificate of Vision Impairment (CVI) formally certifies someone as sight impaired (previously referred to as 'partially sighted') or as severely sight impaired (previously referred to as 'blind'). With the permission of the patient, the CVI is shared, so that the local authority they are ordinarily resident in is able to make contact with them to offer and explain the benefits of registration on a local sight register and to ensure services are accessible as appropriate (Department of Health, 2017). An individual would need to fall into one of the categories below to be eligible for registration:

Sight impaired

- Vision 3/60 to 6/60 and full peripheral field
- Vision up to 3/60 with moderate field contraction, opacities in the media, aphakia but marked field loss
- 6/18 or better visual acuity with marked field loss; for example, a whole half of vision is missing or a lot of peripheral vision is missing

Severely sight impaired

- Visual acuity of less than 3/60 with a full visual field
- Visual acuity between 3/60 and 6/60 with a severe reduction of field of vision, such as tunnel vision
- Visual acuity of 6/60 or above but with a very reduced field of vision, especially if a considerable amount of sight is missing in the lower part of the field

(Shaw & Lee, 2017, Royal National Institute of Blind People [RNIB], 2003).

COMPASSIONATE CARE

The Nursing Associate must be supportive of those they care for with a visual impairment, as it is not always obvious that the individual has a disability. Some individuals will have been blind from birth, some have accidents which result in sight loss and others may have an illness such as diabetes which can lead to sight loss.

Whilst the individual may have a degree of visual impairment, this will depend on the condition; there are numerous types of visual loss and mostly individuals will have some sight or light perception. Only about 4% of those with severe sight impairment in the UK can see nothing at all (BID Services, no date). Thus, it is important to ascertain from the individual what sight they have and how they can best be supported to include them in their care, which can reduce the stigma they may feel or be experiencing (Gibbons & Whitaker, 2017). Altered body image is often difficult to deal with as the face is the first place we look when approaching someone and is a way of recognizing people. With the eyes and visual loss, there may or may not be an obvious defect of the eyes, both of which can cause problems. If there is no obvious defect but the individual has lost vision in the centre of their field, as in macular degeneration, they may appear to be ignoring people as they cannot see the persons face and do not know who they are. If there is an alteration in facial features, for example, after surgery for a tumour, it can cause problems as hiding facial features is more difficult, though prosthetic development means that there is generally a good cosmetic outcome. In both situations there may be support needed for the loss and grief that occurs with visual loss (Gibbons & Whitaker, 2017). Coming to terms with sight loss has been linked to the stages of loss and grief and can lead to social isolation and depression (RNIB, 2017b). Equally, when communicating or helping the individual get from place to place, sighted guiding is needed (RNIB, 2017a) but also ask the person what help they need.

Common sense points to consider

- Say hello and address the person by name; remember non-verbal communication may not be seen. Introduce yourself when you approach and speak directly to the individual.
- If they need help moving around and you are going to guide them, let them take your arm. Do not grab the person's arm. By allowing the person to take your arm they will be slightly behind you and can feel which way you are moving and not feel as though you are dragging them along.
- Inform the person which direction you are going; if there are obstacles, stairs or changes in floor levels, inform them and be clear. Remember you are going to need slightly more space to walk in.
- If you are guiding someone to a seat, place their hand on the back of the seat before they sit down and allow them to explore the chair; wait until they are seated before you leave.
- Do not walk away without saying you are leaving and making sure that they know where they are.

Further advice can be obtained from information sheets and podcasts from the RNIB website.

PHYSIOLOGY OF SIGHT

Light is reflected into the eye at high speeds, with only a small part of the electromagnetic spectrum being visible: the spectrum of visible light (Fig. 38.1).

The refraction is the bending of the light though the cornea and lens to focus the image on the retina (Fig. 38.2).

This image is upside down but very early in life the brain adapts and objects are perceived to be the right way up.

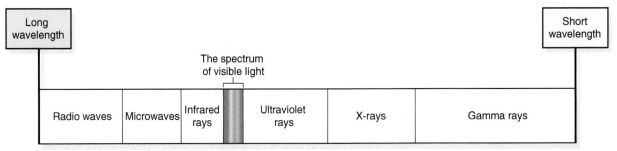

Fig. 38.1 The Electromagnetic Spectrum (Waugh & Grant, 2018).

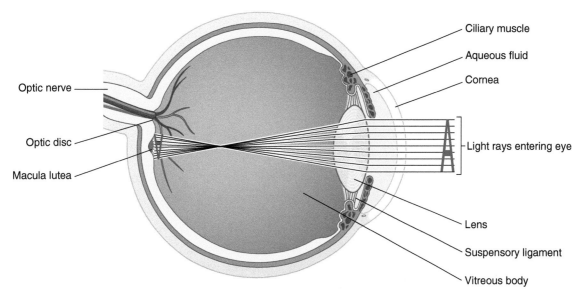

Fig. 38.2 Section of the Eye Showing the Focusing of Light on the Retina (Waugh & Grant, 2018).

The focusing of the light on the central part of the retina is called emmetropia and accommodation refers to the action of the ciliary muscles on the shape of the lens (Fig. 38.3). Abnormal refractions in the eye are corrected using glasses with either a biconvex (hyperopia) or biconcave (myopia) lens (see Fig. 38.3). Myopia is when the focal point of the light refracted though the eye onto the retina is too short (in front of the retina); the eye is too large or there is a greater curvature to the cornea or lens (see Fig. 38.3). Individuals with this vision cannot see objects into the distance (Seewoodhary, 2017).

Hyperopia is when the focal point of the refracted light though the eye onto the retina is too long (behind the retina); the eye is too small or there is an insufficient curvature of the cornea or lens (Fig. 38.4). Astigmatism occurs when the curvature of the refractive surfaces of the eye vary in length and width, often referred to as 'rugby ball-shaped'. Some individuals may not need correction, others may, but head tilting or screwing up the eyes, as with other refractive errors, may indicate the need for assessment.

Accommodation is the ability of the lens in the eye to focus the light on to the retina. This diminishes with age and the eye becomes presbyopic around the age of 40 years. Presbyopia can be corrected using a convex lens in reading glasses.

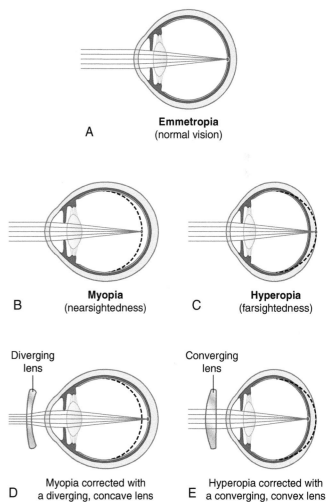

Fig. 38.3 Common Refractive Errors of the Eye and Corrective Lenses (Waugh & Grant, 2018).

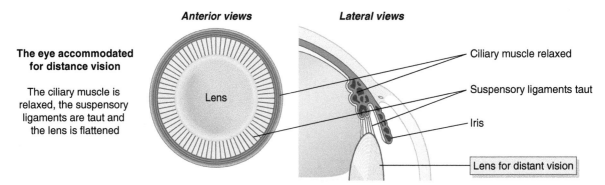

Fig. 38.4 Accommodation: Action of the Ciliary Muscles on the Shape of the Lens, Distance Vision (Waugh & Grant, 2018).

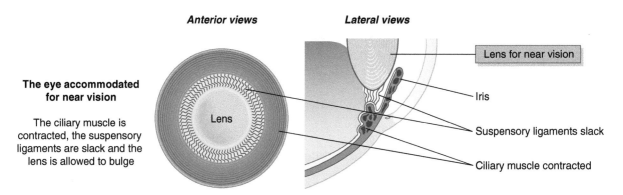

Fig. 38.5 Accommodation: Action of the Ciliary Muscles on the Shape of the Lens, Near Vision (Waugh & Grant, 2018).

Near vision accommodation

See Fig. 38.5.

Distant vision

To focus on an object within about 6 meters, the eye must make some adjustments (accommodate):

- Constrict the pupil, allowing the beam of light to be reduced and pass through the central curved part of the lens
- Movement of the eyes (convergence): light rays enter each eye at different angles; for vision to be clear, the light must stimulate the same point on each retina. The extrinsic muscles of the eye move the eyes in a coordinated way under autonomic control.
- Changing the refractory power of the lens. The thickness of the lens needs to alter depending on the distance of the object from the eyes. The nearer the object, the thicker the lens; this is what is lost with age (presbyopia).
- Distant vision objects at over 6 meters away from the eyes are focused on the retina without any changes to the lens or convergence.

Binocular vision

This enables vision to be three dimensional. As with accommodation, binocular vision allows each eye to see an object from a slightly different angle. These two fields of vision overlap in the centre, with the two images being fused on the cerebrum so that only one image is seen (Fig. 38.6). This enables a more accurate assessment of an object, its distance, height, width and depth. Individuals with one functioning eye lose this and may have difficulty with depth distance. Thus, if an individual has an injury to an eye, they must take care when driving, walking up and down stairs and doing things that require depth perception. Individuals can function with one eye as their brain will adapt over time. Binocular vision develops in the first few years of life but changes to vision can occur up to age 7/8 years of age. Learning to focus and accommodate and use the eyes together can be absent, and it is important that all strabismus are managed and corrected early to prevent amblyopia (reduced vision which is uncorrectable) (Seewoodhary, 2017).

> ### ❗ HOTSPOT
>
> Children and adolescents/younger adults who have headaches or complain of eye strain or are screwing their eyes up a lot should be seen by an optometrist. As we get older, the ability of the lens to accommodate decreases. It is not just at over 40 years of age that accommodation can become difficult; if a person has a slight myopia or hypermetropia, the ability to accommodate when doing lots of studying becomes harder if the person has an uncorrected refractive error.

FUNCTIONAL ANATOMY AND PHYSIOLOGY

In this section the anatomy and physiology of the eye and surrounding structures will be discussed. Fig. 38.7 shows a section of the eye.

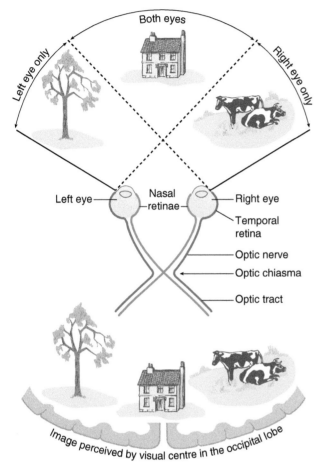

Fig. 38.6 Parts of the Visual Field: Monocular and Binocular (Waugh & Grant, 2018).

The orbit

The eyes are spherical in shape and each is approximately 2.5 cm in diameter. Each eye sees separately but they function as one (Waugh & Grant, 2018) (Fig. 38.8). The orbits are rigid and also contain muscles, nerves, blood vessels and adipose tissue. The orbits have narrow openings to allow these structures to enter and support the functioning of the eye; any inflammation or infection in the orbit can have a devastating effect on vision, causing double vision and loss of visual field (Auld, 2017; Field et al., 2014).

There are seven bones that make up the four walls of the orbit, which help protect eye (Fig. 38.9):

- Frontal
- Maxilla
- Zygoma
- Sphenoid
- Ethmoid
- Lacrimal
- Palatine

Nerve supply for the eye comes from the optic nerve (second cranial nerve) (see Fig. 38.8.).

Blood supply to the eye comes from the internal carotid artery via the ophthalmic artery, which branches off to form the ciliary arteries and central retinal artery. The venous drainage occurs via the central retinal artery and vortex veins (Fig. 38.10).

The extraocular muscles (extrinsic)

There are three pairs of muscles that move the eyes clockwise and anticlockwise and up and down (Fig. 38.11 and Table 38.1). The muscles move both eyes together to support good binocular vision (Field et al., 2014).

The eyelids

These are formed by the upper and lower lids to make a protective layer over the eye, which closes reflexively when a threat is

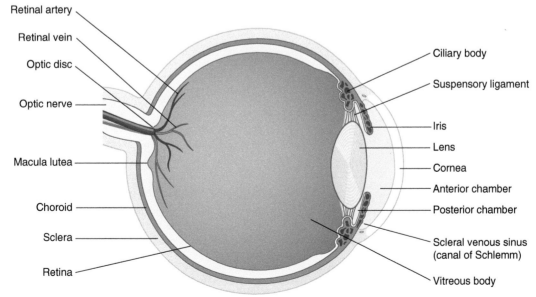

Fig. 38.7 A Section of the Eye (Waugh & Grant, 2018).

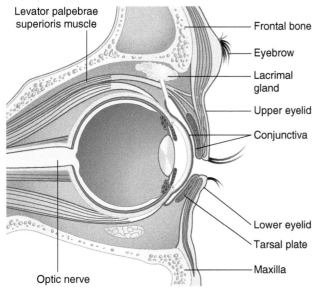

Fig. 38.8 Section of the Eye and its Accessory Structures (Waugh & Grant, 2018).

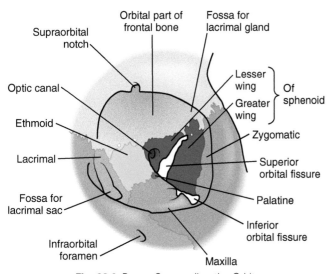

Fig. 38.9 Bones Surrounding the Orbit.

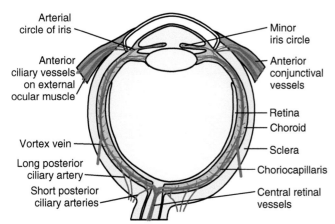

Fig. 38.10 Blood Supply of the Eyeball.

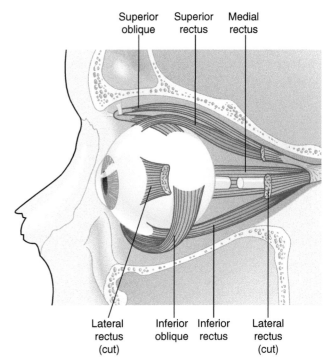

Fig. 38.11 The Extrinsic Muscles of the Eye (Waugh & Grant, 2018).

TABLE 38.1   Extrinsic Muscles of the Eye: Their Actions and Cranial Nerve Supply

Name	Action	Cranial nerve supply
Medial rectus	Rotates eyeball inwards	Oculomotor nerve (third cranial nerve)
Lateral rectus	Rotates eyeball outwards	Abducens nerve (sixth cranial nerve)
Superior rectus	Rotates eyeball upwards	Oculomotor nerve (third cranial nerve)
Inferior rectus	Rotates eyeball downwards	Oculomotor nerve (third cranial nerve)
Superior oblique	Rotates eyeball downwards and outwards	Trochlear nerve (fourth cranial nerve)
Inferior oblique	Rotates eyeball upwards and outwards	Oculomotor nerve (third cranial nerve)

(Reproduced with permission from Waugh & Grant, 2018.)

perceived or the eyelashes are touched. The skin over the eyelids is very elastic; this allows swelling in the event of trauma or infection. The tarsal plate is made of a dense fibrous tissue, providing structure to the eyelid. Tarsal plates are smaller in the lower lids. Within the eyelids are various glands: sebaceous (Zeis) glands, lipid-secreting glands linked to the lash follicles and meibomian glands that are found between the tarsal plate and conjunctiva, all producing sebum and lipids to support the tear film (Field et al., 2014) (Fig. 38.12).

The eyelids have several muscles to support eyelid movement; blink function of the lids moves the tears across the eye to the lacrimal puncta (Field et al., 2014).

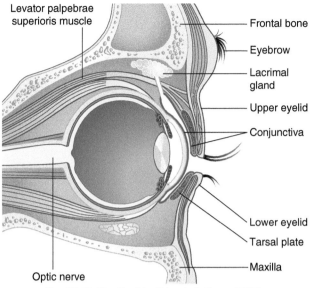

Fig. 38.12 The Eyelids (Waugh & Grant, 2018).

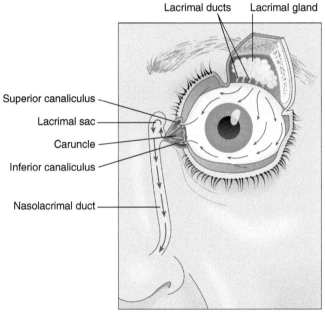

Fig. 38.13 The Lacrimal Apparatus (Waugh & Grant, 2018).

Lacrimal gland

The lacrimal gland is located in the lacrimal fossa of the frontal bone in the upper temporal side of each eye (Fig. 38.13).

The function of the lacrimal system is to produce and drain tears in response to stimulation to keep the eye free from debris. Lacrimation increases when noxious fumes are present (smoke and peeled onions) (Shaw & Lee, 2017). Tears have three layers:

1. Oily layer: helps prevent evaporation of tears, though some will be lost to evaporation.
2. Aqueous layer: to keep the eye hydrated.
3. Mucus layer: to spread the tear film to the eye surface.

The functions of tears are to:

• Lubricate the eye
• Clean away debris
• Keep the surface of the eye smooth to aid refraction though the cornea
• Secretion to protect the eye antimicrobial agent, the enzyme lysozyme and immunoproteins (Shaw & Lee, 2017).

Tear flow

Tears flow from the outer top part of the eye towards the nose, draining via the puncta. The shape and position of the eye support gravity in the drainage of the tears.

> **! HOTSPOT**
>
> Tears are essential to the maintenance of a healthy eye; having a reduced tear film can cause severe problems to the lids, lid margins, conjunctiva and cornea, and thus vision.

The conjunctiva

This is a thin, transparent mucous membrane with a rich blood supply, which lines the upper and lower lids and the globe. The conjunctiva secretes mucin from goblet cells, which form part of the tear film (Shaw & Lee, 2017).

The conjunctiva follows the structure at the front of the eye. Starting at the inside of the lower lid margin, folding back into the fornices of the lower lid, then folding back over the sclera (white of the eye), circling round (not over) the cornea, then folding back into the upper fornices and back along the inside of the upper lid to the lid margin.

The cornea

The cornea is oval in shape and very strong but thin, being approximately 0.52 mm at its centre, thickening to 0.7 mm at the margin (edge). The cornea is made up of five layers:

1. Epithelium is made up of five to six layers of epithelial cells that are continuous with the conjunctiva. This layer will regenerate after trauma.
2. Bowman's membrane is a collagen membrane that does not regenerate and, when damaged, will form a white scar.
3. Stroma makes up 90% of the cornea and is comprised of parallel connective tissue; damage forms white scars.
4. Descemet's membrane is an elastic fibre layer that can regenerate when damaged.
5. Endothelium: this single layer of cells ensures that the stroma is hydrated; they do not reaerate but elongate if damaged.

The cornea has no blood vessels and provides a clear structure for light to pass though and be refracted. Corneal nutrition is supplied by the aqueous and tear film and capillaries at the edge of the cornea (Shaw & Lee, 2017). The cornea also protects the eye and is very sensitive due to the large number of nerves it contains, which lay under the epithelial layer.

The sclera

This is the white part of the eye, made up of collagen fibres. It is very tough and, whilst palpable, is quite inflexible. The four rectus muscles are attached to the sclera and it has a thin elastic layer over it, providing a blood supply; this tissue is known as the 'episclera'.

The uveal tract

The uveal tract is the middle vascular part of the eye and is made up of the iris, ciliary body and the choroid (Fig. 38.14).

Iris

The iris is the pigmented (coloured) part of the eye, the colour of which is genetically determined (Field et al., 2014) (Fig. 38.15). The main function of the iris is to regulate the amount of light entering the eye. Sphincter muscle is circular and constricts the pupil under the control of the short ciliary nerve of the oculomotor nerve.

Ciliary body

The ciliary body has three functions:
1. Secretion of aqueous humour to maintain the anterior chamber
2. Holding the lens in place with the zonules

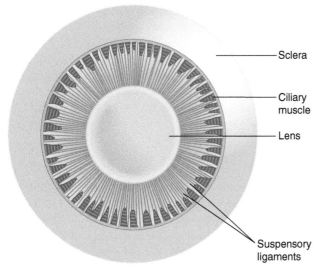

Fig. 38.14 The Lens and Suspensory Ligaments (Waugh & Grant, 2018).

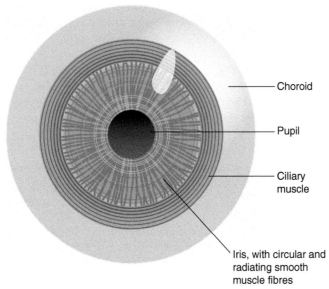

Fig. 38.15 The Choroid, Ciliary Body and Iris (Waugh & Grant, 2018).

3. Accommodation: the ciliary muscle is in the anterior section of the ciliary body, changing the shape of the lens.

The choroid

Lies between the sclera and retina, it extends from the optic nerve to the ora serrata, where it joins the ciliary body. The function of the choroid is:
- To provide nourishment to the outer layers of the retina
- Conduct blood vessels to the posterior part of the eye
- Prevent reflection of light though the retina.

The anterior and posterior chambers, aqueous humour and drainage angle

The posterior chamber is the space behind the iris and in front of the lens. The anterior chamber is the space between the cornea and iris. Both chambers are filled with aqueous humour, a clear fluid produced by the ciliary body (Shaw & Lee, 2017). The drainage angle is found where the cornea and iris meet. It is filled with what is called the 'trabecular meshwork': a spongy network of connective tissue. The canal of Schlemm is contained in this meshwork. These structures help regulate the amount of aqueous humour in the posterior and anterior chambers (Field et al., 2014). The pressure caused in the eye by the fluid is called the intraocular pressure (IOP); normal IOP is 15–20 mm Hg.

> **! HOTSPOT**
>
> Raises in intraocular pressure due to the rigid structure of the eye and the lack of space in the orbit can cause significant visual loss (see glaucoma).

The lens

The lens is a biconcave transparent avascular structure, approximately 9 × 4 mm. It is situated behind the iris and in front of the vitreous humour and held in place by the zonules radiating from the ciliary body. Lens fibres are continuously produced throughout life and the lens grows and becomes more dense as we age. The lens is 65% water and 35% protein, with some trace elements (sodium, potassium and calcium) (Shaw & Lee, 2017). The function of the lens is to refract light onto the retina.

The retina and vitreous humour

The retina is the innermost layer of the eye and is a complex structure. It is filled with photoreceptors, which transmit images though its layers to the optic nerve and on to the brain. The retina has 10 layers. The pars plana is the posterior segment at the posterior region of the ciliary body, situated behind the lens and above the retina. The ora serrata is the junction between the retina and pars plana, where the retina ends. The ora serrata comprises a series of crescent-shaped indentations, making it look like a scallop. The macula is the central part of the retina and the structure of the macula is different from the rest of the retina, with a high concentration of cones (approximately 7 million). The fovea is the central part of the macula and receives nutrients from the choroid. It is an avascular zone, and is the area of the retina that enables fine detailed vision. Rods (approximately 120 million) are found predominantly in the peripheral

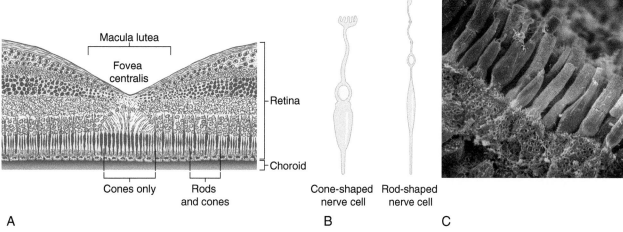

Fig. 38.16 The Retina (Waugh & Grant, 2018).

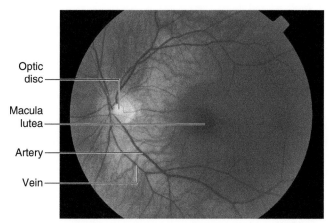

Fig. 38.17 The Retina as Seen Through the Pupil with an Ophthalmoscope. (Waugh & Grant, 2018).

retina and are utilized to see in low levels of light. Fig. 38.16 demonstrates the retina.

The optic disc is a pale, almost circular, area in the posterior pole where the retinal nerve fibres leave and the retinal blood vessels enter and leave the interior of the eye. The optic disc is the part of the optic nerve which can be seen and is about 1.5 mm diameter (Raynel & Brochner, 2017). This is the point in the visual field where there is a blind spot. The retina transmits the light impulses via the optic nerve to the visual cortex, where they are interpreted as sight. Fig. 38.17 shows the retina as seen through the pupil with an ophthalmoscope.

In the posterior part of the eye, the space behind the lens in front of the retina is the vitreous humour. This is a thick gel-like substance containing water and collagen fibres, and is attached at the ora serrata.

Optic nerve pathways

Visual interpretation (what we see) is a learned response that starts at birth and can carry on until the age of around 7 to 8 years. The process of seeing is taken for granted but it is a very complex process. The nerve fibres leave via the optic nerve and fibres relating to left and right fields split at the optic chiasma

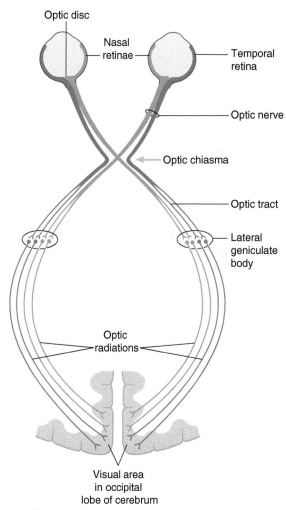

Fig. 38.18 The Optic Nerves and their Pathways (Waugh & Grant, 2018).

(sitting just above the pituitary gland), travelling though the lateral geniculate nucleus to the visual cortex (Fig. 38.18).

As can be seen in Fig. 38.18, the nerve pathways partially cross over. The left visual field is interpreted by the right visual cortex and the right by the left visual cortex.

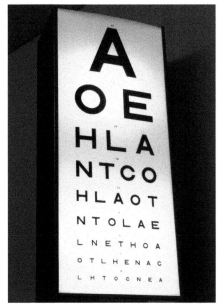

Fig. 38.19 Snellen Chart.

LVA, Left visual acuity; RVA, right visual acuity.

CRITICAL AWARENESS

Due to the length of these pathways, any damage to the brain along these pathways can affect vision and visual fields, for example, haemorrhages (as in strokes), raised intracranial pressure and head injuries. Damage to the visual field may be a neurological rather than an ophthalmic problem, but it may cause a visual field loss (Needham, 2017).

SELECTION OF COMMON CONDITIONS (PATHOPHYSIOLOGY)

Each structure of the eye has specific conditions that can impact on vision, a range of which will be identified in the remainder of this chapter. Watkinson (2014) notes that there are four ocular diseases that cause blindness in the UK. These are:

1. Cataract
2. Chronic open angle glaucoma (COAG)
3. Age-related macular degeneration (AMD)
4. Diabetic retinopathy.

Testing visual acuity

Testing visual acuity is an important aid to diagnosis in ophthalmic practice and this should be tested at each new visit. It is an assessment of acute central vision only. The visual standard for driving is 6/12 on a Snellen chart and reading a number plate at 20 meters with glasses or contact lenses.

The Snellen chart has eight lines of letters (Fig. 38.19). The largest letter is what a normal eye can read at 60 meters, with this distance decreasing as the size of the letters decreases: 36, 24, 18, 12, 9, 6 (normal vision) and 5 meters. Vision is normally tested at a distances of 6 meters, so reading the letter designated 60 with the right eye would be recorded as right visual acuity (RVA) 6/60. Box 38.1 shows how to document visual acuity.

NURSING SKILLS

Vision Testing

Ensure the individual understands the process and the reasons for the vision test. Read the person's notes and make sure that, if glasses are worn for distant vision, they are used during the test.

Equipment

- Snellen test chart, distance vision test (well illuminated)
- Sheridan Gardiner test chart, for those who have difficulty with reading letters but could match letter shapes (Fig. 38.20)
- Pinhole occluder (Fig. 38.21)

Procedure

The procedure should be carried out in line with local policy and procedure.

1. Check the patient's identity, explain the procedure and gain verbal consent.
2. Sit the patient 6 meters from the chart, 3 meters if they are looking into a mirror and the chart is behind them.
3. Make sure the chart is well illuminated.
4. Ensure they are sitting comfortably, with glasses on if worn.
5. Cover one eye with the occluder.

6. Ask the individual to read/identify which letters they see; if using the Sheridan Gardiner test, go down the chart to the smallest letters that can be distinguished.
7. Document and record the line read in the patient's notes.
8. Repeat on the other eye.
9. Document and record the line read in the patient's notes.
10. If the vision is less than 6/12, repeat the process using a pinhole occluder.
11. Document and record the line read in the patient's notes.

After the procedure
Thank the patient and ensure they know what will happen next.

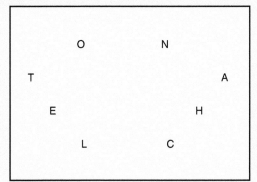

Fig. 38.20 Example of How a Sheridan Gardiner Test Chart Might Look.

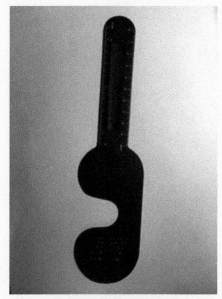

Fig. 38.21 Pinhole Occluder.

THE MEDICINE TROLLEY 38.1

Drug	Drug classification	Reason for administration	Route of administration	Dose	Side effects	Contraindications	Nursing care
Pilocarpine	Miotic	Pupillary constriction Opening drainage channel in the trabecular mesh	Eye drop	Up to 4 times a day Give as prescribed	Blurred vision Smarting Pupillary Block	Pregnancy Breast feeding Acute anti-inflammatory disease conditions where pupillary constriction is undesirable	Eye drop administration Hand washing

(Data from British National Formulary 72, 2016).

⚠ HOTSPOT

It can take longer for the effects of drops to be effective in dark irises; due to the dense pigmentation and dilatation of the pupil may take longer (Shaw & Lee, 2017).

Glaucoma

COAG is the most common registration of blindness in the UK (RNIB, 2017b). There are a number of risk factors associated with this condition and they include:
• Ethnicity (higher risk in African-Caribbean)
• Over the age of 40 years
• Genetic factors (familial link) (Lee, 2017)
• Diabetes mellitus
• Myopia.

To diagnose COAG and related conditions, the National Institute for Health and Care Excellence (NICE) (2017b) suggest that it is important that a full clinical history is taken; this will include noting any familial conditions. A range of tests and investigations will also need to be undertaken.

Signs and symptoms

Glaucoma is sometimes called the 'silent thief of sight', as the individual often has no signs and symptoms until there is a marked loss of visual felid. Thus, having regular eye health checks at the optometrist will identify any issue earlier, particularly if the person is in an at risk category. On examination there may be:
• Raised IOP
• Cupped ophthalmic disc
• Loss of visual field.

Care and treatment

The individual needs to understand the condition, treatment and prognosis and understand that once lost, sight cannot be recovered (NICE, 2017b), with particular emphasis on the need

THE MEDICINE TROLLEY 38.2

Drug	Drug classification	Reason for administration	Route of administration	Dose	Side effects	Contra-indications	Nursing care
Travoprost	Prostaglandin analogue	To reduce intraocular pressure	Drop in the eye	One drop daily preferably in the evening	Blepharitis Blood pressure changes Increased brown pigment in the iris Thickening and lengthening of the lashes Ocular discomfort Conjunctival disorders Corneal erosion transient punctate erosion	Asthma History of significant ocular infections Aphakia Compromised respiratory function	Warn about possible change to iris colour before treatment Eye drop administration technique Hand hygiene Ensure drop kept off the skin as regular contact may trigger hair growth

to take eye drops regularly and for life. The medical therapy in the form of eye drops may have side effects. Some may not suit the individual but they can be changed to prevent side effects.

For primary acute glaucoma In primary acute glaucoma presentation is with rapid decrease in visual acuity, moderate to severe pain and photophobia (aversion to light). The individual should be seen for treatment immediately (Field et al., 2014).

Secondary glaucoma is due to other ophthalmic conditions that will need to be addressed, for example, lens dislocation, cataract, uveitis and trauma.

Medical therapy. Eye drops are the main treatment. There are a wide range of drops but NICE (2017) recommend prostaglandin analogue should be prescribed for those newly diagnosed with early or moderate COAG. It has been identified that if the number of drops and the times at which they are administered impact on the individual's life, having several drops and administration times will help with compliance (Lee, 2017).

There is a balance to be made between the most effective treatment and listening to the individual's needs. Making decision about treatment in partnership with the individual will give ownership and support compliance. Thus, listening and recording any issue is essential; it is often when talking to the person while testing vision that they may tell you how they feel and are coping. Advice about support and where to access it must be available, for example, the International Glaucoma Association and RNIB, particularly if there is visual loss which is registrable (RNIB, 2017b). The fear of sight loss can have an adverse effect and lead to possible depression, which can be prevalent in older people with sight loss (Watkinson, 2014). Fear of sight loss can be all consuming and affect all aspects of life; thus, having practical and emotional support increases confidence and ability to live with this long-term condition.

Inform the individual about the possibility of further treatment if the IOP is not controlled by medical treatment.

Laser therapy. Argon laser trabeculoplasty is where the laser energy is applied to the trabecular meshwork to increase the rate of aqueous outflow, lowering the IOP (Lee, 2017). This procedure is carried out on an outpatient basis. Initial treatment may only take 15 minutes but there may be a requirement for

the IOP to be checked the same day and following day, so these visits need planning.

Surgical therapy. Trabeculectomy is where a channel is created for additional aqueous drainage (Shaw & Lee 2017).

NURSING SKILLS
Instillation of Eye Drops

Explain the procedure and what the drops are for.
Seek consent from the patient to undertake the procedure.

Equipment needed:
- Eye drops/ointment
- Drug chart
- Access to handwashing facilities/alcogel
- Tissues

Procedure:
The procedure should be carried out in line with local policy and procedure, utilizing the Aseptic Non Touch Technique (see Chapter 16 of this text).
1. Ensure all equipment is gathered prior to carrying out the procedure
2. Check patient identity and drug prescription, explain procedure and gain verbal consent
3. Wash hands
4. Ensure a good light source
5. Prepare the eye drops, shake bottle before removing lid
6. Gently hold down the lower lid of the eye the drop is prescribed for
7. Place the drop bottle over the lower fornix but do not touch the eye
8. Instil one drop or 5 mm of ointment
9. If multiple drops, wait 3 minutes before instilling next drop
10. Use alcohol gel between drops
11. Instil any ointment last, inform the patient the vision may be unclear for some time due to the ointment
12. Give patient tissue to dab eye, tell them not to rub their eye
13. Wash/decontaminate hands
14. Dispose of clinical waste and other equipment safely
15. Document and record the procedure in the patient's drug chart/notes

After the procedure
Thank the patient.
Ensure the patient knows what time the next drops are due.

The Nursing Associate should ensure the individual with glaucoma understands their responsibilities and the regulations of the Driver and Vehicle Licensing Agency (DVLA) (NICE, 2017b). The DVLA must be informed if the glaucoma affects one eye and either of the following also apply: if there is a medical condition in the other eye or the person cannot meet the visual standards for driving (Gov UK, 2006).

Cataract

A cataract is an opacity of the crystalline lens in the eye. They may be unilateral or bilateral; if bilateral one eye may have less vision than the other (Fig. 38.22).

There are a number of types of cataracts:
- Congenital
- Age related
- Familial
- Traumatic
- Toxic
- Secondary to existing eye disease
- Associated with systemic disease

Signs and symptoms

Reduction of vision: this includes difficulty in reading small print and difficulty in seeing in the distance, for example, bus numbers or people's faces on the other side of the street. There may be changes to colour vision and glare at night or in bright sunlight (this is known as 'contrast sensitivity').

The choice to have cataract surgery or not must be a partnership between the patient and the clinician. For some individuals, surgery may not be advisable, for example, if there is an underlying medical or ocular condition (Craig, 2017).

Diagnosis/referral for cataract surgery

NICE (2017a) point out that the decision to refer a person with a cataract for surgery should be based on a discussion with the person (and their family members or carers, as appropriate) that includes:
- How the cataract affects the person's vision and quality of life
- Whether one or both eyes are affected
- What cataract surgery involves, including possible risks and benefits
- How the person's quality of life may be affected if they choose not to have cataract surgery
- Whether the person wants to have cataract surgery
- Access to cataract surgery should not be restricted on the basis of visual acuity.

Care and treatment

Treatment is surgical removal of the cataract by phacoemulsification and insertion of an intraocular lens. Cataract surgery is done as a day case under local anaesthetic in the majority of individuals. There are some cases where there may be the need for a general anaesthetic and this will be discussed with the individual's ophthalmologist and anaesthetist (e.g., individuals who cannot lay still for any reason).

Preoperative assessment. This may often take place on the same day as the consultation with the ophthalmologist, when the decision to go ahead with cataract surgery is made (may be known as 'one stop'). At this consultation there will be:
- A full examination of the eye using a slit lamp (Fig. 38.23)
- Pupil examination
- Dilated examination of the cataract and fundus
- Measurement of the IOP.

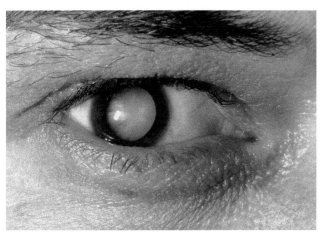

Fig. 38.22 Cataract (Waugh & Grant, 2018).

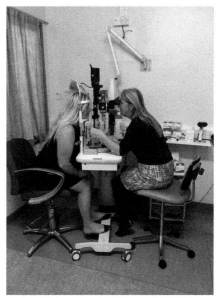

Fig. 38.23 Eye Examination at the Slit Lamp.

Preoperative assessment will also require a complete medical and surgical history to be undertaken to reduce the risk during and postsurgery. This will include:

- Allergies/sensitivities to medications
- Comorbidities, diabetes and macular degeneration, any systemic inflammatory conditions
- Previous surgery which may impact on them lying flat for the duration of the surgery
- Visual acuity with up to date refraction
- Biometry, calculation of the power of the intraocular lens
- Keratometry (measurement of the cornel curvature)
- Family and social support will be discussed to identify any services that may be required and can be put in place so surgery is not delayed
- Exclusion of ophthalmic conditions that may impact on surgery, for example, blepharitis, infections of the cornea, entropion, extropian, trichiasis, and lid infections.

Day of surgery. Local trust policies and procedures must be adhered to for admitting a patient for day case surgery. Specific local trust procedures for preparation for cataract surgery must also be followed and these may include:

- The eye to be operated on is marked
- Check consent and understanding of the procedure
- Dilate the pupil of the eye to be operated on
- Use local policy and procedure with regards to surgical check list.

Postoperative care. After surgery, the patient normally stays in the day surgery unit for 4–6 hours, depending on their condition. Local policy and procedure regarding postoperative assessment should be followed and this will include:

- Bathing the eye
- Examination of the eye.

NURSING SKILL

Bathing the eye

Explain the procedure will ensure the eye is clean before the patient leaves the hospital.

Seek consent from the patient to undertake the procedure.

Equipment needed
- Nonsterile gloves/apron
- Eye-dressing pack
- Extra gauze/cotton wool

Procedure

The procedure should be carried out in line with local policy and procedure, utilizing the Aseptic Non Touch Technique (see Chapter 16 of this text)

1. Check patient identity, explain procedure and gain verbal consent
2. Prepare clean surface
3. Ensure a good light source
4. Ensure all equipment is gathered prior to carrying out the procedure
5. Wash/decontaminate hands
6. Don disposable gloves and apron
7. Open eye pack
8. Use 'no touch' technique to clean the eye

9. Wet gauze or cotton wool and wipe the eye from the nose towards the ear

Note: Ensure cotton wool is wet; if dry, it can leave fibres.

10. Repeat as many times as necessary, never rub the eye, one wipe and discard the gauze cotton wool
11. Remove gloves/apron
12. Wash/decontaminate hands
13. Dispose of used packing and other equipment safely
14. Document and record the procedure in the patient's notes

Important: If both eyes need bathing, wash your hands in-between bathing each eye.

After the procedure

Thank the patient.

Ensure the patient knows what will happen next.

CASE STUDY 38.1.   Jim and Jean

Jim is 67 years old and his wife of 47 years is 65. They have no children but over the years have played an active role in the lives of their community. Jim is a retired accountant, is a member of the Lions and works tirelessly raising money with Jean's support. Jean worked part time as a doctor's receptionist before she retired. They live in a village 15 miles from the nearest town, where there are only four buses a day and one small shop. Two years ago, Jean was not very well and after several months, it was identified she was in renal failure. She is now on renal dialysis and Jim transports her to the hospital for all her appointments.

Jim's father had glaucoma and Jim has always gone for a routine eye test. Otherwise he is in good health and fit as he walks with his dog twice a day.

Visit to the optometrists

Jim has been going to the same optician for the last 20 years, so all his records and previous discussions are available to the optometrist. Prior to the examination by the optometrist, Jim has an automated visual field test and non-contact tonometry as part of his examination due to the glaucoma familial link. Jim is seen by the optometrist and they have a general discussion about the glaucoma tests, with the optometrist identifying that, after the full examination, they will discuss all the results in detail, but the field test and tonometry were similar to last year. The optometrist asked how Jim was generally and how his wife was. Jim identified his wife was doing well on the dialysis and things were OK; they were even thinking of going on holiday. He then hesitated and stopped talking. The optometrist picked up on this and asked if Jim was looking forward to the holiday. Again he was hesitant but then identified he was having trouble seeing in the sunlight and was not keen on driving in the sun, even with sunglasses. He was worried as he did not want to disappoint his wife but did not feel safe driving; he was worried he would lose his license or have an accident. Driving is the only way they get around and to the hospital. Jim was very distressed; the optometrist listened and gave Jim time to compose himself before commencing the eye examination. At the end of the examination, the optometrist discussed his findings with Jim. Jim's vision still met the standard for driving: right visual acuity 6/9 and left visual acuity 6/12 with glasses. This was the first thing he identified, along with the test results and examination of his eyes for glaucoma, which were all normal. There was one area the optometrist indicated he wanted to discuss further with Jim and asked him what he knew about cataracts. They had a discussion about cataracts and the fact that Jim had some thickening of the lens in his left eye.

Diabetic retinopathy

Diabetic retinopathy is one of the leading causes of blindness in the western world, particularly in individuals of working age (Watkinson, 2014). The incidence and progression of diabetic retinopathy is related to the time the individual has had diabetes and the level of control of blood sugar during that time. A delicate network of blood vessels supplies the retina with blood. When those blood vessels become blocked, leaky or grow haphazardly, the retina becomes damaged and is unable to work properly (Diabetes UK, 2017).

Signs and symptoms

The signs and symptoms of diabetic retinopathy are identified in Table 38.2.

Diagnosis

On diagnosis of diabetes, the GP should immediately refer the individual to the local eye-screening service. Perform screening as soon as possible and no later than 3 months from referral and arrange repeat, structured eye screening annually.

Care and treatment

The Nursing Associate should discuss living a healthy lifestyle and maintaining good glycaemic control. (See Chapter 35 for further discussion of diabetes mellitus.) Consideration must be given to the control of hypertension, blood sugar and hyperlipidaemia. Offer advice and support for stopping smoking. It is important that the patient attends all appointments for screening and review; explain the importance of this to the patient.

Explain to the patient that with extensive laser treatment, peripheral visual field may be lost and night vision will be reduced. Thus, when walking around at night, they will need some light so as not to injure themselves as they may be suffering from peripheral neuropathy.

TABLE 38.2	**Signs and Symptoms of Diabetic Retinopathy**		
Stage	**Description**	**Effect of vision**	**Treatment**
No retinopathy	Retina has no abnormal signs.	Normal vision	Retinal screening programme
Background retinopathy/ nonproliferative	The earliest visible change to the retina but it needs to be carefully monitored. The capillaries (small blood vessels) in the retina become blocked, they may bulge slightly (microaneurysm) and may leak blood (haemorrhage) or fluid (exudates).	Normal Vision	Regular review in ophthalmology
Preproliferative retinopathy	Changes to venous vessels with evidence of some blockages bleeding or looping of blood vessels.	Normal vision	Regular review in ophthalmology
Maculopathy	Maculopathy is when the background retinopathy (see above) is at or around the macula. The macula is the most used area of the retina. It provides our central vision and is essential for clear, detailed vision. If fluid leaks from the enlarged blood vessels it can build up and causes swelling (oedema).	Loss of central vision (for reading and seeing fine details)	Laser photocoagulation Anti-VEGF agents (NICE, 2013b)
Proliferative retinopathy	Background retinopathy develops and large areas of the retina are deprived of a proper blood supply because of blocked and damaged blood vessels. This stimulates the growth of new blood vessels to replace the blocked ones. These growing blood vessels are very delicate and bleed easily. The bleeding (haemorrhage) causes scar tissue that starts to shrink and pull on the retina, leading to it becoming detached.	Causing vision loss or blindness	Laser photocoagulation In the late stages there may be a need for surgery Vitrectomy or retinal detachment repair

(Adapted from Diabetes, UK 2017; Watkinson, 2014; Marsden, 2017.)

REFLECTION 38.2

In case study 38.2, what are the options for Karen regarding her vision and driving? Is she legally able to drive?

How, if she was unable to drive, would this impact on her work and life?

Age-related macular degeneration

AMD is the most common cause of sight loss in the developed world. In the UK, more than 600,000 people are affected by AMD, and given the increasing aging population, the incidence of AMD will continue to rise (NICE, 2012). NICE has undertaken a review of macular degeneration and issued a new guideline in 2018. About half of people affected by AMD are registered as visually impaired, although it is important to remember that no matter how advanced the macular degeneration is, it is unlikely that all sight will be lost. There are two types of AMD: dry and wet.

Dry age-related macular degeneration

The dry form of macular degeneration is more common than the wet macular degeneration, affecting approximately 10% of people over 60 years. In this form of macular degeneration, there is no associated vascularization, hence the term 'dry' (Raynel & Brochner, 2017).

Signs and symptoms. The progress of this condition is slow and visual loss is not apparent until significant atrophy has developed. This form of AMD causes thinning of the retinal pigment epithelium (RPE) layer, progressive damage to the photoreceptors and destruction of the central vision if the fovea is involved. Straight lines appear bent; this distortion can be checked using an Amsler grid (Fig. 38.24) or against everyday household grids, such as bathroom tiles or a window frame. Make sure that one eye at a time is used to look at the Amsler grid, as it may only be apparent that one eye is affected when the other eye is closed, due to the brain filling in the gaps, as it were, from what the other eye sees. The patient may find increasing difficulty in reading and seeing objects close up.

Care and treatment. There is currently no treatment for dry AMD. Care is in making the most effective use of the peripheral vision, and eccentric viewing with support from low-vision specialists (Box 38.2). If there is AMD in both eyes but some central

BOX 38.2   Eccentric Viewing

Eccentric viewing is a technique used by people with central vision loss. Also called 'preferred retinal loci', it is a method by which the person looks slightly away from the subject in order to view it peripherally with another area of the visual field.

Eccentric viewing training teaches a person to look slightly to the side so that the blind spot or scotoma is not in their central field of vision. One author describes it as 'not looking at what you want to see' (Macular Society, 2017).

With this training, the patient must learn to control their eye movement and place the object of interest on a particular location of the retina.

The low-vision specialist helps people find the peripheral part of the retina where the tissue is healthy and where they can see or focus the best. This might mean having to look slightly above, below, or to one side of a word to focus on it most clearly.

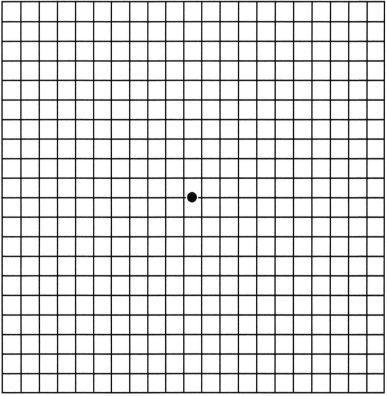

Fig. 38.24 Amsler Grid.

vision remains, then low-vision aids and a good light source may make the best use of the remaining vision. Some rehabilitation support and mobility training will also help the person maintain their independence. For some, the option of a guide dog may be one they wish to explore. The person should be encouraged to stop smoking if appropriate. Eating a healthy diet may also help, as there is some debate as to the use of additional vitamins and antioxidants (Shaw & Lee, 2017).

Wet age-related macular degeneration

This type of AMD is less common but increasing with the aging population, affecting 2% of the population over 60 years. It is aggressive and sight loss can occur rapidly, within weeks (Raynel & Brochner, 2017). It accounts for 80%–90% of all registered blind people with AMD (Watkinson, 2014). There is a reduced ability of oxygen to diffuse though the RPE. Wet AMD is characterized by the development of abnormal choroidal blood vessels and exudative or choroidal neovascularization beneath the RPE. These abnormal vessels expand into the subretinal space and leek blood into the retina, hence the term 'wet'. Due to the leakage of blood, the RPE can detach form Bruch's membrane, causing rapid widespread significant loss of vision.

Signs and symptoms. These may include:
- Sudden loss of central vision
- Flickering flashing lights
- Hallucinatory forms
- Blind spot in the visual field (may only be noticed when the eye not affected is closed)
- Reduction in visual acuity; hard to distinguish between similar letters (e.g., M and N)
- Colour vision is faded/reduced
- Binocular vision and contrast sensitivity can be affected
- Bright light is glaring and uncomfortable or it is difficult to adapt when moving from dark to light environments

- Words might disappear when reading
(Watkinson, 2014; Raynel & Brochner, 2017).
Risk factors for the development and progression of AMD include:
- Smoking
- Increasing age
- High cholesterol
- Family history of AMD
- The presence of AMD in the other eye.

Diagnosis. This is made by taking a detailed patient history and a range of investigations are required, for example:
- Ophthalmic examination with fundal examination
- Optical coherence tomography
- Fluorine angiography.

Care and treatment. Treatment for wet AMD is by intravitreous injection of an anti-VEGF agent, ranibizumab (NICE, 2012), or aflibercept (NICE, 2013a). If one eye only is affected, care should be taken to prevent AMD occurring in the other eye:
- Make the person aware of the signs and symptoms
- Smoking cessation
- Increasing the intake of antioxidants, carotenoids and omega 3 fatty acids through dietary changes, high-dose vitamin and mineral supplementation
- Treatment with statins.

If both eyes are affected:
- Making the most effective use of the peripheral vision; eccentric viewing with support from low-vision specialists
- If some central vision remains, then low vision aids and a good light source may make the best use of the remaining vision
- Rehabilitation support and mobility training will also help the person maintain their independence
- For some the option of a guide dog may be one they wish to explore.

THE MEDICINE TROLLEY 38.3

Drug	Drug classification	Reason for administration	Route of administration	Dose	Side effects	Contra-indications	Nursing care
Ranibizumab	Vascular endothelial growth factor inhibitors	Neovascular (wet) age-related macular degeneration Diabetic macular oedema Macular oedema secondary to retinal vein occlusion Specialist use only	Intravitreal injection	500 µg once a month as prescribed	Allergic skin reaction Anaemia Anterior chamber flare Blepharitis Conjunctivitis Cataract Eye haemorrhage Headache Keratitis Raise intraocular pressure Photophobia Retinal disturbances Uveitis Visual disturbance	Ocular or periocular infection Severe intraocular inflammation	Time to discuss the treatment Time to ask questions

THE MEDICINE TROLLEY 38.4

Drug	Drug classification	Reason for administration	Route of administration	Dose	Side effects	Contra indications	Nursing care
Tropicamide	Mydriatics and cycloplegics	Fundoscopy	Drops to the eye	Consult product literature Follow prescription group directive	Loss of accommodation for 4–6 hours Blurred vision Sensitivity to light	Allergic reaction to any ingredients	Make sure person not driving May need sunglasses or cap with a brim Instruct patient not to operate heavy machinery

THE MEDICINE TROLLEY 38.5

Drug	Drug classification	Reason for administration	Route of administration	Dose	Side effects	Contra indications	Nursing care
Phenylephrine	Mydriatic	Fundoscopy	Drops to the eye	Consult product literature Follow prescription/ group directive 10% dose is not recommended See side effects	Arrhythmias Blurred vision Palpitations Photophobia Tachycardia Myocardial infarction with 10% strength in patients with pre-existing condition	Pregnancy Breast feeding	Make sure person not driving May need sunglasses or cap with a brim Instruct patient not to operate heavy machinery

THE MEDICINE TROLLEY 38.6

Drug	Drug classification	Reason for administration	Route of administration	Dose	Side effects	Contra indications	Nursing care
Cyclopentolate	Antimuscarinics Cycloplegic	Cycloplegia	Eye drops	As prescribed	May sting Toxic systemic reactions can occur in neonates Systemic side effect may occur in children and elderly	Toxic system reaction	Eye drop instillation Hand washing Information related to reason for instillation

(Data from British National Formulary 72, 2016.)

COMMUNITIES OF CARE

Those in Places of Detention

Prisoners receive the same healthcare and treatment as anyone outside of prison and this includes the same ophthalmic care anyone else would need. The treatment is free; however, this has to be approved by a prison doctor or member of the healthcare team.

Prisons do not have hospitals, but many of them will have in-patient beds. The majority of health problems are managed by the healthcare team and this will include the need for eye care. If the prison cannot manage the healthcare issues, then the prison may:

- Request an expert to visit the prison
- Organize treatment in an outside hospital.

The healthcare team can contact the prisoner's family doctor or optician for their records, but this is only if the prisoner agrees to it.

Prisoners can receive specialist support if they, for example:

- Have drug or alcohol problems
- Have HIV or AIDS
- Are disabled or have a learning difficulty.

A prisoner may refuse treatment. However, the healthcare team may choose to give treatment if the prisoner is not capable of making decisions themselves (for example, if they have a mental health condition).

Wherever possible, the healthcare team will discuss this with the prisoner's family first.

LOOKING BACK, FEEDING FORWARD

The purpose of the eyes and visual pathways is to enable us to see the world around us and to live and work with others; vision is the key sense that enables humans to understand the world around us and to support and develop interactions with others. Without sight, individuals are unable to appreciate the world, as it is set up for those who are sighted. This impacts on social and intellectual development in the initial years of life and leads to isolation if visual loss occurs later in life. Both of these can be avoided with good support from families, healthcare professionals, social care and charities. Finding the right support quickly is vital to avoid delay in development and prevent social isolation.

Maintaining eye health is vital and being proactive in preventing visual loss is what healthcare professionals should be encouraging. As with most conditions (cataract being an exception), once vision is lost, it is lost permanently; thus, doing all that is possible to prevent vision loss is vital. Encouraging and highlighting the importance of screening, attending for tests and examinations as required should be a priority, along with helping the individual to maintain a healthy lifestyle.

The Nursing Associate has a crucial role to play in advocating the availability of information that will help support and inform those who need to know how to support and maintain eye health. Having the appropriate knowledge, skills and attitudes, linked with a nonjudgmental approach toward those with visual loss, can help the individual make well-informed decisions that are based on a reliable evidence base. Be mindful that the four most common conditions of the eyes are all linked to aging and because of this the Nursing Associate will be required to offer care to people with visual loss. Consider how you would feel if you could not see and how you would like someone to support and care for you. Take time to find out what the people you care need from you to support them.

REFERENCES

Access Economics, 2009. Future sight loss.1; updated with ONS population estimates for 2017. VISION 2020 the right to sight UK May 2017. Available at: http://www.visionuk.org.uk/download/APDF-ENG170302-VISION-2020-UK-postcard.

Auld, R., 2017. The orbit and extra ocular muscles. In: Marsden, J. (Ed.), Ophthalmic Care, second ed. M&K, Cumbria, (Chapter 23).

BID Services, no date. A guide to working with people with a visual impairment. Best practical guide. Available at: https://www.bid.org.uk/downloads/resources/a-guide-to-working-with-people-with-a-visual-impairment.pdf.

British National Formulary, 2016. BNF 72 September 2016-March 2017. BMJ Group, London.

Craig, S., 2017. The lens. In: Marsden, J. (Ed.), Ophthalmic Care, second ed. M&K, Cumbria, (Chapter 19).

Department of Health, 2017. Certificate of vision impairment explanatory notes for consultant ophthalmologists and hospital eye clinic staff in England. Available at: https://www.gov.uk/government/uploads/system/uploads/attachment_data/file/637590/CVI_guidance.pdf.

Diabetes UK, 2017. Eyes (retinopathy). Available at: https://www.diabetes.org.uk/Guide-to-diabetes/Complications/Retinopathy.

Field, D., Tillotson, J., Whittingham, S., 2014. Eye Emergencies: The Practitioners Guide. M&K, Cumbria.

Gibbons, H., Whitaker, L., 2017. Visual impairment. In: Marsden, J. (Ed.), Ophthalmic Care, second ed. M&K, Cumbria, (Chapter 5).

Gov UK, 2006. Driving eye sight rules. Available at: https://www.gov.uk/driving-eyesight-rules https://www.gov.uk/driving-eyesight-rules.

Lee, A., 2017. The angle and aqueous. In: Marsden, J. (Ed.), Ophthalmic Care, second ed. M&K, Cumbria.

Macular Society, 2017. Living with macular disease. https://www.youtube.com/watch?v=M9BKZvdY7tE.

Marsden, J., 2017. Ophthalmic Care, second ed. M&K, Cumbria.

Needham, Y., 2017. The visual, pupillary pathway and neuro-ophthalmology. In: Marsden, J. (Ed.), Ophthalmic Care, second ed. M&K, Cumbria, (Chapter 24).

NICE, 2012a. National Institute for Health and Care Excellence. Ranibizumab and pegaptanib for the treatment of age-related macular degeneration. Available at: https://www.nice.org.uk/guidance/ta155.

NICE, 2012b. National Institute for Health and Care Excellence. Minimise transmission risk of CJD and vCJD in healthcare settings. Available at: https://www.gov.uk/government/publications/guidance-from-the-acdp-tse-risk-management-subgroup-formerly-tse-working-group.

NICE, 2013a. National Institute for Health and Care Excellence. Aflibercept solution for injection for treating wet age–related macular degeneration. Available at: https://www.nice.org.uk/Guidance/TA294.

NICE, 2013b. National Institute for Health and Care Excellence. Ranibizumab for treating diabetic macular oedema. Available at: https://www.nice.org.uk/guidance/ta274/chapter/1-Guidance.

NICE, 2017a. National Institute for Health and Care Excellence. Cateract in adults - management. Available at: https://www.nice.org.uk/guidance/ng77.

NICE, 2017b. National Institute for Health and Care Excellence. Glaucoma: diagnosis and management. Available at: https://www.nice.org.uk/guidance/NG81.

NICE, 2018. National Institute for Health and Care Excellence. Age related macular degeneration: guidance. Available at: https://www.nice.org.uk/guidance/ng82.

RNIB, 2003. Royal National Institute of Blind People. The criteria for certification. Available at: http://www.rnib.org.uk/eye-health/registering-your-sight-loss/criteria-certification.

RNIB, 2017a. Royal National Institute of Blind People. Guiding a blind or partially sighted person. Available at: http://www.rnib.org.uk/information-everyday-living-family-friends-and-carers/guiding-blind-or-partially-sighted-person.

RNIB, 2017b. Royal National Institute of Blind People. Coming to terms with sight loss. Available at: https://www.rnib.org.uk/recently-diagnosed/coming-terms-sight-loss.

Raynel, S., Brochner, O., 2017. The retina and vitreous. In: Marsden, J. (Ed.), Ophthalmic Care, second ed. M&K, Cumbria, (Chapter 22).

Seewoodhary, R., 2017. Physiology of vision. In: Marsden, J. (Ed.), Ophthalmic Care, second ed. M&K, Cumbria, (Chapter 1).

Shaw, M., Lee, A., 2017. Ophthalmic Nursing. Wiley-Blackwell, Chichester.

Watkinson, S., 2014. Older People with Visual Impairment. M&K, Cumbria.

Waugh, A., Grant, A., 2018. Ross & Wilson Anatomy and Physiology in Health and Illness, thirteenth ed. Elsevier, Edinburgh.

Websites
http://www.rnib.org.uk/.

https://www.glaucoma-association.com/.
https://www.macularsociety.org/about-macular-conditions.
http://www.guidedogs.org.uk/.

39

Musculoskeletal Disorders

Julie I Swann

OBJECTIVES

By the end of the chapter the reader will:

1. Have an understanding of the anatomy and physiology of the musculoskeletal system
2. Understand the relationship between the musculoskeletal system and other body systems
3. Describe how a musculoskeletal disorder (MSD) occurs
4. Understand the physical changes that can occur, which are associated with common disorders of the musculoskeletal system

5. Discuss the treatment options available to patients with an MSD
6. Outline the roles of other healthcare workers involved in patient care and rehabilitation
7. Explain the additional support a Nursing Associate (NA) can offer in addition to contemporary nursing care

KEY WORDS

Joints	Pain	Mobility aids
Bone	Medication	Equipment
Muscle	Surgery	
Inflammation	Rehabilitation	

CHAPTER AIMS

This chapter discusses some musculoskeletal disorders and their treatment, outlining common disorders.

SELF TEST

1. Explain parts of the body MSDs effect.
2. How can the incidence of some MSDs in the general population be reduced?
3. Describe two symptoms of MSDs.
4. List the main groups of medication for MSDs.
5. Explain the difference between arthroscopy and arthroplasty.
6. How can physiotherapy assist patients with an MSD?
7. What ways can Occupational Therapists help patients become more independent in self-care activities?
8. Outline how osteoarthritis (OA) affects a joint.
9. Describe how rheumatoid arthritis (RA) affects joints and other body systems.
10. Describe specific areas that NAs can assist patients to understand how to minimize the symptoms of MSDs.

INTRODUCTION

The first part of this chapter provides an overview of the musculoskeletal system. The wide range of musculoskeletal disorders (MSD) that can occur, their causes and diagnoses are discussed. There is a focus on the treatment of conditions, including the roles of other healthcare professions. Osteoarthritis (OA) and rheumatoid arthritis (RA) are discussed, along with spinal disorders; these are the three most common MSDs.

Patients with an MSD are generally managed by primary care staff, but are referred for outpatient consultations when symptoms are severe. Hospital admission for specialist treatment and surgery, such as joint replacement, may be required. Hospital-based Nursing Associates (NAs) will encounter this client group, particularly within the field of emergency medicine, orthopaedics and rheumatology, or if comorbidities exist with another specialism.

The role of the NA in patient care is discussed in detail within several chapters in this book. Therefore, only specific reference is made in this chapter if specific care is needed, for example postoperatively. However, to ensure the NA has a comprehensive knowledge of the role of rehabilitation staff, this chapter outlines the various roles of healthcare professionals with regards to rehabilitation. This facilitates appropriate referrals and a streamlined approach to patient care.

ANATOMY AND PHYSIOLOGY

Knowledge of how the healthy body works enables practitioners to understand how various disorders can impair function. Therefore, this chapter outlines the anatomy of the musculoskeletal system.

The rigid skeleton consists of 206 bones, divided into the axial skeleton and the appendicular skeleton (Fig. 39.1). Bones provide a firm framework for muscle attachments, enabling the body to move in various directions.

The spinal column

The spinal column consists of 33 vertebrae that allow or restrict movements:

- 7 Cervical
- 12 Thoracic
- 5 Lumbar
- 5 Fused sacral vertebrae form the sacrum
- 4 Coccygeal vertebrae (frequently fused together forming the coccyx)

The primary functions of the spinal column are to:

1. To protect the nervous system and the vital organs of the body (heart and lungs). This role is shared with the ribcage, which also assists with breathing. The spinal column and pelvis encase the digestive and reproductive organs.
2. To support the body and keep it upright.
3. To facilitate motion by providing anchorage points for muscle, tendon and ligament attachment.

Spinal cord

The spinal cord lies within an enclosed cavity at the centre of the spine. Nerve fibres from the spinal cord emerge out of the vertebra. They transmit impulses via peripheral nerves to muscles to activate or inhibit movement. Sensory nerves relay information on touch, pain, deep pressure and limb position back to the brain via the spinal cord. The autonomic system regulates the automatic body systems, including the internal organs. For additional protection, the meninges encase the spinal nerve roots and the spinal blood vessels of the spinal cord, as well as the brain. Chapter 36 discusses the neurological system in detail.

Joints

A joint is the space between two or more bones. The articular surface of a bone has a hard, smooth covering of cartilage to cushion the joint from impact. Many joints have ligaments within a joint capsule to improve joint stability and restrict movement, thus avoiding dislocation, such as at the shoulder, fingers and the knee joint. Muscles around a joint provide additional support.

Some joints are immoveable, for example, the joints between the bones of the skull. Others have only a light range of movement, for example, parts of the spine, and the structure of a joint allows or restricts movement.

Freely moveable joints allow movement. A 'ball and socket joint' permits the greatest range of movement, for example, the hip and shoulder joints. A 'hinge joint' has movement in one plane, for example, the elbow and knee joint.

Moveable joints have a fibrous capsule that contains synovial fluid to lubricate the joint, protect the articular cartilage at the ends of the joints and facilitate smooth movements (Fig. 39.2). The synovium is an inner thin delicate protective lining of a joint capsule. Some joints have additional cushioning, for example, the menisci of the knee and the intervertebral discs of the spinal column.

How the body moves

The end of the muscle attaches to bone by a tendon. Movement occurs when muscles contract on or near a joint. Most are goal-directed voluntary movements, carried out by a group of muscles, not an individual muscle; for example, walking and personal care tasks. Some movements, over time, become automatic, for example: dancing, typing, driving, walking and sports activities.

Involuntary movements are reflexes, for example, the knee jerk reflex. Several neurological conditions present with involuntary movements, for example, strokes, tumours, multiple sclerosis, chronic alcohol abuse, Parkinsonism and some medication (Stamford Medicine, 2018).

DEFINITION AND CLASSIFICATION OF MUSCULOSKELETAL DISORDERS

MSDs affect the ability to move freely, thus impacting on the locomotive system. This includes joints, skeletal bones, muscles, tendons, ligaments, nerves, blood vessels and soft tissues of the human body.

MSDs encompass a wide range of conditions, from minor disorders to major dysfunctions within or around the skeletal bones. MSDs include injury, damage or disorder of the joints or other tissues in the upper/lower limbs or the back (Health & Safety Executive (HSE), 2018). There are over 200 different MSDs, affecting millions of people (adults and children); including all forms of arthritis, back pain and osteoporosis (NHS England, n.d.). MSDs can be classed according to the location (HSE, 2018).

- Upper limb disorders: occur anywhere in the arms, from the shoulder region to the digits.
- Lower limb disorders: occur in the legs, from the hip region to toes. About 20% of all work-related MSDs affect the lower limbs.

MSDs can also be classed as acute or chronic. Many acute conditions are minor, causing transient symptoms. Some acute MSDs are, or become, severe and disabling; for example, injuries sustained in accidents can lead to residual deficits in function and pain with the potential of longer-term joint damage. Chronic conditions also include RA, OA, osteoporosis and associated fragility fractures and other chronic inflammatory conditions.

The International Statistical Classification of Diseases and Related Health Problems 10th Revision (ICD-10 Version: 2016) categorizes all known diseases (World Health Organization, 2016). The diseases of the musculoskeletal system and connective tissue

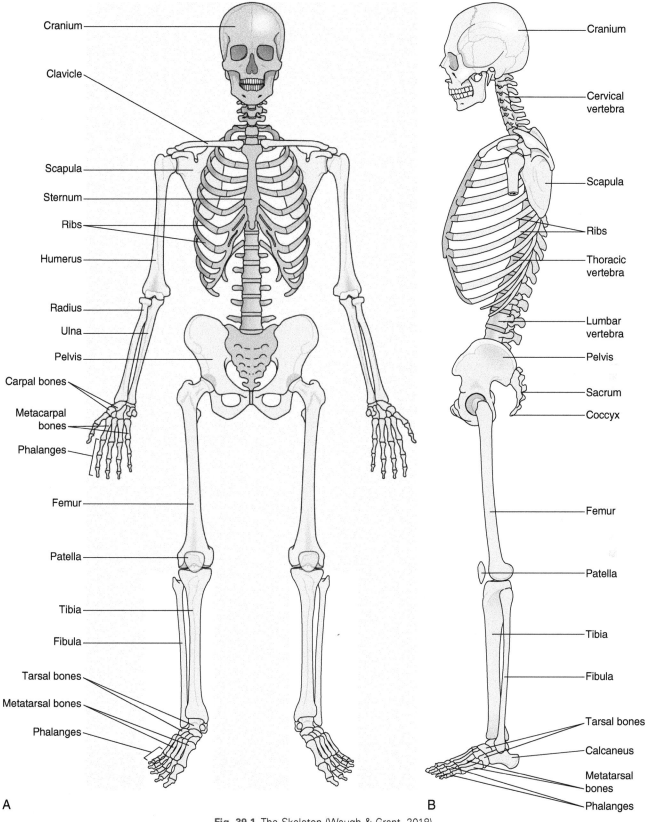

Fig. 39.1 The Skeleton (Waugh & Grant, 2018).

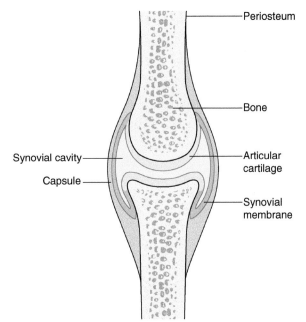

Fig. 39.2 The Basic Structure of a Synovial Joint (Waugh & Grant, 2018).

Periosteum

Bone

Articular cartilage

Synovial membrane

Synovial cavity

Capsule

BOX 39.1.   Diseases of the Musculoskeletal System and Connective Tissue

M00-M25 Arthropathies
- M00-M03 Infectious arthropathies
- M05-M14 Inflammatory polyarthropathies
- M15-M19 Arthrosis
- M20-M25 Other joint disorders

M30-M36 Systemic connective tissue disorders

M40-M54 Dorsopathies
- M40-M43 Deforming dorsopathies
- M45-M49 Spondylopathies
- M50-M54 Other dorsopathies

M60-M79 Soft tissue disorders
- M60-M63 Disorders of muscles
- M65-M68 Disorders of synovium and tendon
- M70-M79 Other soft tissue disorders

M80-M94 Osteopathies and chondropathies
- M80-M85 Disorders of bone density and structure
- M86-M90 Other osteopathies
- M91-M94 Chondropathies

M95-M99 Other disorders of the musculoskeletal system and connective tissue

(From World Health Organization, 2016.)

---

are shown in Box 39.1. Some conditions are very common, whilst others are extremely rare.

ARTHRITIS

Arthritis is a generic name describing inflammation and swelling within a joint, often producing pain, tenderness and stiffness within and around a joint. NHS Choices (2016a) estimate around 10 million people in the UK have arthritis, which affects people of all ages. Some types of arthritis have causes, but for other types the cause is idiopathic (unknown). The type of arthritis is

---

BOX 39.2   Common Work-Related Injuries

- Osteoarthritis in knees, hips, back and fingers.
  Caused by excessive wearing away of cartilage, particularly in floor layers and cleaners.
- Bursitis and repetitive strain injury.
  Tends to affect the upper limbs and is caused by doing repetitive tasks over a prolonged period, particularly if a load is involved. This can also affect knees and hips.
- Vibration exposure, includes:
  - Hand arm vibration syndrome, also called 'vibration white finger', caused by using hand-held power tools.
  - Whole body vibration, which is transmitted through the buttocks or feet when operating machines over rough ground.

(Data from Health & Safety Executive, n.d. and 2018.)

---

diagnosed by looking at the symptoms, supplemented by further investigations, such as x-rays (to identify joint damage) and blood tests.

NHS Choices (2016a) identifies the two most common forms of arthritis as OA and RA; these are focused upon in the next section.

Causes of musculoskeletal disorders

MSDs can be due to a single reason, such as acute injury or infection. Some MSDs are systemic and affect several joints. Many disorders are chronic and disabling. Several MSDs are preventable. Often there is a combination of multifactorial reasons for MSDs occurring, such as:

Moving and handling

Manual handling (HSE, 2018) causes more than a third of all reported workplace injuries, which result in someone being off work for more than 3 days.

Work-related injuries

Prolonged repetitive movements or overuse can lead to musculoskeletal problems, joint damage and degeneration (Box 39.2)

Previous damage or injury

Many musculoskeletal problems affect a joint due to its structure, and joint misalignment can occur if these are not addressed. For example, postural imbalance can lead to back pain. If an articular joint surface is damaged, this can hasten degenerative damage.

Impaired cognition

Impaired cognition due to alcohol, drugs and tiredness can cause accidents. Confusion and perceptual problems can increase the risk of a fall.

Age

The normal ageing process causes some degeneration in a joint, due to 'wear and tear'. Older people are particularly at risk of injury because of reduced bone mass, reduced fitness and unsafe homes (NHS England, n.d.). Ageing affects the articular cartilage of the bone, causing reduced joint flexibility.

Lifestyle factors

Being clinically overweight (body mass index [BMI] 25 or greater), a poor diet, stress, low levels of physical activity or insufficient rest and recovery after illness can contribute to an increased risk of developing musculoskeletal problems.

Incidence of musculoskeletal disorders

MSDs can occur at any age. Musculoskeletal conditions are the most common reason for repeat consultations with a GP, making up to 30% of primary care consultations (NHS England, n.d.). Around one-quarter of adults and around 12,000 children are affected by longstanding musculoskeletal problems, such as arthritis, that limit everyday activities (NHS England, n.d.).

MSDs are the second most common cause of disability worldwide, as measured by years lived with disability, with low back pain being the most frequent condition (Vos et al., 2012).

Disability due to MSDs is estimated to have increased by 45% from 1990 to 2010, in particular OA, and is expected to continue to rise with an increasingly obese, sedentary and ageing population (Vos et al., 2012).

Signs and symptoms of musculoskeletal disorders

The severity of symptoms caused by MSDs varies considerably according to the cause and the location. Generally, symptoms cause swelling and/or pain. Symptoms can be mild or nonexistent, even in the presence of clinical degeneration within the joints.

Swelling can occur inside and outside of a joint capsule. This can be very painful, or painless. A swelling sited near a nerve can compress a nerve and cause neurological impairment, such as weakness or impaired sensation. Swelling can also occur within the muscles, ligaments or soft tissue. Compartment syndrome can arise.

❗ HOTSPOT

Nursing Associates working with acute trauma patients need to be aware of acute compartment syndrome. This is a sudden large painful swelling occurring after a severe injury to the leg. The increased pressure compromises surrounding muscles, blood supply and the nerves. A fasciotomy is the only treatment to prevent ischaemia.

Methods of diagnosis
History

A patient's history and a physical examination help to make a diagnosis, particularly of a degenerative joint condition.

Signs and symptoms

Observable clinical signs and a patient's description of symptoms may be sufficient to make a diagnosis.

Blood tests

Inflammatory conditions, such as RA, can be identified from blood samples, or differential diagnoses ruled out.

TABLE 39.1. Contributing Factors and Intervention	
Obesity	• Advise on healthier eating to reduce calorie input.
Muscle weakness around joint	• Non-weight-bearing exercise can be encouraged, aimed at balance, coordination, flexibility and strengthening.
	• Encourage good seating position.
	• Orthotics and splints can help to support joints.
Occupations	• Avoiding occupations involving heavy repetitive movements, perhaps a change of occupation.
	• Refer for advice on alterative techniques.
Metabolic disorders	• Can predispose a patient (e.g., osteoarthritis can be caused by Wilson disease).

Imaging

Areas of degeneration and subluxation of joints will be visible using x-rays and magnetic resonance imaging scans. This can help to identify if the cause of pain is due to another condition, such as cancer.

Core treatment options

Relief or control of symptoms is the main treatment for all MSDs, in tandem with addressing the cause of the disorder (Table 39.1). NAs will be involved in all aspects of treatment, including prevention.

Prevention
Healthy diet

Overweight patients may be advised to lose weight to prevent a further decline of health. However, some patients may be underweight, identified by a low BMI and observation. Metabolic bone diseases, such as osteoporosis, can be exacerbated by low calcium intake due to a poor diet and being underweight. NAs will need to be aware of these opposing scenarios and encourage healthy eating; referral to the NHS dietician may be needed.

Reducing injury

Risk factors causing MSDs are in every workplace, from commerce to agriculture, health services to construction. An estimated 11.6 million working days a year are lost to work-related MSDs (HSE, 2018).

❗ HOTSPOT

Prolonged lifting and moving of heavy items or repetitive work can cause musculoskeletal problems. NAs must ensure they adhere to the workplace moving and handling guidelines, and not put themselves at risk. Poor moving and handling techniques can cause muscular strain and skeletal problems.

Early diagnosis

Within the last few decades, there have been advances in the early diagnosis of some conditions. Blood tests can identity inflammatory disorders, allowing prompt treatment to improve outcome and prevent disability and further musculoskeletal damage.

Medication

Appropriate and effective management of pain symptoms is essential to ensure the dignity and well-being of all patients. If complete elimination of pain is not possible, effective pain management can help by teaching techniques to reduce awareness of pain. Intervention consists of helping patients to understand why pain symptoms persist. Regular assessment and evaluation of the effectiveness of various treatments and therapies is needed.

The main source of symptom relief is medication, which should be taken on a regular basis, not just when symptoms arise. The type and method of delivery of medication depends on the symptom and individual tolerance. For most MSDs, a combination of pain relief and non-steroidal anti-inflammatory drugs (NSAIDs) is prescribed. Details of medication and side effects can be obtained electronically from MIMS (2018) and the British National Formulary (Joint Formulary Committee, 2017). Medication is generally taken by mouth, as a tablet or in liquid form. Over-the-counter preparations, such as aspirin, paracetamol and ibuprofen can be obtained. These are often cheaper than prescription items, unless the patient is exempt from charges. Many other painkillers can be prescribed, including co-codamol, diclofenac and celecoxib. Pain is discussed in further detail in Chapter 28.

Alternative methods of administering medication are discussed in detail in Chapter 18 on medicine management. NAs should know that medication can be given in various ways, such as directly to the skin, sublingually, inhaled, suppositories (termed 'PR', per rectum), injections and intrathecally.

Combinations of oral analgesia

A combination of painkillers can be more effective than stronger medication. Combinations include co-codamol (paracetamol and codeine), co-dydramol (paracetamol and dihydrocodeine tartrate) and Tramacet (paracetamol and tramadol); the combination selected depends on the nature of the pain experience.

Side-effects of pain killers

Management of severe pain may require the maximum doses of medication, but this can produce considerable side effects and alternative methods of pain relief may need consideration.

> **⚠ HOTSPOT**
>
> Nursing Associates should be aware that if oral pain relief medication of similar ingredients is used, this can lead to an accidental overdose.

Non-steroidal anti-inflammatory drugs

These help to reduce inflammation, swelling and pain. Long-term use of NSAIDs can cause gastrointestinal problems (irritation and bleeding), so they must be used with caution and are contraindicated if stomach ulcers are present. Alternative NSAID creams or gels are rubbed over a painful joint or muscle. The

COX-2-specific NSAIDs have been linked with increased risks of heart attack and stroke.

Corticosteroids

Corticosteroids are effective in controlling inflammation and may have some disease-modifying effects. However, longer-term use or high doses produce side effects. Steroids can cause osteoporosis.

Disease-modifying anti-rheumatic drugs

This medication includes gold, hydroxychloroquine, leflunomide, penicillamine and sulfasalazine. They can reduce pain, swelling and stiffness, but can take a few weeks to be effective.

Immunosuppressant drugs

These disease-modifying drugs suppress the body's defence system: the immune system. They include azathioprine, ciclosporin, cyclophosphamide, methotrexate and mycophenolate. They may produce side effects and need careful monitoring. These are used for conditions that involve autoimmunity, such as RA and lupus.

Biologics drugs

The biologics drugs or 'biologicals', are a type of disease-modifying anti-rheumatic drug (DMARD) that work by treating the underlying condition, rather than a person's symptoms (Arthritis Care, 2017a). They can reduce joint inflammation and are used when there is no response to other disease-modifying drugs. These include adalimumab, etanercept, infliximab, anakinra and rituximab. Anti-tumour necrosis factors (TNFs) suppress the TNF protein, which is produced in excessive amounts in some forms of arthritis, causing inflammation and pain.

Anti-epileptic drugs

These affect nerve activity and reduce oversensitivity in nerves, similar to reducing overactivity of brain cells in patients with epilepsy.

Antidepressants

Pain can produce a low mood. These can improve pain tolerance and sleep quality, if taken before bedtime.

Side effects of medication

Newly diagnosed patients must be made aware of any side effects. Some side effects are short lived; therefore, it is important to give drugs a trial period. Common side effects of painkillers and anti-inflammatory drugs include nausea, vomiting, diarrhoea, ulceration, hearing disturbances, vertigo and hypersensitivity. Other problems may be more specific, such as gastrointestinal problems from NSAIDS, weight gain from anti-epileptics, drowsiness from antidepressants (The British Pain Society, 2015). Opioids can cause constipation, and long-term use can result in haemorrhoids.

Many older people have multiple medical problems and take several medications (polypharmacy) that may react adversely with each other. Cancer Research UK's website (2018) lists the side effects of pain-relieving medications, many of which reduce with time or can be treated effectively.

Some medication, such as azathioprine, ciclosporin, gold, leflunomide, methotrexate, penicillamine and sulfasalazine, can affect the blood and/or the working of the liver or kidney. Patients taking this medication will need regular blood tests and urine checks.

Medication can affect blood pressure, such as ciclosporin and leflunomide, so regular blood pressure checks are required. It is vital that patients are aware of the need for these regular checks.

> ### ⚠ HOTSPOT
>
> Side effects vary according to the medication and the patient's sensitivity. Nursing Associates must be aware of the side effects of medication and report adverse reactions to the prescriber.

Pain management programmes

Those who experience chronic pain may be referred to NHS or private pain management programmes. A multidisciplinary approach is adopted to supplement a medical approach. This includes psychological intervention (such as biofeedback and cognitive therapy), physiotherapy (including manipulation and mobilization), acupuncture and occupational therapy (equipment and alternative techniques). Programmes can include complementary therapies.

Transcutaneous electrical nerve stimulation

Transcutaneous electrical nerve stimulation (TENS) machines pass electrical signals through the spinal cord to block pain signals. They are portable and usually used by a patient under the direction of a doctor or physiotherapist. TENS are contraindicated if a patient has epilepsy, a heart problem or is pregnant.

> ### CRITICAL AWARENESS
> #### TENS
>
> - Ensure medical advice has been sought before a patient uses TENS.
> - TENS machines should not be used if a patient has a pacemaker or another type of electrical or metal implant in their body.
> - Ensure the TENS machine is switched off before the pads are attached to the skin.
> - Pads should be positioned either side of the painful area, at least 2.5 cm (1") apart.
> - Pads should never be placed over:
>   o The front or sides of the neck
>   o The temples
>   o The mouth or eyes
>   o Chest and upper back at the same time
>   o Irritated, infected or broken skin
>   o Varicose veins
>   o Numb areas.
> - Ensure patients know how to control the strength of the electrical impulses.
> - Check that the skin does not become red and irritated, as some patients may be allergic to the pads. Special pads for patients with allergies are available.
> - TENS should not be used when driving or operating machinery, or in a bath or shower.

(Data from NHS Choices, 2018.)

Surgical treatment

A severely affected joint may need surgical treatment (Box 39.3), ranging from injections into a joint to a partial or full joint replacement.

Postsurgery, there may be short-term swelling and pain around the area. After surgery, the treating consultant will discourage a full active range of movement and give clinical guidelines to the patient to prevent dislocation until the surrounding muscles have healed. Maxey and Magnuson (2007) provide evidence-based rehabilitation guidelines for people who have undergone surgery. One aspect of the role of the NA is to reinforce any information provided to the patient. Gradual re-mobilization should be encouraged, as per the treating surgeon's guidelines. After surgery, there is a short period of stiffness, pain and restriction of range of movement.

Wound care is important. A restriction of functional ability results in additional help being required for mobility and/or self-care activities.

> ### BOX 39.3 Surgical Treatment
>
> - **Arthroscopy (fibreoptic surgery)**
>   A fine tube is inserted into the affected joint space to explore the area, inspect and diagnose. Osteophytes and debris can be removed (debridement arthroplasty) and bone, ligaments and cartilage repaired to reduce pain and inflammation. Postprocedure, there can be localized bruising, pain and short-term limitation of movement.
> - **Neurolytic Blocks**
>   This long-term analgesia deliberately blocks the nerve impulses using neurolytic blocks (chemicals such as phenol or a cryogenic block).
> - **Sympathetic Nerve Blocks, Cordotomy or Sympathectomy**
>   This permanently destroys structures involved in pain perception by destroying dorsal nerve roots.
> - **Spinal Cord Stimulation**
>   Electrodes are used on specific nerve pathways to reduce pain. This involves the insertion of a stimulator under the skin, adjusted to a level that adequately controls the pain.
> - **Synovectomy**
>   This is removal of the inflamed joint lining.
> - **Osteotomy**
>   This is partial removal of damaged bone.
> - **Arthrodesis (Surgical Fusion)**
>   Prior to artificial joint replacements, arthrodesis was use to surgically fuse bones. Arthrodesis treats pain and potential deformity of arthritis, particularly the big toe, neck and small joints of the fingers (proximal or distal interphalangeal joints) as this is easier and more reliable than replacing the joints. Bone is harvested from the iliac crest (front of pelvis) as this has only a few muscular attachments.
> - **Arthroplasty (Joint Replacement)**
>   The damaged areas are surgically removed and a prosthesis is inserted to replace the arthritic joint. This provides an improved range of movement and pain relief. Examples are the finger, hip, knee and shoulder joint. Replacement joints are still under development and generally have a lifespan of 15 to 20 years, but this is dependent on individual circumstances and usage (Bird et al., 2006).
> - **Revision surgery**
>   Joint replacements have a life span of 10 to 20 years, but this depends on individual circumstance and the joint replaced. Bird et al (2006) note 'Surgery second time around takes longer and is more complicated than the initial operation. Recovery is likely to take longer too'.

Role of the Nursing Associate in rehabilitation

As part of the rehabilitation process, the NA has a key role to play in helping people with their activities of living. NAs can ensure patient's progress through rehabilitation as well as medical treatment. NAs can support the patient and maximize the input of treatment from physiotherapists and Occupational Therapists.

Addressing the environment

NAs should be aware of any functional restrictions and pay attention to the environment; such as ensuring items around the bed are within reach (e.g., water, call-bell, spectacles, television controls). An assessment of the environment should be carried out according to local policy and procedure.

Maintaining and restoring function

It is important to maintain muscle strength in the muscles surrounding an affected joint; weak muscles can cause further imbalance. Physiotherapy exercises to improve muscle strength around affected joints can be reinforced and good walking patterns emphasized. Prolonged periods of inactivity can increase stiffness and weakness after surgery or a flare-up of an inflammatory condition, such as RA.

Mobility

Mobility aids may no longer be suitable for a patient's needs; for example, it may be the wrong height or postsurgery, a more supportive walking aid may be needed. A flare-up of a hand condition (carpal tunnel syndrome or RA) or surgery may make it difficult to grasp the equipment. NAs may need to ensure correct, safe use of mobility aids.

Increasing independence

By observing and encouraging a patient to be self-managing, NAs can identify the need for equipment on discharge. This ranges from lightweight or long-handled feeding aids and dressing aids, to toilet and bathing equipment. Equipment is sourced via an Occupational Therapist. Morning stiffness is common. Functional abilities may fluctuate from day-to-day, even from morning to night. If patients are helped to identify periods of when they are most mobile, practical activities can be carried out (pacing) and symptoms will reduce.

Joint protection

NAs can reinforce techniques of joint protection to reduce biomechanical factors. This includes using splints and learning alternative techniques (Arthritis Care, 2018). A simple alteration of technique can make an activity easier to do (Swann, 2007).

Joints take less strain if other parts of the body or other muscles can be used to achieve a task, such as using the palm instead of the fingers to grasp, pushing a door open with the arm rather than the hand and using two hands wherever possible, for example, when holding a cup.

Splints

NAs should become familiar with ready-made splints used in their work settings and know how to apply them correctly. Splints help to maintain a functional position and can slow the deformation process, but not prevent it from occurring. Splints can assist in stabilizing bones before or after surgery, such as a cricket splint used on the knee or a neck collar to keep the joints correctly aligned. Hand splints can reduce pain and strain on joints by placing the hand into an optimal position to work (normally 30 degrees of extension). A night resting splint maintains proper alignment of the bones and tendons and eliminates stress on the hands from poor positioning. An external fixator may be applied after surgery to a limb and the pin sites will need cleaning.

A ward or outpatient department may stock splints or a referral to the orthotics or a specialized splint-making department, usually occupational therapy, may be indicated. Occupational Therapists can make custom-made hand splints, whilst innersoles and foot orthosis are made by orthotist.

Care within a patient's home

Additional to providing general nursing care, when working with the district nursing/community nursing services, NAs may change dressings or clean the 'pin-sites' of external fixators or teach patients and carers how to do these tasks. Care must be provided using an evidence base and any care delivered has to be documented in the patient's notes.

Focus on the positive

Unfortunately, many people with MSDs have a limited level of physical activity and restricted mobility. Patients can be helped to focus away from symptoms onto the positive aspects of their lives. Many tasks can be carried out when sitting rather than standing, such as dressing. Within the home, items can be slid across the kitchen surface to avoid lifting.

Avoiding pain cycling

Research shows that people with persistent pain who keep active tend to feel better and can do more (The British Pain Society, 2015). However, wanting to complete a physical activity to the point of unbearable pain results in discomfort or pain the following day and prevents other physical activities being carried out. This is called 'pain cycling'.

REFLECTION 39.1

Think about the ways you can encourage patients (from various backgrounds) to engage in the exercises the physiotherapist has prescribed.

How can you facilitate exercise for patients who have difficulties understanding spoken communication?

If, as part of your role, you have already had to do this, reflect on this important activity and think about the good aspects and the not so good aspects of how you carried this activity.

Are there any physical and human resources you can use to enhance the patient experience?

Reinforcing exercises

Physiotherapy may be arranged, which often includes 'home exercises'. However, patients may need encouragement from an NA to continue prescribed physiotherapy exercises (refer to Reflection 39.1).

Pacing

By forward planning (termed 'pacing'), physically demanding jobs can be spread throughout the week. Patients can spread daily tasks out during the day by alternating a heavier demanding task with a seated, lighter task. NAs can encourage regular breaks to be taken when doing housework and gardening.

Difficulties managing daily life

Referral to social care may be needed for equipment and adaptations. Larger adaptations can be funded using the disabled facilities grant, but eligibility criteria apply. Many high street, mail-order and online outlets are available for smaller items.

Healthcare professionals

Several healthcare professionals can assist patients to adjust to MSDs, and the skills and techniques used by healthcare professionals continue to evolve. As well as helping to improve a patient's function, they can help to reduce problem areas. Their roles are described in Box 39.4; some work in hospitals, the community or in private practice.

REFLECTION 39.2

Reflect on the role of any one of the healthcare professionals in Box 39.4. What is the key function (they may have many); how does the Nursing Associate work along with that healthcare professional in such a way as to ensure that the patient is at the centre of all that is done?

Complementary therapies and other physical exercise

Complementary therapies include aromatherapy, acupuncture, massage, osteopathy, chiropractic treatments and reflexology. These can help to alleviate pain and stiffness. As little or no active involvement is required of the patient, the therapist takes responsibility for control of pain relief, not the patient.

Physical activities such as yoga, tai chi, Pilates and the Alexander technique are useful to strength muscle groups, particularly core muscles around the abdomen and lower back. Techniques aid relaxation and improve flexibility and balance.

Homeopathy and nutritional supplements

As valuable nutrients are lost though certain arthritis medications (Lam & Horseman, 2002), patients may use anti-inflammatory herbs, nutritional supplements or homoeopathic remedies. This should be recorded in medical records, and NAs will need to report this if it has been omitted from records.

CRITICAL AWARENESS

Alternative Therapies

The Nursing Associate should be aware that complementary and alternative therapies may interact with other kinds of medicinal products and blood tests.

OSTEOARTHRITIS

Definition of osteoarthritis

When a joint develops OA, some of the cartilage covering the ends of the bones gradually roughens and becomes thin and the bone underneath thickens (Arthritis Research UK, 2018a). 'Osteo' refers to bone and 'itis' reflects that the joint is red, hot, swollen and painful (inflamed). It is viewed as a metabolically dynamic process, characterized by an imbalance of joint breakdown in association with a maladaptive and insufficient repair process (Kraus & Doherty, 2010).

Signs and symptoms of osteoarthritis

The severity of symptoms varies according to which part of the skeleton is affected. The cartilage, and eventually the joint's articular surface, degenerates. Eventually, bone articulates on bone. One or more joints can become affected, usually with asymmetrical symptoms, for example: one knee and one hip, not both knees.

OA can be mild, even symptomless, or it can cause joint pain, stiffness, swelling, crepitus and disability of varying degrees, which impacts on the patient's abilities and quality of life. OA symptoms can 'wax and wane'; some patients find warmer months or warmer climates reduce symptoms. Stiff joints that worsen with use throughout the day are common.

BOX 39.4. Main Roles of Healthcare Professionals

Chiropractors

Chiropractors are trained in the diagnosis, treatment and prevention of certain mechanical disorders of the musculoskeletal system and their effects on general health. They provide evidence-based, timely and effective assessment, diagnosis and management of certain musculoskeletal disorders. There is an emphasis on manual treatments, including spinal manipulation or adjustment, and on physical and psychosocial rehabilitation.

Clinical psychologists

Clinical psychology aims to reduce psychological distress and to enhance and promote psychological well-being. They work in a wide range of health settings, ensuring that the mental as well as physical health needs of patients are addressed. They provide a bio-psychosocial approach to the care of patients, using methods including psychometric tests, interviews and direct observation of behaviour to assess patients. Assessment may lead to therapy, counselling or advice.

Occupational therapists

Occupational Therapists work across health and social care to promote independence in daily life. They assess, treat and provide information and equipment to assist a person's ability to perform daily tasks and valued life roles. They facilitate successful adaptation to aid occupational independence and promote functional independence. They advise on joint protection (refer 7.18). They provide psychological support in adapting to impairment, dysfunction or disability. Occupational Therapists can smooth patient discharge from hospital, given their unique role at the interface between health and social care.

Orthotist

Orthotists design and fit orthoses to provide support to part of a patient's body to compensate for paralysed muscles, provide relief from pain or prevent physical deformities from progressing.

Osteopaths

Osteopaths specialize in the diagnosis, treatment, prevention and rehabilitation of certain musculoskeletal conditions, including offering guidance on diet, lifestyle and exercise.

Physiotherapists

Physiotherapists look at function and movement and help people to achieve their full physical potential, using physical approaches to promote, maintain and restore well-being. They are first-contact practitioners, able to assess, diagnose and treat a patient without the need for a referral. They also provide specialist, advanced practice in the musculoskeletal field, including helping to realign joints into functional positions and correct poor posture. They provide mobility equipment.

Podiatrists

Podiatrists assess, diagnose and treat foot and ankle pathologies to maintain and enhance locomotion function of the feet and legs; this alleviates pain and reduces the impact of disability. Podiatrists can assist in the management of low back pain and hip and knee problems, utilizing biomechanics (assessment of the function of human motion) by focusing on the lower limbs during activities (such as walking) to help ensure appropriate and effective treatment. Treatment may include specific exercises, the prescription of corrective insoles or orthoses, and advice, especially when related to child development and rheumatological diseases. Biomechanics is also used in the pre- and postsurgical assessment of orthopaedic patients, providing information to help with the selection of an appropriate surgical procedure and treating mechanical back pain. Most podiatrists are qualified to undertake nail and soft tissue surgery and can administer local anaesthetics.

Prosthetist

Prosthetists provide care and advice on rehabilitation for patients who have lost or who were born without a limb, fitting the best possible artificial replacement. They work alongside doctors, nurses, physiotherapists (deals with lower limbs) and Occupational Therapists (deal with upper limbs).

Psychologists

Help may be needed if a patient has post-traumatic stress disorder or an adjustment disorder (stemming from a major alteration in health and lifestyle). Techniques include goal setting, relaxation training and cognitive behaviour therapy to help understand how negative coping mechanisms and stresses can contribute to symptoms and positive coping strategies can be taught.

Radiographers (diagnostic)

Diagnostic radiographers produce images on film and other recording media, using all kinds of radiation. Virtually all people with musculoskeletal conditions will need x-rays, magnetic resonance imaging and other radiographic investigations.

(Adapted from Health Education England, 2018.)

OA affecting the spinal column can cause nerve root compression, resulting in numbness, tingling, reduced muscle power and further limitation of range of movement. If L4/L5 is involved, sciatica, muscle spasm, pain and urinary incontinence may be symptoms.

When hands are affected (Fig. 39.3), grip and dexterity can be severely impaired and affect personal care activities. Fig. 39.4 demonstrates a normal and OA joint in the hand.

OA also affects the larger joints (hips, knees and shoulders) or load bearing joints, particularly in obese people, or if an injury has damaged the articular surface.

REFLECTION 39.3

Take some time to reflect on what body image means and how having a condition such as osteoarthritis may impact on body image.

Incidence

OA is the most common joint disorder. Around 50% of people have OA in one or more of their joints, with around 10% having some disability caused by it. OA has around 8 million sufferers in the UK (NHS Choices, 2016a).

OA most often develops in adults who are in their late 40s or older (NHS Choices, 2016a; Arthritis Care, 2017b). Caucasians have an increased incidence of OA in the hands (Bird et al., 2006). Nodal OA, which affects the hands of middle-aged women, has a familial link (Arthritis Care, 2017b). NICE (2008) mention genetic factors (estimates for hand, knee and hip OA are high at 40%–60%). NICE (2018) also notes constitutional factors (e.g., ageing, female sex, obesity and a high bone density). Women have a higher incidence of OA, particularly in knees and hands (Arthritis Research Care, 2017b), but this may be due to a longer lifespan or occupation.

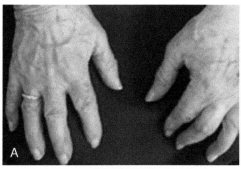
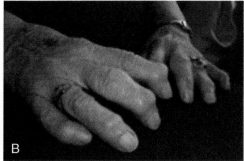

Fig. 39.3 Osteoarthritis in Hands. (A) Early stage. (B) Later stage.

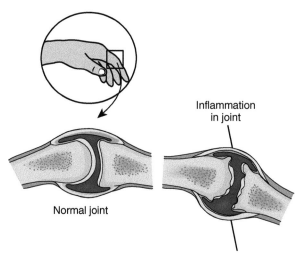

Fig. 39.4 Normal Joint and Joint with Osteoarthritis in Hand (modified from Reed, 2005).

Cause of osteoarthritis

OA is associated with low-grade inflammation (Berenbaum, 2013), but the underlying pathogenic mechanisms are not fully understood and currently there is no curative treatment. OA can be divided into two categories, which helps understand the cause of the condition and risk factors:

Primary osteoarthritis

This is due to excessive degeneration in a previously healthy joint. Kraus & Doherty (2010) note, 'It may also result from normal stresses applied to an inherently compromised joint with abnormal physiology, for example weakened cartilage due to a genetic mutation in collagen II', but the responsible genes are largely unknown.

Secondary osteoarthritis

This develops in previously abnormal joints, such as an injured or deformed joint. Excessive or abnormal biomechanical stresses on tendons and ligaments can cause a mechanical imbalance and a strain on nearby joints, common in athletes, sporting injuries or earlier fractures that have damaged a joint surface. Various practical occupations involve overusing a joint or doing repetitive tasks, including heavy manual workers (construction injury) and some performing artists (dancers and musicians).

Diagnosis of osteoarthritis

X-rays can confirm diagnosis. NICE (2014) advise OA can be diagnosed clinically, without investigations, if a person:

- is 45 years or over and
- has activity-related joint pain and
- has either no morning joint-related stiffness or morning stiffness that lasts no longer than 30 minutes.

Bijlsma et al. (2011), advise there is room for improvement and the development of more specific and sensitive methods for early diagnosis, detailed phenotypic characterization and targeted treatment for the different OA subgroups.

Progression of the condition

Eventually, the articular cartilage thins and erodes. The joint space narrows and is visible on an x-ray. The joint capsule may thicken and produce excessive synovial fluid, causing the joint to become painful and swollen. There can be permanent swellings of the joints, particularly in the hands.

Osteophytes can form adjacent to the joint margins, attempting to repair and protect the joint. These can act as a splint and can fuse the smaller joints naturally; thus, pain levels can reduce, but the process restricts the range of movement. Heberden's nodes and Bouchard's nodes may be present in the hands. Osteophytes can break off, causing more damage to the articular surface, particularly in the knee. Osteophytes can impinge on the nerve around joints or the spine.

Treatment

A detailed assessment is made of the patient's needs, working in partnership to ensure a holistic approach is adopted. Treatment is initially symptom management using medication, such as topical preparations, painkillers or NSAIDs. Strong evidence supports exercise and weight loss for the management of OA (Nelson et al., 2013). If pain levels are high, steroid injections may be suggested.

Changing occupation, leisure or lifestyle can help control the symptoms. A limited level of physical activity will weaken muscles and physiotherapy can assist to strengthen muscles around an affected joint. Mobility equipment and assistive aids, such as bathing aids, perching stools or a stairlift can help. Arthroscopy is used as an investigatory process and a treatment. If the pain is severe and mobility is limited, joint fusion may be advised for smaller joints, or joint replacement. However, addressing the cause of OA can help.

CASE STUDY 39.1 Josiah – Secondary Osteoarthritis

Josiah, aged 55 years, is a single man who lives alone in high-rise city centre tower block. Twenty years ago, he sustained multiple lower limb fractures, including fractures to both tibial plateaus, in an accident when a car reversed into him whilst he was working as a mechanic.

Recently, he developed severe pain in both knees, more pronounced in the left knee. On examination, both knees were slightly swollen with crepitus. X-rays indicated severe degeneration of the tibial plateau of the left knee. Josiah was referred to orthopaedics for consideration of a replacement knee joint and was advised that a knee replacement would last about 20 years before revision surgery is indicated. As Josiah had not received physiotherapy since his original injury, a referral was made for knee-strengthening exercises. Driving was discussed and an automatic vehicle advised. He had difficulty managing the bath and the Nursing Associate referred him to the community Occupational Therapist for bathing aids.

Prognosis

The OA treatment process is one of attempted repair and effectively limits the damage and symptoms in the majority of cases (NICE, 2008). However, many cases of OA are progressive and degenerative. The burden due to OA is anticipated to further increase due to obesity and an ageing population (Vos et al., 2012). Additionally, OA predominantly affects older people, often coexisting with other conditions associated with aging and obesity. There can be other issues due to physical, sensory (poor vision and hearing loss) and psychosocial problems (anxiety and depression). The prognosis and outcome depends on these comorbidities, as much as it does on the joint disease itself. Cartilage changes encourage the deposit of calcium crystals and acute pseudo-gout can develop (Kraus & Doherty, 2010).

RHEUMATOID ARTHRITIS

RA is an autoimmune disease that causes inflammation in joints; the main symptoms are joint pain and swelling (Arthritis Research UK, 2018b). RA is a systemic disease, as it can also occur in other tissues, such as the lungs, heart and eyes.

Symptoms

The protective synovium of the joint capsule thickens and bursae become inflamed; often a pannus is formed. Excess synovial fluid is produced causing swollen joints. RA results in pain, swelling, redness, heat and loss of function (Moots & Jones, 2004) in affected joints, with a resultant loss of strength. The pain experienced can be debilitating and resultant fatigue is common.

RA usually starts with pain and swelling in the small joints of the hands in a symmetrical pattern (i.e., if the wrist is involved, then the opposite wrist will be affected later). Morning stiffness is common.

Arthritis Research (2018b) note inflammation of other body parts can occur, for example lungs and blood vessels, and the membrane around the heart can be affected but this is rare. The meninges may be affected and vasculitis may follow; this may interfere with blood circulation or cause skin ulcers. If the pleura are affected, this may cause shortness of breath.

Cause of rheumatoid arthritis

The exact cause is unknown but thought to be due to impairment of the autoimmune system, causing damage to healthy tissue. The trigger mechanism is unknown, but may be due to a virus, bacteria, air pollution, heavy smoking or a genetic disposition to the disease. Some physicians believe there is a link between stress and RA. Of adults with RA, 80% have what is termed the 'rheumatoid factor', HLA-DR4; this factor is rarely present in the normal population.

Sometimes an inflammation in the joints develops quickly, usually 3–12 weeks after an infection or virus (reactive arthritis) (e.g., influenza, food poisoning or sexually transmitted diseases). Joint swelling and pain generally starts in the knees, ankles or toes; but this is treatable and attacks are usually short-lived. Initially, treatment with antibiotics will tackle the infection or virus that is thought to trigger the condition. Thereafter, treatment is directed to controlling the symptoms.

Incidence and predisposing factors

RA can affect any age, including children (called 'early onset' RA or 'juvenile idiopathic arthritis'). RA affects 1% of the UK population, around 690,000 people (National Rheumatoid Arthritis Society (NRAS), 2014). It often starts between the age of 40 and 60 years (NRAS, 2014). RA appears to be multifactorial. Moots & Jones (2004) state RA is 'likely to be a combination of inherited genes and environmental factors, possibly a virus'.

Gender

Women are three times more likely to be affected than men (NHS Choices, 2016), and often have a remission during pregnancy (Moots & Jones, 2004). Females with a short reproductive life and lower levels of reproductive hormones are at greater risk of RA.

Genes and a genetic link

Studies of identical twins have shown that the disease occurs in both twins in only 30% of cases (Moots & Jones, 2004), yet this is higher than the incidence in the general population. The highest incidence is in Native Americans (5%) and it is far less common in Chinese and Japanese people (0.3%) (Hameed & Akil, 2010). The gene with the greatest contribution towards genetic susceptibility is the major histocompatibility complex (Moots & Jones, 2004).

Environmental factors

The environment is thought to account for 70% of susceptibility to RA (Moots & Jones, 2004), including air pollution and heavy smoking.

Stresses and other medical illnesses

Life stress, obesity, a history of blood transfusions and a lower level of cortisol can increase the risk. Bacterial infection can also trigger RA in those who have risk factors.

Diagnosis

A diagnosis of RA is made when at least four of the following signs and symptoms are present:

- There is evidence of morning stiffness in the joints.
- Arthritis is present in three or more joint areas.
- Joint areas are simultaneously involved.
- Rheumatoid nodules are present.

Abnormal amounts of serum rheumatoid factor and inflammation (elevated erythrocyte sedimentation rate or C-reactive protein) can be detected by a blood test. Blood tests can also reveal if there is anaemia, a common symptom of RA due to a low red blood cell count.

Radiological changes of erosions or unequivocal bony decalcification, localized or adjacent to the involved joint(s), can be identified by x-ray.

Treatment

At present, there is no cure for RA. Early diagnosis facilitates prompt treatment to prevent joint damage and its resultant disability. Treatment, after an in-depth assessment of needs, will depend on the symptoms and the reason for the problems.

Medication

Medication helps to relieve symptoms by reducing inflammation and pain. Over the last few decades, new and effective drugs have improved the longer-term outcomes for patients. A combination of analgesics and NSAIDs is commonly prescribed, such as aspirin, paracetamol and ibuprofen. DMARDs, immunosuppressant drugs and 'biologicals' can suppress the inflammation and slow down the progression. Sometimes steroid injections provide temporary relief.

Surgery

Joint replacement, such as the finger joints, may be recommended to remove pain and increase the range of movement.

> **! HOTSPOT**
>
> Over-straining very inflamed painful joints, including over-exercising, is contra-indicated. This can further weaken joints, and overworking muscles can increase fatigue. Using alternative techniques places less strain on joints.

Progression of rheumatoid arthritis

RA can be a very disabling and painful condition. Several joints can be affected, causing pain, inflammation and swelling, with resultant underuse of the surrounding joints and inevitable muscle weakness.

Due to damage to the synovium, the cartilage is eventually destroyed and the bone itself can be damaged (Fig. 39.5).

The tendon sheaths (tubes in which the tendons move) can also become inflamed, as can the bursae (sacs of fluid that allow tendons and muscles to move smoothly over each other). Swellings can cause compression of nerves and interfere with nerve function, causing numbness, tingling and loss of function. The NRAS (2015) describes rheumatoid nodules (firm subcutaneous lumps made of inflammatory tissue) occurring in 20% of patients with RA, usually around overexposed joints, such as the elbows and fingers.

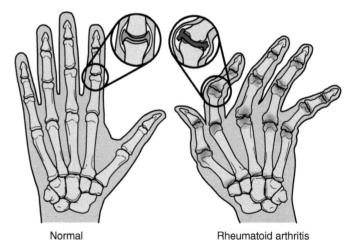

Normal   Rheumatoid arthritis

Fig. 39.5 Normal Hand and Rheumatoid Hand.

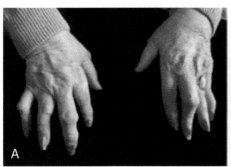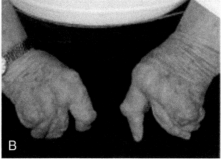

Fig. 39.6 Rheumatoid Arthritis in Hands.

As RA progresses, inflammation causes swollen, painful and misshapen joints, particularly in the hands (Fig. 39.6), knees and feet. In the upper limbs, ulnar drift (the fingers moving away from the direction of the thumb at the knuckle) can occur. Deformed joints decrease the range of movement and mobility, with resultant problems managing activities of daily living. Two common hand deformities are:

• Boutonnière deformity (buttonhole deformity)

This is when the middle joint of the finger bends in a fixed position towards the palm and the outermost finger joint bends excessively outwards, away from the palm.

• Swan neck deformity

This is a bending in (flexion) of the base of the finger, a straightening out (extension) of the middle joint, and a bending in (flexion) of the outermost joint.

CASE STUDY 39.2   Kristen – Rheumatoid Arthritis

Kristen, aged 50 years, had suffered from rheumatoid arthritis for 10 years. Her hands were deformed and very painful in the morning. She had difficulty with aspects of self-care and stair management. The Nursing Associate visited her at home to take blood samples and to check how she was managing. Joint protection advice was provided and Kristen was referred to the Occupational Therapist regarding the provision of a stairlift and adaptations to her property to make access easier.

SPINAL CONDITIONS

Many minor MSDs affect the spine and adjacent structures. These include muscular strain, fractures and inflammation. Often symptoms are acute but transient. Some problems can be due to earlier injuries. Several chronic conditions affect the spine, such as ankylosing spondylosis, cervical spondylosis and OA. Symptoms centre on stiffness, pain and restricted movement.

When the nerves within and around the spinal column are compressed or damaged, the nerve conductivity will be compromised. Patients may report loss of sensation. The exact symptoms vary according to the nerve involved (Fig. 39.7).

Spinal curvature

Many musculoskeletal and other medical conditions can affect the natural curves of the back, causing loss of curvature or exaggerated curvature. Three main curvatures are:

• Kyphosis – an excessive forward curve of cervical vertebrae producing stooped posture.
• Scoliosis – a sideways curve of the spine. Can be hereditary or due to a muscular imbalance stemming from an MSD or neurological condition.
• Lordosis – an exaggerated concave curvature usually in the lower back, which can be due to poor posture, obesity or an MSD.

Often these conditions are symptomless, but physiotherapy can prevent further musculoskeletal problems arising.

Cervical spondylosis

This is a degenerative condition affecting the intervertebral discs and the vertebrae in the cervical spine (neck region) and causes pain, stiffness and weakness (Swann, 2009). Bulging of the intervertebral disc, reduction in the joint space or osteophytes can compress the nerves and cause considerable pain, wasting and weakness of muscles (Swann, 2009). Sensory problems can arise in the hands and legs. MSDs in the back can cause back pain, muscular weakness and loss of function due to problems with nerve conductivity.

Treatment

An assessment of needs is undertaken and care is provided using an evidence base. Rest and medication can help to reduce acute inflammation and pain. Surgical collars may be worn to reduce neck pain, and back corsets can help with lower back pain. It is important that the use of collars is seen as short-term; prolonged use can lead to undue weakening of the muscles in the neck region.

Other forms of treatment include TENS. Back surgery or cervical decompression can help to reduce symptoms and loss of function due to problems with nerve conductivity. There are two main cervical surgical approaches: an anterior approach (Cloward's operation) or a posterior approach.

CASE STUDY 39.3   Rebecca

Rebecca, aged 73 years, lives in a bungalow on the outskirts of the city with her husband, Ted. She had developed pins and needles, with loss of strength and dexterity, in both her arms. This affected her ability to grip and to manage clothing fastenings. An x-ray indicated degenerative disc problems in her cervical region. Cervical decompression was arranged. After an assessment by the Occupational Therapist, small items of equipment were provided to assist Rebecca with dressing and kitchen tasks.

LOOKING BACK, FEEDING FORWARD

This chapter has provided an introduction to MSDs, which have a wide variety of conditions ranging from minor short-term injuries to disabling degenerative long-term problems; some conditions are very painful and disabling.

Additional to providing nursing care, NAs can assist patients to identify factors that have caused problems. Their role may include helping patients to address lifestyle factors that have caused or affected musculoskeletal problems, for example, establishing a healthy diet, increasing physical activity and addressing poor manual handling techniques.

Due to fluctuation of symptoms, additional support may be needed for practical tasks and mobility, and NAs should be aware of this. A patient's level of activity and independence can improve by focusing on positive aspects. NAs can help patients to find easier and less painful ways of managing activities by applying the principles of joint protection.

With a rising life expectancy, MSDs and other degenerative problems are increasing. Therefore, NAs are likely to encounter

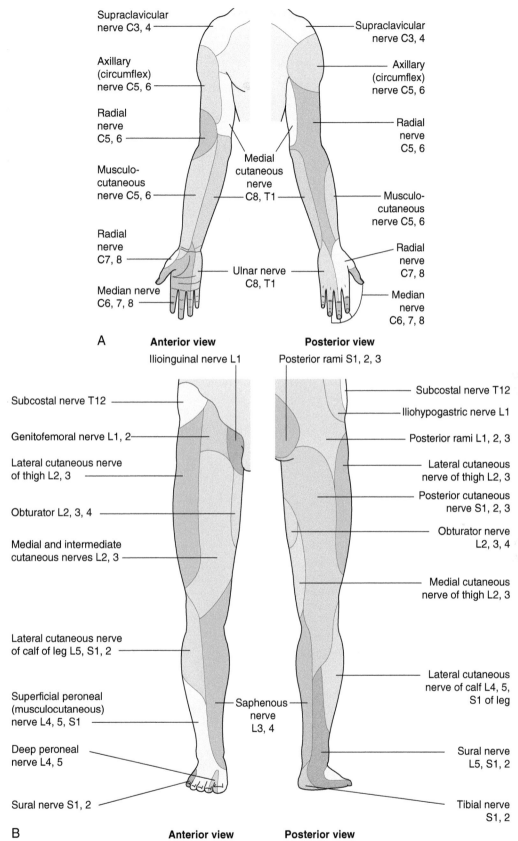

Supraclavicular nerve C3, 4

Axillary (circumflex) nerve C5, 6

Radial nerve C5, 6

Musculo-cutaneous nerve C5, 6

Radial nerve C7, 8

Median nerve C6, 7, 8

Medial cutaneous nerve C8, T1

Ulnar nerve C8, T1

Supraclavicular nerve C3, 4

Axillary (circumflex) nerve C5, 6

Radial nerve C5, 6

Musculo-cutaneous nerve C5, 6

Radial nerve C7, 8

Median nerve C6, 7, 8

A   **Anterior view**   **Posterior view**

Ilioinguinal nerve L1

Posterior rami S1, 2, 3

Subcostal nerve T12

Genitofemoral nerve L1, 2

Lateral cutaneous nerve of thigh L2, 3

Obturator L2, 3, 4

Medial and intermediate cutaneous nerves L2, 3

Lateral cutaneous nerve of calf of leg L5, S1, 2

Superficial peroneal (musculocutaneous) nerve L4, 5, S1

Deep peroneal nerve L4, 5

Sural nerve S1, 2

Saphenous nerve L3, 4

Subcostal nerve T12

Iliohypogastric nerve L1

Posterior rami L1, 2, 3

Lateral cutaneous nerve of thigh L2, 3

Posterior cutaneous nerve S1, 2, 3

Obturator nerve L2, 3, 4

Medial cutaneous nerve of thigh L2, 3

Lateral cutaneous nerve of calf L4, 5, S1 of leg

Sural nerve L5, S1, 2

Tibial nerve S1, 2

B   **Anterior view**   **Posterior view**

Fig. 39.7 (A) The Distribution and Origins of the Cutaneous Nerves of the Arm (Dermatomes); (B) The Distribution and Origins of the Cutaneous Nerves of the Leg (Dermatomes) (Waugh & Grant, 2018).

patients with either a primary presenting problem or comorbidity (other presenting conditions).

Reducing the impact of musculoskeletal orders on a person's quality of life is a significant and important challenge for all healthcare practitioners. NAs can use their insight into a patient's level of abilities to identify additional community help that may be needed.

REFERENCES

Arthritis Care, 2017a. Biologic drugs for rheumatoid arthritis. https://www.arthritiscare.org.uk/do-i-have-arthritis/publications/228-biologic-drugs.

Arthritis Care, 2017b. What causes arthritis? https://www.arthritisresearchuk.org/arthritis-information/conditions/osteoarthritis/causes.aspx.

Arthritis Care, 2018. Protecting your joints. http://www.arthritisresearchuk.org/arthritis-information/daily-life/looking-after-your-joints/protecting-your-joints.aspx.

Arthritis Research UK, 2017. What is rheumatoid arthritis? https://www.arthritisresearchuk.org/arthritis-information/conditions/rheumatoid-arthritis/what-is-rheumatoid-arthritis.aspx.

Arthritis Research UK, 2018a. What is osteoarthritis? https://www.arthritisresearchuk.org/arthritis-information/conditions/osteoarthritis/what-is-osteoarthritis.aspx.

Arthritis Research UK, 2018b. What are the symptoms of rheumatoid arthritis? https://www.arthritisresearchuk.org/arthritis-information/conditions/rheumatoid-arthritis/symptoms.aspx.

Berenbaum, F., 2013. Osteoarthritis as an inflammatory disease (osteoarthritis is not osteoarthrosis!) Osteoarthritis Cartilage 21, 16–21.

Bijlsma, J.W., Berenbaum, F., Lafeber, F.P., 2011. Osteoarthritis: an update with relevance for clinical practice. Lancet 377, 2115–2126.

Bird, H., Green, C., Hamer, A., et al., 2006. Arthritis: Improve your Health, Ease Pain and Live Life to the Full. Dorling Kindersley, London.

British Pain Society, 2015. Understanding and Managing Long-term Pain. https://www.britishpainsociety.org/british-pain-society-publications/patient-publications/.

Cancer Research UK, 2018. Types of pain killers. https://www.cancerresearchuk.org/about-cancer/coping/physically/cancer-and-pain-control/treating-pain/painkillers.

Hameed, K., Akil, M., 2010. Rheumatoid arthritis: Clinical features and diagnosis. In: Adebajo, A. (Ed.), ABC of Rheumatology, fourth ed. Blackwell, Oxford, pp. 71–75.

Health Education England, 2018. Health Careers – explore roles https://www.healthcareers.nhs.uk/eXplore-ROLES.

Health & Safety Executive, 2018. Musculoskeletal disorders (MSDs). http://www.hse.gov.uk/msd/index.htm.

Health & Safety Executive, n.d. Vibration. http://www.hse.gov.uk/msd/index.htm.

Joint Formulary Committee, 2018. British National Formulary (BNF), 20 June 2018. BMJ Publishing/Royal Pharmaceutical Society. https://bnf.nice.org.uk/.

Kraus, V.B., Doherty, M., 2010. Osteoarthritis. In: Adebajo, A. (Ed.), ABC of Rheumatology. John Wiley & Sons (Chapter 9).

Lam, P., Horseman, J., 2002. Overcoming Arthritis. Dorling Kindersley, London.

Maxey, L., Magnuson, J., 2007. Rehabilitation for the Postsurgical Orthopaedic Patient. Mosby Elsevier.

MIMS, 2018. Drug treatment guidelines – June issue. https://www.mims.co.uk (MIMS on-line is free to GPs and nurses – https://www.mims.co.uk/subscribe).

Moots, R., Jones, N., 2004. Your Questions Answered – Rheumatoid Arthritis. Churchill Livingstone, Elsevier.

National Rheumatoid Arthritis Society, 2014. What is RA? https://www.nras.org.uk/what-is-ra-article.

National Rheumatoid Arthritis Society, 2015. Rheumatoid nodules. http://www.nras.org.uk/rheumatoid-nodules.

Nelson, A.E., Allen, K.D., Golightly, Y.M., et al., 2013. A systematic review of recommendations and guidelines for the management of osteoarthritis: The chronic osteoarthritis management initiative of the U.S. Bone and Joint Initiative. Semin. Arthritis Rheum. 43 (6), 701–712.

NHS Choices, 2016a. Arthritis. http://www.nhs.uk/Conditions/Arthritis/Pages/Introduction.aspx.

NHS Choices, 2016b. Recovery – Hip replacement. https://www.nhs.uk/conditions/hip-replacement/recovery/.

NHS Choices, 2018. TENS (transcutaneous electrical nerve stimulation). https://www.nhs.uk/conditions/transcutaneous-electrical-nerve-stimulation-tens/.

NHS England, n.d. Musculoskeletal conditions. https://www.england.nhs.uk/ourwork/ltc-op-eolc/ltc-eolc/our-work-on-long-term-conditions/si-areas/musculoskeletal/.

NICE, 2008. National Institute of Clinical Excellence. Osteoarthritis - National clinical guideline for the care and management of osteoarthritis in adults. Available at: https://www.ncbi.nlm.nih.gov/pubmed/21290638.

NICE, 2014. National Institute for Health and Care Excellence. Osteoarthritis: care and management. Clinical guideline [CG177]. https://www.nice.org.uk/guidance/cg177.

Reed, P., 2005. The medical advisor: Workplace guidelines for disability duration, fifth ed. http://www.dlt.ri.gov/tdi/pdf/Osteoarthritis.pdf.

Stamford Medicine, 2018. Introduction to involuntary movements. https://stanfordmedicine25.stanford.edu/the25/im.html.

Swann, J.I., 2007. Promoting Activity and Independence in Older People. Quay Books, London.

Swann, J.I., 2009. Cervical spondylosis part 1: Osteoarthritis of the cervical spine. British Journal of Healthcare Assistants 3 (2), 81–84.

Vos, T., et al., 2012. Years lived with disability (YLDs) for 1160 sequelae of 289 diseases and injuries 1990–2010: A systematic analysis for the Global Burden of Disease Study 2010. Lancet 380, 2163–2196.

Waugh, A., Grant, A., 2018. Ross & Wilson Anatomy and Physiology in Health and Illness, thirteenth ed. Elsevier, Edinburgh.

World Health Organization, 2016. ICD-10 Version: 2016. http://apps.who.int/classifications/icd10/browse/2016/en#/XIII.

USEFUL ORGANIZATIONS

Arthritis Care
Floor 4,
Linen Court,
10 East Road,
London, N1 6AD
https://www.arthritiscare.org.uk/

Arthritis Research UK
Copeman House, St Mary's Court,
St Mary's Gate
Chesterfield, S41 7TD
https://www.arthritisresearchuk.org

NRAS and Juvenile Idiopathic Arthritis (JIA-at-NRAS)
Ground Floor
4 Switchback Office Park
Gardner Road
Maidenhead
http://www.nras.org.uk
http://www.jia.org.uk/

The British Pain Society
Third Floor
Churchill House
35 Red Lion Square
London, WC1R4SG
https://www.britishpainsociety.org

Abuse May be physical, sexual, emotional or psychological. It may be related to a person's age, ethnicity, gender, sexuality, culture or religion and may be financial, institutional in nature.

Academic referencing Acknowledging the original source you have used both in the body of your work (citation) and also in the reference list.

Accountability To be answerable to yourself and others for your actions.

Acronym An abbreviation formed of the initial letters of other words and then pronounces as a word, i.e. AIDS in an acronym for Acquired Immune Deficiency System.

Activist Someone who involves themselves fully in a new subject, often preferring to learn on the job.

Activities of Living A series of fundamental activities performed by individuals necessary for independent living. The capacity at performing these activities on their own serves as a comparative measure of a patient's independence and determines the level and interventions/assistance required from people or services to achieve each activity.

Acupuncture A method of treating a range of health issues by inserting a number of small needles at strategic points in the body.

Acute conditions These conditions are severe and sudden in onset.

Adherence Adherence literally means a commitment to something. It is used to describe the patient's commitment to a therapeutic intervention, medication for example. Adherence is a term currently used by health professionals as an alternative to the more traditional term compliance. Compliance suggests patients are obliged to follow the instructions of doctors and nurses when in fact they are at liberty to take or reject medical advice.

Adhesions Fibrous bands of scar tissue forming between internal organs and tissues, joining them together abnormally.

Advocacy Pleading a cause on behalf of another, such as a nurse putting forward a case for the better care of a patient or for the patient's desires to be honoured.

Aerosol transmission This occurs when a disease is transmitted via a gaseous suspension of a fine solid or liquid particle.

Agreed ways of working Refers to company policies and procedures.

Alkaline Having a relatively low concentration of hydrogen ions, the opposite to acid.

Amnesia A form of memory loss.

Anaemia Iron deficiency anaemia is caused by a lack of iron, often due to pregnancy or blood loss. It can be treated with prescribed iron tablets and eating iron rich foods. Symptoms can include: tiredness and lack of energy, shortness of breath, pale skin and palpitations. Food rich in iron include: cereals and bread fortified with iron, dark green leafy vegetables, meat and pulses (vitamin C can help the absorption of iron within the body).

Anaesthetic A substance that is used to induce insensitivity to pain.

Anal Fissure An ulcer or tear in the anal canal.

Analgesia An agent (usually pharmacological) that relives pain.

Anaphylactic shock A severe and potentially life-threatening reaction to an allergy. Symptoms can include swollen hands, feet or eyelids, difficulty with breathing and/or collapse and unconsciousness.

Anatomy The science and structure of the body.

Angioedema This is a swelling underneath the skin. It is usually a reaction to a trigger, for example a medication or something the person is allergic to.

Angiogenesis This is a process by which new blood vessel growth is stimulated. To develop beyond a certain size, cancers require oxygen, a blood supply and nutrients. Cancer cells are now known to release chemicals to stimulate vessel growth for this purpose and to continue to grow by developing their own support system.

Angiogram The investigation of the arteries by injecting dye into the blood stream and taking an x-ray so that the internal diameter of the arteries can be viewed.

Ankylosing spondylosis Progressive arthritis that leads to chronic inflammation of the spine and sacroiliac joints. It can also affect other joints and organs in the body, such as the eyes, lungs, kidneys, shoulders, knees, hips, heart and ankles.

Antibiotics These are chemicals that can kill or inhibit the growth of bacteria. They are used to treat bacterial infections.

Antibodies (also known as immunoglobulins, abbreviated Ig) Gamma globulin proteins that are found in blood or other bodily fluids of vertebrates, and are used by the immune system to identify and neutralize foreign objects, such as bacteria and viruses.

Anti-emetic A medicine prescribed to reduce nausea and vomiting.

Antifungal medication Medicine or preparation used to treat fungal infection. There are a number of different antifungal preparations that are used to treat various fungal infections.

Antigen Antigens are proteins found on the surface of foreign invaders or pathogens. These are perceived to be threats by the body which then causes an immune response by producing antibodies to destroy the foreign invader. Human cells have their own antigens which are chemical markers that help the body's cells to identify themselves as 'self' and prevents them from being destroyed.

Anti-psychotic medication A range of medications that are used for some types of mental distress or disorder – can be used to help with severe anxiety.

Anuria Failure of the kidneys to produce urine.

Aorta The main vessel carrying blood away from the heart to the systemic circulation.

Aphakia Absence of the crystalline lens.

Apoptosis Also known as 'programmed cell death'. This process involves a series of intracellular chemical and biological events designed to end the cells life when the cell is old, or when errors are detected.

Appendicular skeleton Bones of the arms and legs.

Appraisal A formal assessment, typically in an interview, of the performance of an employee over a particular period.

Appropriate polypharmacy Concerns the prescribing for a person who has complex conditions or for multiple conditions in those circumstances where medicines use has been improved and where the medicines are prescribed aligned to the best available evidence.

Arthritis and arthropathies Disease(s) affecting joints.

Aspiration A medical term that refers to sucking in a fluid, inhaling of food or fluid into the airways.

Astrocyte The most numerous and diverse neuroglial cells in the CNS.

Atelectasis The collapse of alveoli and small airways.

Atmosphere The air we breathe is an assortment of gases, which are collectively referred to as the atmosphere.

Autocracy Absolute power or control.

Autonomy Independence or self-governance.

Axial skeleton The part of the skeleton that consists of the bones of the head and trunk of a vertebrate.

Axilla The arm pit (axillae two armpits).

Bacillus A genus (group) of rod-shaped bacteria.

Back bench MPs Members of Parliament (MPs) who do not hold ministerial office (the vast majority of MPs) as opposed to Government Ministers and Opposition Shadow Ministers who are known as 'front bench MPs'. The Conservative Party has a Parliamentary organization known as the 1922 Committee that comprises all Conservative back bench MPs.

Basal Metabolic Rate (BMR) The base line energy requirement for the minimal activity of all tissue cells of the body under steady state conditions i.e. just for breathing, blood circulation and tissue repair. Measured in a state of starvation (i.e. 12 hours without eating) so that digestion and absorption does not influence it and in a subject in a state of physical and mental relaxation.

Benchmark A reference standard or basis for comparison.

Bereavement The state of having suffered a loss by death.

Bilateral On both sides.

Biopsy A sample of tissue taken from the body in order to examine it more closely.

Blog This is usually a regularly updated website or web page, often written by an individual. Traditionally these were written in a very informal way; however, more often the blog is used as an assessment tool in universities.

Body Mass Index (BMI) in kg/m² A weight for height indicator. A simple measure that is used as part of nutritional screening tools to classify adults as underweight, overweight or obese.

$$\text{Adult BMI} = \frac{\text{weight in kg}}{(\text{height in m}^2)}$$

Bone marrow Bone marrow is found within the larger bones of the human body. It is a sponge-like substance that can change shape and be mouldable. Its purpose is to produce all three blood cells as lymphocytes, which support the immune system. It's very rich in nutrients, and is even eaten by humans and animals in various cultures.

Boolean logic A type of search using a combination of the words 'and', 'or' or 'not' to achieve a more refined search result.

Bouchard's nodes Osteophytes on the proximal interphalangeal joints. Named after a nineteenth-century pathologist.

Bradycardia An abnormally low heart rate of less than 60 beats per minute.

'Brexit' Brexit is an abbreviation of 'British exit' used to describe the withdrawal of the UK from the European Union.

British National Formulary (BNF) The most widely used source of medicines management information in UK healthcare.

Bursitis Inflammation of the bursa (sac containing synovial fluid that cushions bone).

Cancer staging This is about the size, grade and/or extent (spread) of the primary tumour and whether or not the cancer has spread to another site in the body.

Candour Being honest, open, transparent and frank.

Cannula A thin tube usually inserted into a vein can be inserted into a body cavity to administer medication, drain off fluid, or insert a surgical instrument.

Carcinogen Any substance or radiation that interacts with cellular development and promotes carcinogenesis, the formation of cancer.

Carcinogenesis A process where an accumulation of steps and cellular changes can result in the development of a cancer.

Cardiovascular disease Includes all the diseases of the heart and circulation including coronary heart disease, angina, heart attack, congenital heart disease and stroke. Also known as heart and circulatory disease.

Cartilage A type of connective tissue that contains collagen and elastic fibres. This strong tough material on the bone-ends helps to distribute the load within the joint; the slippery surface allows smooth movement between the bones. Cartilage can withstand both tension and compression.

Cauterization Coagulating blood by the use of heat, cold or chemicals.

Cerebral oedema An abnormal increase in cerebral volume and is one of the secondary complications for patients with traumatic brain injury causing neurological deterioration.

Cerebral spinal fluid Liquid around the brain and spinal cord. The fluid is made by a group of cells, called the choroid plexus, that are deep inside the brain.

Charles Bonnet syndrome People experiencing hallucinations as part of their ocular disease.

Chemotherapy The word chemotherapy literally means 'drug treatment'. It has however come to mean a treatment of cancer by using anti-cancer medicines called cytotoxic medicines (also known as cytotoxic drugs).

Cholangitis Inflammation of the gall bladder.

Chondropathies Disease of the cartilage.

Chromosome In the nucleus within a cell there are 23 pairs of chromosomes which are made of long DNA molecules.

Chronic Long-standing condition.

Chronic alcohol abuse Excessive consumption of alcohol over a long period increases the risk of liver damage, pancreatitis, cancer, neuropathy, diabetes gastrointestinal problems, immune system dysfunction, osteoporosis, heart disease, accidents and injuries. It can affect relationships and employment.

Chronic colonization The repeated presence of a bacteria in a wound which does not usually interfere with healing.

Chronic conditions A condition or disease that is persistent or otherwise long-lasting in its effects or a disease that comes with time.

Chronic obstructive pulmonary disease This is an umbrella term used to describe progressive lung diseases. This disease is characterized by increasing breathlessness.

Cilia Small hair-like structures found on the outer surface of some cells. Cilia vibrate and this causes movement in any fluids covering them.

Clinical pharmacists Professionals who hold a qualification in pharmacology and have experience of working within the healthcare setting. Responsible for dispensing medicines in a quality controlled and safe environment, they can monitor the use of drugs and ensure that where necessary, prescriptions are integrated into care plans. They provide a key role within the general practice and other health care settings to help answer day to day medicine questions from the public and the healthcare team. They can meet with and treat patients directly, helping those with long term conditions manage their medications, and provide ongoing health checks such as blood pressure monitoring.

Clinical supervision The formal process of professional support and learning which enables practitioners to enhance their personal and professional development and competence.

Closed questions Closed questions are those whereby the patient may only respond with a yes or no answer. For example: 'do you feel well today?'

Clostridium difficile Also known as *C. difficile* or 'C. diff.' It is a bacterium that can infect the bowel and cause diarrhoea.

Cognitive Behavioural Therapy (CBT) A talking therapy, which aims to help individuals manage and cope with problems by changing the way they think and deal with situations.

Command Papers Documents that the Government, by Royal command, presents to Parliament for consideration.

Commensal bacteria Bacteria that do no harm to the organism that they inhabit.

Commensals Two living species that are living in close association with each other.

Competence Refers to what individuals know or are able to do in terms of knowledge, skills and attitudes.

Compression bandage A system of layered bandaging which applies levels of pressure to the leg in order to improve circulation.

Conceptualization Forming ideas based on the experience and literature surrounding the subject.

Concussion A diffuse brain injury often resulting in a short loss of consciousness at the time of impact and loss of memory for a short time after the injury. There is no structural damage seen on CT scan.

Confidentiality Protecting personal information. This could include information about patients' life, family, care and treatments, which they would want to keep private.

Conjunctivitis An inflammation or redness of the lining of the white part of the eye and the underside of the eyelid.

Consent This is a voluntary agreement to another person's proposition; where by the person agrees to an act or proposal of another person.

Continuing professional development The way in which a worker continues to learn and develop throughout their careers, keeping their skills and knowledge up to date and ensuring they can work safely and effectively.

Controlled drugs (CDs) Examples: morphine, diamorphine, dexamphetamine and fentanyl.

Contusion The medical term for bruising and consists of areas of haemorrhage, swelling and infarct in the brain, following significant impact often affecting the frontal and temporal lobes.

Copulation Engaging in sexual intercourse.

Coronary artery bypass graft (CABG) A surgical procedure which attempts to restore good blood flow to the heart. A functional cardiac artery is either manipulated to supply blood to a poorly circulated area or a leg vein is used to replace a damaged artery in the heart.

Cor pulmonale Cor pulmonale is the enlargement of the right ventricle as a result of a respiratory disorder.

Cortex Refers to an outer sector.

Costochondritis Inflammation of the cartilage that joins the ribs to the sternum.

Crepitus Creaking, grinding noise.

CRP C-reactive protein – a blood test.

Cryotherapy Treatment using low temperature. Usually refers to the removal of skin lesions by freezing them. The most common product used is liquid nitrogen.

Culture Cultures are medical tests to determine the presence of bacteria growing in bodily fluids, such as blood, sputum, pus and urine.

Cyanosis A bluish hue or tinge visible on the lips and mouth that occurs when arterial oxygen levels are abnormally low.

Cyst An abnormal sac in the body containing a liquid or semi solid substance.

Cytokines Small proteins that act as chemical messengers.

Cytotoxic Toxic to cells. Chemotherapy is drug treatment which is designed to kill cells.

Databases Where data (information) is held in a computer for the purpose of being searched.

Defibrillation A process in which an electronic device sends an electric shock to the heart to stop a very fast, irregular heartbeat and restores normal heart rhythm.

Dehydration This is a condition that results when the body loses more water than it takes in. This imbalance disturbs the usual levels of salts and sugars present in the blood (homeostasis), which can interfere with the way the body functions.

Dentition The number, the type, the arrangement of the teeth.

Dermatologist A medically qualified practitioner who has gone on to specialize in medicine and then further specialize in the diagnosis and treatment of skin disease.

Dermatomes Sensory distribution of a nerve.

DESMOND An acronym which stands for Diabetes Education and Self-Management for Ongoing and Newly Diagnosed people with type 2 diabetes. It is structured and is offered to groups of people with diabetes.

Diagnosis The identification of the nature of an illness or other problem by examination and consideration of the signs and symptoms.

Diaphoresis Profuse or excessive sweating.

Diastole The time period when the heart is in a state of relaxation and dilatation (expansion).

Diathermy A technique involving the production of heat in a part of the body by high-frequency electric currents, to stimulate circulation, ease pain, destroy unhealthy tissue, or cause bleeding vessels to clot.

Differential diagnosis The process of differentiating between two or more conditions which share similar signs or symptoms.

Differentiation The process whereby cells acquire and demonstrate their structural and functional characteristics.

Diffusion The passive movement of molecules or ions from a region of high pressure or concentration to an area of low pressure or concentration until a state of equilibrium is achieved.

Digital Primary Care The move to a paper-free and digital record management has been pioneered within GP practice. Patients can book appointments, request repeat prescriptions and engage with information on line. Patients can utilize online access to elements of their GP held records.

Dilation In the case of eyes refers to making the pupil wider. Instillation of a drug via an eye drop is used to dilate the pupil.

DNA The blueprint containing all the instructions needed for building proteins which tell our cells what to do to build, grow and maintain the human body. DNA is necessary for cell division.

Dorsopathies Conditions affecting the spine.

Dyschezia Difficulty in defaecating, painful defaecation.

Dysphagia Difficulty in swallowing.

Dyspnoea Difficult or laboured breathing.

Dysuria Painful or difficult urination.

Echocardiogram (Echo) An echocardiogram is a test used to assess the heart using ultrasound. A transthoracic echocardiogram is carried out by passing ultrasound waves through the wall of the chest. A transoesophageal echocardiogram is carried out by passing a probe down the patient's oesophagus and sending ultrasound waves to the heart from behind.

Elective admission An elective admission is one that is planned with a pre-arranged date for the delivery of healthcare. The patient is aware of the time and venue, the area of specialty, who will provide their care and how to prepare for their admission in advance.

Electrocardiograph (ECG) The electrocardiograph is a test that looks at the electrical activity of the heart. The ECG is a quick and painless test and can be carried out at the GP surgery or at the hospital.

Electrocoagulation Coagulation of tissue by means of an electric current.

Emesis The sudden expulsion of the gastric contents also known as vomiting.

Emollients These are moisturizing treatments that are applied directly to the skin to soothe and hydrate it. They cover the skin with a protective film and trap in moisture.

Emotional and psychological trauma Emotional and psychological trauma is the result of extraordinarily stressful events that negatively impacts on a person's sense of security, making the person feel helpless.

Empathy Being able to correctly acknowledge the emotional state of another person without experiencing that state oneself, the ability to understand the feelings of another.

Empowerment The participation in decision-making processes in an equal and fair fashion.

Endocrine Glands that release hormones into the blood or other bodily fluids.

Endogenous Originating from within an organism, in instances of endogenous opiates from within the human body.

Energy Energy is derived from the metabolism of carbohydrate, protein and fat. The amount of energy is released as kilocalories (kcals). Fat is the most energy dense nutrient, with carbohydrate and protein providing less than half of this amount of energy.

Enteral nutrition The delivery of nutrients in liquid form directly into the stomach, duodenum or jejunum delivered via a tube or stoma.

Enzyme A protein-based biological catalyst. Enzymes are chemicals found in living systems that alter the rates of chemical reactions and are responsible for drug metabolism.

Epidemiology The study of the distribution and determinants of health-related states or events (this also includes disease) as well as the application of this study in order to control diseases and other health problems.

Epidural Local anaesthetic is injected into the space outside the dura mater of the spinal cord in the lower back region to produce loss of sensation especially in the abdomen or pelvic region.

Epithelium A layer of tissue that lines the outer body and the hollow structures of the body, it is made up of several types of epithelial cells.

Ergonomics The study of people in their working environment.

Erythrocyte Red blood cells. Erythro meaning 'pertaining to red' and cyte meaning 'cell'.

ESR Erythrocyte sedimentation rate – a blood test.

Excoriation Abrading or wearing off of the skin.

Exocrine Glands that secrete chemicals through a duct into an external space.

Expiratory Related to the act of breathing out.

Facet joint A vertebral joint.

Fever A fever is the body's response to fighting infection. An infection causes the release of pyrogens which act on the hypothalamus and release prostaglandins. This resets the internal temperature to a higher level to help fight the bacteria. It also helps support the immune system in fighting the infection.

Fibrin A protein essential for clotting.

Flail chest A life-threatening condition that arises when a section of rib cage becomes detached from the chest wall. Flail chest is normally caused by trauma.

Fracture Also referred to as a break in a bone.

Fragility fracture Results from mechanical forces that would not ordinarily result in fracture called 'low-level' or 'low-energy' trauma, quantified by the World Health Organization as forces equivalent to a fall from a standing height or less.

French gauge The external circumference of a tube measured in millimetres.

Fructose A type of sugar (provides energy).

Gait A manner of walking, stepping or running.

Gaiter area The area extending from just below the ankle to below the knee.

Gametes These are the sex cells. The male gametes are the sperm, and the female gametes are the eggs.

Gender Refers to the socially constructed characteristics of women and men, for example, norms, roles and relationships of and between groups of women and men.

General Sales List (GSL) Medicines Examples: paracetamol 500mg tablets (pack of 8 or 16), Rennie® indigestion tablets and Ibuprofen 200mg tablets (pack of 8 or 16).

Genitalia The male or female reproductive organs.

Gland There are a number of glands all over the body; they have a variety of functions. Some glands make substances that are released, such as saliva or sweat, some produce milk (the mammary glands). Other glands release hormones; they are part of the endocrine system.

Grief An emotional reaction to loss.

Guarding Physical symptom of acute abdominal pain. The muscles of the abdomen go into spasm and become tense, protecting the tender tissues underneath from being disturbed.

Gynaecologist A doctor who specializes in the diagnosis of disorders of the female genital tract and reproductive systems.

Haematocrit The haematocrit (HCT) (also known by several other names including packed cell volume (PCV)) is the volume percentage of red blood cells in blood. It is normally 45% for men and 40% for women.

Haematoma A solid swelling of clotted blood within the tissues – a bruise.

Haemoglobin (Hb) A protein consisting of globin and four haem groups that is found within erythrocytes. It is the primary transporter of oxygen.

Haemoptysis Coughing up blood.

Haemorrhagic diathesis A condition in which there is an unusual susceptibility to predisposition to bleeding.

Half-life The rate of destruction and elimination of a circulating hormone. The shorter the half-life the quicker the hormone levels in the blood will drop once the production of the hormone decreases.

Handler Anyone who is involved in the moving and handing of a patient. The focus of this text is the Nursing Associate but it could be anyone in the multidisciplinary team.

Harm Includes ill treatment (including sexual abuse, exploitation and forms of ill treatment which are not physical); the impairment of health (physical or mental) or development (physical, intellectual, emotional, social or behavioural); self-harm and neglect; unlawful conduct which adversely affects a person's property, rights or interests (for example, financial abuse).

Health education Health education is any combination of learning experiences that have been designed to assist individuals and communities improve their health, this is done by increasing knowledge or influencing attitudes.

Health Education England A public body in England responsible for leadership, on a national level, with regards to training and education within the NHS in England. HEE aims to deliver a better healthcare workforce that is skilled, has the right values and behaviours and delivers care at the right time and in the right place.

Health promotion This is the process of enabling people to increase control over, and to improve, their health.

Heberden's nodes Osteophytes on the distal interphalangeal joints of the hand. Named after a nineteenth-century British Physician.

Histology The anatomical, microscopic study of tissues.

HLA-DR4 A protein on the surface of leucocytes (white blood cells).

Holistic nursing Holistic nursing will focus on the whole health of the patient, as opposed to treating the symptoms of their illness or condition. The patient's environment and mental health are taken into consideration when the Nursing Associate offers care to a person for any reason. The holistic nursing philosophy believes that the patient should not be treated as the sum total of their symptoms, but as a person in need of overall healing.

Homeostasis The tendency of the body to seek and maintain a condition of balance or equilibrium within its internal environment, even when faced with external changes.

Hospice Hospice is both a distinct nursing practice area as well as a philosophy of care for the dying person and their families. It focuses on symptom control and comfort measures as opposed to a cure, and a team approach to meeting the expressed needs of the patient and the family is utilized.

Human papilloma virus (HPV) This is the name for a group of viruses that affect the skin and the moist membranes lining the body.

Humidification The process of making air damp or moist.

Hyfrecation This is where alternating electric current at various voltages is passed through the skin, generating heat and destroying the skin growth.

Hyperextension Extension beyond normal limits.

Hyperkeratosis Hyperkeratosis is thickening of the stratum corneum (the outermost layer of the epidermis), this is often associated with the presence of an abnormal amount of keratin and is also usually accompanied by an increase in the granular layer.

Hypertension High blood pressure (hypertension) is a blood pressure that is or over 140/90 mm Hg each time it is taken, that is, it is sustained at this level.

Hypertrophic scars These are the result of excess collagen being produced at the site of a wound. Hypertrophic scars are red and raised to begin with, prior to becoming flatter and paler over the course of several years.

Hyperventilation Increased respiration rate associated with increased ventilation – increased amounts of air entering the alveoli.

Hyposensitivity Is a lessened or delayed reaction to an allergen in order to minimize or ideally stop signs and symptoms to an allergen.

Hypotension Low blood pressure is a blood pressure that is much lower than usual. It is often defined as systolic blood pressure less than 90 mm Hg or diastolic less than 60 mm Hg.

Hypoventilation Decreased ventilation – lack of air entering the alveoli.

Hypovolaemia Decreased blood volume.

Hypoxia The term used to describe a reduction of oxygen supply at the tissue level or where blood flow to the tissue is not adequate to meet tissue needs.

Ileostomy An artificial opening in the lower abdomen through which part of the bowel evacuates faeces.

Immotile Not capable of moving spontaneously, not moving, lacking the ability to move.

Immunosuppressant agents Medications that reduce the activity of the immune system.

Inclusion Ensuring that people are treated equally and fairly and are included as part of society.

Incubation The incubation period is the time between catching an infection and symptoms appearing. Incubation periods vary, depending on the type of infection.

Induction In relation to human resources this is the initial introduction to work that employees receive. The length is determined by local employers and varies both in length and delivery.

Infarction The reduction of blood supply to a part of the body leading to tissue death.

Information resources An information resource is a resource that provides information – this can be a person, book, journal, recording, video, database or the internet.

Informed consent An agreement to do something or to allow something to happen only after all the relevant facts are disclosed. Informed consent often refers to consent to a medical procedure after the patient has been made aware of all the risks and consequences.

Inspiratory Related to the act of breathing in.

Integrated care Co-ordinated health and social care that is planned and organised around the needs and preferences of the individual, their carers and family. Integration may extend to other services, for example housing, that can offer holistic approaches to address individual circumstances.

Internet search engine An internet search engine is system software that is designed to extract information from the World Wide Web.

Interprofessional A collective term for a team of two or more professions in healthcare, also known as the multidisciplinary team.

Intervertebral discs Act as shock absorbers. A disc is composed of a sturdy collagen exterior and an inner gel-like core.

Intracranial pressure (ICP) A rise in pressure around the brain. It may be due to an increase in the amount of fluid surrounding the brain, for example, there may be an increased amount of cerebrospinal fluid or an increase in blood in the brain as result of injury or a ruptured tumor.

Intravenous Injected directly into a vein.

Introspection Self-examination, reflection.

Intubation The process of inserting a tube, called an endotracheal tube, often through the mouth and then into the airway.

Ischaemia Reduced blood supply to tissue and organs, especially the heart.

Isthmus A piece or strip of tissue connecting two larger parts.

Jargon Terminology used by a profession that is not readily understood by the general population.

Jaundice A yellowish discolouration of the skin, mucous membranes and of the white of the eyes caused by elevated levels of the chemical bilirubin in the blood.

Joint margins Outer edge of joint.

Kilopascal (kPa) 1000 pascals. A pascal is an SI (International System) unit measure of internal pressure. 1 kPa is the equivalent of approx. 7.5 millimetres of mercury (mmHg).

Kinaesthetic A tactile approach to learning; a hands-on approach.

Kyphosis More than 50 degrees of forward curvature of the cervical region.

L4/L5 Vertebrae in the lower back.

Last offices The term relates to the care given to a body after death. It is a process that demonstrates respect for the deceased, focused on respecting their religious and cultural beliefs.

Law The system of rules which a given region, country or community recognizes as governing and regulating the actions of its members and which it may enforce by the imposition of penalties.

Law Lords Senior judges who sit in the House of Lords as Lords Judiciary. When functioning as judges, these peers acted as the highest court of appeal in the UK.

Learning inventories This term describes a profile of your preferred method of learning.

Lesion Any structural change in a bodily part resulting from injury or disease, an injury or a wound.

Lethargy A lack of energy or vigour.

Leucopenia A deficiency of white blood cells in circulation.

Ligament A short tough band of flexible fibrous tissue providing support to bone or other structures, such as the uterus.

Ligation Tying off a blood vessel to stop blood flow.

Load bearing joints Lower spine, hips, knees, ankles and base of the big toe.

Lordosis Inward curvature of the lower back – 'sway back'.

Lymphadenopathy Lymphadenopathy refers to inflammation and enlargement of a lymph node near to the site of an infection. This swelling of the lymph node is due to an increase in the number of lymphocytes within the node which causes engorgement and fluid retention within the node which is palpable on examination.

Maceration This is the softening and breaking down of skin resulting from prolonged exposure to moisture. It is caused by excessive amounts of fluid remaining in contact with the skin or the surface of a wound for extended periods.

Magnetic resonance imaging (MRI) MRI uses a strong magnetic field to 'charge' and influence atoms in tissues, causing them to rapidly spin and behave like atomic magnets. The MRI then records how quickly these atomic magnets return to their normal position. An immune reaction, damaged tissue or swelling affects the speed at which this happens. The MRI image or scan created will show where structures/cells are different from normal.

Makaton A language programme that uses signs and symbols to help people to communicate.

Mastectomy Surgical removal of the breast.

Means testing An official assessment based on how much income a person has in order to determine if they should receive money or services from the government.

Meiosis Involves specifically the reproduction of spermatozoa and ova in embryonic formation.

Meninges Outer covering of the brain and spinal cord consisting of three layers, the pia, arachnoid and dura mater.

Menisci Thin, fibrous cartilage that cushions and protects the knee joint.

Menorrhagia Excessively prolonged or profuse menstruation.

Menses Also known as menstruation, the monthly shedding of the lining of the uterus.

Mental capacity A person's ability to make their own decisions. In relation to health and social care, this means the ability to accept or reject medical/nursing advice and therapeutic input.

Mentor Also so known as supervisors, a nurse who is registered and able to teach and assess Nursing Associates in the clinical area.

Metabolism The process by which the body converts what is eaten and drunk into energy. It is a complex biochemical processes where calories in food and drinks are combined with oxygen to release the energy the body needs to function.

Metastases Secondary cancer sites, caused by metastasis – the spread of cancer from its primary or original site.

Metastatic cancer or a metastasis A cancer that has spread from the part of the body where it started (the primary site) to other parts of the body. The plural is metastases. This is sometimes referred to as 'secondary cancer'.

Midline shift A term used to describe a shift of the midline of the brain (diagnosed from CT scan) where it is no longer in the centre and is the result of pushing or pulling forces from an abnormality in the brain and this causes raised ICP.

Miosis Excessive constriction of the pupils of the eye.

Mitosis The process by which most human cells divide (parent cells) and replicate to make exact copies of themselves (resulting in daughter cells). This is when cancers can form due to mutations occurring within replication.

Monosyllabic Words having only one syllable, such as the word 'no'.

Morbidity Refers to having a disease or a symptom of disease, or to the amount of disease within a population.

Mortality Mortality means death. Mortality data indicates numbers of deaths by place, time and cause.

Motivational interviewing This is a client centered approach to enhancing an individual's intrinsic motivation by encouraging the person to explore and resolve uncertainty. The approach is used by clinicians to support people as they adopt new behaviors.

MRSA *Staphylococcus aureus* bacterium which is resistant to certain antibiotics and can cause life-threatening infections.

Mucoid Mucus, secretions of the glands such as cervical secretion.

Mucopurulent Marked by an exudate (a type of fluid) containing mucus and pus.

Multi-disciplinary team A group of healthcare professionals with different expertise, knowledge and training who are all involved in the care of a patient. In some instances anyone involved in the patient experience, for example, patient, family member, can also be described as a member of the multi-disciplinary team.

Multiple sclerosis A progressive autoimmune neurological condition affecting the myelin sheath surrounding the nerve resulting in loss of nerve conductivity. Movements are affected and sensory problems often occur.

Myelinated A nerve cell having a myelin sheath.

Myocardial infarction Also called a 'heart attack' myocardial infarction is the irreversible death of heart muscle due to a prolonged lack of oxygen supply to the heart.

Myocardium Specialized heart muscle.

Myotomes Muscular distribution of a nerve.

Narrative A spoken (story) or written account of events.

National Insurance Contributions People over the age of 16 who are working or self employed pay a contribution from their earnings to enable entitlement to a variety of benefits, including the basic state pension and access to healthcare.

Negligence Negligence is the breach of a legal duty of care owed to one person by another which results in damage being caused to the first person by the second person.

Nephrotoxic drugs Drugs that are toxic to the nephron and should be used with caution in patients who have problems with their kidneys.

Neutropenia A deficiency of neutrophils (white blood cells) in circulation.

Nitric oxide Nitric oxide (NO) is produced by a number of cells in the body; its production by vascular endothelium is particularly important in the regulation of blood flow.

Non-myelinated A nerve cell in which there is no myelin sheath surrounding its axon.

Non-steroidal anti-inflammatory drugs (NSAIDs) These drugs include ibuprofen, naproxen and diclofenac. These can affect the blood flow to the glomerular and should be avoided if chronic kidney disease is present.

Normal flora Microorganisms that are always present on or in a person and usually do not cause any disease.

Nucleic acid amplification tests A type of test. Technology that is used in the routine diagnosis of Chlamydia trachomatis infections.

Nursing process A scientific method used by nurses to ensure the quality of patient care. This approach is broken down into five separate steps: Assessment, Diagnosing, Planning, Implementation and Evaluation.

Obesity The state of being overweight. A person is defined as being obese when their Body Mass Index (BMI) is over 25.

Objective measurement Measurement that is based on observable fact, for example, the patient's pulse rate is 76 beats per minute.

Objective Structured Clinical Examination (OSCE) An assessment or examination that assesses a student's performance and competency practically.

Objectivity Accounts from the nurse should be factual and not include personal opinions or interpretations. Data is observed (e.g. swelling, redness) or measured (e.g. vital signs, BMI) as well as provide a description of interventions and patient responses to these.

Obstetrics The branch of medicine and surgery that is concerned with childbirth and the care of women giving birth.

Oliguria The term used when urine output is below 0.5mL/kg/hr.

Open questions Open questions are used to encourage the patient to share thoughts, ideas or feelings, promoting discussion between the patient and the nurse. For example: 'how are you feeling today?'

Opioid analgesics Opioids such as morphine are a group of medicines derived from the opium poppy that are commonly used to relieve pain. Other examples include buprenorphine, codeine, diamorphine (heroin) and oxycodone.

Opportunistic infection An opportunistic infection is one that is caused by a microbe that would not normally cause disease in the healthy individual. However, due to the weakened immune system, the microbes are able to take the 'opportunity' to cause disease i.e. become pathogenic.

Opsonisation Opsonisation is a process undertaken by the immune system whereby which foreign cells are coated with a substance to make them more readily accessible to phagocytosis.

Optometrist A healthcare practitioner who is qualified to examine the eyes, prescribe and supply spectacles and contact lenses also called an 'ophthalmic optician'. The optometrist is trained to recognise abnormalities and conditions such as cataracts or glaucoma, and will refer a patient to a GP or a hospital eye clinic for further investigations.

Optometry The study of the eye to detect and prevent defects in vision, ocular disease, eye injury and signs of deterioration in general health such as diabetes and hypertension.

ORIF Open Reduction Internal Fixation refers to a surgical procedure to fix a severe bone fracture. 'Open reduction' means surgery is needed to realign the bone fracture into the normal position. 'Internal fixation' refers to the steel rods, screws, or plates used to keep the bone fracture stable in order to heal the right way and prevent infection.

Osmotic pressure The pressure created by the solutes in a liquid that prevents water from crossing a semipermeable barrier into another area.

Osteoarthritis Degeneration of joint surface.

Osteomyelitis An infection of the bone.

Osteopathy A method of investigating and treating a range of health issues by stretching, manipulating and massaging muscles.

Osteophytes New bone growth.

Osteoporosis Reduced bone density.

Oxygen saturation A term referring to the fraction of oxygen-rich haemoglobin relative to total haemoglobin in the blood. Normal blood oxygen levels are considered 95-100 percent.

Palliate To alleviate or relieve.

Palliative care Palliative care interventions are designed to optimize the patient's ability to live as active and complete a life as possible until their death. A key aspect of palliative care is to alleviate symptoms and maximize quality of life.

Palpitations The feeling of the heartbeat in the chest. The patient may report a fluttering or pounding sensation.

Pancreatitis Inflammation of the pancreas.

Paralytic ileus Obstruction of the intestine due to paralysis of the intestinal muscles. Failure of appropriate forward movement of bowel contents.

Parenteral nutrition (PN) A method of providing nutritional support to an individual whose gastrointestinal tract is not able to absorb sufficient nutrients or is inaccessible. Nutrients are delivered straight into the circulatory system via a dedicated venous catheter.

Parietal Referring to or denoting the wall of the body or of a body cavity or hollow structure.

Parkinsonism Impairment of area of the brain that produces dopamine resulting in symptoms identical to Parkinson disease, but caused by a specific reason e.g. drug overdose, brain trauma.

Parliament The legislature of the UK consisting of the sovereign (monarch), the House of Lords (peers) and the House of Commons (MPs).

Patch In relation to medication a patch impregnated with anaesthesia or strong painkillers.

Pathogen Any disease-producing agent or microorganism.

Pathophysiology The functional changes that occur as a result of a disease or syndrome, the physiology of abnormal states.

Patient Advocate An individual who can verbalize the views or needs of a patient on their behalf.

Perioperative This refers to the three phases of surgery: preoperative, intraoperative and postoperative. The goal of perioperative care is to provide better conditions for patients before operation, during operation and after operation.

Peripheral neuropathy A common side effect of chemotherapy, where the patient experiences tingling and numbness to the fingers and toes.

Peristalsis The wave-like muscular contraction of the digestive tract or other tubular structures (for example, ductus deferens; the fallopian tubes) when their contents are propelled forward.

Personal Development Plan Records information such as agreed objectives for development, proposed activities to meet those objectives and timescales for review.

Person-centred care Care that puts the individual at the centre of their support and goal planning. It takes account the individual's needs, priorities, strengths and preferences. The individual is seen as an equal partner in decisions about their care, to ensure that their needs are met.

Peyronie's disease A condition characterized by a curved penis; the cause is unknown. Thick scar tissue develops and causes the penis to bend.

Phacoemulsification This is technique of extra capsular cataract extraction in which the nucleus of the lens is removed by ultrasonic vibrations and aspirated though a small incision. The outer layers of the lens are retained still attached to the ciliary body. It is in this 'bag' that the new lens is placed.

Pharmacovigilance The ongoing monitoring of the effectiveness and safety of medicines.

Pharmacy (P) Medicines Examples: Small packs of co-codamol 8mg/500mg (paracetamol and codeine combined in one tablet), omeprazole 10mg and mebendazole tablets.

Pheromones Chemicals secreted or excreted triggering a social response in members of the same species.

Philosophy of nursing A philosophy of nursing is a statement that sometimes is written, declaring beliefs, values and ethics regarding the care and treatment of patients.

Physiology The study of normal function in living creatures.

Plagiarism Taking someone else's work and submitting that work as if it is your own without proper referencing or acknowledgement.

Pleura Protective covering of outside of the lungs and lining of the chest cavity.

Pleurisy Inflammation of the pleura.

Pneumotaxic Refers to the regulation of respiratory rate.

Pneumothorax A fully or partially collapsed lung.

Policy A course or principle of action adopted or proposed by an organization.

Polyarthropathies Multiple joint disorders.

Polycystic kidney disease This is an inherited condition in which clusters of cysts develop primarily within the kidneys.

Polymorphic light eruption This is a fairly common skin rash that is exacerbated by exposure to sunlight or artificial ultraviolet (UV) light.

Portfolio A document which contains supportive evidence of professional competencies, accomplishments and skills.

Potassium Potassium is an essential electrolyte that plays an important part in the contracting of skeletal and cardiac muscle cells. It aids transmission of nerve impulses and has an important part in the management of acid-base balance.

Pragmatist A person who approaches things practically and is very focused.

Prescription Only Medicines (POM) A prescription medication is a licensed medicine that is regulated by law to necessitate a medical prescription before it can be obtained, examples include, amoxicillin, ramipril, amlodipine and propranolol.

Prevalence The proportion of a population who have (or had) a specific characteristic in a given time period, usually an illness, a condition or a risk factor such as depression or smoking.

Problematic polypharmacy describes The prescribing of multiple medicines in an inappropriate manner, or where the intended benefit of the medicines are not realized.

Profession A paid occupation which requires specialized knowledge and education.

Prognosis A prediction or an opinion about how someone will recover from an illness or injury.

Proliferate (or proliferation) The rapid increase of something, for example, cancer cells.

Proofreading To read through your work and check and correct errors.

Prophylactic A medicine or course of action used to prevent disease or complications from a condition.

Prostaglandins Lipid compounds that play an important role in inflammation.

Prosthesis An artificial substitute for a missing part, used for functional or cosmetic reasons, or both.

Protocols Also known as 'standard procedures'.

Proto-oncogenes A gene that is involved in normal cell growth. Mutations (changes) in a proto-oncogene may cause it to become an oncogene, which can cause the growth of cancer cells.

Proton pump inhibitors (PPIs) Proton pump inhibitors (PPIs) are a group of medications that are commonly used to treat indigestion, heartburn and peptic ulcers. Common examples include esomeprazole, omeprazole and lansoprazole.

Pruritus Itchy and irritable skin.

Pseudostratified ciliated columnar epithelium Covering or lining of the internal body surface that contains cilia and mucus secreting goblet cells.

Public Bills Public Bills change the law as it applies to the general population and are the most common type of Bill introduced in Parliament. Government ministers propose the majority of Public Bills.

Public health An approach to health that aims to promote and protect the health and well-being of the population by preventing ill health and prolonging life through education, policy making, and research for disease and injury prevention.

Public interest In certain circumstances the rights of confidentiality of a person may be overruled to protect the wider population from potential harm.

Pulmonary circulation The blood vessels carrying blood around the lungs.

Pulmonary embolism Sudden blockage of blood flow through the lungs due to a clot.

Pulmonary rehabilitation Pulmonary rehabilitation is a programme of support, education and exercise devised to enhance breathing and well-being.

Pulse oximetry A non-invasive method for monitoring a person's oxygen saturation. Usually, a glove-like probe is attached to a finger. Light sensors within the probe detect how much oxygen is in the blood based on the way the light passes through the finger.

Pupillary response This is a physiological response that varies the size of the pupil, via the optic and oculomotor cranial nerve.

Pyrexia An abnormally high temperature or fever.

Quality assurance This reflects an organization's guarantee to those who use its services that the product or the services on offer will meet accepted quality standards within that industry. Quality assurance is achieved by identifying what 'quality' means in context (to those using the product or service); identifying methods by which its presence can be ensured and specifying the ways in which it can be measured in order to determine that the organization is conforming.

Quality Assurance Agency An independent agency that checks higher education courses meet required standards.

Radiologist A specialist doctor who interprets x-rays and scans.

Rebound tenderness Pain felt on sudden release of steadily applied pressure on a suspected area of the abdomen.

Reciprocity Mutual dependence, action or influence. The practice of exchanging things with others for mutual benefit.

Recreational drugs These are chemical substances taken for enjoyment, or leisure purposes, as opposed to medical reasons. Alcohol, tobacco and caffeine may also be classed as recreational drugs. Recreational drugs are usually taken to provide pleasure, or improve life in some way. Many recreational drugs are illegal.

Reflector A student who learns through the skill of reflection and contemplation.

Retinopathy Damage to the retina.

Retrospective study A research study that focuses on the past and present. The study examines past exposure to suspected risk factors for the disease or condition.

Revalidation The process all registered nurses, midwives and nursing associates go through to renew their nursing registration with the Nursing and Midwifery Council.

Rheumatoid arthritis Autoimmune inflammatory joint condition.

Safety thermometer The safety thermometer is a tool developed for the NHS by the NHS. This is a point-of-care survey instrument, providing the healthcare provider with a 'temperature check' on harm. The tool can be used with other measures that assess risk or harm.

Salicylic acid This is used for several different skin conditions that are caused by thickened, hard skin, for example warts, psoriasis, scaly skin conditions and some nail infections.

Scoliosis Curvature of the mid-spine.

Scope of Practice This refers to the roles, functions, responsibilities and activities that a registered nurse, registered midwife or nursing associate is educated, competent and has license to perform.

Search parameters Words (code) that are used to narrow the focus of a search.

Self-actualization The realization and fulfilment of one's own potential.

Self-inflicted violence (SIV) The deliberate injuring of one's body as a means of managing with severe emotional and psychological stressors. SIV is usually misunderstood as a highly pathological act or simplistic acting out for attention; however, neither of these viewpoints is precise. This can include, cutting, punching, hitting, burning, bruising, head-banging, picking and scalding one's body.

Sepsis Sepsis is a life threatening response to infection that may lead to tissue damage, organ failure, and death.

Sequelae An abnormal condition resulting from a previous disease.

Slough A form of non-viable tissue which can interfere with wound healing.

Specialist nurses These are nurse practitioners who have been educated to degree level or above and hold specialist knowledge, skills, competencies and experience.

Splenomegaly The enlargement of the spleen.

Sputum Mucus and saliva that is generated by infection in the respiratory tract. Sputum is often expectorated or coughed up by patients with a respiratory infection.

Standard A desired level of performance against which an actual performance is measured.

Stoma An artificial opening, often leading into a hollow space (for instance the throat or the intestines).

Strabismus Misalignment of the eyes, squint.

Stridor A high-pitched breathing noise normally caused by a blocked upper airway.

Sub-cutaneous Applied just under the skin.

Subjectivity Data that is subjective may include statements on how the patient/family say they are feeling or what they say in words, for example 'I am feeling persecuted', and could be used to show how a patient perceives a problem. Subjective information is normally represented within quotation marks (e.g. Mr Smith told me he felt breathless).

Summary of Product Characteristics (SPC) As part of the approval process for marketing medicines, the pharmaceutical company produces a Summary of Product Characteristics (SPC), which provides comprehensive details of the medicine's pharmacological properties and pharmacotherapeutic information. The SPC also includes details of adverse drug reactions associated with the medicine and how its safety profile is being monitored. For most medicines the SPC can be viewed via the electronic medicines compendium website.

Supine Lying face upwards.

SWL Safe working load.

Symmetry Being made up of exactly similar parts facing each other or around an axis, for example, both eyes are symmetrical, the same on each side.

Synapse Junction between two neurons, across which impulses pass by the diffusion of neurotransmitters.

Synovial membrane Specialized connective tissue that lines the inner surface of joints.

Systemic In relation to treatment means treating the whole system.

Systemic circulation The blood vessels carrying blood around the body (except the lungs).

Systole The time period when the heart is contracting. The period specifically during which the left ventricle of the heart contracts.

Tachycardia Refers to a fast resting heart rate. In general, the adult resting heart beats between 60 and 100 times per minute. When an individual has tachycardia, the upper and/or lower chambers of the heart beat significantly faster. When the heart beats too rapidly, it pumps less efficiently and blood flow to the rest of the body, including the heart itself, is reduced. This can lead to significant problems for patients.

Tachypnoea Rapid and usually shallow respiration rate, outside the accepted range for an individual's age, i.e. greater than 20 respirations per minute for an adult.

Tendon Fibrous end of a muscle that attaches muscle to bone.

Theorist A person who learns through understanding theories.

Therapeutic Having a beneficial effect on body, mind and spirit.

Therapeutic range The therapeutic range of a medicine refers to the concentration of the drug required to produce the desired therapeutic effect.

Therapeutic relationships Therapeutic relationships are fundamental to the care of a patient. It incorporates a helping relationship between a nursing associate and the people care is offered to. It is a helpful and equal relationship.

Thoracotomy Incision into the pleural space.

Thrombocytopenia A deficiency of platelets in circulation, which leads to bleeding disorders.

Thrombus A blood clot that is static within the blood vessel (and is normally attached to the blood vessel wall).

Tinnitus A term that refers to noises that can be heard from inside the body. Often this can be a ringing sound but can be a buzzing sound as well.

Tourniquet A tight band placed around an arm or a leg to constrict blood vessels in order to stop blood flow to a wound.

Tracheostomy A surgically created hole through the front of the neck and into the trachea.

Tracheotomy The surgical procedure of creating a tracheostomy.

Transcribed Written text.

Transcutaneous electric nerve stimulation (TENS) machine A small machine that produces an electric current, which is used to stimulate nerves for therapeutic purposes.

Transient Lasting only for a short period of time.

Transvaginal Through or via the vagina.

Trapezius The trapezius muscle is the large muscle between the neck and the shoulder.

Trauma In psychology, psychological trauma is a type of damage to the psyche that occurs as a result of a severely distressing event, such as post-traumatic stress disorder. In physical medicine trauma is injury or damage to a biological organism that is caused by physical harm from an external source, for example a road traffic collision. Major trauma is also injury that can potentially lead to serious long-term outcomes such as chronic pain.

Triage The process of assessing the priority of a patient's treatments based on the severity of their condition. Triage can determine the order and priority of emergency treatment, care and destination for the patient.

Truncation Means to shorten. It is often used when searching database to retrieve words with the same beginning but different ends i.e. adolesc* retrieves adolescent, adolescents, or adolescence.

Tumescence The condition of being swollen.

Tumour Suppressor Genes Genes which control cell division and the rate of cell growth.

Ulceration The process of ulcer formation. An ulcer is the breakdown of surface tissue or mucus membrane on epithelial tissue. Common ulcers include mouth ulcers, stomach ulcers and ulcers within the bowel such as ulcerative colitis.

Ulcerative colitis A form of inflammatory bowel disease which can cause internal swelling, ulcerations, and loss of function of the large intestine.

Unilateral On one side.

Up and down regulation Up regulation occurs when there is an increase in the number of receptors for a hormone, making a cell more responsive to that hormone. Down regulation is associated with a decrease in the number of receptors for a hormone, making a cell less responsive to that hormone.

Values These are a set of personal beliefs and attitudes about truth, beauty, thought, objects or behaviour. Values can be action orientated and often associated with morality and ethics. Values can provide meaning to life and purpose.

Vasculitis Inflammation of the blood vessels.

Vasoconstriction The constriction of blood vessels.

Vasodilation The dilation of blood vessels. Dilation means the lumen of the vessels increase in size.

Venous leg ulcer A long-lasting (chronic) sore that takes more than six weeks to heal.

Verbatim Reproduced exactly either verbally or written as was done originally.

Vertebrae Bones of the spinal column.

Vertigo A sensation of 'whirling' and the loss of balance.

Virtual Learning Environment An internet-based platform that allows the student to interact in various ways with the lectures, tutorial and academic staff.

Visceral Pertaining to an organ of the body. The visceral layer is the layer that is closest to the organ for example; visceral peritoneum – closest to the digestive system organs; visceral pleura – layer closest to the lungs.

Vulnerable Someone who is unable to protect himself or herself from significant harm or exploitation.

Well-being Can be defined as the positive way in which a person feels and thinks about themselves.

Whistleblowing A report by an employee or other about the violation of a service or law.

Wiki A collection of pages on the internet that can be edited by any member of a team.

Wilson disease An inherited disease causing copper to be deposited in various organs of the body.

X-rays Highly penetrating, electromagnetic radiation used to take images of dense tissues for diagnosis. Dense tissue absorbs radiation more than less dense soft tissue.

Page numbers followed by "*f*" indicate figures, "*t*" indicate tables, and "*b*" indicate boxes.